Hazards of Medication

AUTHOR

Eric W. Martin, PhC, BSc, MS, PhD

Director, Professional Communications, Food and Drug Administration, Rockville, MD; formerly: Adjunct Professor, Biomedical Communication, Columbia University; Director, Medical Communication, Lederle Laboratories Division, American Cyanamid; Founder and First President, Drug Information Association; Past President and Fellow, American Medical Writers Association; Fellow, American Association for the Advancement of Science and International Academy of Law and Science.

EDITORIAL BOARD

SECOND EDITION

HAZARDS OF MEDICATION

A Manual on
Drug Interactions, Contraindications, and Adverse Reactions
with Other Prescribing and Drug Information

ERIC W. MARTIN, PhD

Medical Editor
Arthur Ruskin, MD

Clinical Research Editor
Frances O. Kelsey, MD, PhD

Drug Reaction Editor
Edward Napke, MD

Medicolegal Editors
Donald J. Farage, LLD
Don Harper Mills, MD, JD

Patient Response Editor
Stewart F. Alexander, MD

Pharmaceutical Editor
Robert W. Elkas, PhD

Associate Editor
Ruth D. Martin, DSc

J. B. Lippincott Company
Philadelphia and Toronto

Library of Congress Cataloging in Publication Data

Martin, Eric Wentworth.
  Hazards of medication.

  Bibliography: p.
  Includes index.
  1. Drug interactions.   2. Drugs—Toxicology.
I. Ruskin, Arthur.   II. Title.
RM302.M36   1978b   615'.1   78-14265
ISBN 0-397-50389-X

This book was written by Eric W. Martin in his private capacity. No official support or endorsement by the Food and Drug Administration or the Department of Health, Education, and Welfare is intended or should be inferred.

Dedication

To all physicians, biomedical scientists, and other members of the health care team in academia, government, industry, and private practice, who have substantially prolonged the life of man with modern medications; who have placed their professional responsibilities and the welfare of patients above all other considerations whenever they evaluated, developed, manufactured, distributed, prescribed, dispensed, or administered medications; and who have exercised constant vigilance in uncovering, reporting, and overcoming the hazards of medications.

EWM

Preface

The objectives of this volume are three-fold: (1) to alert physicians and other health professionals to the pitfalls facing both patient and prescriber whenever a prescription for medication is written, (2) to present an analysis of the potential hazards inherent in each facet of the entire drug distribution system to the patient, and (3) to provide for ready reference detailed tabulations of interferences in clinical laboratory testing, compatibilities and incompatibilities of intravenous solution additives, adverse drug reactions, drug interactions, and other precautionary information.

The last half of this work comprises the most comprehensive, most thoroughly documented, and most readily accessible information on drug interactions in print. The alphabetical, cross-indexed arrangement of generic and trade names and interactants enables the busy physician to locate instantly the interaction data needed for a prescribed medication. And if the prescriber wishes to delve into a given interaction more deeply, more than 2000 references facilitate entry into the world of scientific and medical literature. The *Table of Drug Interactions* contains the important drug interactions appearing in some 3000 biomedical publications indexed and recorded in the computerized data bases of the National Library of Medicine.

The ten chapters follow in a logical sequence the pharmaceutical and medical links of the American drug distribution chain. A multidisciplinary approach—clinical, pharmacological, and chemical—has been taken throughout. After an introductory overview of the damage and death associated with drug therapy and the major hazards, the inequivalency of medications is discussed. Following these discussions are chapters covering faulty ideas for new drugs, the hazards that can result from improper research, development, manufacturing, distribution, storage, diagnosis, prescribing, dispensing, and administration of drugs as well as defective patient response and medical litigation. The last two chapters on adverse drug reactions and drug interactions include definitions, classifications, mechanisms, effects of the environment, and useful tables.

Concepts, once considered highly radical, are now being widely accepted, including the patient's right to know everything about his case. The consumer of medications has the right to know what they are, exactly how to take them, what they do to the body, what adverse effects they may produce, and what action to take if such effects occur. We hope that the basic information presented in this volume will be passed on to the patient and thus greatly reduce the damage caused by carelessness, ignorance, and faulty body mechanisms. We hope this information will reduce drug mortality rates.

Rockville, MD   EWM

Preface to the First Edition

This volume presents an overview of the numerous therapeutic, biopharmaceutic, legal, and scientific requirements for safe and effective medication of the patient, a major function of the health care system. Delivery of adequate health care is probably the most crucial problem facing mankind. Closely related to this pressing need are others of top priority—population control, elimination of environmental pollution, support of research on critical health problems, and prevention of addiction to alcohol, narcotics, and other dangerous drugs. Because all of these health problems are intimately related to medication of the patient, basic necessities for their solution include adequate regulation of the drug field, efficient dissemination of drug information, and proper utilization of knowledge concerning drug therapy.

But effective control over drug products and adequate distribution of drug information have not consistently accompanied the exponential growth of drug research and development that has occurred since 1930. Misuse and abuse of medications have exacted a staggering toll in needless suffering, time-consuming litigation, economic loss, and destruction of human life. Physicians, often because of lack of adequate information, have not always been able to select optimum medication for their patients or to avoid all harmful drug effects. Adverse drug interactions and other subtle hazards of modern potent drug therapy have created serious problems in medicine today, including permanent injury and death for an appalling number of patients.

Awareness of these problems was deeply intensified by enactment of the 1962 Kefauver-Harris Drug Amendments to the Federal Food, Drug and Cosmetic Act and by the advent of Medicare and Medicaid. Soon after these health care programs were launched, the factors that modify drug efficacy, quality, and safety were spotlighted by leaders in government, industry, and the medical profession. Concern about medication hazards was intensified, and the specter of burdensome litigation began to haunt every medical practitioner, hospital administrator, and pharmaceutical manufacturer.

Data accumulated from the literature and from sources in government and industry have revealed the increasing damage being sustained by patients because physicians lacked adequate information about (1) the many factors involved in developing and delivering safe and effective medications, (2) the precautions that must be taken by all members of the health care team to avoid the numerous hazards to patients inherent in the use of modern potent medications, and (3) the dietary, environmental, hereditary, and other hidden factors that influence patient response to drug therapy.

Under current conditions of rapid change in health care, the potential hazards that exist for physicians and patients have proliferated at every stage of developing, handling, and using medications. The most serious hazards are caused by the following situations which occasionally arise: (1) Irrational concepts for new medications lead to the development of dangerous drug products (see the sulfanilamide, thalidomide and other tragedies). (2) Incompetent drug research and evaluation considerably reduce the efficiency of drug product development and create hazards for test subjects (see the problems created by preclinical and clinical investigators and patients). (3) Poor manufacturing practices result in the production of low-quality and even dangerous drug products (see manufacturing practices and quality control). (4) Improper distribution procedures such as mislabeling and incorrect storage cause drug products to be misused, or to deteriorate, or actually to become highly toxic (see distribution and storage). (5) Errors in prescribing and administering medications and variability of patient response to drug therapy cause perplexing legal and professional problems for the physician and possibly severe injury to patients (see drug interactions diet and drug therapy, environmental factors, enzyme deficiencies, induction, inhibition, and other enzyme anomalies). (6) Undue apprehension about adverse drug reactions and costly litigation causes some physicians to withhold potent lifesaving medications from the patient. (7) Medication of the patient on the basis of cost rather than quality, largely because of a lack of understanding of the biopharmaceutic factors that tend to make chemically identical medications therapeutically inequivalent and sometimes hazardous, lowers the quality of health care.

To ensure delivery of effective, high-quality drug therapy, precautions must be taken at *every* step, beginning with the early stages of *in vitro* testing and animal pharmacology and continuing through clinical research, production, quality control, distribution, prescribing, dispensing, administration, and patient follow-up. Even though every necessary precaution is taken at every stage, however, physicians are often frustrated in their attempts to provide effective therapy because the patient may be subtly influenced by an undetected situation. A weakness such as drug dependence, a genetic flaw such as an enzyme deficiency, an atmospheric pollutant such as a solvent vapor, a food constituent such as a pressor amine, a psychosomatic disturbance, or other hidden element may negate the therapy, or make it hazardous.

In order to alert the physician and his colleagues on the health care team to the large number of frequently obscure factors that influence patient response to drug therapy, this volume includes handy reference tables compiled from the world literature. The tables on adverse drug reactions including drug interactions as well as on IV admixture problems and clinical laboratory interferences are probably the most comprehensive available to date, and hopefully will help the prescriber to avoid many pitfalls.

In general, physicians prescribe drugs carefully, safely, and effectively. But they cannot always avoid the rarely encountered pitfalls that create crises, headlines, and litigation. These unforeseen, often extremely rare events, when they occur for the first time in the unfortunate propositus, should not be used politically, legally, or economically against practitioners or manufacturers. Most members of the health care team are sincerely devoted to their professions and patients and earnestly try not to harm them. They should not be unduly harassed when adverse responses, impossible to foresee, occur. On the other hand, improvements can always be made in patient care. That is why this book was written.

We deeply appreciate the efforts of the contributors listed on page ii, who critically reviewed manuscripts and made numerous helpful comments and suggestions for this volume. Once again we found it particularly rewarding to work with Walter Kahoe, Director of the Medical Publications Division of J. B. Lippincott Company, and his associates, especially J. Stuart Freeman, Jr., the editor, who gave such competent and meticulous attention to our manuscript. We are also grateful for the assistance given us by many other medical and scientific colleagues, particularly Paul H. Bell, Marjorie A. Darken, Vincent F. Downing, Milton W. Skolaut, William G. Stone, Gilbert Wagle, and Hans H. Zinsser.

We hope this book will bring into focus not only the important professional and scientific principles governing drug efficacy, safety, and rational use but also the roles of government, industry, and the biomedical professions in protecting those who give medications and those who receive them.

Montvale, N.J.   ERIC W. MARTIN

Contents

Tables

Hazards of Medication

1 Pitfalls of Medication

Every medication is potentially hazardous. Therefore, safe and effective drug therapy demands profound knowledge of every drug product being prescribed, thorough patient analysis, and adequate patient education. If these three essentials are observed most drug-induced disease and most drug-related malpractice litigation can be avoided.

During the 1960s, at the zenith of misuse of medications in this country, the damage to patients was staggering. One clinical pharmacologist wrote that "one-seventh of all hospital days is devoted to the care of drug toxicity at an estimated annual cost of \$3 billion."[31] Two other authorities wrote that medications cause the death of 140,000 Americans annually.[32] These may have been slightly overstated for the sake of emphasis. Nevertheless, they were indicative of a serious situation and the need for better education of both patients and prescribers concerning the hazards associated with consumption of drug products.*

In the United States during that period some 1,500,000 of the 30,000,000 patients hospitalized annually were admitted *with* adverse drug reactions (ADRs) and about 850,000 of these *because* of such reactions.[1,35] In some hospitals, as high as 20 percent of the patients were admitted because of drug-induced disease. In one general hospital 25 percent of the deaths on the public medical service resulted from ADRs.[3]

In five Boston institutions during a two-year period 31 percent of a large group of hospitalized medical patients experienced ADRs of which 80 percent were major or moderately severe.[14] During a three-month period of surveillance at Johns Hopkins Hospital, 17 percent of the general medical service patients experienced 184 ADRs, or 1.5 ADRs per affected patient, and most of the patients acquired their reactions during hospitalization. Over 30 percent of the hospitalized patients with a reaction acquired another one in the hospital and of this group 22 percent died either from the reaction that resulted in their admission or from one acquired in the hospital.[3,22,23] In one 3½ year study 12.5 percent of all inpatients on a medical service suffered at least one ADR.[39]

However, physicians are becoming much more alert to adverse drug reaction potentials because of the emphasis placed on the hazards of medication during the last ten years.[5] The situation appears to have improved to some extent and the hazards may now at times be somewhat overestimated.[28] The overall mortality for all medical inpatients due to medications is now generally reported to be about 6.5 percent or less.[30,39] In a few recent studies only 1 per 1000 medical inpatient deaths was associated with drug therapy and most of the deaths occurred in patients suffering from severe terminal illnesses (cancer, cirrhosis, leukemia, pulmonary embolism, etc.). Moreover, only 1 per 10,000 of the drug-associated deaths was preventable. Also, the implicated drugs were predominantly IV fluids and potassium chloride.[30] In one carefully studied group of 10,280 *surgical* inpatients, only 2 deaths were drug-related.[29]

---

*The term *drug,* as used in this volume refers to any physiologically active substance used for diagnosis, prevention, or treatment of disease. However, the term is often loosely used to refer to a drug product (capsule, tablet, etc.) as well as a pure chemical (sodium bicarbonate, eucalyptol, etc.).

Unfortunately, precise data that provide accurate benefit-to-risk ratios are still not available for most drugs. The alarming reports of high incidences of ADRs discernible in patients on admission to U.S. hospitals must be evaluated in the context of their mode of collection. Reported incidences, ranging widely from a fraction of 1 to 30 percent, vary with the type of hospital, how "adverse drug reaction" was defined, and how the statistics were compiled.

During this decade we hope that prospective, automated, epidemiologic studies like the Boston Collaborative Drug Surveillance Program[18] and the Registry on Tissue Reactions to Drugs, of the Armed Forces Institute of Pathology, with the continued support of the Food and Drug Administration (FDA) will provide precise and dependable data for specific types of reactions. These can then be attributed to specific drugs and drug categories.

FDA, with the participation of various institutions and hospitals, has spent millions of dollars of taxpayers' money in repeated attempts to develop a useful ADR reporting system, with little success. A major $5 million project at the Kaiser Permanente Foundation was abandoned during the summer of 1970 due to the paucity of useful information obtained over a period of several years. Other such major efforts have been very costly, wasteful, and frustrating to everyone concerned. If an effective ADR reporting program could be established and closely linked with others operated by agencies such as the Kaiser Permanente Foundation, New York Health Insurance Plan, and Washington Group Health, Inc., a statistically significant number of subjects could be followed from the fetal stages until after death,[20] and significant data compiled.

In 1975, the Office of Technology Assessment of the U.S. Congress recognized the seriousness of the adverse drug reaction problem and initiated a nationwide study to provide material for a definitive report. Data were collected during 1976 and a report was drafted in 1977. This may eventually have a beneficial impact on the problem.[37]

Early in 1977 a Commission headed by Senator Kennedy launched a three-year study, largely funded by the Pharmaceutical Manufacturers Association, to examine ADR reporting and arrive at specific recommendations for a national reporting system. Concurrently, FDA, funded by the National Bureau of Standards, began developing pilot systems for postmarketing ADR surveillance. Finally, adequate efforts now seem to be given to the ADR problem.

In order to diminish the hazards of medication, four main types of pitfalls must be avoided—underactivity, overactivity, interactivity, and irrational prescribing. If the desired drug action is absent or too weak or too slow, the patient may suffer needlessly or even lose his life. If the drug action is too intense, the patient may experience toxic reactions with possibly serious or even fatal consequences. If the drug action is modified through interaction with another drug or some other chemical in the environment, the patient may be exposed to one of the many hazards listed in the *Table of Drug Interactions* at the end of Chapter 10. And finally, if medication is incorrectly selected or prescribed the patient may be damaged, or at least inappropriately modified physiologically.

No physician deliberately prescribes medication that produces a toxic reaction in his patient, but too often he does not fully evaluate the possibility of such a reaction before he writes the prescription. The astute prescriber keeps abreast of all possible pitfalls. His major problem, therefore, is how to keep himself well informed on all pertinent factors influencing drug safety and efficacy. This volume represents an attempt to meet this need. It compiles as completely as possible the hazards to the patient that can arise while medications are being manufactured, distributed, prescribed, dispensed, and administered. The dangers of irrational drug therapy thus become more fully appreciated.

IRRATIONAL DRUG THERAPY

Irrational prescribing has injured many patients and too often has been lethal. A major pitfall in prescribing is disregard of the principles of rational medication of the patient.

The major objectives of rational drug therapy, after correct diagnosis of the patient's condition, are to (1) select the most appropriate medication available for that patient, (2) prescribe it with clear directions and full awareness of his specific sensitivities and the potentially hazardous drug reactions and interactions pinpointed by his drug profile, (3) dispense accurately a high quality product, and (4) verify that the patient receives and responds to the prescribed medication in the desired manner. This entails proper education of the patient and follow-up.

Every one of these objectives must be attained if patients are to receive optimum and rational drug therapy.[8,10,13] A basic premise is use of the proper dosage in the specific patient being treated. The skill of the prescribing physician in selecting medications and his knowledge of their physiological actions and inherent side effects as well as required variations in dosage are the keystones of each clinical problem (see page 107). For example, digitalis and its glycosides are some of the most effective drugs in worldwide use. Yet the problems of underdosage, overdosage, intoxication, and acute major rhythm disturbances are seen every day in increasing complexity.[19]

Rational drug therapy avoids undesirable situations by starting only with rational ideas for new drug products, and then implementing these ideas with sound scientific research and development, good manufacturing practices, proper distribution techniques, competent prescribing, dispensing and administration, and finally suitable monitoring of the patient. Every one of these links in the chain of events in the drug delivery system has an important bearing on the competence and effectiveness of medical care whenever drug therapy is an integral part of that care. Accordingly, regulatory agencies such as FDA closely monitor all medications and are constantly on the alert to prevent irrational drug therapies, especially those that present serious hazards to the patient.

But in the final analysis, the patient must depend on the therapeutic knowledge of his own physician and on his own ability to comply with the therapeutic regimen prescribed. Thus thorough knowledge of the patient and individualized attention throughout therapy can increase the probability that the patient will follow instructions and receive maximum benefit with minimum hazard.

OFFICIAL DRUG HAZARDS

Since the 1962 Amendments to the Federal Food, Drug, and Cosmetic Act were enacted, FDA has become much more stringent with regard to claims allowed and precautionary information presented in package inserts.* The Agency now requires that warnings of hazardous situations be clearly stated. These precautionary statements are usually retained in each subsequent revision of the inserts. However, some warnings are dropped whenever additional information demonstrates that the hazards are not as serious as they were originally believed to be.

FDA often requires warnings to be added in revisions of some inserts. Thus in 1977, the Agency published new labeling for estrogens[24,25] that emphasizes (1) the risk of endometrial cancer in estrogen users is up to 14 times greater than in nonusers, (2) the risk of limb reduction abnormalities in fetuses exposed to estrogens is nearly five times the spontaneous rate, (3) gallbladder disease is increased two- to threefold in postmenopausal estrogen users, and (4) other adverse effects—thromboembolic disease, hepatic adenoma, elevated blood pressure, worsened glucose tolerance, and severe hypercalcemia—may occur. A patient package insert must now be supplied with every prescription for estrogenic drug products.[62]

Typical official drug hazards have been documented[5] and they are grouped in package inserts under specific headings: *Contraindications, Warnings, Precautions,* and *Adverse Reactions.* These vary widely with the type of medication.[11]

The value of package inserts as accurate, authoritative, and dependable sources of medical information for the physician has long been questioned. This is because they have often been poorly written, and are incomplete, inappropriately documented, illogically compiled, and inconsistent. Inserts for the same drug product vary in content from one manufacturer to another. Also, unless the physician requests them from a pharmacy or the manufacturer, or purchases original packages of drug products, he may never see the latest inserts. Moreover, most

---

*The original Federal Pure Food and Drug Act of 1906 was concerned with *adulteration and misbranding.* Not until after the sulfanilamide tragedy (page 26) of 1938 was *safety* of drugs made a requirement in the revised Act of that year. And not until the thalidomide tragedy (page 27) was the Act made strict enough to include *efficacy* and many other requirements through enactment of the Amendments of 1962.

practitioners believe that the government should not use inserts to practice medicine and FDA agrees.* For these and other reasons, physicians generally refuse to be restricted in the practice of their profession by such instruments. See *Package Inserts as Legal Documents* (page 82).

During 1976, however, FDA began a thorough review of all inserts. By 1980 it plans to complete class labeling (one insert for certain drug classes that will include comparative data on the members of that class, e.g., tetracyclines), generic labeling (one insert for a drug marketed by more than one drug company, e.g., meprobamate which is sold by some 50 companies), and unique labeling where only one drug in a class exists and is marketed by only one company. These revised inserts are being written by experts under contract to FDA.

Contraindications

An absolute contraindication exists under certain conditions when a particular drug must never be used, otherwise the patient will almost certainly be severely harmed. Fig. 1-1 shows a contraindication which must be heeded or death may occur.

Contraindication

Penicillin should not be used in patients with known hypersensitivity to the drug.

Fig. 1-1

This simple statement and the warning in Fig. 1-2, both of which appear in the labeling of every penicillin product, undoubtedly have saved the lives of many patients and have also been used in lawsuits against physicians who have ignored them. This is also true for the contraindication that sulfonamides must not be used in infants.[6]

Other contraindications are concerned with incipient or active conditions found in the patient and with interactions that may occur when prescribed medications are used with other drug products being taken concomitantly. Examples are certain anti-inflammatory agents in peptic ulcer, barbiturates in porphyria, estrogens in carcinoma, steroids in incipient infections and in active, latent, or questionably healed tuberculosis, and monoamine oxidase inhibitors with sympathomimetics. Hundreds of such contraindications against medication usages that are highly hazardous or life threatening are included in the package inserts.

Warnings

Whenever potent drugs can be particularly dangerous to patients under certain circumstances, warnings are included in the labeling. Such warnings generally pertain to extreme hazards such as those arising from acute hypersensitivity, cumulative and prolonged use, effects on the fetus, and variations in patient response. Fig. 1-2 shows a typical example.

Warning

Serious and occasional fatal hypersensitivity (anaphylactoid) reactions have been reported in patients on penicillin therapy. Although anaphylaxis is more frequent following parenteral administration, it has occurred in patients on oral penicillins. These reactions are more apt to occur in individuals with a history of sensitivity to multiple allergens.

There have been well-documented reports of individuals with a history of penicillin hypersensitivity who have experienced severe hypersensitivity reactions when treated with cephalosporins. Before therapy with a penicillin, careful inquiry should be made concerning previous hypersensitivity reactions to penicillins, cephalosporins, and other allergens. If an allergic reaction occurs, the drug should be discontinued and the patient treated with the usual agents, e.g., pressor amines, antihistamines, and corticosteroids. Serious anaphylactoid reactions are not controlled by antihistamines alone, and require such emergency measures as the immediate use of epinephrine, aminophylline, oxygen, and intravenous corticosteroids.

Fig. 1-2

Despite this warning, fatal reactions have occurred immediately following the ingestion of a penicillin tablet.

---

* Package inserts that since 1961 by law accompany every package of every prescription medication are official regulatory documents written by the manufacturer under the close scrutiny of FDA which must approve every word. They are not promotional brochures as some physicians believe, but are designed to be authoritative prescribing guides with legal implications.

Sometimes a warning is written in capital, boldface or italic type and enclosed in a box when the hazard (e.g., aplastic anemia, hypertensive crisis, Stevens-Johnson syndrome, etc.) is especially serious. Warnings to be directed by the physician to the patient may also be included in package inserts as well as warnings to the physician himself.

FDA, along with consumers, manufacturers and professional groups, is gradually developing patient package inserts to be given directly to patients before they use medications such as estrogens or devices such as intrauterine devices (IUDs) that have potentially serious risks associated with their use. See page 85.

A typical warning for an antibiotic which is useful enough to be prescribed for rickettsial and other serious gram-negative infections in spite of its hazards is given in Figure 1-3. An awareness that chloramphenicol may produce severe blood dyscrasias has undoubtedly saved many lives when suitable medications have been substituted.

Warning

Serious and fatal blood dyscrasias (aplastic anemia, hypoplastic anemia, thrombocytopenia, and granulocytopenia) are known to occur after the administration of chloramphenicol. In addition, there have been reports of aplastic anemia attributed to chloramphenicol which later terminated in leukemia. Blood dyscrasias have occurred after both short-term and prolonged therapy with this drug. Chloramphenicol must not be used when less potentially dangerous agents will be effective, as described in the Indications section. *It must not be used in the treatment of trivial infections or where it is not indicated, as in colds, influenza, infections of the throat; or as a prophylactic agent to prevent bacterial infections.*

Precautions: It is essential that adequate blood studies be made during treatment with the drug. While blood studies may detect early peripheral blood changes, such as leukopenia, reticulocytopenia, or granulocytopenia, before they become irreversible, such studies cannot be relied on to detect bone marrow depression prior to development of aplastic anemia. To facilitate appropriate studies and observation during therapy, it is desirable that patients be hospitalized.

Fig. 1-3

Precautions

Official precautions inform physicians what they must not do under certain circumstances, e.g., high dosage, intensive therapy, prolonged use, or some special condition of the patient. The physician automatically takes precautions in almost every instance where a drug is prescribed in a plan for therapy. Serious situations that may be produced if such precautions are not heeded include addiction, cumulative effects, peripheral vascular collapse, psychic dependence, superinfection, tolerance, withdrawal symptoms, and many others (see below under *Adverse Reactions*). Addiction can be a tragic result with meperidine or methadone; the cumulative effect of digitalis often negates its primary usefulness; peripheral vascular insufficiency or even gangrene can be a serious complication of ergotamine therapy; psychic dependence is too often the aftermath of injudicious or prolonged tranquilizer therapy; superinfection is a major and often lethal complication of immunosuppressives or antimicrobials; and tolerance to narcotics, where use may be mandatory, leads to major management problems. The withdrawal phenomenon following sustained therapy can often be handled better if it is anticipated through the precaution statement.

Figure 1-4 is a typical example of precautions for one category of anti-infectives.

Precautions

Sulfonamides should be given with caution to patients with impaired renal or hepatic function and to those with severe allergy or bronchial asthma.

In glucose-6-phosphate dehydrogenase-deficient individuals, hemolysis may occur. This reaction is frequently dose-related.

Adequate fluid intake must be maintained in order to prevent crystalluria and stone formation.

Fig. 1-4

Adverse Reactions

Every medication can cause unforeseen and undesirable reactions in a certain percentage of patients. These reactions must be avoided if possible, but they often arise unexpectedly because of unknown patient hypersensitivities or idiosyncrasies, interactions with concomitant medication, environmental influences, or improper use of the medication. Examples, in addition to those mentioned above under *Precautions* are anaphylactic shock, blood dyscrasias, carcinogenesis, coma, convulsions, death, hypertensive crisis, gastrointestinal ulceration, kidney and liver dysfunction, mutagenesis, ocular damage, psychoses, severe blood sugar changes, severe hemorrhage, and teratogenesis. Such unfortunate experiences may be the result of *extension effects, side effects,* or *drug interactions.* See Chapter 9.

Awareness of the possibility that such serious reactions can occur must be instilled in every physician. Thus the knowledge that a teratogenic effect may follow the use of a simple and generally safe vaccine if it is injected in early pregnancy will prevent many tragic experiences. Unfortunately, because of a tendency in package inserts to list all minor side effects and extension effects along with serious adverse reactions, inserts do not help the practitioner to locate the serious reactions quickly and thus assist him to administer rational therapy. To alleviate this situation, truly serious reactions to medications will be presented in ready reference tables. (FDA's labeling guidelines provide for this). See Chapter 9 on *Adverse Reactions.*

Fig. 1-5 provides the list of adverse reactions appearing in the package insert for a thiazide diuretic.

Sometimes rare adverse reactions are not recognized until after a large number of patients have used certain medications over a long period of time. And sometimes even after the reactions have been suspected, proof of their existence has been extremely difficult to establish because of a very low incidence. Perhaps oral contraceptives (OCs) provide the best example of this situation. A decade after they were introduced they were being used by many millions of women throughout the world. Then various medical authorities began to caution against prolonged intake of combinations containing potent synthetic hormones. Although these agents were practically 100 percent effective in preventing conception, certain conditions (thromboembolic disorders such as intracranial venous thrombosis and thrombophlebitis as well as myocardial infarction, cancer, and birth de-

---

Adverse Reactions

Gastrointestinal System Reactions: anorexia, gastric irritation, nausea, diarrhea, constipation, jaundice (intrahepatic cholestatic jaundice), vomiting, cramping, pancreatitis.

Central Nervous System Reactions: dizziness, vertigo, paresthesias, headache, xanthopsia.

Hematologic Reactions: leukopenia, agranulocytosis, thrombocytopenia, aplastic anemia.

Dermatologic-Hypersensitivity Reactions: purpura, photosensitivity, rash, urticaria, necrotizing angiitis (vasculitis) (cutaneous vasculitis).

Cardiovascular Reaction: orthostatic hypotension may occur and may be aggravated by alcohol, barbiturates, or narcotics.

Other: hyperglycemia, glycosuria, hyperuricemia, muscle spasm, weakness, restlessness. Whenever adverse reactions are moderate or severe, Metahydrin dosage should be reduced or therapy withdrawn.

Fig. 1-5

fects) were eventually associated with OCs often enough to alert physicians to a possible cause-and-effect relationship. This was particularly true with the sequential type that contained high doses of estrogen. These were voluntarily withdrawn from the market in 1976 by the three manufacturers after FDA pointed out several known and suspected serious disadvantages of the products.[33] Some evidence also suggests that OCs can induce chromosome abnormalities. Carcinogenic, mutagenic, and teratogenic effects must all be considered as possibilities. FDA became so concerned that it now requires every OC prescription to be accompanied by adequate warning literature for the patient.[7] And in 1976-8 the Agency published detailed patient package inserts for OCs as well as revised physician and patient information.[36] Authorities recommend that OCs be discontinued periodically to allow the body to adjust.

The latest warning, to be prominently displayed in OC labeling, was published early in 1978:[36]

"Cigarette smoking increases the risk of serious adverse effects on the heart and blood vessels from oral contraceptive use. This risk increases with age and with heavy smoking (15 or more cigarettes per day) and is quite marked in women over 35 years of age. Women who use oral contraceptives should not smoke."

During the summer of 1970, the American Medical Association and producers of oral contraceptives prepared a patient information booklet giving details on the safety and efficacy of birth control pills and on adverse reactions and contraindications associated with their use. FDA approved the AMA booklet in August, 1970. The document supplements the advice and instructions of the prescribing physician, in accordance with the requirements of an FDA order of June 11, 1970.[7] Brief warning statements, information on family planning, and tables on relative risks of pregnancy and death are included in some of the booklets.

The development of the oral contraceptive brochure with the requirement that it be given directly to the patient was one of the first instances of a government agency exerting a strong influence on medical practice at the physician-patient level. Most health professionals now agree, however, that patients have a right to know what physicians are giving them, what the effects on their bodies will be, and what hazards they face from accepting the therapeutic regimen.

Strong medicolegal overtones were obviously inherent in the forcing of physicians to provide patients with information in the form of written documents. This opened the door to a similar situation with all medications. The action may also connote, unfortunately, lack of confidence that every physician has the ability to make proper judgments in medicating his patients and in applying his knowledge of the hazards of pharmacotherapy.

HAZARDS OF PHARMACOTHERAPY

In addition to the hazards of medication presented in official publications, there are others that arise during the development, production, and distribution of medications, and still others that arise through physician-patient, medication-patient, and drug-drug interactions. Study of the impact of the physician's posture and mannerisms on the patient has been organized into a new discipline known as psychosemantics (kinesics). Medication-patient interactions and their mecha-

nisms are considered under subjects such as therapeutic inequivalency, research and development factors, prescribing factors, clinical laboratory errors, patient response, adverse drug reactions and drug interactions. Interactions among prescribed and self-selected medications and other chemicals introduced into the body at the same time has become one of the most intensively investigated subjects in medicine. Since all of the above must be considered whenever a prescription is written for a patient, questions on the various types of potential hazards should be included in qualifying examinations for licensure to practice medicine.

Among the most significant hazards of pharmacotherapy that prevent attainment of rational therapy objectives are (1) inactivation of medication, (2) unsuitable drug combinations, (3) unfavorable patient response, (4) drug interactions, (5) suicide with drugs, (6) legislative pressure, (7) drug fallacies, (8) inadequate patient education, (9) faulty regulation, and (10) biological unavailability.

Inactivation of Medication

Inactivation of drug products results when one or more of seven faulty situations are not corrected, i.e., when the products are: (1) *formulated* improperly so that vehicles and adjuncts decrease the efficacy of the active ingredients, (2) *manufactured* improperly so that the medication is in a form not suitably released in the body, (3) *packaged, transported* or *stored* improperly so that environmental influences decrease potency, (4) *prescribed* improperly so that the selected therapeutic regimen is ineffective, (5) *dispensed* improperly so that physical or chemical incompatibilities occur or incorrect instructions or packaging are provided (6) *administered* improperly so that the active ingredients do not become biologically available, or (7) *interacted* with other medications, food constituents, or other substances in the patient so that drug effects are nullified.

The factors pertaining to the first six of these unsatisfactory situations influence drug activity up to the moment that the patient receives a medication. They are covered in Chapter 3, *Research and Development Factors;* Chapter 4, *Manufacturing Factors;* Chapter 5, *Distribution Factors;* and Chapter

6, *Prescribing Factors.* The factors pertaining to the seventh situation mentioned above influence drug activity after the patient receives a medication. They are covered in Chapter 10, *Drug Interactions.*

Unsuitable Drug Combinations

Some combinations of drugs are useful, some are not. [2,8,9,13,15,16]

Arguments Pro. FDA has published guidelines for acceptable drug combinations. The following reasons that have appeared in the literature or have been set forth by FDA advisors support the position that certain fixed combinations of two or more drugs in a given dosage form, disparagingly termed shotgun therapy, are sometimes desirable.

1. Combinations are useful when one drug safely potentiates another or otherwise modifies the effects of another so that lower doses will produce the desired degree of effectiveness with lowered incidence of adverse effects. In the treatment of hypertension, combined drug therapy often permits reduction in dosage and circumvents some side effects. [12]

2. One or more ingredients of a drug product may merely give symptomatic relief while the principal ingredient treats some condition. Thus an antitussive administered for cough and cold relief may be combined with an analgesic, an antihistamine, or a decongestant. The patient is thus enabled to conquer his disease and meanwhile is made more comfortable than he would have been with a single drug.

3. Combinations are useful when one drug, e.g., methamphetamine (CNS stimulant) counteracts adverse effects of another, e.g., phenobarbital (drowsiness), and thus permits administration of an effective drug such as an anticonvulsant to a patient who could not otherwise tolerate it. This type of combination is especially useful when no alternative drug therapy exists for that patient.

4. Combinations of some antimicrobial agents are indicated when the ingredients are shown by sensitivity testing to be the drugs of choice for the mixture of organisms present in the infected patient. Combined therapy consisting of penicillin G plus chloramphenicol is the treatment of choice in the initial treatment of children with bacterial meningitis due to *H. influenzae.* A tetracycline plus streptomycin is the most effective treatment for brucellosis. In the treatment of severe infections like bacterial endocarditis caused by enterococci the synergistic combination of penicillin and streptomycin is more effective than single drugs. [12]

5. Combinations of antimicrobial agents are desirable when one of them tends to prevent an overgrowth of organisms or a superinfection caused by another agent or the development of resistant strains. For example, the number of Candida organisms in the stool is reduced by nystatin and amphotericin B. These fungistats have been used concurrently with various antibiotics to prevent fungal overgrowth. Certain combinations of antibiotics delay the emergence of resistant strains in coliform, staphylococcal, and tubercular infections. Thus, tuberculosis, caused by various strains of Mycobacterium, should always be treated with at least two and preferably three antituberculosis agents to suppress the emergence of resistant strains. The emergence of isoniazid-resistant strains is curtailed by concomitant administration of ethambutol. [27]

6. Combinations of antimicrobial agents may be indicated where the cause of a severe life-threatening infection is not identified and immediate therapeutic effects are urgently needed. Parenteral administration is then desirable. But the antimicrobials should be carefully selected on the basis of the most likely diagnosis, and appropriate specimens for culturing should be taken *before* any antibiotics are administered.

7. Combinations may be desirable in the treatment of skin diseases which are commonly caused by both gram-negative and gram-positive bacteria, and in mixed infections of the cardiovascular, respiratory, or urinary system after more than one organism has been identified.

8. Rational combinations of drugs in a single medication are more convenient and less costly than the same drugs prescribed as separate medications. This may be a major reason why about 50 percent of the medications listed in the National Drug Code Directory are fixed-dose combinations. This applies to both prescription and over-the-counter categories.

Arguments Con. The following reasons that have appeared in the literature support the position that products containing combinations of drugs are sometimes not desirable. [4,8]

1. A "fixed dose" combination of anti-infective agents is not useful when it yields no greater therapeutic efficacy than one of the agents used alone, yet presents greater probability of an undesirable drug interaction, or incompatibility, or development of resistant microorganisms. In most infections seldom does more than one microorganism cause the condition and that one is susceptible to treatment with a single drug. FDA and the National Academy of Sciences-National Research Council Drug Efficacy Study in 1969 stated that the use of combinations to treat patients who can be satisfactorily treated by one drug is "irrational, illogical, unscientific, and is a disservice to the patient."

2. A combination of drugs is not desirable when an active ingredient in the combination antagonizes or otherwise adversely inhibits one or more other drugs either present in that combination or in another drug product being given concomitantly.

3. A combination of drugs is not desirable when one active ingredient potentiates one or more other drugs (of that combination or of another drug product being given concomitantly) so intensely that dangerous extension effects or side effects may occur. This is likely to occur when more than one physician is caring for the patient. An excellent example of this has happened when acute thrombophlebitis complicates an orthopedic injury. As one practitioner is attempting to achieve good anticoagulant control with a coumarin derivative, another specialist may all in good faith prescribe an analgesic combination containing aspirin which potentiates the anticoagulant effect and may lead to serious bleeding.

4. A fixed combination of anti-infective agents often does not contain the proper drugs or the proper amounts which will be most suitable for treating mixed bacterial infections associated with many different strains of organisms with highly variable sensitivity patterns. Marked changes in the patterns of microbial sensitivity (susceptibility to anti-infectives) occur constantly. New antimicrobial agents must therefore be developed constantly to overcome new resistant strains that arise.

5. Initial use of an anti-infective combination of drugs may interfere with attempts to identify an etiologic agent.

6. Fixed combinations do not permit flexibility of dosage. The physician is forced to use the combination as it is marketed; he cannot readily tailor the treatment to individual requirements for any one specific ingredient. And he cannot avoid possible drug interactions because he cannot prescribe the drugs at different times.

7. The availability of fixed combinations of anti-infective drugs has led to inappropriate use of these drugs for the treatment of disease states in which the fixed combination is not the treatment of choice. Careless diagnosis and unsuitable therapy may thus be encouraged, and a false sense of security engendered. Moreover, patients may also receive unneeded chemicals which may cause toxic effects or create other problems. All ingredients of a combination may not be required throughout the entire course of therapy and thus the patient may be unnecessarily exposed to possible adverse effects from extraneous medication.

8. The toxicity of one ingredient in fixed combinations of drugs may preclude the use of higher therapeutic doses of another ingredient in that combination.

9. Toxicities that appear for any of many reasons cannot always be definitely associated with any one ingredient. They may be caused by deterioration of one or several of the ingredients, or by patient sensitivity to one ingredient, or by chemical reactions among the active ingredients that occurred during improper storage and handling after packaging, or by other mechanisms.

10. Multiple therapy is seldom required for an infection where only one organism is largely responsible for the disease. Best results are achieved when therapy is directed toward the major pathogen.

The above statements pro and con appear in the literature. Some are contradictory. Therefore the decision whether to use a combination of drugs must be made by the prescriber who uses his best judgment based on his careful analysis of the patient. If a physician does decide to use a combination drug product, he must be thoroughly informed about each ingredient, especially all its potential hazards, including potential unfavorable responses.

Unfavorable Patient Response

The patient may respond unfavorably to medication when it is not properly selected, correctly prescribed, correctly dispensed, or appropriately administered. Or a drug may not become biologically available, or some situation exists in the patient which inhibits the medication, or some environmental factor exerts a deleterious action. So many aspects of patient response require consideration that an entire chapter has been written on the subject. See Chapter 8, *Patient Response.*

Drug Interactions

Drug products may be made dangerously toxic or may be partially or wholly prevented from eliciting the desired response in patients because of interactions with other substances. A monoamine oxidase inhibitor like pargyline (Eutonyl) or tranylcypromine (Parnate) taken concomitantly with any sympathomimetic, like amphetamine or like tyramine present in a strong cheese, can cause a hypertensive crisis and possibly death. Anticoagulants, alcohol, antidiabetics and many other drugs interact adversely with certain other drugs, food constituents, and other chemicals introduced into the body intentionally or inadvertently from the environment. Alteration of drug activity by this means comprises so complex and so significant an aspect of drug therapy that Chapter 10, on *Drug Interactions,* has been devoted entirely to the subject. The *Table of Drug Interactions* at the end of that chapter comprises half of this volume.

Suicide with Drugs

The most common means of attempting suicide in the United States is drug overdosage.[48] Of the thousand suicides a day (1 in 10,000 of the population) around the world perhaps 40 percent (over 10,000 of the 26,400 suicides per year in the US) are accomplished with drugs. Self-inflicted injury is much more common than is generally recognized. Estimates of rates of such injury range as high as

1 in 70 (London, Canada)[46] and of suicide as high as 1 in 770 (rural Fijians).[44]

Suicide, which is widely believed to be underreported, is now eleventh among the leading causes of death in this country (over 12 per 100,000). Among males age 15–34 suicide was second only to accidents as a cause of death in 1974 and the rate doubled among those age 15–24 between 1964 and 1974. The rate did decline slightly during that decade for males over 45 but age 75 and over the rate was still 47 per 100,000. It is higher for women who are much more likely than men to select drugs, probably as a cry for help,[59] rather than an immediately effective tool such as a gun, as a means of self-destruction.

The potential hazard of suicide is particularly high among those who have ready access to drugs on their shelves and are familiar with lethal dosages. Their opportunity for addiction, depression and suicide is considerably increased and very high suicide rates have been documented for dentists, physicians and some other health professionals.* Estimates of narcotic addiction for physicians range from 2 to 100 times that in the general population. More physicians die from suicide in the US than from automobile accidents, plane crashes, drownings and homicides combined. Of the 250 physicians who commit suicide each year, at least 40 percent, or the average number in the graduating class of a US medical school, accomplish it with drugs.[55] In England, every month at least one physician kills himself, 1 in every 50 male physicians eventually takes his own life, and 6 percent of all physicians' deaths under age 65 are from suicide, about the same as from lung cancer. Nearly every English physician who destroys himself uses drugs.[43]

Suicide statistics for England and Wales which are readily available, probably indicate current trends. In those countries during 1963 about 42 percent of the women and 22 percent of the men who killed themselves did so with drugs, and there was a six-fold increase in attempted suicide with drugs between 1955 and 1966.[21] During the next ten years the incidence of self-poisoning with

---

* Preliminary data from an American Cancer Society study indicate that suicide accounts for one of every five deaths among anesthesiologists born in 1920 or later (*US Med,* Nov 15, 1977).

drugs doubled. About 1 in 5 of all medical emergencies were attempted suicides, the second most common reason for emergency admission to hospital beds. Such poisonings accounted for 10 percent of all hospital admissions.[47] By 1977 in one town surveyed there were 1000 such admissions per year, a twenty-fold increase over the past 20 years. Most of the poisonings were in young women in their late teens and early twenties, many with drugs prescribed for others.[53]

Barbiturates and acetaminophen have accounted for most deaths. But a wide array of other drugs are used for self destruction, including some such as colchicine and potassium chloride that may not be considered to be likely tools.[45,48,50] Alcohol, glutethimide, and OTC drugs are the most commonly used. Tricyclic antidepressants, although given to treat depression and prevent suicide, are used to commit an increasing number of suicides. In Birmingham, England this category of drugs accounted for 9 percent of the 1875 suicides recorded in 1974.[58]

Since 1965, hospital admissions per million population due to acute barbiturate poisoning have been declining with declining use of these hypnotics, while those due to other drugs have been increasing, according to a 25-year study of 27,000 suicides with drugs.[54] But because the benzodiazepines and other tranquilizers that have been replacing the barbiturates are less toxic the overall deaths from such poisonings have been declining. Still, barbiturates were instrumental in causing 72 percent of all deaths reported. About 90 percent of these deaths were caused by barbiturates alone and most occurred outside the hospital in the absence of medical care.

About 2 out of 3 people contemplate suicide at some time in their lifetime. Some 15 out of every 100 college students have attempted suicide by age 20. In one undergraduate psychology course 27 percent attempted self-destruction, a third of them with drugs.[51]

Recent statistics for patients are startling. About 60 percent of those who attempted suicide were under medical care and 2 out of 5 used a prescription medication in their attempts. Of those who succeeded 1 out of 6 had seen a physician during the previous 30 days and 1 out of 3 destroyed himself with prescribed medication.[42]

The medical community is obviously deeply involved in the suicide problem. Physicians themselves are likely to be successful in any suicide attempt, not only because they have easy access to potent drugs that are lethal, but also because they are highly knowledgeable about human physiology and anatomy and how to apply the lethal effects of drugs. Psychiatrists, especially, through constantly dealing with suicidal patients are top experts on matters of suicide technique.[52]

Perhaps, also, the proliferation of technical procedures that create a gap between the physician and patient contributes to the suicide problem by deterring development of the trusting relationship that is essential to convey and maintain hope. Quiet confidence attending the prescribing of medication and a warm and understanding concern may help prevent despondency and self destruction.[49]

Legislative Pressure

Some legislators, intent on reaching their goals, have continually attempted to find fault with dedicated government officials and repeatedly required them to testify before specific committees. Although beneficial in some respects, this type of pressure has created an atmosphere of apprehension that has permeated the affected socioeconomic areas. In the health field particularly, since about 1960, tensions thus produced in the Department of Health, Education, and Welfare, especially its regulatory subdivisions, have been transmitted to the industries affected, including the manufacturers of drug products. The resulting disruption of personnel in drug research and development may have robbed patients of needed dependable medications. Political haggling has repeatedly obscured the truth about drug products and sometimes undermined the confidence of physicians and patients in good medications which unfortunately were drawn into the spotlight for use as political levers.

The "democratic process" of attacks and counterattacks, Congressional hearings, informal and formal discussions, suits and countersuits involving the regulatory agencies, pharmaceutical manufacturers, medical practitioners, and related groups has had its merits. In spite of the trauma, publication of the legal argumentation, public testimony, private opinion and scientific data that have been generated year after year has been very revealing and has often eventually brought the truth to light. But Congressional testimony is not disseminated and read as widely as it should be. Also, legislation on medication tends to be poorly written at times because of last-minute action. The "patient consent" provision of the 1962 Amendments to the Food, Drug, and Cosmetic Act was the result of a motion by Senator Javits during the closing moments of Senate consideration of the bill. It had not been discussed in the hearings or debated earlier. Hasty legislative action can be hazardous and disruptive.

Drug Fallacies

In addition, several fallacies about drug products, still being widely circulated, must be disproved for the sake of all patients who depend for their welfare on medications.

Fallacy No. 1. *"Big" pharmaceutical manufacturers produce better products than "little" manufacturers.* This is not necessarily true. The company with more funds for higher salaried employees and more modern equipment certainly has the percentages in its favor. But this alone does not guarantee better products. Much more important are human factors such as attitude, knowledge, loyalty, pride in the company and its products, skill, and the ability to apply backgrounds of training and experience in the creation of valuable drug products. And most important is the proven value of a drug regardless of who makes it.

However, the trend has been for pharmaceutical manufacturing companies, large and small, to be controlled and managed by business men and salesmen who have not been educated and oriented in an atmosphere of professional responsibility. Their ultimate goal is a healthy profit. Many are not deeply concerned about curing patients as the end product of their efforts, or about adverse responses to medications, unless they become involved in litigation concerning one of their drug products or unless they can use medical information as a promotional gimmick.

Fallacy No. 2. *Generic drug products are cheaper than brand name products.* This is not necessarily true.[34] Price is governed by supply and demand and is altered by many variables, including costs of production, quality control, compliance with regulatory laws and regulations, extent of competition, costs of transportation and storage, local economic situations, and various other business and professional factors. Generic products may be sold at the same prices as brand name products or sometimes higher (see the example under *Substitution*, page 94. Either a generic product or a trademarked brand may conceivably be more costly to the patient if he is required to take higher doses because the product has significantly lower bioavailability. Higher dosage may more than offset cost differentials. Also, when a pharmacist receives a generic prescription he may provide any quality of the product called for, whether or not it is equivalent to an established product of certified potency, purity, and quality. Under the new bioavailability regulations and the MAC (maximum allowable cost) program, however, drugs are now required to meet rather rigid and specific bioequivalence requirements for Medicare payments. Thus therapeutic differences between medications are gradually disappearing and the taxpayer is beginning to pay less for drugs under welfare program.[38]

The controversy over prescribing by generic or brand names, which is basically economic in origin, is based on faulty logic. Comparing generic names with brand names is as illogical as comparing flour with bread. *Generic names refer to the pharmacologically active ingredients* of medications whereas *brand names refer to finished drug products.* Thus, tetracycline tablets (generic name) simply means any tablet containing the drug tetracycline as the single active ingredient, whereas Achromycin, Panmycin, Polycycline, Steclin, Tetracyn, etc., refer to specific formulations containing tetracycline plus definite quantities of adjuvants that are used to form the tablet. Generic prescribing permits wide variation in tablet composition and possibly some variation in quality whereas prescribing the product of a specified company restricts the composition to one specific formula.

The complex problem of quality always enters into the creation of a brand name product from a given generic drug by combining that drug with other ingredients and applying sophisticated technologies to arrive at capsules, tablets, suppositories, ointments, and other finished pharmaceutical products. Quality control tests for bioavailability and therapeutic equivalency are now rapidly becoming sufficiently advanced to enable manufacturers to guarantee that all their products will produce the same degree of efficacy as the "same" products of other manufacturers. Marketed products may usually be relied upon as being equivalent both chemically and therapeutically if official standards and appropriate tests are met.

At present, however, even the joint efforts of supplying USP and NF physical and chemical standards in conjunction with FDA good manufacturing standards and its other regulatory controls are not adequate to protect the patient. All three agencies are studying and developing suitable equivalency tests to overcome the deficiency and to reduce the hazards presented by prescribing on the basis of price and not quality. Both physician and patient must, in the final analysis, depend on the reliability of the manufacturer. Meanwhile, dollar savings that have been projected through generic prescribing are being debated. An HEW program known as MAC (maximum allowable cost) limits payment for certain multiple-source drugs through Medicare and other HEW-funded health care programs to the lowest cost at which a drug is widely and consistently available to dispensers.

Fallacy No. 3. *Generic drug products are as good therapeutically as the chemically equivalent brand name products.* This is not necessarily true. Some generic products may be even better than some branded products, but the reverse is very often true also. Names are only labels and do not alter the quality of products. The important factor is how the products are manufactured and handled. The company with outstanding personnel, modern equipment, and an efficient quality control program is much more likely to produce a better product than a company that is poorly staffed and equipped. As a matter of interest, some companies sell basic ingredients used in their own products (branded or generic) to other companies who compound the ingredients into their own products (branded or generic), but this does not necessarily guarantee products of equivalent quality as is shown in Chapter 4, *Manufacturing Factors.* Furthermore, some companies actually manufacture a given product for its competitor. One lot of a given drug product is labeled with its own brand name, while another lot is labeled with the brand name of another distributor. Thus, different lots of the same product, identical in every respect, are distributed under different labeling. This is legally and economically sound through cross-licensing and tends to guarantee therapeutic equivalency.

C. Joseph Stetler, President of the Pharmaceutical Manufacturers Association, succinctly summarized the situation when he testified before Senator Gaylord Nelson's Senate Small Business Monopoly Subcommittee on November 16, 1977:

> There's no magic in brand or generic. . . . There are plenty of little companies that do a quality job. . . . It is our well-established position that the quality of a drug product is dependent on the capability and integrity of its maker, and not on a system of drug nomenclature. . . . quality is independent of brand or generic names; it depends on the credentials of the manufacturer and his commitment to the highest standards in the production of drug products by whatever name he may choose to market them. The issue, therefore, remains one of quality and not simply of nomenclature or price.

On September 2, 1970, FDA made its long expected move to support generic prescribing when it proposed essentially identical wording for indications, contraindications, warnings, precautions, adverse reactions, and administration in the package inserts for five tetracyclines—chlortetracycline, demethylchlortetracycline, oxytetracycline, rolitetracycline, and tetracycline itself.

The wording emphasized the concept of expressing indications in terms of organisms rather than diseases. This concept originated basically from the NAS/NRC Panel on Anti-infectives and was the first step in directing all anti-infective therapy against specific organisms and developing uniform package insert information for closely related medications. These and other objectives are part of a master plan to revise, improve, and update all package inserts for prescription drugs and produce a *National Prescription Drug Compendium* by 1981.

Meanwhile efforts are being made to develop bioavailability testing methods and regulations that will guarantee therapeutic equivalency among all drugs, both generic and brand name, that contain the same active ingredients.

Inadequate Patient Education

Every patient is now considered to be a member of the health care team, for he is usually the one who carries out the therapy.[40] Therefore, he has the right to know what medication the physician is prescribing for him, what it will do to his body, exactly how it should be taken, and its potential hazards. Only when the prescriber explains all of these fully is the patient given his rightful opportunity to receive medical care that is as safe and effective as it can possibly be. See Chapter 6, *Prescribing Factors.*

Faulty Regulation

Either procrastination or undue haste in approving a new drug or in withdrawing one from the market can be harmful to both patients and physicians. The speed with which FDA acts is critical if the heartbreak of injured patients and the trauma of litigation are to be minimized.

Delayed approval of any beneficial new drug year after year can deprive patients of a possibly life-saving product and tremendously increase costs of development. In one period of more than eight years during the 1970s FDA did not approve a single new cardiovascular drug. Introduction of new drugs into the market has become exceedingly difficult. Current regulations covering the approval process now necessitate an average period of ten years for research and development and an expenditure of $15 million by the manufacturer to create a marketable drug product.

Hasty approval of dangerous drugs, on the other hand, can unnecessarily and irreversibly damage patients. Examples include the European-distributed, phocomelia-producing thalidomide and tumorigenic beta-adrenergic blocking pronethalol. A Congressional committee publicly condemned FDA for its hasty approval of one OC.[17]

Delayed withdrawal from the market of a drug whose toxicity outweighs its benefits may expose patients to unwarranted risks. Sometimes the damage and death caused by such a drug can be shocking. Thus, phenformin (DBI, Meltrol), which was being prescribed in 1977 at the rate of nearly 4 million prescriptions a year for 336,000 patients, had been known for nearly 20 years to be a cause of lactic acidosis, a serious condition with a mortality rate of 50 percent. Some estimates of the deaths it has caused run as high as 700 per year.[61] This is not unlikely since alcohol which is so widely consumed potentiates the toxicity. By 1977, FDA itself had filed about 240 reports of deaths from lactic acidosis. The Agency had periodically considered removing phenformin from the market and the Director of the Bureau of Drugs had once actually promised a Congressional committee that the Bureau would do so. But not until Ralph Nader's Health Research Group early in 1977 petitioned the Secretary of HEW to expedite removal did FDA really begin to act. On May 6 of that year FDA published a notice of an opportunity for a public hearing and one was held a week later. Other nations withdrew the drug promptly but the Bureau Director still could not make up his mind whether or not to recommend immediate withdrawal. This can be done by the Secretary of HEW under an "imminent hazard" provision of the Food, Drug, and Cosmetic Act but no Secretary had ever invoked the provision. Finally, when the Bureau of Drugs examined the international statistics it found that an estimated 50 to 700 deaths annually in the US were probably caused by phenformin-associated lactic acidosis. Then the Secretary of HEW acted. He suspended the NDA for phenformin on July 25, 1977 and ordered an end to general marketing of the drug within 90 days (by Oct 23, 1977). Only a comparatively small group of perhaps 3000 carefully selected nonketotic diabetics in whom insulin poses special hardships and for whom the benefits clearly outweigh the risks may be able to obtain the drug.[61]

Other unbelievably prolonged withdrawal actions concern dipyrone,[56] antiobesity agents that are dangerous,[57] Laetrile,[63] and enteric-coated potassium chloride tablets. The background of the serious adverse effects of the latter drug, detailed under *Irrational Ideas* in Chapter 3, appeared in the first edition of this book in 1971. The original reports in the literature date back to 1961 but not until more than 15 years of damage to patients did FDA's Bureau of Drugs begin to act. It published in the *Federal Register* of April 6, 1976 a proposal to remove the drug from the market.[26] Then the Bureau Director and his staff spent more than a year reviewing and digesting the comments received as a result of the proposal. Finally on July 29, 1977 FDA published a notice in the *Federal Register* (effective Aug 8, 1977) withdrawing approval of seven NDAs for oral potassium salt products and all similar products containing 100 mg. or more per unit dosage form of KCl. Controlled release products and solutions, however, were not included, and combination products were still to be considered.[60] Fortunately, most of the responsible manufacturers had voluntarily removed their enteric-coated tablets from the market and replaced them with potassium solutions and slow release tablets. One product (Slow-K), however, began to be associated with ulcerations of the bowel soon after it was introduced. Perhaps FDA will re-examine this drug some day when "sufficient" damage has been done to patients.

Hasty withdrawal of a beneficial drug from the market on the basis of faulty evidence of toxicity can deprive patients of a useful medication. But this is not usually a serious problem since alternatives are generally available. Nevertheless this and the other three types of FDA actions discussed above must be completed at optimum speed. Otherwise medical care in this country suffers. Perhaps current statutory provisions such as those encouraging rapid expansion of administrative "due process" need to be relaxed to some extent so that FDA can act more expeditiously than it does at present.[41]

Biological Unavailability

A drug must be present in a biologically active form at the appropriate site of action in the proper concentration for a suitable period of time in order to provide the patient with an effective medication to which the body mechanisms can respond. When medication is administered to patients so that their bodies are given an opportunity to respond, the medication is said to be biologically available. Of course, if a patient's response mechanisms are faulty or if for some reason they are prevented from reacting to chemical stimuli, the desired effect will not be induced even though the medication is made biologically available. Since the subject has a direct bearing on the therapeutic equivalency of medications, it is treated more com-

prehensively in Chapter 2, *Inequivalency of Medication.*

SELECTED REFERENCES

1. Azarnoff DL: Application of metabolic data to the evaluation of drugs. *JAMA* 211:1691 (Mar 9) 1970. Cluff LE: Problems with drugs. *Proceedings,* Conference on Continuing Education for Physicians in the Use of Drugs, 1969. Simmons HE: Speech delivered to the University of California School of Pharmacy, Sept 10, 1970.
2. Barber M: Drug combinations in antibacterial chemotherapy. *Proc Roy Soc Med* 58:990-995 (Nov) 1965.
3. *Clin-Alert No 2:* Adverse drug reactions. Johns Hopkins Hospital, Jan 12, 1967; *No 1:* Montreal General Hospital and Johns Hopkins Hospital, Jan 12, 1968; *No 45:* Belfast Hospitals, Mar 31, 1969.
4. Conn HE: *Current Therapy,* Philadelphia, Saunders, 1969.
5. Drug Information Association: *Proceedings of the Symposium on Adverse Drug Reactions. Drug Info Bull* 2:63-130 (July-Sep) 1968.
6. *Federal Register* 34:13950 (FR Doc 69-10376) Aug 29, 1969.
7. *Federal Register* 35:9001-3 (FR Doc 70-7293) June 11, 1970.
8. Goodman LS, Gilman A: *The Pharmacological Basis of Therapeutics.* New York, Macmillan, 1975, pp 1095-1105.
9. *Ibid:* p. 1159-1167.
10. Martin EW: *Techniques of Medication.* Philadelphia, Lippincott, 1969.
11. Medical Economics Company: *Physicians' Desk Reference.* Oradell, NJ, Litton Industries, Inc, 1978.
12. Miller LC: How Good Are Our Drugs? Distinguished Lecture delivered Dec. 30, 1969, before the American Association for the Advancement of Science, Boston, Mass. *Am. J. Hosp. Pharm.* 27:366-374 (May) 1970.
13. Modell W: *Drugs of Choice,* St. Louis. Mosby, 1971, pp 133-150.
14. Slone D, Gaetano LF, *et al:* Computer analysis of epidemiologic data on effect of drugs on hospital patients. *Pub Health Rep* 84:39-52 (Jan) 1969.
15. Smith AE: Antibiotic combinations, *FDA Papers* 3:13-14 (June) 1969.
16. Council on Drugs: Fixed-dose combinations of drugs. *JAMA* 213:1172-1175 (Aug 17) 1970.
17. Goldberg DC: Demulen: hastily approved drug. *Science* 170-491 (Oct 30) 1970.
18. Jick H, Miettinen OS, Shapiro S, *et al:* Comprehensive drug surveillance. *JAMA* 213:1455-1460 (Aug 31) 1970.
19. Mahoney RP: Digitalis: continuing problems related to its use. *Hosp Form Manag* 5:8-9 (Mar) 1970.
20. *FDC Reports* 32:26 (Dec 21) 1970.
21. Jones DIR: Self-poisoning with drugs. *Practitioner* 203:73-78 (July) 1969.
22. Ogilvie RI, Ruedy J: Adverse reactions during hospitalization. *Can Med Ass J* 97:1445-1450; Adverse drug reactions during hospitalization. *Ibid* 97: 1450-1457 (Dec 9) 1967.

23. Seidl LG, Thornton GF, Smith JW, Cluff LE: Studies on the epidemiology of adverse drug reactions. III. Reactions in patients on a general medical service. *Bull Johns Hopkins Hosp* 119:299-315, 1966.
24. Estrogens and endometrial cancer. *FDA Drug Bull* 6:18-20 (Feb-Mar) 1976.
25. FDA/HEW: Estrogen and other drugs. Physician labeling and patient labeling for estrogens for general use. *Fed Reg* 40:43108-23 (Sep 29); 47573-8 (Oct 29); 48793 (Nov 5) 1976.
26. FDA/HEW: Certain solid dosage forms of oral potassium salt drug products intended for prophylaxis or treatment of potassium depletion. *Fed Reg* 41:14568-70 (Apr 6) 1976.
27. Grumbach F: Activité antituberculeuse chez la souris de l'ethambutol. *Ann Inst Pasteur* 110:69-85, 1966.
28. Editorial: Deaths due to drug treatment. *Br Med J* 1:1492-3 (Jun 11) 1977.
29. Armstrong B, Dinan B, Jick H: Fatal drug reactions in patients admitted to surgical services. *Am J Surg* 132:643-5 (Nov) 1976.
30. Porter J, Jick H: Drug-related deaths among inpatients. *JAMA* 237:879-81 (Feb 28) 1977.
31. Melmon KL: Preventable drug reactions—causes and cures. *N Engl J Med* 284:1361-8 (Jun 17) 1971.
32. Talley RB, Laventurier MF: Drug-induced illness. *JAMA* 229:1043 (Aug 19) 1974.
33. Sequential oral contraceptives removed from the market. *FDA Drug Bull* 6:26-7 (Jun-Jul) 1976.
34. US Department of Health, Education, and Welfare, Task Force on Prescription Drugs: *Final Report.* Washington, DC, US Govt Printing Office, 1969.
35. Caranasos GJ, Stewart RB, Cluff LE: Drug-induced illness leading to hospitalization. *JAMA* 228:713-7 (May 6) 1974.
36. FDA/HEW: Oral contraceptive drug products: physician and patient labeling. *Fed Reg* 41: 53630-42 (Dec 7) 1976; 42: 27303-4 (May 27) 1977; Requirement for labeling directed to the patient. *Fed Reg* 43:4214-22 (Jan 31) 1978; Physician and patient labeling. *Fed Reg* 43:4223-34 (Jan 31) 1978.
37. Office of Technology Assessment: *Achieving Safer, More Effective, and Less Costly Utilization of Therapeutic Drugs.* US Congress, 1977.
38. FDA/HEW: Reducing the cost of drugs in HEW-funded health programs. *FDA Drug Bull* 6:33 (Aug-Oct) 1976.
39. Caranasos GJ, May FE, Stewart RB, Cluff LE: Drug-associated deaths of medical inpatients. *Arch Intern Med* 136:872-5 (Aug) 1976.
40. Martin EW: Introductory remarks, Joint DIA/AMA/FDA/PMA Symposium on Drug Information for Patients—The Patient Package Insert. *Drug Info J* 11 (Suppl):1-80 (Jan) 1977.
41. Merrill RA: Letter to the editor of *Washington Post*
from FDA General Counsel. *FDC Rep* 38:12-22 (Aug 9) 1976.
42. Motto JA, Greene C: Suicide and the medical community. *Arch Neurol Psychiatry* 80:776-81 (Dec) 1958.
43. Editorial: Suicide among doctors. *Br Med J* 1: 789-90 (Mar 28) 1964.
44. Ree GH: Suicide in Macuata province, Fiji. *Practitioner* 207:669-71 (Nov) 1971.
45. Kaplan M: Suicide by ingestion of a potassium preparation. *Ann Intern Med* 71:363-4 (Aug) 1969.
46. Editorial: Suicide—a world problem. *Lancet* 1:1411 (Dec 25) 1971.
47. Smith AJ: Self-poisoning with drugs: a worsening situation. *Br Med J* 4:157-9 (Oct 21) 1972.
48. Holland J, Massie MJ, Grant C, Plumb MM: Drugs ingested in suicide attempts and fatal outcome. *NY State J Med* 75:2343-9 (Nov) 1975.
49. Motto JA: Hope, suicide, and medical practice. *JAMA* 234:1168-9 (Dec 15) 1975.
50. Heaney D, Derghazarian CB, Pineo GF, *et al:* Massive colchicine overdosage; a report on the toxicity. *Am J Med Sci:* 271: 233-8 (Mar-Apr) 1976.
51. Mishara BL, Baker AH, Mishara TT: The frequency of suicide attempts: a retrospective approach applied to college students. *Am J Psychiatry* 133: 841-4 (Jul) 1976.
52. von Brauchitsch: The physician's suicide revisited. *J Nerv Ment Dis* 162: 40-5 (Jan) 1976.
53. Jones DIR: Self-poisoning with drugs: the past 20 years in Sheffield. *Br Med J* 1: 28-9 (Jan 1) 1977.
54. Johns MW: Self poisoning with barbiturates in England and Wales. *Br Med J* 1: 1128-30 (Apr 30) 1977.
55. Craig AG, Pitts FN: Suicide by physicians. *Dis Nerv Syst* 29: 763-72 (Nov) 1968.
56. FDA/HEW: Drug products containing dipyrone; withdrawal of approval of New Drug Application. *Fed Reg* 42: 30893-4 (Jun 17) 1977.
57. FDA/HEW: Thyroid, digitalis, and related drugs for human use. *Fed Reg* 42: 27262 (May 27) 1977.
58. Brewer C: Suicide with tricyclic antidepressants. *Br Med J* 2: 110 (Jul 10) 1976.
59. Editorial: Recent trends in suicide. *Stat Bull* (Metro Life Ins Co) 57: 5-7 (May) 1976.
60. FDA/HEW: Certain solid dosage forms of oral potassium salt drug products. Withdrawal of approval of New Drug Applications. *Fed Reg* 42: 38644-5 (Jul 29) 1977.
61. FDA/HEW: Phenformin: removal from general market. *FDA Drug Bull* 7: 14-16 (Aug) 1977.
62. FDA/HEW: Progestational drug products for human use: requirement for labeling directed to the patient. *Fed Reg* 42: 37636-48 (July 22) 1977.
63. FDA/HEW: Laetrile: Commissioner's decision on status. *Fed Reg* 42: 39768-806 (Aug 5) 1977.

2 Inequivalence of Medication

Chemically identical medications are not necessarily equivalent therapeutically. Some drug products are less effective than others because of inept research and development, inadequate control of manufacturing processes, improper handling by distributors, improper prescribing, incorrect administration, or abnormal patient response.[1,2,4] Safe and effective medication of the patient with modern, highly potent drug products depends not only on how these products are prepared, packaged, shipped, stored, prescribed, and used, but also on how the body of the individual patient reacts to the medication.

Therapeutic inequivalence of medications may present potential or real clinical hazards.[38]

Factors Influencing Drug Efficacy

A drug elicits the desired biological response in a patient, i.e., is therapeutically effective, only when all the following criteria are satisfied:

1. *Form.* The drug must be in an appropriate biologically active form (salt, ester, ether, metabolite, or other derivative that is utilized efficiently by the body).

2. *Place.* The drug must be released from its dosage form, absorbed, and distributed to the desired site of drug action in the patient (drug receptors in dermatomucosal tissues, gastrointestinal tract, blood and lymph, or a specific tissue, organ, or body system).

3. *Quantity.* The drug must permeate that site in a therapeutically effective concentration in an unbound, pharmacologically active form.

4. *Time.* The drug must reach the site of action promptly enough to meet the patient's therapeutic needs and it must remain at the desired concentration for an appropriate length of time to exert the desired therapeutic effect. Proper timing and concentration are achieved by controlling input (gastrointestinal, parenteral, or dermatomucosal) to offset the output (metabolic destruction and excretion) once the proper blood level has been established. In some instances a "loading dose" is given to achieve that level promptly.

5. *Response.* The patient responds to the drug in the desired and expected manner.

When the first four of these criteria are satisfied, the drug is said to be biologically or physiologically available, i.e., available in the proper form, place and quantity for a long enough time to elicit the desired response in patients with normal reactivity. Patients, however, do not necessarily react to medications in the expected manner. Accordingly, *therapeutic efficacy* depends basically on two major requirements: *biological availability (bioavailability)* and *patient response.* These form the subject matter of two important disciplines concerned with safe and effective medication of the patient: biopharmaceutics and therapeutics.

Biopharmaceutics. This biomedical science is concerned with the effects of formulation on biological availability of drugs. It embraces all the interrelationships between the biological characteristics of the drug product on the one hand and its physical and chemical properties on the other. The science is, therefore, concerned with biological processes such as absorption, distribution, metabolism, storage and excretion of drugs;

with physical and chemical processes such as disintegration, dissolution and dispersion; and especially with the rates (pharmacokinetics) of all of these processes because they govern the rates at which drugs become bioavailable.[47] In the *United States Pharmacopeia XVII* that became official from September 1, 1965, the concept of "physiological availability" was introduced for the first time and a USP-NF Joint Panel on Physiological Availability was activated. During 1969 FDA published (*Federal Register* Doc 69-9980) the requirement to include in each New Drug Application "adequate data to assure the biologic availability of the drug in the formulation which is marketed . . ." These data usually consist of blood levels achieved under rigidly controlled conditions, but because some drugs do not reach sites of action via the blood and some are excreted very rapidly, other criteria are necessary.* A question frequently raised is "What are adequate equivalence data?" Current official drug standards appear to be inadequate.[12] A decade ago Lasagna[21] pinpointed many of the issues and suggested certain guidelines.[21] He asked the following questions:

"How high a peak concentration is 'high enough' for a drug? How fast is 'fast enough' for absorption? How variable can it be? Is a 'peak and valley' drug better than a 'plateau' one? Should a manufacturer's version of a particular generic drug be demonstrated clinically effective prior to approval? Is it ethical to try an unproven version of a generic drug in a patient with a serious disease? Can we rely on new *in vitro* tests, such as those that measure dissolution rate? At what pH should these studies be made? At what temperature? With how large a beaker? At what rate of stirring? Must we at least demand biological performance, with respect to absorption, that mimics closely (how closely?) the performance of the original drug? If so, shall this work be done in animals? If so, in what species? In man? If so, in healthy volunteers, in sick patients or in both? Of what age? . . . Should the tests be single-dose studies or multiple-dose 'equilibrium' studies?"

We still do not have adequate answers to all of these questions and studies to correlate *in vitro* tests, *in vivo* drug level studies, and clinical trials have been underway since the early 1970s. The relative clinical efficacy of chemically identical as well as different drug products will eventually be established by such investigations.

Therapeutics. This medical science is concerned with patient healing and response to various types of treatment. In its broadest sense it embraces all types of therapy including all the techniques of medication. The etiology, diagnosis and treatment of diseases as well as mechanisms of action, precautions, contraindications, warnings, drug interactions, and the adverse effects and other hazards of drug therapy are fundamentals in sound therapeutics. The physician must have up-to-date knowledge in depth about the selection, prescribing, and administration of medication as well as the wisdom to realize when a drug is to be withheld.

The patient benefits when *both* therapeutics and biopharmaceutics are properly applied. Neither one alone insures correct medication of the patient. A carefully formulated, properly preserved, potent, high-quality medication can be rendered worthless when improperly prescribed or administered. And on the other hand, the most skillful physician, even though he employs the very finest techniques of medication, achieves nothing if the drug he prescribes and administers cannot be made available in an active form in the body. Sound scientific and professional practices, both medical and pharmaceutical, are essential for effective medication of the patient.

Throughout the long course of events from research and development of a drug product to the taking of the medication by the patient lie a host of pitfalls anyone of which may prevent a drug from acting in the patient in the desired manner. Because of the multitude of factors that influence drug efficacy and safety, different batches or dosage forms of a given drug product prepared from the same active ingredients, even by the same manufacturer, and made to appear the same in every respect may not have the same degree of biological availability, and therefore may not be therapeutically equivalent.[2,4,20,32,33]

Biological Inequivalence

In an attempt to supply meaningful answers to the many questions concerning bioavailability and therapeutic equivalence, the

---

* This requirement was temporarily rescinded in 1970 before the Regulations became official when it was pointed out the impossibility of fulfilling this requirement until adequate tests are developed.

HEW Task Force on Prescription Drugs* selected the drugs listed in Table 2-1 for scientific examination in 1968. Soon thereafter FDA initiated studies on these drugs in laboratories at Georgetown University, Washington, DC, and the Public Health Service Hospital, San Francisco, CA.[4]

At first glance, Table 2-1 may appear to contain a small number of drugs. Actually, some of these are components of many drug products and dosage forms, some of which are prepared by as many as 100 different manufacturers. Thus this short list of pharmacologically active ingredients represents thousands of different packages of medications on the market. The cost and effort involved in making thorough bioequivalence studies of all drug products with potential bioavailability problems is therefore tremendous.

The drugs were selected for testing because they were (1) *critical,* that is, used to control an important disease or relieve severe, disabling symptoms, (2) dispensed usually in a *solid* rather than a liquid form, (3) *relatively insoluble,* or (4) reported or suspected to have dosage forms *involved in nonequivalence discussions or therapeutic failures.* In testing

---

*Established in May, 1967, upon a directive from President Lyndon B. Johnson. The Report of the Secretary's Review Committee of the Task Force on Prescription Drugs recommended that (1) "FDA continue to develop Reference Standards for generic drugs to assure biological equivalency among drug products" and (2) "The Secretary of the Department of Health, Education, and Welfare be assisted by appropriate Advisory Committees to evaluate drug costs and biologic and therapeutic equivalency."[23]

Table 2-1 Drugs Selected by HEW for Biological Equivalency Studies

Aminophylline	Para-aminosalicylate,
Bishydroxycoumarin	sodium
Chloramphenicol	Phenytoin
Chlortetracycline	Potassium penicillin G
Diethylstibestrol	Potassium penicillin V
Diphenhydramine HCl	Prednisone
Erythromycin	Quinidine
Ferrous sulfate	Reserpine
Griseofulvin	Secobarbital sodium
Hydrocortisone	Sulfisoxazole
Isoniazid	Tetracycline
Meperidine HCl	Thyroid
Meprobamate	Tripelennamine HCl
Oxytetracycline	Warfarin sodium

drugs for bioavailability, FDA often used the drug approved in the original NDA as the Reference Standard since that was the one for which most complete and detailed data were available.

Within a year studies sponsored by FDA and others had pointed out different absorption rates, different bioavailability, or other important inequivalences for different makes of the following: ampicillin, bishydroxycoumarin, chloramphenicol, erythromycin, griseofulvin, isoniazid, nitrofurantoin, oxytetracycline, para-aminosalicylic acid, penicillin G, phenylbutazone, phenytoin, prednisone, quinidine, salicylamide, spironolactone, sulfisoxazole, tetracycline, and tolbutamide.[2,4,15,28]

In some instances FDA stopped certification of a number of drugs sold under generic names and withdrew them from the market when it was shown that they yielded blood levels which were below therapeutic levels and which were far from being equivalent to those yielded by products manufactured by the original patentees or licensees. Even these producers who had had decades of experience and had carefully worked out meaningful control procedures encountered bioequivalence problems. Usually, however, they are now able to insure proper bioavailability.[20,24]

Early in 1971, FDA published a paper on drug investigations that clearly demonstrated that chemically equivalent oxytetracycline HCl capsules were not biologically equivalent. Out of ten generic products that were compared with two lots of Terramycin, used as a reference standard, only three yielded satisfactory serum levels of drug. The other seven yielded levels that averaged only about 50 percent of the Terramycin levels.[30]

Some generic dosage forms (capsules, tablets) were found to remain largely intact after agitation in simulated intestinal fluid for as long as 17 hours.[2,4,19] On the other hand, some generic products were shown to produce higher blood levels more promptly than those yielded by medications with original patents.

During the early 1970s, accumulated evidence indicated that digoxin and digitoxin products made by different manufacturers, and even different batches from the same manufacturer, varied significantly in bioavailability. In 1974 and 1975 FDA implemented digoxin and digitoxin certification programs that included new USP dissolution rate standards based on studies of bioavailability. This assured a high and comparable degree of bioavailability for all marketed digoxin and digitoxin products, but at the same time rendered outmoded the dosages recommended in some textbooks. Use of those dosages, which were appropriate for old, less bioavailable products, could result in dangerous overdosage. Therefore new accurate digoxin labeling was published by FDA in 1976. [39-44]

The quality and therapeutic efficacy of medications obviously depends to a large extent on how each batch of drug product is manufactured rather than on who makes it and how it is named. [3,18,26]

On June 20, 1969, the Commissioner of Food and Drugs spelled out the first FDA protocol and criteria for comparing bioavailability of chemically equivalent oxytetracycline products. During the decade of the 1970s these instructions were modified from time to time as more experience was gained.

In the early 1970s, HEW Secretary Weinberger was determined to cut the $3 billion Medicare expenditures for drugs by initiating generic prescribing and by limiting Federal payments for prescription drugs to "the lowest cost products generally available." He was blocked, however, by the bioequivalence issue since substitution of a less effective drug would raise the problem of lowered quality of medical care. In an attempt "to determine whether or not the technological capability is now available to assure that drug products with the same physical and chemical composition will produce comparable therapeutic effects" a Drug Bioequivalence Study Panel was assembled on April 12, 1974 by the Office of Technology Assessment (OTA), the scientific evaluative body of the US Congress. The Panel's report, [37] submitted three months later, temporarily undercut Weinberger's proposal. OTA's key conclusions were:

1. Present compendial standards and guidelines for Current Good Manufacturing Practice do not insure quality and uniform bioavailability for drug products. Not only may the products of different manufacturers vary, but the product of a single manufacturer may vary from batch to batch or may change during storage.
2. Variations in the bioavailability of drug

products have been recognized as responsible for a few therapeutic failures.
3. A system should be organized as rapidly as possible to generate an official list of interchangeable drug products.

The deficiencies causing therapeutic inequivalences are gradually being rectified. On June 20, 1975, FDA published proposed bioavailability and bioequivalence regulations that with some modification were finalized [36] and in June, 1976 published a list of drugs presenting actual or potential bioequivalence problems. [35] After some overreaction, industry began to cooperate fully in providing the necessary data and the MAC (Maximum Allowable Cost) program was initiated with regulations in August, 1976. A MAC for ampicillin capsules, the first, became effective on June 27, 1977. [46]

Just how much bioavailability testing is necessary for each type of drug, how much the testing adds to the cost of medications, and to what extent the new requirements are decreasing the number of new drugs that are approved can only be determined as the testing programs are designed, implemented, and continually improved. Many years of trial and error will be required to establish therapeutic equivalences adequately.

Therapeutic Inequivalence

Generic equivalence does not guarantee therapeutic equivalence. In an attempt to clarify the discussions about this concept, the Task Force on Prescription Drugs in its Final Report discarded the widely used term *generic equivalents** because it was so controversial [5-11,13,17,22] and it had been given so many different interpretations that its use caused confusion. [14,16] Instead the Task Force used the following terms: [23]

Chemical equivalents—Those multiple-source drug products which contain essentially identical amounts of the identical active ingredients, in identical dosage forms, and which meet existing physicochemical standards in the official compendia.

Biological equivalents—Those chemical equivalents which, when administered in the same amounts, will provide essentially the same biologi-

---

*The term *generic name,* as used in this volume, is defined on page 87.

cal or physiological availability, as measured by blood levels, etc.

Clinical equivalents—Those chemical equivalents which, when administered in the same amounts, will provide essentially the same therapeutic effect as measured by the control of a symptom or a disease.

As a result of the increased attention being focused on nonequivalence of medications, investigators in government, industry, and the universities are developing animal models from which extrapolations to man can be made. Also attempts are being made to utilize specific indicators of nonequivalence, such as degrees of response to antihypertensives, diuretics, hypoglycemics, and anticoagulants. Radioactive tagging is also being tested as an indicator. One long-range goal is to develop improved official *in vitro* tests that

will correlate well with *in vivo* tests and thus obviate as much as possible the need to test for therapeutic efficacy and equivalence in humans.

Factors Causing Therapeutic Inequivalence

The subject of therapeutic equivalence of medications is very complex. Even a quick review of the rapidly growing literature on the subject overwhelms the reader with the variety of pertinent variables. [1,29] The alphabetical lists given in Table 2-2 indicate the multiplicity of factors that govern bioavailability; onset, intensity and duration of action; and therapeutic efficacy and safety of medications.

Optimum medication of the patient demands considerable professional knowledge

Table 2-2 Some of the Factors Governing Therapeutic Inequivalence*

Manufacturing Factors	Pressure of tablet punches	Patient Factors
Additives (adjuncts)	Purity	Absorption characteristics
Adjuvants	Solubility of adjuncts	Adverse reactions
Binders	Solubility of drug	Appearance of medication
Buffers	Solvation	Auto-inhibition of enzymes
Chelation	Stereoisomeric stability	Biotransformation factors
Coating composition	Stereoisomerism	Chelation
Coating thickness	Surface activity	Comcomitant medication
Colors	Surface area	Concurrent disease
Compactness of fill	Surfactants	Deaggregation rate
Complexation	Suspending agents	Disease state
Crystal structure	Uniformity of composition	Dispersion rate
Deaggregation rate	Vehicles	Dissolution rate
Dehydration	Wettability	Dosage regimen
Diluents		Drug half-life
Disintegrators	**Distribution Factors**	Drug interactions
Dissolution rate	Age of drug product	Enzyme deficiency
Emulsifying agents	Deterioration	Enzyme induction
Excipients	Epimerization	Enzyme inhibition
Flavors	Humidity	Excretion rate
Formulation	Inertness of atmosphere	Fasting
Friability of tablets	Moisture, atmospheric	Fluid intake
Granulators	Oxidation	Food intake
Hardness of tablets	Packaging	Hydrolysis rate
Hydration	Radiation	Hypersensitivity
Impurities	Reduction	Inborn metabolic error
Incompatibilities	Stability of ingredients	Metabolism rate
Lubricants	Stereoisomeric shifts	Percentage of drug metabolized
Moisture content	Storage conditions	Permeation rate
Packaging materials	Temperature of environment	pH of body fluids
Particle size	Transportation stresses	Protein binding
pH of drug product		Psychological factors
Polymorphism	**Prescribing Factors**	Site of absorption
Porosity of tablets	Incompatibilities, chemical	Solubility of drug
Potency	Incompatibilities, physical	Temperature of patient
Preservatives	Incompatibilities, therapeutic	
	Techniques of medication	

* This table is merely indicative of the complexity of the problem. Many more factors are given throughout the text. See, for example, pages 250–253.

and experience because so many hidden dangers to the patient must be detected and avoided. Unfortunately, practitioners are not always aware of differences that may exist between different brands of the same drug product or even between different lots of the same dosage form from the same manufacturer. And they are confused by conflicting claims made for generic equivalents.[25] In cases of clinical failure the physician usually prescribes a substitute medication with similar activity, often in the belief that the patient is not responding. How can he respond if for some reason the medication is not bioavailable?

In an attempt to obtain answers to the pressing questions that have arisen in regard to medication efficacy and utilization, FDA developed a National Drug Code.[27] This enabled the agency to develop a vast computerized data bank of facts, including therapeutic equivalence data for every dosage form of every drug product on the American market. (See page 63.)

For purpose of analysis, the factors influencing biological availability, therapeutic efficacy, and safe use of medications are discussed in the next eight chapters under the following subjects: (1) research and development, (2) manufacturing, (3) distribution, (4) prescribing, (5) clinical laboratory testing, (6) patient response, (7) adverse reactions, and (8) drug interactions.

Only if all the key factors mentioned throughout this volume are carefully controlled can a drug product be expected to be therapeutically useful in a given patient. But important questions remain: *Which nonequivalence factors really matter? What degree of nonequivalence is therapeutically significant?*

Until satisfactory answers to these questions are obtained, the Federal Government will undoubtedly continue to purchase its drugs from manufacturers who have carefully established the bioavailability and therapeutic efficacy of their products. It now permits only certain producers to bid because of its past experience with them and because it has knowledge of their facilities for production and quality control.[34] Government purchasers take every possible precaution to make certain that the members of our Armed Services and others who are entitled to government medical services receive effective medications. To ensure this, FDA assumed

responsibility early in 1976 for quality surveillance of all medications purchased by the Department of Defense.

Fortunately, the healing powers of the human body are amazing. Many patients recover with or without prescribed therapy. In non-life-threatening diseases, the course of illness may be shortened or lengthened or not affected at all by the therapy offered. Infections have actually been controlled by withdrawal of all drug therapy.[31] Thus, individual responses in noncontrolled circumstances often give erroneous impressions of value or of hazard. This is one reason why properly conducted research and development is so essential.

SELECTED REFERENCES

1. Blake JB: *Safeguarding the Public.* Baltimore, Johns Hopkins Press, 1970.
2. Castle WB, Astwood EB, Finland M, Keefer CS: White paper on the therapeutic equivalence of chemically equivalent drugs. *JAMA* 208:1171-1172 (May 19) 1969.
3. Crawford JN, Willard JW: *Guide for Drug Manufacturers.* The Food and Drug Directorate, Department of National Health and Welfare, Canada.
4. Drug Information Association: Symposium on formulation factors affecting therapeutic performance of drug products. *Drug Info Bull* 3:116 (Jan-June) 1969.
5. Editorial: Beyond the price tag. *GP* 38:76-77 (July) 1968.
6. Editorial: Brand, generic drugs differ in man. *Medical News, JAMA* 205:23-24, 30 (Aug 26) 1968.
7. Editorial: Brand names. *Br Med J* 1:781-782 (Mar 30) 1968.
8. Editorial: Generic versus brand-named drugs. *Am J Pharm* 139:94-96, 1967.
9. Editorial: Third tradename drug superior. *GP* 38:75 (Oct) 1968.
10. Editorial: Generic drugs and therapeutic equivalence. *JAMA* 206:1785 (Nov 18) 1968.
11. Editorial: The issue of "generic" versus "trade" names. *Int J Clin Pharmacol* 2:1-2 (Jan) 1969.
12. Feinberg M: Drug standards in military procurement. *J Am Pharm Assoc* NS9:113-116 (Mar) 1969.
13. Flotte CT: Editorial. *Md State Med J* 16:33-36 (July) 1967.
14. Friend DG, Goolkasian AR, Hassan WE, Jr, Vona, JP: Generic terminology and the cost of drugs. *JAMA* 209:80-84 (July 7) 1969.
15. Glasko AJ, Kinkel AW, Alegnani WC, Holmes EL: An evaluation of the absorption characteristics of different chloramphenicol preparations in normal human subjects. *Clin Pharmacol Ther* 9:472-483 (Apr) 1968.
16. Goddard JL: The equivalency debate. *J Clin Pharmacol* 8:205-211 (July-Aug) 1968.
17. Hodges RM: Biopharmaceutic equivalency and the role of the Food and Drug Administration. *Am J Hosp Pharm* 25:121-127 (Mar) 1968.

18. Jeffries SB: Current good manufacturing practices compliance—A review of the problems and an approach to their management. *Food Drug Cosmetic Law J*, pp 580-603 (Dec) 1968.

19. Macdonald H, Pisano F, Burger J, *et al:* Physiological availability of various tetracyclines. *Drug Info Bull* 3:76-81 (Jan-June) 1969.

20. Martin CM, Rubin M, O'Malley WE, et al: Comparative physiological availability of "brand" and "generic" drugs in man: chloramphenicol, sulfisoxazole, and diphenylhydantoin. *Pharmacologist* 10 (2):167 (Fall) 1968.

21. Lasagna L: The pharmaceutical revolution; its impact on science and society. *Science* 166:1227-33 (Dec 5) 1969.

22. *Med Trib,* pp 10, 26 (Mar 31) 1969.

23. U.S. Department of Health, Education, and Welfare: *Final Report of the Task Force on Prescription Drugs; Report of the Secretary's Review Committee of the Task Force on Prescription Drugs.* Washington, D.C., 1969.

24. Schneller GH: Hazard of therapeutic nonequivalency of drug products. *J Am Pharm Assoc* NS9:455-459 (Sep) 1969.

25. Sperandio GJ: A look at generic and trade name injectables. *Bull Parent Drug Assoc* 21:153-164, 1967.

26. US Food and Drug Administration: Drugs: current good manufacturing practice in manufacturing, processing, packaging, or holding. *Fed Reg* 34:13553-8, 1969.

27. US Food and Drug Administration: *National Drug Code Directory.* First edition, (Oct) 1969; last edition 1976; Kissman HM: *FDA Papers* 2:26-27, 1969.

28. Varley AB: The generic inequivalence of drugs. *JAMA* 206:1745 (Nov 18) 1968.

29. Wagner JG: *Biopharmaceutics and Relevant Pharmacokinetics.* Hamilton, IL, Drug Intelligence Pub, 1971.

30. Blair DC, Barnes RW, Wildner LE *et al:* Biological availability of oxytetracycline HCl capsules. *JAMA* 215:251-254 (Jan 11) 1971.

31. Price DJE, Sleigh JD: Control of infection due to *Klebsiella aerogenes* in a neurosurgical unit by withdrawal of all antibiotics. *Lancet* 2:1213-1215 (Dec 12) 1970.

32. Wagner JG: Generic equivalence and inequivalence of oral products. *Drug Intell Clin Pharm* 5:115-128 (Apr) 1971.

33. Editorial: Biological availability of drugs. *Lancet* 1:83 (Jan 8) 1972.

34. Shirkey HC: Therapeutic reliability of variously manufactured drugs: generic-therapeutic equivalence. *J Pediat* 76:774-776 (May) 1970.

35. FDA/HEW: *Holders of Approved New Drug Applications for Drugs Presenting Actual or Potential Bioequivalence Problems.* HEW Publication No (FDA) 76-3009, Washington, DC, June, 1976. Updated in 1978.

36. FDA/HEW: Human drugs: procedures for establishing a bioequivalence requirement. *Fed Reg* 40:26164-9 (June 20) 1975.

37. Office of Technology Assessment: *Drug Bioequivalence.* US Government Printing Office, Washington, DC, 1974.

38. Chodos DJ, DiSanto AR: *Basis of Bioavailability.* Kalamazoo, MI, Upjohn Company, 1973.

39. Editorials: Revised digoxin dosage. *FDA Drug Bull* 6:31-2 (Aug-Oct) 1976; Digitoxin reformulation-dosage change. *ibid* 6:39-40 (Nov-Dec) 1976.

40. FDA/HEW: Labeling for digoxin products. *Fed Reg* 41:17755-61 (Apr 28) 1976.

41. Manninen V, Melin J, Härtel G: Serum-digoxin concentrations during treatment with different preparations. *Lancet* II: 934-5 (Oct 23) 1971.

42. Lindenbaum J, Mellow MH, Blackstone MO, Butler VP: Variation in biologic availability of digoxin from four preparations. *N Engl J Med* 285:1344-7 (Dec 9) 1971.

43. Editorial: Bioavailability of digoxin. *N Engl J Med* 285: 1433-4 (Dec 16) 1971.

44. Editorial: Biological availability of drugs. *Lancet* 1:83 (Jan 8) 1972.

45. Dittert LW, DiSanto AR: *The Bioavailability of Drug Products.* Washington, DC, American Pharmaceutical Assoc, 1975.

46. FDA/HEW: Cost limits on ampicillin capsules. *Drug Bull* 7:9 (May-July) 1977.

47. Wagner JG: *Biopharmaceutics and Relevant Pharmaceutics.* Drug Intelligence Publications, Hamilton, IL, 1971.

*Not all drug products are
carefully researched and developed.*

3 Research and Development Factors

Poorly conceived drug research and development programs may create serious hazards for both physician and patient. Unless rather sophisticated studies are carefully designed by competent medical scientists, incorrect conclusions concerning dosage, efficacy and safety can be inadvertently reached and can result in future harm to patients and legal problems for physicians. One of the major reasons for the existence of the Food and Drug Administration which regulates foods, drugs, cosmetics and devices,* is to evaluate the validity of the claims for therapeutic efficacy and safety set forth by various research groups as the end product of their investigations, and to confirm or reject each claim on its own merits.

The major objective of drug research and development is to create medications with high activity, low toxicity, and relatively few side effects. But separation of both toxic and side effects from therapeutic effects within a drug series is never easy and can never be completely accomplished. Side effects are to be expected with some drugs, as for example, mydriasis with anticholinergics. Since the margin of safety between therapeutically effective doses and toxic doses is often narrow, much time and effort are spent in trying to increase this margin, to uncover and study mechanisms of toxicity, and to develop information concerning interactions of chemicals with the biological systems of man.

But better organization and correlation of data on drug toxicity are urgently needed.

The problem of retrieval and evaluation of these data which are widely scattered is receiving considerable attention. The National Library of Medicine with its computer-based National Toxicologic Information Program is actively engaged in locating toxicologic data, including those relating to medications. The Excerpta Medica Foundation, American Chemical Society, and others have also developed very extensive computerized data bases on medicinal toxicity.

IDEAS FOR NEW MEDICATIONS

Fortunately a trend toward rational drug design and testing based on a deeper understanding of medicinal toxicity and activity, especially interactions of specific molecular structures with cellular components (molecular biology), has been developing rapidly since about 1960. A drug with predictable therapeutic utility can now be designed on paper before it is synthesized. Thus, drugs that block essential metabolic processes in infecting microorganisms (the parasite) effectively, but do so much less effectively in the human body (the host), can be visualized and the molecular structures drawn. This was demonstrated when certain pyrimidine antimalarials were found to be several thousand times more toxic to the malarial parasite than to man and certain pyrimidine antibacterials were found to be as high as 100,000 times more active against bacterial enzymes than against human enzymes. [17]

Older methods of development, however, will still continue to be used for many years, especially the following: (1) chemical synthesis of organic compounds followed by rapid

* Comprehensive device legislation has recently been enacted. [80]

24

screening in test tubes and test animals and (2) biosynthesis, whereby substances are introduced into culture media to stimulate microorganisms to produce specific molecular structures or to modify structures of other drugs. These two methods have often yielded valuable new agents which are distinct improvements over naturally occurring or previously synthesized products.

Syntheses are sometimes the result of attempts to improve upon physiologically active natural products that have already been thoroughly investigated subsequent to their isolation from microorganisms, plants or animals. Thus primaquine, which is structurally related to the quinoline moiety of the quinine molecule, was synthesized and found to be the most effective drug available for use against *vivax* malaria.

Systematic testing of synthetic and naturally occurring organic compounds, elucidation of mechanisms of drug action, and specific test methods have been critically reviewed for each of the major drug categories.[35,40] New leads are constantly being sought. Physicians who see patients may recognize a need for a new type of medication or a useful combination of older drugs. The pharmaceutical companies maintain close contact with such practitioners, responsible clinical investigators, and other consultants and often foster brainstorming sessions and seminars as well as sponsor fundamental research by academic, industrial, governmental, and other personnel in the health fields.* These companies also make intensive literature searches with the aid of computers and highly trained reference personnel. When they review compilations of vital statistics, for example, they sometimes discover a need for a drug to control some disease with a high enough incidence or mortality rate to justify the necessary research effort. News reports in the mass media, ideas in correspondence and conversations, and many other sources also frequently supply leads for new medications.[37]

The decision to develop a given drug and its appropriate dosage forms is usually made by a top-level committee composed of scientific and management personnel in a pharmaceutical company. Periodically the committee reviews ideas for new products and establishes research priorities based on need, competition, economic factors, potential market, facilities available, scientific capabilities, and other professional, scientific, and administrative considerations.

As a result of intensified interest in improving research methodology, ideas for new drugs are generally based on sound reasoning. Even if this merely originates in reputed successes of witch doctors in tropical jungles, there is usually some tentative evidence of therapeutic efficacy. Thus, discovery that a special type of paralysis was produced by poison arrows of jungle tribes led to the development of the curare type of neuromuscular blocking agents. Ideas for new medications have repeatedly arisen through examination of natural products derived from animals, plants, and minerals from countries and oceans in all parts of the world.

Evidence of physiological activity in synthetic chemicals is noted during mass screening of tens of thousands of compounds with test animals, sometimes computerized for rapid surveying. Out of the 150,000 substances tested annually by American pharmaceutical manufacturers, only about 10 or 20 show enough activity to justify their development into truly valuable new drugs. The odds against success are roughly 10,000 to 1.

Serendipity and modification of known molecular structures† may at times decrease this ratio somewhat but promises of activity at these early stages must not be relied upon heavily. All new drugs must be based on sound data and rational ideas, otherwise one might be developed that eventually proves to be of little value in therapy or too harmful for use in medications.

---

*The member companies of the PMA budgeted over $1 billion for 1977 for research and development of medications well above 2% of the total research expenditures in the U.S.A. A major manufacturer spends $100,000,000 annually on this phase of its operations.

†Modification of molecular structures, so-called molecular manipulation, can appreciably increase efficacy and safety. Sometimes a minor change can produce dramatic improvements or even produce an entirely different type of activity as when an antihistamine was modified to form chlorpromazine, used to treat anxiety and tension. However, most compounds synthesized and studied in the laboratories of the pharmaceutical manufacturers are never reported in the literature, usually because they appear to have no therapeutic utility, but sometimes because they supply leads which are best not shared with competitors.

Irrational Ideas

Countless illogical, useless ideas for medications date back thousands of years. The older pharmacopoeias include a vast array of incredible ingredients. Powders, jellies, and other preparations were concocted from calcined human bones, crab claws and eyes, dung of the dog and other animals, elk hooves, frog livers, human skulls, incinerated heads of black cats, capon gizzards, powdered precious and semiprecious stones, testicles of the boar and horse, viper skins and so on almost *ad infinitum.*[34] Some of these are still used in various areas of the world where modern therapeutic ideas have not penetrated the gloom of ignorance.

But it isn't necessary to search through musty old tomes. Irrational drug therapy has occurred too often in recent decades, even in our own enlightened country. Less than a century ago album graecum (sunbleached excrement of dogs) was available in powdered form as a drug and was referred to in standard textbooks as late as 1926. In 1904 a widely used medical book for household use described cures for cancer such as chromic chloride in stramonium ointment and Fowler's solution (potassium arsenite). That was just before Federal food and drug laws were enacted and before the American Medical Association began its efforts to protect gullible people from remedies such as watermelon juice, apple juice, and other fake cures for cancer that were prescribed by quacks.[76]

Some drugs have been introduced after available toxicity data should have kept them off the market. As long ago as 1885, Hoppe-Seyler, a founder of modern biochemistry, described the anemia produced in experimental animals with phenylhydrazine. And yet, three years later acetylphenylhydrazine was marketed under the name Pyrodin. Both of these chemicals were found by Heinz in 1890 to produce the Heinz bodies that are diagnostic of drug-induced hemolytic anemias (see page 271). This lack of attention to warning information has persisted down through the decades to recent times.

A few examples of disastrous ideas that led to the creation of harmful medications during recent decades are listed below:

1. Attempts have been made to prolong the action of some parenteral products with the aid of adjuvants or vehicles which are not metabolized or excreted readily by the human body, but which tend to form permanent deposits in the tissues and which may set up foci of irritation and possibly carcinogenic activity. Mineral oil and silicones are typical examples of nonaqueous vehicles that do not meet the official USP requirement that they be of vegetable origin in order that they will be metabolized. However, mineral oil emulsions have been routinely used as vehicles for certain injections (allergenic products, micronized silica sclerosing agent, etc.).

2. Fixed combinations of some drugs, one or more of which cause problems such as hypersensitization or rapid development of resistant organisms, have been prepared. Thus, not only is flexibility of dosage lost, but also the efficacy of a good drug that may be present. See *Unsuitable Drug Combinations* (page 8, Chapter 1).

3. Vehicles for medications have occasionally been selected on the basis of their ability to act as solvents with little or no attention being paid to toxicity. A carefully colored and flavored elixir of sulfanilamide containing 10% of the drug and 72% diethylene glycol (antifreeze) was marketed in 1937 without adequate testing in animals and caused the death of more than 100 children. Even a cursory review of the literature would have revealed that feeding diethylene glycol (3% to 10%) to rats in their drinking water rapidly killed them.[10,14,43] Tragically, this same error was repeated by a chemist in India some 35 years later (1974) when he substituted the same toxic glycol for propylene glycol when compounding an elixir of acetaminophen. Fortunately far fewer deaths than with the first incident resulted (only 16).

4. Enteric-coated tablets of rapidly soluble potassium chloride marketed to replace potassium lost through the action of diuretic medications, and at the same time overcome gastric irritation, have severely injured some patients. Through an escharotic effect, hundreds of patients developed cicatrizing jejuno-ileal ulcerations and perforations of the bowel which usually required surgical intervention. The concept of supplementation with potassium was sound but the resulting highly concentrated depositions of potassium chloride in the intestine were dangerous to the patients.[2,5,7,8,11,20,31-33] Administration of

potassium in liquid form as the bicarbonate, citrate, or other alkalinizing salt minimizes the hazards of intestinal complications. But even the use of improved potassium supplements have caused problems. Slow-K, claimed to release potassium chloride slowly, has produced ulcerations resembling those produced by the enteric coated tablets. Actually, potassium in any form can be hazardous. Hyperkalemia from any cause, whether from overdosage, involution of a postpartum uterus, renal insufficiency, or tissue trauma, may be life-threatening and may contribute to cardiac failure. Kaplan[73] reports a suicidal death after ingestion of a potassium salt.

5. Medications evaluated in the improper species have been very harmful to patients. An outstanding example is thalidomide, the tranquilizer and hypnotic which was synthesized in 1953, patented in 1957, and marketed as Contergan in 1958 in Europe. Studies in mice and other laboratory animals, as well as in man, had shown it had a very low toxicity. It became so popular that by 1961 about 1½ tons a year were distributed. But no prescription was required until April, 1961. About that time, polyneuritis was observed in long-term users and hundreds of pitiful fetal abnormalities, sometimes with complete absence of both arms and both legs (amelia and phocomelia), began to be associated with use of the drug.

On November 26, 1961, in Germany and November 27, 1961, in England thalidomide was withdrawn from the market with warnings on the front pages of newspapers, on radio, and on television, shortly before a paper in *Lancet* by McBride, an Australian, alerted readers to the hazard.[25] The drug appeared to be an excellent compound from the standpoint of efficacy and safety, except for long-term use and in pregnant women, particularly between the 20th and 90th day of gestation. But not until it was finally tested in monkeys and a susceptible species of rabbits were its highly teratogenic effects confirmed. Fortunately, because of the alertness of FDA it was not marketed in this country. In the U.S.A., 29,114 thalidomide tablets were supplied to 1,270 physicians in 39 states for investigational use. The tablets were given to 20,771 patients of whom 3,899 were women of child-bearing age. But the drug was withdrawn so rapidly and efficiently by FDA that

only 9 women who received the drug gave birth to malformed infants. This contrasts dramatically with the results elsewhere. In West Germany alone some 3,000 deformed children live. And as late as 1969 old boxes of thalidomide tablets under a hundred trade names were still lying around in medicine cabinets. Deformed babies were born after old tablets were taken long after the drug was banned.[26]

Its tragic consequences will be visible for decades in the youngsters who began to enter the school systems around the world between 1965 and 1969, mentally alert yet terribly handicapped and presenting exceedingly difficult problems for educators. In Australia, Germany, Brazil, Canada, Great Britain, and elsewhere the drug has caused so much anguish (as high as 20 percent incidence reported among one group of pregnant women who received the drug and 100 percent among those who received it between the third and eighth week after conception)[25] and so much litigation that it will forever remain one of the most dramatic examples of the hazards of medication. In February, 1970, Chemie Grünenthal, the German manufacturer of thalidomide, agreed to pay $27.3 million to 2,300 parents of deformed children after a year and a half of costly litigation. Astra Pharmaceutical Company of Sweden is now paying lifelong compensation to 13 Norwegian children (about $20,000 annually) and to 95 Swedish and 5 Danish children (nearly $120,000 annually). Other companies also lost suits during the 1970s and began compensating victims.

The impact of the phocomeli, numbering in the thousands, of which two-thirds lived, had one beneficial effect. In the future, no drug will be allowed to be recommended for use in women of childbearing age before careful teratologic tests have been conducted in suitable test animals and clinical data have been accumulated to minimize the probability of teratogenicity.[22,23,27,38]

Some benefits may be derived from thalidomide, however. Australians appear to be making some progress in elucidating teratogenicity mechanisms with the aid of the drug.[92]

6. Drugs essentially no more effective than those already available have been developed merely to compete in the market, perhaps a

necessary goal in a highly competitive society. But arguments against marketing a multiplicity of new medications must be made unless a significantly large enough group of patients respond as favorably to each new drug as to the other drugs in its therapeutic category, preferably more favorably. Each new drug should justify its existence by offering some distinct advantage such as greater safety, greater efficacy, fewer side effects, lower toxicity, or lower cost. It should not needlessly compound the opportunities for drug interactions. Sometimes a different route of administration will provide a drug with a distinct advantage. Thus, methotrimeprazine was given orally as a tranquilizer, but parenterally it is a nonnarcotic analgesic. See also *Succedanea,* page 108, for arguments in favor of having several medications with the same uses.

7. Diagnostic drugs with latent toxic effects have damaged patients severely. A classic example was radioactive thorium dioxide (Thorotrast) used in arteriography and visualization of the liver, mammae, and spleen. In spite of warnings by the American Medical Association against its use, diagnosticians continued to administer this chemical which became stored in the body and continued to emit alpha, beta, and gamma rays. Some patients rapidly developed leukocytosis, followed by lymphopenia, leukopenia, hemorrhaging, and death within two weeks. Other patients endured anemia, benign or malignant neoplastic disease, and fragile, necrotic bones for decades after the drug was injected. Malpractice litigation was still being disposed of in the 1970s more than 25 years after medical authorities pointed out hazards of the drug and recommended that its use be discontinued.[47]

Although use of the drug was banned in some countries as early as 1936 (about 11 years after it was first marketed) reports on patients appeared as recently as 1976. Several experienced onset of symptoms (arachnoiditis and myelopathy with bladder dysfunction, deafness, dysphagia, nystagmus, paraplegia with impaired sensation in the buttocks and lower limbs, severe leg pains, and severe muscle weakness) decades after myelography with the drug. One patient died after 24 years of illness. In 1970, a patient developed granuloma on the neck 28 years after percutaneous carotid angiography with thorium dioxide.[70] A 1976 report[74] described a 74-year old man with a hepatoma induced by thorium dioxide received 26 years earlier. Out of over 1,000 patients who received Thorotrast over 400 are still listed at the University of Michigan for follow-up (1978).

Because irrational ideas for drug research have caused harm to patients, and even rational ideas have produced useless or dangerous medications, regulations in many countries now prohibit use of any medication in man unless competent scientists, utilizing the modern techniques of experimental therapeutics, have first thoroughly tested it in lower animals.

EXPERIMENTAL THERAPEUTICS

A future drug product is usually born when a new chemical or a series of new compounds is synthesized, isolated, or otherwise obtained and the chemical structure elucidated. With each new lead the scientist in the laboratory visualizes what his new compound may possibly do to help patients. Does it have some useful effect? If so, is the effect sufficiently pronounced to warrant further investigation? These and similar questions are answered by biological and chemical testing *in vivo* in laboratory animals and by physicochemical testing *in vitro* with laboratory apparatus. Test animals are used to identify drug actions by means of signs, symptoms, and various metabolic, muscular, neural, vascular and other responses. Some drugs that are active *in vitro* are inactive *in vivo* and vice versa.* Some drugs are active both *in vitro* and *in vivo*. But in general, testing or screening *in vivo* with suitable test animals is more likely to demonstrate whether a drug will be active in humans.

Subsequent to screening tests, pharmacological studies in several species of animals are carefully designed to determine acute and

---

* Furazolidone *in vitro,* for example, shows no monoamine oxidase inhibiting activity. In rats, however, the drug is capable of producing 95% inhibition of both hepatic and cerebral monoamine oxidase within 24 to 48 hours after oral administration of 500 mg/Kg. The inhibition is maintained for 10 days in the liver and 2 to 3 weeks in the brain, and is irreversible. The drug is active *in vivo* because it is degraded into the actively inhibiting metabolite 2-hydroxy-hydrazino-ethane.[21]

subacute toxicity and preliminary safety; chronic toxicity and preclinical safety; metabolic pathways, rates and routes of absorption, distribution and excretion; biological availability; pharmacokinetics; mechanisms of action; detoxification routes; and other related data. Studies designed to show whether or not the drug is carcinogenic, mutagenic, or teratogenic are also initiated. And concurrently, both *in vivo* and *in vitro* studies are conducted to determine possible types of efficacy. Depending on use, a drug might be acceptable even if it caused any of the above types of toxicity as long as its efficacy was high enough in some very serious condition, e.g., some anticancer agents and thalidomide in leprosy.

Safety Evaluation

Before any new drug can be clinically tested for the first time in man, a risky act under the best of circumstances, it must always first be tested in the laboratory in several species of animals to establish its pharmacological and toxicological properties.[46] Biophysics, enzymology, radiochemistry, and other disciplines are applied by teams using the scientific method of objective testing and statistical analysis. Adequacy of such preclinical testing is determined by FDA which has published guidelines for animal toxicity studies.[16] Also, for several years FDA has been developing guidelines for clinical testing of specific drug categories.* The agency has also prepared General Guidelines[78] with the collaboration of its Advisory Committees, professional societies, and the Pharmaceutical Manufacturers Association. The latter has also issued its own guidelines for drug sponsors.[79] See Table 3-1.

The drug category, its molecular structure and relationship to other drugs known to produce certain toxic effects, the probable dosage level, route, frequency and duration, and other considerations determine the number and species of test animals, the types and duration of tests, and the observations to be made in order to be reasonably certain the human subjects can satisfactorily tolerate the new drug.† The LD_{50} (lethal dose for 50% of test animals), the ED_{50} (effective dose for 50% of the test animals), the LT_{50} (average lethal time), and the LD_0 (maximum tolerated dose) are obtained in several species of animals to determine acute toxicity by the oral, subcutaneous, intramuscular, intraperitoneal, intravenous, topical, or other appropriate routes.

With the aid of the acute toxicity data, subacute toxicity studies at several dosage levels are conducted for two weeks to two months to determine within rather broad limits the dosages at which physiological effects appear and the upper limits at which the drug can be tolerated without mortality. Based on these data, long-term (chronic) toxicity studies are begun if the pharmacological response continues to be promising.

Pharmacological studies in animals are pursued concurrently with the toxicity studies so that confidence in the probable activity of the drug as well as in its safety is developed prior to any clinical testing.‡ This is always done with the realization that activity and safety in animals are not perfect assurance of the same in man. Potential adverse effects unmasked by high dosages in animals cannot always be extrapolated directly to man. Thus, the possible influence of malnutrition (frequently associated with high-dose studies) on the toxic effects must always be taken into consideration.

Although the pharmacological responses of certain animals to some drugs can often be used with a great deal of confidence to pre-

---

*FDA by June, 1978, published some 15 guidelines for clinical evaluation of *Drugs in Infants and Children* and a variety of specific categories of drugs (anti-anginal, anti-anxiety, anti-arrhythmic, anticonvulsant, antidepressant, antidiarrheal, anti-infective, anti-inflammatory, hypnotic, radiopharmaceutical, etc.). These booklets are available from the Bureau of Drugs gratis. Another 10 guidelines will be available by 1979.

†FDA may require and at times may itself undertake reproductive studies, perhaps beginning in chick embryos and progressing to rats, rabbits, dogs, and primates to verify that the probability of carcinogenic, mutagenic, or teratogenic effects occurring in man is very low. But based only on animal data, definite assurance that these effects will not occur cannot be given.

‡Mathematical models of drug toxicity development have been devised. Assuming a quantal nature of drug-induced damage and a negative binomial distribution of the probability $p(x)$ that death will occur after the xth dose, these models can be used to distinguish between chronic and subacute toxicity, and between reversibly and irreversibly toxic drugs. They also provide a tool for predicting mortality due to drugs.[18]

Table 3-1   General FDA Guidelines for Animal Toxicity Studies*

Category	Duration of Human Administration	Phase[1]	Subacute or Chronic Toxicity[2]	Observations	Special Studies
Oral or Parenteral	Several days	I, II, III, NDA	2 species; 2 weeks	Body weights, food consumption, behavior, hemogram, coagulation tests, liver and kidney function tests, fasting blood sugar, ophthalmological examination, metabolic studies, gross and microscopic examination, others as appropriate.	For parenterally administered drugs: irritation studies, compatibility with blood where applicable.
	Up to 2 weeks	I	2 species; 2 weeks		
		II	2 species; up to 4 weeks		
		III, NDA	2 species; up to 3 months		
	Up to 3 months	I, II	2 species; 4 weeks		
		III	2 species; 3 months		
		NDA	2 species; up to 6 months		
	6 months to unlimited	I, II	2 species; 3 months		
		III	2 species; 6 months or longer		
		NDA	2 species; 12 months (nonrodent), 18 months (rodent)		
Inhalation (General Anesthetics)		I, II, III, NDA	4 species; 5 days (3 hours/day)		
Dermal	Single application	I	1 species; single 24-hour exposure followed by 2-week observation		
	Single or short-term application	II	1 species; 20-day repeated exposure (intact and abraded skin)		
	Short-term application	III	As above		
	Unlimited application	NDA	As above, but intact skin study extended up to 6 months		
Ophthalmic	Single application	I			Eye irritation tests graded doses.
	Multiple application	I, II, III	1 species; 3 weeks daily applications, as in clinical use		
		NDA	1 species; duration commensurate with period of drug administration		
Vaginal or Rectal	Single application	I			Local and systemic toxicity after vaginal or rectal application in 2 species.
	Multiple application	I, II, III, NDA	2 species; duration and number of applications determined by proposed use		
Drug Combinations[3]		I			LD$_{50}$ by appropriate route, compared to components run concurrently in 1 species.
		II, III, NDA	2 species; up to 3 months		

* Adapted from a table by Edwin I. Goldenthal in *FDA Papers* 2 (May) 1968.[16]
[1] Phases I, II, and III are defined in §130.0 of the New Drug Regulations.
[2] Acute toxicity should be determined in 3 to 4 species; subacute or chronic studies should be by route to be used clinically.
[3] Where toxicity data are available on each drug individually.

dict responses of man to those drugs, species variation can cause incorrect conclusions to be drawn and thereby create a hazard to subjects who later receive the same experimental drugs. Biotransformations (oxidations, reductions, hydrolyses, syntheses, etc.), occurring simultaneously or consecutively in animals, cannot always be extrapolated to man because such reactions or combinations of them do not necessarily carry over at the same rate or in the same manner. Such metabolic transformations, mediated by enzymes, may be absent or poorly achieved in a given species while readily accomplished in all others or they may be specific for a given or closely related species while essentially absent in others.

The following illustrate this situation: (1) The cat, unlike man, has little glucuronyl transferase, and it therefore synthesizes glucuronide conjugates at a low level. Thus it detoxifies phenol and naphthylamine mainly by forming sulfates. (2) The rabbit metabolizes sulfonamides differently from man. Thus it forms the metabolic conjugate N^4-acetylsulfadimethoxine from Madribon, whereas man forms the N$'$-glucuronide. (3) The rabbit deaminates amphetamine, but other animals demethylate or hydroxylate the drug. [60,64,65] (4) The dog and man hydroxylate ethyl biscoumacetate, but rabbits de-esterify the drug. (5) Man and many laboratory animals including pigeons (not ducks, geese, hens, and turkeys), produce glycine conjugation. (6) Nearly all animal species acetylate nitrogen and yet the dog cannot acetylate aromatic amines and hydrazides. Thus isoniazid is not acetylated in dogs and is highly toxic to them (polyneuritis), but in monkeys and in man the drug is readily acetylated and toxicity in these species is low. (7) Nalidixic acid at a dose of 50 mg./Kg. is highly toxic in dogs (convulsions), but in man and monkeys the drug is a useful antibacterial agent that is much better tolerated because it is readily detoxified as the glucuronide. [13]

Because of such variations, a drug may appear to be more or less toxic in animals than in man, or possess a widely different duration of action. Thus *in vivo,* hexobarbital is oxidized to hydroxyhexobarbital at different rates so that the half-life in minutes varies as follows: 19 (mouse), 60 (rabbit), 140 (rat), 260 (dog), and 360 (man). Corresponding alterations in sleeping times result. [44] Accordingly, with some drugs for which sensitive assay methods are available, it is desirable from the standpoint of safety to establish metabolic pathways and rates in man at dosage levels below those expected to produce toxicological effects. Even extensive metabolic studies in animals do not always provide a basis for a reliable prediction of what will take place in man.

Safety evaluation in animals attempts to prevent administration to human subjects of investigational drugs which will adversely affect the cardiovascular system, endocrine system, fertility, hematopoiesis, kidneys, liver, metabolic mechanisms, perception, reproduction, and other functions, systems, organs and tissues of the body. Important observations in animal studies include effects of drugs on emesis, fecal and urinary elimination, heart and respiratory rates, motor activity, and survival rates, as well as dose levels, times to produce death, and types of death (circulatory collapse, convulsions, respiratory failure). Crucial data in order of importance for most studies are (1) animal weight curves, (2) hematologic observations, (3) histologic examination of vital organs, and (4) behavior of animals. Other tests and observations are added in specific situations and with certain classes of drugs. The type of animal is often critical. Thus the dog or monkey is most suitable for determination of tolerance to oral medication by means of emetic response, although usually a rodent or possibly another species is added, depending on the drug and its route of administration. In any event, if serious cardiac, renal, or hepatic toxicities or hematopoietic malfunction is evidenced, the research must be terminated unless the adverse effects can be prevented in some way. Seasoned judgment on the part of the investigator is required.

All chemotherapeutic agents have some potential for causing toxic and undesirable reactions, but some molecular structures are more suspect than others. Classic examples of structure-related adverse effects are *addiction* with opiates; *blood dyscrasias* with derivatives of aminophenol (acetanilid) and pyrazolon (aminopyrine); *dermatitides* with bromides and iodides; *habituation* with barbiturates and tranquilizers; *hypersensitivity* reactions with sulfonamides and penicillins;

leukopenia with antineoplastics; and *ortho-static hypotension* with phenothiazines.

Some drugs can cause immediate reactions, e.g., the sudden anaphylactic reactions produced by penicillin. Other drugs may not elicit toxic effects for many months, e.g., the delayed ocular changes with certain psychotropic drugs and endocrine changes with certain anticonvulsant drugs. In fact, some serious toxicities like the reactions to radium or thorium dioxide, may be delayed for many years, even decades. With certain drugs such as estrogens, therefore, animal testing may be prolonged in an attempt to determine delayed toxicities and the number of test animals is increased when rarer types of reactions are suspected. Also massive doses of the drug being tested are given to animals for varying periods of time, not only to unmask potential and latent adverse effects but also to evaluate effects caused by accumulation and to detect changes in metabolism.

The species and number of animals selected and the frequency, levels, and duration of dosage are very important and vary with the category of drug. Some effects are more likely to carry over into man from certain species than from others. Thus, specific strains of mice are used for many drugs, particularly in carcinogenicity studies, dogs for diuretics, dogs and monkeys for estrogens and progestogens, monkeys for psychotropic drugs, etc. In the past, multidose toxicity studies in at least one rodent (mouse, rat, etc.) and at least one nonrodent (dog, etc.) have permitted safe transition of testing from animal to man in the vast majority of cases. But the thalidomide tragedy, which occurred because the drug was not tested in the appropriate animal (page 27), has emphasized the need for special care in the selection of test animals. An extensive compendium of appropriate animal models has been published.[77] It lists references to 352 models that provide organ systems paralleling those in humans. The Institute for Laboratory Animal Resources has initiated an Information Exchange Program on animal models for human diseases. By contacting the office at 2101 Constitution Avenue, Washington, D.C. 20037, data on animal sources, characteristics, and genetic stock as well as literature references may be obtained.

It may never be possible to provide complete assurance of the absence of teratogenicity, carcinogenicity and other serious toxicities before the use of some new drugs in man. Improvements in methodology are constantly being made, however, and studies in nonhuman primates such as the monkey and baboon, as well as comparative drug metabolic studies in animals and man, are helping to refine clinical investigations and improve patient safety. Also, biopharmaceutic data including rates of drug absorption, distribution, metabolism, and excretion are being obtained more and more accurately for each new drug undergoing preclinical testing.

In planning, designing and evaluating metabolic and toxicity studies, erroneous conclusions concerning the safety of a drug can be drawn unless protocols are carefully drawn up and the data generated by the studies are carefully analyzed and interpreted. The pitfalls are numerous and sometimes obscure. Some drugs, for example, can stimulate the metabolism of themselves as well as other drugs administered subsequently. Because of this so-called enzyme induction, metabolites which are rapidly excreted and have low toxicity are formed more and more rapidly with some drugs as a study progresses. As a result, the drug being tested appears to be much less toxic than it really is. Meprobamate, phenacetin, phenylbutazone, steroid hormones, tolbutamide, and many other drugs that stimulate hepatic microsomal enzyme activity can give this false impression. This phenomenon may be a factor to be considered in the evaluation of combinations of drugs or drugs given concomitantly. It can also be an important factor in drug interactions whereby toxicities and pharmacological activities are altered.

Since many drugs, through various interactions, frequently alter the activities of other drugs and sometimes cause undesirable reactions in patients, combinations of drugs must be tested as such even though individually each has been proved to be safe and efficacious. Thus, new diuretics are tested with various cardiac and antihypertensive drugs, antituberculosis drugs with various other drugs in the same category,* and antiepilep-

---

*Tuberculosis is always treated with two or more drug concomitantly to help avoid the development of resistant strains of *Mycobacterium tuberculosis.*

tic drugs with others used for the treatment of epilepsy. Note the very large number of adverse inhibiting, potentiating, synergistic, and other effects of drug interactions which have appeared in the literature in recent years. Imagine how many adverse effects would have appeared if every one had been reported!

Care of Animals

Valid results from drug studies in animals are obtainable only if considerable attention is given to the care of the test animals. Reputable animal pharmacology laboratories employ specialists in animal care who take care of colonies of dogs, guinea pigs, mice, rabbits, rats, and other species. These skilled specialists diligently observe all animals constantly to keep them clean, healthy, and properly housed and nourished. They provide them with water and food under carefully controlled conditions (temperature, humidity and other environmental factors) to obviate variables that may influence the animals and thereby the test results. Much effort has been expended recently to define the term *normal* as applied to animals that have been carefully nurtured for testing purposes.

The National Library of Medicine is developing a major computerized data base of baseline values for test animals. Compilation of such reference data should enhance the precision of experimental therapeutic research.

A seemingly innocent yet very common variable was introduced, for instance, when antibiotics began to be used routinely in the drinking water of some test animals. The effects of ingested antibiotics on the results of some studies may not always be taken into consideration and may not always be readily determinable.

Animal laboratories are now regulated by Federal and state laws and must be licensed by the state in which they are located. The Animal Health Institute and the Public Health Service have been very active in raising the standards for animal care in these laboratories. Manufacturers and others engaged in laboratory animal studies may voluntarily have their laboratories accredited by the American Association for Accreditation of Laboratory Animal Care (AAALAC), Jo-

liet, Illinois. During 1977 the number of accredited facilities reached 340.

The Animal Welfare Act (PL 89-544), enacted August 24, 1966, provided the U.S. Department of Agriculture with authority to develop standards for animal care, handling, transportation and treatment of various laboratory animals. The following year, the Department published minimum standards for adequate veterinary care, feeding, housing, sanitation, separation by species, shelter, watering, and ventilation.[68] A helpful guide was published by the Department of Health, Education, and Welfare.[69] On April 22, 1976, the Animal Welfare Act as amended by Public Law 94-279 was approved. It updated minimum standards for animal care.

Concern for care of the animals begins the minute they are born into a colony or the moment they are captured. Monkeys captured in India, Africa, or elsewhere, are given appropriate care at the collection station, at various holding depots along the transportation routes and, once they have cleared customs, at the laboratories where they are housed. During transit by plane, animal specialists travel with them to make certain that they receive proper care and medical attention. Pharmaceutical manufacturers who use monkey tissues to culture poliomyelitis virus for production of poliovirus vaccine, for example, have spent millions of dollars to build special housing for captured monkeys to simulate their natural environment. For certain other animals they have constructed expensive gnotobiotic housing to maintain them germ-free or in a known state where their microfauna and microflora are completely identified.

It is necessary to protect animals from microorganisms carried by man and vice versa. Some microorganisms found in man, such as staphylococci and streptococci, are highly pathogenic to the guinea pig. And organisms found normally in some animals are highly pathogenic for man. Thus, the B virus of monkeys is not seriously pathogenic for the animals (it merely causes herpes-like lesions), but most handlers have died in spite of all efforts to save them after the virus has been transmitted to them by a bite or a scratch.[58] The same situation holds true for the virus of lymphocytic choriomeningitis carried by mice. It is necessary, therefore, to isolate certain animals like guinea pigs from man while they are in a testing program and to eliminate microorganisms from test animals or at least protect laboratory workers from those that are dangerous.

A comprehensive outline of diseases of laboratory animals, first published in 1969, should be helpful in alerting technicians to those diseases that are particularly hazardous and that may be transmitted from unsuspected sources.[66]

A diseased native in Africa, for instance, can transmit his pathogens to a captured monkey which will carry them to a laboratory colony in some far-distant country, and thence to the laboratory workers. Melioidosis has been diagnosed in a rhesus monkey *(Macaca mulatta)* being used in psychological research at the National Institutes of Health. It has also been diagnosed in the chimpanzee and stump-tailed macaque. Careful control is absolutely essential to protect the health of technicians, the results of tests, and the purity of medications. Deaths may occur among laboratory personnel when control is inadequate.

Suitable species of animals in good health must be cared for properly because data obtained from animal tests must provide a sound basis for tests in humans. But suitable experimental animals are not always available for studying many human diseases or their therapy. Also, investigators who select and utilize the wrong species may make incorrect extrapolations which will actually be hazardous to man. Not only do different species of animals metabolize drugs differently, but they respond differently to diseases. Thus if cats or horses instead of dogs or cattle are used to conduct rabies vaccine studies, the results are unreliable as a guide to the safe and effective use of the virus vaccine in man.

Not only the animals but also the laboratory facilities must be properly selected. Suitable balances and other instruments must be used to keep a continual record of animals weights and the amounts of foods consumed during the periods in which the test animals receive various dosage levels of the drug being studied.

In large studies, such as those being conducted by FDA's National Center for Toxicological Research near Little Rock Arkansas, animal and food weights are recorded and instantly stored in computer memories. Correlations and calculations are made continually and rapidly for tens of thousands of test animals. The animals receive the drug by various routes, orally in the diet, parenterally, etc. Acute toxicity or determination of the lethal dose is obtained in a relatively short period of time whereas chronic toxicity or determination of the effects of various dosage levels over prolonged periods may require observations over a period of many months, sometimes as long as 10 years if the drug happens to be one, like an oral contraceptive, which may be used in each patient over several decades.

Animal care is an exacting science and is basic to sound experimentation and achievement of valid metabolic, biopharmaceutic, pharmacokinetic, and histopathologic results. Faulty animal care can lead to faulty test results and, thereby, faulty conclusions which can create hazards for patients who later receive the drug.

Animal Pathology

The effects of new drugs on animals are analyzed meticulously by all the powerful tools of modern pathology. After observing for grossly apparent pathology, laboratory personnel perform necropsies. They stain, section, and microscopically examine the tissues. In a large research laboratory, technicians prepare and examine as many as 50,000 such histopathology slides annually, and they permanently file the slides for possible future reference in the event problems arise after the drug is marketed. They utilize electron microscopy, photomicrography, and various other methods of medical instrumentation to determine cell and tissue changes. They make hematologic studies, weigh various organs, and otherwise attempt to locate evidence of drug damage. In addition to pathologic evaluation, many laboratories assay tissues for the drug and its metabolites to determine tissue concentration of the test drug. The synovium, for example, has a particular affinity for some drugs whereas cartilage is relatively resistant.

The last preclinical research step is perhaps the most important one of all. It consists of the tabulation, correlation, and complete reporting of all findings in accurate, clear, concise *preclinical research reports.* These help clinical investigators make the transition from animals to man.

CLINICAL INVESTIGATION

After acute and chronic toxicities have been determined, pharmacological actions identified, metabolic pathways elucidated, and other special animal studies as indicated have been carried out, then closely related studies are carefully conducted in consenting patients and volunteers. Because results in animals do not always carry over into man, only clinical testing can firmly establish final valid conclusions regarding human safety and efficacy.[42,60] And because of the many potential errors that can occur in coping with all the known and unknown objective and subjective variables that abound in clinical research, investigators must use proper techniques for *planning* clinical studies, *administering* drugs to humans for the first time, *observing* patient responses (both therapeutic efficacy and undesirable reactions), *evaluating* the results of the studies, and *reporting* the information gained from the clinical research. The pitfalls[9,19,28,36,39,45] have been discussed many times as well as the legal and ethical aspects.[24,30] The World Health Organization has published guidelines on ethical questions involved with drug trials.[93] The primary concern is the *safety* of the subjects used in the studies, and eventually the safety of the general consumer.

From Animals to Man

As soon as the data obtained from the studies of a new drug in animals are adequate to justify preliminary studies in man, certain legal requirements, based on the 1962 Drug Amendments to the Federal Food, Drug, and Cosmetic Act, must be met before clinical testing can be started. The sponsor of the studies, usually a pharmaceutical manufacturer but sometimes an individual physician, files a *Notice of Claimed Investigational Exemption for a New Drug* (see Fig 3-1), also known as an IND, or suitable substitute with the pertinent agencies in the foreign countries where human studies will be conducted. Each investigator must submit to the sponsor evidence in the so-called *Statement of Investi-*

gator that he is competent through experience and training to undertake the given clinical studies. Form 1572 is used for clinical pharmacology (see Fig 3-2) and a similar Form 1573 for clinical trials.

In 1970, FDA published an order in the *Federal Register* (FR Doc 70-10672; Aug. 14, 1970 and 35 FR 9215; June 12, 1970) requiring that 30 days must elapse following the date of receipt of Form 1571 by the FDA before clinical studies are started.

The IND contains full information about the new drug which is about to be tested in man. It includes complete chemical, manufacturing, and quality control information (starting chemicals, new drug composition, dosage form, etc.), results of *in vitro* tests (biological, chemical, and physical); all animal data (pharmacological and toxicological); formulation data; description of human investigations to be undertaken; training and experience of the investigators; copies of informational material supplied to each investigator; and all other preclinical information that will insure its use in man with a high probability of safety. It also includes agreements from the sponsors (1) to notify FDA and all investigators if any adverse effects arise during either animal or human tests, and (2) to submit periodic progress reports.

The sponsor also certifies that *informed consent* will be obtained from subjects or patients to whom the drug will be given. Patient consent forms must be carefully designed to protect the rights and welfare of the subject by revealing the true nature of an investigation (social as well as medical aspects) and by protecting his privacy. But FDA has a right to certain personal information necessary for its regulatory responsibilities. The object is to have subjects participate in medical experiments with full knowledge of the possible risks and consequences, to have them participate voluntarily, and to prevent them from being subjected to the undesired and harmful disclosure of personal information. Every clinical investigator has a moral obligation to submit protocols on investigations in human beings for evaluation, to provide appropriate written consent forms, and to safeguard the patient in every possible way.[54]

Finally, the sponsor makes a definite commitment regarding accountability and disposal of investigational drugs when the stud-

DEPARTMENT OF HEALTH, EDUCATION, AND WELFARE
PUBLIC HEALTH SERVICE
FOOD AND DRUG ADMINISTRATION

Form Approved
OMB No. 57-R0030

NOTICE OF
CLAIMED INVESTIGATIONAL EXEMPTION
FOR A NEW DRUG

Name of Sponsor _____

Address _____

Date _____

Name of Investigational Drug _____

To the Secretary of Health, Education and Welfare
For the Commissioner of Food and Drugs
Bureau of Drugs (HFD-106)
5600 Fishers Lane
Rockville, Maryland 20852

Dear Sir:

　　The sponsor, _____, submits
this notice of claimed investigational exemption for a new drug under the provisions of section 505(i) of the Federal Food, Drug, and Cosmetic Act and §312.1 of Title 21 of the Code of Federal Regulations.

　　Attached hereto in triplicate are:

1. The best available descriptive name of the drug, including to the extent known the chemical name and structure of any new-drug substance, and a statement of how it is to be administered. (If the drug has only a code name, enough information should be supplied to identify the drug.)

2. Complete list of components of the drug, including any reasonable alternates for inactive components.

3. Complete statement of quantitative composition of drug, including reasonable variations that may be expected during the investigational stage.

4. Description of source and preparation of, any new-drug substances used as components, including the name and address of each supplier or processor, other than the sponsor, of each new-drug substance.

5. A statement of the methods, facilities, and controls used for the manufacturing, processing, and packing of the new drug to establish and maintain appropriate standards of identity, strength, quality, and purity as needed for safety and to give significance to clinical investigations made with the drug.

6. A statement covering all information available to the sponsor derived from preclinical investigations and any clinical studies and experience with the drug as follows:

a. Adequate information about the preclinical investigations, including studies made on laboratory animals, on the basis of which the sponsor has concluded that it is reasonably safe to initiate clinical investigations with the drug: Such information should include identification of the person who conducted each investigation; identification and qualifications of the individuals who evaluated the results and concluded that it is reasonably safe to initiate clinical investigations with the drug and a statement of where the investigations were conducted and where the records are available for inspection; and enough details about the investigations to permit scientific review. The preclinical investigations shall not be considered adequate to justify clinical testing unless they give proper attention to the conditions of the proposed clinical testing. When this information, the outline of the

plan of clinical pharmacology, or any progress report on the clinical pharmacology, indicates a need for full review of the preclinical data before a clinical trial is undertaken, the Department will notify the sponsor to submit the complete preclinical data and to withhold clinical trials until the review is completed and the sponsor notified. The Food and Drug Administration will be prepared to confer with the sponsor concerning this action.

b. If the drug has been marketed commercially or investigated (e.g. outside the United States), complete information about such distribution or investigation shall be submitted, along with a complete bibliography of any publications about the drug.

c. If the drug is a combination of previously investigated or marketed drugs, an adequate summary of preexisting information from preclinical and clinical investigations and experience with its components, including all reports available to the sponsor suggesting side-effects, contraindications, and ineffectiveness in use of such components: Such summary should include an adequate bibliography of publications about the components and may incorporate by reference any information concerning such components previously submitted by the sponsor to the Food and Drug Administration. Include a statement of the expected pharmacological effects of the combination.

d. If the drug is a radioactive drug, sufficient data must be available from animal studies or previous human studies to allow a reasonable calculation of radiation absorbed dose upon administration to a human being.

7. A total (one in each of the three copies of the notice) of all informational material, including label and labeling, which is to be supplied to each investigator: This shall include an accurate description of the prior investigations and experience and their results pertinent to the safety and possible usefulness of the drug under the conditions of the investigation. It shall not represent that the safety or usefulness of the drug has been established for the purposes to be investigated. It shall describe all relevant hazards, contraindications, side-effects, and precautions suggested

FD FORM 1571 (11/75)　　　　**PREVIOUS EDITIONS OBSOLETE**

Figure 3-2

by prior investigations and experience with the drug under investigation and related drugs for the information of clinical investigators.

8. The scientific training and experience considered appropriate by the sponsor to qualify the investigators as suitable experts to investigate the safety of the drug, bearing in mind what is known about the pharmacological action of the drug and the phase of the investigational program that is to be undertaken.

9. The names and a summary of the training and experience of each investigator and of the individual charged with monitoring the progress of the investigation and evaluating the evidence of safety and effectiveness of the drug as it is received from the investigators, together with a statement that the sponsor has obtained from each investigator a completed and signed form, as provided in subparagraph (12) or (13) of this paragraph, and that the investigator is qualified by scientific training and experience as an appropriate expert to undertake the phase of the investigation outlined in section 10 of the "Notice of Claimed Investigational Exemption for a New Drug." (In crucial situations, phase 3 investigators may be added and this form supplemented by rapid communication methods, and the signed form FD-1573 shall be obtained promptly thereafter.)

10. An outline of any phase or phases of the planned investigations and a description of the institutional review committee, as follows:

a. Clinical pharmacology. This is ordinarily divided into two phases: Phase 1 starts when the new drug is first introduced into man—only animal and in vitro data are available—with the purpose of determining human toxicity, metabolism, absorption, elimination, and other pharmacological action, preferred route of administration, and safe dosage range; phase 2 covers the initial trials on a limited number of patients for specific disease control or prophylaxis purposes. A general outline of these phases shall be submitted, identifying the investigator or investigators, the hospitals or research facilities where the clinical pharmacology will be undertaken, any expert committees or panels to be utilized, the maximum number of subjects to be involved, and the estimated duration of these early phases of investigation. Modification of the experimental design on the basis of experience gained need be reported only in the progress reports on these early phases, or in the development of the plan for the clinical trial, phase 3. The first two phases may overlap and, when indicated, may require additional animal data before these phases can be completed or phase 3 can be undertaken. Such animal tests shall be designed to take into account the expected duration of administration of the drug to human beings, the age groups and physical status, as for example, infants, pregnant women, premenopausal women, of those human beings to whom the drug may be administered, unless this has already been done in the original animal studies. If a drug is a radioactive drug, the clinical pharmacology phase must include studies which will obtain sufficient data for dosimetry calculations. These studies should evaluate the excretion, whole body retention, and organ distribution of the radioactive material.

b. Clinical trial. This phase 3 provides the assessment of the drug's safety and effectiveness and optimum dosage schedules in the diagnosis, treatment, or prophylaxis of groups of subjects involving a given disease or condition. A reasonable protocol is developed on the basis of the facts accumulated in the earlier phases, including completed and submitted animal studies. This phase is conducted by separate groups following the same protocol (with reasonable variations and alternatives permitted by the plan) to produce well-controlled clinical data. For this phase, the following data shall be submitted:

i. The names and addresses of the investigators. (Additional investigators may be added.)

ii. The specific nature of the investigations to be conducted, together with information or case report forms to show the scope and detail of the planned clinical observations and the clinical laboratory tests to be made and reported.

iii. The approximate number of subjects (a reasonable range of subjects is permissible and additions may be made), and criteria proposed for subject selection by age, sex, and condition.

iv. The estimated duration of the clinical trial and the intervals, not exceeding 1 year, at which progress reports showing the results of the investigations will be submitted to the Food and Drug Administration.

c. Institutional review committee. If the phases of clinical study as described under 10a and b above are conducted on institutionalized subjects or are conducted by an individual affiliated with an institution which agrees to assume responsibility for the study, assurance must be given that an institutional review committee is responsible for initial and continuing review and approval of the proposed clinical study. The membership must be comprised of sufficient members of varying background, that is, lawyers, clergymen, or laymen as well as scientists, to assure complete and adequate review of the research project. The membership must possess not only broad competence to comprehend the nature of the project, but also other competencies necessary to judge the acceptability of the project or activity in terms of instituional regulations, relevant law, standards of professional practice, and community acceptance. Assurance must be presented that neither the sponsor nor the investigator has participated in selection of committee members; that the review committee does not allow participation in its review and conclusions by any individual involved in the conduct of the research activity under review (except to provide information to the committee); that the investigator will report to the committee for review any emergent problems, serious adverse reactions, or proposed procedural changes which may affect the status of the investigation and that no such change will be made without committee approval except where necessary to eliminate apparent immediate hazards; that reviews of the study will be conducted by the review committee at intervals appropriate to the degree of risk, but not exceeding 1 year, to assure that the research project is being conducted in compliance with the committee's understanding and recommendations: that the review committee is provided all the information on the research project necessary for its complete review of the project; and that the review committee maintains adequate documentation of its activities and develops adequate procedures for reporting its findings to the institution. The documents maintained by the committee are to include the names and qualifications of committee members, records of information provided to subjects in obtaining informed consent, committee discussion on substantive issues and their resolution, committee recommendations, and dated reports of successive reviews as they are performed. Copies of all documents are to be retained for a period of 3 years past the completion or discontinuance of the study and are to be made available upon request to duly authorized representatives of the Food and Drug Administration. (Favorable recommendations by the committee are subject to further appropriate review and rejection by institution officials. Unfavorable recommendations, restrictions, or conditions may not be overruled by the institution officials.) Procedures for the organization and operation of instituional review committees are contained in guidelines issued pursuant to Chapter 1-40 of the Grants Administration Manual of the U.S. Department of Health, Education, and Welfare, available from the U.S. Government Printing Office. It is recommended that these guidelines be followed in establishing institutional review committees and that the committees function according to the procedures described therein. A signing of the Form FD-1571 will be regarded as providing the above necessary assurances. If the institution, however, has on file with the Department of Health, Education, and Welfare, Division of Research Grants, National Institutes of Health, an "accepted general assurance," and the same committee is to review the proposed study using the same

Figure 3-2 (Cont.)

procedures, this is acceptable in lieu of the above assurances and a statement to this effect should be provided with the signed FD-1571. (In addition to sponsor's continuing responsibility to monitor the study, the Food and Drug Administration will undertake investigations in institutions periodically to determine whether the committees are operating in accord with the assurances given by the sponsor.)

(The notice of claimed investigational exemption may be limited to any one or more phases, provided the outline of the additional phase or phases is submitted before such additional phases begin. This does not preclude continuing a subject on the drug from phase 2 to phase 3 without interruption while the plan for phase 3 is being developed.)

Ordinarily, a plan for clinical trial will not be regarded as reasonable unless, among other things, it provides for more than one independent competent investigator to maintain adequate case histories of an adequate number of subjects, designed to record observations and permit evaluation of any and all discernible effects attributable to the drug in each individual treated, and comparable records on any individuals employed as controls. These records shall be individual records for each subject maintained to include adequate information pertaining to each, including age, sex, conditions treated, dosage, frequency of administration of the drug, results of all relevant clinical observations and laboratory examinations made, adequate information concerning any other treatment given and a full statement of any adverse effects and useful results observed,

Very truly yours,

together with an opinion as to whether such effects or results are attributable to the drug under investigation

11. A statement that the sponsor will notify the Food and Drug Administration if the investigation is discontinued, and the reason therefor.

12. A statement that the sponsor will notify each investigator if a new-drug application is approved, or if the investigation is discontinued.

13. If the drug is to be sold, a full explanation why sale is required and should not be regarded as the commercialization of a new drug for which an application is not approved.

14. A statement that the sponsor assures that clinical studies in humans will not be initiated prior to 30 days after the date of receipt of the notice by the Food and Drug Administration and that he will continue to withold or to restrict clinical studies if requested to do so by the Food and Drug Administration prior to the expiration of such 30 days. If such request is made, the sponsor will be provided specific information as to the deficiencies and will be afforded a conference on request. The 30-day delay may be waived by the Food and Drug Administration upon a showing of good reason for such waiver; and for investigations subject to institutional review committee approval as described in item 10c above, an additional statement assuring that the investigation will not be initiated prior to approval of the study by such committee.

15. When requested by the agency, an environmental impact analysis report pursuant to § 6.1 of this chapter.

SPONSOR	PER
	INDICATE AUTHORITY

(This notice may be amended or supplemented from time to time on the basis of the experience gained with the new drug. Progress reports may be used to update the notice.)

ALL NOTICES AND CORRESPONDENCE SHOULD BE SUBMITTED IN TRIPLICATE.

3

Figure 3-2 (Cont.)

DEPARTMENT OF HEALTH, EDUCATION, AND WELFARE
PUBLIC HEALTH SERVICE
FOOD AND DRUG ADMINISTRATION
5600 FISHERS LANE
ROCKVILLE, MARYLAND 20852

STATEMENT OF INVESTIGATOR
(Clinical Pharmacology)

Form Approved
OMB No. 57-R0031

TO: SUPPLIER OF THE DRUG: *(Name and address, include ZIP Code)*

NAME OF INVESTIGATOR *(Print or Type)*

DATE

NAME OF DRUG

Dear Sir:

The undersigned, _____,
submits this statement as required by section 505(i) of the Federal Food, Drug, and Cosmetic Act and § 312.1 of Title 21 of the Code of Federal Regulations as a condition for receiving and conducting clinical pharmacology with a new drug limited by Federal (or United States) law to investigational use.

1. A STATEMENT OF THE EDUCATION AND TRAINING THAT QUALIFIES ME FOR CLINICAL PHARMACOLOGY

2. THE NAME AND ADDRESS OF THE MEDICAL SCHOOL, HOSPITAL, OR OTHER RESEARCH FACILITY WHERE THE CLINICAL PHARMACOLOGY WILL BE CONDUCTED

3. If the experimental project is to be conducted on institutionalized subjects or is conducted by an individual affiliated with an institution which agrees to assume responsibility for the study, assurance must be given that an institutional review committee is responsible for initial and continuing review and approval of the proposed clinical study. The membership must be comprised of sufficient members of varying background, that is, lawyers clergymen, or laymen as well as scientists, to assure complete and adequate review of the research project. The membership must possess not only broad competence to comprehend the nature of the project, but also other competencies necessary to judge the acceptability of the project or activity in terms of institutional regulations, relevant law, standards of professional practice, and community acceptance. Assurance must be presented that the investigator has not participated in the selection of committee members; that the review committee does not allow participation in its review and conclusions by any individual involved in the conduct of the research activity under review (except to provide information to the committee); that the investigator will report to the committee for review any emergent problems, serious adverse reactions, or proposed procedural changes which may affect the status of the investigation and that no such change will be made without committee approval except where necessary to eliminate apparent immediate hazards; that reviews of the study will be conducted by the review committee at intervals appropriate to the degree of risk, but not exceeding 1 year, to assure that the research project is being conducted in compliance with the committee's understanding and recommendations; that the review committee is provided all the information on the research project necessary for its complete review of the project; and that the review committee maintains adequate documentation of its activities and develops adequate procedures for reporting its findings to the institution. The documents maintained by the committee are to include the names and qualifications of committee members, records of information provided to subjects in obtaining informed consent, committee discussion on substantive issues and their resolution, committee recommendations, and dated reports of successive reviews as they are performed. Copies of all documents are to be retained for a period of 3 years past the completion or discontinuance of the study and are to be made available upon request to duly authorized representatives of the Food and Drug Administration. (Favorable recommendations by the committee are subject to further appropriate review and rejection by institution officials. Unfavorable recommendations, restrictions, or conditions may not be overruled by the institution officials.) Procedures for the organization and operation of institutional review committees are contained in guidelines issued pursuant to Chapter 1-40 of the Grants Administration Manual of the U.S. Department of Health, Education, and Welfare, available from the U.S. Government Printing Office. It is recommended that these guidelines be followed in establishing institutional review committees and that the committees function according to the procedures described therein. A signing of the Form FD-1572 will be regarded as providing the above necessary assurance; however, if the institution has on file with the Department of Health, Education, and Welfare, Division of Research Grants, National Institutes of Health, an "accepted general assurance," and the same committee is to review the proposed study using the same procedures, this is acceptable in lieu of the above assurances and a statement to this effect should be provided with the signed FD-1572. (In addition to sponsor's continuing responsibility to monitor the study, the Food and Drug Administration will undertake investigations in institutions periodically to determine whether the committees are operating in accord with the assurances given by the sponsor.)

FORM FD 1572 (1/76)   PREVIOUS EDITION MAY BE USED UNTIL SUPPLY IS EXHAUSTED.

Figure 3-2 (Cont.)

---

4. THE ESTIMATED DURATION OF THE PROJECT AND THE MAXIMUM NUMBER OF SUBJECTS THAT WILL BE INVOLVED

5. A GENERAL OUTLINE OF THE PROJECT TO BE UNDERTAKEN *(Modification is permitted on the basis of experience gained without advance submission of amendments to the general outline, but with the approval of the review committee and upon notification of the sponsor.)*

6. THE UNDERSIGNED UNDERSTANDS THAT THE FOLLOWING CONDITIONS GENERALLY APPLICABLE TO NEW DRUGS FOR INVESTIGATIONAL USE GOVERN HIS RECEIPT AND USE OF THIS INVESTIGATIONAL DRUG

a. The sponsor is required to supply the investigator with full information concerning the preclinical investigation that justifies clinical pharmacology.

b. The investigator is required to maintain adequate records of the disposition of all receipts of the drug, including dates, quantity, and use by subjects, and if the clinical pharmacology is suspended, terminated, discontinued, or completed, to return to the sponsor any unused supply of the drug. If the investigational drug is subject to the comprehensive Drug Abuse Prevention and Control Act of 1970, adequate precautions must be taken, including storage of the investigational drug in a securely locked, substantially constructed cabinet, or other securely locked, substantially constructed enclosure access to which is limited, to prevent theft or diversion of the substance into illegal channels of distribution.

c. The investigator is required to prepare and maintain adequate case histories designed to record all observations and other data pertinent to the clinical pharmacology.

d. The investigator is required to furnish his reports to the sponsor who is responsible for collecting and evaluating the results, and presenting progress reports to the Food and Drug Administration at appropriate intervals, not exceeding 1 year. Any adverse effect which may reasonably be regarded as caused by, or is probably caused by, the new-drug shall be reported to the sponsor promptly; and if the adverse effect is alarming it shall be reported immediately. An adequate report of the clinical pharmacology should be furnished to the sponsor shortly after completion.

e. The investigator shall maintain the records of disposition of the drug and the case reports described above for a period of 2 years following the date the new-drug application is approved for the drug; or if no application is to be filed or is approved until 2 years after the investigation is discontinued and the

Food and Drug Administration so notified. Upon the request of a scientifically trained and specifically authorized employee of the Department, at reasonable times, the investigator will made such records available for inspection and copying. The names of the subjects need not be divulged unless the records of the particular subjects require a more detailed study of the cases, or unless there is reason to believe that the records do not represent actual studies or do not represent actual results obtained.

f. The investigator certifies that the drug will be administered only to subjects under his personal supervision or under the supervision of the following investigators responsible to him,

_____

_____

_____

and that the drug will not be supplied to any other investigator or to any clinic for administration to subjects.

g. The investigator certifies that he will inform any patients or any persons used as controls, or their representatives, that drugs are being used for investigational purposes, and will obtain the consent of the subjects, or their representatives, except where this is not feasible or, in the investigator's professional judgment, is contrary to the best interests of the subjects.

h. The investigator is required to assure the sponsor that for investigations involving institutionalized subjects the studies will not be initiated until the institutional review committee has reviewed and approved the study. (The organization and procedure requirements for such a committee should be explained to the investigator by the sponsor as set forth in Form FD-1571, division 10, unit c.)

Very truly yours,

Name of Investigator _____

Address _____

_____

Figure 3-2 (Cont.)

ies are completed or discontinued. An informative paper was published in *FDA Papers.*[81] Table 3-2 shows an outline of a typical IND.

The regulatory agencies in the United States and Canada examine closely the qualifications of the 20,000 investigators who now participate in clinical studies in these countries, and follow the results of the clinical trials through periodic reporting as required by regulations. They may disqualify any investigator if they decide that his credentials are inappropriate for a study or his investigational data are inaccurate, falsified, or otherwise very unsatisfactory. Early in 1970, the regulatory agencies of the United States, Canada and Great Britain agreed to notify each other in advance of regulatory actions with international impact, and the policies and regulations covering clinical research in these countries began to be more uniform.

Table 3-2   Outline of an IND*

1.	Descriptive name	5
2.	Components	53
3.	Composition	55
4.	Source	29
5.	Production standards	77
6.	Preclinical	60
7.	Labeling	58
8.	Investigator qualifications	31
9.	Investigator file	31
10.	Protocol	50
11.	Discontinuance agreement	39
12.	Discontinuance/investigator	41
13.	Commercialization	42
14.	Signature	18

Toxicology and Pharmacology	1. Descriptive name 6. Preclinical 7. Labeling
Chemistry and Manufacturing Controls	1. Descriptive name 2. Components 3. Composition 4. Source 5. Production standards 7. Labeling
Clinical Protocols	1. Descriptive name 7. Labeling 8. Investigator qualifications 9. Investigator file 10. Protocol 11. Discontinuance agreement 12. Discontinuance/investigator 13. Commercialization 14. Signature of sponsor

* Numbered as shown in FD 1571.

But FDA is by far the most stringent. FDA wants all investigational studies that are conducted in homes for convalescents or the mentally deficient, hospitals, orphanages, and other facilities to be subjected to the same type of peer review and evaluation as that required for research work funded by the Department of HEW.* Continuing review and approval of clinical investigation procedures has promoted better monitoring, safer testing, and generation of more reliable data on investigational drugs than existed prior to 1963 when the 1962 Drug Amendments became effective.

Investigators participating in the early critical phases of clinical trials are required by FDA to be highly experienced, have adequate time for research, and have facilities immediately available to take care of any emergency that may arise. They should not begin any clinical trials before they have reached complete agreement with the sponsor concerning their protocol and plans. Personal consultation is essential in addition to the routine paper work and correspondence. FDA uses the 30 day period between IND submission and initiation of trials to determine whether previous animal and laboratory studies have been adequate to justify the proposed trials in man.

Human trials must be stopped by an investigator if any serious toxic effects occur, and he must inform the sponsoring manufacturer who in turn must promptly inform FDA regarding the details. Both sponsor and investigators must keep accurate records and the sponsor must keep FDA fully informed by periodically submitting reports. Hazardous situations such as major adverse reactions and any special precautions required must be transmitted promptly and the patients involved carefully monitored as long as necessary. Legislation making long term monitoring of patients potentially at serious risk mandatory is being pushed by consumer activists.

It is occasionally necessary to conduct clinical investigations in a particular area because some diseases and some types of patients are found only in certain regions of the

___

* More recently, lay members have been added to institutional review boards.

world.* Then, too, some health departments only accept clinical data that have been developed within their own countries.

When selecting new drugs for clinical trial, the investigator considers (1) the need for a new drug in the treatment of the given disease, (2) the risk to the human subjects entailed in administering the drug to them, and (3) the probability that the new drug will make an appreciable contribution to therapy. The physician who is contemplating clinical investigation of a new drug places greatest weight on the potential hazards to his patient and healthy volunteers. He must ask himself, How do the potential hazards relate to the potential efficacy?

The clinician faces many pitfalls in accepting a drug for clinical investigation. He can only expect a limited amount of information from animal studies on some drugs, such as analgesics and antidepressants, with obscure modes of action. He must be alert to inappropriate use of intrinsically sound pharmacodynamic techniques. Thus, the measurement of the abolition of the righting reflex or the potentiation of barbiturate anesthesia in mice as indexes of hypnotic action are not adequately specific. Healthy animals are irrationally used as a basis for predicting the possible action of drugs in diseased human beings. Again, animals are often given the drugs for acute rather than the chronic conditions for which they will be used clinically. Animals often absorb, metabolize, excrete and otherwise biologically handle drugs in a manner different from man.[65] Microsomal enzyme induction, other enzyme situations and drug interactions may differ from animals to man. And, perhaps most important, some highly toxic effects in man cannot be reproduced in animals.[64]

---

*The National Cancer Institute embarked on a worldwide search in 1969 to locate isolated groups of people with special genetic constitutions from whom scientists could obtain tissue specimens to aid in the identification of viruses that may cause human cancer. Volunteers have been found among some Havasupai Indians who have been isolated on the floor of the Grand Canyon for 10 centuries, residents of the island of Saba in the Netherlands Antilles east of the Virgin Islands, Samaritans of Israel, socially isolated since biblical times, people of German descent at Sappada in the Italian Alps who have been isolated by rugged mountains since the thirteenth century, and others.

To arrive at a sound decision whether to accept the responsibility of testing a given drug in humans, the physician must carefully review the data obtained from prior testing in animals and decide upon the relevance of these data to human experimentation by judging the answers to questions like the following. How many species of animals were used? Were they the proper ones for the given medication? How many different tests were applied? Why was each test selected? Were *in vitro* tests confirmed by *in vivo* experiments? Were studies conducted in intact animals as well as isolated organs and tissues? Was the site and mechanism of action demonstrated? What were the results of acute, subacute, and chronic toxicity studies? How long were these studies conducted? Were the biochemical, physiological, pharmacological and toxicological studies adequate? What did they indicate? Which body systems were affected by the drug and how were they affected? Which drugs interact with the new drug, and what adverse effects may be predicted in humans? What are the absorption, metabolism, distribution, and excretion characteristics? What are the therapeutic blood levels and what levels are attained at various time intervals after administration? What information has been obtained on metabolites?[3,12]

These and many other questions must be asked. The answers vary considerably according to the type of medication under study. For some questions, such as those regarding mechanism of action of analgesics and ataractics, no answers may be available. But all available information must be given the clinical investigator. Therefore, close communication between the clinical investigator, the sponsor's monitor of the clinical studies and the research worker who conducted the preclinical studies in animals is essential. All three must understand each other's problems and protocols. Competent pharmacologists and astute clinicians form potent partnerships in drug research.[48,53]

These investigators must constantly resist administrative pressures to conduct animal research programs on new drugs with undue haste; otherwise the drugs may be tested in man prematurely with serious consequences.* Business executives that manage most pharmaceutical companies often know very little about the significance of research data or the dangers revealed by the information generated at the laboratory bench. They concentrate primarily on marketing plans and the urgency of their goals must not be allowed to override the sound professional judgments of the scientists and clinical investigators in laboratories and clinics.

Whenever a physician administers a new drug to man for the first time he takes a calculated risk legally and medically, even with the informed written consent of the subject or his legal representative. He decides whether to take that risk in the light of the patient's condition and the answers he receives to questions like those given above. He particularly wants to determine as accurately as possible how the potential therapeutic value of the new drug relates to its potential for toxicity, how its therapeutic value is likely to compare with established drugs of the same category, and whether the benefit to the patient is likely to be great enough to outweigh the risks being taken.

In order to protect clinical research subjects and ensure that clinical trials are conducted under carefully controlled conditions, FDA was given authority under the 1962 Kefauver-Harris Amendments to monitor bioresearch and establish Good Laboratory Practice.[82-7] In 1967 a Scientific Investigations Staff was established in the Bureau of Drugs to investigate clinical investigators believed to have submitted false patient data or to have conducted research in a manner not affording maximal patient protection.†

---

*Early in 1971, FDA promulgated an Investigational New Drug Regulation that requires manufacturers and investigators to conduct physical examinations every 6 months for a period of 5 years on patients who had received investigational drugs that proved to be more dangerous than had been anticipated. Several companies, were submitting follow-up data to FDA because of serious toxicities such as carcinogenicity discovered in animals on long-term chronic toxicity studies. The INDs were left open to ensure follow-up. The Fountain Committee began studying this problem intensively early in 1971. However, the final regulations had still not been completed by 1978, publication date of this volume.

† This Staff has now been considerably expanded into a Division of Clinical Investigation that is responsible not only for clinical investigation review, but also for the performance of preclinical laboratories and institutional review boards.[86]

Research related injuries were studied by an HEW task force to determine the feasibility of compensating subjects injured in the course of HEW-sponsored research. Data on nearly 133,000 human subjects were obtained from 331 clinical investigators who had received grants for research with patients, donors, and normal volunteers during a three-year period. Of all investigators, 85 (26%) reported at least one patient injury during the period, while 34 percent of those conducting therapeutic research (of direct benefit to the subject) and 15 percent of those conducting nontherapeutic research (not of direct benefit) reported at least one injury. Of the principal investigators conducting therapeutic research 11 percent reported fatalities and 2.5 percent reported permanent disabling injuries. Deaths occurred mostly in patients receiving cancer chemotherapy, but some deaths were caused by dosage error, antibiotic nephrotoxicity, cerebral hemorrhage with anticoagulant therapy, drug withdrawal, and various other adverse drug reactions.

No fatalities were reported for nontherapeutic research. Altogether, only 3.7 percent of the 133,000 subjects suffered injuries and 80 percent of these were trivial. Only about 32 injuries per 100,000 subjects were fatal, and 11 per 100,000 permanently disabling. This compares favorably with the rates of 4 to 5 percent of major injuries and 1.3 percent of fatal injuries in the hospital setting.[90]

A major goal is to reduce these adverse experiences among research subjects to the lowest possible level. The responsible clinical investigator makes certain that he receives from the sponsor of the clinical research adequately informative *preclinical reports* that provide all pertinent data on preclinical testing, including the molecular structure of the new drug, pertinent metabolic data, all available acute, subacute and chronic toxicity data, animal dosages, suggested dose for man, precautionary information, and other necessary pharmacological and toxicological information. He correlates all these data with the *research protocol* and *case report forms* mutually agreed upon and supplied by the sponsor to facilitate his research and reporting. He frequently helps the clinical research *monitor** design these documents so that he is thoroughly familiar with the rationale of the clinical study. He should critically examine the scientific data presented to him by the sponsor before he begins each study with a new drug, to determine what it does and how it does it, how much to give and how to give it, and what actual and potential toxic effects and adverse reactions he might encounter in his patients. His ultimate purpose is to inform himself properly so that he can obtain reproducible data and convert it into reliable information after objective evaluation of patient responses under controlled conditions.

Clinical Protocols

FDA published an Amendment Describing Adequate and Well-Controlled Clinical Investigations (*Fed Reg* 35:3073-4, Feb 17, 1970). The principles presented in that document were developed over a period of years and are recognized by the scientific community as the essentials of adequate and well-controlled clinical investigations. They provide the basis for the determination of whether there is "substantial evidence" to support the claims of effectiveness for new drugs including antibiotics. Each new drug requires an individualized research approach to some extent. The clinical and laboratory data to be sought in accordance with the design of the study tend to vary from any standard checklist of items that might be developed for its particular class of drugs. Nevertheless, according to FDA (*Fed Reg* 35:7250—7253, May 8, 1970) the plan or protocol for the study and the report of the results of the effectiveness study must include the following:

1. A clear statement of the objectives of the study.
2. A method of selection of the subjects that—

a. Provides adequate assurance that they are suitable for the purposes of the study, diagnostic criteria of the condition to be treated or diagnosed, confirmatory laboratory tests

where appropriate, and, in the case of prophylactic agents, evidence of susceptibility and exposure to the condition against which prophylaxis is desired.

b. Assigns the subjects to test groups in such a way as to minimize bias.

c. Assures comparability in test and control groups of pertinent variables, such as age, sex, severity, or duration of disease, and use of drugs other than the test drug.

3. Explains the methods of observation and recording of results, including the variables measured, quantitation, assessment of any subjective response, and steps taken to minimize bias on the part of the subject and observer.

4. Provides a comparison of the results of treatment of diagnosis with a control in such a fashion as to permit quantitative evaluation. The precise nature of the control must be stated and an explanation given of the methods used to minimize bias on the part of the observers and the analysts of the data. Level and methods of "blinding," if used, are to be documented. Generally, four types of comparison are recognized:

a. *No treatment*—Where objective measurements of effectiveness are available and placebo effect is negligible, comparison of the objective results in comparable groups of treated and untreated patients.

b. *Placebo control*—Comparison of the results of use of the new drug entity with an inactive preparation designed to resemble the test drug as far as possible.

c. *Active treatment control*—An effective regimen of therapy may be used for comparison, e.g., where the condition treated is such that no treatment or administration of a placebo would be contrary to the interest of the patient.

d. *Historical control**—In certain circumstances, such as those involving diseases with high and predictable mortality (acute leukemia of childhood), with signs and symptoms of predictable duration or severity (fever in certain infections), or, in case of prophylaxis, where morbidity is predictable, the results of use of a new drug entity may be compared quantitatively with prior experience historically derived from the adequately documented natural history of the disease or condition in comparable patients or populations with no treatment or with a regimen (therapeutic, diagnostic, prophylactic) the effectiveness of which is established.

5. A summary of the methods of analysis and an evaluation of data derived from the study, including any appropriate statistical methods.

Provided, however, That any of the above criteria may be waived in whole or in part, either prior to the investigation or in the evaluation of a completed study, by the Director of the Bureau of Drugs with respect to a specific clinical investigation; a petition for such a waiver may be filed by any person who would be adversely affected by the application of the criteria to a particular clinical investigation; the petition should show that some or all of the criteria are not reasonably applicable to the investigation and that alternative procedures can be, or have been, followed, the results of which will or have yielded data that can and should be accepted as substantial evidence of the drug's effectiveness. A petition for a waiver shall set forth clearly and concisely the specific provision or provisions in the criteria from which waiver is sought, why the criteria are not reasonably applicable to the particular clinical investigation, what alternative procedures, if any, are to be, or have been, employed, what results have been obtained, and the basis on which it can be, or has been, concluded that the clinical investigation will or has yielded substantial evidence of effectiveness, notwithstanding nonconformance with the criteria for which waiver is requested.

6. Standardization of the test drug as to identity, strength, quality, purity, and dosage form in order to give significance to the results of the investigation.

---

*The sponsor's monitor is usually a physician appointed from within a pharmaceutical company to follow and assume responsibility for specified clinical trials. He obtains the clinical investigators, indoctrinates them carefully, and constantly checks on the progress of his assigned clinical studies. In addition, FDA's Division of Clinical Investigation constantly reviews the qualifications of clinical investigators and evaluates the quality of their studies and reports. Falsifications of clinical research data have occurred.

---

* Historical control is acceptable to FDA only when the disease involved has an established, irrevocable course and constant characteristics. In a disease like Meniere's syndrome, for example, which is unpredictable and in which the therapeutic effect of investigational drugs can only be evaluated subjectively, placebo control must be used.

Uncontrolled studies or partially controlled studies are not acceptable as the sole basis for the approval of claims of effectiveness. Such studies, carefully conducted and documented, may provide corroborative support of well-controlled studies regarding efficacy and may yield valuable data regarding safety of the test drug. Such studies will be considered on their merits in the light of the principles listed here, with the exception of the requirement for the comparison of the treated subjects with controls. Isolated case reports, random experience, and reports lacking the details which permit scientific evaluation will not be considered.

Several good reviews on clinical testing and the evaluation of new drugs have appeared. [3, 12, 61, 62, 93-6]

Clinical Investigation Phases

A clinical investigator who undertakes a clinical *trial* or *study* tests a drug product in a *selected* group of individuals. As explained above, the trial must be controlled. It is conducted according to a definite protocol and with the aid of special reporting forms (*case report forms* or *case record forms*). A trial may involve many or few subjects (volunteers and patients), healthy or diseased, and many or few clinics, hospitals, prisons,* private practices, and other institutions.

There are four phases through which complete and continuing clinical investigations proceed. These are outlined below. In general each has its own types of objectives, but at times there may be considerable overlap. Each phase consists of a few to sometimes very many clinical trials conducted by a few to perhaps hundreds of clinical investigators. In any one phase the trials should be organized so that the data obtained from the various trials are uniform and compatible and allow meaningful correlations to be made among all the assembled entries in the case report forms. Throughout Phases I through IV compatibility of reported data must be kept in mind and every step must be carefully planned and closely monitored, so that data from all phases can be correlated and evaluated as a total output of the research.

Proper monitoring of clinical trials is a vital responsibility of every sponsor of a clinical investigation. If the sponsor is a pharmaceutical manufacturer, the physician who is designated as monitor should conduct a com-

prehensive discussion of the research protocol with both preclinical and chemical investigators to make certain that all data and their significance are clearly understood. The monitor should visit the laboratory facilities of the clinical investigator to make certain that the investigator can satisfactorily conduct the necessary chemical, hematologic and other tests, and that both equipment and technique will be acceptable scientifically and professionally. He should have periodic discussions to determine how each trial is proceeding and to detect deviations from the protocol and other problems. He should be aware of any subcontracting of research by the investigator and if this is done assure himself that the secondary investigator is competent and his facilities adequate. If the research deviates from the established protocol or the protocol is poorly designed, doubts may be cast upon the validity of a clinical investigation and the drug's usefulness and safety, and FDA may not approve the drug when the research has been completed.

Phase I Studies. The first time a drug is administered to man, in so-called *initial clinical pharmacology* (Phase I) studies, a few cooperative, carefully examined, healthy volunteers or patients are selected as subjects. After they have given their informed written consent, they are given initially only single doses commensurate with the findings in test animals. The first human doses are usually based upon a fraction of the minimal effective dose per kilogram of dog or monkey since the dog is generally the most sensitive animal in the laboratory and the monkey, being a primate, may be closely related to man in its responses. [36] If these first doses are tolerated, the medication is carefully continued. Studies are conducted during this preliminary clinical pharmacology phase to determine basic data such as the rates of absorption; degree of toxicity to the heart, kidneys, liver, and the hematopoietic, muscular, nervous, vascular, and other important systems, organs, and tissues; metabolism data; drug concentrations in the serum or blood; excretion patterns; and particularly the ability of man to tolerate a physiologically active dose of the drug. All subjects are closely observed for untoward effects and intensive clinical laboratory tests are con-

---

*During 1978 regulations were written to prohibit use of prisoners in any research unless the study will be of health benefit to the prisoners or will have sociological value.

ducted, especially to check for adverse cardiac, hematologic, hepatic, and renal effects.

The investigator should carefully screen subjects about to enter Phases I and II studies to make certain they possess suitable characteristics. Thus Phase I subjects used to evaluate potential hepatotoxicity should have normal values for: complete blood count (CBC), fasting blood sugar (FBS), blood urea nitrogen (BUN), creatinine, urinalysis, transaminase (SGOT, SGPT), alkaline phosphatase, total bilirubin (direct and indirect), prothrombin time, total protein (Gm.%), protein electrophoresis, electrolytes (Na, K, Ca, Cl, CO_2), hepatitis B-antigen (nonA, nonB), platelet count, and reticulocyte count.

If prisoners are used as volunteers in drug studies, certain precautions should be observed. The National Commission for the Protection of Human Subjects of Biomedical and Behavioral Research has published a detailed review with recommendations for research involving prisoners. [88]

Testing in prison volunteers became a hotly debated issue during the 1970s when improprieties and deficiencies were revealed and many states prohibited such research. Legislation, both State and Federal, has been designed to protect prisoners.

In 1978, the Pharmaceutical Manufacturers Association reported that about a third of all pharmaceutical company Phase I studies involved prisoner volunteers. [97] This was at a time when the Secretary of HEW was proposing that all drug research in prisoner volunteers be prohibited. This proposal would be highly detrimental to drug research in this country and would cause US manufacturers to conduct much of their research overseas, claimed PMA.

Phase II Studies. If the Phase I data justify further testing, *expanded clinical pharmacology* (Phase II) studies are started and initial trials on a limited number of carefully supervised patients given the drug for specific disease control or prophylactic purposes. Blood levels at various time intervals, side effects, and additional Phase I data may be accumulated. Small doses are gradually increased until the minimal effective dose is found. All reactions of the subjects are carefully recorded. Preliminary estimates of dosage, efficacy, and safety in man are made. Phase II investigators are either well-qualified practitioners or clinicians who are familiar with the conditions to be treated, the drugs used in the conditions, and the methods of their evaluation. FDA maintains a computerized list of clinical investigators and files their curricula vitae submitted with the INDs.

Phase III Studies. If the Phase II data indicate that the drug has promising properties, a complete report on Phase I studies is submitted to FDA, and if not prohibited, *extensive clinical investigation* (Phase III) trials are begun with the aid of experienced investigators and private practitioners with widely varying experiences. The number of patients used may number only 1,000 or less where carefully designed protocols and reporting forms (case report forms) can elicit adequate data for a New Drug Application.* With immunizing agents and some drugs, however, the patients may number 10,000 or even several hundred thousand where massive trials are necessary to identify very rare, yet serious adverse reactions and other effects. Thus, encephalopathy with pertussis vaccine and paralysis with poliovaccine have been reported only a very few times in the millions of patients who have been immunized with these vaccines.

Pediatric research presents its own particular problems. Lockhart, once a medical officer of FDA, [71] has pointed out several critical ones and has suggested some solutions in a paper "Attitudes of FDA in Drug Evaluation in Infants and Children," presented to the American Academy of Pediatrics in October, 1969. In Phases I and II, for example, consent for use of an investigational new drug must be in writing, whereas in Phase III this is the responsibility of the investigator. After taking into consideration the physical and mental state of the patient, the investigator decides when it is necessary or preferable to obtain consent other than in written form. But can any adult representative of a child give informed consent for that child to be a volunteer subject in a Phase I study? The right of a responsible representative to give such consent began to be challenged in the courts early in 1970. Perhaps the solution is

---

*Subjects for the study must be normal reactors selected and assigned to the appropriate dosage regimens according to sound statistical methods that eliminate bias and placebo effects, e.g., randomization with the aid of Latin squares, etc.

to conduct Phase I studies in adults first, and only if these studies indicate adequate safety to conduct combined Phase I and II studies in subjects of pediatric age who are healthy or have the required disease. Metabolic differences between sick and healthy children, however, must be considered.

More basic pharmacologic information from pediatric research is needed. We know little beyond the fact that iatrogenic disease in the neonate is frequently the result of enzyme immaturity. Infants, especially the premature and newborn, cannot cope well with drugs like chloramphenicol, novobiocin, streptomycin, and sulfonamides. Until drugs have been shown by appropriate pediatric testing to be safe for use in children, they must bear either of these statements on the label: *Not recommended for use in children under 2 years of age due to limited experience in this age group* or *Contraindicated in children under 6 months of age.* So many drugs now bear these statements, because so little specific pediatric research has been conducted with the newer drugs, that there are numerous pediatric patients for whom most modern, clinically approved medications are unavailable unless a physician wishes to prescribe an approved drug for an unapproved use. Shirkey has called these patients therapeutic orphans.

According to the law, drugs cannot be labeled to indicate that they are safe for use in pediatric therapy until they have been clinically evaluated in children. Therefore more pediatric clinical research is needed with both old and new drugs to fill the therapeutic void that exists for pediatric patients. And vast amounts of pediatric clinical data must be pulled out of the files of FDA and the pharmaceutical manufacturers, tabulated, correlated, evaluated, and supplemented where necessary with additional studies. It is hazardous not to have adequate supplies of effective medications available for pediatric use.

In order to develop enough accurate information for patient protection, adequate testing of new drugs usually includes a number of uncontrolled studies to determine dose-response curves and incidence of side effects,[49] as well as an appropriate number of controlled studies.* But more than subjective, testimonial type of data must be obtained.

In the *double blind* type of controlled study, the test drug is given to one group of patients (treatment group) and a placebo or another drug in the same therapeutic category, of identical appearance, is given to another group (control group) of patients having the same characteristics as the treatment group.† Both test drug and placebo (or medication used for comparison) are coded so that neither the investigator's team nor the patients know which is being administered at any given time.

With some drugs, e.g., topical palliative medications in chronic skin diseases, each patient may serve as his own control by the use of different areas of his body. The patient's control and test sites are observed for specific periods of time after application of control and test materials; then the test sites are reversed and the sites are again observed to compare therapeutic and adverse effects. This type of study, so designed that different areas of a patient or patients themselves are alternated between test and control materials, is often called a *crossover* study.‡ In case of serious reactions or other problems, the code for double blind and other controlled studies can be quickly broken by a responsible readily available person who holds the key to the code, often the pharmacist in the hospital. Special tear-off labels are often used. Once the code is broken, however, the study loses its "controlled" status, and most of its value as a supporter of claims may be lost.

The New Drug Application. As soon as chronic toxicity studies in animals have been

---

*The number of controlled studies required depends on the characteristics and incidence of the disease and the spread between the results observed with the test drug and those observed with the placebo or comparison drug during the first few studies conducted. The wider the spread, the fewer the studies needed to prove efficacy.

†No reputable clinical investigator or sponsor of a drug trial will deprive a patient of urgently needed medication. A placebo should only be given when the patient will not be harmed by substitution of a placebo for active medication.

‡If the procedure is repeated with the same patients, as is often necessary with an unpredictable condition like Meniere's syndrome, the study is called a *double crossover.*

completed and all necessary clinical data have been generated, a *New Drug Application* (NDA) containing all research and development data suitably categorized, tabulated, evaluated, and documented is submitted to FDA. This agency by law must approve each new drug before it can be marketed, and it usually spends many months checking the substantiating data and correlating them with submitted labeling.* The agency has stated the following requirements; an NDA must:

1. Provide adequate and complete descriptions of patients with respect to age, sex, weight, and diagnosis of conditions treated.
2. Record accurately the details of drug dosage (amount, frequency, duration).
3. Specify any previous or concomitant therapy the patient receives.
4. Provide baseline pretreatment determinations and obtain subsequent values during the following treatment courses for all appropriate laboratory and clinical examinations pertinent for a given drug.
5. Design case report forms to indicate clearly what signs, symptoms, side effects, and responses were actually sought and what laboratory tests were performed in the study. Statements such as "no side effects" and "laboratory normal" are inadequate and do not allow valid conclusions.
6. Obtain objective measurements of drug response whenever possible. Seriously consider the use of double blind or double blind crossover studies; these are of greatest importance in situations where only a subjective response is available. Clearly separate and identify noncontrolled studies. Minimize them.
7. For the evaluation of combination products, direct specific attention to demonstrating that the combination is better than the individual ingredients alone. This is necessary for several reasons: (*a*) It is not justifiable to expose patients to possible additive side effects of drugs unless there is scientific reason for combining the products. (*b*) Studies comparing the individual ingredients to the combination are indicated in order to evaluate fully possible drug interactions. (*c*) Labeling representing ingredients to be active may not be approved in the absence of substantial evidence that they contribute to the effectiveness of the combination.
8. For the evaluation of sustained release preparations provide data from objective studies demonstrating the characteristics of the release pattern, such as blood and urine levels, as well as clinical observations on the safety and effectiveness of the product.
9. Testimonial-type information as "evidence" of safety and effectiveness, and a large volume of "case histories" presenting conclusions without details of observations made is not *per se* of any significance. However, it is desirable to have each investigator present a concise report stating his impressions regarding the safety and effectiveness of the drug along with any other pertinent observations or recommendations.

The type of clinical data which FDA expects to see in an NDA, the type the law requires, will enable an appropriately qualified observer to render a reasonable and responsible decision that the effectiveness of

the drug will outweigh its hazards when used as labeled. FDA encourages manufacturers to consult it prior to, during, and after clinical trials before the NDA is submitted, in order to improve the content and organization of protocols, case records, clinical summaries, and other components of an application.

Routinely submitted reports include the following tables: investigator-patient distribution, patient age and sex distribution, dosage distribution, duration of therapy distribution, concomitant therapy, adverse effects summary, clinical laboratory test-patient correlation, and correlations of clinical response with investigator, disease, dosage, duration of therapy, coexistant disease, and concomitant therapy.

Special reports include: pathogenic microorganism summary, bacteriological response-pathogenic organism correlation, clinical response-pathogenic organism correlation, clinical response-bacteriological response correlation, plasma blood levels, and others as required by the given drug testing program. Such reports show the number of male and female patients in each age group receiving various dosage levels for varying periods of time with and without concomitant medication. The correlations tabulated reveal relative efficacy and safety of the drug at various dosage levels and durations, in different diseases, and compare the results obtained by different investigators. Additional, more specialized data are collected for antibiotics, diuretics, and certain other categories of drugs. [50-52]

Under certain circumstances, such as the need to comply with FDA requirements based on evaluations of reports of the Drug Efficacy Study Group, the submission of an *Abbreviated New Drug Application* containing designated items of information is sufficient for approval of an application. Specific instructions for submission of abbreviated applications were published in the *Federal Register,* February 27, 1969 (FR Doc 69-2353). [63]

Phase IV Studies. After Phase III studies have been completed and FDA has approved a New Drug Application, *studies on marketed drugs* (Phase IV studies) are often begun in order to add to the store of clinical information about the drug product and to substanti-

---

*FDA intensively studies each NDA. The average elapsed time between submission and approval for applications approved during FY 1976 was about 20 months.

ate new claims so that additional indications will be approved by the agency.

During 1975, Commissioner Alexander M. Schmidt recommended a new Phase IV approval procedure, and early in 1976 Senators Edward Kennedy and Jacob Javits introduced legislation that would expedite new drug approval by means of this new type of procedure. Previously drugs had been approved only after both short-term and long-term safety and efficacy had been shown. Under the new approach drugs in Phase IV are to be made available on a restricted basis to selected physicians, in selected hospitals and geographic areas for specific patients, on a voluntary basis, before chronic studies are completed. In return, accurate complete data on the use of the drug in broad patient populations shall be made available to FDA. This approach overcomes serious deficiencies of the past—lack of information on drug use and nondetection of rare adverse effects prior to general marketing.

Sometimes the most important uses for drugs are discovered some time after they have been investigated for other indications. A good example is acetazolamide, first tested and patented (1951) as a diuretic, then later found to be an effective agent for lowering the ocular tension of glaucoma, and during 1970 reported to prevent and improve attacks of hypokalemic periodic weakness.[55] Phase IV studies may continue indefinitely, as long as useful information concerning prolonged safety and ultimate efficacy is being generated, but each new use being investigated requires a new IND.

Under certain circumstances such as rapid approval of a highly important drug (e.g., levodopa) used in a chronic disease, FDA has required the manufacturer, as a condition of approval, to continue clinical studies to determine whether it induces adverse effects over a prolonged period of time.

The sponsor of drug investigations must immediately report all serious adverse reactions noted by an investigator during any stage of a clinical investigation both to FDA (on Form FD 1639) and to all other investigators involved in clinical studies with an implicated drug. And, when a new drug is marketed, all adverse reactions allegedly or possibly due to the drug that are severe or of greater than usual incidence and that come

to the attention of the manufacturer, must be reported to FDA within 15 working days. All other adverse reactions must be reported every three months during the first year the medication is on the market, every six months the second year, and once a year therafter until FDA publishes an exemption from periodic reporting.* Such "drug experience information" is submitted on FDA Form 1639. However, the agency accepts data from this form as well as certain other types of clinical data as computer printouts. As this practice becomes more widespread, the processing of critical data is being accelerated.

Proper follow-up of each reported adverse reaction is essential. Occasionally a new serious reaction due to a given drug is discovered and appropriate action must be taken promptly. Reactions allegedly caused by medication have been shown on occasion, however, to be nonexistent or due to other causes. See Chapter 9.

In December, 1970, FDA introduced the principle of "imminent hazard." Under its interpretation of this concept, FDA can take steps immediately to correct a public health situation that should be corrected to prevent injury and "that should not be permitted to continue while a hearing or other formal proceeding is being held." The agency can therefore act merely in anticipation of the occurrence of an injury.[67] See *Delayed Withdrawal* (page 14).

The Goal

Drug research in animals and humans is designed to determine approvable therapeutic utility.† To achieve this goal, indications (diseases for which the medication is used), the most effective dosage form (tablet, capsules, syrup, injection, etc.) for each of these indications, and the most suitable dosage required for each disease in each type of patient must be established. Also, the optimum

---

*See for example: Propylthiouracil, methimazole, and iothiouracil sodium; drugs for human use; Drug Efficacy Study implementation. *Fed Reg* 34:5392-5395 (Mar 19) 1969.

†It is doubtful at the present time whether FDA can legally require any manufacturer to develop *relative* therapeutic efficacy data while comparing his product with one already marketed. Testing procedures are largely inadequate to enable investigators to provide such information.

level, frequency, timing, route and duration of dosage, as well as all precautions and contraindications, special hazards and warnings, side effects, adverse reactions, drug interactions, incompatabilities, and all other information about the drug which should be known by the drug therapy team, must be accurately derived. Continuing animal studies provide data which enable the clinical investigator to sharpen the design of his human studies. And vice versa, the clinical studies provide data which enable the investigators in experimental therapeutics to improve the design of their animal studies. Continuing concurrent animal and human studies with constant feedback, if acted on, continually improve drug research programs.

In the final analysis, therapeutic safety, as measured by the spread between the effective dose and the dose at which serious toxic effects begin to appear, may be related to other factors. For example, a drug which is effective in life-threatening situations may be approved if it is the only treatment available, even if it is dangerous to use. In some special cases, routine studies may not be required, subject to FDA concurrence, if the drug is restricted for use in life-threatening conditions. It is evident that a high degree of sophistication, not only in clinical medicine but in the methodology of scientific research, is essential for the development of safe and effective medications. [41,42]

PHARMACEUTICAL DEVELOPMENT

As human studies assume increasing prominence in new drug development, the human data generated should logically be given more and more weight and the animal data less and less weight in evaluating the probable benefit-to-risk ratio for each new medication. However, until we have delved deeper into molecular biology and can predict toxic effects on the basis of chemical reactions and structures we shall continue to evaluate relative safety in laboratory animals.

As soon as animal tests suggest that a useful new drug has been discovered and that a New Drug Application will probably be submitted to FDA for that drug, development of marketable dosage forms, already begun in a preliminary way is accelerated. The many forms in which medication can be made available have been thoroughly discussed. [24] The forms selected are extremely important from the standpoints of safety and efficacy.

Each drug has its own specific peculiarities, but capsules and tablets are the forms of choice for most medications because of their convenience and economy. Liquid forms, especially pleasantly flavored syrups, are usually most suitable for younger children. Drugs that are destroyed in the gastrointestinal tract must be prepared in a form for parenteral use. But with this route there are restrictions. Some drugs may be given by one parenteral route and not by another, and some can be given by only one such route if the proper diagnostic or therapeutic effect is to be achieved. In addition to convenience and proper route of administration, many other factors are involved in the selection of dosage forms, including acceptability to the patient, accuracy and uniformity of dosage, ease of transportation, stability when stored, site of action, biological availability, cost, degree and rate of absorption, rate of spread in the tissues, and the metabolic pathways. These factors influence efficacy, safety, or general usefulness. See Chapter 8.

The most suitable dosage form for each new drug must be selected early, at least before Phase II clinical research is started, because clinical studies must be conducted as nearly as possible with the same dosage units that will eventually be marketed. Only by this means can the final product be certified with confidence to be therapeutically effective. Therefore, concurrently with the later stages of preclinical testing, various dosage forms are developed and studied intensively to determine whether they can be produced so that they will provide uniform, accurate dosage, and will retain their purity, potency, and quality. They must undergo thorough stability testing. This type of testing can be "accelerated" by emphasizing the environmental conditions, e.g., by holding the drug products at elevated temperature and humidity for specified periods of time to simulate what happens when they are held at normal conditions over much more prolonged periods.

From the early stages materials supplied

for clinical investigation by responsible manufacturers are carefully checked and passed through the same type of rigid quality control as that used for marketed products. They are checked for identity, physical and chemical characteristics, limits of impurities, uniformity of content, and correct labeling. They are also assayed to verify the potency, and properly packaged and stored to prevent deterioration.

SOURCES OF ERROR IN DRUG RESEARCH

The literature on experimental therapeutics and clinical research is replete with sources of error which can invalidate studies, lead eventually to inaccurate conclusions, and possibly cause harm to the patient.[50-52] Although most of these errors do not happen frequently enough to cause serious concern, they should be recognized and avoided by all who participate in drug research and development programs. These sources of error can be categorized for convenience under the following headings: (1) errors introduced by preclinical investigators, (2) errors introduced by clinical investigators, and (3) errors introduced by patients.

Errors Introduced by Preclinical Investigators

Scientists undertaking drug research which involves the basic sciences and experimental therapeutics are constantly faced with the problem of avoiding human errors and inaccuracies caused by faulty equipment. Human errors often arise from faulty perception, e.g., misreading of instruments, misinterpretation of test results, misjudgments because of lack of sensitivity of touch, miscalculations, and other faulty functioning where intellect or physical ability are affected by mental attitude (lack of motivation, ennui, disinterest, etc.). Other human errors include improper selection of laboratory animals, improper interpretation of the literature, incorrect evaluation of laboratory data, and inaccurate reporting.

Laboratory errors can easily arise when any instrument is used by the inexperienced technician. In the first place, instruments with the proper degree of sensitivity must be used. Spectrophotometers, colorimeters, and many other instruments must be carefully calibrated. The temperature and humidity of the laboratory must sometimes be critically controlled, also vibration when delicate instruments are to be used. False-positive and false-negative results must be constantly avoided. For example, suitable culture media and proper culture techniques must be used when testing for the absence or presence of specific microorganisms, sensitivities to antibiotics, etc.*

The subject of errors in laboratory procedures is so complex that an entire book can be devoted to it. But it must be understood thoroughly and all possible errors avoided if correct test results are going to be reflected in good medication and patient safety. See Chapter 7.

Errors Introduced by Clinical Investigators

Clinical investigation is a fertile field for human error because so much of it is based on subjective observations, the judgments of individual investigators, and sometimes almost solely on intuition.

FDA frustratingly encounters the same research errors over and over again.[15] The causes of these errors may be categorized as follows: (1) insufficient detail or explanation, (2) faulty planning, (3) incompleteness of studies, (4) obscure objectives, and (5) befuddled communication.

Insufficient Detail. Protocols and reports are unbelievably inadequate at times. A properly prepared protocol should include (1) clearly defined purpose of the study, (2) dosage regimens, including dosage forms, strengths, doses, frequency, timing, duration, and number of patients and controls on each regimen and dosage level, (3) other therapy permitted, (4) criteria for selection and exclusion of cases, (5) plan of the study, including specific observations to be made clinically and tests and analyses to be conducted in the laboratory; pretreatment, treatment, and post-treatment procedures; specific instructions for reporting bacteriologic, radiologic, clinical, and other types of data as needed, (6) case report forms with complete instructions for using them, and (7) suitable check-

---

*Good Laboratory Practices regulations were promulgated by FDA in 1978.

lists for work-ups, patient charts, etc. The protocol should provide such complete and clear guidance that the investigators will abide by the official guidelines for clinical investigation. See also *Clinical Protocols,* page 44.

Faulty Planning. Innumerable times, costly clinical studies have been conducted only to discover upon completion that no base lines were established for critical values.* For example, studies have been set up to evaluate an anesthetic on the basis of vital signs without taking readings of these on the patients prior to use of the drug. How is it possible to know what alteration takes place, if any, in blood pressures, pulse rates, and respiration if no values are obtained for the patients at critical times prior, during, and after use of the investigational medication?

In many types of clinical studies, it is important to make tests for functioning of the liver and other organs. But all too frequently these tests are made only before, or during, or after administration of test medication to the patient and omitted at the other critical times. How can any valid conclusions be drawn in regard to the effects of the medication on the functioning of these organs when such faulty planning exists?

Placebo effects, if not recognized or eliminated by proper planning of studies, are another source of clinical error. In some patients, under certain conditions, placebos produce *placebo responses,* i.e., side effects or other unfavorable responses or various therapeutic effects, occasionally even more intense than those produced by the test medications. Because of psychogenic effects, many patients tend to respond, sometimes adversely and sometimes favorably, whenever they are given any substance they believe to be medication, even when it is physiologically inert. Some studies have shown that women are

twice as likely as men to respond to placebos.[56] Expectation of activity may be induced in patients by suggestion or by the patient's own mental action. Patients so affected, so-called placebo reactors, obscure the true effects of drugs during a clinical trial by reacting abnormally and evidencing effects that cannot possibly be attributed to placebo or medication, and thereby causing the clinical investigator to arrive at false conclusions.[4,39,42]

Improper use of double blind studies is another source of error.[9] When, for example, a corticosteroid is being tested against a placebo, the powerful adrenal suppressive effect becomes an important factor. In fact, abrupt withdrawal may actually be dangerous to the patient. In any event, not only do the patient and physician quickly become aware of which drug is the placebo and which is the active agent, but a medical emergency can be caused by the induced hypoadrenal state. Furthermore, random selection of patients for such studies introduces patients unsuitable for the testing. They may be hyperreactive, hypersensitive, or otherwise unreliable. It is difficult to conduct such studies with powerful, prompt-acting medications without influencing both patients and investigator. Unlike double blind studies with weak, slow-acting drugs, bias is not easily controlled; the drug may have to be withdrawn because of side effects, and incorrect conclusions may be drawn.

Improper delegation of professional duties is another source of error. Situations like the following appear in the literature. A clinical investigator's secretary actually distributed drug and placebo to patients, and after the study was concluded, the investigator discovered that because of faulty randomization, nearly five times as many subjects received the drug as received the placebo.† Bias was introduced and doubts were cast upon the entire clinical trial.[9] Absolute intellectual honesty is essential at each step of the research, not only in the principal investigator

---

*On May 20, 1747, Lind began the first controlled clinical investigation recorded in the literature when he started to evaluate citrus fruits in the treatment of scurvy. Although he clearly revealed his methodology and demonstrated the value of careful observation, controlled experimentation, rigid reliance on fact and logical interpretation, government and industry are still frustrated more than 200 years later by clinical studies that are poorly designed and evaluated. See the paper by Duncan P. Thomas: Experiment versus authority, *N Eng J Med* 281:932-933, 1969.

---

†The nurse on the other hand is a highly valuable participant in clinical research. As Nichols and Glor noted (*Mil. Med.* 133:57-62, 1968), the nurse cares for the patients taking investigational drugs, collects specimens, observes and records pertinent data, and may assist with electronic or electromechanical manipulation of data and the compilation of research reports.

but also in every single person involved with him in the clinical research program.

Other acts that may amount to faulty planning of clinical trials are, (1) testing in the absence of an established reproducible synthesis for a test drug, (2) attempting to test a drug clinically for which chemical controls and the chemical structure have not been established, (3) trying to use double blind studies in Phase I testing, (4) using unsuitable measurements, e.g., axillary temperatures have been reported, (5) administration of two or more investigational drugs to a patient simultaneously (one patient received 19 drugs, 12 of which were investigational), (6) testing drugs in patients who are already receiving other drugs which are affecting the laboratory values and symptoms to be recorded, and (7) testing drugs in patients who have diseases which influence the laboratory values and symptoms to be recorded for the test drug.[15]

Incompleteness of Studies. A common error in clinical studies is a lack of follow-through. In many studies vast amounts of clinical laboratory data are collected from patients or other subjects, and then no corresponding data are obtained either during or after treating the patient with test medication. How can any correlations be made or any conclusions be drawn as to the effects of the medication on the clinical laboratory values?

Another type of incompleteness is due to inadequate design of protocols and case report forms. Some reports defy anyone to interpret them correctly. The elements of the matrix must be logically arranged with headings that are cognate, properly emphasized, and correctly related. The forms must be clear, non-ambiguous, and utilize consistent terminology. Boxes to be checked should request mutually exclusive data which do not conflict or overlap. All essential elements, especially quantity, frequency, timing, and duration of dosage, as well as such important patient characteristics as weight, age, sex, and race must be included. Many times an element (date, weight, etc.) is omitted and later is found to be essential for proper evaluation of a drug. Attention must be paid to detail but a form cannot be made too complex or it will not be completely filled out by very busy physicians, and completeness of reporting is a Federal requirement. Also, separate forms for collecting information on each type of testing should be prepared unless the form is fairly simple and separate and distinct areas can be clearly allocated on the same form. Finally, when the forms are filled out by the investigators, the entries should be made in clearly *legible* handwriting, or better, typewritten.

Valid objections can be raised, of course, against protocols and case report forms that are too detailed and too rigidly structured. The creativity of competent investigators must not be stifled. Enough latitude must be allowed to permit them to inject some of their own originality of thought and observation and thereby improve the content and scope of clinical studies just as long as they report the basic information consistently.

Obscure Objectives. Many clinical studies are designed so that it is very difficult or impossible to understand what is actually being accomplished. FDA has received NDAs containing reference drug names that were unfamiliar to everyone in the agency and the National Library of Medicine and could not be found in any available drug text or reference book. When FDA finally went back to the company that had submitted the NDA, it was discovered that the company didn't know the ingredients of the reference drug names either. Finally, after prolonged searching FDA found that the reference drugs (alinamine, elestol, migrenin, opyato, opystan, pryabital, resochin, sedes, vochin, etc.) were Japanese analgesic products containing aspirin, aminopyrine, barbiturates, codeine, etc.

Another use of obscure terminology sometimes involves the names of tests which are obsolete or seldom or never used because they are too intensive or nonreproducible or have other flaws. The use of such tests as the cadmium, Takata, and Weltmann in modern clinical testing, as reported in one paper, caused the studies to be subjected to unusually intense scrutiny by FDA.[15]

Befuddled Communication. It is amazing how often so-called highly educated individuals show their inability to think and write clearly. Papers, reports, and other research documents blithely present commingled ideas and distorted concepts that defy interpretation. A few examples, taken from research reports that were read by the author during one two-week period, are either meaningless or give an incorrect meaning:

"Patient BM died suddenly at his home and now lives in another town. He has been dropped from the study."

"For a statistical analysis showed that the treated and untreated *rabbits* bore litters whose different birth weights of baby *rats* were not statistically significant."

"The control group consisted of 53 cases with bilateral disease representing 7 investigators and the remaining 130 were from alternate patients."

"There were studies as an anorexiant and in 4 categories of CNS stimulation for psychopathology established with 15 investigators all double blind code comparisons of [drug] versus a placebo."

"There were 5 patients who had drowsiness following a medication found to be [active drug]. Those on B medication as [active drug] had drowsiness (3) or drowsiness with dry mouth (4) and faintness (2) one accompanied by syncope with some decrease of BP yet within normal range and one with weakness. Five patients had side effects listed under placebo two as A only one each of drowsiness and dry mouth. There was one with placebo as A with faint and dizzy in which B or [active drug] was given. To patients on placebo as B medication had one of drowsiness and cne of faintness-weakness."

A great deal of such trash is the result of hasty dictation, hurried typing, and no checking, editing, or proofreading. Typographical errors and omissions are bound to occur under such circumstances. But when clinical research documents transmit information in such a confused fashion, the excellent work of good investigators can be distorted and misinterpreted with consequences that could be hazardous to patients.

Good communication, especially of drug information, is the basic ingredient of competent professional service in any activity concerned with medication. Physicians, nurses, pharmacists, and other health care professionals constantly require dependable drug information that originates with clinical investigators. How do they get it? What do they do with it? How do they get it to those who need it? The answers to these and related questions change constantly, and so these professionals must keep up to date with the latest concepts and also keep their colleagues aware of the latest information in the fields in which they are working. Otherwise patients who receive either investigational or approved drugs will not receive the best available medical care.

During clinical research, it is essential that all drug trials be well designed and the clinical investigator who is studying new drugs in patients be highly experienced in interpreting the protocols, in making adequate and detailed observations, and in evaluating results. If he is not, he may misinterpret his findings and arrive at false conclusions. He may even calculate incorrectly and give a dosage much less or greater than that required by the protocol he is following. As one example, dosage expressed as milligrams per kilogram has been calculated as milligrams per pound, with the result that the patient receives more than double the desired dose. This type of research error can lead to incorrect conclusions concerning toxicity and incidence of side effects, relative safety and efficacy of the medication, and proper dosage. If too high a dose is given in error, a good drug may be abandoned, and if too low a dose is given in error, too high a dose may be recommended for the patient later when the drug is marketed. These situations have arisen a number of times and the errors were corrected only after serious yet unnecessary side effects occurred and the confidence of the physician in a good drug was shaken.

Errors Introduced by Patients

Whether subjects who participate in clinical trials are hospitalized patients or outpatients or healthy volunteers or employees of a pharmaceutical company, the principal investigator who tests the new drugs must carefully supervise them. First of all, he must make certain that the test drug is of high quality at the time the recipient takes it. The drug product must have been stored and preserved properly, not, for example, left in the sunlight or on a window ledge or beside a radiator in the office, the patient's home, or elsewhere.

The investigator must then be certain that the patient receives the correct amount of the medication at the times specified in the research protocol. In the hospital he can usually control this more easily, but with outpatients and volunteers he must often take the word of the test subjects. He can, with some medications, collect urine or blood samples and test for the concentration of drug present to confirm if the medication was taken.* But

---

*In one study, 56% of the children supposedly taking a 10-day course of penicillin were found to have no penicillin in the urine after the third day.[6] FDA is developing, and encouraging others to develop, analytical procedures that can be used to determine the amount of administered drug in the serum, urine, and other body fluids when assurance is necessary that the drug has been taken as prescribed.

a major source of error in clinical studies is failure of the subject to follow directions. He may not take the correct amount at the specified times for the specified duration of time, with proper periods without medication if indicated. He may not take foods and fluids as directed. He may take common household remedies that cause drug interactions. Any deviation from the protocol, no matter how slight, may invalidate a study.

Finally, the investigator must report accurately the effects of the test medication on the recipients. Sometimes, as for example with the prisoner volunteers, they tend to hide adverse effects when they are being paid to participate in clinical investigations, because they don't want to lose the income. And since reporting by patients on the efficacy of test medications is such a subjective procedure, this also can be a major source of error. Emotional factors can strongly influence the patient's judgment, especially with psychopharmacologic agents including psychotomimetics, autonomics, and various neuromuscular agents.

Other sources of error are submission of incomplete specimens, submission in contaminated containers, and improper storage until the specimens are given to the physician for analysis.

The above are just a few of the many errors that can be introduced by test subjects who do not follow the rules when taking investigational drugs. See also page 287 in Chapter 8.

RESEARCH AND DEVELOPMENT RULES

The foregoing sections of this chapter present typical examples of the types of undesirable situations which can arise during research and development with a new drug. It is essential that all personnel responsible for the development of new drug products observe the following rules:

1. Control the Test Drug. Make certain that the drug product used in animal and clinical testing is identical in every respect with (1) the product which will be submitted to FDA for approval and (2) the product that will be marketed. Both of these as well as the test drug, at all stages of research and devel-

opment, must be given by the same routes of administration, have the same chemical structure, crystal structure, particle size, and other characteristics, and the same high level of purity, potency, stability and quality.

Use only fresh drugs when testing in animals or man. Some unstable drugs may undergo degradation or molecular rearrangement if they are allowed to stand in the sunlight, or remain in solution in a warm place or at a destructive pH, or they are subjected to other physicochemical stresses.

Dosage regimens (level, frequency, timing, and duration) at various stages of testing must be comparable and the outer limits noted. Proper numbers and types of subjects must be suitably assigned to appropriate dosage levels. Age, weight, sex, and genetic origin must be suitably assigned in both animal and human studies. Also, concomitant diseases and drugs must be noted and the effects observed. In some studies, geriatric and pediatric as well as normal adult trials will be called for, in others only one or two of these groups will be studied. Both laboratory and human factors must be studiously controlled by proper design of every study.

2. Design Each Study Carefully. Design each study specifically for the therapeutic category of the drug being tested. The amount of clinical laboratory work required and the kind and amounts of data vary with the category. With a hypotensive agent, for example, it is desirable to record pulse rate, cardiac rhythm, hematocrit, plasma volume, and blood volume and pressure; to follow electrolyte balance, secretion of aldosterone, angiotensin, and renin; and to note sodium retention if any, potassium excretion if any, and fluid retention. Renal blood flow and urinary excretion are also useful observations. It may be desirable to make special studies, e.g., determine the effects of the drug on cerebral blood flow and circulation in patients with recent subarachnoid hemorrhage or with intracranial aneurysm, or identify the type of hypertension present. Is it, for example, caused by congenital renal cystic disease or pyelonephritis? Biopsies may be useful if unusual pigmentation of tissues is noted at some stage of testing. Human biopsy may be suggested by animal histopathology.

During the early stages of testing in both animals and man, activities and toxicities sometimes appear that can later be associated with previously undetected, very minute quantities of contaminants such as intermediates, undesired stereoisomers, or other derivatives of the new drug, but not with the new drug in purified form. Alterations in the form of the active ingredient during research and development, such as a shift from a disodium to a monosodium salt, or to an acid, or to an ester or some other derivative, can prevent accurate and valid correlations of data from being made. Any change in experimental design during a study can invalidate that study. Unless rigid control is exercised and a consistent research and development program maintained from the very beginning, the patient may eventually not receive the medication intended, and correct interpretations may not be derived.

3. Inform the Investigators. Make certain that all investigators in each clinical study follow a carefully developed protocol exactly and that they do not delegate their professional duties to nonprofessional personnel. Deviations from directions can invalidate a study and may lead to incorrect conclusions regarding the drug's efficacy and safety, and also to collection of useless data. Supply complete preclinical background information on the drug in an accurate, brief, clear format, and prepare protocols and case report forms with meticulous attention to detail *after* consultation with a competent statistician and with the data processors who will handle the forms. Carefully check with all investigators taking part in a given study to make certain that they fill out the reporting forms completely and carefully, and warn them against giving concomitant therapy that will interfere in any way with the test drug.

4. Inform the Patients. Give precise and specific instructions to the patients (tests subjects) who are to receive an investigational drug so that they are fully aware of all essential aspects of their participation. Make certain they take the medication exactly as directed and, if they are outpatients, that they preserve it under proper storage conditions so that it does not lose its potency or deteriorate during the clinical study. Conduct urinalyses and hematologic studies as necessary to identify the levels of drug present and to insure that the subject has taken the medication.

5. Monitor the Patients. Closely follow every patient to detect degree of efficacy and to observe immediately any adverse effects. Take every precaution to protect patients on investigational drugs and report all serious reactions promptly to the clinical monitor who has the responsibility to report in turn to FDA. Also make certain that the patients provide complete urine samples and otherwise follow the protocol meticulously. Make certain that personality quirks of the patient do not influence the validity of the data collected. Some patients may try to tell the investigator what they think he wants to hear, not what actually occurred.

6. Interpret the Data Correctly. Analyze the clinical data in conformity with the design of the experiment and with full awareness of the degree of specificity and sensitivity of the methods being used. The preciseness of the analytical methodology required varies with the type of data being sought. Check to make certain that the symptoms against which the drug was tested were present, that the protocol was carefully followed, that the patient population was homogeneous and properly representative, that only permitted concomitant therapy was used, that all observations and laboratory tests were made according to plan, and that if the study was double blind, the code was not broken until a final report was prepared. Limit conclusions to those that are supported by the data collected in the study. Separate opinion from fact and identify as such.

7. Distribute the Information. Develop all information possible about a new drug during both animal and clinical trials and promptly *make all data available* to all involved in the research program, including FDA.

8. Improve the Methodology. Constantly seek better and more comprehensive testing methods for evaluating efficacy and safety. We need more specific and more sensitive test systems and we need better descriptions of those now in use. We need to learn how to develop drugs with more specific actions without multiple activities which cause side effects. We need to learn how to predict that certain chemical structures will induce undesirable effects. We must learn to think in terms of total impact of a medication on various types of patients as we develop improved experimental methodologies.

But tools that are available are not always used or if used are not properly applied. In certain types of research, such as diuretic screening in the rat, a sequential probability ratio test has the advantage over nonsequential methods in that testing can be terminated at an acceptable level of significance as soon as enough data have been obtained. Both time and money are often saved in this manner. The same principles can be applied to certain types of clinical studies. We must remain flexible enough to incorporate new procedures into testing programs and new types of tests when indicated. Autoimmune disease, genetically controlled enzyme deficiencies, enzyme induction and inhibition, the structure of drug-receptor complexes, biological availability, distribution patterns of drugs in man, and other pharmacodynamic, pharmacogenetic, and pharmacokinetic considerations urgently require study.

In the final analysis, therapeutic safety, as measured by the spread between the effective dose and the dose at which serious toxic effects begin to appear, must be related to other factors. Thus, a drug which is effective in life-threatening situations may be approved if it is the only treatment available, even if it is dangerous to use. But since it is a hazardous drug its labeling must carry specific and prominent warnings. A few examples of drugs which are required by FDA to have prominent warnings in the package inserts are: carbamazepine, chloramphenicol, chlorpropamide, ethchlorvynol, estrogens, ethotoin, long-acting sulfonamides, methamphetamine, methoxyflurane, paramethadione, pargyline, sodium dextrothyroxine, and succinylcholine chloride injection. There are many others, even including tetracycline, one of the most frequently prescribed drugs in the United States.

Obviously, pharmaceutical research and development requires the application of medical and scientific knowledge in considerable depth if hazards to the patient are to be avoided. As one director of clinical research noted:

New drug investigation, in short, can only be carried out successfully and safely, when one has sufficient knowledge of clinical pharmacology, drug metabolism, biostatistics, and also some understanding of biopharmaceutics and pharmacokinetics.[57]

Modell once succinctly summarized the hazards inherent in new drugs in the following words:

Here, then, is the pattern for disaster with new drugs: a short-sighted view of all effects; faulty experiments; premature publication; too-vigorous promotion; exaggerated claims; and careless use—in brief, a break in the scientific approach somewhere along the line.[59]

Complex interdisciplinary teamwork, extending over a period of seven years on an average, is usually necessary before enough research and development data can be generated to justify the manufacture of a new medication.

SELECTED REFERENCES

1. Alabama Medical Society: Report on drug testing in state prisons. *Drug Res Rep* 12:S34–S45 (Aug 6) 1969.
2. Ashby WB, Humphreys J, Smith SJ: Small bowel ulceration induced by potassium chloride. *Br Med J.* 5475:1409–1412 (Dec 11) 1965; *Br Med J* 5477:1546 (Dec 25) 1965.
3. Barron BA, Bukantz SC: The evaluation of new drugs. *Ann Intern Med* 119:547–556 (June) 1967.
4. Beecher HK: Increased stress and effectiveness of placebos and "active" drugs. *Science* 132:91, 1960.
5. Berg EH, Schuster F, Segal GA: Thiazides with potassium producing intestinal stenosis. *Arch Surg* 91:998–1001 (Dec) 1965.
6. Bergman AB, Werner RJ: Failure of children to receive penicillin by mouth. *N Eng J Med* 268:1334 (June 13) 1963.
7. Billig DM, and Jordan GL: Nonspecific ulcers of the small intestine. *Am J Surg* 110:745–749 (Nov) 1965.
8. Bismuth H, Samain H, Martin E: Les sténoses ulcéreuses du grêle après absorption de comprimés de potassium. *Presse Med* 74:1801–1804 (July 23) 1966.
9. Blank H: Clinical trials, A scientific discipline. *J Invest Derm* 31:235–240 (Oct) 1961.
10. Calvery HO, Klumpp TG: The toxicity for human beings of diethylene glycol with sulfanilamide. *South Med J* 1105–1109 (Nov) 1939.
11. Campbell JR, Knapp RW: Small bowel ulceration associated with thiazide therapy: review of 13 cases. *Ann Surg* 163:291–296 (Feb) 1966.
12. Clinical testing (synopsis of the new drug regulations). *FDA Papers* 1:21–25 (Mar) 1967.
13. Coulston F: Concepts and problems of modern toxicology. Presented to Fifth Annual Meeting, Drug Information Association, Detroit, Mich., (May 26) 1969.
14. Geiling EMK, Cannon PR: Pathologic effects of elixir of sulfanilamide (diethylene glycol) poisoning. *JAMA* 111:919–926 (Sep 3) 1938.
15. Giambalvo JF: Common clinical errors as seen by the FDA. *Drug Infor Bul* 2:4–7 (Jan/Mar) 1968.
16. Goldenthal EI: Current views on safety evaluation of drugs. *FDA Papers* 2:13–18 (May) 1968.

17. Hitchings GH: A quarter century of chemotherapy. *JAMA* A209:1339-1340 (Sep 1) 1969.
18. Janku I: Statistical models of chronic toxicity. *Sensitization to Drugs.* pp 146-151, Amsterdam, Exerpta Medica, 1969.
19. Laurence DR, Bacharach AL: *Evaluation of Drug Activities: Pharmacometrics,* vol 1 and 2. London, Academic Press, 1964.
20. Lawrason FD, Alpert E, Mohr FL, McMahon FG: Ulcerative obstructive lesions of the small intestine. *JAMA* 191:641-644 (Feb 22) 1965.
21. Lechat P, Levy J: Monaminooxidase inhibition by a bacteriostat, furazolidone. *Sensitization to Drugs.* pp 51-56, Amsterdam, Exerpta Medica, 1969.
22. Lenz W: Malformations caused by drugs in pregnancy. *Am J Dis Child* 112:99-106 (Aug) 1966; Thalidomide and congenital abnormalities. *Lancet* 1: 45, 1962.
23. Lenz W, Knapp K: Thalidomide embryopathy. *Arch Environ Health* 5:100-105 (Aug) 1962.
24. Martin EW: *Techniques of Medication.* Philadelphia, Lippincott, 1969; *Dispensing of Medication,* Easton, Pa. Mack Publishing, 1971.
25. McBride WG: Thalidomide and congenital abnormalities. *Lancet* 2:1358 (Dec 16) 1961.
26. Taussig HB: The evils of camouflage as illustrated by thalidomide. *N Eng J Med* 269:92-4 (July 11) 1963; *Medical News-Tribune.* p 9 (Nov 7), 1969; p 2 (Feb 13), 1970.
27. Mellin GW, Katzenstein M: The saga of thalidomide. *N Eng J Med* 267:1184-1193, 1238-1244, 1962.
28. Modell W, Houde RW: Factors influencing clinical evaluation of drugs, with special reference to the double blind technique. *JAMA* 167:2190, 1958.
29. National Academy of Sciences: *Drug Efficacy Study.* Final report to the Commissioner of Foods and Drugs from the Division of Medical Sciences, National Research Council, Washington, DC, 1969.
30. New York Academy of Sciences: New dimensions in legal and ethical concepts for human research. *Ann NY Acad Sci* 169:293-593, 1970.
31. Pomerantz MA, Swenson WM, Economou SG: Jejunal obstruction secondary to enteric-coated potassium chloride therapy. *J Am Geriatr Soc* 14:200-204 (Mar) 1966.
32. Reinus FZ, Weinberger HA, Fischer WW: Medication-induced ulceration of the small bowel. *Am J Surg* 112:97-101 (July) 1966.
33. Roberts HJ: Potassium chloride and intestinal ulceration. *JAMA* 178:965 (Dec 2) 1961; *Am J Gastroenterol* 37:157, 1962; *Lancet* 2:1127 (Nov 27) 1965.
34. Salmon W: *Bate's Dispensatory.* 4 ed., London, W. Innys, 1713.
35. Siegler PE, Moyer JH: *Pharmacologic Techniques in Drug Evaluation.* Chicago, Year Book, 1967.
36. Severinghaus EL: From animals to man *in* Waife SO, Shapiro AP (eds): *The Clinical Evaluation of New Drugs.* New York, Hoeber, 1959.
37. Smith A, Herrick AD: *Drug Research and Development.* New York, Revere Publishing, 1948.
38. Taussig HB: A study of the German outbreak of phocomelia. *JAMA* 180: 1106-1114 (June 30) 1962.
39. Truelove SC: Therapeutic trials in *Medical Surveys and Clinical Trials* (ed: Witts LJ). London, Oxford University Press, 1959.
40. Turner RA: *Screening Methods in Pharmacology.* New York, Academic Press, 1965.
41. U.S. Food and Drug Administration: *FDA Papers,* Jan, 1967 to date.
42. Waife SO, Shapiro AP: *Clinical Evaluation of New Drugs.* New York, Hoeber, 1959.
43. Weatherby JH, Williams GZ: Studies on the toxicity of diethylene glycol, elixir of sulfanilamide-Massengill and synthetic elixir. *J Am Pharm Assoc* 28:12-17 (Jan) 1939.
44. Williams RT: Drug metabolism in man as compared with laboratory animals. *Some Factors Affecting Drug Toxicity.* Amsterdam, Exerpta Medica, 1964.
45. Witts LJ: *Medical Surveys and Clinical Trials.* London, Oxford University Press, 1959.
46. Zbinden G: Drug safety: experimental programs. *Science* 164:643-647 (May 9) 1969.
47. Thorotrast. *Clin-Alert* Nos. 54 and 77, 1963; 59 and 81, 1964; 257, 1965; 160 and 188, 1966; 58, 1967; 146 and 173, 1968.
48. Alstead S, MacArthur JG: *Clinical Pharmacology.* London, Baillière, Tindall & Cassell, 1959.
49. Beecher HK: *Measurement of Subjective Responses.* New York, Oxford University Press, 1959.
50. Gwinn RP, Lees B: *Clinical Investigation for Medical Practitioners.* Lake Bluff, Illinois, Lees Associates, Inc., 1965.
51. Herrick AD, Cattell, M: *Clinical Testing of New Drugs.* New York, Revere Publishing, 1965.
52. Mantegazza P, Piccinini F: *Methods in Drug Evaluation.* Amsterdam, North-Holland Publishing, 1966.
53. Root WS, Hofmann FD: *Physiological Pharmacology.* New York, Academic Press, 1967.
54. Melmon KL, Grossman M, Morris RC: Emerging assets and liabilities of a committee on human welfare and experimentation. *N Eng J Med* 282:427-431 (Feb 19) 1970.
55. Griggs RC, Engel WK, Resnick JS: Acetazolamide treatment of hypokalemic periodic weakness. *Ann Int Med* 73:39-48 (July) 1970.
56. Jick H, Slone D, Shapiro S, Lewis GP: Clinical effects of hypnotics. *JAMA* 209:2013-2015 (Sep 29) 1969.
57. Sanen FJ: General concepts of new drug investigation. *Clin Toxicol* 2:159-164 (June) 1969.
58. Love FM, Jungherr E: Occupational infection with B virus of monkeys. *JAMA* 179:804-806 (Mar 10) 1962.
59. Modell W: Hazards of new drugs. *Science* 139:1180-1185 (Mar) 1963.
60. Koppanyi T *et al:* Species differences and the clinical trial of new drugs: a review. *Clin Pharmacol Ther* 7:250-270 (Mar-Apr) 1966.
61. Anello C: FDA principles on clinical investigations. *FDA Papers* 4:14-15, 23-24 (June) 1970.
62. Finkel, MJ: Investigational and new drugs. What does the FDA expect? Paper presented before the University of Wisconsin IND-NDA Conference, Milwaukee, Wisconsin, Oct 4-7, 1970.
63. Kumkumian CS: The abbreviated new drug application. Paper presented before the University of Wisconsin IND-NDA Conference, Milwaukee, Wisconsin, Oct 4-7, 1970.
64. Perlman PL: Transfer of animal pharmacology and

toxicology data to man. *Drug Info Bull* 4:7-9 (Jan-June) 1970.

65. Hucker HB: Species difference in drug metabolism. *Ann Rev Pharmacol* 10:99-118, 1970.

66. Bivin WS, Bryan JR, Chang J *et al: An Outline of Diseases of Laboratory Animals.* Columbia, Mo. Richard B. Westcott, 1969.

67. *Fed. Reg.* 35:18679 (Dec. 9) 1970.

68. *Fed. Reg.* 32:3270-3282 (Feb. 24) 1967.

69. DHEW/NIH: *Guide for the Care and Use of Laboratory Animals.* Pub No. 77-23, Washington, D.C., 1977.

70. Thorium dioxide: granuloma. *Clin. Alert* No. 158 (June 30) 1970; No. 252 (Oct 21) 1970.

71. Lockhart JD: The information gap in pediatric drug therapy. *FDA Papers* 5:6-9 (Feb) 1971.

72. Boylen JB, Horne HH, Johnson WJ: Teratogenic effects of thalidomide and related substances. *Lancet* 1:552 (Mar 9) 1963.

73. Kaplan M: Suicide by oral ingestion of a potassium preparation. *Ann Intern Med* 71:363-4 (Aug) 1969.

74. Mann NS, Changhry A, *et al*: Hepatoma induced by thorium dioxide. *South Med J* 69: 510-512 (Apr) 1976.

75. Weiss SM *et al:* Gut lesions due to slow—release tablets. *N Engl J Med* 296:111-112 (Jan 13) 1977.

76. AMA: *Nostrums and Quackery,* Vol I (1911) and vol II (1922).

77. Cornelius CE: Animal models—a neglected medical resource. *N Engl J Med* 281:934-44 (Oct 23) 1969.

78. FDA/HEW: *General Considerations for the Clinical Evaluation of Drugs.* US Government Printing Office, Washington, DC 20402, September, 1977.

79. Pharmaceutical Manufacturers Association. *Guidelines for Drug Sponsors in Monitoring Clinical Investigations.* Washington, DC, 1976.

80. FDA/HEW: Implementation of the Medical Device Amendments of 1976. *Fed Reg* 41:22620-1 (June 4) 1976.

81. Gyarfas WJ, Welch A: The IND procedure: assuring safe and effective drugs. *FDA Papers* 3:27-31 (Sep) 1969.

82. Lisook AB: The monitoring of scientific investigation. Presented at the PMA Drug Safety Subsection Meeting, Washington, DC, Mar 12, 1971.

83. Lisook AB: Responsibilities of clinical investigators—FDA viewpoint. Presented at a Symposium on Clinical Pharmacological Methods, Tulane University Medical Center, New Orleans, LA, Mar 24, 1973.

84. Kelsey FO: Peer review in human research: Federal regulations. Bureau of Drugs, FDA, HEW, Nov 5, 1975.

85. Lisook AB: Monitoring of clinical investigations. Presented at 16th Annual International Industrial Pharmacy Conference, Austin, Texas, Feb 23, 1977.

86. Kelsey FO: Biomedical monitoring. *J Clin Pharmacol* 18:3-9 (Jan) 1978.

87. Kelsey FO: Biomedical monitoring by the Food and Drug Administration. New Drug Evaluation, Bureau of Drugs, FDA, Rockville, MD, 1977.

88. The National Commission for the Protection of Human Subjects of Biomedical and Behavioral Research: *Research Involving Prisoners.* DHEW Publication No (OS) 76-131, Bethesda, MD, 1976.

89. The National Commission for the Protection of Human Subjects of Biomedical and Behavioral Research: *Disclosure of Research Information under the Freedom of Information Act.* DHEW Publication No (OS) 77-0003. Bethesda, MD, 1977.

90. Cardon PV, Dommel FW, Trumble RR: Injuries to research subjects. *N Engl J Med* 295:650-4 (Sep 16) 1976.

91. Kelsey FO: Nature, scope and purpose of FDA Bioresearch Monitoring Guidelines. Presented at PMA/FDA Workshop, Arlington, VA, November 22, 1977.

92. Editorial: Postscript to thalidomide. *Lancet* 1:560 (Mar 8) 1975.

93. WHO: Technical Report Series No 403: Principles for the clinical evaluation of drugs, Geneva, 1968.

94. Wheeler LA, *et al:* A general method for optimum drug dose computation. *J Pharmacokinet Biopharm* 4:487-97 (Dec) 1976.

95. Peto R, Pike MC, Armitage P, *et al:* Design and analysis of randomized clinical trials requiring prolonged observation of each patient. I. Introduction and design. *Br J Cancer* 34:585-612, 1976; II. Analysis and examples. *Idem* 35:1-39, 1977.

96. Azarnoff DL, Blackwell B, Goldberg LI, *et al:* Phase I, II, III, and IV investigations—a series of papers. *Clin Pharmacol Ther* 18:629-720 (Nov) 1975.

97. Editorial: FDA readying rules that could virtually end drug testing on prisoners. *PMA Newsletter* 20:1 (Jan 9) 1978.

Every drug product should conform to high standards of identity, potency, purity, and quality.

4 Manufacturing Factors

Every physician and pharmacist has the responsibility to become familiar with the scores of drug manufacturing factors that influence biological availability and therapeutic equivalency of the medications he prescribes or dispenses. Most of these factors are usually considered whenever specifications or standards are being established for dosage forms, but not always. Every prescriber and dispenser of drug products should be fully aware that chemically identical medications may vary considerably in potency, purity and quality in spite of official tests and standards, and enforcement programs of regulatory agencies like FDA.

The first Federal attempt to control drug quality in the United States was enactment of the Import Drugs Act of 1848. Periodically since that date, increasingly more stringent laws have been enacted and implementing regulations promulgated to protect the patient.[1] Almost seven decades before that first drug law was enacted, Schieffelin and Company, the first U.S. pharmaceutical manufacturer, was founded. The pharmaceutical industry then began its long, slow growth, and gradually began to develop drug standards and to introduce the scientific approach. But drug products marketed during the first 150 years of the industry's existence, extending into the 1930's, were largely galenicals extracted from plants and they presented relatively few hazards for the patient. During those early decades most problems arose through adulteration, misbranding, nostrums, and quackery. The first two of these corruptions were corrected through enactment of the Federal Pure Food and Drug Act of 1906 and the last two largely by the efforts of the American Medical Association through educational publications, including its publications of 1911 and 1921, *Nostrums and Quackery.*

Although the age of chemotherapy was introduced in 1909 by Ehrlich with his arsphenamine (Ehrlich 606), compared with recent progress the advances in this field were very slow for nearly three decades. Then, during the 1930s, the scientific approach to drug research began to reap rich rewards. By the late 1950s, after roughly two decades of explosive growth, the volume of prescription drug products had increased tenfold. Prescribing physicians were flooded with as many as 357* new prescription drugs every year. Powerful sales techniques tremendously increased the volume of drugs prescribed. The medications provided, however, were becoming not only more active and beneficial, but also much more hazardous than the herbs and milder medications used earlier. A tragedy with the first of the so-called miracle drugs, sulfanilamide (see page 26), quickly led to the adoption of the Federal Food, Drug, and Cosmetic Act of 1938 which emphasized premarketing safety of drugs, based on scientifically designed animal and clinical studies.

Many valuable categories of medications were successively developed and marketed: antihistamines, antibiotics, corticosteroids, tranquilizers, etc. The pace was rapidly accelerating and was becoming more and more hectic when a few ambitious journalists in publications like the *Saturday Review* began to cast suspicion on the pharmaceutical in-

---

*Peak year was 1955.

dustry, its motivations, and its economics. Like all criticisms, once launched, they became very damaging. Before long, academicians, consumer groups, former employees of both industry and FDA, and politicians quickly joined in attacking a vitally important segment of the American health care team. Although the American pharmaceutical industry leads the world in making contributions to human welfare, nevertheless, because it had grown so rapidly and because the remarkable advances in drug therapy presented new and serious hazards, better controls were needed.[15]

Critics of the drug industry could readily point to (1) inadequacies of preclinical animal research, (2) poor quality of clinical research, (3) inadequate reporting of adverse drug reactions, (4) unfortunate regulatory posture of FDA that legally could only be concerned with adulteration, misbranding, and safety of medications but not efficacy as such, (5) miscellaneous economic, political, and social faults of the drug manufacturing and distribution system. Eventually requests for more legislation were heard and were acted upon rapidly when the thalidomide tragedies (see page 27) were revealed.

The 1962 Kefauver-Harris Amendments to the Federal Food, Drug, and Cosmetic Act gave the FDA broad powers to develop numerous comprehensive and very stringent regulations over practically every aspect of drug research, development, production, quality control, distribution, and use. In fact, the legal network of resulting regulations has become so finely meshed and so tightly drawn that only a very few of the many new drugs emerging from the pharmaceutical research laboratories can now survive the rigid requirements for efficacy and safety to qualify for FDA approval for marketing. Such requirements necessitate years of extensive toxicological and clinical study before final evaluation can be made. Useful drugs may be kept off the market when government drug authorities, acting according to the letter of the law, make particularly severe judgments on New Drug Applications. Nevertheless, by the same token, the probability that a dangerous and undesirable drug will be approved for general use has greatly diminished.

The patient now receives better protection from hazardous medication than at any time in history.* However, the food and drug laws still have not solved a number of urgent problems.[15] We still need (1) better preclinical and clinical drug research, (2) more clinical pharmacology in the medical school curriculum, (3) effective continuing education and greater motivation on the part of the practicing physician to keep abreast of the latest developments and theory in the field of medication, (4) better dissemination of precautionary information about medications, (5) quicker elimination of substandard drugs and drug manufacturers, (6) better appreciation of proper techniques of medication, (7) deeper understanding of the mechanisms underlying patient response, especially inborn errors of metabolism and drug interactions, and (8) elimination of emotion and self-interest as much as possible from controversies among government, industry, and the medical profession so that sound economic, political, professional, and social decisions affecting the patient may be made. Scientific accuracy is fundamental, but these other considerations also may deeply affect the patient and at times may be as important to him as drug standards.

DRUG STANDARDS

Numerous drug standards and specifications which guide the pharmaceutical manufacturer are official, that is, published in the official compendia, the *United States Pharmacopeia* (USP) and the *National Formulary* (NF). Although both of these books are privately owned (the USP first appeared in 1820, the NF in 1888), they were given official status by the Congress of the United States of America under the Pure Food and Drug Act of 1906. Thus, under Federal law all drugs and drug products recognized in these volumes must conform to the *official specifications* (minimum requirements) contained therein for identity, purity, potency and quality. These compendia, which were formerly revised every 10 years and are now revised every 5 years (supplements are issued oftener), contain the most reliable tests and

---

*Significant dates in food and drug law history have been presented chronologically by Taber in *Proving New Drugs* (Geron-X, Inc., Los Altos, CA, 1969).

assays and incorporate the most modern techniques of laboratory evaluation of drugs. In 1975 the United States Pharmacopeial Convention acquired the *National Formulatory* and both the USP and NF were consolidated within the Convention. The goals and philosophy of both volumes had become identical and their contents overlapped considerably.

Some general drug test procedures are not officially recognized in the USP or NF. But drug products which do not appear in the official compendia must still meet rigid specifications established by reputable manufacturers in agreement with FDA.* This agency, in 1963 promulgated updated regulations on *Drugs Current Good Manufacturing Practice in Manufacturing, Processing, Packing, or Holding* and revised these in 1971 and 1977. This was done under authority provided by the 1962 Amendments of the Food, Drug, and Cosmetic Act. FDA periodically inspects† domestic and foreign plants that produce drug products for distribution in the U.S.A. to make certain that each firm meets acceptable standards. Inspectors occasionally uncover manufacturing flaws in compounding, packaging, and labeling. Such flaws can create serious hazards for patients who may receive the wrong medication, the wrong strength, or the wrong dosage form. *Dosage integrity* and *zero critical defects* are now legal demands. Companies without effective, elaborate control procedures may receive unfavorable publicity, be forced to make costly product recalls, and perhaps be closed if FDA inspectors repeatedly discover substandard medications and procedures.‡ Corporate officers and employees may even be criminally charged and convicted regardless of intent. [3,7]

During fiscal year 1977, 350 drug products were recalled from the market, including 268 prescription and 82 OTC drugs. This was a considerable drop from the 927 drug product recalls for 1970. [19]

Some drugs are certified directly by government agencies. For example, antibiotics cannot be legally marketed until certified by FDA after identity, purity, and potency testing by its scientists, and biological products such as vaccines cannot be released for sale until they pass rigid testing by FDA's Bureau of Biologics.

A great deal of confidence has been placed in the standards of the USP and NF since they were first published. They have long insured that a given drug or drug product, when prepared to meet those standards, has the same identity, potency, purity, and quality wherever it is purchased. Confidence in U.S. medications was achieved by this means for more than a century during a period when most of them were botanical in origin and few of them very potent by modern criteria. During the last few decades, however, many medications that have been synthesized are so highly potent and specific that increasingly more rigid controls have become necessary. While chemical and physical testing of drug products is very useful and essential, it has become increasingly more evident that other controls are of vital importance for the protection of the patient. [5,16]

Satisfaction of the USP requirements does not always afford the degree of assurance that one so traditionally associates with the presence of the USP imprint. Thus certain lots of ipecac satisfied compendium specifications for total alkaloid content, but lacked efficacy because the emetic alkaloids, emetine and cephaeline, were replaced in varying degrees with ephedrine. The Drug Efficacy Study panelists and other groups, have repeatedly pointed out that chemical and *in vitro* testing of drug products does not offer ade-

---

*For fiscal year 1978, the FDA budget totaled $282,908,000 of which about two-thirds was earmarked for regulatory activities concerned with human drugs. More than $143 billion of annual trade is in products covered by FDA. More than 110,000 establishments fall under FDA's regulatory jurisdiction; 11,810 of these are involved with drug products. For fiscal year 1979, President Carter proposed an FDA budget of $306 million and 7563 positions.

†Under FDA's Intensified Drug Inspection Program (IDIP), initiated in 1968, a team of four inspectors spent 3 months in each drug manufacturing plant selected for special surveillance because of major noncompliance with Good Manufacturing Practices.

‡In FY 1977, FDA analyzed 1463 batches of drug products, representing 3715 subsamples and 52,602 assays with the aid of automated equipment in its National Center for Drug Analysis in St. Louis, Mo. The Agency

also tested 417 batches of insulin (no rejects) and 20,550 batches of antibiotics (105 rejects) representing more than 250,000 assays in its National Center for Antibiotic Analysis. The categories of products tested vary with the current situation. Major emphasis is placed on the more widely used single active ingredient dosage forms of the more potent organic chemical prescription drugs.

quate evidence that they are clinically equivalent. Generic equivalence, therapeutically, can only be provided by means of suitable biological testing.[9]

Laboratory tests might satisfactorily be substituted for biological tests in man to assure that biological availability and therapeutic equivalence are achieved with specific manufacturing procedures. But, when *in vitro* evaluation or animal tests do not correlate well with pharmacodynamic effects in man, FDA may require clinical tests.[2]

Chemical equivalence does not guarantee therapeutic equivalence.[9] This fact is constantly kept in mind while drug products are being prepared by reputable manufacturers. This is so important that Chapter 2 discusses this in detail. Specific manufacturing factors that affect prescribing and patient response will now be considered.

Until the advent of chemotherapy in 1909 with the classic work of Ehrlich, most medications were given in large doses measured in teaspoonfuls and ounces. But since that time doses have become smaller with the increasing potency of synthetic drugs. Now, the therapeutic dose of some substances is so minute (a fraction of a microgram) that a thousand times that quantity is still invisible to the naked eye, and it must be distributed in many thousand times its weight of adjuncts when it is compounded into medications. Respirators must be worn when processing such drugs because a few fine particles inhaled in the air can be toxic.

But good manufacturing practice demands not only protection of production personnel but also protection of the patient. This requires strict attention to selection of ingredients, formulation, production, and quality control. In general, only aspects of these which have a bearing on the safety and efficacy of medications are discussed in the following sections.

Selection of Ingredients

Raw materials used to manufacture drug products must always be rigidly examined and tested for identity and quality even though they are purchased from a highly dependable supplier. No reputable manufacturer takes anything for granted. Furthermore, he must keep accurate, detailed records of every minute step involved in the production of a medication from the time the raw materials are delivered to the manufacturing plant until the finished product leaves it. Every act during ordering, receiving, testing, weighing, and blending of raw materials and preparing, packaging, and labeling of dosage forms is recorded on special forms with *identifying lot numbers* and the signatures of all key personnel involved.* All possible care is taken to make certain that the proper ingredients have been accurately incorporated into every drug product, and that they are identified so that the entire history of each item can be traced back in the event of some misadventure and any given lot of drug can be quickly recalled from the market if necessary.

Detailed information on the ingredients and the method of compounding of each product must be submitted to FDA as part of the New Drug Application, as well as any changes made thereafter.

FORMULATION FACTORS

Components of drug products consist of physiologically active ingredients compounded or formulated into various dosage forms with the aid of physiologically inactive adjuncts or additives. Variations in formulation procedures for a product modify the dosage required by the patient, the incidence and intensity of side effects, its stability, and its therapeutic efficacy.[4] Because the manner in which a drug product is formulated influences its utility so strongly, preformulation studies are tailored for each new drug. These are designed to determine the factors that influence the efficacy and stability of the active ingredients (e.g., solubility and solubilizing agents; the influence of traces of impurities;

---

*During 1968-69 a *National Drug Code Directory* was developed by FDA in collaboration with many interested groups. Every dosage form of every drug product is now assigned a number which is unique. Thus, for all computer applications from hospital records to Medicare billing, each package of a drug product is identified by lot number and drug code.[12] The first edition of the *National Drug Code Directory*, issued Oct. 15, 1969, contained codes for 12,000 prescription and over-the-counter products marketed by 171 labelers in more than 22,000 package types and dosage forms. The last edition (1976) contained about 53,000 drug product dosage forms marketed by about 2200 labelers. Copies of updated computer tapes of the NDCD are available from the National Technical Information Center, Springfield, VA 22151 and from the Government Printing Office, Washington, DC 20402.

important incompatabilities and degree of compatibility with adjuncts, closures and other packaging components, and processing equipment; and the product's stability characteristics under sterilizing, accelerated shelf life, and other conditions, including photodegradative effects).

A good illustration of how the physiological availability of a drug in a tablet can be greatly modified by only a small change in its formulation was published in 1968. When the amount of a clay binder, Veegum, in a tolbutamide tablet was altered from 50 mg., to 25 mg., the blood levels, degree of depression of blood glucose, disintegration time, and dissolution time were all unfavorably influenced to a marked degree.[13] The absorption rate was appreciably decreased by reducing the quantity of only one adjuvant which served as both binder and disintegrator.

The correct *quantity* of each of the ingredients selected must be homogeneously blended into a batch from which the final dosage is created. A multitude of formulation factors which influence the quality and activity of the completed medication must be carefully controlled during the blending and all other operations. The pertinent factors vary with the active ingredients, adjuncts, and coatings.

Active Ingredients

Active ingredients in drug products must have the proper chemical and physical characteristics.[8] The most suitable *salt* or *ester* or other *derivative* is selected to achieve the desired *solubility* and *stability* characteristics. Every drug product provides examples. Thus, tetracycline for oral use is generally present in capsules as the hydrochloride because that is a relatively stable and readily soluble salt suitable for rapid *intestinal absorption*. The steroid triamcinolone, on the other hand, is often present in ointments for application to the skin as a very slightly soluble derivative, such as the acetonide, when percutaneous absorption is to be minimized or avoided entirely. In intra-articular injections it is present as the highly insoluble diacetate or hexacetonide because prolonged action due to very slow absorption is desired and possible at the given site of injection. Some derivatives also are more stable than others, tend to

form more desirable *crystal structures,* or are more readily pulverized (micronized) to the optimum *particle size* to provide optimum *surface area.* Some drugs are more soluble in the *hydrated* rather than the anhydrous state; when molecules of water are bound with some drugs, they tend to enter the body fluids more readily. A similar situation occurs when they are *solvated,* i.e., when molecules of solvent combine with molecules of the drug. With other drugs the anhydrous or nonsolvated forms are preferable. Some drugs occur in several *polymorphic forms* or *stereoisomers,* one of which is usually the most active and perhaps least toxic.

The purity of the active ingredients is extremely important to the patient who takes the medication. Mere traces of impurities can sometimes cause dangerous sensitivity reactions. Penicillin reactions, for example, have sometimes been found to be due to impurities (degradation products, or protein or peptide from fermentation) in penicillin products, even though they may meet FDA standards. Some patients sensitive to such products are found to be no longer sensitive when the penicillin is more highly refined.[1,6] Other examples of microcontaminants that have been detected are histamine in tetracycline and streptomycin, metaxylidine in lidocaine, and levo-isomers in dextrorotatory drugs. There are literally hundreds of such possibilities.[17,18]

Adjuncts

Adjuncts (additives) sometimes act as *adjuvants,* that is, they improve the activity of a medication by enhancing its antigenic activity or by increasing or decreasing the rate of absorption of its active ingredient from the gastrointestinal tract into the bloodstream, its rate of spread into the tissues, its rate of renal excretion, or some other action. For example, buffering agents are said to increase the absorption of aspirin, hyaluronidase enhances the spread of drugs administered by hypodermoclysis, epinephrine prolongs the action of local anesthetics, probenecid prolongs the blood levels of aminosalicylic acid and penicillin by inhibiting their renal tubular excretion, and globin and protamine prolong the duration of action of insulin. Usually, several of the following types of adjuncts are used in formulating medications: binders, buffers, colors, diluents, disintegrators, flavors, lubricants, preservatives, surfactants, and suspending and emulsifying agents.[8] All must be compatible with the active ingredients.

Binders, sometimes called granulators, are blended with most tablet ingredients to cement them together lightly so that free-flowing *granules* of *proper hardness and size* can be formed. These granules must have characteristics which facilitate their flow into tablet machines and their compression by the tableting dies, after which the binders enable the tablets produced to retain their shape perfectly. If too much binder is used, the dies will form tablets that are too hard, therefore unable to disintegrate readily, and thus unable to release the active ingredient rapidly enough to be effective in the patient. In fact, very hard tablets can pass through the gastrointestinal tract and be excreted essentially intact. See also the effect of *Pharmacodynamic Mechanisms* in Chapter 8.

Buffers are substances that are added to drug products, especially liquids, to maintain a desired pH. So-called buffer systems consisting of acetates, borates, citrates, phosphates, phthalates, and other salts of weak acids mixed with suitable acids or alkalies establish a specific pH and tend to resist changes in that pH. The extent of their ability to resist such changes, known as their buffer capacity, depends on the type and concentration of buffer ingredients present.

The pH of a drug product often has a major influence on its stability, rate of absorption, palatability, and other characteristics. The biological availability of any given drug can therefore be enhanced or reduced, sometimes considerably, by shifts in the pH of its environment. At a pH other than one in the optimum range for that drug, chemical conversions and degradations (hydrolytic, stereochemical, etc.), precipitation as a less soluble product, and other reactions that decrease therapeutic efficacy for the patient may also occur.

The protective effect of proper pH is sometimes astonishing. For example, morphine in solution at a pH less than 5.5 is not affected by boiling for one hour, whereas if the pH is raised until the solution is neutral or even slightly alkaline, morphine is rapidly destroyed by the same treatment. Similarly co-

caine is stable at pH 2 to 5, procaine is stable in very dilute hydrochloric acid, and thiamine hydrochloride solutions below pH 5 can be sterilized in an autoclave. All of these substances, like morphine, are unstable at higher pH.

Some drugs are much more active at certain pH ranges than at others because some are more active in the ionized form while others are more active in the nonionized form. At low pH, for example, benzoic, mandelic, and salicyclic acids are most highly antimicrobial because they are most active in the nonionized form. Thus, 20 times as much sodium benzoate is required at pH 7 as at pH 2.3 to achieve the same preservative effect on liquid medications. The effects of pH on drug absorption and activity are considered in more detail in Chapter 8, *Patient Response.*

Colors, diluents (vehicles or excipients), and *flavors* are adjuncts that are added to medications mainly for purposes of identification, psychological effect on the patient, and dilution of active ingredient for convenience in prescribing. Colors that are appealing improve the *acceptability* of medications, create confidence in their potency, tend to overcome disagreeable tastes, and aid in identification. Diluents and flavors are closely related in their salutary effects on palatability. Actually, a single substance may serve several purposes, e.g., a given solvent may provide a pleasant color and flavor, act as a vehicle which dissolves the drug to form a liquid medication, and perhaps also exert some physiological effects. However, some drugs are finely divided and distributed (emulsified or suspended) in vehicles in which they are insoluble to form liquids or semisolids, e.g., emulsions, suspensions, creams, and ointments. And finally, solid medications often include diluents (excipients or fillers) which are physiologically inert powders that should not influence the patient's response adversely and may even improve efficacy by means of a physical or chemical action. It has been shown that solid fillers (excipients) which are very soluble aid in improving the dissolution and absorption of some medications. On the other hand, fillers or other adjuncts may form molecular complexes with drugs, thereby altering rates and patterns of absorption and distribution in the body, and sometimes substantially affecting the potency of medications.

Disintegrators are adjuncts included in tablets to cause them to break apart readily in the digestive tract and expose the active ingredients to the fluids in the gastrointestinal tract so that dissolution can take place readily. These substances (agar, alginic acid, bentonite, cellulose products such as carboxymethylcellulose and methylcellulose, cation exchange resins, citrus pulp, guar gum, sponge, starch, Veegum, etc.) have a great affinity for water. They swell when moistened and cause tablets to break apart promptly after administration. The speed of penetration of moisture into the tablet is sometimes increased by the addition of surfactants, such as Aerosol OT or MA and sodium lauryl sulfate. The rate of tablet *disintegration* is also considerably influenced by the type and amount of binder, the hardness of the tablet, and the kind of lubricant.*

Lubricants must be added to most tablet formulations to improve the tableting operation. First of all, substances such as boric acid, calcium stearate, lycopodium, magnesium stearate, starch, sugar and talcum function as glidants. They improve the flow of granulations from hoppers into tablet machines so that the punches and dies compress exactly the desired amount of material. Other substances such as cocoa butter, paraffin, soaps and stearic acid function as antiadhesives to prevent compressed tablets from sticking to the dies and punches which create the dosage form by pressure. Lubricants such as calcium and magnesium stearate and talcum reduce the friction between the particles of tablet material during compression and cause the tablet to slip out of the die easily during ejection.

Preservatives are antimicrobials, antioxidants, buffers and other stabilizing chemicals that are included in most formulations of drug products to prevent them from deteriorating as long as possible. *Antioxidants,* which are usually reducing agents, are added to medications to inhibit deterioration through oxidation. Examples are sodium bi-

sulfite, sodium formaldehyde sulfoxylate, and sodium metabisulfite. *Antimicrobials* are added to medications to inhibit the growth of microorganisms. They must be added to multiple-dose vials containing parenterals. Commonly used ones are benzalkonium chloride, benzethonium chloride, chlorobutanol, cresol, phenol, phenylmercuric nitrate, and thimerosal. For dermatomucosal and gastrointestinal preparations, the following are often used: alcohol, benzoic acid, glycerin, methylparaben, phenylmercuric nitrate, propylparaben, and sodium benzoate. *Buffers* are sometimes added to parenterals and other products to stabilize them against changes in pH that could damage the active ingredients (see page 212).

Each of the many types of preservatives available has its own specific applications and range of usefulness. Thus benzoic acid and its esters (*p*-hydroxybenzoates) are widely used as antimicrobials in many drug products. Ethylenediamine, on the other hand, is used in medicine primarily for one purpose, to stabilize aminophylline injection. Maleic acid is used to retard rancidity in fats and oils. Sodium bisulfite, an antioxidant, is used to stablize epinephrine solutions. Sodium formaldehyde sulfoxylate is used as an antioxidant in injections. Sulfur dioxide in solution becomes both a bactericide and fungicide and is used in some injections. Sodium metabisulfite is an antioxidant used to preserve aqueous solutions. The activity of some antioxidants is enhanced by sodium ethylenediaminetetraacetate which chelates metallic ions that catalyze oxidation reactions.

Unless the proper preservative is selected for each given formulation, the preservative itself can be inactivated rapidly in the presence of other ingredients. Thus, the antimicrobial parabens are inactivated by complex formulation with certain gums, surfactants (Tween 80, Myrj 52), and other adjuvants (gelatin, methylcellulose, polyethylene glycol, polyvinylpyrrolidone, etc.).

Antimicrobial preservatives may also be inactivated by contact with various container materials, e.g., rubber affects chlorobutanol and mercurial preservatives. Nylon and polyethylene sometimes decrease the potency of other preservatives, e.g., the nylon barrels formerly used in disposable syringes tended to bind certain phenols, methylparaben, pro-

---

*FDA continually promulgates new regulations to assure proper disintegration of uncoated, film-coated, or plain-coated tablets in gastric fluid and of enteric-coated tablets in intestinal fluid. The Agency works closely with the USP.

pylparaben, and sorbic acid. Inactivation of the preservatives makes a drug product more vulnerable to deterioration.

Also, undesirable effects of some preservatives on the drug products themselves are sometimes encountered. For example, parabens and phenols used as preservatives can cause suspensions of slightly soluble steroids to flocculate. Thus, if the physician dilutes a concentrated suspension of a corticosteroid to prepare an intra-articular injection with a diluent containing one of these widely used preservatives, he can make the parenteral product unsuitable, even hazardous for administration to his patient.

Surfactants (surface active agents) are blended into some drug products to improve disintegration of tablets or the spread and contact of medications (lotions, ointments, ophthalmic solutions, mouth washes, etc.) with body surfaces. But precautions must be taken because some of these agents can inactivate other drug product ingredients. Thus, Tween 20 binds the antiseptic chlorobutanol and Tween 80 binds several other important antimicrobials, e.g., benzalkonium chloride, cetylpyridinium chloride, methylparaben, methylrosaniline, phenolic preservatives, and propylparaben. Tween 80 also binds the ophthalmic anesthetic tetracaine and the mydriatic and cycloplegic dibutoline.

The characteristics of the colors, diluents, flavors and all other types of adjuncts can have a profound influence not only on the psychological aspects of medication but also on the physical, chemical and biological properties of the active ingredients. However, only adjuncts approved by FDA are permitted, and there are many prohibitions. For example, not even a certified dye may be used in any medication to be applied to the eye or the area immediately around it.

Suspending and emulsifying agents are adjuvants used to prepare suspensions and emulsions. Suspensions, consisting of very finely divided, undissolved drugs (suspensoids) dispersed in liquids, usually contain suspending agents (acacia, karaya, tragacanth, and sterculia gum; carboxymethylcellulose, hydroxyethylcellulose, methylcellulose, and other cellulose derivatives; agar, sodium alginate, chondrus, and pectin extracts; bentonite, Veegum, and other inorganic clays and silicates; and Carbopols,

polyoxyl stearates, and other synthetic organic polymers). These agents keep the drugs evenly dispersed and prevent the particles from clumping together and settling.

Emulsions, consisting of very fine droplets of an immisicible liquid (dispersed phase) evenly distributed throughout another liquid (continuous phase), contain emulsifying agents (*carbohydrates* like acacia, agar, carrageenin, honey, methylcellulose, pectin, sodium alginate, sodium carboxymethylcellulose, and sugar esters; *proteins* like casein, egg yolk, and gelatin; *soaps and alkalies* like ammonia and lime waters, castile and soft soaps, and triethanolamine; *alcohols* and *eters* like cetyl, oleyl, and stearyl alcohols, cholesterol and its esters, lecithin, and polyethylene glycol esters; *wetting agents* like dioctyl sodium sulfosuccinate, sodium lauryl sulfate, and sulfated oils; *finely dispersed solids* like certain clays, charcoal, and powdered silica; and *synthetic polymers* like Carbopol, a polymer of acrylic acid, sometimes crosslinked with allyl sucrose to form Carbomer.

For patient safety, both suspensions and emulsions must be stablized by decreasing particle size, increasing viscosity, and controlling concentrations and electrical charges to avoid agglomeration and to obtain uniformity of dosage. Homogenizers, blenders, mills, and various devices are used to decrease the particle size of the dispersed phase, and numerous natural and synthetic gums (hydrocolloids) like those listed above are used to increase viscosity. All adjunvants must be selected on the basis of route of administration, characteristics of other ingredients, dosage, and related factors. Manufacturers are severely limited in their selection of emulsifying and suspending agents for injections, for example, because of increased toxicity by the intravenous, intramuscular, or other parenteral routes. Color, odor, taste, tissue sensitivity, toxicity, and other factors must be carefully considered to provide acceptable and safe medications of the dispersed types.

Coatings

Coatings on dry dosage forms of medication such as capsules, tablets or pills must be added by means of very exacting procedures, some of which date back to the latter part of the ninth century in Europe and the middle of the nineteenth century (roughly one thousand years later) in the U.S.A. The *composition* of the coating, the *thickness, how it is applied* and other elements of the operation greatly influence rates of disintegration, dissolution and absorption in the patient.

Coatings have several important purposes. They mask unpleasant odors and tastes and sometimes provide pleasant flavors. They improve the appearance and thereby make the medications more acceptable to the patient. They protect the active ingredients against the carbon dioxide, moisture, oxygen and various other destructive substances in the atmosphere, including pollutants. They also protect the tender linings of the mouth and stomach against certain caustic, irritating compounds like hexylresorcinol and nauseating drugs like quinacrine and emetine, thus avoiding discomfort, nausea, and vomiting.

Special coatings are purposely applied for special effects. Thus they may cause dissolution and absorption to be rapid to achieve rapid patient response or cause them to be delayed to achieve either prolonged release of medication or protection of the active ingredients from the acid environment of the stomach which is destructive to some biologically active substances. Coatings that avoid disintegration in the stomach are known as enteric coatings since they encourage dissolution and absorption in the enteron, or intestinal tract. Many anthelmintics and intestinal antiseptics are prevented by this means from early dissolution and dilution and perhaps possible destruction before they reach the parasites and infecting microorganisms against which they are being used.

Some authorities have recommended elimination of enteric-coated tablets for all acid-stable substances that cause gastric irritation. Transferring the irritation further down the gut seems to be a poor pharmaceutical solution to the problem. See the disastrous results with enteric-coated potassium chloride tablets (page 26).

A series of coatings (laminations) are sometimes applied one after the other around a central core, each layer containing a different active ingredient so that a series of biological effects occur in the desired sequence. Sometimes the layers are separated by a special coating, perhaps enteric, which releases individual doses according to a predetermined time schedule and permits repeated action of the same medication or timed release of a succession of different medications. The laminations may be made thick or thin and rapidly or slowly soluble for rapid or prolonged action. Thus laminated tablets can be made so that they release medication in the mouth, stomach or intestine or a combination of these at any desired rate at the desired time and location.

Coatings are obviously vital to the patient with respect to dosage, timing, frequency, irritation and other considerations. In fact, not only the ingredients of coatings, but all other ingredients, including those that fall into the foregoing categories of adjuncts, are such important sources of potential adverse effects in the patient that they are subjected to intensive study and are required to be approved by FDA before they can be used in the production of any prescription medications.

PRODUCTION FACTORS

During production of each type of drug product many factors are strictly controlled to make the medication safe and effective for patients. Selection of dosage forms, manufacturing techniques, and quality controls are the major considerations.

Selection of Dosage Forms

The first important step in the preparation of a medication is selection of the form in which individual or multiple doses will be made available. This selection is governed first of all by the routes of its administration, i.e., topical (dermatomucosal), oral or rectal (gastrointestinal), or parenteral. Once the best routes have been established, the next question is whether a solid, semisolid, or liquid dosage form should be manufactured.

Whether a medication is prepared and prescribed as a liquid or solid is important to the patient. Both liquid and solid forms have their advantages and disadvantages. The most commonly used *solid* oral products are tablets and capsules. The most commonly used *liquid* oral products are syrups, elixirs, emulsions, and suspensions. Topical products are made available as liquids (creams, liniments, lotions, pigments, etc.), as semi-solids (ointments, pastes, etc.), or as solids (pencils, plasters, powders, etc.). Parenteral products may be solid (pellets) or liquid (emulsions, solutions, or suspensions). Medications for injection may be supplied in a liquid form, ready for use, in ampuls or vials, or the solid ingredients may be supplied as a sterile powder, ready for reconstitution (solution or suspension) with a suitable sterile liquid vehicle (often sterile distilled water for injection) supplied separately.

Capsules and tablets are convenient and economical to manufacture and distribute. When properly prepared, accuracy of dosage is assured. Because they are in a dry form, they are usually more stable than liquid products and therefore retain their potency longer, especially when stored in a cool, dry place protected from light. They are convenient for the patient to carry and to take. There is no danger of spillage in the purse, automobile, or home. With tablets and capsules, rate of release of medications can be controlled by means of special coatings, beads, cores, granules and layers so that prolonged action can be achieved and fewer doses are required. Thus medication can act throughout the entire period of sleep to control enuresis, epilepsy, infections, migraine, and other conditions without having to awaken the patient.

The major disadvantage of solid oral dosage forms is the multitude of factors that must be rigidly controlled to make certain that they will disintegrate rapidly at the proper location in the gastrointestinal tract, will dissolve readily in the fluids present in that tract, and will be absorbed at the desired rate into the bloodstream. Unless every variable is carefully controlled, wide variations in biological availability and clinical efficacy can occur. See Chapters 2 and 8.

Liquid dosage forms such as elixirs and syrups are not as convenient as capsules and tablets to manufacture and distribute. Breakage, leakage, awkwardness and weight create problems during distribution and storage. Therefore the cost per dose is much higher than with solid dosage forms. Liquids tend to be less stable than dry products because there is more opportunity for hydrolysis, isomerism, racemization, and other types of decomposition and undesirable conversions. Prolonged-action liquid medications are not readily prepared and controlled. The contents of liquids are sometimes undesirable, e.g., the sugar of syrups for diabetics and the alcohol of elixirs for abstainers and alcoholics. On the other hand, liquids do have some major and at times overriding advantages. Most important of all, the drug is already in solution or in a very finely divided state as an emulsion or suspension. There is, therefore, no necessity for disintegration to occur before the medication is made available for dissolution in the fluids of the digestive tract. Also liquids, especially pleasantly flavored syrups for pediatric use, are more convenient since it is much easier to give such a preparation rather than to crush a tablet and mix it extemporaneously with honey or some other product in the home in order to disguise a bitter taste and make it palatable.

Parenteral products with their own particular advantages and disadvantages and special problems and hazards are discussed in Chapter 8. In spite of the hazards and other disadvantages, however, parenteral medications provide the only convenient and promptly effective therapy for the patient who requires immediate response to a drug, perhaps for a life-threatening condition, or for one who cannot or will not take medications by any other route.

Manufacturing Techniques

The manner in which manufacturing processes and procedures are carried out, apart from formulation procedures covered previously, greatly influence the efficacy, safety, and quality of drug products. Potent drugs can be made completely ineffective when improperly compounded into dosage forms. On the other hand their activity can be considerably enhanced by various techniques to the point where toxic effects may appear with the usual dosage, and a lower dose can still produce suitable effects.

p-Aminosalicylic acid (PAS) tablets provide a good illustration of this. One manufacturer sold his brand of these for years with good results until he changed his manufacturing process slightly after he found that only 10% of the PAS was being made available to the patient. However, with the change such a high percentage was then released that toxic effects appeared and problems of acceptablility by both physician and patient arose. It was necessary to revert to the original formulation.[4] In a reverse situation, nitrofurantoin tablets complying in every respect with official standards and the approved New Drug Application caused complaints of nausea, vomiting and general intolerance until the rapid dissolution rate was slowed by changing the formulation.[5]

Another important factor is the selection of the most suitable chemical or physical form of the drug. Perhaps the activity of a drug resides primarily in only one polymorphic form or one stereoisomer or perhaps one of these must be avoided because it is exceptionally toxic. Both in testing and formulating a drug product, it is essential that a suitable form of the investigational drug be used by the clinician, one that is likely to be duplicated when the product is marketed.

Still another factor is compactness. Capsules which are packed tightly make their active ingredients several times less readily available than those which are packed less tightly. Similarly, tablets which are compressed too tightly by the punches and dies of tableting equipment may actually yield little or no medication to the patient. The shape of the dies, characteristics of the granules being compressed, the pressure applied, and other factors must all be rigidly controlled to produce medication which becomes available in the body to the same extent batch after batch. Tablets that are too hard and compact pass through the gastrointestinal tract and are eliminated in the feces undissolved.

Every minute step of each manufacturing procedure must be critically examined, and no step should be taken in producing a drug product unless that step and its results have been thoroughly studied and its impact on the medication thoroughly understood and appreciated. Thus the manner and order in which active ingredients are blended and adjuncts are incorporated, the way the manufacturing equipment is utilized, the accuracy with which humidity, pH, pressure, time, temperature, speed, and other factors are controlled, the manner in which layers and coatings are applied, and a host of other considerations enter into the manufacture of dependable medication that has uniformity of ingredients and equivalent therapeutic efficacy. Even very slight modifications of a process can cause major fluctuations in the efficacy of a drug product.[13] So-called identical products whether they are referred to as chemical equivalents, generic equivalents, or some other kind of equivalents can vary in therapeutic efficacy from batch to batch, sometimes even within the same manufacturing facility. Variations from one company to another represent an even more formidable problem.

Changes in formulation can be hazardous for patients.

QUALITY CONTROL

The pharmaceutical manufacturer is responsible for properly controlling all manufacturing factors and rigidly meeting all official specifications for his drug products so that they conform to established standards. He is bound by legislation to guard zealously against adulteration, cross contamination, decomposition, faulty packaging, label mixups, microbiological contamination, potency variations, and failure to meet all requirements published in the official compendia and official documents of the regulatory agencies. Above all, he must keep complete and flawless records. He cannot wait until he is alerted to poor practices by an FDA order to recall drug products already on the market. His equipment, personnel, facilities, procedures, and supporting services have to be adequate to safeguard the patient and assure the physician that he is prescribing safe and effective medication.

The quality of a medication, according to Elkas of Lederle Laboratories, is determined by the degree to which the following seven criteria exist:

1. *Identity* (correct ingredients, correctly labeled)
2. *Purity* (absence of contaminants)
3. *Potency* (correct quantities of active ingredients)
4. *Stability* (reliable shelf life)
5. *Uniformity* (consistent physical and chemical characteristics)
6. *Efficacy* (biological availability of active ingredients)
7. *Safety* (freedom from unexpected adverse effects)

High quality is built into a drug product by applying three powerful forces at all times: (1) *design for quality,* i.e., proper selection of formulas, methods of compounding, containers, and standards, (2) *conformance to quality*, i.e., meticulous attention to procedures at every stage of manufacture, and (3) *assurance of quality*, i.e., rigid auditing at each step for compliance with Standard Operating Instructions and adherence to Specifications. Apart from management, personnel, and adequate funding, motivation toward a conscientious attitude and optimum selection of equipment, materials, and methods are very important.

Use of suitable test methods for quality control purposes is essential. The Defense Personnel Support Center, which inspects drug contracts for the military and establishes its own high standards, found it necessary to require manufacturers to comply with specifications even additional to those found in official compendia. Upward revision of standards is a continuing process. [5, 16]

Expert committees of the World Health Organization are attempting to accelerate the worldwide dissemination of uniform international specifications for new drugs and drug products. WHO completed a code of good manufacturing practices during 1969 and late the same year recommended that a completely new system of international certification of medications be adopted so that specifications will become widely available at the time a medication is marketed. A delay of up to 10 years may be experienced if dependence is placed on publication of specifications in the *International Pharmacopoeia.* WHO is also augmenting its efforts to provide international chemical reference standards for specific drugs. In the United States, reference standards for 725 drugs (October, 1977) are supplied by the United States Pharmacopeia office at nominal cost to manufacturers and others for control purposes and standardization of assays.

The USP reference standards are prepared through the joint efforts of a large number of laboratories (about 250). The substances from which the Reference Standards are prepared are supplied from commercial sources, often as a contribution at little or no cost. The testing for these is apportioned among about 240 laboratories of the pharmaceutical industry so that none of them test very many standards that they do not provide. About 10 consulting laboratories participate in testing those Reference Standards that require biological assaying. The USP program also depends heavily upon FDA and the Drug Standards Laboratory which test every Reference Standard. The NF program has been combined with that of the USP.

A Pan-American Health Organization committee in July, 1969, succinctly stated the basic considerations when contemplating the establishment of a quality control laboratory for drug products: [10]

"If a drug is defective because it was poorly made, or because it deteriorated before it reached the patient, the doctor's efforts will be obstructed, and the patient may be injured by the drug. These are the public health considerations that underlie the need for drug quality control. . . . A drug testing laboratory will be fully effective only if it has a sufficient number of experienced chemists, bacteriologists, and pharmacologists trained in drug testing work; plus an adequate array of modern testing devices, suitable quarters, and the technical library with current reference texts and journals devoted to drug testing . . . obviously such a laboratory is costly to establish and costly to operate."

Each major pharmaceutical manufacturer spends millions of dollars annually on quality control. A few spend tens of millions. Because of meticulous attention to quality standards, these manufacturers are faced with very few recalls of their products by the FDA. Parke, Davis and Company, for instance, has never had a submitted batch of chloromycetin not certified by the agency.

The major manufacturers developed good manufacturing practices and sound quality control procedures long before they became mandatory under the law. In fact, the FDA largely adopted the practices and standards already in existence when it promulgated its regulations under the 1962 Amendments to the Food, Drug, and Cosmetic Act, and applied them to the more backward, less well equipped segment of the industry. The companies from this segment are the ones that appear time after time on the *FDA Report of Recalls,* undoubtedly because they have not met minimum quality control requirements.

Quality Control Requirements

The official compendia (USP and NF) establish purity and potency tolerances, including minimum potency, limits of foreign substances, ranges for content of active ingredients, official testing and assaying procedures, and limits for specific impurities. They also provide official requirements for uniformity of composition, added substances (adjuncts), identity tests including solubility characteristics, optical rotation, and pH. These and all other specifications for drug products must be related to the specific method of manufacture. And quality control must be rigidly exercised over even the starting chemicals used in syntheses, and then over every material and every step of the manufacturing process, including packaging and labeling. Official requirements for labeling, packaging, preservation, and storage are discussed in Chapter 5.

Control of Bioavailability

Testing for physiological availability is a recent innovation. Testing methods are being developed but the surface of this complex subject has only been scratched. Determinations that appear to be especially important are disintegration and dissolution rates, and blood levels. Attempts to correlate *in vivo* with *in vitro* data are still largely in the experimental stages.

In vitro disintegration and dissolution rates are not likely to be the same as the corresponding *in vivo* rates. But *in vitro* rates are probably a guide to the relative bioavailability of two chemically equivalent drug products. The best guide, however, appears to be blood level data, including peak concentrations of the drug, the rates at which they are reached, and the length of time minimum effective concentrations are maintained. Such data are not significant, of course, for drugs that must reach certain specific areas of the body such as the spinal fluid or a fetus. And, at the present time (1978), high dissolution rates do not necessarily indicate high therapeutic efficacy. Such correlations may be possible with certain types of drugs as more data become available.

FDA Biological Availability Requirements. Biological availability data are needed for all marketed prescription drug products (1) to show whether the various formulations of a given drug (prepared by the same or different manufacturers) are absorbed as well as the original product cleared by the FDA on the basis of clinical trials, (2) to provide baseline data which can serve as a basis for comparison in the event of changes in composition and manufacturing procedures, (3) to provide baseline data for comparing probable therapeutic efficacy of chemically identical medications and of various medications in the same therapeutic category, and (4) to provide the prescribing physician with a sounder basis than he now possesses for selecting medications for his patient.

The FDA set forth a preliminary list of general principles governing biological availability requirements on August 7, 1970, and distributed them to the entire professional staff of the Bureau of Drugs.[14]

1. If possible, *in vivo* tests of comparative absorption should be requested. As an *interim* measure, a simple protocol to show absorption only will be satisfactory. More complex protocols to measure comparability will be developed later.
2. If methodology for assaying the drug is available, a simple protocol to show evidence of a single standard dose of the drug will be designed . . . Consideration should be given to validating the method selected prior to final preparation of the protocol.
3. If methodology for *in vivo* studies is not available but *in vitro* methodology such as disintegration and dissolution tests are available from standard reference sources, such data should be required. Dissolution studies are preferable and should be requested where feasible.
4. If there is no method for assaying the drug in blood, urine or on an adequate physiological basis, the Office of Scientific Coordination* is responsible for initiating studies to develop a method in cooperation with Office of Pharmaceutical Research and Testing. Affected companies will also be requested to undertake such testing.
5. The Office of Scientific Coordination will develop programs to design more complex protocols for a more precise comparision of various products. The Office of Scientific Coordination will (in cooperation with OSE/OPR and DESI) establish the testing required at this time and appropriate guidelines for the firm. All inquiries concerning protocols or planned studies for bioavailability will be transmitted to OSC.

The FDA recognized that the above biological availability guidelines would require periodic updating as the definition of "biologic availability" is clarified, as the agency

---

*After reorganization of the Bureau of Drugs in 1974 the functions of this Office were redistributed and the title was dropped.

learns how to prove the biological equivalence of "identical" medications, and as improved testing for this kind of evaluation and quality control is devised by both the agency and the pharmaceutical industry.

Quality Control Department

Because of the complexity of maintaining consistently high drug product quality under mass production conditions, the manufacturer delegates responsibility for this function to a special group of scientists and technicians who form a Quality Control Department or Section.

A typical organization chart of a quality control department in a large pharmaceutical company is shown in Figure 4-1. A total of four major groups are shown with 12 subgroups and two administrative or staff groups. This chart indicates to some extent the complexity and extent of the quality control activities. The total staff usually numbers several hundred including clerical and secretarial support. The main functions are broadly delineated as follows:

Analytical Development—Develops qualitative and quantitative tests and assay methods for raw materials and finished products where official ones are not available and constantly tries to improve all tests and assays being used in order to achieve greater accuracy more rapidly at lower cost. This group applies automation and electronic equipment whenever possible.

Product Specifications—Establishes specifications for raw materials and finished products in compliance with Federal regulations, compendial requirements, and company standards.

Product Stability—Performs market package shelf-life stability studies of dosage forms under various storage conditions and determines appropriate storage requirements as well as compatibil-

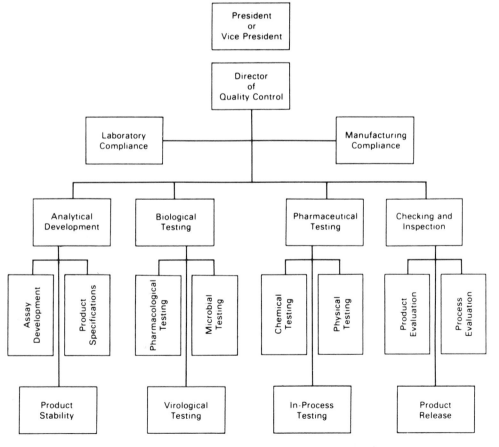

Fig. 4-1. A typical quality control organization chart for a major pharmaceutical manufacturer employing several hundred scientists and technicians in quality control.

ities and incompatibilities of active ingredients with proposed adjuncts and other drugs with which they may be mixed.

Biological Testing—Performs virological, microbial, and pharmacological tests and assays, including: clarity, pyrogen, safety, and sterility of parenterals and infusion and transfusion assemblies; identity, purity, potency, and safety of biological products; biological (animal) assaying of products which do not lend themselves to chemical assay; microbial assaying of antibiotics and several vitamins; and special official biological testing for antibacterial activity, antigenic value, bacterial content, bacteriological purity, biological adequacy (nutritional completeness), depressor substances, nonantigenicity, pressor substances, and toxicity of certain packaging components.

Pharmaceutical Testing—Performs physical and chemical tests and assays on finished drug products to establish identity, potency, purity, and quality. Also conducts in-process testing.

Chemical Testing—Performs physical and chemical tests and assays on raw materials to establish identity, purity, potency, and quality.

Checking and Inspection—Carefully trained inspectors periodically remove samples of drug products from the production lines and subject them to intensive scrutiny and analysis to make certain there are no flaws and that the composition falls within the limits of the established specifications. Representative samples are physically, chemically, and biologically analyzed by standard methods to make certain that every lot of product meets all Quality Control Requirements (page 70).

CURRENT GOOD MANUFACTURING PRACTICES

In 1963, to assure drug product quality, FDA promulgated regulations pertaining to the manufacture, processing, packing, and holding of finished pharmaceutical drugs. These regulations, known as Current Good Manufacturing Practices (CGMP), represented official establishment of the basic features of the drug industry's prevailing "good manufacturing practices" and quality controls. To clarify and strengthen such criteria further and make them more specific, these manufacturing practice regulations were, pursuant to provisions of the Federal Food, Drug, and Cosmetic Act, amended in 1971.

In 1976, the Commissioner of Food and Drugs proposed, in the *Federal Register* of February 13, 1976, to revise the CGMP regulations,[11] to update them in light of current technology, and to adopt more specific re-

quirements better to assure the quality of finished drug products. The revised regulations were published in the *Federal Register* early in the summer of 1978. Copies may be obtained from the Associate Director for Compliance, Bureau of Drugs, Food and Drug Administration, 5600 Fishers Lane, Rockville, MD 20857.

These guidelines are designed to eliminate the hodgepodge of quality control that may be one important reason for variations among supposedly identical medications. A standard system of quality control for drug products has gradually been developed and the quality of American medications is now guarded by essentially one agency, FDA. It even assumed responsibility in 1975 for testing and approving medications for the armed services.

Fortunately and reassuringly, the variation in medications based on official testing is generally small. The typical results shown in Table 4-1 were obtained with 8 categories of drugs (10,000 drug products) collected from hospital and community pharmacies and tested by the FDA. These results are based on chemical and physical tests, however. There are as yet no official, widely accepted standardized tests for therapeutic equivalency of medications. Only relatively few comparative data on tissue and body fluid drug levels, on excretion profiles, and on other pertinent aspects of the clinical equivalency of chemically identical medications are available. The physician who prescribes a medication cannot rely completely on the labeling as an indication of efficacy. He is more likely, under current circumstances, to rely on his own clinical experience and judgment.

Unless suitably educated and properly trained personnel use adequate equipment,

Table 4-1 Typical Results of FDA Testing in 1969[20]

Drug Class	No. of Samples	% Out of Limits
Anticonvulsants	726	0.6
Cardiac antiarrhythmics	917	0.3
Ergot alkaloids	175	5.1
Nitroglycerin	1,343	3.4
Nonsteroid estrogens	679	0.9
Reserpine	968	3.6
Skeletal muscle relaxants	171	0.0
Thiazide diuretics	1,137	1.1

facilities, and procedures to prepare drug products correctly, the patient may not receive dependable and safe medication. If the physician understands this he is careful to specify a definite make of medication for his patient and because the pharmacist knows this he selects a well established and reputable brand when he fills a prescription for his own sick child. Both want to provide drug products which have been prepared by a manufacturer who maintains the most rigid conditions of quality control. They must assume responsibility for protecting the patient who usually cannot judge the quality of medications.

The HEW Task Force on Prescription Drugs has stated, "Only the reputable, professionally and technically proficient manufacturer—large or small—can provide adequate assurance that one lot of therapeutic drug product is as safe and effective as another of the same composition and dosage form."

Of course, the manufacturer cannot completely control how a drug product is handled once it enters distribution channels (see Chapter 5), and the physician must have faith that the drug product he prescribes has been properly protected during distribution and storage at all times. Nevertheless, he does have the responsibility to reassure himself that adequate quality control has been exercised over the drugs he orders. He may accomplish this not only by prescribing by highly regarded brand names of reputable manufacturers, but also by visiting the plants that manufacture the drugs he prescribes. He should also be able to depend on his pharmacist for professional guidance concerning the quality of medications. In fact, pharmacists and nurses as well as physicians should occasionally visit the facilities of the companies whose products they dispense and administer. They may be alarmed to learn that cut-rate drugs may not only be low in price. By cutting corners, their producers may have, of necessity, cut quality, and paid inadequate attention to proper manufacture and distribution.

SELECTED REFERENCES

1. Blake JB: *Safeguarding the Public.* Baltimore, John Hopkins Press, 1970.
2. Castle WB, Astood EB, Finland M, and Keefer CS: White paper on the therapeutic equivalence of chemically equivalent drugs. *JAMA* 208: 1171-1172 (May 19) 1969.
3. Crawford JN, and Willard JW: *Guide for Drug Manufacturers.* The Food and Drug Directorate, Department of National Health and Welfare, Canada, 1969.
4. Drug Information Association: Symposium on formulation factors affecting therapeutic performance of drug products. *Drug Info Bull* 3:116 (Jan-June) 1969.
5. Feinberg M: Drug standards in military procurement. *J Am Pharm Assoc* NS9:113-116 (Mar) 1969.
6. Friend DG, Goolkasian AR, Hassan WE, Jr., Vona JP: Generic terminology and the cost of drugs. *JAMA* 209:80-84 (July 7) 1969.
7. Jeffries SB: Current good manufacturing practices compliance—A review of the problems and an approach to their management. *Food Drug Cosmetic Law J,* Vol. 580-603 (Dec) 1968.
8. Martin EW: *Dispensing of Medication.* Easton, Pa, Mack Publishing, 1971.
9. *Med Trib,* pp 10, 26 (Mar 31) 1969.
10. Pharmaceutical Manufacturers Association: *PMA Newsletter* 11:4 (July 25) 1969.
11. U.S. Food and Drug Administration: Drugs: current good manufacturing practice in manufacturing, processing, packaging, or holding. *Fed Reg* 34: 13553-8 (FR Doc 69-9980; Aug 22) 1969; 36:601-605 (FR Doc 71-638; Jan 15) 1971; revised regulations published in 1978.
12. ———: *National Drug Code Directory.* ed 2 (June) 1970; Kissman, HM: *FDA Papers* 2:26-27 (Dec 1968-Jan 1969) 1968; last edition of NDCD, 1976.
13. Varley AB: The generic inequivalence of drugs. *JAMA* 206:1745 (Nov 18) 1968.
14. Directive on policy respecting biologic availability requirements in abbreviated new drug applications. Memorandum from the director, BuDrugs, FDA, Aug 7, 1970.
15. Dowling HF: *Medicines for Man.* New York, Knopf, 1970.
16. Feinberg M, Cuttler M: USP standards in military drug purchasing. *Drug Intell Clin Pharm* 4:257-259 (Sept) 1970.
17. Stewart GT: Allergenic residues in penicillins. *Lancet* 1:1177-1183 (June 3) 1967.
18. Zollner E, Vastagh G: Uber die Zersetzung des Lidocains. *Pharm. Zentralhalle* 105:369, 1966.
19. *FDC Reports* 32: T&G 2 (Dec 21) 1970.
20. Miller LC: How good *are* our drugs? *Am J Hosp Pharm* 27:366-374 (May) 1970.

5 Distribution and Storage Factors

To ensure correct use, therapeutic efficacy, and safety, medications must be properly packaged, labeled and handled from the moment they are prepared until they are used by the patient. Unless medications are protected from destructive environmental influences, and unless they are accurately identified, carefully transported, and properly stored, the patient cannot receive dependable drug therapy from his physician.

The Distribution Network

The drug distribution network of the United States, astounding in its vast proportions, supplies almost instantaneously any one of some 300,000 different packaged medications including more than 18,000 prescription drug products at practically any location in the country.* About 12,000 pharmaceutical establishments are involved with *human* drug products, including 2900 manufacturers, 1100 repacking and relabeling companies, 200 quality control testing laboratories, 6870 warehouses, distributors, importers, and research laboratories as well as 730 methadone treatment centers. In addition 33 establishments produce biological products, 758 ship blood and blood products in interstate commerce, and 6495 not licensed by FDA collect and ship blood within their home states.

The drug manufacturers alone utilize nearly a quarter of a million employees na-

tionally and internationally (160,000 in the USA), a high percentage of whom are physicians, scientists and technically trained personnel. During 1977 these companies, with a research payroll of over 1.3 billion dollars, distributed worldwide medications valued at more than 15 billion dollars, including 9.4 billion dollars worth of prescription medications at the manufacturer's price level domestically and $6 billion overseas. Ethical pharmaceutical sales worldwide approached $50 billion, with the United States providing the highest percentage of any country.[46]

Distribution of drug products has been rapidly increasing in volume in recent years. During 1977 total sales of prescription medications increased 14%. A total of about 1.5 billion prescriptions were filled in 1977 in 50,000 community pharmacies and other retail outlets and roughly one-third as many again in hospital pharmacies in the United States, with a total of about 2 billion. This number increased at the rate of about 100,000,000 each year between 1970 and 1973 and then began to decline slightly afterwards.† More than 72% of these prescriptions fall into the 10 therapeutic categories shown in Table 5-1.[46]

The great majority of the pharmaceutical companies are merely small repackagers or

---

*Basic pharmaceutical prescription entities number about 2400 but various brands, strengths, and dosage forms multiply this many times. The ratio between single entities and different packages of OTC products is even greater.

---

†The decline was due to a shift in some drug products from R to OTC status, more conservative prescribing and more cautious taking of medications, more tightly controlled and fewer refills, and fewer new drug products. Drug data given in this chapter were taken from recent issues of *American Druggist, Annual Survey Report* of the Pharmaceutical Manufacturers Association, *Drug Topics, FDC Reports,* and similar authoritative sources.

Table 5-1 Leading Therapeutic Categories of 1977

Rx Rank	Therapeutic Category	% of Market
1	Antibiotics	18.3
2	Analgesics	9.3
3	Cough-Cold Rx	8.8
4	Psychotropics	8.7
5	Cardiovasculars	6.3
6	Diuretics	4.4
		55.8

* Table adapted from data published by *Drug Topics,* June 1, 1977.

refinishers of bulk products obtained from large domestic and foreign firms. Most of the prescription drug supply is concentrated in comparatively few firms. Thus, the 127 member firms of the Pharmaceutical Manufacturers Association account for about 93% of all prescription products distributed in the U.S.A.; just 30 of these companies account for more than 70% of these products, 10 for 51%, and 1 company for 7%. Four manufacturers of prescription medications employ more than 15,000 people, and five have global sales for medications of $300 million or more each. Most companies without membership in the PMA distribute over-the-counter proprietary drug products or prescription products under their generic names. Many of these firms distribute only on a regional level, sometimes in one state.[22] About 150 of the larger ones belong to the National Association of Pharmaceutical Manufacturers and about 100 to the Proprietary Association.

The drug distribution network, including its marketing, advertising, and handling procedures, must be constantly and strictly monitored for the sake of the patient's welfare.* Once a drug product leaves a production line it may be transported in the United States by airplane, train, or truck directly to one of the hundreds of thousands of practitioners in the health professions, or to one of

the 7,156 hospitals,† 50,000 retail pharmacies, or 25,000 nursing homes and other extended-care facilities with pharmaceutical service, or be temporarily stored in a warehouse of one of the drug companies or in one of the 4,000 wholesale outlets.

Throughout this vast and complex system, the most important considerations in maintaining the identity, potency, purity, and quality of drug products and their correct distribution, apart from the manufacturing requirements discussed in Chapter 4, are proper packaging, labeling, storage, and preservation, the use of ethical promotional practices that provide adequate and sound professional information, error-free drug distribution in the hospital, and prevention of illegal distribution.

PACKAGING

The official compendia (USP and NF) provide specifications for containers for drug products, volumes, preservatives, storage conditions, label statements, and other official requirements.[1,21] If these specifications and requirements are met, under the usual conditions of handling, distribution, and storage the active ingredients do not deteriorate before the expiration date, and the patient receives a product of acceptable quality. As a further safety precaution the FDA has established maximum limits for certain toxic compounds produced by deterioration of some drugs. Thus they have established limits for epianhydrotetracycline in tetracycline products (*Fed Reg* 34:12286, July 25, 1969).

Container Specifications

Different *official* specifications are given for containers for biologicals, injections, vitamins, and other classes of products.[1,21] Depending on the type of drug present in the

---

*For example, cyclamates, monosodium glutamate, Laetrile, saccharin, the youth drug KH-3 (procaine plus hematoporphyrin), and scores of other products have been subjected to recall, or seizure, or intensive investigation by the FDA over the past decade.

---

†The statistics for the nation's hospitals and skilled nursing homes are impressive. In the past year (1977) there were over 7,100 hospitals registered by the American Hospital Association, with about 1½ million beds; 254,844,000 outpatient visits were made and 36,157,000 inpatients were admitted and cared for by over 3 million employees. Total cost for both inpatient and outpatient services was nearly 50 billion dollars. HEW has distributed comprehensive reports on health manpower in U.S. hospitals.[44]

given dosage form, the container specified for it may be one or a combination of the following: (1) *light resistant,* which protects the contents from the frequencies of light to which they are sensitive, (2) *well-closed,* which merely keeps the contents in the package and prevents dust from entering. (3) *tight,* which keeps the contents in the container, protects them from contamination with solids, liquids, or vapors, and prevents loss through deliquescence, efflorescence, or evaporation, (4) *hermetic,* which is impervious to air or other gases, (5) *single-dose,* which hermetically seals a single dose of a parenteral medication and cannot be resealed and still provide assurance of sterility, (6) *multiple-dose,* which hermetically seals several doses of a parenteral medication and which permits withdrawal of successive doses of the medication without altering its potency, purity, quality, or sterility, or (7) *aerosol,* which hermetically seals medications dissolved, emulsified, or suspended in a propellant or a mixture of a propellant and a suitable solvent under pressure so that when a valve is opened, fine solid particles or liquid mists are provided for application to dermatomucosal surfaces and the cavities that open externally, including the ear, mouth, nose, rectum, respiratory tract, and vagina.

Detailed specifications for glass and plastic containers are published in the USP and NF, including requirements for light transmission. All containers must be properly filled, sealed, and packaged to provide uniformity of content and avoid damage to the contents from contact with air, light, humidity, and other factors. The containers must not react with the medication (highly alkaline glass may cause precipitation and decomposition of alkaloidal and other salts, and corrosive acids like trichloroacetic may be decomposed by alkali). They must be resistant to attack by acid or alkaline chemicals (flakes and spicules of glass loosened from a container can be hazardous in parenteral products). They must protect the medication from certain destructive light frequencies (ascorbic acid, alkaloids, phenothiazines, organometallics, and many other drugs are deteriorated by light). And they must keep the medication sealed from damaging atmospheric constituents. Special closures are available for flasks, jars, vials, and other containers to avoid con-

tamination, deliquescence (absorption of water), efflorescence (loss of water of hydration), and other actions that may cause a drug to change its properties or composition, or cause it to deteriorate so that a hazard is created for the patient. The patient will not receive the intended medication in a pure, potent form if packaging is inappropriate. And in some instances even the safety of the medication is jeopardized.

Safety Closures

Medications in easily opened containers present serious hazards for young children. Some thought-provoking statistics have been compiled by the National Clearinghouse for Poison Control Centers. This agency found that accidental ingestions of medications intended for internal use have accounted for about half of all intoxications reported for children under 5 years of age in recent years. And from data presented at the 1967 Conference on Poison Control held at the University of Mississippi (see the paper by Carter and Brown in the *Proceedings*) the total incidence of reported and unreported major and minor accidental ingestions of toxic substances in this age group can be estimated to be over 3,000,000 per year. Since aspirin accounts for about 40% of the reported accidental ingestions of medications, the total number of all accidental ingestions by very young children numbers hundreds of thousands per year just for aspirin.

To minimize this type of medication hazard, some pharmaceutical manufacturers started to use special safety closures on aspirin containers in 1968. And early in 1970 Senator Moss introduced a bill to make it mandatory to use safety closures on all products containing an ingredient which requires special precautions to protect young children from the serious personal injury or serious illness that may result from handling, using, or ingesting such products. Successive pieces of legislation will undoubtedly be enacted to protect the very young consumer from hazardous medications and also from a large percentage of the 250,000 chemical products now on the market.

Single-Unit Packaging. In a 1969 study, 85% of the hospitals replying to a questionnaire agreed that there are advantages in having unit-dose medication packages. Now, nearly a decade later, unit-dose packaging has become standard practice in most hospitals. Eventually, practically all medications (12 billion doses per year) will be available in this form for United States hospitals and extended-care facilities. Obviously, unit-dose packaging gained in popularity because of the greater safety provided the patient. [7,10,18] For many decades, single-dose ampuls of parenteral products as well as individually wrapped suppositories have been widely used, but now tablets and capsules are individually sealed in tin foil, plastic, and other containers. Certain rectal and vaginal medications are also supplied with special applicators in single-dose containers which can be disposed of immediately after use.

Government regulatory agencies are encouraging the use of this type of packaging because the quality of patient care is improved for a number of reasons:

1. Medication errors are reduced.

2. Contamination of sterile products and equipment is practically eliminated.

3. The time required for dispensing medications is reduced.

4. The time required for administration of medications is reduced.

5. Administration of medications is more efficient. The nurse's time is more efficiently utilized. The handling of medications is cleaner, neater, and less cumbersome.

6. Medication inventory can be controlled more easily and more accurately.

7. Costs of patient care are reduced because the cleaning and sterilizing of containers, syringes, and other equipment is eliminated.

More products should be made available in the unit-dose form by pharmaceutical manufacturers so that eventually as many medications as is feasible will be distributed from production lines to patients without further intervention or manipulation. [2,3]

A distinction must be made between single-unit packaging and unit-dose distribution. Every hospital in the world provides its patients with unit doses, for every medication is reduced to individual doses before it is administered to patients. The important question is when to subdivide a given volume of medication into appropriate dosage units. This can be done at the point of packaging by the manufacturer where efficient control procedures can be utilized economically, or it can be done in the hospital at a point just before the patient receives it, or it can be done anywhere along the distribution chain between these two points. No matter at what stage unit doses are prepared, errors will be less frequent where control is most efficient. But unit doses may vary from patient to patient and single-unit packages are mass produced in a given dosage size. Thus the following definitions [2] have been used as guidelines:

"A *unit-dose* package contains the ordered amount of drug in a dosage form ready for administration to a particular patient by the prescribed route at the prescribed time. A *single-unit* package is one which contains one discrete pharmaceutical dosage form, i.e., one tablet, one capsule, or one 2 ml. quantity of a liquid, etc. A *single-unit* package becomes a *unit-dose* package when the physician happens to order that particular amount for a patient."

FDA favors unit-dose packaging as a general policy. But it may have to relax its labeling regulations somewhat because according to the law all required information must appear on the immediate container which is in direct contact with the drug at all times, and unit-dose packages are too small to accommodate this information.

Experimentation and innovation with the unit-dose packaging concept will continue until it is perfected for hospitals, nursing homes, and various extended-care facilities. Nursing homes in particular, which expanded rapidly at the beginning of the 1970's (1,000 new beds a week), require streamlined systems for patient safety. Automated unit-dose systems now available enable community pharmacies to prepare, transport, and deliver medication systematically to the bedsides of patients in neighboring health care facilities. These automated systems maintain patient drug profiles, supply data for future planning of nursing home layouts and other requirements, reduce the problems of breakage, pilferage, and spillage, provide efficient billing, and check the labeling. [9]

STORAGE

Storage conditions are specified in the USP and NF for each medication which is vulnerable to heat, light, moisture, oxygen, and other environmental factors. [1,21] Storage temperatures were redefined in the 1975 editions of these compendia as follows: *cold place*—one having a temperature not exceeding 8° C (46° F), *refrigerator*—a cold place in which the temperature is held between 2° and 8° C (36° and 46° F), *cool place*—one having a temperature between 8° and 15° C (46° and 59° F), *room temperature*—between 15° and 30° C (59° and 86° F),* and *excessive heat*—temperatures above 40° C (104° F). In announcing the action, the Director of the *National Formulary* pointed out that "the stability—or rather the inherent instability—of many of today's complex and potent drugs requires more rigidly defined storage conditions. The general availability of efficient refrigeration and air-conditioning equipment now makes it possible to provide more carefully controlled storage temperatures for pharmaceutical products at all levels of drug distribution."

When no specific storage conditions or limitations appear in the labeling for a drug product, the official compendia state that "it is to be understood that the storage conditions include protection from moisture, freezing, and excessive heat." Bulk packages of drugs intended for manufacture or repackaging are exempt from official requirements. This exemption may be a hazard. However, the reputable manufacturer or repackager, whatever the source of raw materials, maintains rigidly controlled storage conditions at all stages of production and assumes full responsibility for the quality of his product when he distributes it to a hospital, wholesaler, pharmacy, or physician. When medications are going to be subjected to worldwide distribution under adverse conditions, as in the military, special packaging, stability, and storage requirements must be met.

Unless proper storage conditions are constantly and strictly observed at every point from acquisition of bulk materials to delivery of finished product, the medication may reach the physician's office, hospital, pharmacy, or patient in a deteriorated, subpotent state. This creates a hazard for the patient because if the physician prescribes the usual

dose of a medication in a subpotent state, the desired therapeutic response will not be achieved and adverse effects may be produced by toxic decomposition products. Indeed, after the physician has prescribed and the pharmacist has dispensed a medication, the same care must be taken by all who subsequently handle the medication.

A prescription may be exposed in a sun-baked delivery car to excessive temperatures and "prompt" delivery by the pharmacy may actually mean up to several hours of such unfavorable exposure unless special refrigeration is provided. And either the nurse or the patient may inadvertently leave the medication on a sunny windowsill or near a heater or unstoppered in a humid, possibly even polluted atmosphere. Unfortunately, all too few of the many people involved in the distribution chain are reminded not to do these things, and yet the patients' welfare may depend on how even they handle and preserve their own prescriptions. In general, it is desirable for the physician to tell each patient to keep all medications in a cool place even when the labeling does not provide specific storage instructions.

LABELING

Correct labeling of medications is essential to protect the patient. Incomplete or incorrect labeling can be a major hazard and therefore pertinent Federal regulations are comprehensive and specific. According to the official definition, labeling includes not only the labels on the outside cartons or packages and on the immediate containers, but also the package inserts packed with each container, and brochures and all other literature describing the medical applications of the drug product. But how many physicians closely examine the details of a label or the details in the package insert?

A typical label on the container of a medication available only by prescription should contain (1) generic name† of each drug in the product and the National Drug Code number assigned to the product, (2) the brand name if one is used, (3) amount of each active ingredient per dosage unit, in metric units, and total quantity of drug in the package, (4) route of administration, especially prominent

---

*This refers to *controlled* room temperature, not the widely ranging temperatures which may prevail in a working area.

---

†Nonproprietary or established name. See page 87.

if it is a toxic tablet for topical use only, (5) expiration date, (6) name and address of manufacturer, packer, or distributor, (7) adequate directions for use, often very brief on the label itself, and (8) an identifying logotype or trademark.

To be most useful to practitioners, labeling information for prescription drugs should be orderly and uniform in the sequence and kinds of information presented. For this reason the labeling should contain the information under the following headings in the order as listed. [50]

Description
Actions
Indications
Contraindications
Warnings
Precautions
Adverse Reactions
Dosage and Administration
Overdosage
Drug Interactions
How Supplied
Animal Pharmacology and Toxicology
Clinical Studies
References

FDA makes the last three sections optional. And, in the case of some drugs, headings may be omitted when no applicable information is available.

All of these labeling components have periodically been discussed at great length and some have been the subject of vehement controversy. During the early 1970s the questions of uniform coding of every capsule and tablet and the expiration date and its use were included in discussions on the government's consumer protection program. Because outdated medications have long been shown to possess potentials for severe harm, Federal and state legislators have introduced bills to protect the patient from the hazards of deteriorated drugs. [17] Typical is the legislation proposed by Representative Benjamin Rosenthal early in 1970. He explained that it was designed to

"Prohibit the sale of prescription and over-the-counter drugs, beyond an established expiration date. The Food and Drug Administration has recently expressed concern over the reports that over-aged drugs are sometimes sold to consumers and that consequent drug deterioration may be responsible for some injuries and deaths.

"In 1965, for example, three patients at a New Jersey institution for the mentally retarded died from the ingestion of over-aged carbarsone tablets taken for the treatment of an intestinal disorder. Analysis of the drug showed that over-age had caused a chemical change in the tablet with fatal results.

"Similarly, a large number of deaths and serious injuries documented by the Food and Drug Administration have been traced to the ingestion of out-dated tetracycline, which had undergone a hazardous chemical change. This bill would require an expiration date for drug use—both to the pharmacist and to the ultimate consumer."

To protect the consumer, special statements must appear on the labels and other labeling of certain drugs. Various habit-forming drugs must carry a statement of the quantity and percentage of each active ingredient and the following: *Warning—May be habit forming.* Drugs which are unsuitable for self-medication are labeled with the following legend: *Caution: Federal law prohibits dispensing without prescription.* Such drugs are called legend drugs. When necessary, other warnings must appear on the label or in the package insert or both. Under the headings of Contraindications, Warnings, Precautions, and Adverse Reactions must appear warnings such as those against (1) unsafe use by children, (2) use in conditions where warnings are required to insure against harm, and (3) use in an amount or for a length of time or by a method of administration which may make it dangerous to health.

The labeling of medications must carry a clear indication of therapeutic limitations. Not only must the useful effects be included but also every known harmful or deleterious effect. The labeling must not contain any false or misleading statement regarding the composition of the article or the effects it will produce, or any false or misleading statement regarding any other drug or device. Every available piece of pertinent information must be provided in the labeling to keep the physician, pharmacist, nurse, and patient fully informed so that the drug may be used safely and effectively after the labeling, including the package insert, has been carefully read.*

FDA defines labeling in its regulations, [11,12] as amended March 6, 1969, to be all encompassing, as follows: "Brochures, booklets,

---

*Complete listing on the label of all ingredients in each drug product, including all adjuvants, would enable the physician to avoid some allergic and other adverse reactions when he prescribes.

mailing pieces, detailing pieces, file cards, bulletins, calendars, price lists, catalogs, house organs, letters, motion-picture films, filmstrips, lantern slides, sound recordings, exhibits, literature, and reprints and similar pieces of printed, audio, or visual matter descriptive of a drug and references published for use by medical practitioners, pharmacists, or nurses, containing drug information supplied by the manufacturer, packer, or distributor of the drug and which are disseminated by or on behalf of its manufacturer, packer, or distributor."

The same regulations state, "Advertisements subject to section 502(n) of the Act include advertisements in published journals, magazines, other periodicals, and newspapers, and advertisements broadcast through media such as radio, television, and telephone communication systems."

And to make matters more complex, any product may be legally considered to be a drug product the moment any drug claim is made, even by such innocuous statements as "this baby oil helps or relieves diaper rash."

The regulations promulgated by FDA are extremely detailed. They actually cover such items as the height or area of labels for rectangular, cylindrical and other shapes of containers; the face, size, prominence and positioning of typography; and the use of terminology in labeling and advertising. The regulations even go so far as to require that the established (generic) name be placed immediately after the proprietary (brand) name and that the relationship be clearly shown by the use of a phrase such as "brand of" preceding the established name or by brackets or parentheses surrounding it or by other suitable means. Exact specifications with examples were published in the *Federal Register,* February 21, 1968. [11]

Drug literature must carry "full disclosure," that is, all essential prescribing information included in the package insert.* Many arguments revolved around this requirement as the regulatory agencies became more and more strict, until a regulation was published that required all parts of the labeling to be consistent with the approved pack-age insert. Thus all brochures and other literature supplied to physicians must contain every contraindication, warning, precaution, and adverse effect.

Package Inserts as Legal Documents

The full significance of the drug package insert (official brochure approved by FDA), including its legal implications, slowly became evident during the decade following enactment of the 1962 Kefauver-Harris Amendments to the Federal Food, Drug, and Cosmetic Act. Not only did the insert become a key in regulatory control over the promotion of medications by manufacturers; it also became an important influence in the therapeutic practices of physicians and in various legal proceedings, especially malpractice litigation. Despite the many arguments that have arisen over its place in legal proceedings, the courts of most states recognize it as legally relevant to the responsibility of a physician in his prescribing practices.

The physician is bound by his duty to be fully informed about the composition, mode of action, efficacy, and potential toxicity of any drug before he administers it. Then by his training and experience he has the right to exercise his own independent medical judgment in deciding when and how he will use the drug. His decisions are medically and legally valid if they conform to the acceptable standards of his colleagues. But the package insert may have a direct bearing on those standards. If facts in a lawsuit show deviations from the insert's contents, the defendant-physician may have the burden to justify his conduct. [41,42]

Package inserts contain precautionary statements and warnings concerning certain drugs, e.g., (1) testing for patient hypersensitivity prior to administering them, (2) conducting routine periodic tests such as blood counts during therapy with them, (3) relative and absolute contraindications, (4) specific harmful effects, such as sedative effects in automobile drivers or operators of machinery, and (5) the possibility of occurrence of adverse drug reactions and interactions, and other serious considerations. These warnings tend to relieve the manufacturer of responsibility for adverse effects and intensify the need for physicians to exercise utmost caution in the use of all medications. With any

---

*The package insert is a legal document which now must serve as the basis for all promotional claims. See next section below.

new or potentially hazardous drug, the physician should refer not only to the insert and company literature, but to other available written instructions for use. He should never depend solely on the oral presentations of detail men who may tend to overpromote and thereby possibly cause him to disregard written warnings. [42]

Controversy between the Food and Drug Administration and the American Medical Association arose over deviations by physicians from the indications and dosages given in the package inserts. See pages 3 and 112 for a description of insert content. In April, 1969, the AMA published a discussion on the use of inserts in the courts, [28] and made the following points: (1) The FDA-approved package insert for a particular drug is the result of regulatory activity. (2) Determinations of FDA do not establish standards for medical practice. Such standards are established by the customary practice of reputable physicians. (3) Court actions have established the insert as a legally admissible document which conveys the manufacturer's warnings, but have held it nonconclusive as a standard of medical practice. The AMA cited the following cases:

In a California negligence action involving a patient who had been paralyzed from the waist down following injection of 50 ml. of 70% acetrizoate sodium (Urokon Sodium) for translumbar aortography, when the package insert recommended only 10 to 15 ml, the appellate court made the following statement regarding the evidentiary value of the brochure:

"Thus, while admissible, it [the brochure] cannot establish as a matter of law the standard of care required of a physician in the use of the drug. It may be considered by the jury along with other evidence in the case to determine whether the particular physician met the standard of care required of him. The mere fact of a departure from the manufacturer's recommendation where such departure is customarily followed by physicians of standing in the locality does not make the departure an 'experiment.' " [29]

Similarly, in a later (1961) negligence action against a dentist who had failed to take an adequate medical history before he injected lidocaine and epinephrine into a hypertensive patient who suffered a stroke and died, the appellate court held that the package insert was admissible as evidence that the dentist should have been alerted to the possible dangers, even though it was *not* conclusive to establish proof of standards of care. [30]

In a still later (1968) negligence action against a pediatrician who used an adult dosage form of a combination of procaine penicillin G and streptomycin sulfate (Strep-Combiotic) at more than the upper safe limit in an infant who thereby sustained permanent nerve deafness, the court admitted statements in the package insert ". . . as evidence of a warning which the physician disregards at his peril. Such statements are relevant on the issue of a physician's use of reasonable care where other evidence shows that the drug is, in fact, dangerous to a child." [31]

In April, 1968, the AMA Council on Drugs sponsored a conference with FDA on the package insert and a year later, after the material had been edited and approved by Legal Council for the FDA and the Director of the Bureau of Medicine (now Bureau of Drugs), the AMA published the substance of the conference in a resume using a question and answer format. [32,33] Pertinent statements included the following concepts:

A physician may exercise judgment and use a drug in any manner in which he sees fit in the best interest of his patient. If a physician deviates from the instructions provided in the package insert concerning usage and dosage, or from recommendations provided in the package insert, and an adverse response occurs, the burden of proof may rest upon the physician should the package insert be used in court as evidence of misuse of a drug in a malpractice suit. The package insert may be used as evidence.

Though a physician is free to express his own views concerning a drug and its usage, FDA feels it advisable for physician-authors, who recommend dosages and uses other than those found in the package inserts, to point out these differences and to indicate why such variations are recommended. However, FDA has no jurisdiction over data published in texts or the publication of texts. If a mishap occurs due to misinformation in a textbook, the plaintiff may use the package insert in court, as evidence of a proper use of the drug. A defendant physician may then be required to prove that deviation from recommended usage was proper and justifiable.

Every prescriber of medications should be aware of another legal pitfall. In recent years FDA has required manufacturers of drugs that might be used by children or by pregnant women to include precautionary statements in their inserts sufficient to warn physicians about such usage for these classes of patients. Many drugs have not been proved safe for children; physicians ought to keep this in mind when prescribing. Most package inserts now include the extent of such safety information, if any. The same is true for usage in pregnancy where drugs might have teratogenic effects. In legal proceedings (i.e., malpractice lawsuits) such clear, precautionary statements may carry substantial weight.

Another direct exchange of viewpoints between AMA and FDA was brought about in March, 1970, when a physician wrote to AMA for advice on the use of FDA approved drugs for certain specific conditions in which the medical profession used the drugs but for which use no approval had been given by FDA.[34] Replies from the AMA Law Division and AMA Department of Drugs included the following statements:[35,36]

"The position of the AMA Council on Drugs is that the package insert is part of the labeling of a drug and not a legal restriction on the thoughtful and careful use of a drug by an informed physician. . . . In general, the information or lack thereof contained in the package insert does not place any legal constraints on the prescribing of drugs by physicians. . . . A physician may use any drug that is generally available in and under any condition he may choose as long as this falls within the limits of acceptable, good medical practice."

Six months later, an exchange in *Letters to the Editor* of *JAMA* on these standards was published.[37,38] The Director of the FDA Bureau of Drugs took note of the AMA assumption: ". . . that the physician may regard what is actually a 'new' use, for example for an indication not found in the labeling, as essentially not investigative in nature." In the opinion of FDA, "ideally such a use should be the subject of a Notice of Claimed Investigational Exemption for a New Drug (IND) . . . if the physician uses the drug investigationally on his own, he has really taken upon himself the burden of evaluation of the experience of others with no assurance that he has all the existing data, or that the information he has is soundly based in appropriately designed studies."

The AMA profoundly disagreed and declared that there was no legitimate purpose for the IND procedure, other than to serve as a mechanism by which the manufacturer or comparable distributor of a new drug in interstate commerce may have the necessary testing performed and an NDA approved so that the drug may be marketed. The AMA took the positions: (1) When a physician places himself in the role of clinical investigator under an IND sponsor, he may be legally required to conform to NDA procedure. But a physician in the normal course of his practice is under no compulsion to act as an investigator. (2) By means of the "time wasting" IND procedure, the physician may be supplicating for a privilege of experimentation which may not legally be withheld. The IND procedure perniciously confuses *investigation* within the narrow scope of the Food, Drug, and Cosmetic Act with *experimentation* in the usual sense. (3) A drug might be used strictly according to a package insert and still be used improperly or experimentally by broad definition. (4) The idea that a physician can insulate himself against malpractice suits by engaging in a superficial bilateral ritual with FDA by submitting private INDs, is patent nonsense. (5) There is real danger in the attitude on the part of physicians that something is vaguely illegal or improper about using a drug in some way differing from that of the package insert; this attitude, if it persists, could gradually lead courts in malpractice suits to come to accept the belief.[38]

FDA has stated that the package insert is not intended to instruct the physician in the diagnosis of disease or the recognition of pathological conditions. Neither is it intended to replace the physician's basic medical education in pharmacology or drug therapy. According to FDA, the insert "represents the best source of established information available to the practicing physician regarding the conditions of use under which a drug is considered safe and effective. . . . If a doctor exercises a judgment to prescribe the drug outside the limits of the package insert, he should be aware that the scientific basis for doing so has not been established by data submitted by the manufacturer through the procedures required by law. Investigational new drug procedures cover the use of the drug for conditions other than those in the approved labeling for which there is some rationale,"[40,48,49]

In reality, the package insert, which originates as part of the manufacturer's original New Drug Application, basically reflects the administrative policies of FDA, serves as an informative brochure for the physician apart from the promotional literature of the manufacturer, and to some extent, protects the manufacturer from litigation. It has become a significant legal document for certain restricted evidentiary uses.

However, only the latest edition of any given insert at the time the drug is prescribed may be applicable for the following reasons. (1) The inserts are revised periodically as additional important information becomes available. Most inserts have been revised at least once since 1969 because of the recommendations made by the National Academy of Sciences-National Research Council Drug Efficacy Study panels. The insert is a constantly changing and evolving document, and only the edition current at the time the drug was prescribed is relevant. (2) Important uses for some drugs have not always been included in some inserts (specific usages may be added or deleted from year to year as evidence is presented to and evaluated by FDA). (3) FDA cannot require a pharmaceutical manufacturer to include a new indication for a medication in the insert even if it has been clinically tested and found useful for that indication. (4) No package insert can provide "full disclosure of all known facts pertaining to the use of the drug."[39] To achieve this aim, the insert would become a textbook too large to pack conveniently in the carton used for shipping drug products let alone the individual drug packages. Therefore statements, or the absence of information, or reports of hazards, in either outdated or current editions should carry little or no weight in court. And the physician should not rely solely on the package insert as his source of information on a drug. His own experience in the use of a drug, individual patient response, the benefit-to-risk ratio in each specific case, and the many other factors presented throughout this volume must be considered.

Perhaps for the sake of argument, both FDA and AMA overstated their cases. The truth lies somewhere between the extremes. FDA cannot and should not attempt to impose universal use of the IND procedure every time a physician tries some modification of the drug therapy outlined in the package insert. The manufacturer cannot and should not attempt to use the package insert as a promotional brochure any longer under current regulatory laws and action, even though

he prints it. The judgment and knowledge of the individual physician and not government regulation must determine proper medication of the patient.

Patient Package Inserts

In November 1976 the last of a series of meetings concerning patient package inserts (PPIs) was held in Washington, D.C.[45] Participants and attendees represented nearly all sectors of society and brought with them a myriad of conflicting interests. Some argued against PPIs of any sort, but the rush of consumerism had already foreclosed a retreat. Therefore, the remaining issues dominated the scene: (1) For what drugs should PPIs be prepared? (2) What should these PPIs contain? (3) How shall they be distributed to patients? (4) What will be their legal effect, if any? Though the lack of consensus for any solution prevented the group from establishing clear-cut directions, it was apparent that FDA was already committed to the concept of PPIs and was proceeding on an *ad hoc* basis.

The legal effect of PPIs *vis-a-vis* prescribing physicians will depend greatly on their contents; the contents will depend on their perceived purpose; and according to many, the purpose of PPIs was to comply with supposed patients' rights (i.e., to produce a legal effect). Such circuity made it difficult for anyone to create a framework for problem solving.

Since FDA is burdened with the responsibility to assure the safety, efficacy, and proper labeling of drugs, it would seem reasonable for PPIs to possess characteristics directed primarily toward those goals. *Safety* could be enhanced by informing patients of: (1) Specific circumstances in which the drug should be avoided (i.e., important contraindications). Even though prescribing physicians routinely interrogate their patients about conditions which may contraindicate the use of certain intended drugs, additional disclosures *via* PPIs could reinforce a patient's understanding and avoidance. (2) Specific drug combinations which should be avoided to prevent dangerous interactions (e.g., aspirin and barbiturates for patients on anticoagulation therapy with warfarin). (3) Specific conduct which patients should avoid during certain drug therapy (e.g., driving automobiles and operating machinery while under the influence of sedation-inducing drugs). (4) Specific signs or symptoms which should lead the patient to stop the drug or to call his physician for advice. For less severe side effects (e.g., diarrhea), the PPI could recite the means of self-care.

Efficacy could be promoted by any number of disclosures which should tend to encourage patients to comply with their physicians' directions. For example, many patients require reinforcement to continue taking antibiotic drugs for the prescribed period even though they feel better.

PPIs which are relatively limited to these disclosures could be very helpful and yet not interfere with the prescribing physician's exercise of professional judgment. Such information would supplement and reaffirm the types of disclosures and interrogations required of physicians when embarking on drug therapy for their patients. As a result injuries to patients could be prevented, and the risk of legal liability could be minimized.

However, some advocates want PPIs to serve purposes other than mere safety and efficacy. They want patients to be informed of the officially accepted indications for drugs so that such patients will be able to make more intelligent decisions concerning their own therapy. The reasoning behind this promotion is the alleged frequency with which physicians unnecessarily prescribe hazardous drugs. However, the defect in disclosing indications for usage, except in broad, general terms, is that patients will have to exercise nonexisting medical judgment for their own management. Rather than correcting the problem of unnecessary medication at its source (i.e., physicians' prescribing habits), these advocates are willing to risk having patients suffer major damage through their own efforts.

Consumer-oriented groups have urged acceptance of the patient's "right to know" information about the drugs prescribed for him. Assuming such a right exists and assuming its limits are definable, should the government or drug manufacturers be required to underwrite the expense for an entirely new set of documents when the known information is already available to any patient who wishes to exercise this right? The more utilitarian approach would be to give patients the necessary safety and efficacy data—which

they are capable of using without a medical education—followed by directions for securing additional information if they want more.

As FDA proceeds with PPI development, the tenor of content will become clearer. Physicians ought to keep informed of this progress and be guided accordingly. Regardless of the approach to be taken by FDA, PPIs probably will not exert substantial legal effect on the liability of physicians, particularly if the distribution of these documents rests with manufacturers or pharmacists.

As a matter of fact PPI type of information has been in existence since 1960 when FDA required a special patient warning be printed for isoproterenol (Isuprel, Norisodrine Aerotrol, etc). Shortly thereafter FDA required that PPIs be given to patients when they purchased insulin. The first official relatively complete PPI, however, was that for OCs discussed in Chapter 1. This was followed by PPIs for DES and progestin-only OCs. By 1977 a number were being prepared for the more hazardous drugs.

Hirsh has published a useful analysis of the medicolegal implications of the patient package insert. He points out that patient compliance, "right to know," informed consent, full disclosure, and standards of care are all considerations in PPI development.[52] He concludes:

"Properly utilized, to avoid drug injury and enhance accuracy in compliance, the insert should provide a protective shield for the physician rather than a sword of challenge in the patient's hands."

Mislabeling

Periodically, FDA issues warnings to distributors or the public concerning the mislabeling of packages of drugs. Sometimes the faulty labeling is handled at the manufacturer's level if it is of a minor nature. At other times, however, urgent warnings to the public are needed, as when the wrong drug has been bottled. Thus when bottles labeled Vi-John Brand Castor Oil were found to contain turpentine oil late in the summer of 1970 and the distribution could not be determined because of a lack of coding, FDA was forced to warn all possible consumers by a public announcement. It was hoped that the warning succeeded and few parents forced their children to take turpentine oil under the impression that it was castor oil. Turpentine oil causes clammy skin, colic, cyanosis, diarrhea, headache, depressed and irregular respiration, vertigo, vomiting, and finally coma with albuminuria, glycosuria, and hematuria when ingested in excessive quantities.[41]

Drug Nomenclature

In every discussion of labeling and packaging, questions of nomenclature constantly arise.[11,12] The naming of drug products has created many problems and continual controversy.

Perhaps no other products have such a multiplicity of names, synonyms and other designations as drugs do. Practically every drug has at least one chemical name and also quite often several laboratory designations used during development, generic (common, nonproprietary, public or established), official (USP, NF, USAN), and trademark (brand, proprietary, specialty) names, and, if it has broad distribution, the equivalents of these in many languages in many countries. The resulting confusion in nomenclature has created serious hazards for the patient.[17]

In the literature can be found instances where the same name was applied to two different drugs.*

The *chemical name* is usually the first one assigned to a drug because most modern drugs are pure organic compounds and not crude drugs formed from plant and animal tissues. Identification of modern compounds involves the elucidation of their structures. For example, the molecular structure for thalidomide may be represented as follows:

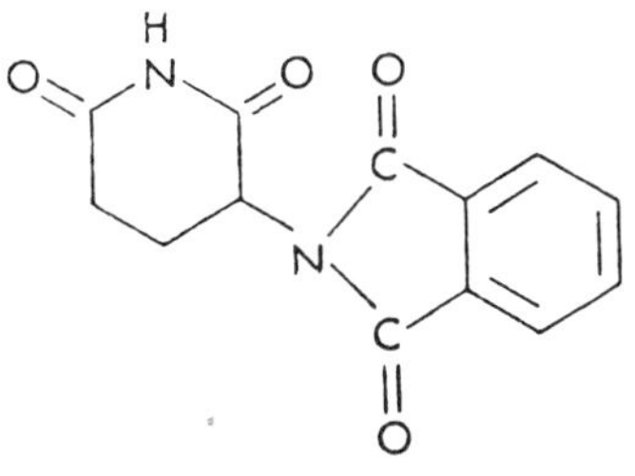

Thalidomide

The *Chemical Abstracts* index name for this structural formula is N-(2,6-dioxo-3-piperidyl)phthalimide, but it has also been designated α-phthalimidoglutarimide; 3-phthalimidoglutarimide; 2,6-dioxo-3-phthalimidopiperidine; N-phthalyglutamic acid imide; and N-phthaloylglutamimide. Rules for naming chemical structures have been well established so that chemists, simply by examining the name, can reproduce the structure and synthesize it in any country of the world. Comprehension of these structures by physicians is particularly valuable in clinical research.

The *laboratory designation* may be a coined name, an abbreviation, or an alphabetical or numeric code. Thus pentaerythritol tetranitrate was known as PETN, pyrilamine as RP 2786, thalidomide as K17, and triamcinolone as CL 19823. Such code numbers and other brief designations facilitate identification and communication among research workers. Sometimes, to make the nomenclature even more complicated, however, pet names are used by a select group of scientists in the laboratory. Such laboratory names may be useful to sophisticated investigators, but they can cause confusion and become a hazard if they are allowed to persist and pass into the general literature.

The *generic name* (common, established, nonproprietary, or public name) is a simplified, shortened name for a drug, often derived from its chemical name. It becomes the established, most frequently used name in the professional literature. Generically, the name of the chemical structure above is thalidomide. In some instances, the nomenclature becomes especially confusing when a given drug has a multiplicity of generic names. For example, pyrilamine, the antihistamine, is also known generically as anisopyridamine, pyranisamine, pyranilamine, and pyraminyl. Most synonymous generic names are rarely familiar to the prescribing physician and therefore only present a hazard by creating confusion when they are used.

The *official name* is the name used as the official title in the USP or NF and is the one name recognized nationally and to a large extent internationally. It is very often the same as the generic name. However, a drug may have several generic names; it can have only one official name. Thus, furazolidone is both the generic and official name for Furoxone.

---

*The tradename Cardoxin is used for the coronary dilator dipyridamole in Israel but for digoxin in Australia. Didion is used in Europe for the antiepileptic ethadione but for the indandione anticoagulant diphenadione in Israel.[51]

Official names are adopted and established by agreement through the mechanism of the United States Adopted Names (USAN) Council, a joint nomenclature committee with representatives from the American Medical Association, the American Pharmaceutical Association, the Food and Drug Administration, and the United States Pharmacopeia. The AMA through its Council on Drugs provides secretarial services.

The USAN procedure is thorough. All manufacturers are encouraged to submit a proposed nonproprietary name (devised according to guiding principles obtainable from the USAN Council) for each of its new drugs (basic chemicals) to the Secretary of the AMA Council on Drugs whenever they plan to undertake Phase III clinical trials or sooner if feasible. When a company submits a suggested name, it should also include its code number, the *Chemical Abstracts* index name, the structural formula (or other accurate means of definition), the general pharmacologic class, intended clinical use, and if available the trademark name of the drug. The suggested official name is reviewed by the USAN Council and its staff and, if necessary, modifications are negotiated with the company to avoid conflicts with other names and to make the name convenient and appropriate. After agreement is reached, the name is submitted to the World Health Organization, the British Pharmacopoeia Commission, and representatives of the FDA, French Codex, Nordic Pharmacopoeia, USP, and NF for review. The names for biologicals are also submitted to the Bureau of Biologics of FDA. If no objections are raised during a 30-day waiting period, the proposed name is adopted and used as the USP or NF title if the drug is admitted to one of these compendia. This official name may or may not be used subsequently by the manufacturer for the drug indicated since for various reasons the drug may not be marketed.

USAN nomenclature, specially identified in reference volumes like the *American Drug Index,* [24] is helping to eliminate a great deal of the confusion in drug nomenclature. FDA recently began to establish its own list of "official" names, but it almost invariably accepts US Adopted Names since it sits on the Council. This tendency to minimize duplication of drug names will be a major step forward in simplifying prescribing for the physician and obviating the hazard to the patient that can be caused by confusing similar names. Synonyms that are not the same as the official name should be discarded.

The *trademark* is a designation (device, name, symbol, or word) which is used by its owner to distinguish its brand of finished marketed product from all others and which is registered in the USA with the US Patent Office. The trademarked name (brand, proprietary, specialty name) is generally established through exclusive use as soon as application for its registration has been made, even before actual registration has been granted. A trademark will not be registered in the United States if it is misleading by implying a virtue or ingredient which is nonexistent. It serves merely to identify the reputation of a manufacturer and the quality of his products. In many foreign countries the use of a trademark is mandatory and approval of a drug product is not granted until a trademark registration has been accomplished.

Confusion in nomenclature has resulted when a company has begun to use a brand name in the later phases of research and then has changed its plans, has not marketed the drug to which the name was first assigned, and has instead assigned the same name to another drug which does reach the market. Confusion also results from the many brand names that sometimes are assigned to the same drug after its patent expires.* Pyrilamine maleate has been sold under some 40 different brand names. Thalidomide was sold throughout the world under more than 50 names, including Contergan, Kevadon, Neurosedyn, Pantosediv, Sedalis, Softenon, and Talimol. For this reason, recall of its dosage forms was extremely difficult. [19] It is now compulsory to use both brand and generic names together in the labeling for American drug products, and over a period of time this practice should eliminate some of the nomenclature hazards.

The greatest hazards resulting from the multitude of synonyms for drugs occur when the physician is prescribing and when hazardous drugs are being recalled from the market. So many names for different drugs

---

* Diethylstilbestrol is sold under more than 70 names.

are the same or so similar in spelling or pronunciation that the physician can very easily prescribe, the pharmacist dispense, or the nurse administer the wrong medication (see Table 6-1 on page 115). Also, if it becomes necessary to order the removal of all of a given dangerous drug from the market, the task becomes almost impossible when it is sold under numerous names in several countries.*

In the future, serious attention will be given to the avoidance of drug names that look alike (homographs) and sound alike (homophones). The coining of synonyms must also be avoided whenever possible. This will eventually eliminate or at least greatly decrease a source of danger to the patient. Also the use of certain chemical prefixes should be avoided when writing prescriptions since they can be confusing to both the prescriber and the dispenser of drug products. One patient received 18 tablets a day instead of 3, when his prescription, written "6-mercaptopurine 50 mg tid", was misinterpreted. Suffixes as well as prefixes may also be confusing since their meaning and use vary widely. They may indicate the action of a drug (SA, i.e., sedative antispasmodic), an ingredient added (Diutensin-R, reserpine added; Cafergot P-B, pentobarbitol added, Anusol-HC, hydrocortisone added), a chemical variant (Delta-Cortef), a clinical trial number (Ciba-1906), a difference in composition (B and O Supprettes No 15A and No 16A), a different drug within a group (Amphotericin B), depot, long acting, or sustained release (Depo-Medrol; TD, timed disintegration), duration of the course of treatment (Ovulen-21), molecular weight (Dextran 45, mol wt 45,000), omission of a product (Atromid-S, sine), particle size (Fulvicin-U/F, ultrafine), repeat action (Butibel-RA; Polaramine Repetabs), a salt (Penbritin-S, sodium salt; Coly-Mycin-S, sulfate), use of a preparation (Meti-Derm), a

vitamin (Betalin-12, B_{12}) or many other characteristics.

Some prefixes have several meanings. Neo may indicate a new type of compound, a new composition, a mixture, or that neomycin is an ingredient. Similar meanings are expressed by a variety of suffixes. Dospan, Duolets, Durules, LA, Repetabs, Retard, SA, Spansules, Sustets, Timespan, TD, etc., signify delayed, sustained, or repetitive release. C may mean vitamin C, carbamate, etc. K may mean vitamin K, potassium salt, etc. The meanings of many alphabetical or numerical prefixes and suffixes are ambiguous and therefore should be avoided because they may be confusing.[25]

PRESERVATION

An expiration date will appear on all drug products if FDA requirements proposed in 1976 eventually are converted into official regulations (see page 74). Very few drug products will maintain their identity, purity, quality, safety, and strength indefinitely, even under optimum conditions.† Aging and ambient conditions often modify molecular structures and thereby impair the drug content. In fact, practically every drug product is adversely affected by *heat*. At higher temperatures cleavage of molecules, formation of undesirable stereoisomers, and other chemical actions are accelerated, especially in the presence of *moisture*. Gas may form and containers explode. Discoloration, precipitation, and degradation may occur. *Freezing* damages containers, and drug products are subsequently exposed to contamination when thawing takes place. Freezing also tends to unstabilize emulsions, suspensions, and products with less soluble ingredients; it may cause deposition and loss of homogeneity. *Light* can be very destructive to some drugs, especially ultraviolet frequencies ranging from 290 mμ to 450 mμ. *Stress* due to agitation, percussion, or pressure may damage certain sensitive drugs like enzymes. Thus,

---

*Davidson,[8] as a member of the *British Pharmacopoeia* Nomenclature Committee, suggested that drugs be registered by brand name and pointed out: "This registration would then entitle the manufacturers to a negotiated period of monopoly for the drug to enable them to recoup their research costs. This concession would be permitted upon the understanding that the brand name would also become the approved name. Thus, on the expiry of the monopoly period, no one would be allowed to market the drug under any other name."

---

†Placing the date of manufacture and an expiration date on the label of drug product and prescription packages is a meaningless act unless the contents are stored properly from time of manufacture to the time of administration of the medication. However, such dating provides valuable information and it should be clearly expressed as month, day, and year, not as a code number.

rapid stirring of some enzyme solutions or excessive pressure of tableting equipment can decrease potency. *Radiation* from some radioactive sources may affect potency since it can enhance oxidation, polymerization, decarboxylation, and other destructive reactions.[14]

In addition to the precautions previously mentioned, many medications include ingredients which tend to resist deteriorating influences. Thus antimicrobials, antioxidants, buffers, and other adjuncts are used in compounding drug products to stabilize the active ingredients (see *Preservatives,* page 000). Particular care must be exercised in selecting preservatives so that a hazard is not introduced through toxicity *per se.* Hypersensitivity to a number of them has been reported.

PROMOTION

Another aspect of distribution which occasionally presents hazards to patients is the manner of marketing medications. This activity, long a controversial subject, includes the use of professional journal advertising, detail men (24,000 professional representatives or salesmen in the US), direct mailings, displays, drug samples, medical information services, scientific exhibits and meetings, and the support of scholarships, fellowships, professional societies, and related efforts. Subsidy and support of professional societies and academic functions with no strings attached are admirable and valuable contributions, especially when small organizations and institutions need help. If the contributions are handled well, the pharmaceutical manufacturer can provide splendid educational services, especially through well-written literature, plant tours, scientific exhibits, and symposia. If handled ineptly, on the other hand, the company may provide biased, inaccurate, misleading, and unscientific information. Highly reputable firms are very careful not to do this but to provide sound services.

Nevertheless, the promotional activities of even a reputable pharmaceutical company, particularly at the time of introduction of a major new product with a high sales potential, are fascinating to observe. Advertising agencies are employed to spend literally millions of dollars to exploit every possible competitive marketing advantage.

One of the first steps is to analyze the current and future *competitive position* and important trends in the pertinent areas of the market. A concerted effort is made to develop a marketing rationale for the new product. What are its *outstanding points* to be emphasized? What are its weak points, to be obscured? What *key phrases* with potent sales impact can be created for use in the various types of promotional effort? Who are the primary *targets,* such as high volume prescribers. How will the sales pitch most effectively reach hospital formulary committees; hospital staffs, including interns, residents and nurses; influential physicians; medical school faculties; military medical officers; pharmacies; public health officers, and other key groups? What is the most appropriate *positioning* for the new medication in the marketplace? Scores of such questions are raised and answered in meticulous detail.

The coordination of the complex marketing effort is a wonder to behold. At every opportunity the promotion reinforces the *image* of the company. For physicians and other health professionals, it emphasizes sophisticated research and development competence, high integrity, and superior quality. For financial analysts, shareholders, and potential merger candidates, it portrays a bright future of growth and increasing wealth.

Carefully timed and beautifully coordinated programs are arranged to have the desired impact on each selected audience at precisely the predetermined time. Publication of clinical papers, presentations at scientific meetings, radio and television interviews with clinical investigators, press releases, indoctrination of detail men and creation of literature for them, preparation of brochures for commercial and scientific exhibits, publication of technical booklets for physicians, massive direct mailings of promotional literature, advertisements in selected medical and paramedical publications, development of special movies, filmstrips, programmed learning documents, speeches, and other communication devices, distribution of samples, catalog sheets, package inserts, compendia, personalized gifts such as scratch pads and imprinted pens, and many other items comprise the modern promotional approach.

The volume of information disseminated by these powerful promotional programs is truly tremendous. And therein lies the potential hazard to those who give and those who take the medication being launched. If the information is unbiased, well balanced, and completely accurate the medication will be used only when it is of value and it will be used correctly. If, on the other hand, the information imparted by high pressure techniques is slanted by improper selection of literature citations, or rendered incorrect because of faulty interpretation of research data, great harm can be done to everyone concerned. Unfortunately, much promotional material is written by journalists and drop-outs from biomedical courses who have acquired very little depth of understanding of the professional and scientific aspects of medication of the patient.

Many of the reputable manufacturers, however, have established medical communication departments with professionals highly trained in biomedical subjects and in communication techniques. These departments compile carefully documented, objective basic documents ("backgrounders") from intramural and extramural research reports generated by research scientists and clinical investigators. These medically oriented documents serve as the basis for the promotional literature prepared by the advertising agencies and by the promotional departments within the companies. After the promotional brochures and related materials have been prepared they are then checked by physicians within the companies before they are allowed to be released. With this type of double control at both the points of origin and release of promotional literature (although it often leads to feuding between conservative medical communicators and sales forces), compliance with government regulations and the caliber of promotional literature has improved significantly.

Promotional factors that are particularly pertinent to patient safety are the use of drug names and the caliber of advertising.

Use of Drug Names

The controversy on the use of brand names versus generic names has raged for many years, and politicians have used some of the verbal contests to their advantage. See *Drug Fallacies* on page 12.

Those who believe in brand names put forth many arguments.[8] The following are the most powerful:

1. The American system of trademark names for specific brands clearly identifies specific marketed products and thereby assures a definite level of reliability and quality.

2. The use of a brand name challenges the owner of that name to live up to its reputation of providing safe, effective, high quality medication.

3. The use of generic names when ordering medications permits any quality of drug product to be supplied, unless of course a reliable manufacturer is specified, which is tantamount to using a brand name.

4. The use of a brand name when prescribing a given medication reduces the hazards of misfilling the prescription and insures that the patient will receive a proper formulation of correct composition, particularly if the product contains more than one active ingredient. If, for example, the physician prescribes Darvon Compound-65, he is fully aware of what his patient should receive in terms of color and size of capsule and will quickly recognize any error in his patient's prescription.

Those who argue in favor of prescribing by generic names put forth the single major argument that the cost to the consumer may be lower. This is a potent and important consideration. However, this premise has been defended with sophistry on the part of people who know almost nothing about the problem. The inner functioning of pharmaceutical firms and the scientific, economic, and professional aspects of drug products themselves should be studied and understood by the proponents of generic prescribing before they take so simple a stand. The hazard of high cost is significant but cannot be equated with the compromising of patient safety and medication reliability.

The proponents of generic prescribing also imply that the generic (chemically) equivalent drug product is therapeutically equivalent. This is not necessarily true and in fact often is not. See page 19.

Legislators must learn the truth firsthand, otherwise they will never be on firm ground no matter which side of the controversy they have decided to take. They should implement this by personal inspection. By visiting a representative spectrum of drug manufacturers, they can correlate much more accurately costs, company image of dependability, and promotional needs including the caliber of advertising.

Caliber of Advertising

The more conservative manufacturers emphasize the educational and professional approaches to the promotion of their drug products. They do not use tactics such as the "blitzkrieg" whereby all salesmen are gathered from all over the country and concentrated on a comparatively small area for intensified high-pressure detailing of a new product to one selected group of physicians. Astute practitioners are not misled but are irritated by such high-pressure sales techniques. Medications, because of their hazards, should not be sold in the same manner as household appliances and other consumer products that do not directly affect health care.

Ideally, the pharmaceutical companies should distribute factual, informative, low-key, well-balanced advertising that avoids exaggeration of efficacy and minimizing of undesirable reactions and other hazards to the patient. They should avoid puffery. They should avoid bombarding and overwhelming busy physicians with a deluge of promotional material, and should make it very clear to the physician that simple reminder advertising must not be confused with carefully documented, well-written professional information. They should avoid slick, multiple-page journal advertisements. They should generally avoid nonprofessional use of gimmicks and enticers such as cocktail parties, golf outings, and uncalled-for gifts.

Advertising claims should be backed up with solid documentation. The *Medical Letter* (Issue No. 212, Feb. 24, 1967) illustrates how careful analysis of the literature of a manufacturer can sometimes show very poor selection for purposes of substantiating claims for a medication. Misleading use of citations can be legally and professionally dangerous for the manufacturer, physician, and patient.

Ultimately, however, it is the physician's responsibility to learn enough factual information about every drug product he uses so that he will prescribe it in the patient's best

interest. To do this, he must consult sources of information which he considers truly reliable, in addition to the promotional literature of the company.

Many physicians look forward to visits from selected detail men at definite visiting hours because these visitors are an important source of new information on drug products. These "reps" are developed into possessors of adequate and reliable information by the reputable companies. They are not trained merely as salesmen but also as dependable sources of drug information for the busy physician, particularly in areas where he has limited access to other sources.* The professional representatives have a major responsibility in safeguarding the patient from the hazards of faulty or incomplete information they may inadvertently implant in the mind of the physician. They must also exercise great care in the distribution of drug samples to keep them out of wrong channels, to prevent their abuse, and to prevent them from falling into the hands of children.

Pharmaceutical manufacturers have largely discontinued routine distribution of drug product samples to physicians and usually provide samples and complimentary stock packages for personal use only on request. Many factors contributed to this change in policy: (1) Sampling procedures bypass normal distribution channels, often cause samples to be received by persons who have no right to possess or use them, and are frequently wasteful. (2) Most physicians really do not want samples and accept them only as a matter of courtesy. (3) Samples often do not serve the useful purpose of starting a patient on a medication until a prescription can be filled or until Medicare and Medicaid can supply the drug because physicians divest themselves of accumulated samples by giving them all to one or two patients. The tolerance of a variety of patients to the drug in a sample cannot then be assessed. (4) Physicians are often faced with special storage, handling, and disposal problems arising when samples are sensitive or dangerous. (5)

---

* As sources of information, they do not attempt to be authorities on medical subjects. They simply supply appropriate literature and refer technical questions to the physicians in the medical advisory departments of their companies. New education and certification plans are being contemplated and may be implemented by 1980.

Hospitals are attempting to control the flow of all drugs and usually do not want samples interfering with their systems.[23] (6) Charitable and other organizations have collected drug samples for distribution through nonprofessional channels.

Through responsible representation of a pharmaceutical manufacturer, detail men can render valuable services to the physician by providing him with the latest prescribing and other information, including experience with adverse reactions and other hazards. Detail men can also render invaluable service to hospitals by providing the professional staffs with the latest drug information and answers to drug distribution problems.

DRUG DISTRIBUTION IN THE HOSPITAL

The hazards to the patient of incorrect dosage because of poor control of the distribution of medications in the hospital was greatly underestimated until about 1960. Some alert hospital administrators and a few physicians and their associates became alarmed at the frequency of medication errors. A vast array of publications on the subject appeared and a number of well-controlled, carefully planned studies were undertaken.[3-6, 16, 18, 20] The results of these studies were so alarming that hospitals of all sizes and in every region began to evaluate the accuracy of their own medication systems and make necessary revisions.

One multidisciplinary research group, subsidized by the US Public Health Service, designed an experimental medication system to reduce the frequency of medication errors at the University of Arkansas Medical Center Hospital. At this teaching hospital with more than 300 beds the system was installed and evaluated during selected periods of 1964 and 1965. Its features included (1) complete centralization within the hospital pharmacy of storage, control, and the preparation for administration of all medications given to patients, (2) editing of every medication order by a pharmacist before it was put into effect, (3) dispensing of all medications in unit-dose form from the pharmacy to the nurse at the time each dose was scheduled to be given to the patient, and (4) automatic handling and checking of all drug records throughout the hospital by remote control from the pharmacy with the aid of electronic data processing and teletype equipment.

Before the system was installed, 31.2% of all doses of medication administered by the nurses were in error. Because of inadequate knowledge of drugs, nurses were repeatedly administering such products as Amphojel, Gelusil, and Maalox interchangeably. Upon close observation they were found to be giving medications by the wrong route, selecting the wrong drug or the wrong dosage form, giving extra doses, omitting doses, injecting IV solutions too fast, misidentifying patients, discontinuing a drug without authorization, and making other errors. About 13% of the errors were due to incorrect timing, more than 5% to incorrect selection of brand of drug product, and 13% to 28 other miscellaneous acts. Nearly half of these miscellaneous acts consisted of mismeasurement, miscalculation, miscounting, or wrong selection and use of medications by the nurses.

After installation of the experimental system, the total error rate dropped from 31.2% to 13.4%, and if errors due to timing and brand selection were deleted, the rate dropped sharply to 1.9%. A great deal of the credit for improvement in medication error rates in hospitals is due those who introduced unit-dose systems (see page 79). But funds are not always available to implement new systems, regardless of how efficient and how urgently needed they may be.

Unfortunately, too, many hospitals are still without the full-time services of a pharmacist. When so many hospitals have inadequate personnel and budgets it is not surprising that drug distribution in them leaves much to be desired.[42]

ILLEGAL DISTRIBUTION

More than 10 billion doses of sedative drugs has been estimated to be the total annual output for the United States. This is the equivalent of about 50 doses for every man, woman, and child in the country. And, much of this supply is in the illicit markets.

In spite of all the efforts of hundreds of thousands of well-motivated scientific and professional personnel who try to provide patients with effective medications, these efforts are occasionally thwarted by a few unethical individuals who engage in such unworthy activities as counterfeiting, substitution, repackaging of outdated or stolen medications and drug samples, and black-marketing of dangerous drugs.

Counterfeiting

Although each manufacturer takes every possible precaution to protect his trademarks and to verify the authenticity of his products in the marketplace in order to protect the patient, he is not always completely successful. Skilled counterfeiters periodically steal dies, plates and other devices, or surreptitiously procure facsimiles of the authentic ones and then proceed to manufacture tablets and other dosage forms that appear like the authentic products in every respect and label them with counterfeit labels. Some of these spurious products are especially hazardous because they may not contain the proper ingredients. In fact, they may contain none of the active ingredient at all. But even if they do, they are not controlled as to identity, purity, potency, or quality. Nobody can know what activity they may have because they are not tested. They undergo no quality control.

Because counterfeiting is a particularly vicious practice and is so extremely hazardous to the patient, some manufacturers now place trace substances in their dosage forms. This enables them to identify their own products and to detect fakes rapidly. Counterfeit medications are also uncovered by means of chemical analyses to determine types and quantities of active ingredients, excipients, and other adjuncts; by microscopic examination of crystal structure; by examination of the characteristic markings from manufacturing equipment; and other techniques.

Substitution

A potentially hazardous, highly unethical practice is substitution of a cheaper, lower quality medication for a high quality one specified or intended by a prescribing physician. Although this happens only occasionally, nevertheless the practice can be so detrimental to the patient's welfare that every effort must be made to root out any person who disgraces himself and his profession in this manner for commercial gain.

Attempts are constantly being made, for economic reasons, to repeal antisubstitution state laws and to achieve legal authorization for substitution of one brand of drug product for another when a prescription is being filled. Although some states have now legalized substitution of generic for brand name products unrestricted substitution can be hazardous for some patients. Because each manufacturer formulates a given drug product differently, the excipients, binders, and other adjuvants as well as the characteristics of the drug itself often vary considerably from one brand to another. Therefore, to patients with allergies, metabolic deficiencies, and special problems of absorption, distribution, and excretion, the brand of product can be a crucial factor in providing safe and effective therapy. When the physician discovers that a specific brand of a medication is well tolerated by a given patient, he wants that one only to be dispensed when he orders it for that patient. The problem of therapeutic equivalency, discussed in Chapter 2, is also a major consideration. The average pharmacist is usually not in a position to make equivalency judgments.[26] Neither is the average physician.

The hazards of substituting similar medication for that prescribed are not always readily appreciated or apparent. Thus, pharmacists have sometimes substituted pilocarpine for atropine in filling prescriptions for eye drops. This does not cause any harm, but the reverse situation can be devastating to the eyes.[27]

Those who urge legislation to permit unrestricted substitution do not understand the hazards involved in not providing the patient with the exact medication ordered, and in removing control of the prescription from the physician who wrote it and placing that control in the hands of the pharmacist. It may become necessary for every physician to tell his patient the brand name of the medication prescribed and to require the pharmacist to label the prescription with that name. Then, any dispenser who substituted would be in the illegal position of mislabeling. Another alternative would be for the physician to dispense his own prescriptions.

A practice closely related to substitution is to collect drug samples that have been distributed to local physicians for promotional purposes and to use them in filling prescriptions.* Not only is it unethical to charge for medication that has been distributed gratis, but unless the expiration date is placed on the samples and they have been stored carefully, the medication may become substandard.

Substitution is somewhat related to prescribing generically without specifying one or several manufacturers. To illustrate by means of personal experience, the author had a prescription filled in a neighborhood pharmacy where he was not known. The prescription called for an antibiotic for a member of his family. After he had paid for the medication, he removed the wrapper and discovered that the product was not the usual well-known brand. He therefore inquired who the manufacturer was and was shown the label of a manufacturer noted for cheap drug products. He then requested that the prescription be filled with the well-known dependable brand. This was done, and the charge *remained the same.*

Another situation occasionally arises that affects tens of thousands of patients. Major cities have bought antibiotics and other medications in very large quantities for the city hospitals, strictly on the basis of price, then have later discovered that the product purchased was substandard. Not only were the expenditures wasted, but indigent and other patients, all of whom are entitled to an adequate quality of medical care, were deprived of proper therapy.

Of course, substitution when properly controlled by hospital policy or by means of specific instructions of a prescriber is accepted by many physicians and hospitals as proper procedure. Some hospital prescription forms now carry a box, which if checked permits substitution of an equivalent medication. The main criterion must always be, however, that the patient is not given lower quality medication if substitution is permitted. This can be achieved only if the hospital pharmacy or the community pharmacy purchases drug products from sources whose quality control is dependable.[43]

Repackaging

The act of buying drugs in bulk from a reputable manufacturer and repackaging and relabeling them with a generic or trademark name is a recognized and respectable enterprise if conducted ehtically and in accordance with Federal and state laws and regulations. On the other hand the practice is reprehensible and dangerous for the patient if stolen or low quality drug products or old samples are repackaged and distributed through this mechanism. It becomes particularly dangerous when there is incorrect packaging and labeling or deteriorated drugs are placed in new packages.

In addition to the possible medical hazards, there are certain economic and ethical considerations which can be detrimental to the patient. Because of the current system of marketing, repackaged drugs often cost the patient many times what he would normally pay for the original brand and at the same time are much more lucrative for the purveyor. But aside from the unfair economics of the practice, particularly questionable are the physician-owned repackaging companies (see page 119). One estimate claims that about 5,000 physicians participate in about 150 of these companies in the United States.[13] This situation creates the great temptation for a physician who is a member both of one of these companies and of a hospital staff to influence the pharmacist to purchase from the repackaging company. Conflict of interests is obvious and the patient is the one who suffers because he does not receive the highest quality medication at lowest possible cost.

These hazards can be minimized if both physicians and pharmacists are meticulous in selecting their source of medications, and particularly in avoiding the black market.

Black-Marketing of Dangerous Drugs

Functioning under strict laws such as the 1970 Controlled Substances Act, which was implemented by regulations that became effective Feb. 14, 1971, the Drug Enforcement Agency (DEA) attempts to control the illegal

---

*This is sometimes done in the name of a charitable or religious organization by personnel not versed in the official requirements for handling, storage, and control.

distribution of depressant, stimulant, and other hazardous drugs.[47] The agency makes every effort to keep amphetamines, barbiturates, narcotics and other potentially dangerous drugs listed in its *Comprehensive List of Controlled Drugs* out of the black market and in proper medical channels to protect consumers from the hazards of improper use. This is extremely difficult in the face of the worldwide problems of drug abuse. The degrading effects of habitual use of lysergic acid diethylamide (LSD), heroin, and numerous other central nervous system agents have been well documented and have created deep concern for the future of our society.

Such drugs have been brought under better control through recent legislation which requires increased record keeping, authorizes official inspection of the drug distribution system, and makes possession of these drugs illegal except under certain specified conditions of medical distribution and use. The law provides, in addition to the usual prescription record keeping requirements, that no prescription for a controlled drug can be refilled more than five times, or dispensed more than six months after the date it is written, under any circumstances. Specific renewal instructions must be given by the prescriber.[47]

The Agency has not always been successful in attaining full control of these drugs. Occasionally dishonest employees of pharmaceutical companies have diverted shipments of these drugs. Sometimes these dangerous drugs have been unwittingly shipped to false addresses. Or they have been hijacked. Or they are manufactured surreptitiously. Many ways have been found by racketeers, addicts, and pushers to obtain supplies.

Proper control of the distribution of such medications at the local, state, and Federal levels had been thwarted by loopholes. For example, on Nov 1, 1969, the Agency regulations concerning exempt narcotics (Class X drugs) went into effect. In accordance with these regulations, only a registered pharmacist is now permitted to dispense these products and he must demand suitable identification, record the date, patient's name and address, time, and the name and amount of the drug purchased, and he must check back to determine whether the purchaser has purchased any Class X drug within the past 48 hours. If for any reason the pharmacist is suspicious, he is supposed to ask the purchaser how he intends to use the drug, and if doubts remain, he should refuse to sell it, even though all legal requirements are met. But there is little or no control over the customer who goes to one pharmacy after another and purchases exempt narcotics in each. It is hoped that with more stringent record keeping, reporting and inspection throughout the distribution system, illicit use will become negligible.

Elimination of illegal distribution of medications can never be completely achieved, however; dishonesty, racketeering, and the desire to prey on those who are ignorant and ill will always be present to some extent in our society. The best approach appears to be rigid control over all stages of the distribution of controlled drugs and other hazardous medications from the moment they are manufactured to the time they are prescribed by the physician and taken by the patient.

SELECTED REFERENCES

1. American Pharmaceutical Association: *The National Formulary XIV.* Easton, PA Mack Publishing, 1975.
2. American Society of Hospital Pharmacists: Guidelines for single-unit package of drugs. *Am J Hosp Pharm* 24:79 (Feb) 1967.
3. Barker KN: Pediadose. *Am J Hosp Pharm* 27:132–135, 1970.
4. ———: The effects of an experimental medication system on medication errors and costs. *Am J Hosp Pharm* 26:324–333 (June) 1969.
5. Barker KN, Kimbrough W, Heller W: The medication error problem in hospitals. *Hosp Form Management* 1:29 (Feb); 36 (Mar) 1966.
6. Bohl JC, McLean WM, Meyer F, Phillips GL, Scott WV, Thudium VF: The medication system. *Am J Hosp Pharm* 26:316–317 (June) 1969.
7. Brauninger JC: Unit dose—A marketing report. *Bull Parent Drug Assoc* 23:243–244 (Sep-Oct) 1969.
8. Davidson JO: Brand names controversy. *Pharm J* 199:548 (Nov 25) 1967.
9. Drugs for nursing homes: new system said to minimize errors. *Drug Topics* (Oct 27) 1969.
10. Durant WJ: Unit dose packaging—user requirements and practices. *Bull Parent Drug Assoc* 23:237–243, 1969.
11. *Fed Reg* 33:3217–3218 (Feb 21) 1968.
12. *Fed Reg* 33:10283 (July 18) 1968; *Fed Reg* (Mar 6) 1969.
13. Hassan WE: Physician-owned repackaging companies. *Drug Topics* 28: (Oct 13) 1969.

14. Martin EW: *Dispensing of Medication.* Easton, Pa., Mack Publishing, 1971.

15. Martin EW: *Techniques of Medication.* Philadelphia, Lippincott, 1969.

16. Meyers RM: Centralized unit dose system in a community hospital. *Lippincott's Hosp Pharm* 5:6-11 (Feb) 1970.

17. Pharmaceutical Manufacturers Association: *Newsletter* 12:3 (Mar 27) 1970.

18. Single unit packaging and the unit-dose system. *Am J Hosp Pharm* 27:113, 1970.

19. Taussig HB: The evils of camouflage as illustrated by thalidomide. *N Engl J Med* 269:92-94, 1963.

20. Turco S: One hospital's approach to unit dose packaging: a review of currently available methods. *Lippincott's Hosp Pharm* 5:12-22 (Feb) 1970.

21. United States Pharmacopeial Convention,: *The United States Pharmacopeia XIX.* Easton, PA, Mack Publishing, 1975.

22. US Department of Health, Education, and Welfare: *The Drug Makers and the Drug Distributors,* Washington, DC, Task Force on Prescription Drugs, 1969.

23. Why Roche stopped routine MD sampling. *Am Drug* 161:32 (Jan 12) 1970.

24. Billups NF: *American Drug Index.* Philadelphia, Lippincott, 1977.

25. Compound names for drugs. *Drug Ther Bull* 8:9-10 (Jan 30) 1970.

26. Editorial: Repeal of antisubstitution laws. *Drug Intell Clin Pharm* 4:115 (May) 1970.

27. Smith HE: Warning from ophthalmologist. *Utah Digest* p. 12 (Nov) 1969.

28. Anderson BJ: Package inserts as evidence. *Law and Medicine. JAMA* 208:589-590 (Apr 21) 1969.

29. *Salgo* vs *Leland Stanford, Jr., University Board of Trustees,* 317 P 2d 170, 1957.

30. *Sanzari vs Rosenfeld,* 167 A 2d 625, 1961.

31. *Koury vs Follo* (158 SE 2d 548, 1968).

32. AMA Council on Drugs: Notes on the package insert. *JAMA* 207:1335-1338 (Feb 17) 1969.

33. Editorial: The package insert. *JAMA* 207:1342 (Feb 17) 1969.

34. Unfug HV: Nonapproved uses of FDA-approved drugs. *Questions and Answers, JAMA* 211:1705 (Mar 9) 1970.

35. Anderson BJ: Discussion of question from Unfug. *Questions and Answers, JAMA* 211:1705 (Mar 9) 1970.

36. Hayes TH: Discussion of question from Unfug. *Questions and Answers, JAMA* 211:1705 (Mar 9) 1970.

37. Simmons HE: Investigational exemption procedure for new drugs. *Letters, JAMA* 213:1902 (Sep 14) 1970.

38. AMA Department of Drugs: Investigational exemption procedure for new drugs. *Letters, JAMA* 213:1902-1904 (Sep 14) 1970.

39. Committee on Drugs, American Academy of Pediatrics: "Therapeutic orphans" and the package insert. *Pediat.* 46:811-813 (Nov) 1970.

40. Belton EDeV: The package insert—our final product. Paper presented before the University of Wisconsin IND-NDA Conference, Milwaukee, Wisconsin, Oct 4-7, 1970.

41. Mills DH: Physician responsibility for drug prescription. *JAMA* 192:460-463 (May 10) 1965.

42. ———: Physicians and drug brochures. *Penn Med* 64-67 (Feb) 1969.

43. Board of Trustees, American Pharmaceutical Association: A white paper on the pharmacist's role in product selection. *JAPhA* NS11:181-199 (April) 1971. An overview of the antisubstitution laws and the American Pharmaceutical Association's advocacy of their amendment relative to drug product selection.

44. Losee GJ, and Altenderfer ME: *Health Manpower in Hospitals.* Washington, DC, Division of Manpower Intelligence, Bureau of Health Manpower Education, National Institutes of Health, US Department of Health, Education, and Welfare, 1970.

45. *Proceedings* of Joint DIA/FDA/AMA/PMA Symposium on Drug Information for Patients—The Patient Package Insert. *Drug Info Bull* 11:51-5 (Jan-Mar Suppl) 1977.

46. *Factbook 77.* Pharmaceutical Manufacturers Association, Washington, DC, 1977.

47. Regulations Implementing the Comprehensive Drug Abuse and Control Act of 1970. *Fed Reg* 36:4928-66 (Mar 13) 1971.

48. FDA/HEW: Use of drugs for unapproved indications: your legal responsibility. *FDA Drug Bull* (Oct) 1972.

49. FDA/HEW: Legal status of approved labeling for prescription drugs; prescribing for uses unapproved by the Food and Drug Administration. *Fed Reg* 37:16503-5 (Aug 15) 1972.

50. FDA/HEW: Labeling for prescription drugs used in man. Proposed format for prescription drug advertisements. *Fed Reg* 40:15392-9 (Apr 7) 1975.

51. Allan FN: The problem of multiple names for drugs, in *Use and Misuse of Antimicrobial Drugs.* CENTO, Ankara, Turkey, 1976.

52. Hirsh HL: Patient package insert. *Lawyers' Med J* 6 2d(3): 227-37 (Nov) 1977.

6 Prescribing Factors

A well-written prescription is tangible evidence of the physician's professional competence and when written and given to the patient in the proper manner is highly reassuring and thereby partially therapeutic in itself. Even if the prescription is not written but is telephoned to a pharmacy, the medication that results from the act of prescribing can have a salutary psychological impact on the patient if it is labeled and packaged in a suitable manner.

Ideally, a prescription is the end point of astute diagnosis and thoughtful selection of the best medication available for the condition diagnosed. Occasionally a tentative diagnosis is made over the telephone. Time and distance, or economic and work circumstances, or home and family responsibilities often make it impossible and impractical for a physician to see every patient each time before prescribing. In some instances, prescribing by telephone is unavoidable and very often the physician is thoroughly familiar with the patient's medical history. It is then quite feasible to prescribe or renew a prescription by this means intelligently, effectively, and safely.

However, it can be very hazardous for a physician to diagnose and prescribe by telephone when he is attempting to treat an individual who is unknown to him, or one who has a new and different medical condition even though he has treated him previously for an unrelated problem.

The patient, as well as the physician, must recognize the hazards of diagnosis and prescribing at a distance when the physician is not familiar with existing problems that can result in serious adverse reactions to drug therapy. The public must recognize and understand this situation and not be annoyed or alienated by the physician who is reluctant to prescribe in an unfamiliar setting. In most instances the physician should carefully examine the patient before prescribing any medication. And, after selecting the appropriate medication, he should give both verbal and written directions to the patient to make certain that dosage instructions are accurately and clearly communicated. [20,72]

Proper prescribing technique enhances the efficacy and safety of medications. Major considerations are correct evaluation of the patient, avoidance of errors in clinical laboratory testing, careful analysis of disease and patient characteristics, proper informing of the patient, rational selection of suitable medication, careful writing of the prescription, proper dispensing and administration of the medication, and appropriate monitoring of the patient during and in some instances subsequent to the course of medication.

The physician who prescribes a highly toxic drug like methotrexate and then goes on vacation without arranging for careful monitoring of the patient should not be surprised to learn on his return that his patient has died. One physician who did that lost a $600,000 malpractice suit. The hazards of not following a patient closely enough are particularly serious if he or she has suicidal intentions. Teitelbaum and Ott described a fourth attempt at suicide by injection of a syringeful of elemental mercury (17.75 Gm.). Debridement and the drainage of a sterile abscess reduced the size of the depot and chelation therapy with BAL and penicillamine controlled serum mercury levels. But follow-up was impossible because the patient upon discharge successfully committed suicide in his fifth attempt by placing a plastic bag over his head. [82]

EVALUATING PATIENTS

The first step in treating a patient is to evaluate him properly. What is the problem presented by this particular patient with his own unique set of characteristics, signs, and symptoms? What are his inherited weaknesses? What are his rare phenotypical traits? His allergies? His anomalies? What drugs are safe for him to take?

The physician, calling upon his knowledge and experience, delves into the patient's history, examines him physically, and determines what laboratory tests and other ancillary examinations are also appropriate to establish his diagnosis. In difficult problems he may require expert consultation or he may refer the patient to a specialist. But he never gives advice or treatment or prescribes medication without first making a careful diagnosis, for he is fully aware that selecting medication for any patient without adequate insight is fraught with many pitfalls.

Approaching the Patient

Before he can safely prescribe, the physician must carefully determine through adroit questioning not only the disease present but also the patient's activities, deficiencies, and environment. Important factors such as pregnancy, psychological state, and pertinent contraindications must be detected. How the physician approaches his patient may be critical. The subject of kinesics, the psychological impact of the physician's facial expression, manner, and his movements in general, is receiving increasing attention. One editorial [11] pointed out:

"Although therapy is ordinarily thought of as deriving from symptom analysis and diagnosis, as indeed it should when it is to be specific, there is more to it than that. In their first contact, by the nature of the physician's manner and manners, the patient may obtain reassurance, which is beneficial, or little reassurance, which is hurtful."

The influence that unspoken feelings such as anger, anxiety, guilt, and helplessness on the part of physicians can have upon a patient is dramatically emphasized by the case history of a 10-year-old boy who underwent quadruple amputation and who attempted suicide after removal of his last remaining extremity. A highly stressful situation and a breakdown in communications, arising from constant interservice discord among attending and house staff concerning the amputations, delayed provision of proper attention and reassurance for the patient for several days and resulted in deep depression. The boy's feeling of abandonment was so deep that he refused to eat, pulled out his intravenous tubing, and threw himself from his bed in an attempt to land on his head so "I can die." Resnik points out: "What the physician says or omits, what he masks or lets appear upon his face, what inflection he chooses— these signals can be perceived by patients. . . . We should remember how sensitive to our own conflicts are our patients and often, how narrow is the margin by which we are therapuetic." [88]

By presenting an attitude and an image that inspire confidence, his sincere interest in his patient becomes readily apparent. Most physicians do not realize that they function simultaneously as medical doctors and psychiatrists. Goldfarb says that "an error . . . physicians slip into is to become so preoccupied with physical and laboratory diagnosis and pharmacologic or physical therapy as to miss the extraordinary helpfulness of the word or gesture." The psychological aspects of prescribing are often very important in obtaining a suitable patient response. [4, 11, 80]

Some physicians are beginning to appreciate the impact of religion on the outcome of therapy. A new medical school being completed in 1978 is built on the belief that "prayer puts the person who needs healing in position to be healed." One surgeon engenders a cooperative attitude in emergency situations by asking seriously injured patients to pray for him to perform a successful operation. [104]

Because of the sensitive physician-patient relationship, a patient may be psychologically traumatized by a physician's chance remark even when the patient is anesthetized. A physician who underwent surgery to correct a broken nose suffered excruciating pain and developed severe headaches over a ten-year period whenever he inhaled air through his nose. During the operation the surgeon had said: "Whenever air is inhaled, he'll have sharp pains and severe headaches." Hypnotherapy resolved this particular situation. But many other patients have also reacted adversely after recovery from anesthesia when surgeons have said things during the operations that could be construed to be derogatory or have acted in a manner that was considered to be objectionable. Anesthesia may not block out hearing, and subliminal impacts can be very strong in patients whether they are in coma or wide awake once a deep physician-patient relationship is established. [78]

The Multiple Therapy Problem

Once the physician has made good contact with his patient, some of the most important questions that he can ask and ones that are easily overlooked are concerned with both prescription and over-the-counter drug products being taken concomitantly.

Which medications have you taken recently?

Which medications are you now taking?

Are any other physicians treating you?

Are you allergic or sensitive to any drugs or foods?

Even though a busy practitioner sees many patients a day, he must nevertheless take time to obtain the answers to every important and relevant question, otherwise he may be deemed professionally and legally negligent and may possibly be forced to defend himself against a malpractice lawsuit. [1,5] Only by being acutely aware of what drugs are in the patient's body and only by making certain that his prescription will not conflict with concomitant therapy provided by a colleague or with self-administered medication can the physician safely provide his patient with effective drug therapy. Physicians often overlook interactions between prescribed medications and the readily available and frequently used nonprescription medications such as cough syrups, sedatives, laxatives, and remedies used to palliate the common cold (containing analgesics, antihistamines,

sympathomimetics, exempt narcotics, etc.). Physicians are also sometimes placed in an impossible situation when drugs are not immediately and correctly recorded on the patient's medical record. Only when the physician has a complete drug profile on his patient can he safely prescribe.

Self-medication with over-the-counter products, many of which are combinations of drugs, severely complicates the physician's prescribing problem. Of the nonprescription drug products listed in the National Drug Code Directory, fifty percent are combinations, twenty percent contain five or more active ingredients, and some contain ten or more.

Typical of the multiple therapy problem is that of a female patient, age 35, who required hospitalization when she developed cardiac insufficiency from the following drug regimen.

One physician prescribed ethchlorvynol (Placidyl) 500 mg. and chlorprothixene (Taractan) 100 mg. The patient then saw another physician who, unaware that she was taking these medications, also prescribed Placidyl 500 mg. sodium pentobarbital (Nembutal) 100 mg. and tranylcypromine (Parnate) 10 mg. A few months later she saw a third physician who prescribed thioridazine (Mellaril) 10 mg. and Nembutal 100 mg. At the same time she revisited one of her other physicians and he prescribed glutethimide (Doriden) 0.5 Gm., Placidyl 500 mg., and Nembutal 100 mg. She also visited still another physician at the same time and was given imipramine hydrochloride (Tofranil) 25 mg. Later she received prescriptions for 40 Taractan 25 mg., 15 Placidyl 500 mg., and 50 meprobamate (Equanil) 400 mg. Refills for the prescriptions were authorized often enough so that within a little over 2 weeks she had in her possession 160 Taractan 25 mg., within a month 90 Placidyl 500 mg., and within 70 days 450 Equanil 400 mg.

When she was hospitalized, the patient was treated for her drug-induced cardiac insufficiency with another drug, digitoxin 0.2 mg. [15]

Some large medical centers, such as the Los Angeles County-University of Southern California Medical Center with 700 full-time physicians, have computerized their prescriptions to evaluate prescribing practices and avoid inappropriate prescriptions. At the LA—USC center a committee of five physicians and two pharmacists concluded that the following situations resulted in inappropriate prescriptions: (1) inappropriate quantities of drugs by single prescription, (2) inappropriate amounts of individual drugs in the possession of patients as a result of multiple prescriptions, and (3) inappropriate concurrent prescriptions. Computer analysis pinpoints such abuses and hazards. Thus one patient, who was found to have received more than 100 prescriptions for tranquilizers and hypnotics in a nine-month period, had apparently been authorized to receive 1,130 chlorpromazine hydrochloride spansules 50 mg., 2,018 trifluoperazine tablets 10 mg., and 661 amobarbital sodium capsules 200 mg.[32] Computer applications in medical centers are being developed to check on prescription refill programs (refill eligibility, maximum amounts that may be prescribed, inappropriate concurrent prescriptions) and to recall drug information (data on dosage forms, therapeutic indications, warnings on toxicity, and previously encountered adverse drug reactions).

In obtaining such data, physicians who practice medicine and hospitals which have service functions encounter gray areas of responsibility. These must be resolved in each specific situation to achieve optimal prevention of drug abuse, interactions, and reactions through efficient analysis of disease and patient history.[38,44]

Analysis of Disease and Patient

After the physician learns his patient's drug history, he must utilize his own judgment based on his knowledge and experience because every patient presents a unique combination of biochemical, physiological, and psychological characteristics. Every patient is a delicately balanced, highly sensitive, complex organism which is often strongly affected by congenital, emotional, environmental, and hereditary factors. Accordingly, medication must be individualized. Fortunately, this is not as difficult as it appears. Patient response, being a biological phenomenon, is not very precise. Rather wide ranges in the dosage of most medications will achieve the desired effect. With only a comparatively few drugs is it necessary to titrate and gradually adjust a critical dosage until it meets the requirements of a specific patient. This is done, for example, with certain anti-

coagulant, anticonvulsant, antineoplastic, cardiovascular, hypoglycemic, and muscle relaxant agents. But whether the dosage of a given medication is critical or not, adequate analysis of both the disease and the patient is essential since the response of a patient to his medication is basically governed by the nature of his disease and his own inherent characteristics.

DISEASE CHARACTERISTICS

The extent of a diagnostic work-up, as was pointed out on page 99, depends on the judgment of the physician. He takes into consideration the appearance of the patient, his temperament, history, environment, probable seriousness of the condition, and many other components. The thoroughness of the analysis depends to a large extent on the etiology and how difficult it is to determine.

Etiology

Determination of the cause of a disease is basic to rational drug therapy. The hazards to the patient are very real in many situations of undetermined or incorrectly identified etiologic agents. Many examples can be given. If certain strains of streptococci which are causing an infection are not identified and the drug therapy which is prescribed is not adequate, rheumatic fever or glomerulonephritis may develop. If a malignancy is not detected early, a patient may unnecessarily lose his life. If a husband harbors the organisms responsible for his wife's trichomoniasis, no amount of therapy will cure her until he is treated also. A patient with quiescent tuberculosis, if not identified as such and if treated with corticosteroids or live virus vaccines, may experience a serious exacerbation of the disease.

If the etiologic agent for a disease is a microorganism, it is often desirable to characterize it fully. Its sensitivity to various antimicrobial agents, for example, is useful information, for it enables the physician to attack the organism more specifically. When he combines this type of knowledge with critical analysis of his patient, he avoids many pitfalls. The hazards associated with inadequate identification of etiologic agents are numerous and are intimately associated with patient characteristics.

PATIENT CHARACTERISTICS

The patient as a whole must be understood if he is to be treated effectively and rationally.[4] In the following sections are discussed the more important patient characteristics which influence patient safety and upon which the physician bases his judgments when selecting medication and specifying the *individual effective dose*. The characteristics are discussed in the following order: age, environment, heredity, sex, temperament, weight, and history.

Age

The three major age groups of patients, (young children, older children and adults, and the elderly) often react differently to some drugs and require different dosages. On a weight basis, young children and the elderly often require lower doses of a number of medications such as central nervous system agents, hormones, narcotics, sulfonamides, and those that affect fluid and electrolyte balance, because of greater sensitivity or lower tolerance. In the young, some medications have dramatic effects on normal development. A very young girl, for example, may be caused to menstruate years before she normally should if medication she takes is contaminated with an estrogenic hormone. Some hormones can greatly affect the development of children. On the other hand, the young can be highly resistant to some drugs and require comparatively higher doses. Infants appear to be able to tolerate higher doses of convulsant drugs per unit of body weight than adults, and as a matter of interest, since it is related, they can withstand more severe electrical shocks than adults. In general, young children require relatively larger doses than adults of drugs affecting the undeveloped higher cortical centers.

Toxic effects which are accentuated or found only during the perinatal period and early infancy may result from (1) *immature enzyme processes* which do not act on the drug like the mature processes of the adult, (2) *different disposition of the drug* by the body, e.g., different absorption, distribution,

metabolism, detoxification, and excretion patterns, (3) *differences in response of cells and organs* to the drug, e.g., sensitives inherent in the immature tissues, (4) *drug-induced alteration of biochemical distribution,* e.g., altered distribution of substances originating in the body, such as bilirubin, enzymes, and hormones, and (5) *drug-induced alteration of developmental processes,* e.g., bone, hematopoietic, and emotional development.[24]

The effects of immature enzyme systems have been studied mostly in animals. However, some enzymes have been studied extensively in man. Cholinesterase at birth is at a low level. For this reason procaine and related local anesthetics, succinylcholine, and other esters cannot be handled as well by the young as by adults. The enzyme reaches its maximum levels at puberty and these then decrease with advancing age. Levels are lower in females. The levels increase with increasing body weight and thickness of subcutaneous fat. They are also higher after a meal and in nephrosis.[79]

The following results are worth considering when infants and young children are being medicated. Methemoglobinemia is readily produced by nitrites and by anesthetics related to procaine when there is a deficiency of methemoglobin reductase and diaphorase in erythrocytes. Hypoprothrombinemia is readily induced by coumarin derivatives and other drugs that inhibit prothrombin formation in the presence of a prothrombin deficiency. Hemolysis occurs with synthetic vitamin K substitutes and some quinones when there is a deficiency of glutathione (reduced state) in erythrocytes. Jaundice is readily induced when chloramphenicol, novobiocin, streptomycin, and sulfonamides compete for metabolic and serum protein binding pathways if there is a deficiency of bilirubin conjugating enzymes. Many other examples of serious conditions resulting from inadequate enzyme activity have been reported in animals or man. They should sound a warning to pediatricians. See Enzyme Deficiencies in Chapter 8.

The effects of drug-induced alteration of the distribution of substances in the body may also be deterimental in the neonate. Thus novobiocin, salicylates, sulfadimethoxine, and sulfisoxazole displace bilirubin from its albumin-bound form causing it to cross the blood-brain barrier and produce kernicterus. See Chapter 8.

Patients from the geriatric population that now numbers about 25 million in the United States, more than 10 percent of the total population, also require special consideration when they are being evaluated and when medications are being selected for them. Aging brings about alterations in the blood, endocrine and nervous systems, number and structure of cells, vasculature, and tissues in general. Mutations may produce antigenic protein or faulty lymphoid cells and this may result in autoimmune diseases. If mutations disrupt cell division, uncontrolled growth (cancer) may be induced. Circulation, metabolism, and other physiological functions may be disrupted.[77] The glomerular filtration rate is often appreciably decreased and the half-life of digoxin, kanamycin, and other drugs may be more than doubled, even though serum creatinine levels remain normal because of diminished production.[101]

Because of these changes due to aging, the potential hazards of some drugs is much greater for geriatric patients. Thus, the elderly are particulary susceptible to bleeding episodes after IV administration of heparin. In women over age 60, there is a 50% risk of bleeding, whereas in women under 60 the risk drops to 14%. In men, the increased risk is 19% and 10% respectively. Bleeding into the hip and groin occurred with unusual frequency in one group of elderly women described by Vieweg *et al.* Contributing factors however, may have been congestive heart failure and gluteal injections of various drugs, including digoxin, meperidine hydrochloride, and morphine sulfate.[89,90] Some potent drugs like phenylbutazone should be avoided completely in the senile patient. Other drugs like benzodiazepines (Librium and Valium) and tolbutamide (Orinase) must be administered with care because the elderly are particularly sensitive to them.

Potential hazards exist when the geriatric patient may possibly over-react, under-react, or respond abnormally to medication because of alterations in their psyche or soma. Extensive infiltration of connective tissue with advancing age, for example, decreases total viability or reactivity of the body mass and therefore necessitates a corresponding reduction in drug dosage.[85] But the literature is far from being in agreement on the changes in response to drugs that take place with aging.[86]

Emotional response may also be abnormal and associated with decreased ability to be attentive, and to comprehend, perceive, remember, and respond. Impaired attitudes and intellectual capacity to receive and act upon medical information and specific directions may create serious problems. Custodial care may be necessary to prevent abuse or misuse of prescribed medications. Such care may be mandatory where poor morale, low socioeconomic levels, mental illness, and faulty ethnic and religious values are adversely influencing good adjustment to aging.

A conservative approach to prescribing for the elderly patient must be maintained until his interactions with his medication, other human beings, and the environment have been carefully evaluated.

Environment

Many conditions of the patient can be traced to environmental factors, including those that are associated with particular seasons, residential or work areas, modes of transportation, diet, clothing, or contact with specific animal, human, mineral, or vegetable substances. Allergies and respiratory distress can be associated with dusts, feathers, hairs, plants, pollens, pollutants, and other allergens in the atmosphere and in the home and work areas. Systemic, dermal, gastrointestinal, and respiratory conditions are caused by contact with food and water constituents and contaminants, household products, pesticides, and other chemicals. The type of work and recreation govern contact with all the above as well as many other items. Any change in the location and environment must therefore be noted promptly.

Medication hazards may arise if chemicals in the environment interact with medications used in or on the body. These chemicals may also exacerbate conditions caused by any of the environmental factors that affect the body. The effects of medications may be markedly altered if the physiological equilibrium is unbalanced by altitude, cold, heat, humidity, sunlight, vibrations, and other stresses. Electrolyte imbalance, hypervolemia, hypovolemia, phototoxic reactions, and many other undesirable situations can arise, sometimes suddenly and unexpectedly, as a result of environmental influences.

Heredity

Susceptibility to some medications varies from one race to another. Chinese and Negroes are less susceptible than Europeans to the mydriatic effect of cocaine, ephedrine, and certain other drugs.[71] Ethnic origins may also be indicators of idiosyncrasies. A classic example is the increased susceptibility to hemolytic anemia found in 100 million Greeks, Iranians, Negroes, Sardinians, Sephardic Jews, and certain other races because of an inherited deficiency of glucose-6-phosphate dehydrogenase and other enzymes in their erythrocytes. This is the reason why primaquine causes anemia in some races. It is also the basis for a special FDA requirement since August 25, 1969, that sulfonamides carry the special precaution shown on page 5. *Inborn errors of metabolism* due to enzymatic defects and gene mutations are continually being uncovered. See Enzyme Deficiencies in Chapter 8.

Sex

The female patient, in general, appears to react more strongly to most medications and to suffer a higher incidence of adverse effects than the male. A lower dosage is therefore often indicated. There are a number of special precautions for the female. During menstruation, purgatives or even gentle cathartics are contraindicated because they may increase the menstrual flow. During pregnancy, all medications except vitamins and other drugs employed in prenatal care should be avoided if possible. The uterus or the fetus may be adversely affected (see the damaging drugs in Table 8-2 and described on page 258. Many drugs cross the placental barrier, e.g., sulfonamides which may cause kernicterus in the newborn. Some drugs are also excreted in the mother's milk and may affect the breast-fed infant. See Tables 8-2 to 8-5 on pages 258 to 262.

Temperament

Sensitive, frail, high-strung, hypochondriacal, perhaps neurotic individuals may report more placebo reactions from medications and may tend to experience more actions and reactions which are figments of the imagination. Those with emotional problems must be given special consideration. The selection of medications for such patients is often difficult and dosage may have to be reduced because of psychogenically induced hyperactivity. In such patients the dissemination of information about adverse drug effects and the use of potent package inserts must be carefully controlled.

Patients who lead an inactive life and tend to be constant invalids also usually require lower doses of medication than the robust, very active athlete or laborer who is powerfully built, even though they weigh the same.

Weight

In general, aside from the special situations discussed in the preceding paragraphs, the heavier the patient the larger the dose and vice versa. However, the composition of the body is very important. Since dosage should be based on active tissue, the amount of bone, fat, and fluid strongly affects the dosage calculation, as these substances play little or no part in metabolizing the drug or actively responding to it. A strong, active 200-pound man who has large muscles, a medium bone structure, and essentially no fat will usually require a great deal more medication than an obese, edematous, 200-pound woman with a heavy skeleton.

History

In taking the patient's history the factors discussed under Age, Environment, Heredity, Sex, Temperament, and Weight are usually noted. In addition, previous and concurrent diseases, previous and concomitant therapy, tolerances, and adverse reactions to medications are carefully determined. The information obtained may preclude the use of certain medications and certain routes of administration. In hemophilia, for example, intramuscular injections are contraindicated. Albinos and patients with fair, sensitive skins, notably red-headed individuals, are prone to phototoxic and other hypersensitivity reactions. Some individuals inherit a predisposition for death from anesthetics. Some inherit the tendency to suffer from certain

diseases, e.g., cancer, diabetes, and cardiac conditions. Patients with a history of hypothyroidism are frequently sensitive to narcotics and sedatives.

Patients with certain inherent characteristics may develop a sensitivity to some drugs. Thus, those with congestive heart failure frequently become more sensitive to coumarin anticoagulants and require less of the medication. See page 276 for other types of patients who are particularly resistant to these anticoagulants.

The checklist of idiosyncrasies and hypersensitivities is very long, indeed. But all possible hazardous situations must be fully considered when selecting a medication and specifying its dosage so that the proper response in a patient is achieved with safety. The physician must obtain all the information he needs for competent prescribing and then in turn properly inform the patient.

INFORMING THE PATIENT

Once the physician has arrived at a diagnosis, perhaps with the aid of carefully evaluated clinical laboratory data, he must then advise his patient, or his patient's family. In certain cases the emotional status of the patient may cause the physician to modify his conversation concerning the condition uncovered. He may wish to defer full disclosure until he has verified an apparently incurable malignancy or some other psychologically traumatic situation, or until he finds a more appropriate time. Nevertheless, as Annis has stated[2]:

"The patient has the right to be informed about his illness and the medication prescribed. The information is invaluable when the patient changes physicians. It is advisable that patients with allergies know what is being prescribed. Specific information on the label helps prevent mix-ups between two or more drugs being taken at the same time, or between medications being taken by different members of a family."

An editorial in the *Journal of the American Medical Association*[14] points out the need to inform the patient fully about the medication prescribed for him:

"When a physician prescribes a drug, he has an obligation to warn the patient about the drug's potential for causing adverse reactions, especially the more serious ones. For example, the possibility of drowsiness resulting from an antihistamine can be serious for an automobile driver.... For some patients the physician has a similar responsibility to warn about the dangers of over-the-counter drugs. Consider the ubiquitous aspirin ... for patients with peptic ulcer or various bleeding tendencies it can be dangerous, and they should be instructed to refrain from use.

"There are instances when information to the patient must be quite explicit. For example, when prescribing a thiazide diuretic, some physicians advocate copious amounts of orange juice as a means of counteracting the potassium-depleting effect of the drug. It should be made clear that the instruction means *orange juice* and not one of the popular substitutes that contains sodium but no potassium."

FDA Commissioner Alexander M. Schmidt, during the Joint DIA/AMA/FDA/PMA Symposium on Drug Information for Patients—The Patient Package Insert[105] stated: "*The patient's right to know* has been persuasively argued by articulate proponents, and indeed it has become a recognized and important principle of our lives. ... a consumer has the right, indeed the obligation, to know what medicine he or she is taking, why, what good or bad effects might result from it, and what he or she should do to insure the best possible therapeutic result."

See also the discussion on *informed consent* under Clinical Investigation in Chapter 3. The physician must make certain that the patient fully understands any serious risks and consequences associated with use of a given drug whether it is being used in an investigation or in routine practice.

A good example of poor communication that resulted in faulty informing of a patient appeared in the *New England Journal of Medicine*:[12]

"To: Chief, Nursing Service
"Name of Individual Involved:
  Smith, John
"Mr. Smith on 14 April 66 was given some liq pHisoHex soap so he could take a shower before going (sic) to surgery. Instead of taking a shower c̄ pHisoHex he drank it. Because he didn't go to surgery on 14 April Mr. Smith was given some more liq pHisoHex so he could take a shower before going to surgery, but instead he drank it again. There was another person with Mr. Smith this AM when the aide gave him the pHisoHex and heard me tell him to take a shower c̄ the pHi-

soHex soap. This AM the patient complained that the medicine made him vomit to the doctor."

A similar situation with a more toxic product could have been fatal. Most patients need to be carefully instructed because they are highly vulnerable to the hazards of misunderstanding professional directions and they are not fully aware of the dangers of administering medications to themselves.[3]

Hazards of Self-Medication

From ancient times man has always had the urge to medicate himself, and this has always been permissible and relatively safe— until the advent of chemotherapy. With the resulting increase in the potency of drugs and the number of prescriptions being written, the hazards of self-medication have increased astronomically.

Now there are other dangers in addition to well-known ones like taking cathartics in the presence of an inflamed appendix, or using cantharides[96-98] as an aphrodisiac. Such practices have caused many injuries and deaths through the centuries. But in recent decades, literally millions of injuries have been caused by the almost unbelievably potent drugs that have been synthesized. And many of these drugs are not restricted to prescriptions. Some are available to the layman in over-the-counter products designed specifically for self-medication after self-diagnosis. Thus, the unwary purchaser has a vast spectrum of unrestricted medications which he can take concurrently with one another and with any others that are prescribed for him. The potential exists for an almost infinite number of drug interactions to occur and they do. In fact, medications are often prescribed for drug reactions caused by drug interactions that are misdiagnosed by the prescriber because he is unaware of the patient's drug profile and he may be only one of several practitioners seeing the same patient.

But other hazards apart from biochemical damage exist with over-the-counter medications. If taken during pregnancy, they may cause abnormalities in the offspring. They may mask the symptoms of a serious disease or delay it long enough to allow it to progress to a stage where it cannot be controlled. Also, laymen can become habituated to some household medications that they believe to be innocuous. When prolonged, such habituation sometimes results in undesirable conditions which may or may not be irreversible. Certain headache remedies containing central nervous system depressant bromides are sometimes taken every day for years and can cause bromism with mental and neurological disturbances, dermatitis, and symptoms sometimes simulating those of encephalitis, cerebral tumor, general paresis, multiple sclerosis, uremia, and other diseases. Even aspirin, often believed to be harmless by the layman, has caused many cases of gastrointestinal hemorrhage, especially when taken concurrently with alcoholic beverages.

Because of its common use, aspirin is apparently not regarded by many people as a drug and they consume it freely without being aware of its hazards. Gastrointestinal hemorrhaging in adults has caused particular concern. But now that frequent excessive fetal exposure to the drug has been demonstrated, its use during pregnancy is also causing concern. In 26 (9.5%) of 272 consecutively delivered infants at the University of Alabama Medical Center, the average salicylate level in the umbilical serum ranged from 1.2 to 10.9 mg./100 ml. Since circulating salicylate may significantly depress albumin-binding capacity, the levels may be a consideration in the management of hyperbilirubinemia of the newborn.[49]

Thus, physicians when writing prescriptions or pharmacists when dispensing them must be mindful of interactions that can occur not only between concurrently prescribed medications, but between them and self-administered ones. To remember all possible drug interactions for every medication prescribed is an impossible task, beyond the capacity of the human brain. But this problem is being solved with the aid of electronic computers. Pertinent information from patient records in hospitals, pharmacies, and physicians' offices can be stored in computer memories for instantaneous retrieval and correlation. Steps are being taken to make such information nationally and internationally available so that eventually wherever the patient goes he will be protected from medication hazards and all physicians will be aided in selecting medications for the patient.

Pharmacists help physicians improve drug therapy by maintaining patient medication records, reviewing patient drug profiles, alerting prescribers to possible adverse drug reactions, designing clinical research protocols, and executing medication research programs, including retrospective and prospective analyses of the epidemiology of drug interactions. Drug therapy is also being improved by integrating medical, dental, pharmacy, and nursing schools. The closer interprofessional relationships thus engendered tends to enhance the quality of academic instruction, clinical research with medications, and professional services in general, including optimum selection of medications.

SELECTING MEDICATIONS

The physician often finds it necessary to select one drug product from a large number available for a given indication.* Does he do this on the basis of past experience with a few of the products? Is he influenced by recent discussions with detail men? Is he guided by information he has recently obtained by attending meetings, or listening to recordings, or reading professional journals, or discussing cases with his colleagues? How much is he influenced by the constant barrage of arguments concerning medications among leaders in medicine, government, and industry?

Knowledge about drug therapy changes so rapidly that much of what is learned during any given year cannot be used as a basis for medical practice a few years later. New uses for old medications are constantly being discovered and many uses once enthusiastically endorsed by authorities are found to be dependent merely on placebo effects. Masses of opinions expressed by colleagues verbally and in the literature must be continually sifted and evaluated as new drugs replace old ones.

Whatever his sources of information, the physician must nevertheless make a decision based on (1) characteristics of the patient and

his environment, (2) correct diagnosis, (3) the desired drug action, (4) the regimen that will be tolerated and effective, and (5) possible drug reactions and interactions. He must also take into consideration the problem of achieving biological availability of the selected medication in his specific patient and be able to make sound judgments concerning the therapeutic equivalency of the various medications from which he makes his selection.

Faulty Selection

In selecting particularly potent and dangerous medications, the physician often wisely seeks consultations with colleagues in his specialty. Unwise selection of medications can create serious problems. Friend[99] has noted four types of faulty selection.

1. *Dangerous drugs for trivial conditions*— Highly toxic drugs like chloramphenicol have been used in conditions like a minor sore throat and infections on "hammer toes," sometimes with fatal results.

2. *Unnecessary medication*—Antibiotics that are strictly antibacterial have been used in viral infections, and have thus subjected the patients to such unnecessary potential hazards as development of resistant strains.

3. *Unwise selection of drugs*—Chloramphenicol given for a sore throat can result in death. This is an unnecessary risk since in some individuals the drug induces irreversible aplastic anemia. A "shot of penicillin" for a head cold is another example of improper use of medication, as is penicillin for mumps.[29]

4. *Drugs useless for the given condition*— One patient died after being given a tablet of ampicillin for a painful elbow. He actually had gout and the medication was useless for that condition.

The HEW Task Force on Prescription Drugs listed the following types of irrational prescribing in its *Final Report.* (1) Use of drugs without demonstrated efficacy. (2) Use of drugs with an inherent hazard not justified by the seriousness of the illness. (3) Use of drugs in excessive amounts, or for extended periods of time, or inadequate amounts for inadequate periods. (4) Use of a costly duplicative or "me-too" product when an equally effective or less expensive drug is available.

---

*As many as several hundred new drug products, mostly combinations of drugs, were introduced annually prior to 1962, but in recent years only a dozen really new drug products have been introduced annually and perhaps half of these represented truly significant improvements in therapy. During FY 1977 (ending June 30, 1977), FDA approved 19 new drug entities.

(5) Use of a costly combination product when equally effective but less expensive drugs are available individually. (6) Simultaneous use of two or more drugs without appropriate consideration of their possible interaction. (7) Multiple prescribing, by one or several physicians for the same patient, of drugs which may be unnecessary, cumulative, interacting, or needlessly expensive. [63]

The economic hazards can be challenged in that they may be based on false logic and on political needs. A "me-too" product must usually be introduced at a highly competitive price level. Also, combinations of medications are usually cheaper for the patient than the same drugs purchased in separate dosage forms. The other hazards, however, are real and must be considered in determining benefit-to-risk relationships.

Benefit versus Risk

The medication selected for the patient should not be more hazardous than the disease to be treated. This sound principle of drug therapy causes physicians constantly to ask incisive questions, like the following: Should the health measure be continued? Should the drug be abandoned? Smallpox vaccination provides an excellent illustration of the basic issue. This viral disease has been essentially eradicated in nearly every country through rigid immunization programs. Although the preventive program was highly successful, however, it bore some hazards for those who were inoculated.

In the weekly report for the week ending Sep. 13, 1969 (*Morbidity and Mortality*, Vol. 18, No. 37), the National Communicable Disease Center* reported that during 1968 an estimated 5,594,000 primary vaccinations and 8,574,000 revaccinations were administered to residents of the United States. A total of 572 complications (accidental infection, eczema vaccinatum, generalized vaccinia, postvaccinial encephalitis, and vaccinia necrosum) occurred, with 9 deaths. This was an incidence of 74.7 complications per million primary vaccinations (over half in children under the age of 5 years) and 4.7 complications per million revaccinations (mostly in persons over the age of 10 years). In the

_____
*Renamed Center for Disease Control during 1970.

United States the incidence of these serious complications of smallpox vaccination (average of 7 deaths per year) [67] far outweighed the consequences of smallpox itself (no cases among American residents since 1949). Smallpox vaccination was therefore discontinued even for foreign travel in most countries.

Smallpox has now been eradicated worldwide except for one epidemiologic unit consisting of Ethiopia, Kenya, and Somalia in Eastern Africa. In that area 3234 cases were reported during January 1 to December 6, 1977. The last known case in Ethiopia occurred on August 9, 1976, the last in Kenya February 5, 1977, and the last in Somalia on October 26, 1977. During the dry season, January through April, 1978, World Health Organization epidemiologists intensified their efforts to ensure that all foci had been detected. [105]

Succedanea

Alternative medications (succedanea) that may be substituted for another with equivalent properties are essential in the practice of medicine because no two patients may react in exactly the same manner to a given drug product. In fact the same drug product given at different times may not even produce the same effect in the same patient. Alternatives must be available also when the patient reacts adversely to one or more drugs in a given category or fails for some reason to respond adequately.

Take, for example, an antibiotic. The physician prescribes the usual dose of one of the tetracyclines in which he has great confidence because of earlier satisfactory experiences, perhaps in the same patient with the same infection, e.g., gonorrhea. But perhaps the patient exhibits an allergic reaction; he may have developed a hypersensitivity to the drug during his last treatment with it. Or perhaps he has picked up a strain of gonococcus which is resistant to the antibiotic. (Some organisms actually adapt so well to antimicrobials that they proliferate better in their presence). Or his job takes him outdoors in bright sunshine most of every day where he may be apt to sustain a phototoxic reaction. Or he is taking other medication such as an antacid containing calcium which tends to prevent absorption of tetracyclines. In these situations the physician will shift to another antibiotic or another type of antimicrobial with the desired activity.

It may sometimes happen, if a drug is withdrawn from use long enough, that strains resistant to it may gradually disappear and eventually the drug will become useful once again. Nevertheless, newer antimicrobials must be constantly developed to replace older ones that have engendered resistance.*

These are just a few of the many reasons why a physician finds it necessary to give a substitute to replace a drug which is not acting well in his patient at a given time. Even though it has worked well for him in most of his patients in the past, and probably will continue to do so, for his adversely affected patient he is nevertheless compelled to find a substitute. Physicians therefore find it necessary to become thoroughly familiar with several medications for each indication and all pertinent medical information. Pharmaceutical manufacturers usually provide enough different products in each therapeutic category to provide the physician with adequate flexibility of drug therapy and with more information than he can possibly digest and retain.

HAZARDS OF INADEQUATE MEDICAL INFORMATION

The quality of all drug therapy depends largely on the quality of the drug information received by the prescriber. Up-to-date, complete, accurate data are essential if patients are to be treated safely and effectively. Every physician who writes a prescription for drug products must know exactly what they are, what they do, how to give them and what pitfalls to anticipate.

Inadequate Communication

Many hazardous situations for the patient are caused by inadequate communication of

information about medications.* Precautionary information sometimes does not reach the practitioner who needs it soon enough. Perhaps it remains buried in the literature and is not reported because of incomplete review or incompetent searching. Occasionally when someone becomes aware of a serious situation caused by some type of therapy, he cannot or will not transmit a warning quickly enough. A language barrier, unfamiliar or confusing terminology (see page 115), a multiplicity of names (see page 87), or some other hindrance may exist. Hiding unfavorable information may prevent an economic loss or legal action or loss of professional prestige or anger on the part of the patient and his family or some other problem.

Many examples of the hazards of inadequate communication can be given. For instance, faulty communications between nurses and patients cause lawsuits. The following typical situation has been slightly altered for ethical reasons, but it is a true representation of what can happen when there is a language barrier, when medication records are inadequate, or when a medication nurse or other adequate supervision has not been established. Patient records should be updated immediately after the medication has been selected for the patient. Otherwise the dose may be repeated in error, the patient injured, and litigation instituted.

A female patient underwent elective surgery successfully and soon after she regained consciousness was given 15 mg of morphine parenterally by a nurse who then continued on her rounds. About 10 minutes after the injection was given, a second nurse appeared and began to prepare the patient for another injection. The patient protested and tried to explain that she had already received medication. The nurse could not understand English very well and insisted that the patient submit to a second injection of morphine. The respiratory depressant effects of the double dose of opiate added to those of the anesthetic

*It is of interest, however, that for several years the three most frequently prescribed drugs in the U.S. have been tetracycline, phenobarbital, and penicillin G potassium, two of which are antibiotics. Overprescribing and misuse of antibiotics by physicians in this country plus OTC indiscriminate sale of antibiotics and overuse as prophylactics by prostitutes abroad has resulted in serious worldwide problems (resistant gonococci and other dangerous organisms).

*Most physicians are conscientious and make every effort to keep abreast of the most important therapeutic information affecting their own specialty. Besides, they use only a comparatively few drugs with which they become thoroughly familiar. The problem of incompleteness of information arose about 1950 when the information explosion occurred with a subsequent breakdown in coordinating the flow of biomedical information at all levels, nationally and internationally.

used in the operation resulted in respiratory failure and cardiac arrest. Heroic measures, including heart massage and stimulants saved the patient's life, but the traumatic experience she endured was unnecessary. The patient sued the hospital.

The problem of communication, not only between nurse and patient, but also among physician, pharmacist and patient is being resolved in part with the aid of patient package inserts (see page 85).

Serious consequences can occur when communication between physicians, pharmacists, and nurses is faulty. Accurate prescribing, dispensing and administration of medications demands precise, complete and accurate transfer of instructions at every step of patient care. Unfortunately communication, comprehension and conscientiousness leave so much to be desired at times that truly serious errors are made. In some parts of the country one out of every seven physicians is sued for malpractice, negligence or some other reason. Often lawsuits are incurred because of an adverse drug reaction that the physician could have avoided if he had been aware of information that was available, and if his directions had been correctly followed. [5,9,12,13,18]

The physician should read the nurse's notes carefully, even though he may think they are incorrect, to alert him to possible patient injury. Plaster casts, restraining belts, medications, and other items have too often been involved in litigation because the nurse's notes and verbal information were not heeded promptly and appropriate action taken.

Unless precautionary and toxicity information on medications is received and acted upon promptly; unless prescribing, dispensing and administering directions are communicated accurately; and unless drug interactions and adverse effects are communicated rapidly and preferably worldwide, many patients are harmed and some die. Complete, up-to-date information is an essential ingredient of patient safety and welfare.

A thorough description of a medication includes comprehensive information about its molecular structure, physical and chemical properties, and dosage forms and strengths available; its therapeutic and pharmacologic category, mode of action, and indications; routes of administration and dosage for each indication; and all contraindications, warnings, precautions, and adverse reactions. The well-informed prescriber is familiar with all of these for each drug product he uses. Moreover, he knows where to locate pertinent literature, including brochures, illustrations, microforms, photocopy, reproductions, reprints, and other substantiating information for every prescription he writes, every paper he submits for publication, and every lecture he gives. Only by being on such solid ground can he do his best for his patients, his students and his colleagues, and avoid costly and time-consuming litigation.

Drug Efficacy Study

An effort with legal implications which has had an impact on drug information is the so-called Drug Efficacy Study. During the years 1966-69 all prescription drugs marketed in the United States between 1938 and 1962 were thoroughly reviewed for efficacy by 30 panels of experts gathered through the National Academy of Sciences-National Research Council under a contract signed in May, 1966, with the Food and Drug Administration. This Federally sponsored project has completed its evaluation of an estimated total of 2,824 reports and 10,000 claims for 4,349 different pharmaceutical preparations [94] marketed by 237 pharmaceutical manufacturers. Periodically, the *Federal Register* carries notices of changes in authorized claims resulting from Drug Efficacy Study Implementation (DESI). By about 1980 the project will cover every prescription medication, new as well as old. As a result of this very extensive effort, drug literature is being materially changed. [102]

The FDA goal of publishing all initial announcements of efficacy in the *Federal Register* by July 1, 1971 was hindered by several pharmaceutical manufacturers who challenged FDA on its findings in the courts. To avoid undue delay, FDA promulgated its regulations defining what is meant by an adequate and well-controlled clinical investigation. This provides a mechanism for measuring the adequacy of clinical data offered in support of a company's request for a hearing and for summarily disposing of any request that failed to establish legally sufficient grounds for a hearing. See page 44.[94]

It is now illegal for many drugs to be promoted for certain indications that were formerly carried in their package inserts and other literature, in some instances for many years. Many drugs were removed from the market between 1969 and 1977. Some 50 drug categories were involved. A *Table of Drug Categories Classified Ineffective* with dates of the *Federal Register* in which notice of NDA withdrawal was published may be obtained from Prescription Drug Compliance Branch, Bureau of Drugs, FDA, Rockville, MD 20857.

Some products reviewed were voluntarily withdrawn, others were not, and legal contests were initiated. A few of the DESI items remained on the market after the formula was altered or the wording of the package insert was modified to include more meaningful precautionary information and more complete dosage instructions.

DESI is believed to be a preliminary step toward the development of a *United States Prescription Drug Compendium* designed to provide physicians with a complete and authoritative source of prescribing information on prescription drug products marketed in the United States.[34] Considerable controversy arose over the determination of responsibility for the design and source of the compendium.

Similar major reviews were also begun for nonprescription (OTC) drug products and biologics. The results of all of these studies are being computerized and eventually health professionals will be able to depend on the safety and efficacy of every type of drug product on the market as well as the drug information disseminated.

Sources of Medical Information

Drug information sources have been frequently reviewed in the literature. To keep abreast of his field, the physician must find some means to cull from nearly 2 million scientific and technical articles published each year in the 35,000 scientific periodicals of the world the comparatively small amount of crucial information which pertains to him and his practice. The alert practitioner copes with this problem by attending meetings and regularly reading selected publications that cover subjects in which he is most deeply interested. And he routinely sees a few of the most informative detail men from selected pharmaceutical companies. Also, he obtains answers to questions about specific drug products by contacting the medical advisory (professional service) departments of these companies. In addition, he subscribes to medical tape recordings and views medical movies. He often consults pharmacists and drug information centers.

Competent therapy with modern medications demands that the physician keep abreast of the latest prescribing facts so that he does not unnecessarily take chances with the safety of his patients.* Accordingly, he usually maintains personally or has access to enough unbiased sources of medical and drug information to keep him current on the comparatively few drugs he uses in his own particular specialty. Some of the more useful and more widely used sources are books, periodicals, meetings, manufacturers, pharmacists, and societies.

Books. In addition to the standard textbooks used in the medical schools such as *The Pharmacological Basis of Therapeutics, Cecil-Loeb Textbook of Medicine* and others, the practitioner requires the latest editions of a few supplemental volumes devoted to the general practice of medicine, to the medical sciences, and to the economic, political, and social aspects of medicine. He is forced to make a very critical selection because some 2,000 medical books are published annually in the United States. The following supplemental volumes are some of the most widely used: AMA *Drug Evaluations, Current Diagnosis, Current Therapy, Drugs of Choice, Hazards of Medication, American Drug Index, Physicians' Desk Reference, The Merck Manual,* and the *United States Dispensatory.*

Periodicals. Although about 6,000 medical publications are published regularly around the world (1,500 of these in the United States alone), the average physician can keep abreast of information in his own field if he

---

* A safety factor for patients is the conservative attitude of the average practicing physician. He does not readily switch from medications which he has learned to use well and which he has found in his own experience to be safe and dependable.

subscribes to a few carefully selected journals and scans them promptly for papers of interest to him. In some information areas, physicians and scientists have found that about 50 journals adequately cover all the latest advances because there is so much duplication and so many papers that clutter up the literature without making a contribution.

The following periodicals are some of those most widely read by physicians.*

American Heart Journal
American Journal of Obstetrics and Gynecology
American Journal of Ophthalmology
American Review of Respiratory Disease
Anesthesiology
Annals of Allergy
Annals of Internal Medicine
Archives of Dermatology
Archives of Internal Medicine
Archives of Neurology and Psychiatry
Archives of Ophthalmology
British Journal of Anesthesia
British Journal of Diseases of the Chest
British Journal of Ophthalmology
British Medical Journal
Clin-Alert
Clinical Medicine
Clinical Pharmacology and Therapeutics
Clinical Symposia
Clinical Toxicology Bulletin
Current Medical Digest
Current Research in Anesthesiology
Diseases of the Chest
FDA Drug Bulletin
Journal of the American Medical Association
Journal of Experimental Therapeutics
Medical Clinics of North America
New England Journal of Medicine
Obstetrics and Gynecology
Pediatric Clinics of North America
Pediatrics
Pharmacology for Physicians
Postgraduate Medicine
Surgery, Gynecology, and Obstetrics
The British Journal of Clinical Practice
The Lancet
The Medical Letter
The Practitioner

---

*In a continuing effort to provide more information about drugs and new developments, FDA began publishing a journal, *FDA Papers* in January, 1967, and *Current Drug Information,* a newsletter for physicians, in April, 1970. This newsletter was replaced by the *FDA Drug Bulletin* in 1971. It now is sent free to 1,000,000 physicians and other health professionals and students. It has the highest readership of any medical publication. *FDA Papers* became *FDA Consumer.*

Meetings. Local, national, and international meetings and conventions of professional societies and various other types of smaller meetings such as hospital staff meetings, closed-circuit television conferences, seminars, symposia, and workshops, as well as reports of these meetings in medical news media, often provide the latest medical information, long before it is published in text books. The exchange of very recently acquired information at these gatherings, the "invisible college," is one of the best methods of keeping current. No better way has yet been found to uncover recent advances made by fellow medical practitioners and scientists. A major danger to patients arises, however, when self-appointed lay guardians of the public attend medical conferences and report alarming statistics, taken out of context, to the public. The apprehensions aroused by public misinformation and improperly emphasized information on subjects such as alcohol, aspirin, cancer, cholesterol, contaminated foods (mercury and salmonella), cyclamates, dyes, monosodium glutamate, oral contraceptives, penicillin, and tolbutamide will never be completely allayed.[100]

Manufacturers. The manufacturers of drug products continually disseminate information about their products by means of many media (see page 90). The physician should make certain he has the latest package insert for each medication he prescribes. He can obtain these from the local pharmacy or directly from the manufacturer. They provide him with dependable, albeit highly condensed information officially approved by FDA under standardized headings in this order: Description, Actions, Indications, Contraindications, Warnings, Precautions, Adverse Reactions, Dosage and Administration, Overdosage (where applicable), How Supplied, and sometimes Animal Pharmacology and Toxicology, Clinical Studies, and References. This order, with the proviso that "in the case of some drugs special warnings may be required to appear conspicuously in the beginning of the labeling for special attention of physicians for the safety of patients," was established by a 1969 statement of FDA policy[17] regarding labeling.

FDA has emphasized that the three main purposes of package inserts are: (1) to make essential information on medications available to physicians and patients, (2) to provide a tool for educating physicians, and (3) to provide a factual basis and limitations for the promotion of medications. Unfortunately, the only professional persons who are certain to have access to the package circulars without fail are the pharmacists. See Package Inserts as Legal Documents (page 82).

Pharmacists. Since the curricula in accredited colleges of pharmacy have been extended to 5 and 6 years with emphasis on pharmacology and biopharmaceutics, many pharmacists in community and hospital practice have become excellent sources of dependable drug information. A few maintain large files of reference literature and up-to-date libraries. Some work with computerized drug information.

In the larger hospitals and medical complexes drug information centers have been established to provide answers to medical and scientific inquiries from professional staffs. These centers publish bulletins and newsletters that serve as alerting services (new therapies, medication hazards, revised policies, etc.) and as a means of continuing education, especially when tied in with therapeutic conferences. The head of the drug information center usually serves as the secretary of the Pharmacy and Therapeutics Committee which selects the medications used in the hospital and publishes the Hospital Formulary. Members of the staff of the center are often involved in the drug research activities of the hospital. They compile adverse drug reaction reports, handle the clinical investigation reporting and Investigational New Drug paperwork, and even occasionally identify areas of drug investigation that should be considered.

Information experts in the drug information center store essential information and retrieve it expeditiously. Critical data, such as hypersensitivities and drug interactions are extracted from patient records for future reference and stored methodically either by manual methods such as file cards or by more sophisticated mechanized and computerized methods. Some centers use suitably designed forms to record the details of inquiries in a standardized format for computer input. Then by means of random access the data can be almost instantaneously retrieved and correlated when needed at any time in the future. This approach tends to safeguard the patient from serious, life-threatening adverse drug reactions and interactions, and when these do occur, provides the attending physician with urgently needed information about antidotes and other controls. By tying small hospitals to computer centers in large hospitals such vital life-saving information is being made more widely available.

Some of the larger pharmaceutical companies like Hoffmann-LaRoche have established a team of pharmacists on 24-hour call to handle emergency phone calls pertaining to drug products. In addition one or two of the senior medical staff are always available for consultation. When a drug product is involved in a medical crisis, on-site visitations are made by company medical experts, and sometimes in serious situations outside consultants are retained. By these means FDA is given accurate and complete information, and manufacturers, practitioners, and hospitals have records which provide them with legal protection.

Societies. Many of the county, state, and national medical societies provide information for their members. The American Medical Association develops packages of information, sometimes in the form of questions and answers, on key questions, e.g., LSD. AMA is well equipped with a reference service which exhaustively keeps abreast of the medical information reported in several hundred selected journals, but it does not conduct exhaustive literature searches in answer to inquiries. It provides key references to physicians and thereby leads them into the most informative literature. If a question justifies the time and effort, AMA calls on its consultants, but it does not practice therapeutics.

A recent breakdown of questions received by AMA revealed that 27 percent were on specific disorders treated with a specific drug, and most of the remaining requests for information were concerned with adverse effects of drugs. The largest number of requests involved a specific side effect caused by a specific drug. It is evident that most physicians are primarily concerned about the safety and efficacy of the medications they prescribe.

With all of these sources available, the average practitioner can readily obtain all the information he needs on medications (much more readily than for other hazardous chemicals) and can conveniently keep abreast of the latest developments in one or two narrow fields. However, unlike his predecessors, he does not have the time to cover the whole field of medicine or remain competent in many specialties at the same time. He does well if he can see patients in a few medical areas and write prescriptions that will have optimum efficacy for them.

WRITING PRESCRIPTIONS

Before the practitioner of medicine writes a prescription, he sorts out in his mind all known facts about his patient's history and physical and emotional status; any diseases identified, with their etiology and preferred treatments available; his patient's medications, past, present and future; and environmental or hereditary factors which might influence the prescribed medication, including congenital conditions, hypersensitivities, and idiosyncrasies. He must then avoid making any errors when writing the prescription.

Errors in Prescribing

The art of prescription writing has been thoroughly discussed from various viewpoints in a number of standard textbooks.[33] Most physicians know how to write prescriptions, but often neglect some of the points given below under Rules for Prescribing. All are essential from the standpoint of patient safety.

The legal pitfalls for the physician, of course, extend far beyond the 17 precautions listed below. Because he has the ultimate responsibility for proper care of his patients, he is nearly always held responsible for the acts of his nurses, his laboratory assistants, and for all others who come under his direction in clinic, hospital, or office. However, in a crucial 1968 decision, a hospital was held liable for the negligence of a registered nurse who administered an injection postoperatively to a seven-year-old patient, struck the sciatic nerve, and caused a permanent foot drop. The Colorado Supreme Court refused to hold the surgeon liable for the nurse's negligence, but applied the principle of *respondeat superior* to the hospital and held it, as the employer, liable for the negligence of its agent.[9]

Nevertheless, every decision the prescribing physician[16] makes must be correct. Is the treatment necessary? Is it the proper one under the given circumstances? Has he taken all possible precautions to determine hypersensitivities, idiosyncrasies, concomitant medications, etc.? Is the diagnosis based on adequate testing? Has he selected the proper dosage regimen? Has he varied from standard practice? Has he obtained informed consent if required? There are so many pitfalls for the modern practitioner and it is so easy to bring legal action that it is not astonishing that in some areas of the country, e.g., southern California, the number of lawsuits brought against physicians has been more than doubling every 15 years.[42] It behooves every physician, therefore, to abide by strict rules for prescribing.

Rules for Prescribing

The following rules for prescribing medication should be constantly kept in mind.

1. Communicate clearly. Remember that you are transmitting an important medication order. Many drug product names sound alike or look alike when telephoned or handwritten rapidly. They perhaps differ by only one letter (see Table 6-1 on page 115).[61] Poorly enunciated, ambiguous speech and illegible writing cause the wrong medication to be dispensed.

2. Place the decimal point in the proper place. A shift of one place to the right causes the patient to receive 10 times the dose intended. This error has also been fatal. A shift of one place to the left causes the patient to receive 1/10 of the intended dose. This also can have serious consequences.

3. Use *Gm.* for gram and *gr.* for grain when specifying quantity, or better yet, carefully spell out grain and dot the *i*. If grams are given instead of grains, the patient receives roughly 15 times the dose intended. This error has been fatal. The introduction of *g* for gram in the 1970 editions of the USP and NF may lead to confusion and errors. Fortunately, only the Metric System will be used soon for all doses of medication.

4. Provide all essential information for the pharmacist. A serious delay in filling an urgently needed prescription may occur if you forget to specify strength or quantity, or omit

Table 6-1 Confusing Names of Medications*

Acetanilid / Cedilanid	Ananase / Orinase	Bontril / Vontril	Daricon / Darvon	Disophrol / Isuprel	Ertron / Eutron	Hycodan / Hycomine	Medomin / Metamine	Orenzyme / Parenzyme	Preceptin / Pro-Ception
Acidil / Actifed	Anavac / Anavar	Butabarbital / Butobarbital	Darcil / Diuril	Diuril / Doriden / Dolantal / Dolantin / Dilantin	Esimil / Estynil / Estomul / Ismelin / Isomel	Imferon / Infron	Menacyl / Midicel	Ornade / Orinase	Prednisone / Prednisolone
Acusol / Aquasol	Apresoline / Priscoline	Butabel / Butibel	Decagesic / Equagesic	Dolonil / Polanil	Ethamide / Ethionamide	Indocin / Lincocin	Mepergan / Meprobamate	Pabalate / Robalate	Protamide / Protamine
Aerolone / Aralen / Arlidin	Aralen / Arlidin	Butagesic / Butigetic	Detla-Dome / Deltasone	Donnagel / Donnatal	Felsol / Feosol / Fer-in-Sol / Festal	Iberol / Ipral	Mephyton / Merataran / Metreton	Pabamide / Pavabid	Quadrinal / Quatrasal
Afrodex / Azotrex	Atarax / Enarax / Marax	Calamine / Calomel	Demerol / Deprol / Dicumarol	Donnazyme / Entozyme	Folbesyn / Fulvicin	Ilomel / Isomel / Isordil / Isuprel	Methedrine / Methergine	Pantapon / Parafon	Quinidine / Quinine
Agoral / Argyrol	Auralgan / Otalgine	Calcidin / Calcidrine	Demerol / Temaril	Doriden / Doxidan	Fostex / pHisoHex	Kaon / Kao-Con	Methiscol / Meth-i-sol	Papaverine / Pavatrine	Sigmagen / Signemycin
Alcohol / Alkalol	AVC / HVC	Calurin / Saluron	Desoxyn / Digitoxin	Duracton / Taractan	Garamycin / Terramycin	Karidium / Pyridium	Modane / Mudrane	Paregoric / Periogesic	Sparine / Sterane
Aldomet / Aldoril	Aventyl / Benadryl	Chloromycetin / Chlor-Trimeton	Dexameth / Dexamyl	Duragesic / Duo-gesic	Gevral / Gevrine	Kwell / Quell	Myleran / Milicon	Paremycin / Terramycin	Surbex / Surfak
Aldoril / Elavil	Bentyl / Benylin	Compazine / Compacillin	Diafen / Delfen	Dyrenium / Serenium	Glaucon / Glukor	Lasix / Labstix	Nico-Span / Nitrospan	Periactin / Taractan	Temaril / Tepanil
Alidase / Elase	Clistin / Twiston	Consol / Konsyl	Dialose / Dialose Plus / Dialog	Ecotrin / Edecrin / Medaprin	Haldol / Holdrone / Halodrin	Levophed / Levoprome	Nilevar / Noludar	Persantine / Persistin / Trasentine	Terfonyl / Tofranil
Ambenyl / Ambodryl / Amvicel / Aventyl	Benuron / Enduron	Coumadin / Kemadrin	Diazide / Thiacide	Effergel / Effersyl	Hormonyl / Hormonin	Lidaform / Vioform	Norlutate / Norlutin	Phantos / Thantis	Vigran / Wigraine
Amodrine / Amonidrin	Benylin / Betalin	Daprisal / Tapazole	Dicyclomine / Dyclonine	Ephedrol / Tedral		Lotusate / Peritrate	Orabiotic / Otobiotic / Urobiotic	Phenaphen / Phenergan	
Ampicillin / Compocillin	Bicillin / V-Cillin		Digitoxin / Digoxin / Dipaxin			Mebaral / Mellaril / Medrol	Oracon / Oreton	Placidyl / Plaquenil	
	Bonacal Plus / Donnatal Plus								

* Adapted from a table compiled by Benjamin Teplitsky, VA Hospital, Brooklyn, N.Y.,[61] and from other sources.

your narcotic registration number, for example. Patients have sometimes endured agonizing pain unnecessarily because of such delays.

5. Provide all essential information for the nurse. Indicate dosage form, dose, frequency, timing, route, duration, and other instructions clearly. Patients are too often given the wrong dosage. Especially in the prison environment, proper medication of patients appears to be very difficult. In one small study less than 10 percent of the prescriptions examined had been taken correctly by the prisoners. [60]

6. Never prescribe medication unless it is absolutely needed. Don't satisfy the whims of a patient who says, "I want to have a shot of penicillin for my cold," or "I want to try drug X that I read about in *Reader's Digest.*" Indoctrinate as necessary, and always be conservative when prescribing.

7. Know your patient's condition thoroughly before prescribing and consider it in relation to the prescribed medication. Be able to justify its use.

8. Prescribe only medication with which you are thoroughly familiar. Thoroughly study authoritative literature on the products you use. In particular, never prescribe any drug unless you have thoroughly studied every known contraindication, warning, precaution, and adverse reaction, as well as all administration and dosage information given in the physician's package insert. This helps you to avoid malpractice litigation and protect your patient.

9. Specify a dependable brand of each drug product prescribed. One safe way to do this is to specify a brand in which you have developed confidence. If you use a generic name, be sure to specify one or several companies in whom you have confidence; otherwise the prescription can legally be filled with a quality of medication lower than what you wish your patient to have. Permissive prescribing can be hazardous.

10. Avoid overprescribing which is costly to the patient and creates hazards when excess medication remains in the house. Warn the patient against using leftover medication for a later condition or recommending and giving it to another person.

11. Give the patient full and precise instructions and make certain he clearly understands them. Provide printed instructions when the details of administration and dosage are especially complex. [20] Tell him what he is taking, and when advisable, make certain that the prescription label carries the name of the medication, an expiration date, and full instructions. "Take as directed" is an abomination unless printed instructions accompany the prescription.

12. Warn every patient when necessary against the hazards of taking other medication simultaneously. Briefly explain what may happen if certain conflicting drugs are taken at or about the same time.

13. Monitor patients carefully to determine whether the medication is taking effect and also whether there are any adverse effects. Request each patient to keep you full informed. In some situations, it may be desirable to warn a patient, calmly without creating apprehensions, about the possibility of an adverse reaction when a particularly dangerous drug has to be administered. One physician was held liable because he failed to advise a bus driver, for whom he had prescribed an antihistamine, about possible drowsiness and to warn the driver not to operate a vehicle. [3] In situations where informed consent must be obtained, give the same amount of information about risks and benefits as would be given by any prudent physician practicing in the same or a similar community under the same circumstances. Never treat a patient without proper consent. All that a patient needs to do to be awarded damages for any injury suffered is to prove that he did not give proper consent. [7]

14. Continue medication for an appropriate period of time. Some drug therapies, once started, must be continued for a minimum period of time. Thus, tetracycline should be continued for one to three days beyond the time when the characteristic symptoms of an infection have subsided; otherwise resistant organisms may develop and a serious relapse may occur. In acute staphylococcal infections, for example, tetracycline should be given for 10 to 14 days.

15. Stop drug therapy as soon as possible. Unnecessarily prolonged use of medication increases the hazards of drug interactions and other possible adverse effects on the body.

16. Maintain accurate patient records. [74,75] Be certain to list all medications taken, past and present, and carefully record any hyper-

sensitivities, idiosyncrasies, or other special situations that must be avoided in the future. For your protection, in case of litigation, make a note in the patient's record that you inquired about these special situations. The pharmacist and the nurse, also, have the grave responsibility to be alert and give proper information to the physician whenever they review patient records and encounter possible hazards due to interactions that might arise because of multiple drug therapy, including self medication. The physician should keep a copy of every prescription he writes, preferably a carbon copy for his own files to be sure that his copy is identical to the one he gives to the patient. He should also follow up telephoned prescriptions with written ones and keep carbon copies for his files.

17. Avoid prescribing several medications simultaneously unless they are absolutely necessary, are therapeutically compatible, do not cause undesirable drug interactions, and can have their dosages properly adjusted. It may be necessary in some instances of rational multiple therapy to prescribe active agents independently rather than in fixed combination. See, for example, the discussions on page 100 and in Chapter 10.

One of the most important of the above rules is number 11: Give the patient full and precise instructions and make certain he clearly understands them.

Instructions to the Patient

What the patient does with prescribed medication can influence its efficacy dramatically. Either he can provide a favorable situation for the drug or he can do the opposite and lessen its effectiveness even to the point of inactivating it completely. Some medications work best on an empty stomach, some on a full stomach, some with large quantities of water or other fluids. With some drugs the amount of fluid is immaterial. Many medications interact with certain foods and drugs which inhibit, potentiate, or decrease their therapeutic activity. Some drugs must be maintained at a therapeutic level in the blood for certain minimum periods of time, sometimes even after the patient feels he has recovered, as was pointed out in Rule 14 above. The patient must be thoroughly instructed as to the manner of using the medication, whether hypodermically, orally, rec-

tally, vaginally, or via some other route. The patient must also be instructed as to the amount of medication, as well as the frequency, duration, and timing of the dosage.

Patients are sometimes given a printed sheet of paper containing recommendations for proper handling of medications. The following is typical:

1. Give or take medications only as prescribed by a medical authority. Do not rely on the advice of a friend or on what you read in the newspapers and other lay publications.

2. Read the entire label carefully before giving or taking any medications.

3. Do not give or take medications in the dark.

4. Do not keep more than enough medication for one day or one night on the bedside table.

5. Do not keep two or more different medications together on the bedside table. Confused by sleep, the patient may take the wrong one.

6. Pour liquid medications from the side of the bottle opposite the label to avoid dripping over the label and obscuring directions.

7. Keep all medications in a locked medicine cabinet.

8. Discard all old outdated medications promptly. Toxic substances may develop in those that have deteriorated.

In addition to the above list of recommendations, patients are sometimes given a list of specific warnings and reactions with pertinent ones checked. Examples are:

1. This medication may color the urine green ☐, blue ☐, red ☐, . . .

2. Alcoholic beverages taken with this medication may cause undesirable effects.

3. Aspirin products taken with this medication may cause undesirable effects.

4. The following foods taken with this medication may be harmful: beer, cheese, figs, pickled herring, . . .

Such instructions are usually supplied by the dispenser of the prescribed medication.

DISPENSING MEDICATIONS

In the United States, where more than 2 billion prescriptions are filled a year, accuracy is essential. The correct drug, correct dosage form, correct amount, correct strength, and correct labeling, including correct directions must be provided. Errors can be and have been fatal. Carefully trained dispensers of medication who check and double-check each other make essentially no serious errors. Also, prepackaged prescriptions and unit-dosage packaging under rigidly controlled conditions by manufacturers has obviated many errors. On the other hand, the use of technicians and other personnel not fully qualified presents definite hazards, and if they are permitted to perform some of the duties of pharmacists they must be rigidly supervised by professionals at all times.

In one case of criminal negligence wherein dispensing duties were delegated to unqualified individuals, two patients in a hospital died when sodium nitrite solution was dispensed instead of Phospho Soda. In another case, an administrative nurse (assistant director of the nursing service) administered parenteral digoxin which was five times the strength of the oral medication intended. The three-month-old patient died. In yet another case, a patient died when fluid *extract* of ipecac was dispensed instead of the *syrup* by an unqualified person. In all three instances judgments were found against the hospitals involved.[76] The literature cites innumerable other cases involving criminal and civil tort liability where licensed pharmacists did not dispense or licensed nurses did not administer the proper medications.

Cleanliness is another key word in dispensing. Not only the drugs and drug products must be kept free of contamination of every type, but all equipment and working areas must be kept scrupulously clean and neat. Orderly arrangement of medications and their ingredients is essential to prevent errors in dispensing, loss of confidence in the prescription facility, and hazards for the patient.

Every physician should periodically pay unannounced visits to all pharmacies where his prescriptions are being filled and all nursing stations where his medications are being handled. He should inspect for cleanliness, neatness, and adequacy of facilities and personnel. If any unsatisfactory situation is ever encountered, he should immediately make suggestions for improvement directly to the chief pharmacist. If these are not followed, he should notify the appropriate authorities and try to prevent the medications for his patients from being handled there until the situation is taken care of one way or another. The welfare of his patients is at stake.

Mail Order Prescriptions

The practice of dispensing by mail can be detrimental to the patient. Because of the pitfalls this presents, distribution of prescriptions through the mail has been restricted. Federal regulations specifically prohibit use of the mails for narcotic prescriptions. In addition, mail order pharmacies are expressly forbidden by the statutes of 11 states and they are expressly allowed in only one. Legislation is pending in other states because most state Boards of Pharmacy believe that they cannot properly supervise such distributors. However, the use of mail orders for prescriptions is increasing substantially under the guise of association, club, or society sponsorship. If such sponsors assume the responsibility for dispensing medications, they must be prepared to face all the ethical, legal, and professional problems that may arise through both state and Federal actions and regulations. And there are some problems that they can never overcome.

In emergencies, patients cannot tolerate the time lag of several days which is normal for mail order prescriptions, especially if they have a severe, life-threatening infection or other serious condition. Even without the existence of an emergency, it is safer for any given patient to take his prescriptions to a pharmacy where he has routinely had prescriptions filled, because more and more pharmacies are keeping patient records so that they can keep track of patient hypersensitivities and idiosyncrasies and detect potential hazardous drug interactions and give the prescriber and patient adequate warnings.

Requirements for writing and handling prescriptions vary from state to state. In Massachusetts, by law, the physician must prescribe by generic name, even if he includes a brand name. The pharmacist is free to select the brand when a generic name is used, and he is not required to place the name on the prescription label. Patented drugs are excluded from the state formulary used as a basic prescribing tool. These and other practices and regulations vary as state borders are crossed. Therefore the hazards to the patient of substitution and inadequate information exist in some states and not in others. This is a major reason why ordering prescriptions by mail from another state may not guarantee the same quality of service that is available locally.

Physician-Controlled Medications

The United States government has estimated that in recent years about 10 percent of all patients purchased their drug products from physicians. By extrapolation from government data, it can be estimated that physicians control or own about 3,500 of the 52,000 pharmacies in this country.[63] Also, some own nursing homes, hospitals and other health care facilities with pharmaceutical services.

Although convenience, emergency situations, and the need for such service in isolated areas have been cited as major reasons for dispensing by physicians and for the existence of physician-owned pharmacies, there are obvious disadvantages to this system. Patients do not have free choice as to where they will have their prescriptions dispensed. Aside from lack of competition that normally tends to keep prices under control, unless the physician engages the professional services of a pharmacist, the patient is at the mercy of someone neither trained to dispense nor to preserve medications properly so that they remain fresh and potent. Even if surveys are conducted sometime in the future to determine whether the number of errors committed by dispensing physicians are minimal and whether their prescription prices compare favorably with those in the surrounding community pharmacies, there still remain the obvious risk of over-prescribing and the ethical consideration of conflict of interests when the physician is both prescriber and dispenser. Even if he does retain the services of a well-qualified pharmacist, the latter is not likely to be in a position to act freely and objectively in pointing out what appears to him to be prescription errors. In any event the entire situation is fraught with hazards for the patient,[63] and it is basically unethical for a physician to own and operate a pharmacy.

Somewhat related to the above situation is the physician-owned repackaging company. The potential for conflict of interests and patient exploitation is so obvious that the Judicial Council of the American Medical Association made the following declaration in 1967:

"It is unethical for a physician to be influenced in the prescribing of drugs or devices by his direct financial interest in a pharmaceutical firm or other suppliers. It is immaterial whether the firm manufactures or repackages the products involved. It is unethical for a physician to own stock or have a direct financial interest in a firm that uses its relationship with physician-stockholders as a means of inducing or influencing them to prescribe the firm's products. Participating physicians should divest themselves of any financial interest in firms that use this form of sales promotion. Reputable firms rely on quality and efficacy to sell their products under competitive circumstances, and not upon appeal to physicians with financial involvements which might influence them in their prescribing.

"Prescribing for patients involves more than the designation of drugs or devices which are most likely to prove efficacious in the treatment of a patient. The physician has an ethical responsibility to assure that high-quality products will be dispensed to his patient. Obviously, the benefits of the physician's skill are diminished if the patient receives drugs or devices of inferior quality. Inasmuch as the physician should also be mindful of the cost to his patients of drugs or devices he prescribes, he may properly discuss with patients both quality and cost."

When some repackaging companies were found to be selling drug products relabeled with their own name at 13 times the price charged by some other firms for exactly the same products from the same supplier, the Federal government pointed out that there was no valid reason to accept them under any Federal drug program.[63] No mention was made, however, of the potential hazards to the patient of improper packaging and incorrect labeling (see Chapter 5, *Distribution and Storage Factors*).

Rules for Dispensing

The physician depends on the pharmacist for proper support in many ways—proper handling of the patient and his prescriptions, keeping the medications of prescribers readily available, and having at his fingertips all needed information about these medications. Commandments have been written many times for prescription practice.[64] Some of the most useful are:

1. Allow only a qualified dispenser to handle the prescription from the time the written order is received until it is dispensed and the finished medication is ready for the patient.

2. Reinforce the physician's professional approach with appropriate attitude toward the patient and proper communication with him.

3. Avoid making any comments that are derogatory about the medication or the physician who prescribed it. Do not divulge information that only the physician should discuss with his patient.

4. Check for incompatibilities, dosage out of usual range, and possible drug interactions by referring to the patient's records. Call the physician immediately if any problems are detected.

5. Dispense in a quiet, professional atmosphere that will engender confidence in the facility, the personnel, and the medication.

6. Dispense the medication in a clean, neat package, carefully labeled after double-checking the name on the label with the patient to reinforce the fact that the therapy has been individualized for him. Also advise the patient about any special precautions to take and situations to avoid.

7. Label the prescription with the patient's full name; physician's name; prescription identification number; the name, quantity and strength of the drug unless exempted by the prescriber; date of issue; expiration date of all time-dated medications; name and address and telephone number of the pharmacy or hospital issuing the prescription; name or initials of dispenser; and complete and clear directions for use. Affix *Shake Well, External Use Only, Refrigerate, Keep Out of Reach of Children,* and similar precautionary labels as necessary. It is desirable to place the lot or control number and the name of the manufacturer on the original prescription order.*

8. Do not engage in a dispute over prices, but calmly explain why the price is high if it is above average.

9. Emphasize any special storage conditions necessary to preserve the prescription and explain why it has an expiration date and what will happen if it is not stored properly or it is used after the expiration date.

10. Make certain the patient has any necessary accessories such as droppers, eye cups, absorbent cotton, and other aids.

11. Make available special services, such as special phone numbers and delivery service, especially to the aged and infirm.

A major service rendered by the physician's associates is the providing of accurate, clear information about medications. In recent years, physicians have encouraged nurse's aides, practical nurses, and pharmacists to have closer contact with patients in clinical settings. The pharmacist, in particular, functions as a drug therapy consultant and keeps patient records which enable him to alert the attending physician to possible problems. He can also provide detailed information about each drug, including composition, dosage, and routes of administration.

Prescription Record System

A Prescription Record System should be maintained by every pharmacy to avoid duplication of drug therapy, administration of conflicting medications, and dangerous simultaneous use of interacting drugs. The system should record the following in a simple, easily maintained format.

1. *Patient Data*—Name, address, telephone number, chronic diseases, and known allergies, drug sensitivities, and idiosyncrasies.

2. *Prescription Data*—Prescription number, the name, strength and quantity of medication dispensed, the initials of each pharmacist who dispensed the prescription with date dispensed, directions for use, and cost to the patient.

Current levels of effective prescribing and of proper use of medications leave much to be desired. We are far from experiencing optimum return for current expenditures for drug therapy. For the sake of better patient health and welfare, we are introducing drug utilization review programs so that effective standards that will minimize irrational prescribing can be developed and established. Every hospital staff physician and pharmacist should become involved in correlating and analyzing drug data in patient records.[73]

---

*The American Society of Hospital Pharmacists has compiled *Guidelines Relative to the Safe Use of Medications in Hospitals.*

The pharmacist, with the aid of good record keeping, should be the first to know when a suicidal patient is stock-piling a drug product such as a barbiturate which he may be obtaining from several physicians. He should be fully alert to all potential hazards, such as use of a given medication over too long a period of time and he should note for permanent reference whenever an adverse drug reaction occurs, particularly when idiosyncrasy or hypersensitivity is involved.[92]

But neither consultant nor practitioner can depend completely on either experience or literature alone and be absolutely certain that the prescribed drug will be adequately safe and effective in any given patient. Experiences can be fortuitous, the literature can be incorrect, and even judgment can be faulty occasionally. In the final analysis, everyone concerned with medication of the patient must assume certain probabilities and act accordingly. The manner in which a drug product is administered is particularly critical to the patient.

ADMINISTERING MEDICATIONS

Far too many errors have been made in the administration of medications. Some error is inevitable in all human performance, but surveys indicate that up to 30 percent of all doses of medications given in some hospitals, where quality of drug therapy should be at the highest level, were either incorrect or harmful.[28] The major hazards lie in the nurse's interpretation of the physician's prescribing instructions and in the nurse's incorrect implementation of the prescribing.[28,57] Errors increase rapidly as the volume of prescriptions increases and when more than six prescriptions are being received by the same patient concurrently, administration of medication becomes inefficient.[83] See the discussions in Chapter 9 and Chapter 10.

A major contributing factor is a shortage of competent, well-trained, experienced nurses. During 1977, out of about 2 million persons in the active nursing personnel force of the United States about 1,200,000 were registered nurses of which 750,000 were active. The balance were licensed practical nurses, nurse's aides, orderlies, attendants, and homemakers-home health aides. Many of the latter groups who are not trained nurses, sometimes even assistants in the physician's office with only a high school education, are allowed to give injections and fulfill other patient care responsibilities. This situation will probably be intensified for some years as the demand for nurses continues to increase. Obviously, to improve the error situation, utilization of personnel and systems of health care must be improved. Hospitals are particularly vulnerable because they can be held responsible for the acts of nurses.[9]

Admittedly, many of the errors made by nurses such as a slight variation from the desired time schedule, omission of a dose, and failure to give the full dose either because too little liquid was poured into the medicine glass or too small an amount of a parenteral product injected, or a dosage form below the strength specified was used are not basically harmful to the patient. But on the other hand, increasing the frequency of dosage, prolonging administration beyond the specified period of time, giving too large a dose by selecting the wrong strength or administering too much, giving the wrong medication, giving the medication by the incorrect route or at a harmful rate, injecting in an improper manner or at the wrong site,[55,56,59,65,66] and many other related acts can be very dangerous for the patient.[6,8,13,21-23,25,27,31,35,36,48,69]

Some of the rules given for prescribing (page 114) and dispensing (page 119) apply to nurses. For example, a shift in the decimal place in calculating the volume of a parenteral to be injected can be tragic. Potent drugs have caused the death of patients when given in tenfold dose. Digoxin, for example, with a usual adult maintenance dose of 0.25 mg., has caused death when given in a dose of 2.5 mg. to an adult, and the same drug has caused death when 0.25 mg. was given by the nurse to an infant instead of the 0.025 mg. dose prescribed. Attempts are constantly being made to prevent such tragedies. In the well-managed hospital, a medication nurse is charged with the responsibility of supervising the dispensing of all medications from the various nursing stations to the individual patients. In the physician's office, the home of the patient or the hospital, dosage instructions are properly given in writing, reiterated verbally, and at times reinforced by sign language. Legibility of all written instructions is essential.

Rules for Administering

A recommended method for handling and checking medications before they are administered to patients in the hospitals, consists of the following rules and steps.[33,84]

1. Do not administer any medication without a prescription order signed by a physician, except in a real emergency. If medication has to be given without written authority, record it immediately on the standard record form and have it certified by the physician within 24 hours.

2. Do not, as a general rule, prescribe prospectively. The *date commenced, date given,* and *date prescribed* should be synonymous.

3. Make certain that the prescription order is legibly written in English, and clearly understood. Do not *assume* anything. Do not carry out any orders when there is any doubt as to the instructions; check with the supervisor or prescribing physician.

4. Know the medication to be administered—its method of preparation, composition, dose, mathematical calculations underlying the dosage, method of administration, desired effect, potential adverse effects, and proper antidotes.

5. Record the prescription order permanently on a standard form (file card or prescription sheet) which is used as a medicine list to avoid transcription errors. Avoid confusing abbreviations. Use only well understood ones like IM (intramuscular), INHAL (inhalation), IV (intravenous), PR (rectal), SC (subcutaneous), SL (sublingual), and TOP (topical). Write the others in full. Make special provisions for drugs such as anticoagulants and insulin that create special problems when the dose requires frequent adjustment. Some physicians prefer forms that record the diet, and that separate medications to be given regularly from those that are to be given only once, as well as parenteral from other types of medications.

6. Prepare a medication card for every medication ordered. Use red cards for narcotics and single and *stat* doses. Always check the card, which should be initialed by the nurse who prepared it, against the file card and prescription order book in which the original prescriptions are filed. Check the name of the patient, name of the medication, route, date, and time carefully. Always use the metric system of dosage.

7. Clearly identify the patient in all records and at all times. Enter the name, age, room number, physician in charge, and the names of the drugs to which the patient is sensitive.

8. Check the medication card against the drug label at least three times: (a) before removing the drug from the shelf, (b) before pouring and counting, and (c) when returning the drug to the shelf. Have a witness double check the dispensing and administration of dangerous drugs, particularly the identity of the drug, calculation of dosage, the measured dose, and the identity of the patient.

9. At the bedside, identify the patient by checking the medication card against the name on the wrist band and the name on the bed card, and by asking the patient to state his name.

10. Make certain that the prescribed dose has not already been administered by another nurse.

11. Administer only medications that were personally checked out for the patient and double check with the prescriber as necessary regarding calculations and identity of the product.

12. Remain at the bedside until the required dose of the medication has been taken by the patient. Do not leave medication at the bedside, except upon written order of the physician.

13. *Immediately* after the medication has been given, enter the fact in the patient's record card, also enter any unusual situations such as absence of the patient, refusal to take the medication, etc. Never make such entries prior to administration of the medication.

14. Do not return to the stock bottle any unused medication that has been poured or counted into a medication cup. Discard it.

15. Observe the patient carefully for a sufficient length of time (at least 30 min)* for adverse drug effects and report undesirable reactions according to the hospital regulations.

---

* Anaphylactic reactions to penicillin, for example, have not occurred for half an hour after the drug was given.

16. Always conform to the latest hospital regulations on handling emergency drugs, narcotics and dangerous drugs (anticoagulants, barbiturates, digitalis, etc.), controlling medicine cabinets and keys, ordering medications from the pharmacy, distributing and storing medications, and administering parenterals, internal and external liquids, and other special medications, including additives to IV fluids.

The three main principles covered by the above rules are (1) the prescription is the focus of the checking system, (2) drugs should not be administered without written prescriptions, except in a real emergency, and (3) meticulous care must be taken in order to administer the proper drug to the proper patient in the proper manner.

The U.S. Department of Health, Education, and Welfare has developed and is gradually establishing higher standards for professional care in nursing facilities receiving Federal funds for Medicare patients. As stricter standards relating to physician coverage, nursing care, dispensing and administration of drugs, medical records, planning and supervision of diet, fire protection and safety, sanitation, and environment are incorporated into regulations, improvements in medication accuracy will undoubtedly be realized, as well as a reduction in the frequency of litigation involving medications and medical practice.[91]

Some physicians have attempted to supervise and closely control the dispensing and administration of medications through group practice in their own clinics, but this concept has the disadvantages noted under Physician-Controlled Medications (page 119) and litigation continues to be voluminous.

HAZARDS OF LITIGATION

Whenever a patient suffers a consequential adverse drug effect, the physician is haunted by the spector of malpractice litigation. The legal theory most frequently involved in such suits is negligence. Occasionally, lack of informed consent will be of significance.

Complexity of the Problem

Cases which illustrate the diversity of situations which have led to lawsuits against practitioners include fractures induced by insulin shock therapy, injury resulting from radioactive cobalt therapy given subsequent to mastectomy, paralytic poliomyelitis following vaccination, nerve injury and cardiac arrest resulting from the use of spinal and local anesthetics, injury resulting from puncture of the dura during epidural anesthesia, excessive dosage with morphine following surgery, and loss of limbs when analgesics were given for gangrene diagnosed as tetanus.[62]

A patient with a family history of cancer developed the disease after a physician prescribed diethylstilbestrol for her for three years. Another patient developed serious abscesses at the site of injection of liver extract after continued use. Another, after receiving medication for pain, left the physician's office without a warning that it might make him drowsy. He went to sleep at the wheel of his car, ran off the road, and was killed. A bus driver experienced a similar problem and ran into a car. A child died from aplastic anemia as a result of chloromycetin therapy and the physician had not warned the parents of the danger. In all of these cases the physicians were held liable.[29]

Individual responses due to unique combinations of patient characteristics, environmental influences, drug interactions, physical and chemical incompatibilities, and variations in biological availability of drug products in the patient are some of the factors to be considered by those who prescribe and administer medications. In fact, the subject of adverse drug reactions and interactions has become so complex with the advent of more and more effective and potent drugs that it has become a subspecialty of medicine.

Every prescriber of medication, no matter what his specialty, repeatedly encounters unexpected, unpredictable, unfavorable, and, on rare occasions, violent responses to medication. The rarer types of adverse reactions are sometimes not identified until many thousands of patients have received a drug. On the other hand, once a reaction is clearly identified, the incidence sometimes seems to increase rapidly because physicians are alerted and it is then noted more frequently.

The physician is constantly confronted with the fact that adverse experiences tend to destroy good physician-patient relationships and, if severe, frequently lead to recriminations and legal actions which seek compensation for the injury. Even a simple diagnostic test can lead to a lawsuit, inasmuch as it is difficult to explain to an irate patient that a given reaction was caused by a drug interaction with the food eaten, or by some rare idiosyncrasy or hypersensitivity, or indirectly by some pollutant in the inhaled air. The doctrine of *caveat emptor* does not apply when the patient pays the physician for services, including written prescriptions for medication. [62]

Proof of Negligence

Some of the types of negligence with which physicians are charged include the following acts and omissions: (1) treatment of a condition with a drug not suitable for the condition, (2) failure to note a history of allergy to the drug administered, (3) use of improper injection technique, (4) failure to stop treatment with a drug as soon as a reaction occurs, and (5) failure to provide adequate therapy to counteract a reaction when it occurs.

Even failure to prescribe a needed medication constitutes negligence. Thus, a physician who treated a patient with a broken leg was sued when he failed to prescribe an antimicrobial after a controllable infection developed under the cast and the necrotic leg could not be saved. The orthopedic specialist who was called in to amputate the limb testified in court that the administration of a suitable antibiotic would have been in accordance with the standard practice of medicine.

In Daniels versus Hadley Memorial Hospital the decedent was given penicillin in the emergency room of the hospital for abrasions received in a fall from a bicycle at 9:05 AM. At 9:30, after leaving the hospital, he was discovered in its parking lot in anaphylactic shock, and was rushed back to the emergency room. General resuscitation efforts were started as soon as he was back in the emergency room, but negligence was found in the hospital personnel's failure to give an intravenous injection of epinephrine until 9:42 AM. [106]

In any court of law the plaintiff's attorney is always required to establish a cause-and-effect relationship by a preponderance of the evidence. Thus, in a case of drug allergy the following questions are often asked of the physician: When did the patient first have contact with the suspected ingredient? What was the source of the ingredient? When was the eruption or reaction first noticed, and in what parts of the body? How and during what time did the eruption or reaction spread? What prior skin condition did the patient have? What prior allergies did he have? What drugs, foods, and other products did the patient use before, during and after the time of exposure to the suspected allergen? Were suitable tests performed to determine patient sensitivity? How, when, and by whom were they done? What did they show? If no such tests were done, why not? [16]

The attorney must also establish a proper time relationship between exposure to the agent and the onset of reaction. Evidence must also be submitted to show that other users have previously had allergic reactions to the same product, in order to establish causation and to show that the offending ingredient is injurious. [51-53]

The determination of drug-induced permanent impairment or permanent disability, and the ratings for these are of major legal significance to the patient, attending physician, manufacturer of the implicated drug, and the insurance carrier. A valuable series on this subject, prepared by the AMA Committee on Rating of Mental and Physical Impairment, has been published in the AMA *Journal* beginning in 1958.

Whenever litigation is commenced, the questions asked of the prescribing physician go to the very heart of his medical reasoning. Why did the complication or error occur? Was it the result of negligence, or was there a certain probability that it would occur? Were you (or your employee) competent to administer the medication which is alleged to have caused the complication? Should you have expected it to occur? Did you take steps to prevent it? How long did it take you to recognize its presence? Did you handle it properly as soon as you recognized it?

The physician's defense, at times, may include one or more of the following theories: (1) that the patient was not injured by the medication, or by a complication, or by lack of proper care, (2) that he or his employee did not cause the injury, and (3) that he or his employee was not negligent. [39-43,53,54]

To protect himself, every physician must give his patients all necessary warnings and other important precautionary information, in accordance with the knowledge he possesses.[3] And manufacturers of drugs, to protect themselves, must provide physicians with complete information, especially through the package inserts which the courts have held to be the major source of drug information provided to physicians by the producers of medications. Once the manufacturer fulfills his responsibility through full disclosure to the physician, the latter almost automatically becomes the main legal target.[32,50] Ignorance of drug reactions is no defense when so much literature is available from government, industry, and private sources.[18,26,37,45-47]

The increasing involvement of physicians in drug related litigation was emphasized by Gossett, president of the American Bar Association in 1969[104] and by Curran of Harvard Medical School.[54] Gossett said:

"What is of special concern here, of course, is the extent to which the strict liability doctrine is being extended to physicians by recent court decisions. That such an extension is occurring is well known to all of us. Not long ago the trend of the decisions was to impose the greatest risk of liability on the drug manufacturer. But more recently, as you know, the warning procedures adopted by manufacturers have tended to shift a large share of that responsibility to the marketers of drugs and to physicians who prescribe them. In consequence, as we all know, physicians have been confronted with the need for more elaborate testing measures, greater precision in diagnosis, record-keeping, and the exercise of a high degree of care in obtaining informed consent from patients for the use of potentially harmful drugs, whether of an experimental or an established nature. Devising routine procedures to guard against liability thus has come to be of the greatest importance to the individual practitioner."

Added to the legal burdens of physicians was the elimination of the "locality rule", beginning in 1968.‡ Back in 1880 a Massachusetts court§ had declared:

"It is a matter of common knowledge that a physician in a small country village does not usually make a specialty of surgery, and however well informed he may be in the theory of all parts of his profession he would, generally speaking, be but seldom called upon as a surgeon to perform difficult operations. He would have but few opportu-

nities of observation and practice in that line such as public hospitals of large cities would afford. The defendant was applied to, being the practioner in a small village, and we think it was correct to rule that he was bound to possess that skill only which physicians and surgeons of ordinary ability and skill practicing in similar localities with opportunities for no larger experience ordinarily possess; and he was not bound to possess that high degree of ardent skill possessed by eminent surgeons practicing in large cities and making a specialty of the practice of surgery."

But in 1968 another Massachusetts court reversed that holding. The plaintiff had sustained numbness and weakness of her left leg following delivery of a baby on October 4, 1958 at St. Luke's Hospital in New Bedford, Mass. During delivery the specialist in anesthesiology administered an "excessive" dose of pontocaine (8 mg. in 1 ml. of 10% glucose) intraspinally. The court held that the conduct of the specialist, practicing in a city of 100,000 slightly more than 50 miles from Boston, one of the medical centers of the nation, was measurable not by the skill and ability of physicians in New Bedford but by the skill of the average member of the profession practicing the specialty, taking into account the advances in the profession and medical facilities available, and that instruction to the contrary was reversibly erroneous.

Within a year after the Massachusetts case was decided, 15 states had also rejected the 1880 decision. In these states, practitioners in any locality, rural or urban, no matter whether they are meagerly equipped or they have access to highly sophisticated instrumentation, are expected to possess the same high degree of competence and skill. The hazards of not taking adequate precautions to guard against liability are steadily becoming more ominous.

Although the trend is definitely away from the locality rule, it has not been eliminated in all states. In some it is still law and in others there is uncertainty. Almost all states have dropped the locality rule in cases of physicians who are board certified, since national examinations and standards govern certification.

Human Experimentation

Inherent in the nature of most physicians is the desire to push the frontiers of medicine forward by trying new techniques of drug

---

‡ *Brune v. Belinkoff*, 235 N.E. 2d 793 (Mass. 1968).
§*Small v. Howard*, 128 Mass. 131, 136 (1880).

therapy, exploring new uses for available medications, and testing new drugs not yet approved by the Food and Drug Administration. But such experimentation presents serious legal pitfalls, especially if a physician gives a patient assurance that he will be cured. This has happened occasionally and it places the physician in the awkward position of making a guaranty.

Legal pitfalls abound whenever physicians conduct human studies, especially with new drugs. Because the laws and regulations governing human experimentation are so comprehensive and exacting, every prospective investigator finds it necessary to spend many hours studying pertinent documents in order to avoid legal problems. Even the use of methadone in addiction is legally an investigational use, according to a 1970 FDA ruling. See pages 35-57 in Chapter 3.

In attempts to form suitable guidelines for human experimenters, numerous codes and statements have been prepared including the Oath of Hippocrates, the Declarations of Geneva and Rome, the Principles of Medical Ethics of the American Medical Association, the Nuremberg Code of Medical Ethics, the International Code of Medical Ethics of the World Medical Association, the Declaration of Helsinki, and the Regulations of the Food and Drug Administration. [19,30]

Codes of ethics in all spheres of human endeavor are merely detailed extensions of the Golden Rule. The relationships between doctor and patient, investigator and subject, and between all other professionals and those they serve are always highly honorable if the Rule is followed: "Whatsoever ye would that men should do to you, do ye even so to them."

A hundred years ago Claude Bernard wrote:

"The principle of medical and surgical morality, therefore, consists in never performing on man an experiment which might be harmful to him to any extent, even though the result might be highly advantageous to science, i.e., to the health of others."

However, imaginative experimentation is indispensable to the progress of medical science. If all forms of treatment were actually withheld until everything was known about them, physicians might not even be prescribing aspirin or performing appendectomies today. Clinical research with drugs always involves varying degrees of risk to the patient who agrees to be a test subject. The only way to eliminate risk completely is to abandon all medical practice and all medical research. Obviously, unimpeded suffering, rampant illness, and premature death would then prevail. [10]

Ultimately, evaluation of every type of medication for humans can only be made by means of trials in human subjects. Hence, clinical investigation is an essential element of drug research, and to some extent also of drug therapy. The prescriber who explores and understands the clinical research data substantiating his use of medications, and the legal and ethical considerations discussed above, feels secure when he administers drug therapy. He is in a position to select the most appropriate medications for his patients and to evaluate their response accurately. He is also well aware of the potential errors in diagnosis and follow-up that he can make if the drugs he uses can interfere with clinical laboratory testing.

SELECTED REFERENCES

1. American Medical Association: *Professional Liability and the Physician,* pamphlet issued by the Committee on Medicolegal Problems, 1963.
2. Annis ER: *Med. Trib.* 10:26 (Mar 31) 1969.
3. Anon: Explain ℞ side effects, attorneys warn physicians. *AMA News* p 17 (Oct 7) 1968.
4. Atchley DW: Patient-physician communication, *Cecil-Loeb Textbook of Medicine,* Philadelphia, Saunders, 1967.
5. Barr DP: Hazards of modern diagnosis and therapy—The price we pay. *JAMA* 159:1452, 1955.
6. Birch CA: Intramuscular injections and gas gangrene. *Br Med J* 2:242 (Apr 27) 1968.
7. Chayet NL: Technical assault and battery. *N Engl J Med* 276:514 (Mar 2) 1967; *The Citation* 14:145 (Feb 28) 1967.
8. Cohen SM: Accidental intra-arterial injection of drugs. *Lancet* 2:361-371 (Sep 4) 1948.
9. Curren WJ: Quality standards of hospital care—Who is legally liable? *N Engl J Med* 280:316 (Feb 6) 1969; Bernardi v Community Hosp Assoc, 443 p. 2d 708 (Col., 1968).
10. DeBakey ME: Medical research and the golden rule. *JAMA* 203:574-575 (Feb 19) 1968.
11. Editorial: Art of therapy. *JAMA* 211:1002 (Feb 9) 1970.
12. ———: Clean inside and out. *N Engl J Med* 281:853 (Oct 9) 1969.

13. ——: Gas gangrene from adrenaline. *Br Med J* 1:721 (Mar 23) 1968.

14. ——: Inform the patient. *JAMA* 211:654 (Jan 26) 1970.

15. ——: The case of the overdrugged patient. *Chain Store Age* 45:76-79, 1969.

16. Farage DJ: Judicial allergy to claims for allergic reactions, presented at an Institute on Personal Injury Litigation, held by the Southwest Legal Foundation, Dallas, Texas, Nov 5-6, 1964.

17. *Federal Register,* Doc 69-11461, (Sep) 1969.

18. Food and Drug Administration, U.S. Department of Health, Education, and Welfare: *FDA Clinical Experience Abstracts* Vol 15, 1966 to date; *FDA Reports of Adverse Reactions to Drugs* Vol 66, 1966 to date.

19. Food and Drug Administration, U.S. Dept. Health, Education, and Welfare: *Federal Food, Drug and Cosmetic Act* including Drug Amendments of 1962 with Explanations, Chicago, Commerce Clearing House, 1962.

20. Fox LA: Written reinforcement of auxiliary directions for prescription medications. *Am J Hosp Pharm* 26:334-341 (June) 1969.

21. French JH: Iatrogenic sciatic palsy. *Syllabus,* University of Colorado Medical Center, Annual General Practice Review, Denver, Colo (Jan. 7-13) 1962.

22. Gammel JA: Arterial embolism. *JAMA* 88:998-999 (Mar 26) 1927.

23. Gilles FH, French JH: Postinjection sciatic nerve palsies in infants and children. *J Pediat* 58:195-204 (Feb) 1961.

24. Goldstein SW: *Development of Safer and More Effective Drugs,* Washington, D.C., American Pharmaceutical Association, 1968.

25. Hanson DJ: Intramuscular injection injuries and complications. *GP* 27:109-115 (Jan) 1963.

26. Harris HW, *et al:* Registry of adverse drug reactions. *JAMA* 203:31-34 (Jan 1) 1968.

27. Harvey PW, Purnell GV: Fatal case of gas gangrene associated with intramuscular injections. *Br Med J* 1:744-746 (Mar 23) 1968.

28. Hoddinott BC, Gowdey CW, Couter WK, *et al:* Drug reactions and errors in administration on a medical ward. *Can Med Ass J* 97:1001-1006 (Oct 21) 1967.

29. Holder AR: Physician's liability for drug reactions. *JAMA* 213:2143-2144 (Sep 21) 1970.

30. Ladimer I, Newman RW: *Clinical Investigation in Medicine: Legal, Ethical, and Moral Aspects.* Boston University Law-Medicine Research Institute, 1963.

31. Lee WH, Stallworth JM: Sciatic nerve injury due to intragluteal injection of tetracycline HCI, followed by acute arteriospasm of the lower extremity: Report of case. *Angiology* 9:63-66, 1958.

32. Maronde RF, Burks D, II, Lee PV, *et al:* Physician prescribing practices, *Am J Hosp Pharm* 26:566-573 (Oct) 1969.

33. Martin EW: *Dispensing of Medication.* Easton, Pa., Mack Publishing, 1971; *Techniques of Medication,* Philadelphia, Lippincott, 1969.

34. ——: United States compendium of drugs. *Lex et Scientia,* The International Journal of Law and Science 6:49-53 (Jan-Mar) 1969.

35. Matson DD: Early neurolysis in the treatment of injury of the peripheral nerves due to faulty injection

of antibiotics. *N Engl J Med* 242:973-975 (June 22) 1950.

36. Mazzia VDB, Mark LC, Binder LS, *et al:* Radial nerve palsy from intramuscular injection. *NY State J Med* 62:1674-1675 (May 15) 1962.

37. Meyler L: Side effects of drugs as reported in the medical literature of the world, Vols I, II, III, IV, V, and VI. *Excerpta Medica.* New York, Excerpta Medica Foundation, 1957-1966.

38. Mills DH: Allergic reactions to drugs. *Calif Med* 101:4-8 (July) 1964.

39. ——: Malpractice and the administration of drugs. *Med. Times* 93:657-662 (June) 1965.

40. ——: Medical lessons from malpractice cases. *JAMA* 183:1073-1077 (Mar 30) 1963.

41. ——: Medicolegal responsibilities in physician-laboratory relations. *Texas J Med* 61:865-866 (Dec) 1965.

42. ——: Medicolegal responsibilities of practitioners to assure optimal therapeutic performance of drug products in patient care. *Drug Info Bull* 3:92 (Jan-June) 1969.

43. ——: Physician responsibility for drug prescription. *JAMA* 192:460-463 (May 10) 1965.

44. ——: Soliciting drug information from newly admitted patients. *Hospitals* 39:75-76 (Mar 16) 1965.

45. Miller AB, *et al: Physician's Desk Reference to Pharmaceutical Specialties and Biologicals* ed 22, Oradell, New Jersey, Medical Economics, 1968.

46. Moser RH: Diseases of Medial Progress. *N Eng J Med* 255:606, 1956; *Clin. Pharmacol. Ther.* 2:446, 1961.

47. Norman PS, Cluff LE: Adverse drug reactions and alternative drugs of choice in Modell W: *Drugs of Choice.* St. Louis, Mosby, pp. 30-47, 1966.

48. Ogilvie RI, Ruedy J: Adverse drug reactions during hospitalization. *Can Med Assoc J* 97:1450-1457 (Dec 9) 1967.

49. Palmisano PA, Cassady G: Salicylate exposure in the perinate. *JAMA* 209:556-558 (July 28) 1969.

50. Peeler RN, Kadull PJ, Cluff LE: Intensive immunization of man: Evaluation of possible adverse consequences. *Ann Int Med* 63:44-57 (July) 1965.

51. Personal Injury, Vol 3A. *Drugs and Druggists.* Matthew Bender, 1965.

52. Product Liability, Vol. 3. *Drugs and Druggists.* Legal Aspects, Matthew Bender, 1967.

53. Proof of Facts. *Am. Jur.* (see "Drugs" in General Index), Lawyers Co-op Pub. Co., 1965.

54. *Res Ipsa Loquitur, Trial of Malpractice Cases.* Chap. XV, Matthew Bender, 1966; Curran, WJ: Difficulties of proof in malpractice cases—Informed consent and *res ipsa loquitur. N Engl J Med* 281:1283 (Dec 4) 1969; 282:36-37 (Jan 1) 1970.

55. Rubbo SD, Gardner JF: Intramuscular injections and gas gangrene. *Br Med J* 2:241-242 (Apr 27) 1968.

56. Schreinberg L, Allensworth M: Sciatic neuropathy in infants related to antibiotic injections. *Pediat* 19:261-265, 1957.

57. Schimmel EH: The hazards of hospitalization. *An Int Med* 60:100-110, 1964.

58. Seneca H: Nephrotoxicity from cephaloridine. *JAMA* 201:146-147 (Aug 21) 1967.

59. Shaw EB: Transverse myelitis from injection of penicillin. *Am J Dis Child* 111:548-551 (May) 1966.

60. Smith MC, Hopper CB: Pharmacy service in prison hospitals. *Am J Hosp Pharm* 26:36-40 (Jan) 1969.
61. Teplitsky B: *Am Prof Pharm* 34:30-31 (Apr) 1968.
62. Tozer FL, Kasik JE: The medical-legal aspects of adverse drug reactions. *Clin Pharmacol Ther* 8:637-646 (Sep-Oct) 1967.
63. U.S. Department of Health, Education, and Welfare: *The Drug Prescribers.* Washington, DC, Task Force on Prescription Drugs, 1968.
64. Walsh RA: For prescription practice—ten commandments. *J Am Pharm Assoc* NS5:536-537 (Oct) 1965.
65. Williams B: Intramuscular injections and gas gangrene. *Br Med J* 2:242 (Apr 27) 1968.
66. Wilson GD, Hillier WF: Post injection paralysis. *South Med J* 45:109-113 (Feb) 1952.
67. Lane JM, Ruben FL, Abrutyn E, et al: Deaths attributed to smallpox vaccination 1959 to 1966, and 1968. *JAMA* 212:441-444 (Apr 20) 1970.
68. Hunter-Crain I, Newton KA, Westbury G, et al: Use of vaccinia virus in the treatment of malignant metastatic melanoma. *Br Med J* 2:512-515 (May 30) 1970.
69. Barker KN: The effects of an experimental medication system on medication errors and costs. *Am J Hosp Pharm* 26:324-333 (June) 1969.
70. National Communicable Disease Center: Follow-up smallpox—Federal Republic of Germany. *Morb Mort* 19:234-235, 240 (June 20) 1970.
71. Sollmann T: *A Manual of Pharmacology.* Philadelphia, Saunders, 1957, p 506.
72. Shilling JG: Patient instruction by written communication. *J Am Pharm Assoc* NS6:632-634 (Dec) 1966.
73. Rucker TD: The need for drug utilization review. *Am J Hosp Pharm* 27:654-658 (Aug) 1970.
74. Cain R: Patient record systems. *J Am Pharm Assoc* NS4:164-166 (Apr) 1964.
75. Rosner MM: Maintaining family records on drug sensitivities. *J Am Pharm Assoc* NS4:169-172, 175 (Apr) 1964.
76. Archambault GF: Legal considerations relative to drug distribution in hospitals. *Hosp Form Manag* 3:30-32 (Dec) 1968; 4:31, 40 (Sep) 1969.
77. U.S. Department of Health, Education, and Welfare: *Working with Older People,* PHS Publication No 1459, Vol I-IV, 1970.
78. Is your anesthetized patient listening? *JAMA* 206:1004 (Oct 28) 1968.
79. Kalow W: *Pharmacogenetics.* Philadelphia, Saunders, 1962, p 71.
80. Goldfarb AI: Doctor-patient role makes psychiatrists of all physicians. *Geriat* 25(4):45 (Apr) 1970.
81. Fisher TL: Casts. *Can Med Assoc J* 100:684 (Nov 29) 1969.
82. Teitelbaum DT, and Ott JE: Elemental mercury self-poisoning. *Clin Toxicol* 2:243-248 (Sep) 1969.
83. Vere DW: Errors of complex prescribing. *Lancet* 1:370-373 (Feb 13) 1965.
84. Crooks J, Clark CG, Caie HB, et al: Prescribing and administration of drugs in hospital. *Lancet* 1:373-378 (Feb 13) 1965.
85. Mann DE: Biological aging and its modification of drug activity. *J Pharm Sci* 54:499-510 (Apr) 1965.
86. Lasagna L: Drug effects as modified by aging. *J Chron Dis* 3:567-574 (June) 1956.
87. *FDC Rep* 43:5 (May 11) 1970.
88. Resnik HLP: Suicide attempt by a 10-year-old boy after quadruple amputations. *JAMA* 212:1211-1212 (May 18) 1970.
89. Vieweg WVR, Piscatelli RL, Houser JJ, et al: Complications of intravenous administration of heparin in elderly women. *JAMA* 213:1303-1306 (Aug 24) 1970.
90. Jick H, Slone D, Borda IT, et al: Efficacy and toxicity of heparin in relation to age and sex. *N Engl J Med* 279:284-286, 1968.
91. Standards for payment for skilled nursing home care. *Fed Reg* 34:9788-9790 (FR Doc. 69-7402) 1969; 35:6792-6795 (70-5147) 1970.
92. Wertz DL, Fincher JH, and Smith HA: Why use a prescription record system? *Iowa Pharm* 15:18-19, 23 (May) 1970.
93. Mullen SA: Liability for transfusion hepatitis. *JAMA* 213:467 (July 20) 1970.
94. Bryan PA, and Stern LH: The drug efficacy study, 1962-1970. *FDA Papers* 4:14-17 (Oct.) 1970.
95. *FDC Reports* 32: T&G 10 (Dec 14) 1970.
96. Craven JD, and Polak A: Cantharidin poisoning. *Br Med J* 2:1386-1388, 1954.
97. Presto AJ, and Muecke EC: A dose of Spanish fly. *JAMA* 214:591-592 (Oct 19) 1970.
98. Nickolls LC, and Teare D: Poisoning by cantharidin. *Br Med J* 2:1384-1386 (Dec 11) 1954.
99. Friend DG, Panelist, Drug Interaction Symposium, Hartford, Conn., May 6, 1970. Sponsored by the University of Connecticut School of Pharmacy, Connecticut State Pharmaceutical Association, and Connecticut Society of Hospital Pharmacists.
100. Herrell WE: Panic in the public. *Clin Med* 77:14-17 (Dec) 1970.
101. Hansen JM, Kampmann J, and Laursen H: Renal excretion of drugs in the elderly. *Lancet* 1:1170 (May 30) 1970.
102. Ineffective drugs. *FDA Papers* 5:13-16 (Feb) 1971.
103. Curran WJ: Legal responsibility for actions of physicians' assistants. *N Engl J Med* 286:254 (Feb 3) 1972.
104. Winslow JE: Introduction to *Better Health and Miracle Living* by Oral Roberts. Oral Roberts Evangelistic Assn, 1976.
105. Drug Information Association: *Proceedings* of the Joint DIA/AMA/FDA/PMA Symposium on Drug Information for Patients—The Patient Package Insert, 1977.
106. Daniels v Hadley Memorial Hospital. 566 F 2d 749 (CA DC) 1977.
107. Gossett WT: Address before the 1969 National Medicolegal Symposium jointly sponsored by the American Medical Association and the American Bar Association.
108. Editorial: Smallpox surveillance—worldwide. *Morb Mort Wkly Rep* 27:8 (Jan 6) 1978.

7 Hazards of Errors in Clinical Laboratory Testing

A major hazard in medication of the patient is overdependence of the physician on clinical laboratory data accepted without question or careful interpretation. Because laboratory procedures have limitations of accuracy, faulty values are sometimes reported. Based on these spurious values, wrong conclusions can lead to incorrect diagnosis, followed by faulty prescribing and irrational therapy with serious potential hazards for the patient.[1,5]

Faulty clinical laboratory test results are caused by a variety of situations that may or may not be under the control of the physician. The clinical and metabolic state of the patient and substances within the patient are often responsible.[21,76] Wirth and Thomson made an important contribution when they reported that a high value for catecholamines in one of their specimens was actually due to the presence of previously administered methyldopa rather than to adrenal pathology. They thereby prevented a patient from undergoing unnecessary major surgery, and the pathologist and his staff from receiving unjustified criticism.[40]

False values may be reported from a laboratory not only because of such chemical interferences, but also because of inferior laboratory technique, equipment failure, and biological and physical interferences. Faulty interpretation, however, as well as faulty results may have serious consequences for the patient. Yet no standard medical textbooks or reference works mention the problem that is created and its significance in drug therapy.[10,13,23,26-29,35,65,69-71]

INFERIOR LABORATORY TECHNIQUE

Analyses of specimens submitted to clinical laboratories depend upon chemical reactions with functional groups in chemical structures, upon the separation and measurement of specific ions, upon the electronic, manual, or mechanical measurement of physical characteristics, and upon other biological, chemical and physical procedures. But the accuracy achieved with these analytical procedures can be markedly influenced by aging of specimens; by contaminants (certain medications and their metabolites, oxidizing or reducing substances, etc.); dissolved oxygen; light; moisture; shifts in line voltages, in pH, and in temperature; and by a host of other variables if they are not detected and controlled by suitable means. The effects of interfering substances and of controlling variables should be assessed in the development, selection, and use of clinical laboratory testing methods and procedures.[6,7,9,40,68]

Prolonged experience with modern laboratory procedures is essential before a technician can be depended upon to report acceptable results. Adjusting pH, chromatographing, cooling, distilling, extracting, filtering, heating, measuring, mixing, pouring, separating, standardizing reagents, transferring, using instruments, weighing, and performing scores of other operations must be done skillfully to avoid losses, contamination, incorrect reading, and other defects of technique that cause inaccuracies. The following examples of faulty technique are typical of many that have been published. If the serum-salt mixture obtained during a serum proteinbiuret test is shaken too vigorously, the albumin is denatured and false colorimetric readings are obtained. If the glassware used for collecting specimens is not absolutely clean and the distilled water used for dilution of samples is not absolutely free from sodium and potassium, flame photometer readings for these elements can be seriously in error. It is unbelievable that a container used to collect a specimen for electrolyte determinations is sometimes rinsed in tap water first, but this has been done. [12, 15, 20, 25]

Cleanliness, accurate timing, frequent calibration of instruments and checking of reagents, gentle manipulation of sensitive materials, and use of control charts, control serums, highly specific test methods, suitable buffers, and other controls tend to minimize laboratory errors. Competent laboratory personnel not only use good technique but in addition they are always on the alert for hemolysis, lipemia, normal physiological variations in the patient, drug interferences, old or unstable specimens, and other less readily discernible influencing factors.

Hemolysis, which transfers constituents such as the enzymes lactic dehydrogenase and serum glutamic oxaloacetic transaminase to the serum and which interferes with tests for bilirubin, potassium, and sulfobromophthalein, should be avoided by prompt centrifugation to remove the cells as soon after collection of the specimen as possible. Lipemia, which occurs after a meal containing lipids and which interferes with colorimetric determinations, may be avoided by collecting the specimen after a fasting period.

EQUIPMENT FAILURE

In addition to paying such strict attention to pitfalls and technique, laboratory technicians must be constantly on the alert for equipment failure. [6, 7, 9, 20, 40]

Flame photometers, spectrophotometers, and other instruments used to examine blood, urine, and other specimens must be accurately calibrated in the laboratory in the environment where they are to be used. And they must be recalibrated periodically, especially if there is any change in an assay or

testing procedure or any change in the environment. The effects of shifts in temperature, humidity, and electric current, of changes in reagents, standards, or parts of instruments, and all other influencing factors must be eliminated with suitable blanks, recalibrations, or other control measures that eliminate variables. Unless sensitive, delicate instruments are used with meticulous care and handled by competent personnel, the laboratory values obtained can vary considerably from the true values.

Modern diagnostic clinical laboratories are being computerized and equipped with automatic analyzers.* With the aid of such mass production technology, and with competent supervision, these laboratories can accurately and rapidly perform several thousand determinations an hour on minute specimens of blood or urine. And as many as 20 simultaneous determinations can be made on a single specimen. Even complicated tests can be completed rapidly on small samples. For example, the assay of urinary alkaline phosphatase developed by Hardy of Beecham Laboratories as a sensitive indicator of early renal tubular damage (before histological evidence appears) entails predialysis to remove inhibitors and naturally occurring phenols, then incubation with substrate and activator, and finally postdialysis to remove protein and colored contaminants. In spite of its complexity, the assay, which is said to be a reliable indicator of drug safety, can be performed at the rate of 40 samples per hour, and only 0.6 ml of urine is needed for a determination.

Regardless of how advanced the methodology and equipment may be in a given laboratory, however, spurious results may be encountered, such as the false SGOT elevation induced by PAS in an AutoAnalyzer due to an inadequately specific coupling technique, [60] and globules of pHisoHex used as a perineal prep which were falsely reported as "red blood cells too numerous to count." [8] Technicians have a vital responsibility to the physician and to the patients whose samples

---

*Small, manual analyzers complete with liquid reagents are also available from a number of firms for performing tests rapidly in the physician's office so that prompt diagnoses can be made.

they are examining to detect such problems. But unfortunately they are not always made aware of the consequences of false reporting. This is the reason why more and more physicians, competent to judge technique, are directing clinical laboratories, and why exchange of information between clinicians on the one hand and clinical laboratory personnel on the other is being encouraged. As such communication improves, interpretations of test results will tend to become more accurate and the undesirable consequences of biological (especially pharmacological), chemical and physical interferences will tend to be eliminated.

BIOLOGICAL INTERFERENCES

Biological interferences may be the result of *immunological, pharmacological,* or *toxic* actions of medications or other chemicals in the patient. Examples are plentiful. Diuretics and certain steroids alter the concentrations of electrolytes in the blood and urine. Morphine, methyldopa, and other drugs elevate catecholamine levels in the blood. Probenecid decreases uric acid levels in the blood. Heparin depresses aldosterone secretion.[57] Penicillin increases 17-ketosteroid excretion.[53] A nasal decongestant containing phenylpropanolamine (Ornade Spansules) induces hypertension (bp 240/120) which responds positively to the phentolamine test for pheochromocytoma. Bismuth and gold salts, monoamine oxidase inhibitors, phenothiazines, and other drugs with hepatotoxic activity tend to produce abnormal values for alkaline phosphatase, cholesterol, cephalin flocculation, and other liver function tests (see Table 7-5). Phenothiazines also interfere with tests for pregnancy. Methyldopa, cephalothin, and other drugs interfere with the Coombs test and thus pose hazards in proper cross matching of blood for transfusion purposes.[6,17,48,49,51,52,54,55]

A number of interferences have been encountered in making skin tests. Antihistamines interfere with tests for allergies and they may mask hypersensitivities. Oral contraceptives may interfere with immune responses, and therefore may interfere with (depress) tuberculin skin test sensitivity. Live attenuated rubella and measles virus vaccines also interfere with tuberculin hypersensitivity

testing. False negative BSP results may be recorded when protein-bound BSP is excreted in the presence of marked proteinuria.[46,47]

Prothrombin time and the tendency to hemorrhage may be increased by (1) suppressing vitamin K synthesizing organisms in the intestinal tract with antimicrobial agents, (2) sequestering the oil-soluble vitamin in nonabsorbed mineral oil used as a cathartic, thus preventing absorption, (3) decreasing hepatic synthesis of prothrombin, (4) inhibiting metabolism of anticoagulants, and (5) displacing anticoagulants from protein binding sites (see Chapter 10 on *Drug Interactions* for explanations of these types of interferences).

Prothrombin time and the tendency to hemorrhage may be decreased by (1) administering vitamin K, (2) improving its absorption, (3) increasing hepatic synthesis of prothrombin, (4) inducing the rate of metabolism of anticoagulants, and (5) binding anticoagulant drugs.

Thyroid function tests may give faulty readings in the presence of drugs that alter the rate of metabolism (enzyme inducers or inhibitors), excite or depress the central nervous system (CNS stimulants, sedatives, etc.), uncouple phosphorylation from oxidation (salicylates), and interfere with iodine uptake, its bio-transformation into organic iodine, release of thyroid hormone into the blood, protein binding of this hormone, amount of proteins that bind the hormone (sex hormones), or its displacement from binding sites (salicylates).[68]

Liver function tests may yield elevated readings with hepatotoxic drugs that cause liver damage (see Table 7-5). Jaundice and intrahepatic cholestasis may occur. Both the damage and the jaundice are usually reversed by discontinuing the medication. The icterus index may be lowered when barbiturates stimulate the enzymatic glucuronidation of bilirubin and lower its serum level.[68]

Biological interferences may also be the result of altered biochemical activity *in vitro*. Fluoride may be added to a specimen to prevent enzymatic breakdown of a constituent such as glucose but the inhibiting fluoride may interfere with the enzymatic determination of other constituents. Certain drugs may also act as enzyme inhibitors. Thus, BUN determinations may be seriously inaccurate if the enzyme urease used in the test is significantly inhibited by a fluoride additive or some medication in the blood. Uric acid values determined with uricase, glucose values determined with glucose oxidase, and other values determined with the aid of other enzymes may be highly inaccurate unless inhibition of the enzymes by additives, medications, and proteins in the specimens is avoided.

Among the many substances that cause interferences in the enzymatic determination of glucose are (1) fluoride and chloride at low pH which inhibit peroxidase in the *o*-toluidine colorimetric method, (2) shift in pH during protein precipitation, (3) heavy metals introduced by protein precipitation reagents, (4) peroxides released from whole blood by acid or by reactions with or by ion exchange resins, (5) reducing agents such as ascorbic acid, bilirubin, catechols, cysteine, glutathione, thymol, and uric acid, (6) oxidizing agents such as chlorine and light, (7) impurities in the glucose oxidase preparation such as amylase and maltase. [1,66]

PHYSICAL INTERFERENCES

Physical interferences are often encountered in colorimetric, fluorometric, or photometric determinations. Thus, colors are imparted to the urine by the anthelmintic dithiazanine iodide (blue) and the urinary analgesic phenazopyridine hydrochloride (orange-red). The vitamin riboflavin, carrots, and other foods containing yellow pigments will elevate the values reported for an icterus index if they are ingested by a patient just prior to the withdrawal of a specimen for the determination (see Tables 7-4 and 7-5). In the performance of arterial dilution curves with indocyanine, heparin preparations containing sodium bisulfite reduce the absorption peak of the dye in the blood and should therefore be avoided. Heparin containing benzyl alcohol interferes in the fluorometric determination of plasma corticosteroids. [58] Spironolactone interferes in the measurement of plasma 11-hydroxycorticosteroids. [56] In spectrophotometric and colorimetric determinations selection of the optimum wavelength may be critical. Thus, selection of the

wavelength of 460 mμ rather than the 420 mμ sometimes specified for determining bilirubin in the serum tends to avoid elevation of the reading by traces of hemoglobin.

CHEMICAL INTERFERENCES

The most frequently encountered sources of error in clinical laboratory testing are interfering chemicals, including drugs and food constituents taken by the patient for whom tests are being conducted. Hundreds of examples of chemicals that can cause false positive (or abnormally high) or false negative (or abnormally low) clinical laboratory test values, or prevent a given laboratory method from working properly are listed in Tables 7-1 to 7-7. Both physician and technician, as well as the pharmacist and nurse if they are involved, must try to prevent such interferences from producing false results.

The presence of a drug, contaminant, or other substance that causes false test results is often completely unsuspected by the technicians or the physician. Boucher *et al.* provide an interesting example of detection of an obscure interfering chemical in a specimen. Despite pretreatment with Amberlite resins, samples of blood withdrawn through indwelling venous Intracath catheters were found to have PBI values falsely elevated 20-50 mcg. per 100 ml. The cause of the false-positive values was found to be iodine leached from the iodine-containing plastic used to manufacture the "radiopaque" catheters. [4]

Ubiquitous chemicals are often unsuspected causes of false clinical laboratory results. For example, *chelating* (sequestering) *agents* such as ethylenediamine tetraacetic acid (Edathamil, EDTA, Versene) and derivatives such as calcium disodium edetate (Calcium Disodium Versenate) decrease or give false-negative values for serum calcium. These agents are widely used in many drug products to prevent discoloration and oxidation caused by traces of some metals, to improve filtration of the products, to stabilize ascorbic acid, hyaluronidase, and other medications, and to improve cleansing of manufacturing equipment. In addition they are used as antidotes in lead poisoning and as an experimental treatment for urinary calculi, hypercalcemia, and calciferous corneal deposits.

Some drugs contribute an *element* being determined. Thus, the iodine content of radiographic contrast media interferes with protein-bound iodine determinations. Drugs also interfere through *oxidation* or *reduction* reactions. Thus ascorbic acid, penicillin, streptomycin, and many other drugs react with copper sulfate in the Benedict test for glucose. Especially noteworthy are the opposite results obtained with different *methods*. Elevated or false-positive glucose readings are obtained in the presence of ascorbic acid when the Benedict method is used and the opposite, that is, decreased or false-negative readings, are obtained with the same drug when the oxidase method is used. The same holds true for other substances such as hydrogen peroxide and hypochlorites. [2,6,7,12,15]

Some drugs produce *metabolites* that interfere with certain tests. To illustrate, any aspidium absorbed from the gastrointestinal tract yields a metabolite that produces a false-positive glucose value with the Benedict test; penicillin and tolbutamide yield metabolites that produce false-positive values for protein in the urine; and quinine yields a metabolite that produces elevated readings for catecholamines in the urine.

Some of the most widely used medications interfere with an appreciable number of tests. [19,45] Tetracyclines, for example, may interfere with laboratory values for albumin, amino acids, bilirubin, catecholamines, glucose, and estrogens in the urine, and values for alkaline phosphatase, bilirubin, BSP, cephalin flocculation, cholesterol, glucose, NPN, phosphate, potassium, SGOT, SGPT, WBC, and thymol turbidity in the blood. Thiazide diuretics may interfere with the values for calcium, creatine, creatinine, glucose, hemoglobin and uric acid in the urine, and BUN, calcium, chloride, glucose, hemoglobin, RBC, thrombocytes, and WBC in the blood. Other commonly used substances that interfere with various tests are ascorbic acid, bananas, corticosteroids, nicotinic acid, PAS, penicillin, phenothiazines, salicylates, and sulfonamides. [6,7,14,38,40,67]

Some drugs interfere with test results through enzyme induction or inhibition (see pages 371 and 373). Thus, prolonged use of phenytoin increases hepatic metabolism of metyrapone (Metopirone) and interferes with the use of this agent in the pituitary function test. Since metyrapone is an inhibitor of the enzyme 11-beta hydroxylase which is active in the synthesis of aldosterone, cortisol and corticosterone, the agent tends, in the normal individual, to decrease plasma concentrations of these substances and increase the precursors which are measured as 17-hydroxycorticosteroids (17-OHCS) and 17-ketogenic steroids (17-KGS). Decreasing the activity of the test agent with the enzyme inducing phenytoin lessens the enzyme inhibiting effect of the agent and readings for 17-OHCS and 17-KGS are lower than they should be. Since this is the effect produced in patients with hypopituitarism (lack of ACTH stimulation), the low readings in a normal patient may be thus misinterpreted. Also by means of enzyme induction, phenytoin interferes with the dexamethasome suppression test, as diagnostic of Cushing's syndrome. [15,59]

Cross et al. [11] drew attention to the large number of drug products that may be involved in a given type of interference despite the fact that only one drug is the interfering chemical. They cite the false-positive or elevating effect of formaldehyde on catecholamine values. Because methenamine liberates formaldehyde, a large number of urinary medications (Azolate, Azomandelamine, Donnasep, Hexatone, Hiprex, Lithitroll, Mandalay, Mandechlor, Mandelamine, Mandex, Mesulfin, Proklar, Renelate, Urised, Urital, Uritone, Urolitia, Uropeutic, Uro-phosphates, Uroqid, etc.) may incorrectly indicate a probable diagnosis of pheochromocytoma because they may cause catecholamine readings of up to 100 times normal. Lipman published a list of medications containing alcohol which interferes with some clinical laboratory tests. [80] Reeme has compiled a list of 52 medications containing glyceryl guaiacolate, an antiasthmatic drug that interferes with the 5-hydroxyindoleacetic acid (5-HIAA) test for the presence of serotonin (5-hydroxytryptamine). [32-34,63] He recommends withdrawal of medications for 48 to 72 hours prior to collection of urine for this test for carcinoid tumors. [32] Abnormal values are also frequently caused by physical and chemical effects of drugs in the patient and by drug-induced iatrogenic diseases. [11,24, 36,37]

The long list of drugs given in Table 7-5 may cause an increased or false positive BSP test because they may produce hepatotoxicity, alter liver function, or produce jaundice or hepatitis. Some of the drugs (e.g., barbiturates, isocarboxazid, meperidine, morphine, and radiopaque media may increase BSP retention by competing for the same excretion mechanism. Radiopaque media may interfere for as long as a week after administration for radiological diagnosis of biliary tract disease. Marked proteinuria may give rise to a false negative BSP reading through excretion of protein-bound BSP in the urine. Also, if the patient has not fasted, false negative results may be obtained because of increased hepatic blood flow which results in increased excretion of BSP from the blood via the bile. [55]

For some tests the list of interferences is very long. Probably hundreds of drugs and other chemicals, if introduced into the body, interfere with the determination of glucose and almost all of them give an elevated or false-positive reading. The same is true for albumin in the urine as an indicator of renal function. Since albuminuria occurs in congestive heart failure, infectious diseases, and renal disease, elevated values can be dangerously misleading.

Tables 7-1 to 7-8 (pages 140-199) summarize biological, chemical, and physical interferences that have been reported in the literature. An attempt should always be made to avoid the addition of substances that will affect test values and to isolate the substance being determined as much as possible from all interfering constituents of the specimen before making a determination. Additives such as anticoagulants, ammonium oxalate, sodium citrate, and disodium EDTA decrease blood pH whereas potassium and sodium oxalates elevate it. Proper selection of anticoagulants and preservatives for specimens, therefore, is critical.

Attempts have been made to compile computerized lists of all effects of drugs on clinical laboratory tests [74] and to prepare critical reviews of the original literature on the subject. [75-7,81] Attempts also have been made to evaluate statistically the probabilities for the problems arising from false laboratory values. [50] Obviously, when multiple drug therapy is administered, the difficulty of interpreting test results correctly is increased many times.

FAULTY INTERPRETATION

Correct interpretation of clinical laboratory test results is often very difficult because so many factors must be kept in mind, not only all the interferences and other sources of error mentioned above, but also the normal variations and abnormal responses in patients.* Many of the factors are beyond the control of the physician even though he must sometimes depend almost completely on test results to guide him in selecting appropriate medication for his patient.

Interfering substances derived from diet and drug therapy can usually be eliminated by withdrawing all foods and drugs for an appropriate period of time before specimens are obtained. Most dietary constituents can be eliminated by fasting from early evening until late morning or noon of the following day. But there are exceptions. Meat, for instance, must be avoided for several days before the feces are tested for occult blood, and a number of interfering drugs may be present in the body fluids for several days or longer.

More care must usually be taken in avoiding the effects of medications than the effects of foods. Some drugs like ACTH, probenecid, salicylates and steroids that substantially alter uric acid levels in the blood should be discontinued for several days to a week prior to removal of a specimen for uric acid determination. But drugs with very long half-lives, such as certain organic intravenous radiopaque iodine compounds that influence PBI readings for years, often cannot be discontinued long enough before a test. Lipiodol and iophendylate (Pantopaque) may affect PBI values for 9 or 10 years. Offspring born several years after the mother received a radiopaque iodine compound (Teridax iophenoxic acid) were found to have extremely high PBI

---

*Thus, no test for glycosuria is a certain diagnosis for diabetes. Persons without diabetes but with a low renal threshold for glucose may excrete appreciable quantities of it, whereas a person with diabetes but with a high threshold may excrete no detectable quantities. Only blood sugar determinations are confirmatory, in conjunction with a glucose tolerance test.

levels, as well as the mother. This phenomenon does not occur with all iodine-containing diagnostics, but allowances must often be made for their effects on the clinical test values. [42,43,65]

The effects of drugs on biochemical values may be altered by dosage level and concomitant therapy. A common but rarely considered example is the variation in the effect of aspirin on test results. At lower dosage levels, it tends to cause uric acid retention and elevate values for the serum level, whereas at doses above 3 Gm. per day the drug becomes uricosuric and the reverse is true. However, the uricosuric action of aspirin and other salicylates at high doses (5 Gm. per day) is reversed by phenylbutazone therapy. And, interestingly, the uricosuric action of probenecid (Benemid) and sulfinpyrazone (Anturane) is inhibited by large doses of aspirin, and urates are retained.

The aging of a specimen may seriously affect the clinical test values through chemical reactions. The following important situations illustrate this problem. The ammonia (NH_3) content of a blood specimen increases at the rate of 0.3 mcg. per 100 ml. per minute at 23°C (room temperature).* And blood glucose decreases at the rate of 15 mg. per 100 ml. of blood per hour at 37°C (body temperature) when it is allowed to stand for a period of time before analysis. Obviously chemical action alters ammonia and glucose and possibly other values when specimens are allowed to stand for a period of time before analysis. [6,7]

Temperature variations also affect test values. Usually, changes in values for most constituents tend to be prevented as the temperature is reduced, but not always. One exception is the pH of blood, which increases 0.015 units per degree decrease in temperature from body temperature. Turbidity and flocculation test values are also influenced by temperature, but not always in the same direction. For instance, values for thymol turbidity decrease and for phenol turbidity in-crease as the temperature is raised from 15°C to body temperature. Refrigeration and freezing are recommended by various authorities for the preservation of specimens. But sometimes neither refrigeration nor freezing are necessary and sometimes neither should be used when certain constituents are to be determined. Thus, some lactic dehydrogenase isoenzymes (elevated in myocardial infarction) are stable at room temperature (20-25°C) but are labile at 4°C. And serum proteins can be denatured by freezing. They should be merely refrigerated (about 4°C). Obviously the temperature at which specimens are stored is an important consideration. [6,7,9,14,39]

Wide variations in normal biochemical values from one individual to another are often noted. Therefore, base lines for each individual would be useful for reference purposes since individual patterns usually remain fairly constant, but these data are seldom available before disease strikes. Then, too, certain values fluctuate in every person because of diurnal, nocturnal, or seasonal influences and because of the effects of the patient's age, postural changes, sex, and other factors.

Diurnal variation (circadian periodicity) in the levels of iron, 17-ketosteroids and uric acid in the serum as well as in the urinary excretion of catecholamines and 17-hydroxycorticosteroids and the fecal excretion of urobilinogen have been noted. Hansen and others have described diurnal patterns for ACTH, adenosine phosphates, amino acids, blood glucose, glucagon, growth hormone, insulin, iron, nucleic acids, serum free fatty acids, and tyrosine transaminase. Even the gastric secretory response to the common stimuli of alcohol, histamine, and food vary from day to day in any one individual. Thus difficulty may be encountered in interpreting a histamine test for gastric secretion of hydrochloric acid unless antihistamines are used with a dose of histamine large enough to produce maximum parietal cell output of acid. [18,61,62,64,65]

But these diurnal patterns may be altered by degree of activity and emotional disturbances. Exercise can affect serum levels of glucose, lactic acid, and proteins. Psychic adversities can have a powerful impact on the

---

* Room temperature is an inaccurate designation as it varies from one laboratory to another and from one country to another. Laboratory temperature in the United States averages 25°C but actually ranges between 20°C and 30°C, while in China, according to the literature, "room temperature" is reported at 40°F.

body and precipitate psychosomatic disorders with resultant biochemical changes in the body. Emotional disturbances can affect serum cholesterol, glucose, and hydrocortisone values. The levels of serum cholesterol may vary as much as 200 mg. per 100 ml. or 100% from one day to the next in persons under stress conditions. [1,15,22]

To make interpretation of test results even more difficult the periodicity of circadian patterns is reversed by reversal of the day-night living schedule, by altering the length of the rest-activity pattern, by dissociating waking from the onset of light, by certain depressive illnesses, and by central nervous system diseases associated either with impairment of consciousness or an impaired hypothalamic-limbic system. Nevertheless, all variations in the normal individual should be taken into consideration when his specimens are tested in the clinical laboratory and the results evaluated. Otherwise the consequences can be hazardous for him. [6,7,14,40,62]

Multiphasic testing presents some complex and difficult problems when used in mass screening programs. Incorrect interpretations thus mass-produced can lead to needless expense and undesirable responses due to the administration of inappropriate or unnecessary medication. Whenever a single laboratory result is inconsistent with the remainder of the clinical data, interpretation must always be guarded. About half of a group of healthy subjects receiving laboratory tests may show one or more abnormal values due solely to chance. No test has the proper degree of sensitivity to identify all individuals with an abnormal condition or to yield negative findings consistently for all normal individuals. There is always appreciable overlapping of ranges for abnormal and normal values even when age, race, sex, and other pertinent variables are taken into consideration. Also, the distinction between healthy and diseased persons is not sharply defined, and the exact effect of medications on test values is still in some instances a moot point.

Agreement on the extent to which medications influence clinical laboratory test results has not been unanimous. In one survey, comprising 2,532 adult hospital admissions and 1,904 instances of medication, abnormal test results in patients with and without disease, and receiving or not receiving medication, were computerized and the incidences evaluated. The admission multiphasic screening battery of tests consisted of alkaline phosphatase, calcium, cholesterol, creatinine, fasting serum glucose, glutamic oxaloacetic transaminase, phosphorus, urea nitrogen, and uric acid. Statistical analyses of the correlations indicated that (1) very few medications affected the test results in this particular population, (2) medications affected the test results only to a minimal extent or only in a few unusually idiosyncratic patients, and (3) combinations of medications were without effect. [44] Obviously, more data must be carefully collected under rigidly controlled conditions to confirm or disprove the large body of information on chemical interference that has been reported. Numerous questions can be raised. How much dependence can be placed on the test results reported from each given laboratory? Which medications definitely affect clinical laboratory test results? Which tests? And to what extent? What is the true clinical significance of each abnormal test result? Was the correct dose given? Was specimen withdrawal timed correctly? Was the patient fasting as directed? Were all the guidelines given on pages 137–138 carefully followed?

And which reference data are to be used in interpretating results? Some papers on clinical laboratory testing present correlations of test results with disease conditions that are in direct conflict with most of the other clinical literature. Statements can be found to the effect that serum copper levels are *elevated* in Wilson's disease, serum iron binding capacity is *decreased* in the presence of low serum iron levels, decreased serum cholesterol values are noted in *hypothyroidism,* plasma cholesterol is *decreased* by the action of ACTH, mineral oil *promotes* the absorption of vitamin K, etc. Moreover, normal values used for reference vary from one reference book to another and from one laboratory to another. [10,16,21,23,35,68]

The foregoing facts emphasize the necessity of evaluating the results of laboratory tests in the light of *all* factors present which are known to alter normal values. [14] Although clinical laboratory values are some of the most critical diagnostic indicators, they frequently depart from the norm not only because of well understood influences but also because of some that are not always readily recognized. [1-8,19,21,26,38] Although the variations from correct test values caused by the problems discussed in this chapter are large enough to cause faulty diagnosis, a great deal of investigation remains to be carried out to determine the true effects on patient diagnosis and therapy. To increase sensitivity of case identification in mass multiphasic testing programs, computers are being used to evaluate individual laboratory results against values obtained for an optimum range of health rather than against so-called "normal ranges" as they are presently derived. Many of the serious consequences of faulty interpretations can thus be avoided. [41,44,67]

SERIOUS CONSEQUENCES

The consequences to the patient, physician, or litigant can be serious if a physician (general practitioner, specialist, or forensic consultant) receives a faulty laboratory report or he misinterprets the test results. Perhaps a normal blood cholesterol is reported instead of a very high one, a very high BMR or radioactive iodine uptake instead of a normal one, no increase of blood bilirubin for a patient with obstructive jaundice, no elevation of SGOT in the presence of myocardial infarction, arsenic in the blood when none is actually present, lead absent in a victim of lead poisoning, or no organisms identified in a patient with a potentially fatal infection. Hundreds of potentially serious situations involving electrocardiography, hematologic and histologic techniques, microbiological methods, microscopy, and physical and chemical testing may arise. Patients may be given incorrect medication when the physician places too much dependence on clinical laboratory results. That faulty results are reported all too frequently has been demonstrated in several countries by sending identical samples for testing to a number of laboratories simultaneously and then comparing the reported values and readings. The comparisons are often very disheartening and alarming.

The literature on the effect of various conditions and substances on the results of clinical laboratory testing has been reviewed by several authors and lengthy tables of literally hundreds of interfering substances have been published (see Tables 7-1 to 7-7). Most of the interfering chemicals elevate the laboratory values or cause false-positives, but most of the interferences can be eliminated by withdrawing all food and medication for 12 to 24 hours before taking a specimen for a test. A serious problem is always present, however. All values must be related to so-called normal ranges which are sometimes broad. It is often difficult to be certain whether a given value determined in a given clinical laboratory should be considered normal or abnormal. This problem is to some extent due to the nature of the base lines established for the patient, but it is largely due to variations in laboratory technique, not only between laboratories but also between personnel in the same laboratory. [5,10,12,13,15,16,20,22,23,25,35]

To promote the development and use of national and international standards that are needed for proper activity and operation of clinical laboratories, the National Committee for Clinical Laboratory Standards (NCCLS) was formed in 1968. This nonprofit organization, composed of representatives of governmental, industrial, and professional organizations, prepares written specifications for (1) biological and chemical reagents and reference materials, (2) reference methods and procedures, (3) operating methods (4) controls for equipment, and (5) other applicable matters. The resulting NCCLS Standards are reviewed at three-year intervals and updated if necessary.

A list of organizations which offer short-term training in clinical and public health laboratory procedures has been compiled by the National Center for Disease Control, Atlanta, Georgia.* Some of the courses, offered as continuing education, are made available at no cost to the student, in an attempt to upgrade the caliber of clinical laboratory testing.

RULES FOR CLINICAL LABORATORY TESTING

How physicians obtain and handle specimens for clinical laboratory analysis, how technicians subsequently process these speci-

---

*For information write to Education Specialist, Laboratory Division, National Center for Disease Control, Atlanta, Georgia 30333.

mens, and how physicians interpret the test results influence the accuracy of each diagnosis. The pitfalls present at each step may be largely avoided if both physicians and technicians abide by the following rules.

1. Obtain an appropriate specimen paying particular attention to procedure, size, and source. Avoid interferences from diet and medication by requiring a suitable fasting period and a period of abstention from medication (a week or more) prior to withdrawal of the specimen.

2. Avoid contamination in obtaining the specimen. Use perfectly clean, dry glassware, syringes, and other equipment cleansed with distilled water and sterilized when necessary. When testing for alcoholic content of the blood, for example, withdraw the blood specimen very carefully to avoid contamination of the blood with the alcohol used to cleanse the withdrawal site.

3. Seal the specimen immediately in a suitable container that affords protection from air, condensation, evaporation, light, and other influencing factors to which it is sensitive while it is being transported to the clinical laboratory.

4. Add appropriate anticoagulants, preservatives, and other substances as necessary. Select those that do not interfere with the laboratory tests to be performed.

5. Lable the container clearly with name and address of both patient and physician, also the date and time specimen was obtained.

6. Analyze the specimen as soon as possible to avoid alteration of the constituents, or store under specified suitable conditions until analysis is begun.

7. Use the most specific analytical method available and allow only competent technicians to make the determinations with the aid of accurate instrumentation that provides reproducible results.

8. Record the analytical results for each specimen methodically and accurately to avoid errors in reporting.

9. Report the results accurately, completely, and promptly. Double-check calculations and hold an exact duplicate of the report on file.

10. Interpret the results in terms of patient's activities, environment, diet, medication, normal variabilities (age, sex, and diurnal, nocturnal, postural, and seasonal variations), and the other influencing factors that must be considered.

11. Refer to Tables 7-1 to 7-7, keeping in mind that the interferences listed have been reported in the literature but that all of them do not necessarily occur during every test to a degree that is significant. Also, other interferences are constantly being discovered. Keep abreast of these by consistently reviewing publications that concentrate on this type of information. The following are very useful:

Clin-Alert
Clinica Chimica Acta
Clinical Chemistry
Drug Intelligence and Clinical Pharmacy
Excerpta Medica
Hospital Formulary Management
Index Medicus
International Pharmaceutical Abstracts
The Medical Letter

Physicians who make certain that these rules are followed, who understand the interferences in clinical laboratory testing, and who make the final interpretation in the light of all pertinent factors, are consistently more accurate in their diagnoses and hence more often achieve satisfactory patient response to medications. Laboratory procedures, nevertheless, represent merely an extension of a carefully compiled history and a carefully performed physical examination and are not a substitute for these basic procedures. [67]

Tables of Clinical
Laboratory Interferences

Note: The interferences with clinical laboratory tests, collected from the literature and tabulated in the following pages, may not occur or may occur to varying degrees depending on the test method used, concentrations, temperature, and other factors. Also, even slight modification of a test method may eliminate the effect of an interfering drug.

Table 7-1　Interferences in Clinical Chemistry of Blood[6,7,11,12,13-16,20,25,40,65,68,72-78,81]
(Values for Serum Unless Otherwise Stated)

Laboratory Tests (Conditions Detected)	Normal Values and Significance of Abnormal Values	Causes of False-Positive or Elevated Values (+)	Causes of False-Negative or Decreased Values (−)
Acid Phosphatase (Abnormal erythrocytic and prostate gland functions; prostatic carcinoma with metastases)	0.5–5 Babson Read units 0–0.4 units, Bodansky 0.5–2 units, Gutman & Gutman method (total) Elevated in carcinoma of the prostate and occasionally in acute myelocytic leukemia	Androgens (in females) Carcinoma of female breast (metastatic) Clofibrate Clotting process Hemolysis Prostatic massage	Aging of specimen Fluorides Oxalates Phosphates Alcohol Aminocaproic acid (Amicar) Clofibrate (Atromid-S)
Albumin	See Protein below		
Aldolase (Abnormal muscular and other conditions)	Elevated in muscular dystrophy, dermatomyositis, hepatic disease, and leukemia, etc.	Alcohol Aminocaproic acid (Amicar) Clofibrate (Atromid-S)	
Alkaline Phosphatase (Abnormal bone growth and hepatic function; biliary cirrhosis; healing fractures; hyperparathyroidism; obstructive jaundice; occlusion of hepatic duct; osteitis deformans; rickets; space-occupying lesions of the liver)	1.0–3.5 Babson Read units 0.8–3 Bessey Lowrey units per 100 ml.; up to 10 in infants (rapid bone growth) 1.0–4.0, adult; 5.0–12.0, children; Bodansky units 2.8–8.6 units, Shinowara, Jones, Reinhart method 3–13 units, adult; 15–20, children; King Armstrong method 0.8–2.3 units, adult; 2.8–6.7, children; Sigma method Elevated in bile duct obstruction, hepatitis or other hepatocellular diseases; congestive heart failure, intra-abdominal bacterial infections, Hodgkin's disease, myeloid metaplasia, hyperthyroidism, osteoblastic disease, osteomalacia; regional enteritis, rickets, tumor metastases, ulcerative colitis. Decreased in hypothyroidism and growth retardation.	Acetohexamide Aging of specimen Albumin infusions from human placentas Allopurinol Anabolic agents Androgens Chlorpropamide Colchicine Erythromycin Gold salts Hemolysis N-hydroxyacetamide Indomethacin Lincomycin Methyldopa (Aldomet)* Oxacillin Penicillamine Pertrofane Phenothiazines	Albumin infusions from venous blood Fluorides Oxalates Phosphates Placebo* Vitamin D

Placebo*
Procainamide
Progestin-estrogen oral
  contraceptives
Sulfobromophthalein (BSP)
Thiothixene
Tolazamide
Tolbutamide

Amino Acids
(Abnormal amino acid metabolism by the liver)

3.5–6.0 mg. amino acid nitrogen per 100 ml. of plasma

Elevated in acute yellow atrophy of the liver, hepatitis, and occasionally in eclampsia. Decreased in nephrotic syndrome, pneumonia, and following severe injury

ACTH
Aging of specimen
Bismuth
Blood (laked)
11-Hydroxysteroids
Serum
Sulfonamides
Uric acid

Epinephrine
Insulin

Ammonia
(Abnormal liver function, protein metabolism)

40–70 μg. per 100 ml. whole blood determined as NH_3-N, (Conway)

Elevated in liver insufficiency or in liver bypass by means of a portacaval shunt

Acetazolamide
Aging of specimen
Ammonium chloride
Barbiturates
Chlorthalidone (Hygroton)
Exercise
Filter paper
Furosemide (Lasix)
Hemolysis
Heparin (some samples)
Hyperalimentation
Ion exchange resins
Lipomul (oil inj.)
Mercurial diuretics
Methicillin
Narcotics
Oral resins
Thiazide diuretics
Urea

Acetohydroxamic acid (AHA)
Diphenhydramine (Benadryl)
Kanamycin (Kantrex)
Lactobacillus acidophilus
  (Lactinex)
Lactulose
Levodopa
Neomycin
Potassium salts
Sodium salts
Sorbitol

*Substances with an asterisk in this table reportedly influence the test but further study is needed to determine the exact effect and the mechanism of action.

Table 7-1 Interferences in Clinical Chemistry of Blood *(continued)*
(Values for Serum Unless Otherwise Stated)

Laboratory Tests (Conditions Detected)	Normal Values and Significance of Abnormal Values	Causes of False-Positive or Elevated Values (+)	Causes of False-Negative or Decreased Values (−)
Amylase (Abnormal pancreatic function; acute pancreatitis; acute diseases of the salivary gland; ectopic pregnancy; perforated peptic ulcers; peritonitis; renal insufficiency)	40–120 Somogyi units, saccharogenic or amyloclastic method 60–160 units, iodometric method 160 units, Caraway method Elevated in acute pancreatitis and obstruction of pancreatic duct, mumps, and occasionally in renal insufficiency; decreased in hepatitis, pancreatic insufficiency, and occasionally in eclampsia	Alcohol (gross intake) Aminosalicylic acid (PAS) Azathioprine (Imuran) Chlorides Chlorthalidone Codeine Corticosteroids Cyproheptadine (Periactin) Ethacrynic acid (Edecrin) Fluorides Furosemide Histamine Hyperalimentation Indomethacin Isoniazid Lipemia Meperidine (Demerol) Methacholine Methanol intoxication Methyldopa Morphine Oral contraceptives Oxyphenbutazone (Tandearil) Pancreozymin Pentazocine (Talwin) Phenformin (DBI) Rifampin (Rifadin, Rimactane) Radiopaque contrast media Salicylates Salicylazosulfapyridine (Azulfidine) Saliva Sodium diatrizoate Sulfamethizole Tetracycline Thiazide diuretics	Citrates Fluorides Oxalates

Barbiturates

See Table 7-3. Either the dithizone or diphenylcarbazone method is used for either serum or urine.

Bicarbonate

(Abnormal acid-base balance)

(See also Carbon Dioxide Combining Power and Carbon Dioxide Content)

(As CO_2 content): 24–29 mEq. per liter or 55.65 vol. %
Elevated in metabolic alkalosis due to ingestion of excessive amounts of sodium bicarbonate, protracted vomiting with subsequent loss of potassium, and in respiratory acidosis due to pulmonary emphysema or hypoventilation. Decreased in metabolic acidosis due to diabetic ketosis, starvation, persistent diarrhea, renal insufficiency and salicylate toxicity. Also decreased in respiratory alkalosis due to hyperventilation

Aldosterone
Viomycin

Metformin
Phenformin
Triamterene

Bilirubin (& Icterus Index)

(Abnormal liver function—excretion; depth and progress of jaundice)

Total 0.0–1.5 mg. per 100 ml.
Direct 0.0–0.3 mg. per 100 ml. (conjugated)
Elevated in chronic and acute hepatitis and biliary tract obstruction, drug toxicities, erythroblastosis fetalis, jaundice, hemolytic disease, kernicterus, and Gilbert's disease
Some substances such as dextran produce turbidity in methods where methanol is present (Malloy-Evelyn). Some substances such as carotene, hemoglobin, and novobiocin as well as a condition such as lipemia interfere with absorbance in spectrophotometric (icterus index) methods.

Acetohexamide
Aging of serum (opacity)
Anabolic agents (conjugated)
Androgens (conjugated)
Ascorbic acid
Aspidium (if absorbed)
Carotene
Carrots
Chlordiazepoxide
Dextran 75
Epinephrine
Ethoxazene*
Erythromycin (conjugated)
Hemoglobin (icterus index)
Hemolysis
Indomethacin
Isoniazid
Isoproterenol
Levodopa
Lipemia
Lipochromes

Alcohol
Barbiturates
Caffeine
Chlorine (contaminant)
Citrates
Dextran
Ethoxazine
Hemoglobin (competition for nitrite, Malloy-Evelyn method)
Light
Phenazopyridine (atypical color gives interference)*
Placebos (reported)*
Protein
Theophylline
Urea

[143]

Table 7-1 Interferences in Clinical Chemistry of Blood *(continued)*
(Values for Serum Unless Otherwise Stated)

Laboratory Tests (Conditions Detected)	*Normal Values and Significance of Abnormal Values*	*Causes of False-Positive or Elevated Values (+)*	*Causes of False-Negative or Decreased Values (−)*
Bilirubin (& Icterus Index) *(continued)*		Menadiol Na Diphosphate (large doses) Mercaptopurine Methanol (impure) Methyldopa Monoamine oxidase inhibitors Nitrofurantoin Novobiocin (yellow metabolite) Oxacillin Phenazopyridine (color)* Phenothiazines Phytonadione Pipobroman Placebos* Pyrazinamide Radiopaque contrast media Riboflavin Sulfonamides Triacetyloleandomycin Trifluperidol Vitamin K, K₁ (large doses in newborn) Yellow pigments in foods Xanthophyll	
Blood Urea Nitrogen (BUN) (Abnormal renal function—glomerular filtration and tubular reabsorption)	10–15 mg. per 100 ml. whole blood (diacetyl monoximine method)[a] 8–25 mg. per 100 ml. whole blood (urograph method) 0.2–2 Gm. per 100 ml. serum (nitrogen micro-Kjeldahl method) Elevated in chronic gout, malignancy, myocardial failure, nephritis, nephrosclerosis, oliguria caused by CCl₄ or HgCl₂ poisoning, postoperative urinary suppression, pyelonephritis, renal corti-	Acetohexamide Acetone[c] Alkaline antacids P-aminosalicylate[d] Amphotericin B Antimony compounds Arsenicals Bacitracin Blood (whole) Capreomycin Cephaloridine (high doses)	Chloramphenicol[b] Dextrose (glucose) infusions Fluorides Fluphenazine* Mercury Compounds (glassware)* Nitrofurantoin* Pregnancy Sodium azide[a] Spironolactone (aldactone, etc.)

cal necrosis, renal failure, renal insufficiency, renal tuberculosis, suppuration, urinary tract obstruction, increased nitrogen metabolism from dehydration or GI bleeding, and in decreased renal blood flow due to shock, adrenal insufficiency or congestive heart failure. Decreased in hepatic failure, nephrosis, pregnancy, and cachexia

Chloral hydrate[e]
Chlorobutanol
Chlorthalidone
Citrulline[a]
Colistimethate sodium
Creatinine[c]
Dextran[d]
Doxapram
Ethacrynic acid
Fluphenazine*
Furosemide
Gentamycin
Guanethidine
Guanochlor
Hemolysis
Hydantoin[a]
Impure urease
Indomethacin
Kanamycin
Lipomul (oil inj.)
Methicillin (may cause azotemia)
Methyldopa (Aldomet, Aldoril)
Methylurea[a]
Methysergide
Nalidixic acid
Neomycin
Nitrofurantoin*
Pargyline
Phenylurea[a]
Polymixin B
Radiopaque contrast media (may cause azotemia)
Streptokinase-streptodornase
Sulfonamides[d]
Sulfonylureas[a]
Thiazide diuretics
Triamterene (Dyrenium)
Vancomycin (may alter)

Streptomycin[b]
Thymol

[a] Fearon method
[b] Urease with phenol-hypochlorite reaction
[c] Urease with Nessler's reagent
[d] Dimethylaminobenzaldehyde reaction

Table 7-1 Interferences in Clinical Chemistry of Blood (continued)
(Values for Serum Unless Otherwise Stated)

Laboratory Tests (Conditions Detected)	Normal Values and Significance of Abnormal Values	Causes of False-Positive or Elevated Values (+)	Causes of False-Negative or Decreased Values (−)
Bromide (Abnormal ratio of chloride to bromide)	0.5–1 mg. per 100 ml. of blood Elevated above 17 mEq. per L. in bromide intoxication, e.g., bromism	Hemolysis	
Bromsulphalein (BSP) Retention (Abnormal excretory capacity of liver, in absence of jaundice)	Less than 5% retention after 45 minutes Elevated in hepatocellular disease, chronic hepatitis, cirrhosis, and in anemia, heart failure, thyrotoxicosis and infectious diseases which reduce liver function	Abdominal surgery (recent)* Amidone Anabolic steroids Androgens Antifungal agents Aspidium (if absorbed) Barbiturates (increased retention) Biliary fistula (draining)* Bilirubin (excessive amounts) Chlorpropamide Chlortetracycline (Aureomycin) Choleretics Clofibrate Clomiphene citrate Dehydrocholic acid (Decholin) Estrogens Ethoxazene (Serenium) Florantyrone Halogen compounds Hemolysis Heparin Iopanoic acid (Telepaque) Isocarboxazid (Marplan) Kanamycin* Iodine radiopaque media Lipemia Malaria with hepatic engorgement* Meperidine (Demerol) Metaxalone Methadone (Dolophine)	Albuminuria Ascites Barbiturates (increases hepatic excretion) Kanamycin* Nonfasting state Phenazopyridine (pink acid solu.) Placebos* Proteinuria Radiopaque contrast media*

Methotrexate
Methyldopa (Aldomet)*
Methyltestosterone (impaired hepatic function)
Morphine
Norethandrolone (Nilevar)
Novobiocin
Oral contraceptives
Oxacillin
Pancreatitis (acute)*
Phenazopyridine (Pyridium)
Phenolphthalein
Phenolsulfonphthalein (PSP)
Placebos*
Probenecid (Benemid)
Progestin-estrogen oral contraceptives
Radiopaque contrast media*
Stress situations*
Sulfonamides
Tolbutamide
Triacetyloleandomycin

Bilirubin (titrimetric)*
Citrates
Copper*
Delayed separation of serum
Edathamil (EDTA, edetates) in photometry
Fluorides
Hemolysis*
Heparin
High bilirubin*
Incompletely dissolved calcium oxalate
Insufficient heat
Insulin
Iron*
Laxatives (excessive use)
Lipomul (oil inj.)
Magnesium (no effect at acid pH)
Methicillin

Calcium
(Abnormal calcium or bone metabolism)

1-11.5 mg. per 100 ml. or 4.5-5.7 mEq./L. Elevated in hyperparathyroidism, multiple myeloma, osteolytic diseases, and vitamin D excess. Decreased in Cushing's syndrome, hypoparathyroidism, malabsorption syndromes, steatorrhea, and vitamin D deficiency

Anabolic hormones (associated usually with certain carcinomas)
Androgens (associated usually with certain carcinomas)
Alkaline antacids
Ammonium oxalate
Bilirubin (photometric)*
Calcium salts (tap water)*
Calcium soaps
Copper*
Cork stoppers
Dihydrotachysterol
Estrogens
Filter paper
Hemolysis
High bilirubin*
Iron*
Magnesium
Nonfasting state
Parathyroid inj.

Table 7-1 Interferences in Clinical Chemistry of Blood *(continued)*
(Values for Serum Unless Otherwise Stated)

Laboratory Tests (Conditions Detected)	Normal Values and Significance of Abnormal Values	Causes of False-Positive or Elevated Values (+)	Causes of False-Negative or Decreased Values (−)
Calcium *(continued)*		Potassium Progestins Sodium (in photometry) Sulfobromophthalein (BSP) Thiazide diuretics (early in therapy) Vitamin D Zinc*	Oxalates (photometry) Phosphates (photometry & EDTA methods) Protein (photometry) Sodium polystyrene sulfonate Sulfates (photometry) Zinc*
Carbon Dioxide Combining Power (Abnormal acid-base balance. See also Bicarbonate and Carbon Dioxide Content)	24–34 mM. per liter or 53–76 vol. %, volumetric method Elevated in metabolic alkalosis due to ingestion of excess sodium bicarbonate, and protracted vomiting leading to potassium deficit. Also elevated in respiratory acidosis due to pulmonary emphysema, or hypoventilation. Reduced in metabolic acidosis due to diabetic ketosis, starvation, persistent diarrhea, renal insufficiency or salicylate toxicity. Also decreased in respiratory alkalosis due to pulmonary hyperventilation	Anticoagulants* Nitrofurantoin* Potassium oxalate (anticoagulant)* Sodium fluoride (anticoagulant)*	Anticoagulants* Edathamil (EDTA) Nitrofurantoin* Potassium oxalate (anticoagulant)* Sodium fluoride (anticoagulant)*
Carbon Dioxide Content (Abnormal acid-base balance. See also Bicarbonate and Carbon Dioxide Combining Power)	24–34 mM. per liter or 53–76 vol. %, manometric method Elevated and decreased in same conditions as cited above under Carbon Dioxide Combining Power	Nitrofurantoin* Salicylates (compensation for initial respiratory alkalosis)	BAL Lipomul (oil inj.) Methicillin (may cause azotemia) Nitrofurantoin* Salicylates (initially, a respiratory alkalosis)

Cephalin Flocculation

(Abnormal liver function—protein synthesis. See also Table 7-5.)

0 to 2+ flocculation in 48 hrs., Hangar method

Elevated in hepatocellular injury, chronic liver disease. Test is not very specific but may be of value in differential diagnosis of hepatocellular damage—elevated—and obstruction where it is decreased

Ampicillin (alters time)*
Bacterial contamination
Carphenazine*
Chlorpropamide
Erythromycin (weak)
Ethosuximide
Florantyrone
Fluphenazine
Glassware (heavy metals or strong acids)
Indomethacin
Kanamycin*
Light
Lincomycin (may give weak)
Metaxalone
Methsuximide
Methyldopa (Aldomet)
Nicotinic acid (large doses)
Oxacillin*
Pargyline*
Penicillamine
Placebo
Temperature (> or <25°C)
Thiabendazole
Tolbutamide

Ampicillin (alters time)*
Carphenazine*
Kanamycin*
Oxacillin*
Pargyline*
Placebo*

Chloride

(Abnormal acid-base and electrolyte balance)

570–620 mg. per 100 ml. or 98–106 mEq./L.

Elevated in renal insufficiency, decreased O_2 at high altitudes, anxiety states, excessive salt intake, fever, hysteria, nephrosis, renal tubular acidosis, and dehydration. Decreased in adrenal cortical dysfunction, chronic respiratory acidosis, diabetic acidosis, adrenal insufficiency and metabolic alkalosis

Acetazolamide
Ammonium chloride
Boric acid (toxicity)
Bromides
Chlorides (contaminants)
Corticosteroids
Ion exchange resins (therapy)
Oxyphenbutazone
Phenylbutazone
Potassium chloride
Protein
Saline infusions
Silver nitrate loss
Triamterene
Saline infusions (excessive)

ACTH
Diuretics (excessive)
Ethacrynic acid
Hemolysis
Mercurial diuretics
Steroids
Thiazide diuretics

Table 7-1   Interferences in Clinical Chemistry of Blood *(continued)*
(Values for Serum Unless Otherwise Stated)

Laboratory Tests (Conditions Detected)	Normal Values and Significance of Abnormal Values	Causes of False-Positive or Elevated Values (+)	Causes of False-Negative or Decreased Values (−)
Cholesterol [6, 7, 14, 30, 68] (Abnormal lipid metabolism, liver function. See also Table 7–5.)	Total 160–200 mg. per 100 ml.; Free 20–25% of total, Crawford method. Elevated in xanthomatosis, hypophysectomy, pancreatitis, hypothyroidism, poorly controlled diabetes, nephrotic syndrome, chronic hepatitis, obstructive jaundice, biliary cirrhosis, hypoprotein-emia and hyperlipemia. Decreased in acute hepatitis, hyperthyroidism, acute infections, anemia, malnutrition, tuberculosis, terminal cancer, and starvation	ACTH (usually) Alcohol Aminopyrine (Pyramidon)* Anabolic agents Androgens Bile salts* Bilirubin Bromides Chlorpromazine Corticosteroids Epinephrine Ether Hemoglobin Heparin Levodopa Lipemia (Lipomul inj.) Metandienone Norepinephrine (Levarterenol) Oral contraceptives Paramethadione Penicillamine (Cuprimine) Phenothiazines Pregnancy Protein Salicylates* Trimethadione Tryptophan Vitamin A Vitamin D*	Aluminum nicotinate (Nicalex) Aminosalicylic acid (PAS) Androsterone Antidiabetics Ascorbic acid Bile salts* Chlortetracycline Cholestyramine resin Clofibrate (Atromid-S) Colchicine Cortisone Dextrothyroxine (Choloxin) EDTA Estrogens Glucagon Haloperidol Heparin Insulin Kanamycin (Kantrex) Metyrapone (Metopirone) Neomycin (Mycifradin) Nicotinic acid Nitrates and nitrites Oxalated plasma Paromomycin Pentylenetetrazol (Metrazol) Phenformin (DBI) Salicylates Sitosterols (Cytellin) Sodium dextrothyroxine (Choloxin) Thiouracil Thyroid (thyroxin, etc.) Vastran Forte Water (contaminating H₂SO₄)

Copper
(Abnormal copper metabolism)

Adult male: 70–140 μg. per 100 ml.
Adult female: 85–155 μg. per 100 ml.
Children: 27–153 μg. per 100 ml.
Newborn: 12–67 μg. per 100 ml.
Elevated in rheumatoid arthritis, pregnancy, cirrhosis of the liver, myocardial infarction, schizophrenia, tumors, and severe infections. Decreased in Wilson's disease, hypothyroidism, dysproteinuria of infancy, kwashiorkor, sprue, and nephrotic syndrome

Cobalt
Iron
Needles (hypodermic, containing Cu)
Nickel
Oral contraceptives

Cortisol (Hydrocortisone)
(Abnormal steroid production)

Adult male: 9–28 μg./100 ml.
Adult female: 8–25 μg./100 ml.
Depressed in Addison's disease and hypopituitarism. Highly elevated in Cushing's syndrome (not all), extreme stress, acute pancreatitis, and eclampsia. Moderately elevated in burns, infections, and surgery. Slight elevation in first trimester of pregnancy, severe hypertension, and virilism.

Benzyl alcohol
Spironolactone

Creatinine
(Abnormal glomerular filtration)

0.7–1.5 mg. per 100 ml. whole blood
Elevated in acute and chronic renal insufficiency and urinary tract obstruction. Value below 0.8 mg. per 100 ml. is of no significance

Amphotericin B
Ascorbic acid
Bromsulphalein (also for creatine)
Chromogens (noncreatinine) of erythrocytes
Clofibrate
Colistin
Dextrose
Diabetes (glucose and acetone)
Diacetic acid
Heat
Kanamycin
Levulose
Lipomul (oil inj.)
Mannitol
Methicillin
Methyldopa (Aldomet)*

Methyldopa (readily oxidized, interferes with determination by alkaline picrate method)*
Viomycin

Table 7-1 Interferences in Clinical Chemistry of Blood (continued)
(Values for Serum Unless Otherwise Stated)

Laboratory Tests (Conditions Detected)	Normal Values and Significance of Abnormal Values	Causes of False-Positive or Elevated Values (+)	Causes of False-Negative or Decreased Values (−)
Creatinine (continued)		Protein Phenosulfonphthalein (also for creatine) Pyruvate Streptokinase-streptodornase Triamterene	
Glucose (Fasting) (Abnormal carbohydrate metabolism; diagnostic for diabetes mellitus) See also the interferences in Table 7-3. Some of those shown for urine may also be applicable to serum.	80–120 mg. per 100 ml. whole blood, Folin Wu method 50–90 mg. per 100 ml. whole blood, Somogyi Nelson method 50–90 mg. per 100 ml. whole blood, oxidase method (GO-POD/on serum) Elevated in adrenocortical hyperactivity, chronic hepatic dysfunction, eclampsia, epilepsy, general anesthesia, diabetes mellitus, hyperpituitarism, hyperthyroidism, and intracranial trauma. Decreased in adrenal insufficiency, functional hypoglycemia, hyperinsulinism, hypopituitarism, hypothyroidism, pancreatic tumors, poisoning that destroys hepatic cells, and occasionally in hepatic insufficiency	Acetazolamide ACTH (corticotropin) Aluminum nicotinate Anabolic agents Arginine Aspirin BAL (initially, toxic doses) Caffeine Chlorthalidone Clopamide Corticosteroids Creatinine (ferricyanide method) Dextran Dextrothyroxine Diazoxide Diphenylhydantoin Diuretics Epinephrine Estrogens Ethacrynic acid Ferrous ascorbate Furadantin Furosemide (in diabetic) Glucuronic acid Glutathione Heparin Hexoses (Galactose, Mannose) Hypochlorite (GO-POD)	Acetaminophen (Tylenol) Acetohexamide (overdosage) Aging of sample Alcohol Ascorbic acid (GO-POD) Amphetamine poisoning Anabolic steroids Asparaginase BAL (after initial elevation in toxic doses) Benzene (toxicity) Bilirubin Caffeine Carbutamide Chlorpropamide (overdosage) Carbon tetrachloride (toxicity) Chloroform (toxicity) Ethacrynic acid Formaldehyde (GO-POD and o-toluidine) Glutathione (GO-POD) Haloperidol (Haldol) Homogentisic acid (GO-POD) Insulin (overdosage) Levodopa MAO inhibitors Metformin (overdosage) Pargyline

Phenazopyridine (Pyridium in GO-POD)
Phenformin
Phosphorus (toxicity)
Potassium chloride
Potassium oxalate
Potassium para-aminobenzoate (prolonged use)
Propoxyphene (Darvon)
Propranolol (Inderal)
Salicylates
Sulfaphenazole
Tetracyclines (may contain ascorbic acid)
Tolazamide
Uric acid (GO-POD)

Indomethacin
Isoniazid (excessive doses)
Lithium carbonate
Morphine
Nalidixic acid
Nicotinic acid
Oxazepam
Pentoses
Phenolphthalein (Ex-Lax)
Phenothiazines
Physostigmine
Progestin-estrogen oral contraceptives
Quinethazone
Reserpine
Saccharides (lactose, maltose, etc.)
Sympathomimetics
Thiabendazole
Thiazide diuretics
Triamterene
Tricyclic antidepressants
Trioxazine
Uric acid (ferricyanide method)

Glucose Tolerance
(Differential diagnosis for diabetes mellitus)

Diabetic curve: Peak high with slow return to fasting level
Hepatic disease: Peak high with rapid return to below fasting level in 3–4 hours
Hyperinsulinism: Normal with exaggerated fall to hypoglycemic level
Addison's disease: Flat, then drop to hypoglycemic level

Corticosteroids (impaired glucose tolerance)*

Corticosteroids (impaired glucose tolerance)*
Diurnal variation (decreased in afternoon)
Estrogens (decrease tolerance)
Nicotinic acid and derivatives (resembles diabetic curve)
Progestin-estrogen oral contraceptives (decrease tolerance)

Iron and Iron-Binding Capacity
(Abnormal erythrocytic function)

Total: 300–360 μg. per 100 ml.
Unsaturated: 150–300 μg. per 100 ml.
Serum iron elevated in excess iron administration, hemochromatosis, hemolytic diseases, hemosiderosis, liver disease,

Chloramphenicol
Diurnal variation (morning high)
Fluorides*
Hemolysis
Iron dextran (Imferon)—iron

ACTH
Diurnal variation (afternoon low)
Fluorides*

[153]

Table 7-1 Interferences in Clinical Chemistry of Blood (continued)
(Values for Serum Unless Otherwise Stated)

Laboratory Tests (Conditions Detected)	Normal Values and Significance of Abnormal Values	Causes of False-Positive or Elevated Values (+)	Causes of False-Negative or Decreased Values (−)
Iron and Iron-Binding Capacity (continued)	and multiple transfusions. Decreased in iron deficiency anemia, malignancy, nephrotic syndrome, pregnancy, chronic infections, and some other chronic diseases in which low serum iron levels are found. Binding capacity elevated in presence of low serum iron or iron deficiency anemia; decreased in presence of high serum iron, hemochromatosis, malignancy, nephrotic syndrome	Oral contraceptives Oxalates* Tungstates*	Iron dextran—iron-binding capacity Oxalates* Tungstates*
Lactate (Lactic Acid)		Isoniazid Alcohol Phenformin (DBI, Meltrol—may be fatal) Epinephrine Sodium bicarbonate infusions Glucose infusions dl-Lactate infusions (under certain conditions) Metformin (may be fatal) Streptozotocin	Lactate infusions (under certain conditions) Methylene blue Morphine
Lactic Dehydrogenase (Abnormal liver function—transaminase)	30–120 units, Cabaud Wroblewski method Elevated in myocardial infarction, cancer metastatic to the liver, cirrhosis, acute hepatitis, obstructional jaundice, pulmonary embolism, and pernicious anemia	Contact with clot Hemolysis Temperature	Clofibrate Oxalates Temperature
Lipase (Acute pancreatic necrosis, carcinoma of pancreas, pancreatitis)	0–1.5 Cherry-Crandall units/ml. serum. Elevated in acute pancreatic necrosis (acute hemorrhagic pancreatitis) with high mortality rate.	Bilirubin	Hemolysis Incorrect buffer

Lipids (total) (Abnormal fat metabolism, pancreatic function)	360–765 mg. per 100 ml. plasma. Elevated in diabetes mellitus, nephrotic syndrome, xanthomatosis and biliary cirrhosis	Filter paper	Cholestyramine resin Estrogens
Magnesium		Lithium carbonate Magnesium compounds	Alcohol, ethyl Aldosterone Ammonium chloride Amphotericin B Calcium gluconate Calcium salts Ethacrynic acid (Edecrin) Insulin Mercurial diuretics Neomycin Oral contraceptives Thiazide diuretics
Nonprotein Nitrogen (NPN) (Abnormal renal function. See also above for BUN and Creatinine)	25–40 mg. per 100 ml., micro-Kjeldahl method. Elevated in renal insufficiency, nephritis, urinary tract obstruction. Decreased in renal blood flow due to shock, adrenal insufficiency, hepatic failure, and occasionally in congestive heart failure	Acetophenetidin (azotemia) Amphotericin B (prolonged adm.) Capreomycin Edathamil (EDTA) Filter paper (containing NH_3) Kanamycin Lipomul (oil inj.) Methicillin (azotemia) Neomycin Nitrofurantoin* Polymyxin Sulfonamides Sulfuric acid (containing NH_3) Temperature (increasing) Tetracyclines Vitamin D	Nitrofurantoin*

Table 7-1   Interferences in Clinical Chemistry of Blood *(continued)*
(Values for Serum Unless Otherwise Stated)

Laboratory Tests (Conditions Detected)	Normal Values and Significance of Abnormal Values	Causes of False-Positive or Elevated Values (+)	Causes of False-Negative or Decreased Values (−)
Paper Electrophoresis (Abnormal lipid metabolism)	Total lipids in serum: 400–800 mg. per 100 ml. Phospholipids: 150–380 mg. per 100 ml. Cholesterol: 115–340 mg. per 100 ml. Neutral fat: 25–150 mg. per 100 ml. Free fatty acids: 0.3–0.8 mEq./L. (Hyperlipoproteinemia in acute alcoholism, acute pancreatitis, atherosclerosis, diabetes mellitus, glycogen storage disease, myxedema, nephrotic syndrome, pancreatitis, and pregnancy. Hypolipidemia in acanthocytosis, liver disease, malabsorption syndrome, starvation, and Tangier disease	Increased drying temperature (albumin increased) Iodinated contrast media (patterns uninterpretable)	Increased drying temperature (globulins decreased)
pH (Acute metabolic acidosis, alkalosis, chronic respiratory acidosis, hyperventilation)	pH 7.40 elevated in alkalosis to >7.45 with a fall in total plasma CO_2 to <24 mEq. per liter. Caused by hyperventilation due to CNS lesions, fever, hepatic coma, hypoxia, salicylate intoxication, etc., or by metabolic alkalosis due to excessive use of sodium bicarbonate, potassium depletion, and loss of acid—vomiting, etc. Decreased in acidosis, e.g., in diabetes, excessive chloride—$CaCl_2$, NH_4Cl—and impaired renal excretion of acid—acute tubular necrosis, chronic glomerulonephritis, chronic pyelonephritis	Exposure to air Potassium oxalate Sodium oxalate Temperature	Acetazolamide Ammonium chloride Ammonium oxalate Anaerobic storage (37° C) Calcium chloride EDTA Hemolysis Methyl alcohol Paraldehyde Salicylates Sodium citrate
Phosphate (Inorganic Phosphorus) (Abnormal parathyroid function, bone metabolism, intestinal absorption, malnutrition and renal function)	5 mg. per ml. (children) 2.7–4.5 mg. per 100 ml. (adult) Elevated in renal insufficiency, hypoparathyroidism, hypervitaminosis D, hyperinsulinism, nephritis, pyloric obstruction, renal insufficiency, and uremia. Decreased in hyperparathyroidism, hypo-	Aging of specimen Alkaline antacids Detergents Healing of fractures Hemolysis Heparin Lipomul (oil inj.) (azotemia)	Aluminum hydroxide Anesthesia, general (chloroform, ether, or ethylene) Citrates Epinephrine (Adrenalin) Insulin

vitaminosis D, osteomalacia, malabsorption syndrome, idiopathic steatorrhea, lobar pneumonia, myxedema, neurofibromatosis, rickets, renal tubular abnormalities, and Fanconi syndrome

Mannitol*
Methicillin (azotemia)
Pituitrin
Tetracyclines
Vitamin D

Mannitol
Nonfasting state
Oxalates
Parathyroid inj.
Tartrates

Potassium (K)

(Abnormal electrolyte balance and muscular activity; capability of muscle to contract)

3.8–5.1 mEq. per liter

Elevated in renal insufficiency, adrenal insufficiency, circulatory failure, damaged cell membranes, shock, hypoventilation, too rapid administration of potassium salts. Decreased in hyperventilation, IV glucose and saline therapy prolonged, starvation, excessive loss from persistent vomiting or diarrhea, malabsorption syndrome, unusual renal loss secondary to hyperaldosteronism, adrenal cortical hyperfunction, and in renal tubular damage or defect

Amiloride
Aminocaproic acid (Amicar)
Anticoagulants containing K
Antineoplastic agents
Arginine
Calcium
Carbacrylamine resin
Cephaloridine (reported toxicity)
Cigarette smoke
Contact with clot
Copper
Epinephrine (initial transient rise)
Hemolysis
Iron
Isoniazid
Lipomul (oil inj.)
Mannitol
Metformin
Methicillin (azotemia)
Penicillin G potassium
Phenformin
Protein
Spironolactone (Aldactone)
Succinylcholine (Anectine)
Triamterene (Dyrenium)
Urea*
Venous stasis

Acetazolamide
ACTH
Aminosalicylic acid (rare)
Ammonium chloride
Amphotericin B
Carbenicillin (Geopen, Pyopen)
Carbenoxolone (Duogastrone)
Chlorthalidone (Hygroton)
Corticosteroids
Corticotropin
Dextrose infusions (without electrolytes)
Dichlorphenamide
Diuretics, oral
Edathamil (EDTA)
Epinephrine (after initial rise)
Ethacrynic acid (Edecrin)
Furosemide (Lasix)
Glucagon
Glucose
Insulin
Laxatives (excess use)
Lithium carbonate
Licorice
Methazolamide (prolonged use)
Penicillin G sodium
Phosphates
Polymixin B
Salicylates
Sodium phytate
Sodium polystyrenesulfonate
Sulfates
Tetracyclines (degraded)
Thiazide diuretics
Urea*
Viomycin

[157]

Table 7-1 Interferences in Clinical Chemistry of Blood *(continued)*
(Values for Serum Unless Otherwise Stated)

Laboratory Tests (Conditions Detected)	Normal Values and Significance of Abnormal Values	Causes of False-Positive or Elevated Values (+)	Causes of False-Negative or Decreased Values (−)
Protein (Various disease states which characteristically alter the concentration of the total protein or the albumin, globulin or fibrinogen fractions). The interferences for the *Biuret reaction* and *dye binding procedures* (HABA) differ. Unless specified, Biuret applies or both apply. With electrophoresis penicillins and radiopaque contrast media may cause variable results.	Total protein: 6.4–8.0 Gm. per 100 ml., Weischselbaum method Albumin: 3.9–4.6 Gm. per 100 ml., Reinhold method Globulin: 2.3–3.5 Gm. per 100 ml. **Albumin** elevated in dehydration, hemoconcentration, and shock; decreased in exercise, glomerulonephritis, hepatic insufficiency, malabsorption syndrome, malnutrition, neoplastic diseases, and protein loss through hemorrhage and proteinuria as in nephrosis. **Globulin** elevated in acute infectious diseases, biliary cirrhosis, cirrhosis of the liver, hemochromatosis, hepatic disease, and neoplastic diseases; decreased in agammaglobulinemia and malnutrition. **Fibrinogen** elevated in glomerulonephritis, infectious diseases, and nephrosis; decreased in accidents of pregnancy, hepatic insufficiency	Bilirubin (Biuret) Bromsulphalein Clofibrate Dextran (Biuret) Hemoglobin Hemolysis Heparin (HABA) Lipemia Mercuric chloride Penicillin (massive doses) Phenazopyridine (Pyridium) Salicylates Sulfobromophthalein (BSP) Tolbutamide X-ray contrast media	Ammonium ion Bilirubin (HABA) Dextran (hemodilution) Penicillin (HABA) Posture Pyrazinamide Salicylate (HABA) Sulfonamides (HABA) Unstable biuret reagent Violent and prolonged shaking
Serum Glutamic-Oxaloacetic Transaminase (SGOT) (Acute myocardial infarction; biliary obstruction; cirrhosis; infectious mononucleosis; infectious serum hepatitis; pancreatitis)	Up to 40 units, Reitman and Frankel Up to 36 units, Babson Elevated very high in acute hepatitis and obstructive jaundice, moderately in chronic hepatitis, neoplastic diseases metastatic to the liver, and in cirrhosis of the liver. Serum glutamicpyruvic transaminase is greater than the serum glutamic-oxaloacetic transaminase in extrahepatic obstruction, acute and toxic hepatitis. Serum glutamic-oxaloacetic transaminase is greater than the serum	Acetaminophen Acetoacetic acid Amantadine p-Aminosalicylate Ampicillin (Polycillin, etc.) Anabolic agents Androgens Ascorbic acid Cephalothin Chloroquin Clofibrate (Atromid-S) Cloxacillin	Salicylates*

glutamic-pyruvic transaminase in cirrhosis of the liver, intrahepatic neoplasms, and in hemolytic jaundice

Colchicine
Cycloserine
Desipramine
Erythromycin
Ethionamide
Gentamycin
Guanethadine analogs
Hemolysis
N-Hydroxyacetamide (toxicity)
Ibufenac
Indomethacin
Isoniazid
Leukocytes (spinal fluid)
Levodopa
Lincomycin
Lipemia (alcoholic)
Methotrexate
Methydopa
Nafcillin
Nalidixic acid
Opiates
Oxacillin (Prostaphlin)
Para-aminosalicylic acid (PAS)
Phenothiazines
Placebo
Polycillin
Progestin-estrogen oral
    contraceptives
Prostaphlin
Salicylates*
Stibocaptate
Sulfamethoxazole
Thiabendazole
Thiothixene
Triacetyloleandomycin

Serum Glutamic-Pyruvic Transaminase (SGPT)

(Abnormal liver function, enzyme activity. See also Serum Glutamic-Oxaloacetic Transaminase and Table 7-5)

Up to 35 units, Reitman-Frankel method
Elevated very high in acute hepatitis and obstructive jaundice, moderately in chronic hepatitis, cirrhosis of the liver, and neoplastic diseases metastatic to the liver. Serum glutamic-pyruvic trans-

Anabolic agents
Androgens
Clofibrate
Cycloserine
Desipramine
Erythromycin (lauryl salt)

Salicylates*

Table 7-1   Interferences in Clinical Chemistry of Blood (continued)
(Values for Serum Unless Otherwise Stated)

Laboratory Tests (Conditions Detected)	Normal Values and Significance of Abnormal Values	Causes of False-Positive or Elevated Values (+)	Causes of False-Negative or Decreased Values (−)
Serum Glutamic-Pyruvic Transaminase (SGPT) (continued)	aminase is greater than serum glutamic-oxaloacetic transaminase in extrahepatic obstruction, acute hepatitis and toxic hepatitis. Serum glutamic-oxaloacetic transaminase is greater than the serum glutamic-pyruvic transaminase in cirrhosis of the liver, hemolytic jaundice, and intrahepatic neoplasms	Ethionamide Gentamycin Guanethedine analogs Hemolysis N-Hydroxyacetamide Ibufenac Indomethacin Isoniazid Lincomycin Lipemia Methyldopa (Aldomet) Phenothiazines Progestin-estrogen comb. oral contraceptives Pyrazinamide Salicylates* Stibocaptate Thiothixene Triacetyloleandomycin	
Sodium (Abnormal body water distribution)	138–148 mEq./L. (flame direct method) Elevated in central nervous system trauma or disease, dehydration, and hyperadrenocorticism. Decreased in adrenal insufficiency, renal insufficiency, renal tubular dysfunction, uncontrollable diabetes, unusual losses as in diarrhea, intestinal fistula, physiological response to trauma, burns or hyperhydrosis	Anabolic agents Anticoagulants containing Na Boric acid (toxicity) Calcium Copper Corticosteroids Detergents Excess saline Glucose* Iron Mannitol Methyldopa Oxyphenbutazone Phenylbutazone Potassium	Carbacrylamine resin Diuretics (oral) Ethacrynic acid Glucose* Hemolysis Heparin Laxatives (excessive use) Mercurial diuretics Paracentesis Phosphates Quinethazone Spironolactone Sulfates Triamterene Urea*

Progestin-estrogen oral
  contraceptives
Protein
Rauwolfia alkaloids
Urea*

Albumin (high)
Heparin
Oxalated plasma
Temperature increase

Thymol Turbidity
(Abnormal liver function, protein synthesis. See also Table 7-5)

0.0 to 4.0 units, MacLagan
Increased or positive in hepatocellular damage, especially in infectious hepatitis. Negative in obstructive or hemolytic jaundice

Bilirubin
Cephalothin
Chlorpropamide
Erythromycin (weak)
Florantyrone
Hemoglobin
Indomethacin
Lincomycin
Lipemia
Nalidixic acid
Penicillamine
Tolbutamide
Triacetyloleandomycin

Transaminase

See *Serum Glutamic-Oxaloacetic Transaminase (SGOT)* and *Serum Glutamic-Pyruvic Transaminase (SGPT)* above.

Urea Nitrogen

See *Blood Urea Nitrogen (BUN)* above.

Uric Acid [6,7,14,31,75,76,78]
(Abnormal purine metabolism, renal excretion; diagnostic for gout)

Males: 2.1–7.8 mg. per 100 ml.
Females: 2.0–6.4 mg. per 100 ml.
Elevated in chronic eczema, chronic nephritis, eclampsia, gout, lead poisoning, leukemia, pneumonia, polycythemia vera, and renal insufficiency. Decreased in acute hepatitis, occasionally

Acetazolamide
Adrenocorticosteroids (in leukemia)
Alcohol (acute ingestion)
Aluminum nicotinate
Aminophylline
Angiotensin (Hypertensin)
Antihypertensives (Hyperstat, Inversine, etc.)
Anti-infectives (Garamycin, Myambutol)

Acetohexamide
ACTH
Aging of specimen
Alcohol (chronic ingestion)
Allopurinol
Anticoagulants, coumarin
Aspirin (large doses)
Azathioprine (Imuran)
Azauridine
Azoserine
Benziodarone
Chlorine[a]
Chlorprothixene (Taractan)
Cincophen

[161]

a Phosphotungstate colorimetric method.

Table 7-1 Interferences in Clinical Chemistry of Blood *(continued)*
(Values for Serum Unless Otherwise Stated)

Laboratory Tests (Conditions Detected)	Normal Values and Significance of Abnormal Values	Causes of False-Positive or Elevated Values (+)	Causes of False-Negative or Decreased Values (−)
Uric Acid *(continued)*		Ascorbic acid	Clofibrate (Atromid-S)
		Aspirin (usual dose)	Corticosteroids
		Atromid-S	Dicumarol
		Azathymine	Ethyl biscoumacetate
		Blood, whole	Fenoprofen
		Busulfan	Glucose
		Caffeine	Glyceryl guaiacolate
		Coffee	Griseofulvin (Grifulvin, etc.)
		Chlorthalidone	Halofenate
		Diamox	Lithium carbonate
		Diazoxide	Mannitol
		Diuretics, oral (thiazides, Edecrin, Hygroton, Hydromox, Lasix, Dyrenium, mercurials, quinazolines)	Methotrexate
			Phenindione
			Phenylbutazone (Butazolidin)
			Piperazine
		Epinephrine	Potassium oxalate
		Ergothioneine	Probenecid
		Ethacrynic acid	Radiopaque contrast media
		Ethambutol (Myambutol)	Salicylates (large doses)
		Formaldehyde[b]	Saline infusions
		Furosemide (Frusemide, Lasix)	Sodium oxalate
		Gentamicin	Sulfinpyrazone
		Gentisic acid	Triamterene*
		Glutathione	
		Ibufenac	
		Levodopa	
		Light (reagent)	
		Lipomul (oil inj.)	
		Mecamylamine (Inversine)	
		Mercaptopurine	
		Mercurial diuretics (Mersalyl, etc.)	
		Methicillin (azotemia)	
		Methotrexate	
		Methyldopa	
		Nicotinic acid	
		Nitrogen mustards	

Norepinephrine (Levophed)
Pempidine
Phenacetin[a]
Phenothiazines
Potassium ion[a]
Pyrazinamide
Quinethazone
Reducing substances
Salicylates (in lower doses and
  with phenylbutazone or
  uricosurics, e.g. probenecid,
  sulfinpyrazone)
Quinethazone (Hydromox)
Sympathomimetics (Adrenalin,
  Hypertensin, Levophed, etc.)
Theophylline[a]
Thiazides
Triamterene
Vincristine

[b] Uricase method. Formaldehyde inhibits uricase. Low results when added as a preservative. High results when unknown compared with standards containing formaldehyde.

Table 7-2 Interferences in Hematologic Testing [6, 7, 11, 12, 14-16, 40, 65, 75]

Laboratory Tests (Conditions Detected)	Normal Values and Significance of Abnormal Values	Causes of False-Positive or Elevated Values (+)	Causes of False-Negative or Decreased Values (−)
Bleeding Time (For normal blood coagulation factors and hemostatic mechanisms)	Duke: 1-3 minutes Ivy: 2-4 minutes Elevated or prolonged in systematic vascular disease and thrombocytopenic purpura Variable in nonthrombocytopenic purpura and hypoprothrombinemia	Dextran Pantothenyl alcohol and derivatives Streptokinase-streptodornase	
Coagulation Time (For the composite action of all the plasma factors of coagulation acting simultaneously)	Lee White method: 6-10 minutes Howell method: 10-30 minutes Often poorly correlated with the thrombocyte count and bleeding time since so many variable and often uncontrollable factors are or can be involved Elevated or increased in any disease in which there may be an absence of or very small amounts of any of the essential components, in hemophilia, fibrinolytic diseases and anticoagulant therapy	Anticoagulants Tetracyclines	Corticosteroids Epinephrine
Coombs Tests (Typing) (For detection of antibody-coated erythrocytes, or RH factor)	Positive agglutination confirms presence of antibody on the erythrocytes Positive in hemolytic anemia, erythroblastosis in the newborn and following hemolytic transfusion reactions	Amphotericin B (Fungizone) Cephaloridine Cephalothin Chlorpropamide (Diabinese) Cyclophosphamide (Cytoxan) Diphenylhydantoin (Dilantin) Ethosuximide (Darontin) Hydralazine (Apresoline) Indomethacin (Indocin) Isoniazid (INH) Levodopa Mefenamic acid (Ponstel) Mephenytoin (Mesantoin) Methadone (Dolophine) Methyldopa (Aldomet)	

Methysergide (Sansert)
Oxphenisatin
Penicillin G
Phenacetin
Phenylbutazone (Butazolidin)
Quinine, quinidine
Rifampin (Rifadin, Rimactane)
Tolbutamide (Orinase)

Globulin
Lipemia
Posture

Erythrocyte (RBC) Count and/or Hemoglobin
(For normal erythropoiesis)

Adult male: 5 million per cu. mm. equivalent to 15–16 Gm. % hemoglobin
Adult female: 4.5 million per cu. mm. equivalent to 13–15 Gm. % hemoglobin
Elevated in polycythemia vera; decreased in the various anemias

Acetaminophen
Acetophenazine maleate
Acetophenetidin
Aminosalicylic acid
Amphotericin B
Antimony compounds
Antineoplastic agents
Arsenicals
Chloramphenicol
Diiodohydroxyquin
Doxapram
Ethosuximide
Furazolidone
Glucosulfone
Haloperidol
Hydantoin derivatives
Hydralazine
Hydroxychloroquine sulfate
Indomethacin
Isoniazid (rare)
MAO inhibitors (Isocarboxazid, etc.)
Mefenamic acid
Mepacrine (quinacrine)
Mephenoxalone
Mercurial diuretics (prolonged use)
Metaxalone
Methaqualone
Methsuximide
Nitrites
Nitrofurantoin (rare)
Novobiocin

[165]

Table 7-2 Interferences in Hematologic Testing (continued)

Laboratory Tests (Conditions Detected)	Normal Values and Significance of Abnormal Values	Causes of False-Positive or Elevated Values (+)	Causes of False-Negative or Decreased Values (−)
Erythrocyte (RBC) Count and/or Hemoglobin (continued)			Oleandomycin Oxyphenbutazone Paramethadione, trimethadione Penicillamine Penicillin Phenacemide Phenobarbital (rare) Phenylbutazone Phytonadione (large doses in infants) Posture Primaquine Primidone Pyrazolone derivatives Pyrimethamine Radioactive agents (large doses) Sulfonamides Sulfones Sulfonylureas (oral hypoglycemic agents) Thiazide diuretics (rare) Thiocyanates Thiosemicarbazones Triacetyloleandomycin Triethylenemelamine Trimethadione Tripelennamine Urethan Vitamin A (excess dose and use)
Leukocytes (For normal leukopoiesis)	Average: 8,000 per cu. mm Range: 5,000 to 10,000 Elevated normally during digestion and in	Allopurinol (hypersensitivity) Aminosalicylic acid (eosinophilia) Ampicillin (eosinophilia)	Acetaminophen Acetohexamide Acetophenetidin

Leukocytes

pregnancy; pathologically elevated in inflammations, fevers and anemias

Atropine (in children)
Barbiturates (vinbarbital, talbutal)
Capreomycin (eosinophilia)
Cephalothin (eosinophilia)
Chlorpropamide (eosinophilia)
Cloxacillin (eosinophilia)
Desipramine, imipramine (eosinophilia)
Diethylcarbamazine
Digitalis (rare)
Diphenhydramine*
Epinephrine (eosinophilia)
Erythromycin
Florantyrone (in patients with preexisting liver disease) (eosinophilia)
Gold compounds (eosinophilia)
Hydantoin derivatives (eosinophilia)
Iodides (eosinophilia)
Isoniazid (eosinophilia)
Kanamycin (eosinophilia)
Methicillin (eosinophilia)
Methyldopa (eosinophilia)
Methysergide (eosinophilia)
Nalidixic acid (eosinophilia)
Novobocin (eosinophilia)
Phenothiazines (eosinophilia)
Potassium iodide (eosinophilia)
Ristocetin (eosinophilia)
Stibocaptate (antimony)
Streptodornase-streptokinase (eosinophilia)
Streptomycin
Sulfonamides
Sulfonamides (long-acting) (eosinophilia)

Allopurinol (hypersensitivity)
Aminoglutethimide
Aminopyrine
Aminosalicylic acid
Amodiaquin
Antineoplastic agents
Antipyrine
Bismuth
Carbimazole
Cephalothin
Chloramphenicol
Chlordiazepoxide
Chloroquine
Chlorpropamide
Chlorprothixene
Chlorthalidone
Cloxacillin
Colistin
Corticosteroids (reported for prednisolone)
Desipramine, imipramine
Diazepam
Dichlorphenamide
Diethazine
Diiodohydroxyquin
Diphenhydramine*
Dipyrone
Ethacrynic acid
Ethoxzolamide
Furosemide
Glaucarubin
Glucosulfone
Gold compounds
Haloperidol
Hydantoin derivatives
Hydralazine
Hydroxychloroquine
Idoxuridine (in high conc.)
Indandione derivatives (oral anticoagulants)

*Substances followed by an asterisk reportedly influence the test but further study is needed to determine the exact effects and the mechanism of action.

Table 7-2 Interferences in Hematologic Testing *(continued)*

Laboratory Tests (Conditions Detected)	Normal Values and Significance of Abnormal Values	Causes of False-Positive or Elevated Values (+)	Causes of False-Negative or Decreased Values (−)
Leukocytes *(continued)*		Tetracyclines (prolonged use) (eosinophilia) Triamterene (eosinophilia) Trifluperidol (eosinophilia) Vancomycin (eosinophilia) Viomycin (eosinophilia)	Indomethacin Iothiouracil MAO inhibitors Mefenamic acid Mepacrine (quinacrine) Mepazine Mephenesin Meprobamate Mercurial diuretics (rare) Metaxalone Methampyrone Methazolamide Methicillin sodium Methimazole Methocarbamol Methsuximide Methyldopa Methylthiouracil Methyprylon (metabolite) Methysergide Metronidazole Novobiocin Oleandomycin Oxacillin Oxandrolone Oxazepam Oxyphenbutazone Paraldehyde Penicillamine Phenothiazines Phenylbutazone Potassium perchlorate Primaquine Primidone Procainamide Propylthiouracil Pyrathiazine (prolonged use) Pyrazolone derivatives

Pyrimethamine
Quinine
Radioactive agents
Ristocetin
Sulfonamides
Sulfonylureas (oral
  hypoglycemic agents)
Sulthiame
Thiabendazole
Thiazide diuretics (rare)
Thiosemicarbazones
Thiothixene
Triethylenemelamine
Tripelennamine
Vitamin A (prolonged use)

pH

(Acute metabolic acidosis, alkalosis, chronic respiratory acidosis, hyperventilation)

pH 7.40 elevated in alkalosis to >7.45 with a fall in total plasma CO_2 to <24 mEq. per liter. Caused by hyperventilation due to CNS lesions, fever, hepatic coma, hypoxia, salicylate intoxication, etc., or by metabolic alkalosis due to excessive use of sodium bicarbonate, potassium depletion, and loss of acid—vomiting, etc. Decreased in acidosis, e.g., in diabetes, excessive chloride—$CaCl_2$, NH_4Cl—and impaired renal excretion of acid—acute tubular necrosis, chronic glomerulonephritis, chronic pyelonephritis

Exposure to air
Potassium oxalate
Sodium bicarbonate
Sodium oxalate
Temperature

Acetazolamide
Ammonium chloride
Ammonium oxalate
Anaerobic storage (37° C)
Calcium chloride
EDTA
Hemolysis
Methyl alcohol
Paraldehyde
Salicylates
Sodium citrate

Prothrombin Time

(Prothrombin activity in the bloodclotting mechanism; hepatic parenchymal damage; vitamin K deficiency)
Note: Many drug interactions alter prothrombin time. Refer to the section on *Anticoagulants* in the Table of Drug Interactions, Chapter 10. Suppression of vitamin K synthesis with antibiotics, prevention of absorption of the vitamin through its sequestration in mineral oil used as a cathartic, suppression of hepatic synthesis of prothrombin, al-

Level: 20 mg. per 100 ml.
Time: 11.5–12.5 seconds (inversely proportional to level)
Decreased in vitamin K deficiency, hepatic diseases, biliary disease, and often in hemorrhagic diseases of the newborn

ACTH
Alcohol (large quantities)
Amidopyrine
Anabolic steroids
Antibiotics (broad spectrum)
Anticoagulants (oral)
Barbiturates
Benziodarone
Cholestyramine resin
Clofibrate (unpredictable)
Diphenylhydantoin
Heparin

Antibiotics
Antihistamines
Barbiturates
Chloral hydrate
Clofibrate (unpredictable)
Corticosteroids
Digitalis
Diuretics
Edathamil
Glutethimide
Griseofulvin
Hydroxyzine (Vistaril)

Table 7-2 Interferences in Hematologic Testing (continued)

Laboratory Tests (Conditions Detected)	Normal Values and Significance of Abnormal Values	Causes of False-Positive or Elevated Values (+)	Causes of False-Negative or Decreased Values (−)
Prothrombin Time (continued) teration of the rate at which anticoagulants are metabolized, and displacement of anticoagulants from protein binding sites (active and inactive) with indomethacin, oxyphenbutazone, salicylates, sulfonamides, and other drugs are examples of drug effects on prothrombin time.		Hydroxyzine Indomethacin Iothiouracil Lipomul (oil inj.)* Mefenamic acid Metandienone Metaproterenol (abnormal)* Methimazole Methyldopa* Methylthiouracil Mineral oil (excessive ingestion) Oxyphenbutazone Para-aminosalicylic acid (PAS) Phenylbutazone Phenyramidol Phosphorus (toxicity) Propylthiouracil Quinidine Quinine Salicylates (>1 Gm. per day) Sulfonamides (oral) Thyroid hormones Vitamin A	Lipomul (oil inj.)* Metaproterenol (abnormal)* Methyldopa* Mineral oil Progestin-estrogen combinations (oral contraceptives) Pyrazinamide Salicylates Sulfonamides Vitamin K Xanthines (caffeine, theophylline, etc.)
Sedimentation Rate (For normal body reaction to injury or disease)	Wintrobe, Male: 3–5 mm. in 1 hr. Female: 4–7 mm. in 1 hr. Rapid rate in acute infections, toxemias, fevers, nephrosis, shock, liver disease. Decreased or slow in polycythemia, congestive heart failure, allergic conditions and sickle cell anemia	Dextran Methyldopa Methysergide Penicillamine Trifluperidol Vitamin A	

Thrombocytes
(For normal mechanism of blood co-agulation)

Brecher Cronkite method: 200,000 to 500,000 per cu. mm.
Rees Ecker method: 150,000 to 450,000 per cu. mm.
Elevated often in polycythemia vera. Decreased in most leukemias and in thrombopenic purpura

Acetazolamide
Acetohexamide
Aminosalicylic acid
Amphotericin B
Antazoline
Antimony compounds
Antineoplastic agents
Arsenicals
Brompheniramine maleate
Chloramphenicol
Chloroquine
Chlorthalidone
Colchicine
Ethacrynic acid
Ethoxzolamide
Gold salts
Iothiouracil sodium
Lipomul (oil inj.)
Mefenamic acid
Methazolamide
Methimazole
Methyldopa
Oxyphenbutazone
Penicillamine
Phenindione (indane derivative)
Phenylbutazone
Propynyl-cyclohexanol carbamate
Pyrimethamine
Quinidine sulfate
Quinine
Ristocetin A & B
Salicylates
Smallpox vaccine
Sulfadimethoxine
Sulfonyl ureas (oral hypoglycemic agents)
Thiazide diuretics (rare)

Table 7-3 Interferences in Clinical Laboratory Testing of Urine [6,7,11,12,14-16,40,65,68,75]

Laboratory Tests (Conditions Detected)	Normal Values and Significance of Abnormal Values	Causes of False-Positive or Elevated Values (+)	Causes of False-Negative or Decreased Values (−)
Acetoacetic Acid (Impaired fat metabolism) Acetest, Ketostix, etc. (nitroprusside) tests are sensitive and have interferences shown. Gerhardt Test (ferric chloride) less sensitive	Up to 2 mg./100 ml. normal. Ketonuria (acetone, acetoacetic acid, β-hydroxy-butyric acid) occurs in uncontrolled diabetes mellitus, fever, toxic states, following anesthesia, in cachexia, and vomiting of pregnancy	Ether anesthesia Levodopa Methyldopa Paraldehyde Phenazopyridine (Pyridium) Phenothiazines Phenolsulfonphthalein (PSP) Phenothiazines (Gerhardt Test) Phenylpyruvic acid Sulfobromophthalein (BSP) Salicylates (Gerhardt Test)	
Acetone (Impaired fat metabolism)	1.7 to 42 mg. total ketone bodies as acetone/100 ml. normal, depending on test method. Positive in diabetes mellitus and starvation. See more complete discussion under *Acetoacetic Acid*.	BSP (Bromsulphalein) Ether anesthesia Inositol and methionine Insulin (overdose) Isoniazid (toxicity) Levodopa Metformin Methionine Phenformin PSP (Phenolsulfonphthalein)	
Albumin	See Protein below		
Amino Acids (Impaired amino acid metabolism; gout; liver disease; Wilson's disease)	0.5 Gm. N_2 in 24 hr. Elevated in Fanconi's syndrome, gout, Hartnup disease, inborn errors of amino acid metabolism, leukemia and Wilson's disease	ACTH Cortisone 11-hydroxycorticosteroids Sulfonamides Tetracyclines (degraded)	Epinephrine Insulin

Barbiturates
(Poisonings, suicide, overdosage)

False positives are encountered at high or toxic levels of the drugs listed. Either the dithizone or diphenylcarbazone method is used

Chlordiazepoxide (Librium)
Chlorpheniramine (Chlor-
    Trimeton, etc.)
Diazepam (Valium)
Glutethimide (Doriden)
Meperidine (Demerol)
Methyprylon (Noludar)
Phenytoin (Dilantin)
Tin (in filter paper at times)
Tolbutamide (Orinase)

Salicylate (spectrophotometric)

Benzidine
(Renal damage; blood in the urine. See also RBC or Hemoglobin below)

Absent (no blood in urine)
Present in acute glomerulonephritis, py-elonephritis, collagen disease, lipoid ne-phrosis, or other renal damage

Bacteria
Bromides
Copper
Ferricyanides
Filter paper
Formalin
Iodides
Iron salts
Methyldopa
Nitric acid
Oxidizing agents
Permanganates
Pus
Sulfobromophthalein (BSP)

Ascorbic acid
Tetracyclines (containing
    ascorbic acid)

Bile
(Impaired liver function)

Negative (absent)
Present in biliary obstruction and hepato-cellular disease

Chlorzoxazone
Thymol

Bilirubin
(Impaired liver function. See also Table 7-5)

Absent or up to 0.3 mg. per 100 ml.
Elevated in biliary obstruction, hepatitis, hepatocellular disease, neonatal jaun-dice, and hemolytic disease due to Rh and ABO incompatibilities
Drugs such as ethoxazene and phenazo-pyridine interfere with the Ictotest color

Acetophenazine (Tindal)
Chlorprothixene (Taractan)
Ethoxazene (Serenium)
Flufenamic acid (Arlef)
Fluphenazine (Prolixin, etc)
Mefenamic acid (Ponstel)
Perphenazine (Trilafon)
Phenazopyridine (Pyridium)
Phenothiazines

Table 7-3 Interferences in Clinical Laboratory Testing of Urine (continued)

Laboratory Tests (Conditions Detected)	Normal Values and Significance of Abnormal Values	Causes of False-Positive or Elevated Values (+)	Causes of False-Negative or Decreased Values (−)
Blood Occult See *Benzidine* in this table and Table 7-7.		Bacteria (peroxidase, old specimens) Bromides Iodides Iron salts Methyldopa Sulfobromophthalein	Ascorbic acid Tetracyclines
Calcium (Impaired calcium metabolism)	2.4–20.0 mEq. per 24 hr. Elevated in hyperparathyroidism, excess intake of vitamin D and lysis of the bone in metastatic neoplasms. Decreased in hypoparathyroidism, osteomalacia and steatorrhea	Cholestyramine resin Dihydrotachysterol Nandrolone (in some cancer patients) Parathyroid inj. Vitamin D	Alkaline urine (pH increased) Sodium phytate Thiazide diuretics Viomycin
Catecholamines (Impaired adrenal medulla function; muscular dystrophy, myasthenia gravis).	Epinephrine: under 10 μg. per 24 hr. Norepinephrine: under 100 μg. per 24 hr. Total: 30–100 μg. per 24 hr. depending on method Elevated in pheochromocytoma or extra medullary chromaffin tumors and occasionally in malignant hypertension Tumors may cause an elevation of *metanephrines* (hydroxycatecholamines), the metabolites of catecholamines, e.g., in pheochromocytoma. The specific interferences for metanephrine tests are chlorpromazine (+), imipramine (+), and methylglucamine (−)	Adrenalin type drugs Alcohol, ethyl Aminophylline Antihypertensive drugs (some) B-complex vitamins (high dose) Caffeine (coffee) Carbon tetrachloride Chloral hydrate? Chlorpromazine Epinephrine Erythromycin? Exercise Formaldehyde (fluorescence method) Hydralazine* Hypertensive drugs Imipramine (Tofranil, etc.) Isoproterenol Levodopa	Familial dysautonomia Formaldehyde Guanethidine (Ismelin) Hydralazine* Malnutrition Methenamine (Hingerty method) Methylglucamine (Renografin, Renovist) Radiopaque iodine media Reserpine

		Thiazide diuretics

Methenamine (inhibit
fluorescence of added
standard)
Methyldopa (Aldomet)
Myasthenia gravis
Nicotinic acid
Nitroglycerin
Progressive muscular dystrophy
Quinidine
Quinine
Riboflavin
Salicylates
Sympathomimetics
(amphetamines, ephedrine,
phenmetrazine, etc.)
Tetracyclines
Vigorous exercise

Creatine & Creatinine
(Impaired muscle physiology and renal function—glomerular filtration)

Adult male: Creatine 0–50 mg.; Creatinine 25 mg. per Kg.
Adult female: Creatine 0–100 mg.; Creatinine 21 mg. per Kg.
Elevated in excessive catabolism, muscular dystrophies, myasthenia gravis, starvation, hyperthyroidism and certain febrile diseases. Decreased in hypothyroidism and renal insufficiency

Acetoacetic acid
Acetone
Aminohippurate
Androgens
Ascorbic acid
Corticosteroids
Fructose
Glucose
Methyldopa
Nitrofuran derivatives
Phenolsulfonphthalein (PSP)
Protein
Pyruvate
Sulfobromophthalein (BSP)

Crystals
(Impaired kidney function)

Usually present are crystals of phosphates, uric acid, calcium carbonate, ammonium urate, and sodium urate
Elevated in kidney damage, atrophy of the liver, and cystinuria

Acetazolamide
Aminosalicylic acid
Formalin (urea precipitate)
Sulfonamides
Thiabendazole

*The substances followed by an asterisk reportedly influence the test but further study is needed to determine the exact effects and the mechanism of action. Some effects are pharmacological, some chemical.

Table 7-3 Interferences in Clinical Laboratory Testing of Urine (continued)

Laboratory Tests (Conditions Detected)	Normal Values and Significance of Abnormal Values	Causes of False-Positive or Elevated Values (+)	Causes of False-Negative or Decreased Values (−)
Diacetic Acid (Impaired pancreatic function and carbohydrate metabolism)	Absent Present in starvation and diabetes mellitus	Acetate* Antipyrine* Cyanate* Phenol* Phenothiazines Salicylates Sodium bicarbonate*	Acetate* Antipyrine* Cyanate* Phenol* Sodium bicarbonate*
Diagnex Blue (Impaired gastric function—free hydrochloric acid)	25–50 degrees or test value in excess of 600 mcg. Azure A excreted Hypochlorhydria: 300–600 μg. Achlorhydria: less than 300 μg. Elevated in duodenal ulcer. Decreased in achlorhydria, gastritis, and often absent in gastric carcinoma	Aluminum salts Atabrine Barium Calcium Congestive heart failure* Dehydration* Intestinal malabsorption* Iron Kaolin Kidney and liver disorders* Magnesium Medications with K or Na Methylene blue Nicotinic acid Phenazopyridine* Quinacrine (mepacrine) Quinidine Quinine Riboflavin Subtotal gastric resection	Caffeine sodium benzoate Congestive heart failure* Dehydration* Insufficient stimulation by caffeine sodium benzoate Intestinal malabsorption* Kidney and liver disorders* Phenazopyridine* Pyloric obstruction
Estrogens (Impaired ovarian function)	Female: 4–60 μg. per 24 hr. Male: 4–25 μg. per 24 hr. Elevated in prepuberty; may indicate ovarian tumor, pituitary or hypothalamic lesions, or certain types of adrenal tumors.	Meprobamate Phenolphthalein Prochlorperazine* Tetracyclines* Vitamins*	Cascara (−estradiol) Cortisone (−estradiol) Hydrochlorothiazide (destroys estriol) Prochlorperazine*

Decreased in ovarian failure or pituitary deficiency; falling levels in late pregnancy may be indicative of abnormal placental function

Senna (-estrone)
Stilbestrol (-estradiol, estriol)
Tetracyclines*
Vitamins*

Glucose (Benedict's)
(Impaired carbohydrate metabolism)

Absent
Present in diabetes mellitus, renal glycosuria, ingestion of sugars containing glucose, after prolonged fasting, in poisonings due to carbon monoxide, mercuric chloride, morphine, etc. Glucosuria must be differentiated from pentosuria. Also emotional hyperglycemia, pancreatitis, pheochromocytomas, cerebral lesions (encephalitis, fractures, tumors, and vascular accidents) must be considered as they may provoke glucosuria

Acetanilid
Amino acids ($\pm$)
Aminopyrine
Aminosalicylates
Amygdalins
ANTU rodenticide
Ascorbic acid (high doses)
Aspidium oleoresin (if absorbed)
Aspirin
Bismuth salts
Carbamazepine (Tegretol)
Carbon tetrachloride
Carinamide
Cephalosporins (cephalothin, cephaloridine, cephalexin)
Chloral betaine (Beta-Chlor)
Chloral hydrate (Noctec, Somnos, etc)
Chloramphenicol
Chloroform
Chlortetracycline
Cinchophen
Corticosteroids
Corticotropin
Creatinine
Dextrothyroxine (Choloxin)
Edathamil (EDTA)
Ephedrine (large doses)
Epinephrine
Estrogens (potentiate glucosuria from hydrocortisone)
Ethacrynic acid
Ether
Formaldehyde
Fructose
General anesthetics
Glucagon
Gluconates

Ascorbic acid (Combistix)
Sulfanilamide

Table 7-3 Interferences in Clinical Laboratory Testing of Urine *(continued)*

Laboratory Tests (Conditions Detected)	*Normal Values and Significance of Abnormal Values*	*Causes of False-Positive or Elevated Values (+)*	*Causes of False-Negative or Decreased Values (−)*
Glucose (Benedict's) *(continued)*		Glucosamine	
		Glucosides	
		Glucuronic acid (glucuronates)	
		Growth hormone	
		Hippuric acid	
		Homogentisic acid	
		Hydrocortisone (glucosuric effect potentiated by estrogens)	
		Hydrogen peroxide	
		Hypochlorites	
		Indican	
		Indomethacin	
		Isoniazid	
		Levodopa (Clinitest)	
		Ketone bodies	
		Lithium carbonate	
		Menthol	
		Metaproterenol	
		Metaxalone (Skelaxin)	
		Methenamine (Hiprex, Mandelamine)	
		Methyldopa	
		Methyprylon (Noludar)	
		Morphine	
		Nalidixic acid (NegGram)	
		Neocinchophen	
		Nicotinic acid	
		Nitrofurans (reducing metabolites)	
		Nucleoproteins	
		Oxalic acid	
		Oxazepam	
		Oxytetracycline	
		Paraldehyde	
		Penicillins (high doses)	
		Phenacetin	
		Phenols	
		Phenothiazines (long term)	
		Phloridzin	

Probenecid (Benemid)
Prolonged boiling
Protein
Pyrazolone derivatives
Quinethazone
Radiopaque media
Reducing sugars (fructose,
  galactose, lactose, maltose,
  rhamnose, ribose)
Saccharoids (glucuronic acid,
  glutathione, ergothioneine)
Salicylates
Streptomycin
Strychnine
Sulfathiazole
Sulfonamides
Tetracyclines (degraded)
Thiazide diuretics
Trioxazine
Turpentine
Uric acid
Uronates
Vaginal douches (some contain
  glucose)
Vaginal suppositories (containing
  reducing substances)
Xylose

Hydrogen peroxide | Ascorbic acid
Hypochlorites | Gentisic acid
Trimetozone (Trioxazine) | Levodopa
| Meralluride (Mercuhydrin)
| Phenazopyridine (Pyridium)
| Salicylates

Glucose (Oxidase Method)

Gualac
Occult blood. See also *RBC or Hemo-*   See *Benzidine* above.
globin, below)

Hematest
(Occult blood)   Negative
                                  Positive in renal damage. See Benzidine,
                                  Guaiac and RBC or Hemoglobin tests

Bacterial

[179]

Table 7-3 Interferences in Clinical Laboratory Testing of Urine *(continued)*

Laboratory Tests (Conditions Detected)	Normal Values and Significance of Abnormal Values	Causes of False-Positive or Elevated Values (+)	Causes of False-Negative or Decreased Values (−)
Homovalinic Acid (HVA) (Evaluation of function of adrenal medulla)	HVA elevation suggests presence of tumors such as ganglioneuromas and neuroblastomas.		Acetylsalicylic acid Salicylic acid Unidentified metabolite
Human Chorionic Gonadotropin (HCG) (Pregnancy test)	HCG in the urine of a pregnant woman neutralizes the antiserum to HCG and HCG-coated particles (latex or erythrocytes) do not agglutinate in test.	Oral contraceptives Pentylenetetrazol (Metrazol) Phenothiazines (Sparine, Thorazine, etc). Protein	
17-Hydroxycorticosteroids (Impaired adrenal function)	Males: 3–10 mg. per 24 hr. Females: 2–6 mg. per 24 hr. Elevated in adrenal adenomas, adrenal cortical carcinoma, adrenal hyperplasia, severe hypertension and thyrotoxicosis. Decreased in Addison's disease and panhypopituitarism	Acetone Ascorbic acid Acetazolamide* Chloralhydrate Chlordiazepoxide Colchicine Cortisone Dextroamphetamine* Digitoxin* Erythromycin Ethinamate Etryptamine Hydroxyzine (Atarax) Meprobamate Methenamine Paraldehyde Penicillin G? Phenazopyridine* Phenothiazines Potassium iodide Quinine Sprionolactone Trioleandomycin	Acetazolamide* Chlorpromazine (Thorazine) Dexamethasone Dextroamphetamine* Digitoxin* Pentazocine (Talwin) Prochlorperazine (Compazine) Progestin-estrogen oral contraceptives Promethazine (Phenergan) Propoxyphene (Darvon) Reserpine (Serpasil) Salicylates

5-Hydroxyindoleacetic Acid (5-HIAA)
(Carcinoid tumors)

2–8 mg. per 24 hr.
Elevated in presence of carcinoid tumors
Following administration orally of 5-hydroxytryptamine, urinary 5-HIAA provides a measure of MAO inhibition

Acetaminophen
Acetanilid
Aspirin
Bananas
Caffeine
Fluorouracil
Glyceryl guaiacolate
Melphalan (Alkeran)
Mephenesin
Methocarbamol (Robaxin)
Methamphetamine (Methedrine)
Phenacetin
Phenmetrazine (Preludin)
Serotonin (in foods)

Alcohol
Chlorpromazine
p-Chlorophenylalanine (Fenclonine)
Corticotropin
Formaldehyde
Heparin
Isoniazid
Keto acids
Levodopa
Methenamine (Mandelamine, etc)
Methyldopa
Monoamine oxidase inhibitors
Phenothiazines
Tricyclic antidepressants

Ketone Bodies

See *Acetone, Acetoacetic Acid,* and *Phenyl Ketone*

17-Ketosteroids & 17-Ketogenic Steroids
(Impaired adrenal function and male gonadal function)

Males: 7–25 mg. per 24 hr.
Females: 5–15 mg. per 24 hr.
Children: 0.8–11.3 mg. per 24 hr.
Elevated in testicular tumors, adrenalcortical carcinoma and hyperplasia, female hirsutism, and lutein cell tumor of the ovary. Decreased in Addison's disease, panhypopituitarism, nephrosis, and gout

Acetone
Cephalosporins
Chlordiazepoxide*
Chlorothiazide*
Chlorpromazine
Cloxacillin
Cortisone*
Dextroamphetamine (±)
Ethinamate (Valmid)
Etryptamine (Monase)
Glutethimide (Doriden)
Meprobamate
Methyprylon*
Nalidixic acid
Paraldehyde*
Penicillin G
Phenaglycodol
Phenazopyridine*
Phenothiazines
Prochlorperazine (±)

Chlordiazepoxide*
Chlorothiazide*
Cortisone*
Dexamethasone
Dextroamphetamine (±)
Glucose
Glutethimide (±)
Methyprylon*
Metyrapone
Paraldehyde*
Phenazopyridine*
Prochlorperazine (Compazine)*
Progestin-estrogen comb. (oral contraceptives)
Propoxyphene
Pyrazinamide
Quinine*
Radiopaque media (Conray, Duografin, etc.)

Table 7-3 Interferences in Clinical Laboratory Testing of Urine (continued)

Laboratory Tests (Conditions Detected)	Normal Values and Significance of Abnormal Values	Causes of False-Positive or Elevated Values (+)	Causes of False-Negative or Decreased Values (−)
17-Ketosterolds & 17-Ketogenic Sterolds (continued)		Quinine* Secobarbital* Spironolactone Troleandomycin Urinary chromogens	Reserpine (Serpasil) Seccbarbital*
Metanephrines	See *Catecholamines.*		
Occult Urine Casts (Renal disease)	Absent (urine is normally quite clear) Elevated or present in glomerular inflammation, degenerative renal disease, or infection	Antimony compounds Arsenicals Bacitracin Capreomycin Chloroguanide Colistimethate Edathamil (EDTA) Isoniazid Melarsopral Methicillin Neomycin Paramethadione Trimethadione	
Phenolsulfonphthalein (PSP, Phenol Red) (Impaired kidney function—tubular excretion)	40–60% eliminated during first hour 20–25% eliminated during second hour Abnormal retention indicates renal insufficiency	Anthraquinones (Cascara, etc.) Bile BSP (Bromsulphalein) 1,8-Dihydroxyanthraquinone (Danthron) Dyes Ethoxazene (Serenium) Hemoglobin Novobiocin Phenazopyridine (Pyridium) Phenophthalein Probenecid Sulfinpyrazone* Sulfobromophthalein (BSP)	Alkali (excess) Carinamide (Staticin) Diuretics Iodopyracet (Diodrast) Penicillin Salicylates Sulfinpyrazone* Sulfonamides Thiazide diuretics

Phenyl Ketone (Phenylpyruvic Acid)
(Impaired amino acid metabolism; deficiency of phenylalanine hydroxylase)

0.3–3.3 mg. per 100 ml. of specimen
Elevated in phenylketonuria, an error in phenylalanine metabolism associated with lack of skin and hair pigmentation, and mental retardation

Bilirubin (high conc.)*
Histidine metabolites (β-imidazolepyruvic acid, a rare deficiency of enzyme histidine α-deaminase)
Levodopa
Phenothiazines
Salicylates

Bilirubin (high conc.)*
Phenothiazines*
Phosphates
Salicylates*

Porphyrins (Fluorometric method)
(Abnormal porphyrin and pigment metabolism)

Uroporphyrins 10–30 μg. per 24 hr.
Elevated in hepatic or erythropoietic porphyria, moderately in porphyrinuria, also in infectious hepatitis, obstructive jaundice, infections, alcoholic cirrhosis, lead poisoning, and following ingestion of many chemicals

Acriflavine
Alcohol
Antipyretics
Barbiturates
Chlorpromazine
Ethoxazene
Green vegetables (phylloerythrogen)
Phenazopyridine (Pyridium)
Phenylhydrazine
Procaine
Sulfonamides
Tetracycline with phenazopyridine

Pregnancy Test

See *Human Chorionic Gonadotropin*

Protein (as albumin)
(Impaired renal function; nephritis; renal amyloidosis, neoplasms, or tuberculosis)

0–0.1 Gm. per 24 hr.
Elevated in increased glomerular permeability, renal disease or damage, cardiovascular disease such as congestive heart failure, infectious diseases, chemical poisoning by arsenic, lead, mercury, etc., ureteral obstruction, CNS diseases such as brain tumor, cortical damage and epilepsy, very high protein diet, and violent physical exertion
Note: The false-positive column contains many nephrotoxic drugs that induce or exacerbate proteinuria.

Acetazolamide (Diamox)
Alkaline urine (highly buffered, Combistix)
Aminophylline
p-Aminohippurate (PAH)
Aminosalicylic acid
Amphotericin B
Antimony compounds
Arsenicals
Bacitracin
Bismuth triglycollamate
Capreomycin
Carbarsone

Table 7-3 Interferences in Clinical Laboratory Testing of Urine *(continued)*

Laboratory Tests *(Conditions Detected)*	*Normal Values and Significance of Abnormal Values*	*Causes of False-Positive or Elevated Values (+)*	*Causes of False-Negative or Decreased Values (−)*
Protein (as albumin) *(continued)*		Carbon tetrachloride	
		Carinamide	
		Cephalosporins (cephalothin, cephaloridine)	
		Colistimethate (Coly-Mycin)	
		Contrast media (radiographic)	
		Corticosteroids	
		Dextrans	
		Dihydrotachysterol	
		Dithiazanine	
		Doxapram	
		Edathamil (EDTA)	
		Ethosuximide	
		Gentamicin	
		Gold salts	
		Griseofulvin	
		Iron sorbitex	
		Isoniazid	
		Jaundice	
		Kanamycin	
		Levodopa	
		Lipomul (oil inj.)	
		Lithium carbonate	
		Mefenamic acid (Ponstel)	
		Mercuric chloride	
		Metaxalone (Skelaxin)	
		Methenamine (large doses)	
		Methicillin (Staphcillin)	
		Methsuximide	
		Neomycin	
		Nephrotoxic drugs	
		Paraldehyde	
		Paramethadione (Paradione)	
		Penicillamine (Cuprimine)	
		Penicillin (massive doses)	
		Phenacemide	
		Phenazopyridine (Pyridium)	
		Phenindione (Hedulin)	

Phenylbutazone (Butazolidin)
Phosphorus
Polymixin B
Probenecid (Benemid)
Pyrazolone derivatives
Radiopaque contrast media
Salicylates (overdosage)
Salyrgran Theophylline
Streptomycin
Sulfisoxazole (Exton's)
Sulfonamides
Sulfones
Suramin
Tetracyclines (degraded)
Theophylline sodium glycinate (high doses)
Thiabendazole (Mintezol)
Thiosemicarbazones
Thymol
Tolbutamide (Orinase)
Trimethadione (Tridione)
Turpentine
Viomycin
Vitamin D
X-ray contrast media

RBC or Hemoglobin
(Kidney, bladder and urethra damage, or severe hemolytic reactions. See also Benzidine and Guaiac, above)

Absent

Presence may indicate acute glomerulonephritis, infection, kidney damage, drug toxicity, tumors of kidney, bladder or urethra; presence of hemoglobin *per se* is indicative of sickle cell crisis and acute or severe hemolytic reactions

Aminosalicylic acid
Amphotericin B
Bacitracin
Chloroguanide
Colchicine
Corticosteroids
Coumarin derivatives
Cyclophosphamide
Gold salts
Indomethacin
Kanamycin
Lipomul (oil inj.)
Mandelic acid derivatives
Mefenamic acid
Mephenesin
Mersalyl theophyline
Methenamine

Table 7-3 Interferences in Clinical Laboratory Testing of Urine (continued)

Laboratory Tests (Conditions Detected)	Normal Values and Significance of Abnormal Values	Causes of False-Positive or Elevated Values (+)	Causes of False-Negative or Decreased Values (−)
RBC or Hemoglobin (continued)		Methicillin Oxyphenbutazone Phenindione derivatives Phenylbutazone pHisoHex Phosphorus Phytonadione Polymyxin B Probenecid Proguanil Pyrazoline derivatives Sulfonamides Sulfones Suramin Thiazide diuretics Viomycin	
Specific Gravity (Impaired renal function—tubular reabsorption and concentration)	1.015–1.025 Increased or elevated in diabetes mellitus, marked fluid restriction, febrile diseases, acute glomerulonephritis, lipoid nephrosis and eclampsia. Decreased in collagen diseases, pyelonephritis and hypertension	Dextran Radiopaque contrast media	
Uric Acid (Impaired purine metabolism and renal function)	250–750 mg. per 24 hr. Decreased in gout, leukemia, polycythemia, a lead intoxication, starvation, certain acute infections, and toxemia of pregnancy	ACTH Ascorbic acid Bishydroxycoumarin 11-Hydroxycorticoids Mercaptopurine Methyldopa (Aldomet) Probenecid Salicylates (>3 Gm. per day) Sulfinpyrazone Theophylline Triamterene	Acetazolamide Allopurinol Aspirin Ethacrynic acid Methyldopa* Salicylates (low dosage) Thiazide diuretics

Urobilinogen
(Impaired liver function)

Up to 1.2 Ehrlich units per 2 hr. (Watson Method)
Not above 3 mg. per 24 hr.
Elevated in impaired liver function and hemolytic jaundice. Decreased or absent in complete biliary duct obstruction

Increase	Decrease
Acetone	Bile*
Afternoon (diurnal variation)	Chloramphenicol (large doses)
Aminosalicylic acid	Formalin*
Antipyrine	Light
Bilirubin	Procaine*
BSP (Bromsulphalein)	Smog (ozone)
Chlorophyll	Sulfonamides*
Chlorpromazine	Urotropin*
Constipation	
Formalin*	
Hemolysis	
5-Hydroxyindoleacetic acid	
Indole	
Phenazopyridine	
Procaine*	
Radiographic contrast media	
Sulfonamides	
Urotropin*	

Vanilmandelic Acid (VMA)
(Impaired adrenal medulla function—endogenous catecholamines)

1.8-10.8 mg. in 24 hr.
Elevated in pheochromocytoma or extra-medullary chromaffin tumors and occasionally in malignant hypertension

Increase	Decrease
p-Aminosalicylic acid[a]	Anileridine*
Anileridine[a]	Bananas*
Bananas[a]	Clofibrate[b]
5-Hydroxyindoleacetic acid[a]	
Methenamine mandelate[a]	
Methocarbamol[a]	
Nalidixic acid[b]	
Phenolsulfonphthalein (PSP)[a]	

[a] Diazotized p-nitroaniline colorimetric method.
[b] Pisano spectrophotometric method.

Table 7-4   Interferences in Coloration of the Urine [3, 6, 7, 11, 12, 14-16, 40, 65, 73, 76, 79, 83]
as an Indicator of Pathologic Conditions

Pathologic Conditions Indicated by Coloration of the Urine

Pathologic Conditions	*Colors Produced in Urine*
Alkaptonuria (homogentisic acid)	Dark brown to brownish black
Biliuria	Brown or yellowish, yellow foam
Blackwater fever	Dark red to brown or black
Cholera	Bluish green
Chyluria	Milky
Hemolytic anemia (urobilin)	Red to brown
Hematuria	Red to dark brown or black (smoky)
Hepatopathy	Greenish tint
Intestinal disease (indigo compounds)	Blue (indicanemia)
Jaundice	Greenish-yellow (bile pigments)
Malignant melanoma (melanin)	Brown to black
Nephropathy	Greenish tint
Phenoluria	Olive green to brownish black
Porphyria (porphyrins)	Brownish burgundy red*
Typhus	Bluish green

Substances Interfering with Coloration of the Urine

Interfering Substance	*Colors Produced in Urine*
Acetanilid	Yellow to red
Acetophenetidin (metabolite)	Yellow (dark brown to wine color)
Alcohol	Lightens color
Aloin	Red brown to yellow pink (alkaline urine), yellow brown (acid urine)
Aminopyrine	Red brown
Aminosalicylic acid (PAS)	Discoloration (no distinctive color)
Amitriptyline (Elavil)	Blue green
Anisindione (Miradon)	Orange (alkaline urine), pink to red-brown
Anthraquinone laxatives	Reddish (alkaline urine)
Antipyrine	Yellow to red brown
Azuresin (Diagnex Blue)	Blue or green
Beets	Red
Benzene	Red brown
Carbon tetrachloride	Red brown
Carrots	Yellow
Cascara	Yellow brown (acid urine), yellow pink (alkaline urine), darkens to brown to black on standing
Chloroquine (Aralen)	Rust yellow to brown
Chlorzoxazone (Paraflex)	Orange to purple red
Cincophen	Red brown
Creosote	Dark green
Cresol	Dark color on standing
Danthron (Dorbane)	Pink to red
Deferoxamine mesylate (Desferal)	Reddish
Dihydroxyanthraquinone (Danthron)	Pink to orange (alkaline urine)
Dinitrophenol	Red brown
Diphenylhydantoin	See *Phenytoin* below
Dithiazanine hydrochloride	Blue
Doan's kidney pills	Greenish blue
Emodin†	Pink to red to red brown (alkaline urine)
Ethoxazene (Serenium)	Orange to red
Ferrous salts	Black
Fluorescein IV	Yellow-orange

* Occasionally varies from pale pink to black. The urine may be yellow when freshly voided, but develops a color on standing.
† Emodin is 1,3,8-trihydroxy-6-methylanthraquinone. The major cathartic constituents of cascara, senna, and Danthron are closely related. These urine coloring substances are found in many combination products (Dorbantyl, Doxidan, Modane, Senokap DSS, etc.).

**Table 7-4   Interferences in Coloration of the Urine
as an Indicator of Pathologic Conditions** *(continued)*

Substances Interfering with Coloration of the Urine *(continued)*

Interfering Substance	*Colors Produced in Urine*
Furazolidone (metabolite)	Brownish or rust yellow
Indandiones	Orange (alkaline urine)
Indomethacin (Indocin)	Green (biliverdinemia)
Iron-sorbitex (Jectofer)	Dark to black on standing
Lead (chronic)	Red brown
Levodopa (Dopar, Larodopa)	Dark
Mercury (chronic)	Red brown
Methocarbamol (Robaxin)	Dark brown, black or green on standing
Methyldopa (Aldomet)	Dark (red to black) on standing
Methylene blue (Urised, etc)	Greenish yellow to blue
Metronidazole (Flagyl)	Dark brown
Naphthol	Dark color on standing
Nitrobenzene	Dark color on standing
Nitrofurantoin & derivatives	Brown or rust yellow
Pamaquine naphthoate (Plasmoquine)	Rust yellow or brown
Phenacetin	See Acetophenetidin
Phenazopyridine (Pyridium)	Orange red to red brown (HNO_3 turns orange to pink)
Phenindione (Danilone, Hedulin)	Reddish-brown to pink, orange in alkaline urine
Phenolphthalein	Pink to red to magenta (alkaline urine), yellow brown (acid urine)
Phenolsulfonphthalein (PSP)	Red (alkaline urine)
Phenols	Dark green to brownish black (darkens on standing)
Phenothiazines	Pink to red brown
Phensuximide (Milontin)	Pink to red to red brown
Phenyl salicylate	Dark green
Phenytoin (Dilantin)	Pink to red to reddish brown
Picric acid	Yellow to red brown
Porphyrins	Burgundy red, darkens on standing
Primaquine phosphate	Rust yellow to brown
Pyrogallol	Brown to black (darkens on standing)
Quinacrine HCl (Atabrine)	Yellow (deep yellow upon acidification)
Quinine & derivatives	Brown to black
Resorcinol	Dark green to greenish blue, darkens on standing
Rhubarb	Yellow brown (acid urine), yellow pink (alkaline urine), darkens to brown to black on standing
Riboflavin	Yellow
Rifampin (Rifadin, Rimactane)	Red to orange
Salicylazosulfapyridine (Azulfidine)	Orange yellow (alkaline urine)
Salol	Dark color on standing
Santonin	Bright yellow (NaOH changes to pink or scarlet)
Senna	Yellow brown (acid urine), yellow pink (alkaline urine), darkens on standing
Sulfonamides	Rust yellow or brown
Sulfonethylmethane (Trional)	Red
Sulfonmethane (Sulfonal)	Red brown
Tetralin	Greenish blue
Thiazosulfone	Pink to red
Thymol	Greenish blue
TNT (trinitrotoluene)	Red brown
Tolonium (Blutene)	Blue green
Triamterene (Dyrenium)	Bluish color (pale blue fluorescence)
Warfarin sodium (Coumadin)	Orange

Table 7-5 Drugs That May Affect Liver Function Tests [6,7,11,12,14-16,30,40,65,68]

The following drugs have been reported "to be hepatotoxic," "to produce changes in liver function" or "to cause jaundice or hepatitis." They should, therefore, be kept in mind for the possibility of altering one or more of the following tests:

Urine: Bilirubin—increased or false-positive
Serum: Alkaline phosphatase increased or false-positive
Bilirubin (icterus index) increased or false-positive
Blood glucose decreased or false-negative
BSP increased or false-positive*
Cephalin flocculation increased or false-positive
Cholesterol decreased or false-negative
Icterus index—see *Bilirubin* above
SGOT and SGPT increased or false-positive
Thymol turbidity increased or false-positive

Acetohexamide	Guanoxan	Perfenazine
Acetophenazine	Haloperidol	Pertofrane
Acetophenetidin	Halothane	Phenacemide
Allopurinol	Hydrazine compounds	Phenazopyridine (Pyridium)
Aminosalicylic acid	Ibufenac	Phenothiazines
Amodiaquin	Imipramine	Phenindione
Amphotericin B	Indandiones (anticoagulants)	Pheniprazine
Anabolic agents (Nilevar *et al.*)	Indomethacin	Phenolsulfonphthalein (PSP)
Androgens (testosterone *et al.*)	Iopanoic acid (Telepaque)	Phenylbutazone
Antimony compounds	Iproniazid	Phenytoin
Arsenicals	Isocarboxazid	Phosphorus (toxicity)
Aspidium oleoresin	Isoniazid	Polythiazide
Barbiturates	Lincomycin	Probenecid (Benemid)
Benziodarone	MAO inhibitors	Procainamide
Bismuth	Mepacrine (quinacrine)	Prochlorperazine
Carbon Tetrachloride	Mephenytoin	Progestin-estrogen comb.
Carbutamide	Mercaptopurine	Progestogens
Carfenazine	Metahexamide	Promazine
Chloramphenicol	Methandienone	Promethazine
Chlordiazepoxide	Metaxalone	Propylthiouracil
Chlormezanone	Methimazole	Pyrazinamide
Chlorothiazide	Methotrexate	Quinethazone
Chlorpromazine	Methoxalen	Sulfafuragole
Chlorpropamide	Methoxyflurane	Sulfamethoxazole
Chlorprothixene	Methyldopa	Sulfamethoxypyridazine
Chlorzoxazone	Methyltestosterone	Sulfonamides
Cincophen	Methyl thiouracil	Sulfones
Clofibrate	Morphine	Testosterone
Colchicine	Nicotinic acid derivatives	Tetracyclines (prolonged use or
Cyclophosphamide	Nitrofurans	high dose)
Cyclopropane	Norethandrolone (Nilevar)	Thiacetazone
Cycloserine	Norethisterone	Thiamazole
Desipramine	Norethynodrel	Thioguanine
Diphenylhydantoin	Novobiocin	Thioridazine
Ectylurea	Oleandomycin	Thiosemicarbazones
Erythromycin estolate	Oral contraceptives	Thiothixene
Estrogens	Oxacillin	Tolazamide
Ether	Oxazepam	Tolbutamide
Ethionamide	Oxyphenbutazone	Tranylcypromine
Ethotoin	Para-aminosalicylic acid (PAS)	Triacetyloleandomycin
Ethoxazene (Serenium)	Paraldehyde	Trimethadione (rarely)
Fluphenazine	Paramethadione	(prolonged use)
Glycopyrrolate	Pargyline	Trioxsalen
Gold compounds	Pecazine	Uracil mustard

* Drugs that increase BSP retention include anabolic steroids such as norethandrolone (Nilevar), barbiturates, estrogens, ethoxazene (Serenium), iopanoic acid (Telepaque), morphine, phenolsulfonphthalein (PSP), and probenecid (Benemid). Drugs that give low BSP results include phenazopyridine (Pyridium).

Table 7-6 Interferences in Testing Cerebrospinal Fluid [6,7,11,12,14,15,40,65,75]

Laboratory Tests (Conditions Detected)	Normal Values and Significance of Abnormal Values	Causes of False-Positive or Elevated Value*	Causes of False-Negative or Decreased Value†
Proteins (Inflammation or infection of the central nervous system)	Total protein 20–45 mg.% equivalent to very slight turbidity (Pandy qualitative tests) Elevated or increased in meningitis, dementia paralytica, arthropod encephalitis, acute poliomyelitis, tumors of the brain or cord, or CNS infection, e.g., neurosyphilis	Acetophenetidin p-Aminobenzoate p-Aminosalicylate Chloramphenicol Chlorpromazine Epinephrine 5-Hydroxyindoleacetic acid 5-Hydroxytryptophan Imipramine Oxytetracycline Penicillin Phenacetin Salicylates Serotonin Streptomycin Sulfonamides DL-Thyronine Tryptophan Tyramine Tyrosine	Albumin

* Determined by Folin-Ciocalteu method except for the bilirubin interference which is encountered with the sulfosalicylic or trichloroacetic turbidimetric method.
† Determined by sulfosalicylic acid turbidimetric method.

Table 7-7   Interference In Testing the Stool [3, 6, 7, 11, 12, 14–16, 40, 65]

Laboratory Tests (Conditions Detected)	Normal Values and Significance of Abnormal Values	Causes of False-Positive or Elevated Values (+)	Causes of False-Negative or Decreased Values (−)
Benzidine or Guaiac Test (Occult blood in stool)	Normally absent (negative for color formation with benzidine or guaiac) Presence of blood may be diagnostic for inflammatory, neoplastic, or ulcerative diseases of the gastrointestinal tract. See *Occultest* below.	Bacteria Boric acid (toxicity) Bromides Colchicine (toxicity) Iodides and iodine Iron, inorganic Meat in the diet Methyldopa Oxidizing agents (excreted in urine) Plant constituents in diet Sulfobromophthalein (BSP)	Ascorbic acid (high doses) Tetracyclines containing ascorbic acid

		Substances Interfering with Coloration of the Stool	Colors Produced in the Stool by the Interfering Substances
Color Changes [3, 6, 14, 72] (Dietary intake, or diagnostic for biliary obstruction or gastrointestinal bleeding)	Normal color: brown (due to presence of urobilin and stercobilin) Light brown: milk diet Dark brown: high meat diet Black: blood Clay colored: biliary obstruction	Antacids (Aluminum hydroxide, etc.)	Whitish discoloration or speckling
		Anthraquinones	See *Senna* and the footnote below
		Antibiotics, oral	Green-grey (impaired digestion)
		Anticoagulants (excess dose)	Pink to red to black (resulting from internal bleeding)
		Anti-inflammatory drugs	See *Indomethacin, Oxyphenbutazone,* and *Phenylbutazone* below
		Bismuth salts (Bistrimate, Milibis, etc.)	Black
		Charcoal	Black (coloration)
		Dihydroxyanthraquinones	Brownish staining
		Dithiazanine (Delvex)	Green to blue
		Hematinics	See *Iron Salts* below

Heparin — Pink to red to black
Indocin (indomethacin) — Green (biliverdinemia)
Iron salts (ferrous sulfate, etc.) — Black (oxidized iron)
Mercurous chloride — Green
Oxyphenbutazone (Oxalid, Tandearil) — Pink to red to black (GI bleeding)
Phenazopyridine (Azo Gantanol, Azo Gantrisin, Pyridium) — Orange red (Dye)
Phenylbutazone (Azolid, Butazolidin) — Pink to red to black (GI bleeding)
Pyrvinium (Povan, Vanquin) — Red (Dye)
Rhubarb* — Yellow to brown
Salicylates — Pink to red to black (resulting from internal bleeding)

Santonin — Yellow
Senna* — Yellow-green to brown
Tetracyclines (glucosamine potentiated syrup form) — Red

	Causes of False-Positive or Elevated Values (+)	Causes of False-Negative or Decreased Values (−)
Occultest (Occult blood in stool detected by peroxidase-like activity with o-tolidine) Normally absent (when present, amount of blood is proportional to intensity of color and time of appearance) Blood present in inflammatory, neoplastic, or ulcerative conditions of the gastrointestinal tract, e.g., duodenal, gastric or peptic ulcer or lesions, esophageal bleeding, gastric or intestinal carcinoma, biliary or hepatic disease, hemorrhaging of respiratory passages, blood dyscrasias, etc.	Bacteria Plant residues Meat in diet Plant constituents in diet See also other possible interferences under *Benzidine Test* above.	Ascorbic acid Tetracyclines containing ascorbic acid
Trypsin (Pancreatic insufficiency) Normal value: 4+ at 1:10 or higher dilutions Absent or reduced in pancreatic insufficiency. Decreased in premature infants	Bacteria	

* Cathartics containing Danthron, emodin., and other anthraquinone derivatives may stain the rectal mucosa brown. This includes mixtures like Dorbantyl, Doxidan, Modane, Senokap DSS, etc. as well as simple products like Dorbane, Doxan and Senokot.

Table 7-7 Interference in Testing the Stool (continued)

Laboratory Tests (Conditions Detected)	Normal Values and Significance of Abnormal Values	Causes of False-Positive or Elevated Values (+)	Causes of False-Negative or Decreased Values (−)
Urobilinogen (Anemias, certain malignancies, liver disease)	40–280 mg. per day; usually 100–250 mg. per day Decreased in inactivity, complete lack of food, e.g., inanition, in all cases of hypochromic anemia, some cases of hyperchromic anemia, and in low grade infection. Increased in fever, Hodgkin's disease, leukemia, pernicious anemia, and half the time in polycythemia vera		Antibiotics

Laboratory Tests (Conditions Detected)	Normal Values and Significance of Abnormal Values	Causes of False-Positive or Elevated Values (+)	Causes of False-Negative or Decreased Values (−)
Protein-bound Iodine (PBI) (Abnormal thyroid function; measure of circulating thyroxin)	3.5–8 μg. per 100 ml. Elevated in hyperthyroidism, thyroiditis, and pregnancy. Reduced in hypothyroidism, myxedema	Barbiturates Barium sulfate Bromides Bromsulphalein* Catheters (Intracath) Chlormadinone (Lormin) Clofibrate Cod liver oil Corticosteroids Dextrothyroxine (Choloxin) Diiodohydroxyquin (Diodoquin, Floraquin, etc.) Dimethisterone Dithiazanine (Delvex) Erythrosine Estrogens Ether, anesthetic* Gallamine triethiodide (Flaxedil) Inorganic and organic iodides Iodinated albumin Iodinated glycerol Iodinated water (drinking) Iodine containing compounds: amebicides, anthelmintics, antidandruff preparations, antiseptics, antithyroids (iothiouracil, etc.), diuretics, iodinated oils, cough mixtures, gargles, ointments, oral disinfectants, lotions, Lugol's solution, I[131] labeled diagnostics, radiographic contrast media (Pantopaque iophendylate, Telepaque iopanoic acid, etc.), antiasthmatics, Floraquil vaginal suppositories, Neopentil, some	Acid (2N HCl) ACTH* p-Aminobenzoates Aminoglutethimide p-Aminosalicylic acid (PAS) Anabolic agents Androgens Antithyroid drugs (methimazole, etc.) Barbiturates Bromsulphalein* Chlorates Chlorpromazine Chlorpropamide Cobalt Corticosteroids* o, p-DDD Diazo dyes 2,4-Dinitrophenol Diphenylhydantoin (phenytoin, Dilantin) Disulfiram Ethionamide (Trecator) Fluorides Gentisate Glucocorticoids Gold sodium thiosulfate Hydrochlorothiazide? Isoniazid Liothyronine (Cytomel) Lithium carbonate Mephenytoin Mercurial diuretics Methimazole Methylthiouracil Para-aminobenzoic acid (PABA)

*Substances followed by an asterisk reportedly influence the test but further study is needed to determine the exact effects and the mechanism of action.

Table 7-8 Thyroid Function Tests *(continued)*

Laboratory Tests (Conditions Detected)	Normal Values and Significance of Abnormal Values	Causes of False-Positive or Elevated Values (+)	Causes of False-Negative or Decreased Values (−)
Protein-bound Iodine (PBI) *(continued)*		toothpastes, suntan preparations, vitamin-mineral products, etc.	Para-aminosalicylic acid (PAS)
		Iodochlorhydroxyquin (Clioquinol, Vioform)	Penicillin
		Iodophors	Phenothiazines
		Iothiouracil (Itrumil)	Phenylbutazone (Butazolidin)
		Isoniazid	Propylthiouracil (antithyroid drugs)
		Isopropamide	Reserpine
		Methysergide maleate (Deseril, Sansert)	Resorcinol
		Metrecal	Salicylates (high dose)
		Mouthwashes	Sodium nitroprusside
		Nessler's reagent	Soybean milk substitute
		Perphenazine (prolonged use)	Sulfonamides
		Potassium iodide	Sulfonylureas
		Providone-iodine (Isodine, even topically) See above	Testosterone
		Progestin-estrogen oral contraceptives, (Enovid, Ortho-Novum, Provest, etc.)	Thiazide diuretics
		Pyrazinamide	Thiocyanates
		Radiopaque contrast media	Tolbutamide
		Sulfobromphthalein (BSP) due to iodine contamination	Triiodothyronine
		Suntan oil	
		Tetraiodofluorescein (in pink capsules)	
		Thyroid hormones (thyroxine, etc.)	
		Tubing (Intracath)	
		Undecoylium chloride-iodine (even topically)	
		Vitamins A & D (cod liver prep.)	

Thyroxine-binding Globulin (TBG)
(Abnormal thyroid function)

12–20 μg. thyroxine per 100 ml. Elevated in myxedema, normal pregnancy, and estrogen, iodide or thiouracil therapy. Decreased in thyrotoxicosis and nephrosis.

Chlormadinone	Anabolic agents
Progestin-estrogen oral contraceptives	Androgens
	Phenylbutazone (Butazolidin)
	Phenytoin (Dilantin)
	Salicylates

Triiodothyronine (T₃) Uptake
(Abnormal thyroid function; more reliable for hyperthyroidism)

Males: 11–19% uptake
Females: 11–17% uptake
Elevated uptake in hyperthyroidism, nephrosis, liver failure, pulmonary insufficiency and anticoagulant therapy. Reduced uptake in hypothyroidism and estrogen therapy

ACTH (conflicting reports)*	ACTH (conflicting reports)*
Aminoglutethimide	Antithyroid drugs (propylthiouracil, methimazole, etc.)
Anabolic agents	BAL
Androgens	Chlordiazepoxide
Anticoagulants, oral	Corticosteroids*
Barbiturates	Estrogens
Chlorpropamide	Iothiouracil
Contraceptives, oral	Ipodate (Oragrafin)
Corticosteroids*	Methylthiouracil
Coumarin derivatives	Perphenazine (prolonged use)
o,p'-DDD	Progestin-estrogen oral contraceptives
Dextrothyroxine (Choloxin)	Propythiouracil
Diazo dyes	Sulfonylureas
Dicumarol (coumarins)	Thiazide diuretics
2,4-Dinitrophenol	
Diphenylhydantoin (Dilantin)	
Gentisate	
Heparin	
Ipodate	
Penicillin	
Phenylbutazone	
Salicylates (high doses)	
Sulfonamides	
Tolbutamide	

Thyroxine (T₄) Test
(Anion exchange ceric arsenite method)

Dextrothyroxine	Aminoglutethimide
Estrogens	Androgens
Iodine	Barbiturates
Iodoalphionic acid (Priodax)	Chlorpropamide
Iopanoic Acid (Telepaque)	o,p'-DDD
Oral contraceptives	Diazo dyes
	2,4-Dinitrophenol
	Diphenylhydantoin (phenytoin)
	Ethionamide
	Gentisate

Table 7-8 Thyroid Function Tests (continued)

Laboratory Tests (Conditions Detected)	Normal Values and Significance of Abnormal Values	Causes of False-Positive or Elevated Values (+)	Causes of False-Negative or Decreased Values (−)
Thyroxine (T₄) Test (continued)			Iothiouracil (Itrumil) Oxyphenbutazone (Tandearil) Penicillin Phenytoin (Dilantin) Phenylbutazone (Butazolidin) Salicylates Sulfonamides Tolbutamide (sulfonylureas) Triiodothyronine
Thyroxine (T₄) Test (By CPB-competitive protein binding)		Dextrothyroxine Estrogens Oral contraceptives	Androgens Chlorpropamide o,p′-DDD 2,4-Dinitrophenol Gentisate Iothiouracil (Itrumil) Penicillin Phenytoin (Dilantin) Phenylbutazone (Butazolidin) Salicylates
Radioactive Iodine (RAI) Uptake		Chlorpromazine Lithium carbonate Procyclidine	p-Aminobenzoate p-Aminosalicylate (PAS) Antithyroid drugs (methimazole, propylthiouracil, etc.) Barium sulfate Bromides Chlordiazepoxide (Librium) Chlorpheniramine Clofibrate Corticosteroids Corticotropin (ACTH) Diiodohydroxyquin (Diodoquin, Floraquin, etc) Dithiazanine iodide

Indocyanine
Iodides
Iodinated drinking water
Iodinated glycerol
Iodine preparations
Iodine, inorganic
Iodine, organic
Iodochlorhydroxyquin
  (Vioform)
Iothiouracil (Itrumil)
Isoniazid
Isopropamide iodide (Combid,
  Darbid)
Lithium carbonate
Methantheline bromide
  (Banthine)
Perphenazine (Trilafon)
Phenylbutazone (Butazolidin)
Radiopaque contrast media
Resorcinol
Salicylates
Sodium nitroprusside
Sulfonamides
Sulfonylureas?
Vitamin A

SELECTED REFERENCES

1. Aaron H et al: Drugs and other factors interfering with reliability of blood chemistry determinations. *Med Let* 9: 59-60, Issue 223 (July 28) 1967.
2. ———: Effects of drugs on the PBI and T_3 uptake. *Med Let* 9:82-84, Issue 229 (Oct) 1967.
3. Block LH, Lamy PP: These drugs discolor the feces or urine. *Am Prof Pharm* 34:27-29 (Feb) 1968.
4. Boucher BJ, Godfrey, JM, Mace P: Another contaminant affecting serum-protein-bound-iodine. *Lancet* 2:1133-1134 (Nov 22) 1969.
5. Bradley SE: Laboratory findings in the blood and urine in health and disease. *Med Clin N Am* 29:1314, 1945.
6. Caraway WT: Chemical and diagnostic specificity of laboratory tests. *Am J Clin Path* 37:445-464 (May) 1962.
7. ———: Sources of error in clinical chemistry. *Standard Methods of Clinical Chemistry,* Vol 5, New York, Academic Press, 1965.
8. Ceremsak, RJ, Sanderson E: Perineal prep with pHisoHex, a source of error in urinalysis. *Am J Clin Path* 45:225-228 (Feb) 1966.
9. Harris AH, Coleman, MB: Processing specimens, pp. 71-88, *Diagnostic Procedures and Reagents.* New York, American Public Health Association, 1963.
10. Conn HF: *Current Therapy.* Philadelphia, Saunders, 1968.
11. Cross FC, Canada AT, Davis NM: The effect of certain drugs on the results of some common laboratory diagnostic procedures. *Am J Hosp Pharm* 23:234-239 (May) 1966.
12. Davidsohn I, Henry JB: *Todd-Sanford Clinical Diagnosis.* ed 14, Philadelphia, Saunders, 1969.
13. Eastham RD: *Biochemical Values in Clinical Medicine.* Bristol, England, John Wright, 1967.
14. Elking MP, Kabat HF: Drug induced modification of laboratory test values. *Am J Hosp Pharm* 25:485-519 (Sep) 1968.
15. Frankel S, Reitman S, Sonnenwirth AC: *Gradwohl's Clinical Laboratory Methods and Diagnosis.* ed 7, Saint Louis, Mosby, 1970.
16. Goodale RH: *Clinical Interpretation of Laboratory Tests.* Philadelphia, Davis, 1964.
17. Gralnick HR, Wright LD, Jr., McGiniss MH: Coombs' positive reactions associated with sodium cephalothin therapy. *JAMA* 199:725-726 (Mar 6) 1967.
18. Hansen ÅP, Johansen K: Diurnal patterns of blood glucose, serum free fatty acids, insulin, glucagon and growth hormone in normal and juvenile diabetes. *Diabetologia* 6:27-33, 1970.
19. Hansten PD, Owyang E: Effects of drugs on clinical laboratory results. *Am J Hosp Pharm* 25:298-301 (June) 1968.
20. Henry RJ: Principles and techniques. *Clinical Chemistry.* New York, Hoeber, 1964.
21. Hicks JT: Drugs affecting laboratory values. *Hosp Form Manag* 2:19-21 (Dec) 1967.
22. Hollander JL: *Arthritis and Allied Conditions.* ed 7, pp. 563-573, Philadelphia, Lea & Febiger, 1960.
23. Lakeside Laboratories: *Clinical Norms.* Butler, New York, Francis Roberts Agency, 1961.
24. Lazerte GD, et al: False positive urine tests due to drugs. *Northwest Med* 63:106-108, 1964.
25. Levinson SA, MacFate RP: *Clinical Laboratory Diagnosis.* Philadelphia, Lea & Febiger, 1961.
26. Meyers, FH, Jawetz E, Foldfien A: *Review of Medical Pharmacology.* Los Altos, Cal., Lange, pp. 647-663, 1968.
27. Miller SE: *A Textbook of Clinical Pathology.* Baltimore, Williams & Wilkins, 1966.
28. *Modern Drug Encyclopedia.* ed 11, New York, Reuben H. Donnelley, 1970.
29. Moser RH: *Diseases of Medical Progress.* Springfield, Ill. Thomas, 1969.
30. Narduzzi JV, et al: Laboratory indices in clofibrate therapy of juvenile-onset diabetes. *Clin Pharmacol Ther* 8:817-838 (Nov-Dec) 1967.
31. Nivet M, Marcovici J, et al: Decrease in serum uric acid levels after oral administration of benziodarone. *Drug Digests from the Foreign Literature* 3:3-236 (No 5) 1967-1968.
32. Reeme PD Glyceryl guaicolate and 5-hydroxyindoleacetic acid. *Hosp Form Manag* 5:15-16 (Feb) 1970.
33. Sjoerdsma A: A clinical and laboratory feature of malignant carcinoid. *Arch Int Med* 120:936-938, 1958.
34. Sjoerdsma A, Terry L, Udenfriend, S.: Malignant carcinoid, a new metabolic disorder. *Arch Int Med* 99:1009-1012 (June) 1957.
35. Sunderman FW, Boerner F: *Normal Values in Clinical Medicine.* Philadelphia, Saunders, 1950.
36. U.S. Department of Health, Education, and Welfare: *FDA Clinical Experience Abstracts,* vol 15-31, Washington, DC, Food and Drug Administration, 1966-1970.
37. *FDA Reports of Adverse Reactions to Drugs,* vol 66-70, Washington, DC, Food and Drug Administration, 1966-1970.
38. Waalkes T, et al: Serotonin, norepinephrine, and related compounds in bananas. *Science* 127:64, 1958.
39. Winsten S: Collection and preservation of specimens. *Standard Methods of Clinical Chemistry.* vol 5, New York, Academic Press, 1965.
40. Wirth WA, Thomson RL: The effect of various conditions and substances on the results of laboratory procedures. *Am J Clin Path* 43:579-590 (June) 1965.
41. Files JB, Van Peenen HJ, Lindberg DAB: Use of "normal range" in multiphasic testing. *JAMA* 205:94-98 (Sep 2) 1968.
42. Shapiro R: The effect of maternal ingestion of iophenoxic acid on the serum protein-bound iodine of the progeny. *N Engl J Med* 254:378-381 (Feb 23) 1961.
43. Jankowski JJ, Feingold M, Gellis SS: Effect of maternal ingestion of iophenoxic acid (Teridax) on protein-bound iodine: report of a family. *J Pediat* 70:436-438 (Mar) 1967.
44. Van Peenen HJ: The effect of medication on laboratory test results. *Am J Clin Pathol* 52:666-70 (Dec) 1969.
45. Hunninghake DB: Drug interactions. *Postgrad Med* 47:71-75 (June) 1970.
46. Arnason BG: Is the tuberculin skin test sensitivity depressed by oral contraceptives? *JAMA* 212:1530 (June 1) 1970.

47. Editorial: Oral contraceptives and immune responses. *JAMA* 209:410 (July 21)1969.

48. Carstairs KC, Breckenridge A, Dollery CT, *et al:* Incidence of a positive direct Coombs test in patients on α-methyldopa. *Lancet* 2:133–135 (July 16) 1966.

49. Croft JD, Swisher SN, Jr, *et al:* Coombs-test positively induced by drugs. *Ann Intern Med* 68:176–187 (Jan) 1968.

50. Schoenberg BS: The "abnormal" laboratory result; problems in interpreting laboratory data. *Postgrad Med* 47:151–155 (Mar) 1970.

51. Fass RJ, Perkins RL, Sallow S: Positive direct Coombs tests associated with cephaloridine therapy. *JAMA* 213:121–123 (July 6) 1970.

52. Molthian L, Reidenberg MM, and Eichman MF: Positive direct Coombs test due to cephalothin. *N Engl J Med* 277:123–125, 1967.

53. Bower BF, McComb R, Ruderman M: Effect of penicillin on urinary 17-ketogenic and 17-ketosteroid excretion. *N Eng J Med* 227:530–532, 1967.

54. Duvernoy WFC: Positive phentolamine test in hypertension induced by a nasal decongestant. *N Engl J Med* 280:877 (Apr 17) 1969.

55. Possible sources of error in bromsulphalein test. *Drug Intell* 2:313 (Nov) 1968.

56. Wood LC, Richards R, Ingbar SH: Interference in the measurement of plasma 11-hydroxycorticosteroids caused by spironolactone administration. *N Engl J Med* 282:650–653 (Mar 19) 1970.

57. Majoor CLH: Aldosterone suppression by heparin. *N Engl J Med* 279: 1172–3 (Nov 21) 1968.

58. Werk EE, Theiss KE, *et al:* Interference of heparin containing benzyl alcohol in the fluorometric determination of plasma corticosteroids. *J Clin Endocrinol Metab* 27:1350–1352 (Sep) 1967.

59. Jubiz W, Meikle W, *et al:* Failure of dexamethasone suppression in patients on chronic diphenylhydantoin therapy. *Clin Res* 17:106 (Jan) 1969.

60. Glynn KP, Carfaro AF, Fowler CW, *et al:* False elevations of serum glutamic-oxalacetic transaminase due to para-aminosalicylic acid. *Ann Int Med* 72:525–527 (April) 1970.

61. Freigin RD, Haymond NW: Circadian periodicity of blood amino acids in the neonate. *Pediatrics* 45:782–791 (May) 1970.

62. Krieger DT: Factors influencing the circadian periodicity of adrenal steroid levels. *Trans NY Acad Sci* 32:316–329 (Mar) 1970.

63. Pedersen AT, Batsakis JG, Vanselow NA, *et al:* False-positive tests for urinary 5-hydroxyindoleacetic acid. *JAMA* 211:1184–1186 (Feb 16) 1970.

64. Kay AW: Effect of large doses of histamine on gastric secretion of HCl. *Br Med J* 2:77–80 (July 11) 1953.

65. Damm HC, King JW: *Handbook of Clinical Laboratory Data.* Cleveland, Ohio, Chemical Rubber, 1965.

66. Fales FW: Glucose (enzymatic), in Seligson D: *Standard Methods of Clinical Chemistry,* p. 102. New York, Academic Press, 1963.

67. Talso PJ: Symposium on advances in laboratory diagnosis, *Med Clin N Am* 53:1–236 (Jan) 1969. A collection of 19 review papers by physicians in the Chicago area.

68. Lubran M: The effects of drugs on laboratory values. *Med Clin N Am* 53:211–222 (Jan) 1969.

69. Goodman, LS, Gilman A: *The Pharmacological Basis of Therapeutics.* ed 4, New York, Macmillan Co, 1970.

70. Wintrobe, MM, Thorn GW, Adams, RD *et al:* *Harrison's Principles of Internal Medicine.* New York, McGraw-Hill, 1970.

71. Beeson PB, McDermott W: *Cecil-Loeb Textbook of Medicine.* ed 12, Philadelphia, Saunders, 1967.

72. Lipman AG: Drug-induced coloration of the feces. *Mod Med* 44:79 (May 1) 1976.

73. Lipman AG: Drug-induced coloration of the urine. *Mod Med* 44:83 (Apr 15) 1976.

74. Young DS, Pestaner LC, Gibberman V: Effects of drugs on clinical laboratory tests. *Clin Chem* 21: 1D–432D (Apr) 1975.

75. Caraway WT, Kammeyer CW: Chemical interference by drugs and other substances with clinical laboratory test procedures. *Clin Chim Acta* 41:395–434 (Oct) 1972.

76. Forman DT, Young DS: Drug interference in laboratory testing. *Ann Clin Lab Sci* 6:263–71 (May–Jun) 1976.

77. Knoben JE, Anderson PO, Watanabe PS: *Handbook of Clinical Drug Data.* Hamilton, IL, Drug Intelligence Publications, 1973.

78. Lipman AG: Hyperuricemia and serum uric acid test changes induced by drugs. *Mod Med* 44:101–2 (Aug) 1976. (No references.)

79. Knoben JE, Anderson PO, Watanabe PS: *Handbook of Clinical Drug Data.* Hamilton, IL, Drug Intelligence Publications, 1973.

80. Lipman AG: Alcohol content of commonly used drugs. *Mod Med* 45:43–4 (Jun 30) 1977.

81. Hansten PD: *Drug Interactions.* Philadelphia, Lea & Febiger, 1976.

82. Djahanbakhch O, et al: Thyroid function tests and oral contraceptives. *Br Med J* 1:1413 (May 28) 1977.

83. Package insert information, 1971.–1978.

84. Ahlberg CD: Interference in the fluormetric quantitation of urinary 5-hydroxyindoleacetic acid by aspirin. *Biochem Pharmacol* 20:497–500, 1971.

8 Patient Response

Patient response to medications varies with the interplays that occur among a multitude of disease, environmental, medication, and patient factors. These are now understood well enough to eliminate *unforeseeable* as a valid excuse in many instances when patients manifest adverse responses. The latter can be largely eliminated if official statements about contraindications, warnings, precautions, and adverse reactions are heeded. In fact, so much information on the hazards of medication has now been accumulated that the physician may often be held accountable if adverse effects injure his patients.

Unfortunately, undue concern about potential toxic or adverse reactions may delay or prevent the use of a possibly life-saving drug. The multitude of published warnings and precautions together with the possibility of a malpractice action often deter the physician from prescribing a potentially effective medication. The same inhibitions also lead to requests for many additional laboratory tests and additional consultations. These tremendously increase the cost incident to the prescribing of the medication. If the physician is thoroughly familiar with a given drug, has read and understood all of the pertinent warnings, contraindications and precautions, and has meticulously heeded them, he should not be held accountable if severe reactions occur because of rare, anomalous conditions that cannot be detected.

However, to minimize the probability of enduring the frustrations of litigation, the physician should always become thoroughly familiar with the current medical literature on a drug before prescribing it. Careful evaluation of every patient and his disease,

skillful prescribing, proper administration and appropriate follow-up are all essential to insure optimum therapeutic results. If safety or efficacy appears to be questionable or if adverse reactions occur, the physician should immediately re-examine the factors influencing the patient's response and adjust the therapy accordingly. [105]

It is imperative that the physician avoid falling into the trap of treating a specific disease with medication A which causes adverse reaction No. 1, which is treated with medication B which causes reaction No. 2, which is treated with medication C which causes reaction No. 3, etc. This "domino effect" establishes what Moser refers to as a "melancholy chain of misadventures." [8] We must keep constantly in mind the realization that once a drug or other chemical is administered to a patient his soma or psyche may never be the same again.

At times, the possibilities of major, serious, and even potentially life-threatening reactions must be accepted when treating or preventing an already existing life-threatening illness, or preventing a serious disease from developing. In such a situation, when adverse reactions occur they must be accepted as being as much a hazard of the original disease as of the medication. [79] The physician must use his own best informed judgment in making the final decision for use or nonuse of any drug or treatment. But informed judgment does not necessarily relieve him of responsibility or guarantee avoidance of all pitfalls since medicine is not an exact science. [210]

Many physicians feel that once they have made a decision on the use or nonuse of any medication, based on adequate information, they should not be held further responsible. They believe that litigation that has veered in the direction of complete accountability will inevitably interfere with medicine and lower its standards of professional practice. If they are correct, this trend may create one of the greatest hazards to the patient that could possibly exist, i.e., the hazard of withholding a life-saving medication that could have been given, but was not used because of the hazard of later legal action.

It is unlikely, however, that the law will be unfair to physicians who are sued. They will probably nearly always receive an objective hearing,* but they will often be held accountable if they persistently (1) apply inadequate diagnostic procedures, (2) prescribe and administer unsuitable medications, or even appropriate ones improperly, (3) use a drug in categories of patients known to react adversely to that drug, (4) fail to act promptly to counteract serious adverse drug reactions, (5) provide incorrect drug information or directions for use, or (6) provide inadequate follow-up of patient response to medication.

FACTORS INFLUENCING PATIENT RESPONSE

Response of the patient to medication, the final step in drug therapy, is strongly influenced by: (1) the *medication factors,* including biological availability, therapeutic inequivalency, and the other biopharmaceutic factors discussed in the first five chapters, (2) the *disease factors,* including disease characteristics discussed in Chapter 6, and (3) the *patient factors,* including the patient characteristics discussed in Chapter 6, the techniques of medication, mechanisms of drug therapy, and other factors discussed in this Chapter, the adverse drug reactions discussed in Chapter 9, and the drug interactions discussed in Chapter 10. The state of the patient's psyche may also play a role and psychosomatic influences may be important

*This is basically true. However, in such adversary proceedings a major effort is directed toward minimizing or preventing the effective presentation of the opponent's evidence. Actually, the relative legal competence of the opposing attorneys and arbitrary decisions by insurance companies to settle at any given stage of the litigation are often overriding factors controlling the outcome.

considerations in patient response to medications.[62] Many adverse reactions originate in the mind of the patient or of his lawyer.

The efficacy of any medication depends on (1) the status of the defense mechanisms of the patient and their capacity to return to normal with or without medication, (2) the presence or absence of congenital abnormalities such as enzyme deficiencies, (3) the status of the absorptive, digestive, excretory, metabolic, neurohumoral and other functions, (4) the inherent capacity of the drug, if it is an anti-infective, to inhibit or kill pathogenic microorganisms without inducing the emergence of resistant strains, (5) the inherent capacity of the drug to act at receptors to produce specific desired effects without hazardous adverse effects, (6) the distribution characteristics of the drug, including the extent and tenacity of its binding to receptor sites, proteins, and other constituents of the body, (7) the effects of interacting drugs or other chemicals that modify the action of the prescribed drug in the body, and (8) the adroitness with which the prescribing physician determines, evaluates, and utilizes his knowledge of the patient's absorption, metabolism, excretion, and the other characteristics discussed on pages 246 to 286.[6,106,119]

So many combinations of disease, environmental, medication, and patient factors influence response that no two patients react to any given chemotherapy in exactly the same manner nor to the same degree. Patients may respond rapidly to some drugs. Anesthesia occurs immediately with Pentothal IV, diuresis in minutes with furosemide (Lasix), and tetany is dramatically reversed with calcium IV. On the other hand, patients may respond slowly, after a long lag period, to some diuretics, hormones, and anti-infectives in resistant conditions. But identical medication in identical dosage for the same disease may vary widely in the response obtained in two seemingly similar patients. Although most patients respond favorably to officially approved medications, a certain number out of any large group receiving a drug product experience unexpected and undesirable reactions, a few unforeseeable, but nearly all preventable. Apart from biopharmaceutic factors, these adverse responses largely stem from hazardous techniques of medication (improper *routes and sites of administration* and unsuitable *dosage regimens*), from alterations in *pharmacodynamic mechanisms* that occasionally may not yet be fully understood and controllable, from *errors made by the patient* (see page 287), and from *dietary* and *environmental factors* (see page 384). A potential for *hazardous responses* (see page 288) is always present. [131]

ROUTES AND SITES OF ADMINISTRATION

The route of administration strongly influences the efficacy and safety of some medications. Thus chloramphenicol sodium succinate is not effective when injected intramuscularly, but is effective intravenously. Poliovirus vaccine (live, oral, attenuated) must not be injected, but must be given orally to allow the virus to multiply in the intestinal tract and thereby stimulate the appropriate body mechanisms to produce an active immunity. Some injections must be given by the subcutaneous route only, e.g., attenuated live mumps virus vaccine. Some must not be given intravenously, e.g., oleandomycin, triamcinolone hexacetonide suspension, and immune serum globulin. Some may be given by many routes, e.g., oxytocin by the buccal, IM, IV, and IV infusion routes, but only one route at a time. Death may result if topical thrombin is injected intravenously or allowed to enter a large blood vessel. [114,168]

In studies with aspirin, the form of the medication (tablets given orally or rectally, suspension orally, or suppositories rectally) did not affect the relative proportions of urinary excretion products (unchanged drug and the metabolites salicyluric acid and salicyl glucuronides). However, absorption rate, half-life, and excretion rate varied appreciably with dosage form and especially the route selected. Absorption was slower and more erratic and recovery of salicylate from the urine was significantly less with the rectal than with the oral route. Also the half-lives were significantly longer and rate constants significantly smaller for total salicylic and salicyluric acids with tablets or suspensions given rectally than with tablets orally or suppositories rectally. [23]

Choice of the site where medication is placed via one of the routes of medication, based on accurate knowledge of drug effect on given tissues, is a major consideration in assuring that a given drug therapy will be safe and effective. An escharotic agent applied to an eye may destroy it. Drugs that are safe and effective at one site may be less effective or ineffective or more toxic at another. A drug like polymyxin B that does not readily enter the cerebrospinal fluid must be injected intrathecally to treat patients with meningitis due to *Pseudomonas aeruginosa*. Some drugs are absorbed only at certain sites. The hazards of every medication must be considered in relationship to both the route and site of administration selected. [114]

Routes of medication may be classified into three major categories: (1) dermatomucosal, (2) gastrointestinal, and (3) parenteral. For purposes of this discussion, these are defined as follows. *Dermatomucosal* routes include the topical, percutaneous, and transmucosal routes of medication via all dermal sites on the outer covering of the body (skin, its appendages, and the external ear) as well as all mucosal sites in cavities that open externally (eye, nose, mouth, throat, and the externally accessible passages of the genitourinary and respiratory tracts). *Gastrointestinal* routes include oral and rectal entry to the sites of the alimentary canal (esophagus, stomach, intestines and anal canal). *Parenteral* routes include the intradermal, subcutaneous, intramuscular, intrathecal, intravenous, intra-articular and the other routes of injection into sites of the body lying between the dermatomucosal and gastrointestinal surfaces. All routes of medication carry hazards to the patient, and the exact site of administration selected is very important in assuring safety and efficacy. [91]

DERMATOMUCOSAL ROUTES

Medications are usually applied to dermatomucosal surfaces merely to treat the surface tissues and produce strictly local effects. The precautions to be taken vary with the area to be treated.

Dermal Route

Some substances are percutaneously absorbed from certain types of liquid vehicles and ointment bases, through the skin into the deeper tissues and body fluids where they may exert systemic effects. Sometimes such effects are desired, but sometimes they are harmful and thus dermal medications and other toxic chemicals that are absorbed can be hazardous.

Many attempts have been made to evaluate, improve, and control dermal medications. At various times attempts were made to introduce medications intentionally into the body percutaneously by inunction. Mercurial medications, for example, were once massaged into the axillae for syphilis, and periodically, hormone preparations have been introduced for "rejuvenating" and other effects. Such procedures are not currently considered to be acceptable medical practice.

Other procedures are recognized. Airtight, occlusive dressings (thin, pliable polyethylene sheets) are occasionally used over applications to improve and prolong the contact of some drugs (e.g., corticosteroids) with the skin and certain lesions. Deeper penetration into the dermal lesions is afforded, but substances that produce undesirable systemic effects through percutaneous absorption must be avoided. With some conditions, occlusive dressings that provide anaerobic conditions may be dangerous.

Substances such as dimethylsulfoxide (DMSO) and squalene have purposely been added to dermal applications to improve percutaneous absorption of some drugs. But such devices and additives present their own specific toxicologic problems, and because the rate of entry of medications is highly unpredictable the percutaneous route is very unreliable. Skin thickness, amount of pressure applied during application, amount of sebum present, composition of vehicles, length of time the medication remains in contact, pH, dermal lipid content, and other chemical and physical variables influence both the amount of medication that is absorbed and its rate of passage through the outer surface. Also, medication tends to pass through abraded surfaces much more readily than through intact skin. The percutaneous route therefore, in our present state of knowledge, does not appear to be practical for administering precise doses of most medications to achieve definite systemic effects. See, however, examples on page 250 of a few newer dosage forms that give promise of changing this situation.

Note—In the interest of brevity and clarity, the precautionary statements in the following sections on routes and sites of administration, beginning with the ear, are largely presented in direct discourse.

Ear. The external ear, including the external auditory meatus and the ear drum, is the only externally opening body cavity that is lined with epidermal tissue. The ear is therefore considered under the dermal route.

Touch the sensitive dermal linings of the ear very gently, if it is necessary to contact them. The introduction of medications by means of any device can easily cause serious damage if the device is handled roughly or incorrectly. A syringe placed into the ear at the wrong angle is one of the many such situations to be avoided. Do not use very hot or very cold fluids in the ear as these produce excessive stimulation of the semicircular canals. Do not use water as a vehicle for ear drops to be applied to the external auditory canal as this may be detrimental to the epithelium. Do not apply drops or syringe the ear if the tympanic membrane is injured. Avoid insufflation of powders of low solubility and impaction of ointments into the tympanic recess and against the tympanic membrane. To cleanse the canal of the newborn, use smoothly tipped droppers and oil warmed to 37° C. or slightly above. Remember the anatomical relationships of an infant vary from those found in adults and the ear canal of an infant is extremely delicate.

Mucosal Routes

Absorption through the mucous membranes is much more reliable than through the skin. Medications are therefore sometimes administered by the buccal, respiratory, and rectal routes to achieve systemic effects. Typical examples are nitroglycerin administered sublingually and amyl nitrite inhaled as a vapor in angina pectoris, anesthetics and sedatives administered by rectal installation in preparation for surgery, and drugs like aminophylline, amphetamine, cyclopentamine and ergotamine applied in aerosol inhalations. Such mucosal applications to obtain systemic effects are widely accepted.

But special precautions must be taken when medications are applied to the mucous linings of body cavities that open externally—the eye, nose, mouth, throat, and the genitourinary and respiratory tracts, since treatment of these sites present special hazards for the patient.

Eye. Use properly buffered, isotonic, sterile ophthalmic solutions free from insoluble particles and gently drop them from a short distance to avoid trauma. Or use high quality ophthalmic ointments that are fresh, homogeneous, and free from grittiness. Make certain each patient avoids cross-contamination by using only the eye medications prescribed for himself. To help insure continuing sterility and efficacy of treatment, do not allow the tips of droppers to touch the eye or any other surface. If an eye cup (the least desirable device) is used, cleanse around the eye thoroughly before each use and sterilize the cup after each use to avoid carrying an infection from one eye to another or from the surrounding skin into the eye. Do not use an eye bath when there is a copious discharge, but wash with an undine. Do not apply medications to a recently wounded eye with absorbent cotton, as sterility cannot be maintained. Do not apply ice-cold or excessively hot medication directly to the eye lids.

Special precautions are required with certain ophthalmic medications.[69] For instance, check the ocular pressure before instilling medications such as mydriatics. The presence of glaucoma is a contraindication to dilatation of the pupil. Also, the use of powerful cycloplegics like atropine may prevent patients from performing some visual tasks for as long as two weeks, unless counteractive medication is applied. Overuse or overduration is especially hazardous with sympathomimetics (may even exacerbate myocardial infarct) and with corticosteroids (systemic absorption).

Do not permit subconjunctival injections to be performed by anyone other than an ophthalmologist thoroughly trained in the technique.

Nose. Use only bland fluids in the nose because the mucosae are very sensitive. If nasal medications are to be applied in aqueous vehicles these should be buffered, isoionic and isotonic with the nasal fluids, and have a specific gravity near 1.020. Nasal drops are useful when they can be applied gently and directly to the area to be treated, but the intricate nasal passages can only be reached completely by means of a gas or a very finely divided aerosol.

Do not use medications such as oils that interfere with ciliary motion except when specifically indicated for their emollient or other appropriate action. Generally use only water-miscible emulsions, jellies and ointments when prolonged medication is desirable, as these cling to the surface without interfering seriously with the cilia. Do not routinely use nasal medications with an oily base as the hazards of aspiration are always present. Do not use alcohol or glycerin in the nose unless very highly diluted, because of the prolonged watery discharge that ensues.

Except in special instances, e.g., in ulceration or after an operation, avoid insufflation of powders, because inhaled particles may be irritating to the lungs. Also, particles on the sensitive nasal membranes act as foci of irritation.

When irrigating the nose with quantities of fluid under pressure (preferably by gravity), be very careful to avoid possible infection of the middle ear through entry of the fluid via the eustachian tube. To avoid patient discomfort and even worse, do not allow anyone but a well-trained operator to administer irrigations that may enter the paranasal sinuses. Also avoid entry of the fluid into the larynx and bronchi by instructing the patient to breathe through his mouth. Stop the irrigation if he has a compulsion to swallow. Avoid frequent and continued application of antiseptics, astringents, decongestants and irritants, including menthol and volatile oils. Do not use alkaline washes during the early dry stage of coryza as they tend to increase the swelling of the membranes. Constant washing away of mucus with various medications may lead to catarrhal conditions, paralysis of the cilia, and possible loss of sense of smell. Avoid frequent and continued use of silver preparations as these occasionally cause argyria.

Undesirable and sometimes hazardous systemic effects may be produced by both prescription and over-the-counter nasal applications. Through overuse or use in sensitive patients, decongestant drops and sprays containing phenylephrine, for example, may affect the cardiovascular system causing elevated systolic and diastolic blood pressures, reflex bradycardia, peripheral resistance, and other effects on the vasculature. Also repeated decongestion is often followed by the "rebound" effect of dilation which may cause a condition worse than the original. Such widely used prescription and proprietary medications by law must carry appropriate warnings against overuse. Unfortunately, patients often ignore these warnings as completely as they ignore the warnings on cigarettes.

Mouth. Avoid, if possible, application of medication with a disagreeable taste to the oral mucosa. Also avoid toxic substances that can be absorbed readily through the mucous linings.

Instruct patients not to eat or drink for a specified period after applying medications in the mouth so that the therapeutic agents will remain in constant contact with the tissues as long as possible. Constant secretion of saliva and repeated involuntary swallowings severely limit the period of effectiveness of applications in the mouth. This is one reason why the mouth cannot be sterilized. Reproduction of microorganisms proceeds faster than mouth washes can destroy them during the relatively short time the medications are active. This is especially true when the organisms have become established in abscesses and other lesions below the surface of the oral tissues. In such situations incision, drainage, and use of systemic antimicrobials may be necessary.

Throat. The precautions to be taken in medication of the throat are similar to those just given for the mouth. In addition, apply throat irrigations with care to avoid choking and use only in adults. Do not medicate the throat with drugs that will be harmful if swallowed and do not rely on gargling to medicate an infected throat, especially in children. This procedure often does not adequately carry the medication even to the anterior areas of the fauces. It is often futile to attempt to treat the larynx alone if infections exist concurrently in the nasal pharynx and sinuses. If laryngitis is secondary to these infections they must also be treated to effect a cure.

Genitourinary Tract. The precautions for medication of this tract may be categorized according to three main structures: bladder, urethra and vagina.

Bladder irrigation is useful in cystitis, hemorrhage and other conditions where blood and clots must be removed. But the procedure may aggravate the distress and pain of the patient if the cystitis is at an acute state. Take aseptic precautions and introduce catheters slowly only after thoroughly lubricating them with a water-soluble lubricant. When catheterization is difficult because of stricture or prostatic hypertrophy it may be facilitated by injecting warm sterile oil into the urethra. Always avoid overdistention of the bladder. Preferably irrigate by the gravity method. If a syringe is used always inject slowly and gently. Remember that some inflamed bladders cannot hold more than perhaps 10 ml. of fluid nor tolerate complete emptying without severe pain. When necessary, prevent excessive pain by administering an analgesic.

Over-eager use of the catheter in accident patients with posterior urethral injury does more damage than it provides information, according to J. P. Mitchell, consultant urological surgeon at the Royal Infirmary, Bistol.* Thoughtless use of a catheter can convert a contusion into a partial rupture or a partial rupture into a complete transection. A partially ruptured urethra can still guide a catheter into a ruptured bladder, draw off urine, and lead to the belief that there is no damage despite a small hole in the anterior wall. Preferably, make a diagnosis on the basis of the triad: blood on the external meatus, inability to pass urine, and ultimate retention of urine. Avoid catheterization if at all possible and make every effort to preserve the residual strand of tissue in partial ruptures to protect the patient from a severe stricture subsequent to examination. [12]

The precautions for medication of the urethra depend on whether the drugs are applied locally, orally or parenterally. In applying medication locally with an urethral syringe, expel all air from the syringe before beginning the injection and have the patient urinate to cleanse the passage as much as possible. Avoid excessive pressure especially with an inflamed and swollen urethra and be certain to prevent entry of material into the bladder in situations where this is contraindi-

---

*Symposium at Stoke Mandeville Hospital, Aylesburg, England, May, 1970.

cated. Use only mild preparations warmed to approximately body temperature or slightly above. The mucous membranes of the urethra (like the upper portions of the urinary tract, the ureters, and renal pelvis) readily absorb some medications, especially if trauma is present, as this increases absorption. Do not inject any medication into the traumatized urethra that cannot safely be injected intravenously.

Vaginal medications may produce toxic effects if they are absorbed through the mucosa. Antiseptic mercury bichloride tablets inserted in the vagina and a potassium permanganate douche used as an abortifacient [61] have caused death. Some drugs penetrate the membranes so readily that they can be administered for systemic effects by this route. Nevertheless, certain deep-seated vaginal infections are best treated with oral or parenteral anti-invectives. In deep-seated trichomoniasis, for example, metronidazole (Flagyl) is given orally to both the consort and the female patient.

Whenever bleeding or raw surfaces are present in the vagina, use aseptic techniques. Appropriate douches or irrigations may be effective, but avoid accidental introduction of fluid into the uterus; use a syringe with a nozzle that has openings on the sides and not at the tip. Do not use hot douches or strong pressure if bleeding is present. Do not apply paints and tampons in serious, acute, inflammatory conditions that require surgery or other treatment. Use of medicated tampons in minor conditions may convert neurotic individuals into more confirmed invalids by focusing their attention on a trivial situation. For vaginitis (candidiasis, trichomoniasis, and other infections and inflammatory conditions) carefully select the appropriate cream, douche, insufflation, jelly, ointment, pigment, suppository or tampon containing suitable antiseptics, astringents, deodorants, detergents, or other medications. Some medical authorities do not recommend frequent douching in healthy women, certainly no oftener than twice a week as it may interfere with the normal cleansing and antimicrobial action of the vaginal secretions.

The precautions for oral and parenteral treatment of the genitourinary tract are discussed under *Gastrointestinal Routes* and *Parenteral Routes* below.

Respiratory Tract. Use a coarse spray to dislodge nasal and pharyngeal secretions and a finely subdivided spray to medicate the larynx and bronchi. A very finely subdivided spray (1-5μ droplets) generated by a nebulizer is required to reach the alveoli and tissues of the lower respiratory tract.

When using readily absorbed potent medications like soluble corticosteroids remember that the respiratory tract affords almost direct access to the blood, only slightly inferior in absorptivity to an intravenous injection. The externally opening surfaces of the lungs present a thoroughly vascularized, enormously absorbent surface which is highly sensitive to irritants and receptive to suitable medications, particularly if they are in the gaseous state and soluble in the tissue fluids. Examples of such medications are amyl nitrite, mixtures of oxygen and carbon dioxide, vinyl ether, nitrous oxide and the drugs mentioned on page 341.

Avoid application of any medications to the lungs over too extended a period and avoid concentrations which are irritating, especially in inflammatory conditions of the tract. *Apply medications to the sensitive tissues of the tract gently and properly diluted.* Steam inhalations are useful if properly applied, but do not allow the patient to contact hot vapors, especially steam, directly at close range. This can scald sensitive surfaces. Allow only warm vapors to be inhaled and do not smother the patient with covers over the head and the vaporizer. A child, especially, must have very gentle treatment or the results can be disastrous. And do not expose tissues to cold air soon after a warm inhalation.

In all respiratory tract therapy try to use sprays and vapors which have pleasant odors. Consider suitable combination therapy when indicated. It may be desirable to use an inhalation containing agents that provide both systemic and local effects.

Important causes of dermatomucosal problems in general are too frequent washing on the one hand and dryness on the other. Various douches, irrigations and lavages can interfere with normal functioning of mucous membranes if applied too frequently and some lotions can have a drying effect if repeatedly used on the skin. The mucous membranes of the body cavities, through natural secretions or ciliary motion, cleanse themselves normally and tend to remain healthy with only very little artificial assistance. Pollutants, humidity and other environmental factors are often crucial etiologies and sometimes have serious effects. Health authorities claim that most respiratory conditions are usually caused by: (1) low humidity in wintertime housing and (2) irritants in industrialized atmospheres. Both injure the nasal mucosa, predispose the tissues to invasion by microorganisms, and present other possible hazards to patients receiving drug therapy.

GASTROINTESTINAL ROUTES

Both the peroral route at the upper end of the gastrointestinal tract and the rectal route at the lower end are associated with special hazards.

Peroral Route

The peroral administration of medication promptly provides the desired effects if the biopharmaceutic and therapeutic factors previously discussed are properly controlled. It is usually the safest systemic route, largely because injection injuries are avoided. However, because there are so many factors to be controlled this route is often the least dependable. Unless the capsules, tablets and other solid dosage forms prescribed are of high quality, deaggregation and dissolution followed by absorption and dispersion in the body fluids will not occur sufficiently fast or in the proper manner to achieve the desired therapeutic response. Lack of activity presents its own particular hazard.

On the other hand, sudden high concentrations of medications which are made suddenly available in the gastrointestinal tract can be hazardous. Enteric-coated dosage forms of rapidly soluble salts may severely damage the intestines as was pointed out for enteric-coated potassium chloride tablets on page 26. Also high serum levels may be quickly achieved through rapid absorption at sites of such high concentration of drug and thereby intensify side effects. Oral dosage requires adjustment in accordance with the make of drug product. This was pointed out for PAS on page 69.

As a general rule, for efficient absorption and distribution of systemically active drugs prescribe peroral medications in forms that are readily soluble in the body fluids. Insoluble ones can form enteroliths and may not be absorbed. Even relatively harmless products like psyllium hydrophilic mucilloid may become involved in intestinal obstruction when a patient overdoses himself. Some basic drugs are readily soluble as acid salts (e.g., hydrochloride or phosphate of tetracycline), some acidic drugs as alkali salts (e.g., potassium or sodium salts of barbiturates and sulfonamides), and some as the base or the naturally occurring principle (e.g., caffeine alkaloid and digitalis glycosides). Some drugs become increasingly more soluble and more active as they are more and more finely subdivided.[298] Note the principles covered below under Absorption and Distribution.

Prescribe irritating substances well diluted to prevent damage to the mucosa. Do not prescribe caustic or irritating substances in powder form unless well diluted with an inert substance or taken with copious quantities of water. Avoid excessive or prolonged use of alkalies in the gastrointestinal tract. Alkalosis may ensue and be very harmful, especially in cardiac patients with congestive heart failure.

Avoid prescribing drugs that interact to form explosive mixtures such as carbonates and acids. If a patient is damaged by such a mixture he may take legal action against both the prescriber and the dispenser of the medication. Avoid prescribing highly toxic medication in mixtures that deposit a sediment and require shaking before taking. The resuspended drugs may not be homogenously distributed and very high, perhaps dangerous doses, can be received as the last portions of the medication are consumed. An alert and knowledgeable pharmacist can help in circumventing such problems.

When introducing medications by gavage, observe closely for coughing, choking, or embarrassment of any type. The tube may enter the trachea. Check for correct entry by noting the absence of any air current at the end of the tube and by withdrawing some of the gastric contents with the aid of a syringe to establish positioning in the stomach. If suction is applied it must be very gentle. In severe vomiting and other gastric conditions, when intubation is desired but no contact with the stomach is permissible, a duodenal tube may be used to administer medications.

Rectal Route

Before resorting to rectal medication of patients with proctitis or other conditions that may make the rectum exceedingly sensitive, perform a digital examination to determine to what extent the patient may have difficulty in retaining any medications administered. Adjust the rectal dose in accordance with the specific drug. Some drugs should be given in lower doses, others in higher doses than the usual quantities given orally. Thus the rectal dose for a digitalis product may be 25% higher than the oral dose. For various drugs it may be anywhere from one half to twice as much, depending on the medication and condition of the patient. This type of dosage information should be made available by the manufacturer of the given drug and should be based on both pharmacodynamic and clinical studies.

PARENTERAL ROUTES

The most frequently used routes of injection are the subcutaneous, intramuscular, and intravenous in order of increasing hazard to the patient. Reports on injection injuries with these routes have continually appeared in the literature since the latter parts of the 19th century, and since 1927 have rapidly increased in frequency of appearance. Bones, muscles, nerves, and blood vessels are sometimes injured by hypodermic needles and serious damage may then be sustained by patients. Examples of these and other injuries produced by improper techniques of parenteral administration are numerous.[91]

The following conditions, as reported in the medical literature, have been produced by improper parenteral injection technique: abscesses, anesthesia, arteriolar spasm, cysts, edema, foot drops, hematomas, hypoesthesia, muscular dystrophy, numbness in the extremities, necrosis with sloughing, paralysis, pedal growth arrest, peripheral neuritis, periostitis, transverse myelitis, vasospastic disease, and wrist drop.

Medications associated with injection injuries, as reported in the medical literature, include alcohol, analgesics, antipertusis rabbit serum, caffeine sodium benzoate, chloramphenicol, digitoxin, emetine, erythromycin, gamma globulin, iron dextran, meperidine, mercurial diuretics, morphine, pancreatic substances, paraldehyde, penicillins, phenobarbital, promazine, propylene glycol, quinine, salts of arsenic, bismuth, calcium and mercury, streptomycin, sulfonamides, tetanus antitoxin and toxoid, tetracyclines, typhoid vaccine, vitamin preparations, and many others. However, because a certain drug has been associated with an injection injury does not necessarily implicate that drug. Improper selection of medication, dosage or procedure may actually be the cause of the damage to the patient. Repeated IM administration of almost any drug can cause abscesses, necrosis, or atrophy.

Muscle Damage

Injection of a drug into a muscle may or may not quickly provide appropriate blood levels safely. It will if the drug is in solution in a suitable vehicle and is promptly absorbed with minimal trauma into blood vessels at the proper site of injection. It will not if the vehicle is irritating, or the injection technique is incorrect, or the drug precipitates from solution because of the pH of the tissue fluids, or the drug is in a repository form. When the drug is intentionally localized at the site of injection and its rate of solution retarded by some means to obtain a prolonged effect, irritation may be more intense and blood levels may be attained much more slowly than when it is administered in an appropriate oral dosage form to obtain a rapid, immediate effect. However, an intramuscular injection is usually more rapid in its action than an oral dose if the drug is in a suitable vehicle. Even suspensions of microcrystalline particles of a drug can be rapidly and safely absorbed from a muscle if the crystals are readily soluble in the tissue fluids. By varying the vehicle and the derivative of the drug (ester, salt, ether, etc.) the rate of release of the medication at the injection site can be varied widely, from almost immediate dispersion with least amount of damage to the muscle to highly prolonged and very slow release with greater risk of damage. However, prolonged release does not necessarily imply that the patient will be harmed.

Reports in the literature have described injuries to the deltoid, gastrocnemius, infraspinous, serratus anterior, supraspinous, trapezius and other muscles, caused by nerve injury or direct effect on the muscle. Apparently, all injections into muscles cause some trauma. Even properly injected sterile saline solutions can cause lesions which may persist for several days. IM lesions vary in intensity and character with the volume, speed, and depth of injection and with the type of medication. Slowly absorbed, irritating, vasoconstricting drugs like epinephrine can cause serious problems. Some drugs may cause necrotic lesions that take several weeks to heal in spite of good injection technique.

Nerve Damage

Published reports describing intraneural lesions caused by inadvertent injection of neurotoxic medications into nerves, and extraneural compression caused by injecting too close to a nerve, are not uncommon. The axillary, cervical, cutaneous, lateral femoral, peroneal, radial, sciatic, suprascapular, tibial, the fifth and sixth cervical roots, and other autonomic and motor nerves have all been mentioned. Any nerve near the site of injection is a vulnerable though inadvertent target.

Damage to the common peroneal nerve can cause foot drop which may be mistaken for the paralytic condition caused by poliomyelitis. A similar paralysis, wrist drop, may be caused by injection too close to the brachial nerve plexus, and particularly into the radial nerve. Injury to the sciatic nerve, which is most readily sustained by squirming, struggling infants but which also occurs occasionally in adults, can cause atrophy and paralysis of the lower leg muscles. Such paralysis may occur immediately after faulty injection, or be delayed for a week or more. It may be reversible or permanent. The buttock should never be used as an injection site in infants or young children as they have only thin layers of subcutaneous tissue and muscle separating the skin from the nerves to be avoided in this region. The vastus lateralis is the preferred site for young children.

Injection injuries to nerves occur much too frequently and can be disastrous. In one country alone (Germany) about 70 cases of nerve injury were reported to insurance companies over one five-year period. How many patients around the world suffer such injuries in one year? How many occur that are not reported? As computerized reporting becomes more complete, more accurate statistics for such questions are becoming available.

Vascular Damage

Damage to blood vessels because of incorrect injection technique has occasionally been reported. Unintentional perforations of arteries may cause bleeding into the surrounding tissues and drugs that are inadvertently introduced into cutaneous arteries have induced ischemia and excruciating pain. Accidental intra-arterial injection of secobarbital (Seconal) into the antecubital space has produced immediate, severe, burning pain that radiated into the hand and was followed by muscle edema and necrosis (Volkmann's ischemic contracture).[108] Injection into deep arteries may also produce embolism. Always carefully guard against extravasation. And remember that inadvertent IV or IA injection can cause gangrene, anaphylaxis, or death.

When making any type of intravenous injection, exercise caution. Even when care is taken to inject slowly an in the proper site, some drugs, notably aniline derivatives, nitrobenzenes, phenylhydrazines, and sulfonamides, may induce intravascular hemolysis of erythrocytes. The hemolysis is particularly severe with some drugs in the presence of glucose-6-phosphate dehydrogenase deficiency, or when an autoimmune reaction occurs, e.g., an erythrocyte-drug combination becomes antigenic, or when the reducing systems in the erythrocytes (glutathione, etc.) become overloaded by constant challenge with the drug. This overloading becomes more likely in renal insufficiency, as the uremia also tends to lower the glutathione content.

Intravenous Injection. Injection of a drug in solution directly (but slowly!) into a vein with force from a syringe or other injector is the fastest and surest way to achieve a desired drug level in the blood and to make the drug biologically available in the patient's cardiovascular system. The drug in the serum must, however, contact the appropriate receptor sites where the required activity is to be initiated. It must cross the various membranal barriers and spread to the target tissues before the blood level can bear a significant relationship to biological availability.

Intravenous Infusion. The introduction of a fluid medication into a vein by gravity produces blood levels in a manner different from that of the usual intravenous injection. With infusion of a fixed concentration of a drug at a steady rate, drop by drop, the blood level gradually increases and when plotted forms a concave increasing and finally asymptotic curve that reaches the desired limiting value (the maximum attainable level with the given prescribed dosage). Once this value has been reached, a definite rate of input of drug exactly offsets for all practical purposes an equivalent rate of output due to excretion and metabolism. The exact level of this maintenance dose must be carefully gauged by the attending physician to avoid overdosage or inadequate dosage.

Hypodermoclysis. The introduction of large volumes of parenteral fluids containing electrolytes such as sodium chloride or other medications into loose subcutaneous tissue requires that special precautions be taken. Use only high quality isotonic, sterile fluids of suitable pH. Do not permit overdistention of the tissues with too rapid a flow because this is painful. The rate of administration should not exceed that of an intravenous infusion.

Shut off the flow occasionally to permit even normal distention to subside. Consider the addition of a local anesthetic to relieve pain and hyaluronidase to increase the rate of absorption of fluid. And check for hypersensitivity to any medications that are added. The application of warmth and gentle massage decreases any distress and facilitates absorption. Generally do not use hypodermoclysis in a patient who is in shock, or one with local edema induced by a damaged heart, or with a low serum protein level. Usually limit the input of fluid to 3 or 4 liters in 24 hours.

Use of hypodermoclysis has greatly declined since the introduction of convenient plastic containers for infusions.

Intravenous Additives

The literature contains many warnings about the hazards of improperly prepared intravenous medications. The use of any drug for parenteral therapy demands detailed and accurate information regarding its suitability for such therapy and its physical, chemical and pharmacological properties. Before preparing or using parenterals, read the package circular carefully, particularly in regard to the control of drug concentration, use of additives, maintenance of proper pH, elimination of pyrogens, and avoidance of incompatibilities. [130]

Closely supervise the addition of medications, buffers, and other substances to any nutrient or electrolyte solutions or other fluids to be administered by intravenous infusion or hypodermoclysis.

Control the drug concentration in the parenteral fluid very carefully. Concentrations that are too high can produce sclerosing or thrombosing or hemolytic effects with many medications. Some drugs (e.g., sodium morrhuate, sodium psylliate and sodium tetradecyl sulfate) are intentionally used for sclerosing vessels but when used to produce this effect must be injected slowly by proper technique because of the danger of anaphylaxis and of extension of a thrombus into the deep venous system. Accidental injection of sclerosing solutions into the deep veins rather than into the superficial varicosities has caused gangrene and amputations have been necessary when death of limbs occurred.

Do not use a drug additive if it adversely affects the pH, causes formation of crystals, or precipitates other particulate matter, produces a gas, destroys the clarity, or interacts with an intravenous preparation or modifies it in any way that may cause loss of effectiveness or make it unsafe for parenteral use. Also, scrupulously avoid trace impurities and microorganisms in drug additives and their containers as well as in the intravenous fluid itself. Prepare all intravenous additives in a sterile place, certainly not extemporaneously in congested nursing units under poor environmental conditions that permit the presence of interactants. [208] Allow only a pharmacist experienced in handling parenterals to prepare IV admixtures. A pharmacy-centralized IV additive program has many advantages, including better control and patient safety. [283]

Carefully review drug interaction potentials. Avoid such undesirable ones as reversal of epinephrine pressor effects with Dibenzyline HCl and the potentiation of succinylcholine chloride with neostigmine bromide. Use with caution compatibility charts and tables, such as the typical ones shown in Tables 8-1 and 8-1A.* Variations in brands may substantially alter the data. Also, take into consideration the effects of light, radiation, temperature, and container and closure materials, in addition to the effects of the other factors previously mentioned.

The vehicle used for an IV admixture may also strongly influence stability of the additive. Thus, the decomposition of ascorbic acid is accelerated in vehicles that do not contain dextrose and the decomposition of thiamine is accelerated in vehicles that contain bisulfite. [283] Some admixtures must be used promptly before they decompose.

Avoid the addition of medications to blood to be used for transfusions. Antihistamines, oxytocin, and certain other drugs should not be added to blood to be used for transfusion, according to the American Association of Blood Banks *(Standards for a Blood Transfusion Service,* Chicago). [3] Such additives make use of the blood for different patients questionable. Also compatibility of these drugs with so complex a substance as blood, is unpredictable, and if a transfusion reaction occurs, its cause in some cases may be impossible to determine when medication is also present.

Maintain the pH of intravenous fluids near 7.4, the pH of blood. Chemical thrombophlebitis may be caused by large volumes of parenteral solutions with a pH too far from that of the blood, even by IV dextrose solution with a pH of 5 or slightly higher. [24] But many variables governing pH, such as aging, autoclaving time, container materials, and source of water are difficult to evaluate and control. Because of the problems, the USP allows a wide range of pH for injections. Thus the pH

of official injections often varies from one batch to another, even from the same manufacturer. This frequently makes it impossible to duplicate results with additives.

Chemical, physical, or therapeutic incompatibilities caused by additives in intravenous solutions can create many hazards for the patient. One report lists 118 drugs that cause problems in parenterals. Some of these react with as many as 20 other drugs or adjuncts. [115] A chart of incompatibilities for 61 frequently used intravenous additives was published in 1966, [284] and since then many publications on the subject have appeared. [279-296,307] Abbot Laboratories, Baxter Laboratories, and other manufacturers have prepared useful charts which are available on request.

A study was made of 270 of the 11,000 unique combinations (in 2's, 3's, and 4's) that can be made with the 24 drugs most commonly prescribed in the hospital. The investigators found that 8.5% of the possible combinations of just two drugs in 5% dextrose solution possessed physical incompatibilities. Also, chemical as well as physical incompatibilities can occur not only between drugs and other chemicals, but also between drugs and the containers in which they are placed. [283] Rubbers and plastics may cause many problems, including alteration of physical properties, chemical reactions, leaching, permeation, and sorption.

The magnitude of the problem was emphasized by Latiolais, of the Ohio State University Hospitals, who pointed out that based on an average US daily census in short-term general hospitals of 550,000 patients, 137,500 parenteral admixtures are administered per average patient day, if data obtained in his hospitals are projected nationally. Therefore, about 50 million admixtures are probably administered annually in the United States. No one can accurately determine at the present time how many of these admixtures present incompatibilities and interactions that are hazardous for the patient. According to one estimate, 28 man years would be required to develop chemical incompatibility data comparable to just the physical incompatibility data published by Abbott Laboratories as the result of the 10,000 tests made by them. [287]

Carlin found that 68% of the intravenous solutions administered at the University of

---

*These tables present the more common compatibilites and incompatibilities. The subject has now become so extensive that entire treatises are devoted to it, some in loose-leaf form for constant updating. Cutter Laboratories provides such a service for an annual fee.[307]

Illinois Hospital contained at least one additive, 20% contained two, 6% three, and 6% four or more.[283] At the Clinical Center of the National Institutes of Health about 50% of all IV solutions administered contained additives. Of those with additives, 58% contained one drug, 27% two, 9% three, and 6% four or more. At University Hospital, University of Michigan, about 70% of all IV fluids contained added drugs; 24% contained two, 14% three, and 32% four or more. Studies at other hospitals yielded similar findings.[285]

Table 8-1   Compatibilities and Incompatibilities of IV Additives[115,120,280,284-295]*

Additives	Compatibilities	Incompatibilities
Acetazolamide (Diamox)	Standard IV fluids.†	Protein hydrolysate (Amigen).
Achromycin	See Tetracycline HCl.	
ACTH	See Corticotropin.	
Aerosporin	See Polymyxin B Sulfate.	
Albamycin	See Novobiocin Sodium.	
Albumin, human	Dextrose 5% in saline or in water, invert sugar solutions, lactated Ringer's injection, normal saline, Ringer's injection, sodium lactate (⅙ M) injection.	Protein hydrolysate (Amigen).
Alcohol, benzyl	Chloramphenicol (Chloromycetin) sodium succinate.	
Alcohol, ethyl	Dextrose, invert sugar, and sodium chloride injections, protein hydrolysate.	Lactated Ringer's injection, Plasmanate, Ringer's injection.
Alkaloidal salts		Alkalies, iodides.
Aminocaproic acid (Amicar)	Standard IV fluids except sodium lactate.	Protein hydrolysate, sodium lactate.
Aminophylline	Standard IV fluids.	Acid solutions (precipitation), anileridine (Leritine) HCl, ascorbic acid, codeine phosphate, dimenhydrinate (Dramamine), fructose solution (color change), hydroxyzine (Vistaril) HCl, invert sugar solution (color change), levorphanol (Levo-Dromoran) tartrate, meperidine (Demerol) HCl, methadone HCl, oxytetracycline (Terramycin) HCl, phenobarbital (Luminal) sodium, phenytoin (Dilantin) sodium, procaine (Novocain) HCl, prochlorperazine (Compazine) edisylate, promazine (Sparine) HCl, promethazine (Phenergan) HCl, protein hydrolysate (Amigen), vancomycin (Vancocin) HCl, vitamin B complex with ascorbic acid.

* Because the tables of compatibilities and incompatibilities published in the literature often disagree on certain information, this table serves only as an alerting device until the pharmacist retests the data under his own specific conditions, including brand of IV fluids and additives, concentrations, container materials, order and rate of mixing, pH, temperature, and other variables.

† The standard IV fluids are dextrose (various strengths) in saline (various strengths) or in water, invert sugar 10% in saline or water, lactated Ringer's injection, Ringer's injection, sodium chloride injection, and sodium lactate (⅙ M) injection.

Table 8-1 **Compatibilities and Incompatibilities of IV Additives** *(continued)*

Additives	Compatibilities	Incompatibilities
Ammonium chloride	Dextrose 2½% to 10% in water or isotonic saline or ½ strength saline, invert sugar 5% or 10% in water or saline, lactated Ringer's injection, Ringer's injection, sodium lactate (⅙ M) injection.	Anileridine (Leritine) HCl, codeine phosphate, levorphanol tartrate (Levo-Dromoran), methadone HCl, sulfisoxazole (Gantrisin) diethanolamine.
Amobarbital sodium (Amytal)		Anileridine (Leritine) HCl, cephalothin (Keflin) sodium, codeine phosphate, diphenhydramine (Benadryl) HCl, hydrocortisone sodium succinate (Solu-Cortef), hydroxyzine (Vistaril) HCl, insulin (aqueous), levarterenol (Levophed) tartrate, levorphanol (Levo-Dromoran) tartrate, meperidine (Demerol) HCl, methadone HCl, procaine (Novocain) HCl, streptomycin sulfate, tetracycline HCl, vancomycin (Vancocin) HCl.
Amphotericin-B (Fungizone)	Heparin sodium, hydrocortisone (Solu-Cortef) sodium succinate. Dilute with sterile water for injection without a preservative or 5% dextrose injection of pH above 4.2 (buffer if necessary). If protected from light, the drug is stable for 3 days at room temperature in the dextrose 5% and 6 weeks if kept refrigerated.[286]	Diphenhydramine (Benadryl) HCl, nitrofurantoin (Furadantin) sodium, normal saline, penicillin G (K or Na), preservatives (e.g., benzyl alcohol causes precipitation), saline solutions, tetracycline HCl. Protect amphotericin-B solutions from light and always administer alone.
Ampicillin sodium (Amcill-S, Omnipen-N, Penbritin-S, Polycillin-N, Totacillin-N)	Dextrose in saline or water, 10% invert sugar, sodium chloride injection, sodium chloride injection, sodium lactate (⅙ M) injection. The reconstituted drug in NaCl injection, loses about 10% potency after 7 days if kept refrigerated and about 9% in 24 hr. at room temperature.[286]	Protein hydrolysate. Do not use as an additive with other drugs. The higher the concentration of ampicillin the faster is its rate of degradation in solution.
Amytal	See Amobarbital.	
Angiotensin (Hypertensin)	Dextrose 5% in water, sodium chloride injection.	Protein hydrolysate.
Anileridine HCl (Leritine HCl)		Aminophylline, ammonium chloride, amobarbital (Amytal) sodium, chlorothiazide (Diuril) sodium, heparin, sodium, methicillin (Staphcillin) sodium, nitrofurantoin (Furadantin) sodium, novobiocin (Albamycin) sodium, pentobarbital (Nembutal) sodium, phenobarbital (Luminal) sodium, phenytoin (Dilantin) sodium, sodium bicarbonate, sodium iodide, sulfadiazine sodium, sulfisoxazole (Gantrisin) diolamine, thiopental (Pentothal) sodium.
Antihistamines		Radiopaque contrast media
Apresoline	See Hydralazine HCl.	
Aqua Mephyton	See Phytonadione.	

Table 8-1   Compatibilities and Incompatibilities of IV Additives *(continued)*

Additives	Compatibilities	Incompatibilities
Aramine	See Metaraminol Bitartrate.	
Ascorbic acid	Erythromycin (Ilotycin) glucoheptonate, menadiol sodium diphosphate (Synkayvite), potassium chloride (40 mEq./l.) and vitamin B complex—in dextrose 5% in saline or water, invert sugar solutions, normal saline, protein hydrolysate, lactated Ringer's injection, Ringer's injection, sodium lactate (⅙ M) injection.	Aminophylline, chloramphenicol (Chloromycetin) sodium succinate, chlordiazepoxide (Librium), conjugated estrogens (Premarin), dextran, phytonadione (Aqua Mephyton) penicillin G (K or Na), vitamin B₁₂.
Aureomycin	See Chlortetracycline.	
Bacitracin		Polyethylene glycols inactivate the antibiotic.
Barbiturates	See Pentobarbital and Phenobarbital.	Phytonadione (Aqua Mephyton)
Bejectal	See Vitamin B Complex with C.	
Bemegride (Megimide)	Do not add to infusion fluids. May inject through Y-tube of administration set.	
Benadryl	See Diphenhydramine HCl.	
Blood (whole)	See recommendation of the American Association of Blood Banks (page 213).	Dextrose solutions (clumping of cells causes transfusion reactions), levarterenol (Levophed) bitartrate, metaraminol (Aramine) bitartrate,‡ phytonadione (Aqua Mephyton).‡
Calcium chloride	Hydrocortisone sodium succinate (Solu-Cortef), methicillin (Dimocillin, Staphcillin) sodium, nitrofurantoin (Furadantin) sodium in normal saline, oxytetracycline (Terramycin) HCl, penicillin G (K) buffered, phenobarbital sodium, tetracycline HCl, vitamin B complex with C.	Cephalothin (Keflin) sodium, chlorpheniramine (Chlor-Trimeton) maleate, chlortetracycline (Aureomycin) HCl, nitrofurantoin (Furadantin) sodium in dextrose solutions, sodium bicarbonate, tetracycline HCl.
Calcium disodium edetate (calcium disodium edathamil, calcium disodium ethylenediaminetetraacetate, Calcium Disodium Versenate)	Normal saline.	Dextrose 5% in saline or water, invert sugar solutions, lactated Ringer's injection, protein hydrolysate (Amigen), Ringer's injection, sodium lactate (⅙ M) injection.
Calcium Disodium Versenate	See Calcium Disodium Edetate.	
Calcium glucoheptonate	Dextrose 2½% to 10% in water or sodium chloride injection or halfstrength saline, invert sugar 5% or 10% in saline or water, lactated Ringer's injection, Ringer's injection, sodium ascorbate, sodium chloride injection, sodium lactate (⅙ M) injection, vitamin K preparations.	Cephalothin (Keflin) sodium, tetracyclines.

‡ Dilute therapeutic dose with a large volume prior to infusion.

Table 8-1   Compatibilities and Incompatibilities of IV Additives *(continued)*

Additives	Compatibilities	Incompatibilities
Calcium gluconate	Chloramphenicol (Chloromycetin) sodium succinate, heparin sodium, hydrocortisone sodium succinate (Solu-Cortef), methicillin (Dimocillin, Staphcillin) sodium, oxytetracycline (Terramycin) HCl, Penicillin G (K) buffered, phenobarbital sodium, tetracycline HCl, vitamin B complex with C (Bejex) in standard IV fluids.	Cephalothin (Keflin) sodium, magnesium sulfate, novobiocin (Albamycin) sodium, prochlorperazine (Compazine) edisylate, sodium bicarbonate,§ streptomycin sulfate, tetracyclines.
Carbazochrome (Adrenosem) salicylate		Antihistamines (inactivate), oxytetracycline (Terramycin) HCl, tetracycline HCl.
Cedilanid-D	See Deslanoside.	
Cephalothin sodium (Keflin)	Betalin Complex FC, blood (whole), blood serum, casein hydrolysate, chloramphenicol (Chloromycetin) sodium succinate, Darrow's solution, dextran 6%, dextrose 5%, ethyl alcohol 5%, heparin sodium, hydrocortisone sodium succinate (Solu-Cortef), 10% invert sugar solution, lactated Ringer's injection,§ levarterenol (Levophed) bitartrate, lidocaine (Xylocaine) HCl, methicillin (Dimocillin, Staphcillin) sodium, nitrofurantoin (Furadantin) sodium, penicillin G (K) buffered, phenobarbital (Luminal) sodium, potassium chloride, prednisolone-21-phosphate (Hydeltrasol), procaine (Novocain) HCl, Reticulogen, Ringer's injection, sodium bicarbonate, sodium chloride injection, sodium lactate, vitamin B complex with C, vitamin K. Administer solutions within 24 hours after preparation. The pH should be between 4 and 7.	Alkaline earth metals, amobarbital (Amytal) sodium, calcium chloride,‖ calcium glucceptate, calcium gluconate, chlorpromazine (Thorazine) HCl, chlortetracycline (Aureomycin) HCl, colistimethate sodium (Coly-Mycin M) injection, diphenhydramine (Benadryl) HCl, erythromycin (Ilotycin) glucceptate (10 mg/ml or above) and lactobionate,‖ kanamycin (Kantrex) sulfate, oxytetracycline (Terramycin) HCl, polymyxin B sulfate (Aeroporin), penicillin G (K or Na salt), pentobarbital (Pentothal) sodium, phenytoin (Dilantin) sodium,‖ prochlorperazine (Compazine) edisylate, protein hydrolysate, tetracycline HCl, vitamin B complex with ascorbic acid (but see Betalin Complex FC under Compatibilities). In general, drugs of high molecular weight are incompatible.
Chloramphenicol sodium succinate (Chloromycetin)	Ascorbic acid, benzyl alcohol, calcium gluconate, cephalothin (Keflin) sodium, colistimethate (Coly-Mycin) sodium, hydrocortisone sodium succinate (Solu-Cortef), heparin sodium, kanamycin (Kantrex) sulfate, levarterenol (Levophed) bitartrate, methicillin (Dimocillin, Staphcillin) sodium, nitrofuran-	Acid (<pH 5.5) and alkaline (>pH 7.0) solutions, ascorbic acid (Parke, Davis brand), erythromycin (Ilotycin) glucoheptonate, erythromycin (Erythrocin) lactobionate,* hydrocortisone sodium succinate (Solu-Cortef), hydroxyzine (Vistaril) HCl, Lyo B-C Forte with vitamin B_{12}, novobiocin (Albamycin) sodium,

§ Dependent on the concentration of the additive, and the interfering ion (Ca, Mg, Sr, etc.)
‖ Precipitate forms after several hours.
* Dependent on the concentration of the additive.

Table 8–1   Compatibilities and Incompatibilities of IV Additives *(continued)*

Additives	Compatibilities	Incompatibilities
Chloramphenicol sodium succinate (Chloromycetin) (continued)	toin (Furadantin) sodium, potassium penicillin G, protein hydrolysate (Amigen), streptomycin sulfate, vitamin B complex with C, in standard IV fluid. Dissolve first in sterile water for injection.	oxytetracycline (Terramycin) HCl, phenytoin (Dilantin) sodium, promazine (Sparine) HCl, promethazine (Phenergan) HCl, polymyxin B (Aerosporin) sulfate, procaine (Novocain) HCl, prochlorperazine (Compazine) edisylate, sulfadiazine sodium, 25%, tetracycline HCl, tripelennamine (Pyribenzamine) HCl, vancomycin (Vancocin) HCl, vitamin B complex preparations.§
Chlordiazepoxide (Librium)		Ascorbic acid.
Chlorothiazide sodium (Diuril)	Dextrose 2½% to 10% in normal or half-strength saline or water, invert sugar 5% or 10% in saline or water, lactated Ringer's injection, Ringer's injection, sodium chloride injection, sodium lactate (⅙ M) injection.	Aminosol solutions, anileridine (Leritine) HCl, codeine phosphate, insulin (aqueous), Ionosol-B with 5% dextrose (precipitate forms after several hours), levarterenol (Levophed) bitartrate, levorphanol (Levo-Dromoran) tartrate, methadone HCl, morphine sulfate, procaine (Novocain) HCl, prochlorperazine (Compazine) edisylate, promazine (Sparine) HCl, promethazine (Phenergan) HCl, streptomycin sulfate, Surbex-T with dextrose 5% (cloudy or precipitate), tetracycline HCl, vancomycin (Vancocin) HCl.
Chlorpheniramine maleate (Chlor-Trimeton)		Calcium chloride, levarterenol (Levophed) bitartrate, pentobarbital (Nembutal) sodium.
Chlorpromazine HCl (Thorazine HCl)		Paraldehyde, penicillin G (K) buffered, pentobarbital (Nembutal) sodium, phenobarbital (Luminal) sodium, vitamin B complex with C.
Chlortetracycline HCl (Aureomycin)	Dextrose 5% in saline or water, invert sugar solutions, normal saline.	Alkaline solutions, ammonium chloride, amphotericin-B (Fungizone), calcium chloride, cephalothin (Keflin) sodium, chloramphenicol (Chloromycetin) sodium succinate, colistimethate (Coly-Mycin) sodium,‖ dextran, dextrose 5% in Ringer's injection, heparin sodium, hydrocortisone, Ionosol-B with dextrose 5%, lactated Ringer's injection, polymyxin B (Aerosporin) SO₄, potassium penicillin G in 5% dextrose in water, promazine (Sparine) HCl,# protein hydrolysate (Amigen, Aminosol), Ringer's injection, sodium lactate (⅙ M) injection, sodium methicillin (Dimocillin, Staphcillin).

§ Dependent on the concentration of the additive.
‖ Precipitate forms after several hours.
Incompatible in 5% dextrose injection.

Table 8-1 Compatibilities and Incompatibilities of IV Additives *(continued)*

Additives	Compatibilities	Incompatibilities
Chlor-Trimeton	See Chlorpheniramine Maleate above.	
Codeine phosphate		Aminophylline, ammonium chloride, amobarbital (Amytal) sodium, chlorothiazide (Diuril) sodium, heparin sodium, methicillin (Dimocillin, Staphcillin) sodium, nitrofurantoin (Furadantin) sodium, novobiocin (Albamycin) sodium, phenytoin (Dilantin) sodium, pentobarbital (Nembutal) sodium, phenobarbital (Luminal) sodium, sodium bicarbonate, sodium iodide, sulfadiazine sodium, sulfisoxazole (Gantrisin) diolamine, thiopental (Pentothal) sodium.
Colistimethate sodium (Coly-Mycin)	Chloramphenicol (Chloromycetin) sodium succinate, diphenhydramine (Benadryl), HCl, heparin sodium, kanamycin (Kantrex) sulfate, methicillin sodium, oxytetracycline (Terramycin) HCl, penicillin G K) buffered, phenobarbital (Luminal) sodium, polymyxin B (Aerosporin) sulfate, tetracycline HCl, vitamin B complex with C.	Chlortetracycline (Aueromycin) HCl, cephalothin (Keflin) sodium, erythromycin (Erythrocin) lactobionate, hydrocortisone sodium succinate (Solu-Cortef), kanamycin (Kantrex) sulfate.
Compazine	See Prochlorperazine Edisylate.	
Coramine	See Nikethamide.	
Corticotropin (ACTH) aqueous	Standard IV fluids.	Novobiocin (Albamycin) sodium, protein hydrolysate, sodium bicarbonate.
Cortisone acetate (Cortone Acetate)		Invert sugar solutions, lactated Ringer's injection, protein hydrolysate, Ringer's injection, sodium lactate (1/6 M) injection.
Coumadin	See Warfarin Sodium.	
Cyanocobalamin	Standard IV fluids.	Protein hydrolysate.
Cyclophosphamide (Cytoxan)	Cyclophosphamide in sodium chloride injection is stable for at least 4 weeks if kept refrigerated.[286]	
Decadron Phosphate	See Dexamethasone 21-Phosphate.	
Decholin Sodium	See Sodium Dehydrocholate.	
Demerol	See Meperidine HCl.	
Deslanoside (Cedilanid-D)	Dextrose 2½% to 10% in isotonic or half-strength saline or water, invert sugar 5% or 10% in saline or water, lactated Ringer's injection, Ringer's injection, sodium lactate (⅙ M) injection.	Protein hydrolysate. Do not mix with infusion fluids, but may inject through Y-tube of administration set.

Table 8-1   Compatibilities and Incompatibilities of IV Additives *(continued)*

Additives	Compatibilities	Incompatibilities
Desoxyn	See Methamphetamine HCl.	
Dexamethasone 21-phosphate (Decadron)		Prochlorperazine (Compazine), edisylate, vancomycin (Vancocin) HCl.
Dexpanthenol (Ilopan, pantothenyl alcohol)	Dextrose 5% in saline or water, invert sugar in saline or water, lactated Ringer's injection, Ringer's injection, sodium chloride injection.	Protein hydrolysate.
Dextran	Dextrose in saline or water solutions, invert sugar solutions, Ringer's injection, sodium chloride injection, sodium lactate ($\frac{1}{6}$ M) injection.	Ascorbic acid, chlortetracycline (Aureomycin) HCl, phytonadione (Aqua Mephyton, Konakion), protein hydrolysate.
Dextrose		Kanamycin (Kantrex) sulfate, novobiocin (Albamycin) sodium, warfarin sodium (Coumadin), vitamin B$_{12}$, whole blood.
Dihydromorphinone HCl	See Hydromorphone HCl.	
Dilantin	See Phenytoin Sodium.	
Dilaudid	See Hydromorphone HCl.	
Digitoxin	Do not add to infusion solutions. May inject through Y-tube of administration set.	Protein hydrolysate (Amigen).
Digoxin	Do not add to infusion solutions. May inject through Y-tube of administration set.	Protein hydrolysate (Amigen).
Dimenhydrinate (Dramamine)	Dextrose solutions, invert sugar solutions, lactated Ringer's injection, Ringer's injection, sodium chloride injection, sodium lactate ($\frac{1}{6}$ M) injection.	Alkaline solutions (cloudiness), aminophylline, ammonium chloride, amobarbital (Amytal) sodium, diphenhydramine (Benadryl) HCl, heparin sodium, hydrocortisone sodium succinate (Solu-Cortef), hydroxyzine (Vistaril) HCl, pentobarbital (Nembutal) sodium, phenobarbital (Luminal) sodium, phenytoin (Dilantin) sodium, prochlorperazine (Compazine) edisylate, promazine (Sparine) HCl, promethazine (Phenergan) HCl, protein hydrolysate, thiopental (Pentothal) sodium.
Dimocillin	See Methicillin Sodium.	
Diphenhydramine HCl (Benadryl)	Dextrose 2½% to 10% in water or saline or half-strength saline, invert sugar 5% or 10% in water or saline, lactated Ringer's injection, normal saline, Ringer's injection, sodium lactate ($\frac{1}{6}$ M) injection, methicillin sodium, penicillin G (K) buffered, polymyxin B sulfate (Aerosporin), tetracycline HCl, vitamin B complex with C.	Amobarbital (Amytal) sodium, amphotericin B (Fungizone), cephalothin (Keflin) sodium, pentobarbital (Nembutal) sodium, phenobarbital (Luminal) sodium, phenytoin (Dilantin) sodium, protein hydrolysate (Amigen), secobarbital (Seconal) sodium, thiopental (Pentothal) sodium.

Table 8-1   Compatibilities and Incompatibilities of IV Additives *(continued)*

Additives	Compatibilities	Incompatibilities
Disodium edetate (disodium edathamil, disodium ethylenediaminetetraacetate, disodium versenate)	Dextrose 5% in saline or water, lactated Ringer's injection, Ringer's injection, sodium chloride injection, sodium lactate (⅙ M) injection.	Protein hydrolysate (Amigen).
Disodium versenate	See Disodium Edetate.	
Diuril	See Chlorothiazide Sodium.	
Dolophine	See Methadone HCl.	
Dramamine	See Dimenhydrinate.	
EDTA	See Disodium Edetate.	
EDTA calcium	See Calcium Disodium Edetate.	
Ephedrine sulfate	Do not add to infusion solutions. May inject through Y-tube of administration set.	Alkaline solutions (precipitate free base), hydrocortisone sodium succinate (Solu-Cortef), pentobarbital (Nembutal) sodium), phenobarbital (Luminal) sodium, thiopental (Pentothal) sodium.
Epinephrine HCl (Adrenalin HCl)	Standard IV fluids.	Alkaline solutions (precipitate free base), chlorpromazine (Thorazine) HCl, cyclopropane, dextrose 5% in water, hyaluronidase, mephentermine (Wyamine) sulfate, novobiocin (Albamycin) sodium, potassic saline injection (Darrow's solution), procaine (Novocain) HCl (color change), protein hydrolysate (Amigen), sodium chloride injection (color change), warfarin (Coumadin) sodium. #
Ergonovine maleate	Standard IV fluids. Do not add to infusion solutions. May inject through Y-tube of administration set.	Protein hydrolysate (Amigen).
Ergotrate	See Ergonovine Maleate.	
Erythrocin lactobionate	See Erythromycin Lactobionate.	
Erythromycin gluceptate (Ilotycin Gluceptate, Ilotycin Glucoheptonate)	Dextrose solutions in saline or water, invert sugar solutions, lactated Ringer's injection, Ringer's injection, sodium chloride injection, sodium lactate (⅙ M) injection. Most stable at pH 6 to 8. Inactivated rapidly at pH 4 and below.	Bacteriostatic water for injection (preservatives), chloramphenicol (Chloromycetin) sodium succinate, heparin sodium, kanamycin sulfate (Kantrex) with 10 mg./ml. or more of the erythromycin, novobiocin (Albamycin) sodium, pentobarbital (Nembutal) sodium, phenobarbital (Luminal) sodium, phenytoin (Dilantin) sodium, prochlorperazine (Compazine) edisylate, protein hydrolysate (Amigen), streptomycin sulfate, tetracycline HCl.
Erythromycin lactobionate (Erythrocin Lactobionate)	Aminophylline, diphenhydramine (Benadryl) HCl, hydrocortisone sodium succinate (Solu-Cortef),	Ascorbic acid, cephalothin (Keflin) sodium (ppt in several hours), chloramphenicol (Chlo-

Incompatible in 5% dextrose injection.

Table 8-1   Compatibilities and Incompatibilities of IV Additives *(continued)*

Additives	Compatibilities	Incompatibilities
Erythromycin lactobionate (Erythrocin Lactobionate) (continued)	methamphetamine (Desoxyn) HCl, methicillin (Dimocillin, Staphcillin) sodium, Modumate, nitrofurantoin (Furadantin) sodium, penicillin G (K), pentobarbital (Nembutal) sodium, polymyxin B sulfate (Aerosporin), potassium chloride, prednisolone sodium phosphate (Hydeltrasol), prochlorperazine (Compazine) edisylate, promazine (Sparine) HCl, sodium bicarbonate, sodium iodide, sulfisoxazole (Gantrisin) diethanolamine. A 5% stock solution in sterile water for injection (stable for 2 weeks when refrigerated) may be diluted with dextrose or sodium chloride injections, or invert sugar in water, or other commercially available IV fluids.[293] Extremely dependent on pH. Most stable at pH 6 to 8. Inactivated rapidly at pH 4 and below.	romycetin) sodium succinate, colistimethate sodium (Coly-Mycin; hazy), heparin sodium (hazy); metaraminol (Aramine) bitartrate, protein hydrolysate (Amigen), sodium chloride solutions (special order of mixing required), sodium salts of macromolecules of biological origin (e.g., antibiotics), tetracycline HCl, vitamin B complex with C.
Estrogens, conjugated (Premarin)	Dextrose in saline or water, invert sugar in saline or water, sodium chloride injection.	Ascorbic acid, lactated Ringer's injection, protein hydrolysate, Ringer's injection, sodium lactate (⅙ M) injection.
Ethamivan (Emivan)	Dextrose in saline or water, sodium chloride in injection.	Invert sugar in saline or water, lactated Ringer's injection, protein hydrolysate, Ringer's injection, sodium lactate (1/6 M) injection.
Fibrinolysin (human) (Cutter)		Dextrose 10% solutions, metaraminol (Aramine) bitartrate, promazine (Sparine) HCl, protein hydrolysate (Amigen).
Fibrinolysin (human) (Merck)		Oxytocin (Pitocin), promazine (Sparine) HCl, thiopental (Pentothal) sodium.
Folbesyn	See Vitamin B Complex with Ascorbic Acid.	
Fungizone	See Amphotericin B.	
Furadantin	See Nitrofurantoin Sodium.	
Heparin sodium (Liquaemin, Panheprin, etc.)	Dextrose in saline or water solutions, invert sugar solutions, lactated Ringer's solution, Ringer's solution, sodium chloride injection, sodium lactate (⅙ M) injection. Compatible for 24 hours with amphotericin B (Fungizone), Bejectal with C, calcium gluconate, cephalothin (Keflin) sodium, chloromycetin, (Chloramphenicol) sodium succinate, chlorotetracycline (Aureomycin) HCl, colistimethate (Coly-Mycin) sodium, dimenhy-	Anileridine (Leritine) HCl, codeine phosphate, dimenhydrinate (Dramamine), erythromycin (Ilotycin) gluceptate and (Erythrocin) lactobionate, hyaluronidase, hydrocortisone sodium succinate (Solu-Cortef), hydroxyzine (Vistaril) HCl, kanamycin (Kantrex) sulfate, levorphanol (Levo-Dromoran) tartrate, meperidine (Demerol) HCl, methadone HCl, novobiocin (Albamycin) sodium, penicillin G (K), polymyxin B sulfate

Table 8-1 Compatibilities and Incompatibilities of IV Additives *(continued)*

Additives	Compatibilities	Incompatibilities
Heparin sodium (Liquaemin, Panheprin, etc.) (continued)	drinate (Dramamine), lincomycin (Lincocin), methicillin (Dimocillin, Staphcillin) sodium, nafcillin (Unipen) sodium, nitrofurantoin (Furadantin) sodium, oxytetracycline (Terramycin) HCl, potassium chloride, promazine (Sparine) HCl, sulfisoxazole (Gantrisin) diethanolamine, tetracycline (Achromycin) HCl.	(Aerosporin), prochlorperazine (Compazine) edisylate, promethazine (Phenergan) HCl, protein hydrolysate, streptomycin sulfate, tetracycline HCl, vancomycin (Vancocin) HCl.
Histamine diphosphate	Dextrose in water solution, invert sugar solutions, lactated Ringer's injection, Ringer's injection.	Sodium chloride injection, protein hydrolysate.
Hyaluronidase (Alidase)	Standard IV fluids.	Epinephrine (Adrenalin) HCl, heparin sodium, protein hydrolysate.
Hydeltrasol	See Prednisolone Sodium Phosphate.	
Hydralazine HCl (Apresoline)	Dextrose 2½% to 10% in water or normal saline or half-strength saline, invert sugar 5% or 10% in water or saline, lactated Ringer's injection, Ringer's injection, sodium chloride injection, sodium lactate (⅙ M) injection.	Protein hydrolysate (Amigen). Color change occurs when hydralazine is added to dextrose 10% in lactated Ringer's injection, or 10% fructose in saline or water.
Hydrocortisone sodium succinate (Solu-Cortef)	Dextrose 2½% to 10% in water or normal saline or half-strength saline, invert sugar 5% or 10% in water or saline, lactated Ringer's injection, Ringer's injection, sodium chloride injection, sodium lactate (⅙ M) injection, amphotericin B (Fungizone), calcium chloride, cephalothin (Keflin) sodium, erythromycin (Erythrocin) lactobionate, heparin sodium, penicillin G (K) buffered, polymyxin B (Aerosporin) sulfate.	Amobarbital (Amytal) sodium, chloramphenicol (Chloromycetin) sodium succinate, colistimethate (Coly-Mycin) sodium, dimenhydrinate (Dramamine), ephedrine sulfate, heparin sodium, kanamycin (Kantrex) sulfate, metaraminol (Aramine) bitartrate, methicillin (Staphcillin) sodium, novobiocin (Albamycin) sodium, oxytetracycline (Terramycin) HCl, pentobarbital (Nembutal) sodium, phenobarbital (Luminal) sodium, prochlorperazine (Compazine) edisylate, promazine (Sparine) HCl, promethazine (Phenergan) HCl, protein hydrolysate, Surbex-T with dextrose 5% (ppt in several hours), tetracycline HCl, vancomycin (Vancocin) HCl, vitamin B complex with ascorbic acid.§ The succinate precipitates if Solu-Cortef is not diluted first before adding to dextrose 5% in normal saline with another drug of acid pH such as Aramine.
Hydromorphone HCl (Dilaudid, dihydromorphinone HCl)		Sodium bicarbonate, thiopental (Pentothal) sodium.

§ Dependent on the concentration of the additive.

Table 8-1 Compatibilities and Incompatibilities of IV Additives *(continued)*

Additives	Compatibilities	Incompatibilities
Hydroxystilbamidine isethionate		Heparin sodium
Hydroxyzine HCl (Vistaril)		Aminophylline, amobarbital (Amytal) sodium, chloromycetin (Chloramphenicol) sodium succinate, dimenhydrinate (Dramamine), heparin sodium, penicillin G (K or Na), pentobarbital (Nembutal) sodium, phenobarbital (Luminal) sodium, phenytoin (Dilantin) sodium, sulfisoxazole (Gantrisin) diolamine, vitamin B complex with ascorbic acid.
Hykinone	See Menadione Sodium Bisulfite.	
Ilopan	See Dexpanthenol.	
Ilotycin	See Erythromycin Gluceptate.	
Insulin (aqueous)	Standard IV fluids.	Amobarbital (Amytal) sodium, chlorothiazide (Diuril) sodium, nitrofurantoin (Furadantin) sodium, novobiocin (Albamycin) sodium, pentobarbital (Nembutal) sodium, phenobarbital (Luminal) sodium, phenytoin (Dilantin) sodium, sodium bicarbonate, sulfadiazine sodium, sulfisoxazole (Gantrisin) diolamine, thiopental (Pentothal) sodium.
Iodides		Alkaloidal salts, anileridine (Leritine) HCl, metals, mineral acids.
Isoproterenol (Isuprel)	Standard IV fluids.	Protein hydrolysate.
Kanamycin sulfate (Kantrex)	Dextrose 5% in water, sodium chloride injection. Chloramphenicol (Chloromycetin) sodium succinate, colistimethate (Coly-Mycin) sodium, penicillin G (K) buffered, polymyxin B (Aerosporin) sulfate, sodium bicarbonate, tetracycline HCl, vitamin B complex with C (Bejex). To avoid incompatibilities administer kanamycin separately from other antimicrobial agents.	Cephalothin (Keflin) sodium, colistimethate sodium (Coly-Mycin), dextrose, heparin sodium, hydrocortisone sodium succinate (Solu-Cortef), methicillin (Dimocillin, Staphcillin) sodium, nitrofurantoin (Furadantin) sodium, pentobarbital (Nembutal) sodium, phenobarbital (Luminal) sodium, phenytoin (Dilantin) sodium, prochlorperazine (Compazine) edisylate, protein hydrolysate, sulfisoxazole (Gantrisin) diolamine. Do not mix kanamycin physically with other antibiotics.
Kappadione	See Menadiol Sodium Diphosphate.	
Keflin	See Cephalothin Sodium.	
KMC	See Polyionic Solutions.	
Konakion	See Phytonadione.	
Lactated Ringer's injection		Amphotericin B (Fungizone), calcium disodium edetate (Versenate), chlortetracycline (Aureomycin) HCl, cortisone (Cortone) acetate, ethamivan (Emivan),

Table 8-1 **Compatibilities and Incompatibilities of IV Additives** *(continued)*

Additives	Compatibilities	Incompatibilities
Lactated Ringer's injection (continued)		ethyl alcohol, histamine diphosphate metaraminol (Aramine) bitartrate, oxytetracycline (Terramycin) HCl, sodium bicarbonate, thiopental (Pentothal) sodium.
Leritine HCl	See Anileridine HCl.	
Levallorphan (Lorfan) tartrate		Methicillin (Dimocillin, Staphcillin) sodium, phenytoin (Dilantin) sodium, sulfisoxazole (Gantrisin) diethanolamine.
Levarterenol bitartrate (Levophed)	Dextrose 5% (protects against oxidation) in saline or water, invert sugar solutions, lactated Ringer's injection, Ringer's injection, sodium lactate (⅙ M) injection. Do not administer in sodium chloride injection.	Amobarbital (Amytal) sodium, chlorothiazide (Diuril) sodium, chlorpheniramine (Chlor-Trimeton) maleate, nitrofurantoin (Furadantin) sodium, novobiocin (Albamycin) sodium, pentobarbital (Nembutal) sodium, phenobarbital (Luminal) sodium, phenytoin (Dilantin) sodium, protein hydrolysate, sodium bicarbonate, sodium iodide, streptomycin sulfate, sulfadiazine sodium, sulfisoxazole (Gantrisin) diolamine, thiopental (Pentothal) sodium. Do not administer in normal saline.
Levophed	See Levarterenol Bitartrate.	
Levorphanol tartrate (Levo-Dromoran)		Aminophylline, ammonium chloride, amorbarbital (Amytal) sodium, chlorothiazide (Diuril) sodium, heparin sodium, methicillin (Staphcillin) sodium, nitrofurantoin (Furadantin) sodium, novobiocin (Albamycin) sodium, phenytoin (Dilantin) sodium, pentobarbital (Nembutal) sodium, phenobarbital (Luminal) sodium, sodium bicarbonate, sodium iodide, sulfadiazine sodium, sulfisoxazole (Gantrisin) diolamine, thiopental (Pentothal) sodium.
Librium	See Chlordiazepoxide.	
Lincocin	See Lincomycin HCl.	
Lincomycin HCl (Lincocin)	Dextrose 5% in water, sodium chloride injection. Penicillin G may be compatible under certain conditions.	(Dilantin) sodium, protein hydrolysate.
Lytren	See Polyionic Solutions.	
Magnesium sulfate	Dextrose in saline or water solutions, invert sugar solutions, lactated Ringer's solution, Ringer's solution, sodium chloride injection, sodium lactate (⅙ M) injection.	Calcium gluconate-glucoheptonate, novobiocin (Albamycin) sodium, procaine (Novocain) HCl, sodium bicarbonate, protein hydrolysate.

Table 8-1   Compatibilities and Incompatibilities of IV Additives *(continued)*

Additives	Compatibilities	Incompatibilities
Mannitol	Sodium chloride injection.	Erythrocytes (agglutination and irreversible crenation if mannitol and blood are mixed in a drip set or if the drug is infused too rapidly into a vein). Never mix hypertonic solutions of mannitol in an administration set. Administer intravenous mannitol solutions at a carefully controlled slow rate.
Megimide	See Bemegride.	
Menadion sodium bisulfite (Hykinone)	Do not add to infusion solutions. May inject through Y-tube of administration set.	Phenytoin (Dilantin) sodium, promazine (Sparine) HCl.
Menadiol (Menadione) sodium diphosphate (Kappadione, Synkayvite)	Dextrose in saline or water solutions, invert sugar solutions, lactated Ringer's injection, Ringer's injection, sodium chloride injection, sodium lactate (⅙ M) injection.	Alkaloids, anileridine (Leritine) HCl, codeine phosphate, levarterenol (Levophed) bitartarte, levorphanol (Levo-Dromoran) tartrate, meperidine (Demerol) HCl, metals, methadone HCl, mineral acids, procaine (Novocain) HCl.
Meperidine HCl (Demerol)	Do not dissolve in infusion fluids. May inject through Y-tube of administration set. Inject very slowly. This method is not recommended.	Aminophylline, amobarbital (Amytal) sodium, heparin sodium, methicillin (Staphcillin) sodium, morphine sulfate, nitrofurantoin (Furadantin), pentobarbital (Nembutal) sodium, phenobarbital (Luminal) sodium, phenytoin (Dilantin) sodium, protein hydrolysate, sodium bicarbonate, sodium iodide, sulfadiazine sodium, sulfisoxazole (Gantrisin) diolamine, thiopental (Pentothal) sodium.
Mephentermine (Wyamine)	Dextrose in water or saline, sodium chloride injection.	Protein hydrolysate.
Mercaptopurine sodium (6-purinethiol, Purinethol)	Mercaptopurine sodium in sodium chloride or dextrose 5% injection is stable for at least 7 days if kept refrigerated. [286]	
Metaraminol bitartrate (Aramine Bitartrate)	Dilute with a large volume of isotonic saline injection or dextrose in saline or water before infusion.	Hydrocortisone sodium succinate (Solu-Cortef), invert sugar, lactated Ringer's injection, methicillin (Dimocillin, Staphcillin) sodium, penicillin G (K or Na), phenytoin (Dilantin) sodium, protein hydrolysate (Amigen), Ringer's injection, sodium lactate injection, sodium methicillin (Staphcillin), thiopental (Pentothal) sodium,# warfarin (Coumadin sodium.#
Methadone HCl (Dolophine)		Aminophylline, ammonium chloride, amobarbital (Amytal) sodium, chlorothiazide (Diuril) sodium, heparin sodium, meth-

Incompatible in 5% dextrose injection.

Table 8–1   Compatibilities and Incompatibilities of IV Additives *(continued)*

Additives	Compatibilities	Incompatibilities
Methadone HCl (Dolophine) (continued)		icillin (Staphcillin) sodium, nitrofurantoin (Furadantin) sodium, novobiocin (Albamycin) sodium, pentobarbital (Nembutal) sodium, phenobarbital (Luminal) sodium, phenytoin (Dilantin) sodium, sodium bicarbonate, sodium iodide, sulfadiazine sodium, sulfisoxazole (Gantrisin) diolamine, thiopental (Pentothal) sodium.
Methamphetamine HCl (Desoxyn)	Inject directly into a vein or into the tubing of an IV solution.	Do not use in any intravenous infusion.
Methicillin sodium (Dimocillin, Staphcillin)	Calcium chloride, calcium gluconate, cephalothin (Keflin) sodium, chloramphenicol (chloromycetin) sodium succinate, colistimethate (Coly-Mycin) sodium, diphenhydramine (Benadryl) HCl, erythromycin (Erythrocin) lactobionate, heparin sodium, penicillin G (K) buffered, polymyxin B sulfate (Aerosporin), prednisolone sodium phosphate (Hydeltrasol), sodium bicarbonate, vitamin B complex with C. Suitably buffered methicillin sodium in sodium chloride injection or dextrose 5% injection is stable for at least 7 days if kept refrigerated. [286]	Anileridine (Leritine) HCl, codeine phosphate, hydrocortisone sodium succinate (Solu-Cortef), kanamycin (Kantrex) sulfate, levallorphan (Lorfan) tartrate, levorphanol (Levo-Dromoran) tartrate, meperidine (Demerol) HCl, metaraminol (Aramine) bitartrate, methadone HCl, oxytetracycline (Terramycin) HCl, prochlorperazine (Compazine) edisylate, promethazine (Phenergan) HCl, protein hydrolysate, sodium bicarbonate, tetracycline HCl, vancomycin (Vancocin) HCl. Methicillin is extremely unstable in acid media.
Methylphenidate HCl (Ritalin)	Dextrose saline or water solutions, invert sugar solutions, lactated Ringer's injection, Ringer's injection, sodium chloride injection, sodium lactate (⅙ M) injection.	Alkaline solutions (strong), barbiturates, phenytoin (Dilantin) sodium.
Metrazol	See Pentylenetetrazol.	
Modumate solution	Dextrose 5% in saline or water, invert sugar solutions, lactated Ringer's injection, Ringer's injection, sodium chloride injection, sodium lactate (⅙ M) injection.	Dextrose 20% solutions, thiopental (Pentothal) sodium.
Morphine sulfate	Do not add to infusion fluids. May inject through Y-tube of administration set.	Aminophylline, amobarbital (Amytal) sodium, chlorothiazide (Diuril) sodium, heparin sodium, meperidine (Demerol) HCl, methicillin (Staphcillin) sodium, nitrofurantoin (Furadantin) sodium, novobiocin (Albamycin) sodium, phenobarbital (Luminal) sodium, phenytoin (Dilantin) sodium, sodium bicarbonate, sodium iodide, sulfadiazine sodium, sulfisoxazole (Gantrisin) diolamine, thiopental (Pentothal) sodium.

Table 8-1   Compatibilities and Incompatibilities of IV Additives *(continued)*

Additives	Compatibilities	Incompatibilities
Nafcillin sodium (Unipen)	Standard IV fluids. Add sodium bicarbonate injection to prevent precipitation.	Surbex-T in 5% aqueous dextrose solution (addition of sodium bicarbonate prevents precipitation, after several hours, of the penicillin but solution still hazy).
Neo-Synephrine HCl	See Phenylephrine HCl.	
Nikethamide (Coramine)	Dextrose in saline or water, invert sugar solutions, lactated Ringer's injection, Ringer's injection, sodium chloride injection, sodium lactate (⅙ M) injection.	Protein hydrolysate.
Nitrofurantoin sodium (Furadantin)	Dextrose solutions, invert sugar solutions, lactated Ringer's injection,** Ringer's injection, saline solutions containing ascorbic acid and vitamin B complex, or calcium chloride or tetracycline HCl,# sodium chloride injection, sodium lactate (⅙ M) injection. Cephalothin (Keflin) sodium, chloramphenicol (Chloromycetin) sodium succinate, penicillin G (K) buffered, prochlorperazine (Compazine) edisylate. Do not dilute with injections containing phenol or paraben preservatives.	Aminosol solutions, ammonium chloride, amphotericin B (Fungizone), anileridine (Leritine) HCl, codeine phosphate, dextrose in lactated Ringer's solution, dextrose solutions containing ascorbic acid and vitamin B complex, calcium chloride or tetracycline HCl, codeine phosphate, Inpersol solutions, insulin (aqueous), Ionosol B with dextrose 5%, kanamycin (Kantrex) sulfate, levarterenol (Levophed) bitartrate, levorphanol (Levo-Dromoran) tartrate, meperidine (Demerol) HCl, methadone HCl, polymyxin B sulfate (Fungizone), prochlorperazine (Compazine) edisylate, preservatives (parabens and phenols), procaine (Novocain) HCl, protein hydrolysate, streptomycin sulfate, Surbex-T with dextrose 5%, tetracaine (Pontocaine), tetracycline HCl in dextrose solution), vancomycin (Vancocin), vitamin B complex with C (in dextrose solutions). Protect infusion bottles containing nitrofurantoin from sunlight and ultraviolet light.
Novobiocin sodium (Albamycin)	Administer in sodium chloride injection. Solutions must be kept above pH 6. Do not use dextrose solutions.	ACTH (aqueous), ammonium chloride, anileridine (Leritine) HCl, calcium gluconate-glucoheptonate, chloramphenicol (Chloromycetin) sodium succinate, codeine phosphate, dextran in saline, dextrose 5% injection, epinephrine (Adrenalin) HCl, erythromycin (Ilotycin) glucoheptonate, fructose, heparin sodium, hydrocortisone sodium succinate (Solu-Cortef), insulin (aqueous), invert sugar, lactated Ringer's injection, levarte-

** Some tables list lactated Ringer's injection as incompatible. Concentration and other factors may govern this.[284]
# Incompatible in 5% dextrose injection.

Table 8–1 Compatibilities and Incompatibilities of IV Additives *(continued)*

Additives	Compatibilities	Incompatibilities
Novobiocin sodium (Albamycin) (continued)		renol (Levophed) bitartrate, levorphanol (Levo-Dromoran) tartrate, magnesium sulfate, methadone HCl, procaine (Novocain) HCl, protein hydrolysate, sodium lactate, streptomycin sulfate, tetracycline HCl, vancomycin (Vancocin) HCl, vitamin B complex with ascorbic acid.
Novocain HCl	See Procaine HCl.	
Ouabain	Do not add to infusion solutions. May inject through Y-tube of administration set.	
Oxacillin sodium (Prostaphlin)	Dextrose in saline or water, invert sugar in saline or water, sodium chloride injection.	Protein hydrolysate.
Oxytetracycline HCl (Terramycin)	Ringer's injection and other standard IV fluids. Calcium chloride and calcium gluconate (said to be compatible, but some authorities state that calcium should be avoided), colistimethate (Coly-Mycin) sodium, polymyxin B sulfate (Aerosporin). Hazy solution produced with dextrose in lactated Ringer's injection.	Aminophylline, amphotericin B (Fungizone), cephalothin (Keflin) sodium, chloramphenicol (Chloromycetin) sodum succinate, heparin sodium, hydrocortisone sodium succinate (Solu-Cortef), lactated Ringer's injection, methicillin (Staphcillin) sodium, penicillin G (K or Na), pentobarbital (Nembutal) sodium, phenobarbital (Luminal) sodium, phenytoin (Dilantin) sodium, polymyxin B (Aerosporin), prochlorperazine (Compazine) edisylate, protein hydrolysate, sodium bicarbonate, sodium lactate, sulfisoxazole (Gantrisin) diolamine.
Oxytocin (Pitocin)	Dextrose in saline or water solutions, invert sugar solutions, lactated Ringer's injection, Ringer's injection, sodium chloride injection, sodium lactate (⅙ M) injection.	Protein hydrolysate, sodium warfarin (Coumadin).
Panmycin	See Tetracycline HCl.	
Papaverine HCl	Dextrose in saline or water solutions, invert sugar solutions, lactated Ringer's injection, Ringer's injection, sodium chloride injection, sodium lactate (⅙ M) injection.	Protein hydrolysate.
Paraldehyde		Chlorpromazine (Thorazine) HCl.
Penicillin G (K or Na salt) buffered	Reconstitute with water for injection prior to addition to IV fluids. Dextrose in saline or water solutions, invert sugar solutions, lactated Ringer's injection, Ringer's injection, sodium chloride injection, sodium lactate (⅙ M) injection. Compatible in dextrose solutions with calcium chloride, cephalothin (Keflin) sodium, chloramphenicol	Acid media, amphotericin B (Fungizone), ascorbic acid, chlorpromazine (Thorazine) HCl, chlortetracycline (Aureomycin) HCl, heparin sodium, hydroxyzine (Vistaril) HCl, metaraminol (Aramine) bitartrate, oxytetracycline (Terramycin) HCl, phenytoin (Dilantin) sodium, prochlorperazine (Compazine) edisylate, promazine (Sparine)

Table 8-1   Compatibilities and Incompatibilities of IV Additives *(continued)*

Additives	Compatibilities	Incompatibilities
Penicillin G (K or Na salt) buffered (continued)	(Chloromycetin) sodium succinate, colistimethate (Coly-Mycin) sodium, diphenhydramine (Benadryl) HCl, kanamycin (Kantrex) sulfate, lincomycin (Lincocin), methicillin (Dimocillin, Staphcillin) sodium, nitrofurantoin (Furadantin) sodium, phenobarbital (Luminal) sodium, polymyxin B (Aerosporin) sulfate, vitamin B complex with C. Compatible in dextrose, dextrose-saline, or saline with hydrocortisone sodium succinate (Solu-Cortef) and sulfisoxazole (Gantrisin) diethanolamine. Compatible with chloramphenicol (Chloromycetin) sodium succinate, ephedrine sulfate, erythromycin (Erythrocin) lactobionate, heparin sodium, potassium chloride, promethazine (Phenergan) HCl, sodium bicarbonate, and sodium iodide in standard IV fluids.	HCl,# promethazine (Phenergan) HCl, protein hydrolysate, tetracycline HCl, thiopental (Pentothal) sodium,# vancomycin (Vancocin) HCl.
Pentobarbital sodium (Nembutal)	Do not add to infusion solutions. May inject through Y-tube of administration set. Ephedrine sulfate, hydrocortisone sodium succinate (Solu-Cortef), sodium bicarbonate.	Anileridine (Leritine) HCl, cephalothin (Keflin) sodium, chlorpheniramine (Chlor-Trimeton) maleate, chlorpromazine (Thorazine) HCl, codeine phosphate, diphenhydramine (Benadryl) HCl, ephedrine sulfate, erythromycin (Ilotycin) glucoheptonate, hydrocortisone sodium succinate (Solu-Cortef), hydroxyzine (Vistaril) HCl, insulin (aqueous), levarterenol (Levophed) bitartrate, levorphanol (Levo-Dromoran) tartrate, meperidine (Demerol) HCl, methadone HCl, oxytetracycline (Terramycin) HCl, phenytoin (Dilantin) sodium, prochlorperazine (Compazine) edisylate, promazine (Sparine) HCl,# promethazine (Phenergan) HCl, protein hydrolysate, sodium bicarbonate, streptomycin sulfate, succinylcholine chloride, tetracycline HCl, vancomycin (Vancocin) HCl.
Pentothal sodium	See Thiopental Sodium.	
Pentylenetetrazol (Metrazol)	Do not add to infusion fluids. May inject through Y-tube of administration set.	
Phenergan	See Promethazine HCl.	

Incompatible in 5% dextrose injection.

Table 8-1 Compatibilities and Incompatibilities of IV Additives *(continued)*

Additives	Compatibilities	Incompatibilities
Phenobarbital sodium (Luminal)	Dextrose solutions, invert sugar solutions, lactated Ringer's injection, Ringer's injection, sodium chloride injection, sodium lactate (⅙ M) injection. Calcium chloride, calcium gluconate, colistimethate (Coly-Mycin) sodium, penicillin G (K) buffered, polymyxin B sulfate (Aerosporin).	Alcohol 5% with dextrose 5% (color change), anileridine (Lerittine) HCl, cephalothin (Keflin) sodium, chlorpromazine (Thorazine) HCl, codeine phosphate, dimenhydrinate (Dramamine), diphenhydramine (Benadryl) HCl, ephedrine sulfate, erythromycin (Ilotycin) glucoheptonate, hydrocortisone sodium succinate (Solu-Cortef), hydroxyzine (Vistaril) HCl, insulin (aqueous), kanamycin (Kantrex) sulfate, levarterenol (Levophed) bitartrate, levorphanol (Levo-Dromoran) tartrate, meperidine (Demerol) HCl, methadone HCl, methylphenidate (Ritalin) HCl, oxytetracycline (Terramycin) HCl, phenytoin (Dilantin) sodium, procaine (Novocain) HCl, prochlorperazine (Compazine) edisylate, promazine (Sparine) HCl, promethazine (Phenergan) HCl, streptomycin sulfate, tetracycline HCl, tripelennamine (Pyribenzamine) HCl, vancomycin (Vancocin) HCl.
Phenylephrine HCl (Neo-Synephrine HCl)		Phenytoin (Dilantin) sodium.
Phenytoin sodium (Dilantin)	Dilute only with the diluent supplied, buffered to pH 12. Do not dilute further in an infusion solution.	Aminophylline, anileridine (Leritine) HCl, chloramphenicol (Chloromycetin) sodium succinate, codeine phosphate, diphenhydramine (Benadryl) HCl, erythromycin (Ilotycin) glucoheptonate, hydroxyzine (Vistaril) HCl, insulin (aqueous), kanamycin (Kantrex) sulfate, levarterenol (Levophed) bitartrate, levorphanol (Levo-Dromoran) tartrate, meperidine (Demerol) HCl, metaraminol (Aramine) bitartrate, methadone HCl, oxytetracycline (Terramycin) HCl, penicillin G (K or Na), pentobarbital (Nembutal) sodium, phenobarbital (Luminal) sodium, phytonadione (Aqua Mephyton, Konakion), procaine (Novocain) HCl, prochlorperazine (Compazine) edisylate, streptomycin sulfate, sulfisoxazole (Gantrisin) diolamine, tetracycline HCl, vancomycin (Vancocin) HCl, vitamin B complex with ascorbic acid.

Table 8-1   Compatibilities and Incompatibilities of IV Additives *(continued)*

Additives	Compatibilities	Incompatibilities
Phytonadione (Aqua-Mephyton, Konakion, vitamin K)		Ascorbic acid, barbiturates (depends on pH), barbituric acid, dextran, phenytoin (Dilantin) sodium, vitamin B_{12}.
Pitocin	See Oxytocin.	
Plasmanate (Human plasma proteins)		Ethyl alcohol, protein hydrolysate.
Polycycline	See Tetracycline HCl.	
Polyionic solutions (KMC, Lytren, Polysal, etc.)	Compatibility often governed by pH (Range for polyionic solutions 4.4 to 6.1).	Sulfadiazine sodium (pH 9.25 at room temperature), sulfisoxazole (Gantrisin) diolamine (pH 7.70 at room temperature). Polyionic solutions at pH 4.5 slowly produce precipitate of Gantrisin 1:250 to 1:500 solution at room temperature; pH 6 to 7 at 20°C or lower also incompatible.
Polymyxin B sulfate (Aerosporin)	Dextrose 5% in water. Colistimethate (Coly-Mycin) sodium, diphenhydramine (Benadryl) HCl, erythromycin (Erythrocin) lactobionate, hydrocortisone sodium succinate (Solu-Cortef), kanamycin (Kantrex) sulfate, methicillin (Staphcillin, Dimocillin) sodium, oxytetracycline (Terramycin) HCl, penicillin G (K) buffered, phenobarbital (Luminal) sodium. Vitamin B complex with C.	Cephalothin (Keflin) sodium, chloramphenicol (Chloromycetin) sodium succinate, heparin sodium, nitrofurantoin (Furadantin) sodium, chlortetracycline (Aureomycin) HCl, prednisolone sodium phosphate (Hydeltrasol), protein hydrolysate, tetracycline HCl.
Polysal	See Polyionic Solutions.	
Potassium chloride	Dextrose in saline or water solutions, lactated Ringer's injection, Ringer's injection, sodium chloride injection, sodium lactate (⅙ M) injection.	Protein hydrolysate.
Prednisolone sodium phosphate (Hydeltrasol, Prednisolone-21-phosphate sodium); Prednisolone sodium succinate (Meticortelone)	Prednisolone sodium succinate in sodium chloride or 5% dextrose injection is stable for at least 12 days if kept refrigerated.[286] Cephalothin (Keflin) sodium, erythromycin (Erythrocin) lactobionate, heparin sodium, methicillin (Dimocillin, Staphcillin) sodium, penicillin G (K) buffered, tetracycline HCl, vitamin B complex with C.	Calcium gluconate-glucoheptonate, polymyxin B sulfate (Aerosporin), prochlorperazine (Compazine) edisylate.
Premarin	See Estrogens, Conjugated.	
Preservatives (Parabens or Phenols)		Do not use bacteriostatic water for injections, containing parabens or phenols, to dilute nitrofurantoin (Furadantin) sodium or amphotericin-B (Fungizone).
Procainamide (Pronestyl)		Phenytoin (Dilantin) sodium.

Table 8-1   Compatibilities and Incompatibilities of IV Additives *(continued)*

Additives	Compatibilities	Incompatibilities
Procaine HCl (Novocain HCl)	Dextrose in saline or water solutions, invert sugar solutions, lactated Ringer's injection, Ringer's injection, sodium chloride injection, sodium lactate (⅙ M) injection.	Aminophylline, amobarbital (Amytal) sodium, chloramphenicol (Chloromycetin) sodium succinate, chlorothiazide (Diuril) sodium, magnesium sulfate, nitrofurantoin (Furandantin) sodium, novobiocin (Albamycin) sodium, phenobarbital (Luminal) sodium, phenytoin (Dilantin) sodium, protein hydrolysate, sodium bicarbonate, sodium iodide, sulfadiazine sodium, sulfisoxazole (Gantrisin) diolamine, thiopental (Pentothal) sodium.
Prochlorperazine edisylate (Compazine)	Alphaprodine (Nisentil), anileridine (Leritine) HCl, atropine sulfate, chlorpromazine (Thorazine) HCl, codeine sulfate, dextrose 2½% to 20% in isotonic or half-strength sodium chloride injection or water, dihydroergotamines (DHE 45), epinephrine 1:1000 in sodium lactate (⅙ M) injection, invert sugar 5% or 10% in saline or water, levallorphan (Lorfan), 50% magnesium sulfate, meperidine (Demerol) HCl, mephentermine (Wyamine) sulfate, methadone HCl, morphine sulfate, procaine (Novocain) HCl, propantheline bromide (Probanthine), PVP 3.5%, pyridoxine (vitamin B₆), Ringer's injection, scopolamine, sodium chloride injection, succinylcholine chloride.	Aminophylline, amobarbital (Amytal) sodium, antibiotics ("mycins"), barbiturates, calcium gluconate - glucoheptonate, chloramphenicol (Chloromycetin) sodium succinate, chlorothiazide (Diuril) sodium, cyanocobalamin (Rubramin), dexamethasone (Decadron) sodium phosphate, dimenhydrinate (Dramamine), erythromycin (Ilotycin) glucoheptonate, heparin sodium, hydrocortisone sodium succinate (Solu-Cortef), kanamycin (Kantrex) sulfate, meralluride (Mercuhydrin) sodium, methicillin (Staphcillin) sodium, nitrofurantoin (Furadantin) sodium, phenytoin (Dilantin) sodium, oxytetracycline (Terramycin) HCl, paraldehyde, penicillin-G (K or Na), pentylenetetrazol (Metrazol), pentobarbital (Nembutal) sodium, phenobarbital (Luminal) sodium, sulfisoxazole (Gantrisin) diolamine, tetracycline (Achromycin) HCl, thiopental (Pentothal) sodium, vancomycin (Vancocin) HCl, vitamin B complex with ascorbic acid. Do not mix with other drugs in a syringe. Slight yellow discoloration does not alter potency (10 mg. colors 1 liter of lactated Ringer's injection).
Promazine HCl (Sparine)	Dextrose in saline and water solutions, invert sugar solutions, lactated Ringer's injection, Ringer's injection, sodium chloride injection, sodium lactate (⅙ M) injection.	Aminophylline, chloromycetin (Chloramphenicol) sodium succinate, chlorothiazide (Diuril) sodium, chlortetracycline (Aureomycin) HCl, dimenhydrinate (Dramamine), heparin sodium, hydrocortisone sodium succi-

Table 8-1   Compatibilities and Incompatibilities of IV Additives *(continued)*

Additives	Compatibilities	Incompatibilities
Promazine HCl (Sparine) *(continued)*		nate (Solu-Cortef), menadione sodium bisulfite (Hykinone), penicillin G (K or Na), # pentobarbital (Nembutal) sodium, # phenobarbital (Luminal) sodium, phenytoin (Dilantin) sodium, sodium bicarbonate, # sodium warfarin (Coumadin), # sulfisoxazole (Gantrisin) diolamine, # thiopental (Pentothal) sodium. #
Promethazine HCl (Phenergan)	Dextrose in saline and water solutions, invert sugar solutions, lactated Ringer's injection, Ringer's injection, sodium chloride injection, sodium lactate (⅙ M) injection.	Aminophylline, chloramphenicol (Chloromycetin) sodium succinate, chlorothiazide (Diuril) sodium, dextran, dimenhydrinate (Dramamine), heparin sodium, hydrocortisone sodium succinate (Solu-Cortef), methicillin (Dimocillin, Staphcillin) sodium, nitrofurantoin (Furandantin) sodium, penicillin G (K or Na salt), pentobarbital (Nembutal) sodium, phenobarbital (Luminal) sodium, phenytoin, (Dilantin) sodium, protein hydrolysate, sulfisoxazole (Gantrisin) diolamine, thiopental (Pentothal) sodium, vitamin B complex with ascorbid acid.
Protein hydrolysate (Amigen, Aminogen, Aminonat, Aminosol, Lacotein, etc.)		ACTH, aminophylline, chlortetracycline (Aureomycin) HCl, deslanoside (Cedilanid-D), digitoxin (Crystodigin, Purodigin), digoxin (Lanoxin), epinephrine HCl, ergonovine (Ergotrate) maleate, hydralazine (Apresoline) HCl, meperidine (Demerol) HCl, metaraminol (Aramine) bitartrate, nitrofurantoin (Furadantin) sodium, novobiocin (Albamycin) sodium, pentobarbital (Nembutal) sodium, plasma proteins (Plasmanate), thiopental (Pentothal) sodium. Do not add other drugs to protein hydrolysate solutions.
Pyribenzamine	See Tripelennamine.	
Pyridoxine HCl	Protein hydrolysate, standard IV fluids.	
Ringer's injection		Amphotericin B (Fungizone), ethyl alcohol, calcium disodium edetate (Versenate), cortisone (Cortone) acetate, ethamivan (Emivan), histamine diphosphate, sodium bicarbonate, thiopental (Pentothal) sodium.

Incompatible in 5% dextrose injection.

Table 8-1 Compatibilities and Incompatibilities of IV Additives *(continued)*

Additives	Compatibilities	Incompatibilities
Ritalin	See Methylphenidate HCl.	
Secobarbital sodium (Seconal Sodium)		Anileridine (Leritine) HCl, codeine phosphate, diphenhydramine (Benadryl) HCl, ephedrine sulfate, erythromycin (Ilotycin) glucoheptonate, hydrocortisone sodium succinate (Solu-Cortef), insulin (aqueous), levarterenol (Levophed) bitartrate, levorphanol (Levo-Dromoran) tartrate, methadone HCl, phenytoin (Dilantin) sodium, procaine (Novocain) HCl, streptomycin sulfate, tetracycline HCl, vancomycin (Vancocin) HCl.
Sodium bicarbonate	Dextrose in saline or water or 2.5% in half-strength lactated Ringer's injection,‡ Ringer's injection, sodium chloride injection, sodium lactate ($\frac{1}{6}$ M) injection. Cephalothin (Keflin) sodium, kanamycin (Kantrex) sulfate, methicillin (Dimocillin, Staphcillin) sodium, penicillin G (K) buffered, pentobarbital (Pentothal) sodium, tetracycline HCl.	ACTH (aqueous), alcohol 5% with dextrose 5% (color change), anileridine (Leritine) HCl, calcium chloride, calcium gluconate, codeine phosphate, insulin (aqueous), levarterenol (Levophed) bitartrate, levorphanol (Levo-Dromoran) tartrate, magnesium sulfate, meperidine (Demerol) HCl, methadone HCl, methicillin (Staphcillin) sodium, oxytetracycline (Terramycin) HCl, pentobarbital (Nembutal) sodium, procaine (Novocain) HCl, promazine (Sparine) HCl,‡‡ protein hydrolysate, lactated Ringer's injection, Ringer's injection, sodium lactate ($\frac{1}{6}$ M) injection, streptomycin sulfate, tetracycline HCl, thiopental (Pentothal) sodium, vancomycin (Vancocin) HCl, vitamin B complex with ascorbic acid.
Sodium chloride injection (NaCL 0.9%)		Amphotericin B (Fungizone), levarterenol (Levophed) bitartrate. Use 5% dextrose in water or saline instead of normal saline to protect these drugs against oxidation and loss of potency.
Sodium dehydrocholate (Decholin Sodium)	Dextrose solutions in saline or water, sodium chloride injection.	Dextrose 10% in lactated Ringer's injection or saline, invert sugar 10% solutions, protein hydrolysate.
Sodium iodide	Dextrose in saline or water solutions, invert sugar solutions, lactated Ringer's injection, Ringer's injection, sodium chloride injection, sodium lactate ($\frac{1}{6}$ M) injection.	Alkaloids, anileridine (Leritine) HCl, codeine phosphate, levarterenol (Levophed) bitartrate, levorphanol (Levo-Dromoran) tartrate, meperidine (Demerol) HCl, metals, methadone HCl, mineral acids, procaine (Novocain) HCl, protein hydrolysate.

‡ Sodium bicarbonate is reported to be incompatible in lactated Ringer's injection, Ringer's injection, and sodium lactate injection,[284] but this has been questioned.[291]

‡‡ Incompatible in 5% dextrose injection.[284]

Table 8-1   Compatibilities and Incompatibilities of IV Additives *(continued)*

Additives	Compatibilities	Incompatibilities
Sodium lactate	Dextrose in saline or water solutions, invert sugar solutions, lactated Ringer's injection, Ringer's injection, sodium chloride injection, sodium lactate (⅙ M) injection.	Sodium bicarbonate.
Sodium warfarin	See Warfarin Sodium.	
Solu-Cortef	See Hydrocortisone Sodium Succinate.	
Sparine	See Promazine HCl.	
Steclin	See Tetracycline HCl.	
Streptomycin sulfate		Amobarbital (Amytal) sodium, calcium gluconate-glucoheptonate, chlorothiazide (Diuril) sodium, erythromycin (Ilotycin) glucoheptonate, heparin sodium, levarterenol (Levophed) bitartrate, nitrofurantoin (Furadantin) sodium, novobiocin (Albamycin) sodium, pentobarbital (Nembutal) sodium, phenobarbital (Luminal) sodium, phenytoin (Dilantin) sodium, sodium bicarbonate, sulfadiazine sodium, sulfisoxazole (Gantrisin) diolamine.
Succinycholine chloride (Anectine)	Dextrose in saline or water solutions, invert sugar solutions, lactated Ringer's injection, Ringer's injection, sodium chloride injection, sodium lactate (⅙ M) injection.	Pentobarbital (Nembutal) sodium, protein hydrolysate, thiopental (Pentothal) sodium. One paper states that lactated Ringer's injection, Ringer's injection, and sodium lactate (⅙ M) injection are incompatible.[289]
Sulfadiazine sodium		Ammonium chloride, anileridine (Leritine) HCl, chloramphenicol (Chloromycetin) with 25% concentration of sulfadiazine, codeine phosphate, fructose solutions, insulin (aqueous), invert sugar solutions, lactated Ringer's injection, levarterenol (Levophed) bitartrate, levorphanol (Levo-Dromoran) tartrate, meperidine (Demerol) HCl, methadone HCl, polyionic solutions, procaine (Novocain) HCl, sodium lactate injection, streptomycin sulfate, tetracycline HCl, vancomycin (Vancocin) HCl.
Sulfisoxazole diethanolamine (Gantrisin, sulfisoxazole diolamine)	Dextrose in saline or water solutions, invert sugar solutions, lactated Ringer's injection, Ringer's injection, sodium chloride injection, sodium lactate (⅙ M) injection.	Ammonium chloride, anileridine (Leritine) HCl, codeine phosphate, hydroxyzine (Vistaril) HCl, insulin (aqueous), kanamycin (Kantrex) sulfate, levallorphan (Lorfan) tartrate, levarterenol (Levophed) bitartrate, levorphanol (Levo-Dromoran) tartrate, meperidine (Demerol)

Table 8-1   Compatibilities and Incompatibilities of IV Additives *(continued)*

Additives	Compatibilities	Incompatibilities
Sulfisoxazole diethanolamine (Gantrisin, sulfisoxazole diolamine) (continued)		HCl, methadone HCl, oxytetracycline (Terramycin) HCl, phenytoin (Dilantin) sodium, polyionic solutions (pH<4.5 or>6 at 20°C or lower), prochlorperazine (Compazine) edisylate, promazine (Sparine) HCl,# promethazine (Phenergan) HCl, streptomycin sulfate, tetracycline HCl, thiopental (Pentothal) sodium,# vancomycin (Vancocin) HCl.
Surbex-T with dextrose 5%		Chlorothiazide (Diuril) sodium, hydrocortisone sodium succinate (Solu-Cortef), levarterenol (Levophed) bitartrate, nafcillin (Unipen) sodium, nitrofurantoin (Furadantin) sodium, pentobarbital (Pentothal) sodium, sodium warfarin (Coumadin; haze or precipitate in several hours).
Synkayvite	See Menadiol Sodium Diphosphate.	
Terramycin	See Oxytetracycline HCl.	
Tetracycline HCl (Achromycin, Panmycin Polycyclin, Steclin, Tetracyn, etc.)	Dextrose in saline or water, invert sugar solutions, lactated Ringer's solution,§§ Ringer's solution,§§ sodium chloride injection, sodium lactate injection (⅙ M).§§ Very stable in solutions of low pH. Calcium salts (acid pH), colistimethate (Coly-Mycin) sodium, diphenhydramine (Benadryl) HCl, kanamycin (Kantrex) sulfate, vitamin B complex with C.	Amobarbital (Amytal) sodium, amphotericin B (Fungizone), calcium salts (ppt in alkaline to neutral), cephalothin (Keflin) sodium, chloramphenicol (Chloromycetin) sodium succinate, chlorothiazide (Diuril) sodium, erythromycin (Ilotycin) glucoheptonate and (Erythrocin) lactobinate, heparin sodium (Panheprin, etc.), hydrocortisone injections, hydrocortisone sodium succinate (Solu-Cortef), methicillin (Staphcillin) sodium, nitrofurantoin (Furadantin) sodium# (compatible in normal saline), novobicin (Albamycin) sodium, penicillin-G (K or Na), pentobarbital (Nembutal) sodium, phenobarbital (Luminal) sodium, phenytoin (Dilantin) sodium, polymyxin B (Aerosporin) sulfate, prochlorperazine (Compazine) edisylate, protein hydrolysate riboflavin (photooxidation), sodium bicarbonate, sodium chloride 5% (color change), sulfadiazine sodium, sulfisoxazole (Gantrisin) diolamine, thiopental (Pentothal) sodium,# warfarin (Coumadin) sodium,# vitamin B complex (inactivation of TC).

§§ Compatible with calcium in these solutions because of the low pH.
# Incompatible in 5% dextrose injection.

Table 8-1   Compatibilities and Incompatibilities of IV Additives *(continued)*

Additives	Compatibilities	Incompatibilities
Tetracyn	See Tetracycline HCl.	
Thiamine HCl	Standard IV fluids.	Protein hydrolysate.
Thiopental sodium (Pentothal Sodium)	Use reconstituted solution within 24 hours. Reconstitute only with dextrose 5% in water, sodium chloride injection, or water for injection. In dextrose 5% in water, compatible with chloromycetin (Chloramphenicol) sodium succinate, chlortetracycline (Aureomycin) HCl, ephedrine sulfate, hydrocortisone sodium succinate (Solu-Cortef), nitrofurantoin (Furadantin) sodium, oxytocin (Pitocin), pentobarbital (Nembutal) sodium, phenobarbital (Luminal) sodium, potassium chloride, sodium bicarbonate. pH must remain very alkaline or precipitation of thiopental occurs.	Acidic solutions anileridine (Leritine) phosphate, codeine phosphate, dextrose 10% with sodium chloride, doxapram (Dopram), diphenhydramine (Benadryl) HCl, ephedrine sulfate, insulin (aqueous), lactated Ringer's injection, levarterenol (Levophed) bitartrate, levorphanol (Levo-Dromoran) tartrate, meperidine (Demerol) HCl, metaraminol (Aramine) bitartrate,# methadone (Dolophine) HCl, Modumate, penicillin G (K or Na),# procaine (Novocain) HCl, prochlorperazine (Compazine) edisylate, promazine (Sparine) HCl,# protein hydrolysate (Amigen, Aminosol), Ringer's injection, sodium bicarbonate, succinylcholine chloride, sulfisoxazole (Gantrisin) diolamine,# tetracycline HCl,# thiopental (Pentothal) sodium.‖ ‖
Thorazine HCl	See Chlorpromazine HCl.	
Tripelennamine HCl (Pyribenzamine (HCl))	Sodium chloride injection.	Chloramphenicol (Chloromycetin) sodium succinate, pentobarbital (Pentothal) sodium, phenobarbital (Luminal) sodium, phenytoin (Dilantin) sodium, protein hydrolysate.
Tubocurarine chloride	Standard IV fluids.	Protein hydrolysate.
Unipen	See Nafcillin Sodium.	
Vancocin	See Vancomycin HCl.	
Vancomycin HCl (Vancocin)		Aminophylline, amobarbital (Amytal) sodium, chloromycetin (Chloramphenicol) sodium succinate, chlorothiazide (Diuril) sodium, dexamethasone (Decadron) sodium phosphate, heparin sodium, hydrocortisone sodium succinate (Solu-Cortef), methicillin (Dimocillin, Staphcillin) sodium, nitrofurantoin (Furadantin) sodium, novobiocin (Albamycin) sodium, penicillin-G (K or Na), pentobarbital (Nembutal) sodium, phenobarbital (Luminal) sodium, phenytoin (Dilantin) sodium, prochlorperazine (Compazine) edisylate, sodium bicarbonate, sulfadiazine sodium, sulfisoxazole (Gantrisin) diolamine, vitamin B complex with ascorbic acid.

Incompatible in 5% dextrose injection.
‖ ‖ Incompatible in 10% dextrose with sodium chloride and in lactated Ringer's injection.

Table 8-1   Compatibilities and Incompatibilities of IV Additives *(continued)*

Additives	Compatibilities	Incompatibilities
Vistaril	See Hydroxyzine HCl.	
Vitamin B$_{12}$	Dextrose in saline or water solutions, invert sugar solutions, lactated Ringer's injection, Ringer's injection, sodium chloride injection, sodium lactate (⅙ M) injection.	Ascorbic acid, dextrose, phytonadione (Aqua Mephyton, Konakion), sodium warfarin (Coumadin), # vitamin B complex with ascorbic acid.
Vitamin B complex with ascorbic acid (Folbesyn, Bejectal)	Calcium chloride, calcium gluconate, dextrose in saline or water solutions, invert sugar solutions, lactated Ringer's injection, Ringer's injection, sodium chloride injection, sodium lactate (⅙ M) injection. Colistimethate sodium (Coly-Mycin), diphenhydramine (Benadryl) HCl, heparin sodium, kanamycin (Kantrex) sulfate, penicillin G (K) buffered, polymyxin B sulfate, prednisolone-21-phosphate (Hydeltrasol), sodium bicarbonate.	Aminophylline, cephalothin (Keflin) sodium, chloramphenicol (Chloromycetin) sodium succinate,§ chlorpromazine (Thorazine) HCl, hydrocortisone sodium succinate (Solu-Cortef),§ hydroxyzine (Vistaril) HCl, nafcillin (Unipen) sodium, nitrofurantoin (Furadantin) sodium (in dextrose solutions; compatible in saline), novobiocin (Albamycin) sodium, oxytetracycline (Terramycin) HCl, phenytoin (Dilantin) sodium, prochlorperazine (Compazine) edisylate, sodium bicarbonate, tetracycline (inactivated by riboflavin through photo-oxidation), vancomycin (Vancocin) HCl, vitamin B$_{12}$, warfarin (Coumadin) sodium.‖
Vitamin K$_1$	See Phytonodione.	
Warfarin sodium (Coumadin Sodium)	Do not add to infusion fluids. May inject through Y-tube of administration set.	Ammonium chloride, dextrose, epinephrine (Adrenalin) HCl,# fructose, invert sugar, lactated Ringer's injection, metaraminol (Aramine) bitartrate,# promazine (Sparine) HCl,# tetracycline HCl,# vitamin B$_{12}$,# vitamin B complex with ascorbic acid.
Water for injection, bacteriostatic	See Preservatives.	

\# Incompatible in 5% dextrose injection.
§ Dependent on the concentration of the additive.
‖ Precipitate forms after several hours.

Table 8-1 presents a compilation of compatibilities and incompatibilities for common IV additives. The basic information it contains should be transferred to file cards or other convenient form for rapid reference. It should be kept up-to-date and revised constantly as new data become available.

The collected data, however, must be used primarily as an alerting device. Until much more investigation of incompatibility mechanisms has been completed, we cannot know exactly the influence of components of dilu-

ents, concentration of additives, order of mixing, temperature, and other factors known and unknown. This explains why the literature makes conflicting statements.

Most incompatibilities encountered are physical or chemical in nature but some, such as the antagonism between heparin and penicillin, may be pharmacological. Some, such as the destructive effect of ascorbic acid in a tetracycline product on penicillin, may not be readily discernible. A number of important incompatibilities give no outward evidence that they are present.[283]

Table 8-1A   IV Additive Stability [283-289, 293, 295]

Additive	Duration of Compatibility in Infusion Solutions (Hours)*						
	A5-D5	D5-E	D5-S	D5-W	ME	NS	W
Erythromycin (Erythrocin) Lactobionate			6	12	12	24	24
Heparin Sodium			72	72	72	72	72
Hydrocortisone Sodium Succinate (Solu-Cortef)		24	24	24	24	24	24
Metaraminol (Aramine) Bitartrate			48	48	48	48	48
Nicotinic Acid			72	72	72	72	72
Penicillin G Potassium	6			6	24	12	24
Pentobarbital (Pentothal) Sodium			48	48	48	24	24
Sodium Pantothenate			72	72	72	72	72
Tetracycline (Achromycin) HCl			24	24	24	24	24
Vitamin B$_1$ (Thiamine HCl)		†	72	72	72	72	72
Vitamin B$_2$ (Riboflavin)			72	72	72	72	72
Vitamin B$_6$ (Pyridoxine HCl)			72	72	72	72	72
Vitamin B$_{12}$ (Cyanocobalamin)			72	72	72	72	72
Vitamin C (Ascorbic Acid)			48	48	12	48	48

* A5-D5: alcohol 5% dextrose 5%; D5-E: 5% dextrose in electrolyte solution; D5-S: 5% dextrose in saline; D5-W: 5% dextrose in water; ME: multiple electrolyte solution; NS: normal saline; W: water for injection.
†To be used immediately after admixture.

Contamination

Hazards to the patient may arise from contamination of injection sites, parenteral medications, and equipment. The introduction of *Clostridium welchii* deeply into the gluteal region by means of a contaminated syringe or needle has produced gas gangrene and led to the death of the patient. The buttock is a particularly dangerous site from the standpoint of injection because of its constant exposure to rectal flora. With this site, aseptic technique must be used after proper scrubbing with iodine tincture or a powerful antiseptic in 70% alcohol. All injection areas must be sterilized before inserting a needle, but special care must be taken with areas near the anus.[57]

The development and use of disposable equipment is decreasing the hazards due to contamination. Catheters, needles, syringes, transfusion apparatus, and other presterilized, inexpensive and expendable items are now available from reliable sources. But problems constantly arise. It was discovered, for example, that ethylene oxide failed to sterilize certain types of disposable syringes with recesses between the plunger head and the barrel where the gas could not penetrate sufficiently to destroy the spores of *C. welchii*. Ionizing radiation from a cobalt-60 source finally solved this problem.

Another problem is contamination introduced by the medication itself. Rigid sterility testing does not guarantee that the contents of every package of a parenteral product are sterile. Such testing is of necessity approached through representative sampling procedures because the drug product is rendered useless for sale by the tests. An occasional contaminated ampul, vial, or flask therefore may remain undetected and be released for distribution. This is a relatively rare occurrence under good quality control procedures, but a dangerous situation arises whenever any nonsterile medication is added to a parenteral fluid. Since large volumes of intravenous fluid can be contaminated in this manner, it is essential that purchases of parenteral additives be made from reliable sources, and that experienced pharmacists be consulted.

A biological product like an immunizing agent or a blood replenisher may be contaminated at its source of supply. The risk of transmission of diseases such as viral hepatitis via these parenteral products varies from no risk with gamma globulin to high risk with fibrinogen* and UV exposed plasma pooled from many donors. The highest risk is incurred, of course, during direct transfusion of blood.

Meticulously observe aseptic precautions in giving all types of injections. Avoid or eliminate contamination of parenteral products at the source of supply and in ampuls,

---

* Fibrinogen, because of the high risk, was withdrawn from the market in 1978.[308]

flasks, and vials during withdrawal or transfer from the original container. And maintain sterility of all equipment used in parenteral dosage regimens.

Policies and Procedures

The main characteristics of an acceptable IV program in the hospital are:

1. Good Housekeeping. All IV additives and admixtures should be stored in appropriate containers under suitable conditions of temperature in a clean, neat manner, properly labeled as to cautions, contents, expiration date, strength, and other necessary information.

2. Aseptic Addition. Additives should be placed in IV solutions under aseptic conditions in an environment maintained clean with the aid of laminar air flow, air filters, positive pressure, etc. Some IV fluids are excellent culture media.

3. Strict Attention to Precautions. The administration of IV medications entails varying degrees of risk to the patient. That risk is particularly serious with this type of therapy because once a drug is injected or infused into the blood stream, it cannot be withdrawn and its effects remain until it is excreted, metabolized, or counteracted. The following precautions, therefore, must routinely be observed with IV medications. Those who handle IV therapy must make certain that:

(a) The identity of the medication, the dose, and the route and rate of administration are correct.

(b) All physical, chemical, and pharmacological incompatibilities are avoided.

(c) The most suitable vein is selected for injection or infusion or the most appropriate site for hypodermoclysis.

(d) A tourniquet is not left on an extremity during repeated attempts to insert a needle into a vein. This increases extravasation from damaged veins.

(e) Varicose veins are not used for injection as medication may pool and then subsequently be released rapidly from the dilated vessels.

(f) Infusion needles are firmly anchored and properly taped in place to obtain uninterrupted flow of solution.

(g) Only a physician injects certain types of medications, e.g., those with a potential for an immediate severe adverse reaction, those whose dosage must be carefully controlled according to the patient's response, those with a narrow gap between the therapeutic and toxic doses, and those that may cause sloughing if extravasation occurs. Examples include cytarabine, methylphenidate, nitrogen mustard, and tubocurarine chloride.

(h) Multiple medications are given separately at different times, and by different routes when undesirable physical and chemical interactions may occur.

(i) IV additives are handled under rigidly controlled conditions.

(j) Orders for IV additives are written not only on fluid balance charts, but also on prescription order forms that are checked by the clinical pharmacist who warns the prescriber if he detects any problems.

(k) Drugs are not added to aminoacids, blood, or emulsions containing fats or oils.

(l) Written protocols and policies are maintained for all matters pertaining to safety of the patient receiving parenteral therapy, including (1) personnel permitted to administer parenteral therapy in the various routes and in various volumes, (2) personnel permitted to administer certain types of parenteral medications, (3) recommended routes, sites, and rates for various parenteral medications, (4) procedure for handling IV orders, including duration and labeling, (5) method of using various types of parenteral equipment and, (6) action to be taken when allergic reactions, extravasation, transfusion reactions, and other emergencies occur.

(m) Records are compiled and kept up-to-date. They include useful administrative and professional information such as number of venipunctures performed, who performed them and at what hours, number of IV additives for each drug category, nursing performance data, percentage of infusions requiring additives, and data from patient charts.

(n) Responsibilities of physicians, pharmacists, nurses and other personnel in regard to ordering, control, and delivery of parenteral medications are clearly defined, physical facilities and equipment are specified and closely re-examined periodically, and standard operating procedures are kept up-to-date in writing.

The above policy and procedures should be approved by both the Pharmacy and Therapeutics Committee and the Nursing Service.

DOSAGE REGIMENS

After both route and site of administration have been decided upon, the most appropriate dosage regimen of the selected drug must be tailored to the individual patient to achieve the desired effect as precisely as possible with minimum adverse effects. Dosage form, strength, frequency, rate, timing, and duration must be considered in relation to the status of the patient's absorption, distribution, metabolism, and excretion mechanisms and his gastrointestinal, hepatic, renal, and other pertinent organ functions.[74] The extent of the evaluation of these mechanisms and functions of the patient depends on the nature of the drug, its toxic potential, its known therapeutic effects, and the state and character of the disorder being treated.

As a general guide, *usual doses* are included in the official compendia (USP and NF). These doses are based on the amount of drug usually required to produce a satisfactory diagnostic, prophylactic or therapeutic response in a 70 Kg. adult following administration in the manner indicated at the time intervals designated. More precise official dosage information is provided in the package inserts. These indicate the weight of drug to be given per Kg. of body weight and they sometimes state the different dosage to be used in the pediatric (12 years and under), adult (up to 65), and geriatric patient. The optimum dosage varies with acid-base balance, fluid and electrolyte balance, genetic status, pathological state, temperature, and many other factors.[103,104]

To determine and to take into consideration all variables that affect dosage regimens is beyond the realm of practicality for both the manufacturer and the physician. In the pharmaceutical industry, however, the trend is definitely in the direction of more extensive and more expensive studies to arrive at more nearly optimum strengths, frequencies, rates, timing and duration of dosage for each medication.

Dosage Form

The dosage form selected by the physician depends on the condition of the patient, nature of the disease, types of medication available, and other factors.[74,91,104] The patient and disease factors used in diagnosis and discussed in Chapter 6 must be carefully considered, but certain other factors affecting patient response must also be considered, including psychological impact (color, flavor, odor, taste, viscosity, etc.) and techniques of medication.[91]

Although peroral solid and liquid preparations are the most convenient, economical, and usually the least distressing forms for administering systemic medications, they have limitations and must be used with certain special precautions. A very young child cannot readily swallow capsules and tablets and may choke if they are given to him, unless they are soft, flavored, and chewable. A pleasantly flavored syrup is usually the safest and most pleasant vehicle for the very young patient, but if he is vomiting, use the parenteral or rectal route. Pediatric antinauseants, for example, may be effectively administered in rectal suppositories. Besides nausea and vomiting, other conditions that contraindicate the use of oral medication in patients of all ages are aphagia algera, circulatory stasis, cleft palate, coma, delirium, dysphagia, fractured jaw, malabsorption, psychosis, shock, and uncooperative behavior. In a fulminating or life-threatening condition, prompt medication of the patient parenterally may be essential.

Liquid oral medications generally act promptly, are usually homogeneous and easily administered, and mask the disagreeable tastes of some drugs. Occasionally they lack stability or deposit a sediment either of which may lead to inaccurate dosage. Also, uniform doses may be difficult to pour when the medication is highly viscous or a suspended drug is unevenly distributed. These problems may be overcome by proper prescribing and compounding but capsules or tablets, because they are more acceptable than liquids, are the dosage forms usually prescribed to administer medication orally to the adult.

Do not use the oral route if the medication adversely disturbs digestion or severely irritates the gastrointestinal mucosa, if it is absorbed too slowly because of circulatory stasis, if any other contraindication noted above is present, or if an effect is urgently required in an emergency. In these situations consider either a parenteral or another transmucosal route.

If a medicated external application is desired, select one with the type of base or vehicle that prevents absorption if only a local effect is desired, or one that facilitates penetration if a systemic effect is required. Proper consistency at skin temperature, freedom from irritating particles, emollient and protective actions, and cosmetic acceptability are other important considerations.

Strength

Ideally, the strength of capsule, tablet, injection, or other manufactured dosage form is determined by the amount of drug required to provide blood and tissue levels in each patient with his own specific characteristics and disease. Obviously, this is possible only within rather broad ranges due to manufacturing economics and patient variability. Nevertheless, in spite of the practical limitations, an attempt is made to determine the optimum strength of each medication on the basis of the half-life of the drug, the shape of dosage-response curves, and the drug level (minimum effective concentration) that must be maintained at appropriate sites in the body if the patient with his many variable and individual characteristics, is to be treated effectively.

The strengths of dosage forms that are made available should permit flexibility of dosage. If only large units are marketed precise adjustment of dosage is impossible or very difficult, and frequency of dosage cannot be adjusted to convenient or most effective intervals. Tablets may be broken apart and the contents of capsules removed, but such procedures are inconvenient and lead to inaccurate dosage. Since pediatric doses of tablets and capsules are often lacking, however, powdering tablets and distributing the contents in honey or a preserve often cannot be avoided.

Frequency

Each medication should ideally be given at a time interval that will provide the desired drug concentration at the appropriate site for an appropriate length of time. It is necessary to determine the optimum between many small doses given frequently and a few large doses given infrequently. If a medication is given too frequently, excessive concentrations may build up, remain for prolonged periods, and possibly cause adverse effects that could otherwise be avoided. If it is not given often enough the drug concentration may not remain high enough to produce the desired effect. Figure 8-1 shows a typical pattern of blood levels versus a series of doses of a drug. The frequency or *rhythm of drug administration* that is proper is governed by the rates at which the drug is absorbed, distributed, made biologically available, metabolized, and excreted, also by the condition of the patient, the nature of the disease being treated, the dosage form and strengths available, the technique of administration, the presence of other drugs and other chemicals in the body and other pertinent biological, chemical, and physical factors.

Some medications must be given special consideration. Thus, an antituberculosis drug may be given most effectively only once a day in a comparatively large dose that produces a peak blood level well in excess of the minimum inhibitory concentration for the strain of *Mycobacterium* present. Apparently, some slowly growing organisms are more vulnerable to antimicrobials when they are in the most actively growing state. Therefore, large doses are spaced at greater intervals so that actively growing tubercle bacilli are destroyed by each dose, and the remaining organisms are given time to recover from the bacteriostatic impact of the drug and become

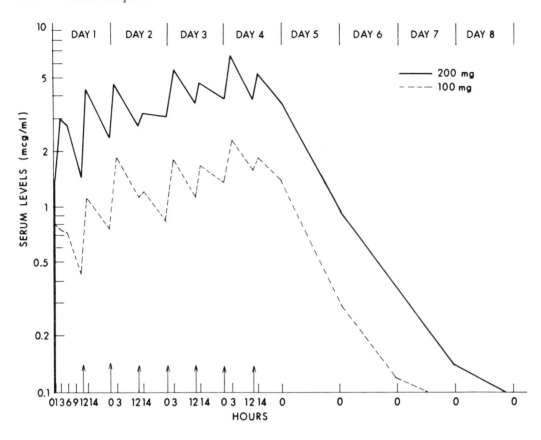

Fig. 8-1. Blood level curves with repeated doses of a medication. Average serum levels of an antibiotic in man after oral administration of 100 mg. and 200 mg. doses every 12 hours for 4 days.

vulnerable to its possible bactericidal action at the next dose.

Some drugs, if given on a chronic or sub-acute basis, require special adjustment when they are being withdrawn otherwise distressing and perhaps hazardous symptoms appear. Abrupt withdrawal of thiothixene (Navane), an antipsychotic drug, may cause severe delirium in chronic schizophrenic patients. Abrupt withdrawal of anticonvulsant drugs may bring on status epilepticus. Abrupt withdrawal of barbiturates may bring on convulsions. And unless the frequency and size of dosage of corticosteroids are gradually decreased after treating a patient, withdrawal may exacerbate previous symptoms. The effects of the relative adrenocortical insufficiency induced may require carefully regulated reinstitution of the therapy during periods of stress (surgery and trauma).[114,227]

One of the most hazardous situations oc-

curs with sudden withdrawal of propranolol from patients with stabilized angina pectoris. This may markedly increase the severity and frequency of the angina. In some instances myocardial infarction, serious arrhythmia, or sudden death has occurred.[306]

Rate

The rate (frequency and size of dose) at which a drug is made biologically available to a patient has an important bearing on safety. For safe and effective use of every medication it is essential that the correct rate of intake be maintained to attain the correct concentration at the proper site for the optimum duration of time; not too long to overmedicate and possibly have adverse results, not too short to undermedicate and have inadequate results; just long enough to accomplish the desired therapeutic effect with minimal complications.

Rate, like frequency, also depends on the patterns of absorption, metabolism, distribution, and excretion. Some drugs must not be introduced rapidly into the blood, especially in an IV injection. They may precipitate in the serum, or coagulate the blood, or cause the formation of a dangerous thrombus. Or they may act too rapidly and thereby cause a serious drug reaction which is avoidable with slower administration. Intravenous administration of a barbiturate too rapidly may depress respiration so severely that oxygen, intubation, and artificial respiration may be necessary. And in hypersensitive patients laryngeal or pharyngeal spasm may occur. Analeptics, cardiac stimulants, and intravenous fluids may be required if the overdosage is considerable. The hazards of incorrect technique of administration have been thoroughly reviewed.[91]

Duration

Duration of drug action is an exceedingly important factor to be considered in connection with patient safety. If a patient experiences a serious drug reaction from a medication which is slowly metabolized or slowly excreted, adverse effects cannot be readily reversed and may continue to be severely intensified to the point where permanent injury or possibly loss of life may result. Thus with long-acting sulfonamides, serious reactions such as the Stevens-Johnson syndrome cannot be brought under control quickly and the consequences have sometimes been tragic. Closely monitor both dosage and blood levels after administering prolonged action, highly toxic medications, particularly if liver damage decreases the rate of metabolism or kidney damage decreases the rate of excretion. Be prepared to use suitable agents to counteract the action of the drug, enhance its metabolism, and otherwise neutralize its toxic effects, as well as aid the body defenses.

The duration of a given concentration of a given drug in a given tissue is governed by a combination of many factors, including the following: (1) *The rate at which the drug reaches the target tissue.* This depends on the rates of intake and distribution which in turn depend on the amount of drug given, the dosage form, route of administration, the site and rate of absorption and dispersion, patterns of distribution, solubility in body fluids, drug binding, tissue storage, condition of the patient (activity, temperature, etc.) vascular flow rates, and other factors. (2) *The frequency of dosage.* This may vary from continuous administration as during hypodermoclysis or intravenous infusion, to periodic individual doses, and infrequently administered repository types of medication where one dose may provide adequate response for several weeks. (3) *The excretion rate.* This varies with the clearance of metabolites and unchanged drug via one or more of the eight routes mentioned under *Excretion* (page 284). (4) *The mode and rate of metabolism.* This varies with pH, concentration, microsomal enzyme induction, temperature, and other factors that influence enzymatic activity. In addition to rate of metabolism, the relative amounts of less active, inactive, and more active metabolites produced strongly influence duration of appropriate drug activity.[121]

The duration of a given concentration of drug at a given site is therefore the result of numerous offsetting factors, such as absorption and transport that tend to increase concentration, or metabolism and excretion that tend to decrease concentration.

Administering a drug with inappropriate duration of action can be hazardous. Thus parenteral heparin is the drug of choice to affect thrombogenesis when fast action (peak response IV, 10 min.; duration IV, 1-3 hours, duration SC, 4-6 hr.; duration IM, 2-3 days) is needed, but is not the most suitable agent for therapy lasting more than 36 hours because of its side effects (alopecia, diarrhea, erythema, fever, osteoporosis, etc.). The antivitamin K coumarin derivatives (acenocoumarol oral, peak 24-48 hr., duration 2 days; bishydroxycoumarin oral, peak 36-72 hrs., duration 4-7 days; cyclocumarol, peak 36-48 hrs., duration 15-20 days, ethyl biscoumacetate oral, peak 18-30 hrs., duration 2 days; warfarin sodium oral, SC or IV, peak 12-36 hrs., duration 3-5 days) may be substituted, or possibly the indandiones. The selection largely depends on how rapidly peak activity must be achieved and what duration of action is required. Since the indandiones are reported to be associated with blood dyscrasias, dermatitis, fever, hepatitis, nephropathy, and paralysis of accommodation, the coumarin anticoagulants are usually preferred. [109]

Although duration of action is primarily governed by the size of the dose, attempts to achieve prolonged drug action by giving massive doses of any drug is basically unsound and usually hazardous. Other methods such as the formulating of drug products to slow rates of absorption, inactivation, or excretion are preferred.

The duration of the need for each therapeutic dosage regimen must also be considered. Serious complications may occur if dosage is not sufficiently prolonged when treating infections with beta hemolytic streptococcus and other virulent organisms. On the other hand, adverse reactions may be experienced when medication is administered over an unnecessarily prolonged period. [25] Anti-inflammatory analgesics used for arthritis and rheumatism like indomethacin, mefenamic acid, and phenylbutazone often cannot be administered for prolonged periods and require particularly close supervision of the patient because they have the potential to produce serious toxicity and possibly fatal responses. [110] Some drugs are so toxic that they should not be administered for more than a few days at a time. [97]

Timing

Many medications are more effective if they are given at a specific time, in relation to the following: (1) *Other medication.* If possible or feasible, when several drugs must be used simultaneously, give them at different times to avoid or minimize interactions. (2) *Meals.* Meals influence tolerance to some drugs, and the activity and toxicity of many. The effects of diet are discussed on page 384. (3) *Sleep patterns.* Generally give sedatives long enough before bedtime to achieve adequate somnifacient effect at the proper time. Avoid stimulants. (5) *Diurnal, nocturnal and seasonal variations.* When desirable, administer drugs to coincide with appropriate levels of hormones and other constituents of the body with diurnal and nocturnal patterns. Different amounts of some medications are required by night and by day since microsomal metabolizing enzymes appear to be more active during periods of light. Blindness and artificial light can alter this rhythm.

Directions for timing the doses of a medication must be communicated carefully to make certain that they are properly understood. Four times a day may mean four times during the daytime, e.g., at 8 am, 12 noon, 4 pm and 8 pm. It may also mean 4 times in 24 hours, e.g., at 8 am, 2 pm, 8 pm and 2 am. The former is usually meant in the hospital, but not always. The different blood levels maintained by the two different timings may be a significant factor in overcoming a severe infection or other serious condition.

Although only a few illustrations are given above, almost countless warnings and precautions, automatically heeded in developing most plans of therapy, can be recalled. They range from the proper timing of antiallergenic therapy with respect to seasonal patterns of dissemination of pollens and other allergens, to the administration of a CNS stimulant to an astronaut at precisely the proper length of time before an emergency landing.

PHARMACODYNAMIC MECHANISMS

Conservative drug therapy is designed to strengthen the vital powers of the patient's own defensive mechanisms. Therefore, always administer the smallest amount of the least potent drug that will achieve the desired therapeutic effect. Also, avoid multiple drug therapy unless it is specifically and definitely indicated. Overmedication and self-medication pose a serious threat to national health, particularly in the presence of polluted air and water, inappropriate diet, sedentary living, and other undesirable conditions.

No prescriber can ignore the roles of environment, drug interactions, genetic influences, personal habits, and psychosomatic disorders without taking unnecessary risks when selecting medication for his patient. Sometimes air purification, application of heat and cold, hydrotherapy, orthopedic aids, physiotherapy, special diets, and other secondary measures are needed to supplement or even possibly replace medications. Combinations of medications, psychotherapy and secondary measures may be administered with minimum hazard to the patient if pertinent pharmacodynamic principles are understood and fully appreciated. And inherited anomalies such as enzyme deficiencies and abnormal intake, distribution and excretion mechanisms may be the source of super-susceptibilities to medication and rare adverse drug reactions.

The concept of reacting drug molecules with specific receptors in body cells, tissues, organs, and systems to modify function is a rational route to therapy. The objective is to achieve a desired preventive, diagnostic or therapeutic effect safely by means of chemical modification of specific biochemical mechanisms of the body. Its constituents are constantly undergoing dealkylation, deamination, decarboxylation, demethylation, hydrolytic cleavage, hydroxylation, oxidation, reduction, sulfoxidation, transamination, transmethylation and the other biotransformations which occur in normal enzyme-mediated anabolic and catabolic processes. These complex processes that continuously build and destroy tissues and yield energy for somatic and mental activities may be reinforced by appropriate medications to correct an existing malfunctioning, or to prevent one from occurring.

Drugs that are introduced among the complex, delicately balanced, sensitive body components and mechanisms may be identical with normal body constituents (e.g., ACTH, epinephrine, insulin) and replace or supplement them when they are not present in sufficient quantities for normal functioning. Other drugs may not be identical, merely structurally related so that they mimic natural products, sometimes producing more potent or more specific effects. Still others may be antimetabolites or blocking agents that interfere with the reactions of the natural somatic chemicals, or displace them in enzyme systems, e.g., the antifolates in neoplastic processes, and the anticholinesterases in abnormal neurohumoral synaptic transmission of nerve impulses.

Regardless of their mechanism of action, when administering drugs to man, we must consider their impact on the total organism. Each category of drugs bears its own special hazards. Thus, electrolyte imbalance is a possible hazard with diuretics, deafness with certain antimicrobials, respiratory depression with narcotics and general anesthetics, drug dependence with CNS agents, extrapyramidal symptoms and drowsiness with phenothiazines, photosensitivity with some tetracyclines, and adrenal suppression with corticosteroids. Therapy that is healing in one part of the body may be disastrous in another part. A drug that effectively treats one condition may activate another. Because so many pharmacodynamic and biopharmaceutic factors are involved, we must avoid highly potent medications, combinations of drugs, and high dosages whenever possible. [50] As the primary objective, we must assist the patient to maintain his own healthy homeostasis and to balance anabolic and catabolic processes amidst the influences of the environmental, emotional, and other known and unknown, tangible and intangible factors. Achievement of that objective connotes well defined limits for the homeostatic indicators that denote the state of the internal organism.

The adult, who is stabilized and is functioning normally with or without medication, is able to cope with all the intellectual, physical, and psychological demands made upon him. But the homeostatic ideal is rarely achieved for prolonged periods in any man because he is constantly being besieged and *dis*-eased by a vast number of biological, chemical, emotional, and physical stresses. His inherited and acquired defensive capabilities must constantly ward off an enormous number of potential disorders. Rational use of medications, therefore, implies fortification of these defenses, not replacement of them. We must not allow them to atrophy through disuse, oversupport, or suppression.

Although our knowledge of how drugs act in the body and how the body functions is incomplete we must nevertheless always attempt to administer precisely the type and amount of medication that enables the body to approach gradually and maintain *homeostasis*. And we must follow as necessary drug *intake, distribution, metabolism, action,* and *excretion.* The impacts of these six processes on patient response under normal and abnormal conditions are briefly reviewed below. The abnormal responses induced by special situations arising from drug interactions are covered in detail in Chapter 10.

Homeostasis

Major shifts in homeostatic indicators such as cerebral blood flow, electrolyte concentrations, fluid ratios, glucose concentrations, pH, vital signs and weight, from abnormal pretreatment values towards normal ones, may indicate that medication being administered is restoring the body to normal functioning, and that the patient is responding well. On the other hand, shifts in values away from normal may indicate that the medication is exerting an adverse physiological effect, or that a new disease is appearing. Whether the medication is functioning safely and effectively, or is inducing an adverse reaction, or a new disease is developing must be determined promptly.

During follow-up of patients on medication, variations from normal ranges of some or all of the above indicators may be highly significant, depending on the nature and degree of illness and the mode and intensity of therapy. The values may indicate acidosis or alkalosis, excess or deficiency of potassium, sodium or other electrolytes, hypovolemia or hypervolemia, increased or decreased anabolic or catabolic effects, inflammatory or hypersensitivity reactions, critical cardiovascular, hepatic, or renal pathology, or other abnormal conditions. Prompt detection of these is essential for safe medication of the patient, for they may indicate the existence of a serious adverse drug reaction or interaction that must be corrected promptly.

Dynamic shifts in patients must be carefully monitored. Rapid drop in temperature from very high levels to near normal must be achieved promptly. But a rapid drop in blood pressure obtained with a potent antihypertensive may be dangerous due to sudden decrease of coronary, renal or cerebral perfusion. Always carefully select proper rate of medication to achieve a moderate rate of return to healthy homeostasis. The goal is constancy of the internal milieu amidst the inconstancy of the external environment.

Many pitfalls are encountered with certain medications. Growth of resistant organisms, habituation, hypersensitivity, interactions with concomitantly administered drugs or tolerance can occur. Because of these and other problems, a medication may become either too hazardous or insufficiently active for the patient and must be discontinued. Replacement therapy must then be instituted.

pH

The pH of specific fluids in various vessels, tissues, and tracts is one of the most important variables in the body. It strongly influences such crucial functions as gastrointestinal hydrolysis, absorption, transport, metabolic processes, and excretion patterns of medications. The pH of a local area of the body or of the body fluids *in toto* may be altered. Large quantities of sodium bicarbonate taken orally can cause general alkalosis whereas a medication like alkaline eye drops applied topically usually only elevates the pH locally. Some drugs may produce a general acidosis, and agents like ammonium chloride, ascorbic acid, citric acid, lysine hydrochloride and methionine can acidify the urine, whereas a medication like an acidic vaginal douche usually only lowers the pH locally. [103]

The local activity of antimicrobials and certain other drugs usually varies with the pH. For urinary tract infections, methenamine mandelate, nitrofurantoin, and tetracyclines are most active when the urinary pH is 5.5 or less. On the other hand, chloramphenicol, kanamycin, neomycin, and streptomycin are most active as urinary antimicrobials in an alkaline medium. [35] However, some antimicrobials are not strongly influenced by pH. Nalidixic acid, for example, is an effective bactericidal agent over the entire urinary pH range. [114]

The role of pH in drug interactions is discussed under Mechanisms of Drug Interactions in Chapter 10, and its role in pharmacodynamics is explained in the following sections of this chapter under Intake, Distribution, Metabolism, Drug Action and Excretion.

Pharmacokinetic studies demonstrate the rate and completeness of these five aspects of drug therapy, provide concentration curves for drugs and metabolites in blood, urine and other body fluids, and evaluate shifts caused by interfering drugs and other stresses. The development of useful predictive mathematical models, the solution of complex pharmacokinetic problems with the aid of these models and analog and digital computers, and the integration of these studies with cybernetics are modern developments in the theory and practice of drug therapy.[218]

DRUG INTAKE

Patient response to medication is markedly influenced by rates, routes, and sites of intake. Any abnormality of dermatomucosal or gastrointestinal absorption, or any interference with absorption mechanisms, or any change in the site or method of parenteral administration may seriously affect the efficacy of medication.

Intake orally, rectally, and at other mucosal sites is altered by (1) the percentage of drug released and its rate of release from a tablet, suppository, ointment or other dosage form, (2) the rates of miscibility and dissolution of the drug in the fluids bathing the absorbing membranes, and (3) the rates of absorption from the site of application. These rates are dependent on the functional state of the tract or organ and barrier membranes, as well as duration of contact. The physical and chemical properties of a drug and its formulation also markedly influence rate and amount of intake from any site of application. Each molecular structure is absorbed at certain sites and not at others. Some drugs are absorbed quickly, others slowly. Sometimes only minor modifications of the biopharmaceutic factors or the biological properties of tissues that control intake patterns can produce significant variation in patient response.[82]

Drug Release

Patient response is strongly influenced by the *percentage of drug released* from a dosage form. If a given drug product, formulated so that it makes available only 50% or less of its active principles at the site of absorption, is reformulated so that it releases all of its active principles at that site, at least double the usual amount of drug is then provided. The patient may then absorb a much higher dosage and may possibly sustain adverse responses due to the excessive intake. On the other hand, if reformulation decreases the amount of drug available, there may be fewer adverse effects, but perhaps inadequate efficacy.

Alteration of the *rate of release* of active principles from a given medication and the rates of dissolution in ambient body fluids markedly influence the intensity and duration of the patient's response. These rates as well as rates of absorption and dispersion are governed largely by the biopharmaceutic factors previously discussed. Too rapid a release can cause adverse reactions due to excessively high peak blood levels; to slow a release may not permit the attainment of minimum effective blood levels.

Miscibility and Dissolution

The rapidity with which a drug passes from its dosage form, after disintegration and deaggregation if a solid dosage form is used, and dissolves in the mucosal fluids plays a very important role in drug intake. Solution occurs rapidly if the drug and its vehicle are readily miscible with the body fluids, if the excipients, binders, and other adjuvants dissolve rapidly, if the pH permits the drug to be present in a soluble state, if there is adequate natural fluid present to dissolve the drug, and if other drugs or other chemicals that interfere with the solubility of the drug administered are avoided.

The importance of the dissolution rate in determining the rate of absorption and the blood levels of drugs has been discussed widely since it was discovered that the USP disintegration test left much to be desired as a manufacturing control. Several investigators found that some tablets on the market were clinically ineffective, although they met USP requirements. They began to study the factors influencing the dissolution rate more intensively and found that particle size was particularly important as well as the factors mentioned in the preceding paragraph. See also Chapter 2.

During the 1970s considerable effort by the USP, FDA and manufacturers resulted in better control of dissolution rate and improved apparatus for its determination. Correlations between dissolution and bioavailability may one day resolve bioequivalence problems.

With increasing fineness of particles there were increasing blood levels in one thorough study with phenacetin. The mean maximum plasma concentration of the drug ranged from 1.4 mcg. per ml. with coarse particles

($>250\mu$ diameter) to 13.5 mcg. per ml. with fine particles ($<75\mu$) in either suspensions or tablets. As the fineness increased so also did the central nervous system effects. [298,299]

Intake Routes and Rates

Rates (pharmacokinetics) of drug release, intake, distribution, receptor binding, metabolism, and excretion are influenced strongly by the *route* of medication. Each of the three main routes (dermatomucosal, gastrointestinal, and parenteral) has its own characteristic absorption and diffusion patterns.

Dermatomucosal Intake. Dermal and mucosal medications, since they are primarily applied to obtain local rather than systemic effects, are usually not considered in the context of absorption, distribution, drug action, metabolism, and excretion. Notable exceptions are medications that can be absorbed through the eye, mouth, nose, rectum, respiratory tract, urethra, and vagina. Their rate and extent of absorption are governed by concentration of drug, pH, amount of friction, vehicle, condition of the tissues, and many other factors operating at the site of absorption. The amount of drug absorbed through these external surfaces can be an important factor in the appearance of unexpected systemic effects and drug interactions. See Chapter 10.

Since the late 1970s drug manufacturers have been developing special dosage forms that permit drugs to be introduced into the body percutaneously and transmucosally. Progestasert intrauterine contraceptive devices (IUDs) provide progesterone over a prolonged period. Ocusert Pilo-20 and 40 are clear oval devices containing pilocarpine. They are inserted into the upper or lower cul-de-sac of the eye where the drug diffuses into the membranes and exerts its miotic, antiglaucomatous action for 2 to 7 days. Nitro-Bid Ointment containing nitroglycerin 2 percent in a special lanolin base is spread over the chest, abdomen or anterior thighs where the drug is absorbed through the skin and promptly exerts its prolonged vasodilator effect for the relief or prevention of anginal attacks. Other products of this general type are being developed. [114]

Gastrointestinal Intake. Oral medication must overcome many hurdles to produce the desired patient response. Each dose must be swallowed and carried to the specific site of absorption for the given drug, dissolved, absorbed across membranes, and distributed to the site where it can exert its action. There are appreciable time lags at each step and therefore oral medication may not elicit maximum response in a patient for many minutes or even hours after it is swallowed.

If for some reason the patient is unable or unwilling to swallow, the oral route is eliminated. If, however, the medication is swallowed and it enters the stomach, the drug must still be released from the dosage form before it becomes available for absorption into the body. In a liquid preparation such as a flavored syrup or elixir, the drug is already in solution or suspension and is immediately available for absorption if the vehicle is miscible with the gastric fluid. But in a solid preparation such as a tablet or capsule, the drug is released for absorption only after the product disintegrates and deaggregates in the ambient fluid and the drug is leached from the adjuvants and dissolved.

Dissolution may be complete or incomplete or it may not occur in the stomach at all, depending on the characteristics of the specific formulation, and the contents and functional status of the stomach. A tablet that is compressed too tightly, or made too hard through improper formulation and thereby rendered highly insoluble, or purposely enteric coated to prevent it from disintegrating in the stomach, or formulated to prolong its rate of drug release, may pass from the stomach into the intestinal tract essentially unaltered. If improperly formulated it may pass through the entire gastrointestinal tract with little or no absorption and be eliminated practically intact in the feces. The time lag between swallowing and complete passage into the intestines varies with the activity and age of the patient, the environmental situations, the motility of the patient's stomach, the viscosity, volume and composition of its contents, emotional influences, timing with respect to food intake, posture, influence of concomitant medication, and other factors.

Both gastric emptying time and the stability of drugs in the gastric fluid have a marked effect on drug absorption. But even if the ingested drugs dissolve in the gastric fluids, and even if they are stable in the gastric contents, they may or may not be readily absorbed in the highly acidic stomach. Its low pH inhibits absorption of many medications, particularly basic ones, and thus delays their absorption. Furthermore, onset of action may be unduly delayed if they are not absorbed in the stomach, if gastric emptying time is prolonged, and if they are only slowly absorbed in the intestine because of pH, problems with pancreatic or biliary secretion, or the composition of the medication.

Gastrointestinal absorption of a drug is accomplished largely by means of passive transport across its epithelial lining. This lining varies from stomach to small intestine to large intestine macroscopically, but microscopically the external covering of the gastric rugae or the intestinal circular folds with their millions of villi is a thin monocellular layer of columnar epithelial cells. These are covered by thin lipoprotein membranes that contain pores filled with aqueous fluid. The rate of absorption is controlled by the rate of transport through the cells of the membrane. And this rate is governed by the intake factors listed below, basically by electrochemical and osmotic gradients and the other key mechanisms discussed under Transport (page 254).

Lipid-soluble drugs diffuse across the lipoid layer of the membranes from the tract into the cell and from the cell into the lamina propria of the mucosa at a rate proportional to the relative concentrations of drug on each side of the membrane. If the concentrations become equal, the passive transport ceases. But the flow of vascular fluids as well as drug binding, storage, metabolism, and excretion remove the drug from the site of absorption and the process continues until the drug is all absorbed, degraded in the intestines, or fecally eliminated. [82]

Water-soluble drugs filter in solution through the pores in biological membranes at a rate proportional to the relative electrochemical, hydrostatic, osmotic and pH gradients on either side of the membrane. Most inorganic ions and small water-soluble molecules with diameters less than 4Å and molecular weights below 200 can be transported via this route.* But highly ionized, lipid-insoluble drugs, with higher molecular weights

are largely or totally unabsorbed. Drugs like magnesium sulfate that have only very slightly absorbable ions are almost completely unabsorbed, and drugs like cholestyramine and barium sulfate, that are insoluble in both lipids and water, are completely unabsorbed.

Absorption of certain polar drug molecules and certain organic ions is accomplished by *active* transport mechanisms. Thus specialized processes transport amino acids, bile salts, certain antimetabolites, glucose, pyrimidines, sugars, tyrosine, certain cardiotonics, 5-substituted uracils, and various other compounds. Such processes have limited capacities, they are highly specialized, they require energy to function, and they transport with the aid of carrier complex formation. See Transport (page 254).

Whether a given drug is nonabsorbed, or absorbed completely or partially, slowly or rapidly, intact or modified, by one mechanism or another, depends on a host of intake factors.

Some of the more important gastrointestinal intake factors to be considered are the following: active transport mechanisms; amount of fluid and food in the tract; adjuvants that prolong action or influence absorption; agglomeration tendency; anion or cation combined with the drug base or acid; blood supply to the villi and the gastric mucosa; buffer capacity of the medication; capability of the absorbing membrane to transport the given drug molecules; chemical or physical interaction; coating characteristics of capsules, pills, and tablets; coating of the absorption site with lipoids or mucoids; complexation; composition of the vehicle, including carriers; concentration of the drug at the site of absorption; deaggregation rate; degree of ionization; diffusion characteristics and constants; disintegration rate; dissolution rate; energies of solvation; extent of vascularization, vasodilation, or vasoconstriction; flow rates of blood and lymph; gradients across absorption membrane (electrochemical, hydrostatic, osmotic); ionic charge and its strength; lipid-water partition coefficient; local tissue irritation and tolerance; molecular structure including shape, size, and steric configuration of the drug molecules; morphology of absorbing membranes (cells or surfaces); motility of the gastrointestinal

---

*The diameters of the pores range up to 40Å in the capillary epithelium.

tract; pH at the site of absorption; pk_a of the drugs; particle size; polarity, shape, size, and stability of the ionized and non-ionized forms of the drug; porosity of the absorbing membrane; polymorphic form; rate of release of drug molecules from the crystalline matrix; rate of removal of drug after it has been absorbed; size and nature of crystals and particles (amorphous, microcrystalline, micronized, etc.); solubilizing agents; solvent drag; solvolyzing rate; stability of the drug; surface area of both drug particles and absorption site; surface activity of the drug; surface tension of dissolution fluid; thermodynamic stability of the crystalline form; thickness of the absorbing membrane; viscosity of liquid medications, viscosity of the ambient fluid; wettability of the drug; width of intercellular channels; and numerous other formulation and physiological factors influencing the patient-drug intake relationship.[7,15,16,40,43,82,122,124,127,132,151,161-163]

Absorption from the tract may be enhanced by (1) removing interfering molecules or ions (tripalmitin enhances tetracycline absorption by removing Ca ions), (2) introducing carriers to facilitate diffusion (phosphatopeptide is a carrier for quaternary ammonium drugs), (3) depressing motility (anticholinergics thereby tend to prolong contact with absorbing membranes), (4) altering secretory function (reserpine increases secretion of gastric acid), (5) enhancing blood supply to the villi and gastric mucosa (ethanol thereby enhances gastric absorption of barbiturates), and (6) producing many other types of enhancing drug interactions (see Chapter 10).

Enhanced absorption, however, does not necessarily translate into enhanced therapeutic efficacy. Chelation of iron with ethylenediaminetetraacetic acid considerably enhances absorption of the metallic ions but these are so firmly held after absorption that they are not readily released for utilization by the body. The potential value of complexation for improving the absorption, solubility, and stability of medications requires further investigation.[82]

Absorption from the tract may be hindered by (1) drug binding with mucin (quaternary ammonium drugs plus mucopolysaccharides), (2) elevating or lowering pH (weakly acidic drugs tend to diffuse across membranes to regions of higher pH, whereas weakly basic drugs tend to do the opposite, (3) complexation with other drugs or other chemicals (tetracycline forms complexes with aluminum, magnesium, calcium, etc.), (4) increasing gastrointestinal motility (cholinergic stimulants accelerate emptying time), (5) biotransformations in the absorbing mucosa, and (6) many other drug interactions (see Chapter 10).[119]

The rate of absorption may be strongly influenced by the pH produced by the medication at its site of absorption. However, diminishing the pain of injection or of application to sensitive tissues such as those of the eye, ear, nose, and throat, and increasing the stability of the medication by using an appropriate pH may also be important considerations. Therefore a drug product may have to be designed so that its pH is an optimum compromise of the pHs that provide optimum activity, maximum stability, and least amount of pain.

Unexpected deviations in absorption rates may occur. Although we might expect the weak acids, pentobarbital and phenobarbital, and also alcohol, the absorption of which is independent of pH, to be absorbed largely in the stomach, before reaching the intestine, this does not take place. Because the absorbing surface of the intestinal mucosa is so vastly greater than that of the stomach, the rate of absorption is 10 to 20 times that of the stomach. Although the rate per unit area is greater in the stomach than in the intestine, more of these drugs are absorbed in the intestines than in the stomach.[82]

Many drug biotransformations take place in the intestinal mucosa. Thus, intestinal glucuronide conjugation, hydrolytic cleavage of amides, esters, glycosides, and other compounds, and various other metabolic processes may be accelerated or decelerated by inducers or inhibitors of the specific drug metabolizing enzymes. Any such changes in rates of biotransformation during absorption may have a significant impact on absorption rates and patient response to drugs, especially if they are administered in small doses, or if they are slowly released from formulations and slowly absorbed. Also any alterations of the active transport of amino acids, glucose, sodium ions, water, and other substances may influence drug absorption and therefore response. Tetracycline, for example, is more rapidly absorbed in isotonic sodium chloride solution than in water and this potentiating effect is decreased by inhibitors of sodium ion transport such as ouabain and possibly by certain other cardiac glycosides, cathartics, diuretics, and hormones. [82]

Sometimes the reasons for modification of absorption rates are not readily identified. Thus, the absorption rate of a medication is sometimes purposely prolonged with various adjuvants such as gelatin and carboxymethylcellulose. But the rate may be markedly increased and overdosage result from the crumbling or chipping of these medications by rough handling during transportation. Also, the rate of absorption may vary for some reason that is not obvious without careful study. For example, the rate of absorption may depend on the rate of gastrointestinal solution, which may depend on the rate of hydrolysis, which may depend on the polymorphic form. A sequential dependency of this type was demonstrated for chloromycetin palmitate. [124] And finally, different areas of the gastrointestinal tract absorb different drugs at different rates. Thus atropine sulfate, chloral hydrate, methylene blue, morphine sulfate, and sodium salicylate are absorbed more rapidly rectally than orally.

When too many of the absorption factors enumerated above are unfavorable for a given orally administered drug, it will not be adequately absorbed. It may then require parenteral administration for the production of systemic effects or it may simply be used topically in the gastrointestinal tract. Thus, mercurial diuretics are given parenterally because they are poorly absorbed when given orally. Unabsorbable antimicrobials like furazolidone and succinylsulfathiazole may serve as intestinal disinfectants. And sensitive drugs like penicillin G, N-nitrosoureas, and streptozoticin that are highly unstable at the pH of the tract require special handling. Enteric coating or appropriate timing with respect to food intake may help prevent destruction in the stomach and facilitate their oral administration. But parenteral administration is usually the most appropriate remedy for faulty absorption. [43]

Parenteral Intake. Injection of a medication directly into the body circumvents all the above problems of absorption. Only biopharmaceutical considerations and the problems of distribution to sites of action, excretion, and metabolism, remain. [7] The major hazard to the patient is damage to bones, muscles, nerves and vessels that may be sustained by improper placement of the hypodermic needle (see page 211).

Additives may markedly alter response to parenteral medications by altering rates of absorption from the tissues into the capillary bed. Estrogenic hormones tend to reduce the spreading of injected medication by decreasing the permeability of connective tissue, and thus to decrease the rate of capillary absorption. This effect is produced either by administered estrogens or by increased endogenous estrogen such as occurs during pregnancy. The practical value of epinephrine when used with local anesthetics is well known. By locally restricting the terminal capillary bed, arteries, arterioles, and venules the drug depresses the flow of blood through the absorbing area and thereby slows absorption and prolongs local contact and action of the local anesthetics. [132]

The enzyme hyaluronidase, although its chemical composition is not well defined and its exact mechanisms of action are still in doubt, is widely used for increasing the fluidity of the ground substance of connective tissue, and thus increasing permeability and spread of injected medication. Because a larger total area of capillaries is then exposed to the medication, its rate of absorption is increased. Apparently the enzyme depolymerizes the hyaluronic acid which normally swells in the interstitial fluid to form the viscous gel that fills the spaces between the cells and the network of fibrils and chains of protein molecules that comprise the connective tissue. The enzyme may also increase capillary permeability, although this effect may be due to impurities like histamine. Increased permeability caused by such impurities would tend to cause edema and offset its absorption-promoting effect. [132]

Various hormones (cortisone, prednisone, and other adrenal glucocorticoids) increase the rate of subcutaneous absorption and enhance blood levels of parenteral medications. This effect is possibly the result of the anti-inflammatory and anti-edematous effects that reduce the production of edema fluid and accelerate its absorption. Also the content of histamine and 5-hydroxytryptamine in the skin and connective tissue is reduced. Antihistamines, by blocking the edema-producing effects of histamine and 5-hydroxytryptamine, also tend to enhance absorption. And diuretics, by reducing edema, also improve the perivascular flow of fluids from the extravascular toward intravascular and thus also enhance absorption. However diuretics apparently do not produce this effect in normally hydrated patients.[132]

The ultimate criterion for all medications, regardless of route of intake, dosage form or formulation, is therapeutic efficacy. However, guaranteeing identity, purity, potency, and quality by means of chemical and physical testing is not enough. Even guaranteeing adequate intake by establishing minimum blood levels as an index of biological availability does not assure the prescribing physician that a minimum standard of efficacy will be met. Specifications for medications should include minimum requirements for distribution to specified receptors, including rate, concentration, and duration of contact.

DRUG DISTRIBUTION

As soon as a drug is injected or absorbed into the body it begins to be actively or passively distributed from the site of entry. Its rate of distribution depends on (1) flow rate in the artery, vein, or lymphatic vessel if it is injected or absorbed into one of these, (2) physical factors such as miscibility, solubility, surface tension, and viscosity, especially if it is injected extravascularly and directly into muscular, subcutaneous, or other tissues, and (3) active and passive mechanisms that govern transport across membranes that enclose vessels, fluid reservoirs, organs, tissues, cells, cell nuclei, and other cellular components. Concepts of drug distribution currently being explored and further elucidated are briefly discussed below. Modification of any of the transport mechanisms described may induce significant changes in patient response to a medication.[7, 15, 43, 122, 127, 151, 162, 167]

As previously mentioned, a drug to be safe and effective must be in the right form, in the right concentration, and at the right place for an adequate length of time. If any one of these requirements is not met, the drug may not become adequately biologically available. Even a high blood level does not translate necessarily into therapeutic activity. Although the total concentration of a drug in the plasma may be relatively high, the concentration of unbound drug may be below the threshold necessary to induce a therapeutic response. In one investigation, the hypotensive action of diazoxide, which is highly bound to plasma constituents, disappeared in the presence of a high total plasma concentration. The plasma half-life (26 hours) greatly exceeded the duration of its hypotensive effect (4 to 8 hours). It can be dangerous to extrapolate from total plasma levels of drug to therapeutic efficacy.[134]

Furthermore, an antimicrobial may be exquisitely formulated into a high quality medication with superb therapeutic and biopharmaceutic properties so that anti-infective levels of highly active unbound drug are attained in the blood. Yet these levels will not cure an infection of the meninges if the drug does not reach the cerebrospinal fluid, or of the joints if it does not reach the synovial fluid. And these levels may damage the fetus if they reach the placental fluid. Some drugs produce useful levels in one body fluid and not in others. Cephaloglycin (Kafocin), after oral administration, produces useful antibacterial activity in the urine against some strains of *Escherichia coli, Klebsiella,* indolenegative *Proteus,* and *Staphylococcus,* but it is not therapeutically active in the serum.[229]

Rates and routes of *transport,* distribution *barriers* such as the placental and central nervous system barriers, and drug *binding, storage,* and *redistribution* from sites of action modify total distribution patterns and may strongly affect drug safety and efficacy.

Transport

Drugs are transported across membranes by means of active transport, convective absorption, facilitated or passive diffusion, phagocytosis, and pinocytosis. Abnormalities of any of these processes may result in unsatisfactory patient response.

For purposes of analysis the body fluids may be divided into the following compartments: (1) vascular fluids of the cardiovascular and lymphatic systems, (2) that part of the interstitial fluid that bathes these vascular systems, parenteral drug depots, and semipermeable membranes covering organs, tissues and cells, (3) that part of the interstitial fluid that is isolated in reservoirs (transcellular fluid) that can only be reached by direct injection or transport across barrier membranes, such as amniotic fluid (placental barrier), aqueous fluid of bones, cartilage and tendons, aqueous humor of the eye, cerebrospinal fluid (blood-CSF barrier), extracellular fluid of the brain, (blood-brain barrier), endolymph of the ear, luminal fluid of the thyroid, and synovial fluid of the joints, (4) intracellular fluid, and (5) extrasomatic reservoirs of fluid such as those in the gastrointestinal tract and urinary tubules, ureters and bladder. The first three compartments comprise the total extracellular fluid. The last (fifth) compartment is actually outside the body proper.

The blood plasma, which is bounded by the cardiovascular walls and the walls of the erythrocytes, leukocytes and platelets, is the most efficient transport medium for drugs. It carries them rapidly to all vascularized tissues and to receptor, metabolic and excretory sites. The lymph also plays a role in drug distribution. It is the major route for cholesterol, fatty acids, proteins, and other large molecules. Although readily absorbed drugs like *p*-aminosalicylic acid and tetracycline are absorbed only in small percentages via the lymph under normal conditions, these percentages may be increased by stimulating the flow of lymph with agents like tripalmitin. Also drugs that are absorbed via the lymph gain access to the cardiovascular system without passing through the liver first, and they therefore circumvent metabolism prior to some circulation in the blood.

Lymph capillaries are located in the capsule and septa of the liver, fascial planes of muscles, gastrointestinal villi (lacteals), genitourinary and respiratory linings, myocardium, omentum, peritoneum, pleura, skin, subcutaneous tissues, and walls of the abdominal cavity. Through confluence, the small vessels repeatedly form larger ones until they form the large right lymphatic and thoracic ducts that empty into the right and left subclavian veins respectively. However, only about 1% of a salt injected subcutaneously passes through the thoracic duct. Nearly all of it passes by direct hematogenous absorption into the blood capillaries

locally at the site of injection. Also the circulation of drugs is much slower via the lymph (1 to 1.5 ml./min. in the thoracic duct) than via the blood (more than 3000 ml./min. in the capillaries during exercise). Lymphatic circulation of the entire albumin requires nearly a day whereas complete cardiovascular circulation requires only a few minutes.[132,219]

Nevertheless, a drug injected merely superficially into the skin soon reaches lymph nodes because the skin is so abundantly supplied with lymphatic vessels and the flow of lymph from skin to nodes is relatively rapid. A drug is also usually diffused promptly from a subcutaneous injection site because the lymph capillaries are so permeable that complete interchange of plasma proteins and drug occurs dozens of times in 24 hours, even though the molecules may be very large. The permeability can be increased even more by chemical stimulation (especially histamine), mechanical stimulation (including massage), sunlight, and warmth to such a degree that essentially no barrier remains between the lymph in its vessels and the surrounding interstitial fluid.[132,219]

Transport from one compartment to another depends basically on permeability properties and driving forces prevailing across the compartment membranes. Controlling variables include (1) *membrane area* accessible for transport, (2) *mobility* which depends largely on size, shape, and solubility of the penetrating drug molecules or ions, membrane charge, and diameter of the pores in the membranes, (3) *concentration* of drug at the opposite sides of the membrane, (4) *cross section area* of the membrane at points of transport, (5) *compartment volumes* on opposite sides of the membrane, and (6) *driving forces* such as pH and osmotic (chemical potential) gradients, lipid:water partition coefficients, hydrodynamic pressure gradients (bulk flow) across a compartment boundary such as a vascular wall, electrical potential (H^+ ionic) differences across the boundary (electro-osmosis), etc.[132] Depending on the net effects of the various driving forces, the diffusion flux may be accelerated (as with superimposed forces), diminished, nonexistent, or reversed (counter-current diffusion).

Ions or molecules may be transported actively against chemical, physical, or electrochemical gradients (pumped uphill) by utilizing electrical membrane forces or metabolic pumping via chemical, energy consuming intervention. Other mechanisms that are energy consuming may also participate. Thus, active transport (carrier mediated or facilitated transport) may function with the aid of some special compound which circulates within the membrane. This compound reversibly binds the drug to be transported on one side of the membrane, carries it across to the other side, releases it, and recycles for more drug. [128]

Patient response to drugs may be modified by shifts in the foregoing variables and mechanisms, and especially any alteration of (1) membrane accessibility through coating or destruction, (2) molecular mobility or concentration through physical or chemical action that changes the drug molecule or size of the membrane pores, (3) compartment volumes through dehydration or other hypovolemic or hypervolemic influences, or of (4) hydrodynamic gradients through changes in blood pressure and flow, metabolism and excretion rates, obesity patterns, etc. Thus if capillary perivascular flow is from intravascular outward to extravascular as in edema, absorption of a subcutaneous injection from tissue fluid into the vessels is adversely affected.

Although many drugs may pass freely throughout the extracellular fluid once they have entered it, distribution tends to be uneven throughout the body. Drugs vary widely in their degree of binding to protein and other body constituents. There are several reasons why distribution to adrenals, liver, lungs, spleen, various parts of the brain, and to other organs varies widely. Some drugs become perferentially stored in certain tissues. Some drugs cannot pass across certain barrier membranes and therefore cannot readily enter certain transcellular reservoirs. And rates of transport across some membranes such as the placental and blood-brain barriers vary widely.

Distribution Barriers

Many drugs and other substances in the blood, lymph and interstitial fluid do not cross some membranes like the blood-brain barrier and the placental barrier. Some do,

and as a result create problems, like kernicterus with sulfonamides that displace bound bilirubin, hypoglycemia with sulfonylureas taken during pregnancy, etc. There are indications that some drugs, e.g., clofibrate, may actually tend to accumulate in the fetus and since the fetal enzyme system is not sufficiently developed to excrete the drug, such drugs may cause serious congenital problems. Barbiturates, which were shown to accumulate in the fetus of experimental animals, may severely decrease fetal respiration. A dose of a barbiturate that caused 50% decrease in the maternal respiration rate caused 85% decrease in the fetal rate (unrelated to hypoxia). [225]

Drug Reactions in the Fetus and Neonate

Studies of the maternal and fetal placental blood and the exchange of various molecules and ions across the amniotic membranes have been conducted *in utero* and in isolated tissues. The placenta was found to possess a highly selective absorbing capacity. Small molecules (mol. wt. < 1000) appear to pass readily by simple diffusion in both directions, but larger molecules either do not pass or they are transported across the barrier membrane by other active processes. Constituents of the human fetus, absorbed from the mother or synthesized *in situ*, may be transferred to and from the maternal circulation by the pumping actions of the fetus and the uterus or an enzymatic "pumping" mechanism. [225]

Drugs that cross the placental membranes do so primarily by means of simple diffusion. Thus ionized drugs and those with a very low lipid:water partition coefficient, like glucuronides, quaternary ammonium ions (except ganglionic blocking agents like hexamethonium) and succinylcholine* are not significantly transported to the fetus. On the other hand, nonionized drugs with a high lipid:water partition coefficient like alcohol, alkaloids, anesthetic gases, atropine, barbiturates, chloramphenicol, chlorpropamide, phenytoin, salicylates and sulfonamides are readily

---

*Tubocurarine does not appear to cross the placenta in significant amounts. Reports on suxamethonium are conflicting. Gallamine and decamethonium cross the placental barrier but they are apparently safely used during the delivery of infants. [225]

Table 8-2 Drugs That Cross the Human Placental Barrier and That May Endanger the Fetus

Drugs	Adverse Effects
Acetophenetidin	Methemoglobinemia [251]
Alphaprodine (Nisentil)	Fetal respiratory depression [270]
Amethopterin (methotrexate)	Abortion; anomalies; cleft palate [238,239,243,248,265]
Aminopterin	Abortion; anomalies, cleft palate [238,239,243,248,265]
Ammonium chloride	Acidosis [265]
Analgesics	See Acetophenetidin, Heroin, Morphine
Anesthetics (volatile)	Depressed fetal respiration [225]
Androgens	Advanced bone age; clitoral enlargement; labial fusion; masculinization [240,241,248,251,265]
Anesthetics	See Mepivacaine
Antibacterials	See Chloramphenicol, Nitrofurantoin, Novobiocin, Streptomycin, Sulfonamides, Tetracyclines
Anticoagulants	See Bishydroxycoumarin, Sodium Warfarin, etc.
Antineoplastics	See Aminopterin, Busulfan, Cyclophosphamide, Methotrexate
Barbiturates	Depressed respiration [225]
Bishydroxycoumarin (Dicumarol)	Fetal death and intrauterine hemorrhage [113,238,265]
Bromides	Neonatal skin eruptions (bromoderma) [225]
Busulfan (Myleran)	Cleft palate [238,239,243,248]
Cannabis	Possible teratogen [302-3]
Chloral hydrate (large doses)	Fetal death [225]
Chlorambucil (Leukeran)	Abortion; anomalies [265]
Chloramphenicol (Chloromycetin)	Fetal death; gray syndrome [238,239,241,253,254,265]
Choroquine (Aralen)	Thrombocytopenia [265]
Chlorpromazine	Neonatal jaundice, mortality? and prolonged extrapyramidal signs [114]
Chlorpropamide (Diabinese)	Prolonged neonatal hypoglycemia [170,243]
Cholinesterase inhibitors	Muscular weakness (transient) [251]
Cortisone	Cleft palate [248,255]
Cyclophosphamide (Cytoxan)	Defects of extremities; stunting; fetal death [238,239,243,248]
Cyclopropane	Neonatal respiratory depression [225,269]
Dextroamphetamine sulfate (Dexedrine)	Transposition of vessels? [244,249]
Ergonovine maleate	Poland anomaly [301]
Estrogens (stilbestrol, etc.)	Advanced bone age; clitoral enlargement, labial fusion; masculinization [225,240,241,256,265]
Ether	Neonatal apnea [225]
Ethyl biscoumacetate (Tromexan)	Fetal death; neonatal hemorrhage [114,238,265]
Ganglionic blocking agents	Neonatal ileus [265]
Heroin	Initial neonatal addiction, neonatal death; respiratory depression [238,239,265]
Hexamethonium (Bistonium) bromide	Neonatal ileus; death [225,250]
Influenza vaccination	Increased anti-A and B titers in the mother [265]
Iodides	Goiter [20,58,92,111,238,241,258]
Iophenoxic acid (Teridax)	Hypothyroidism; retardation [212]
Iothiouracil (Itrumil)	Neonatal goiter [20,58,92,111]
Isoniazid (INH, Nydrazid)	Retarded psychomotor activity [247,257]
Levorphanol (Levo-Dromoran)	Fetal respiratory depression [272]
Lithium carbonate	Neonatal goiter [133]
Lysergic acid diethylamide (LSD)	Chromosomal damage; stunted offspring [242,302-3]
Mecamylamine (Inversine)	Fatal neonatal ileus [225,273]
Mepivacaine (Carbocaine)	Fetal bradycardia; neonatal depression [245,251]
Methadone	Fetal respiratory depression [271]
Methaqualone (Quaaludes)	Teratogenic
Methimazole (Tapazole)	Neonatal goiter; hypothyroidism; mental retardation [20,58,92,238,265]
Methotrexate	Abortion; anomalies, cleft palate [238,239,243,248,265]
Morphine	Initial neonatal addiction; respiratory depression, neonatal death [238,239,265]
Nicotine (smoking)	Small neonates [238,255]
Nitrofurantoin (Furadantin)	Fetal hemolysis [238,239,265]
Nitrous oxide (anesthetic)	Inhibits fetal respiratory movement [225]

**Table 8-2   Drugs That Cross the Human Placental Barrier
and That May Endanger the Fetus** (continued)

Drugs	Adverse Effects
Novobiocin (Albamycin)	Hyperbilirubinemia [238,239,265]
Oral anticoagulants	See Bishydroxycoumarin and Sodium Warfarin
Oral progestogens (Norlutin, Lutucylol, Pranone, Progestoral)	Clitoral enlargement, labial fusion; masculinization [240,241,251,256,265]
Paraldehyde (large doses)	Respiratory depression [225,230]
Phenmetrazine (Preludin)	Multiple anomalies (skeletal and visceral) [238,248,255]
Phenobarbital (in excess)	Neonatal hemorrhage and death [265]
Phenylbutazone (Butazolidin)	Neonatal goiter
Podophyllum	Fetal resorption; deformities [238]
Potassium iodide	Cyanosis; goiter; mental retardation, respiratory distress [238,241,258]
Progestogens	See Oral Progestogens
Propylthiouracil	Neonatal goiter, hypothyroidism, mental retardation [20,58,92,238,259,265]
Quinine	Deafness; thrombocytopenia [252,265]
Radioactive iodine	Congenital goiter, mental retardation, hypothyroidism [251,265]
Radiopaques	See Iophenoxic Acid, etc.
Reserpine	Nasal block, respiratory obstruction [241,255]
Salicylates (aspirin)	Neonatal bleeding; [265] severe hypoglycemia?
Serotonin	Multiple anomalies (organs and skeleton) [238]
Smallpox vaccination	Fetal vaccinia [265]
Sodium warfarin (Coumadin, Panwarfin, Prothromadin)	Intrauterine hemorrhage, fetal death [113,238]
Streptomycin	Hearing loss; micromelia; multiple skeletal anomalies; 8th nerve damage [238,243,265]
Sulfonamides (long acting)	Kernicterus; hyperbilirubinemia; acute liver atrophy; anemia [225,238,247,254,265]
Sulfonylureas (Diabinese, Orinase, etc.)	Neonatal goiter; prolonged neonatal hypoglycemia
Tetracyclines	Discolored teeth, inhibited bone growth, micromelia, syndactyly [240,241,254,265]
Thalidomide (see page 27.)	Hearing defects; phocomelia; death [238-240,264,265]
Thiazides (Chlorothiazide, Methyclothiazide, etc.)	Neonatal death, thrombocytopenia [241,260]
Thiouracil	Hypothyroidism; neonatal goiter, mental retardation [265]
Tolbutamide (Orinase)	Congenital anomalies [240,261] and prolonged neonatal hypoglycemia [170,243]
Tribromoethanol	Depressed fetal respiration [225]
Vitamin A (large doses)	Cleft palate; congenital anomalies; eye damage; syndactyly [248,262,263]
Vitamin D (large doses)	Hypercalcemia; mental retardation [252]
Vitamin K analogs (large doses)	Hyperbilirubinemia; kernicterus [240,241,255,264,265]

transported from the maternal plasma to the fetal circulation, and may adversely affect the neonate. (See Table 8-2).

Drugs that cross the placental barrier have been implicated in a wide range of fetal abnormalities and neonatal iatrogenic diseases (see Tables 8-2 to 8-4). But drugs affect the fetus in only 3 to 5% of cases despite the fact that 92% of pregnant women are given at least one drug by their physician. And no one is certain exactly what causes malformations in humans or in most instances whether an abnormality has been caused by a drug. Practically no neonates are perfect; essentially all have at lease some minor abnormal-

ity. Actually, the normal neonate is an anomaly. Much more investigation is urgently needed, therefore, to determine how often cause and effect relationships truly exist in cases where drugs have been associated with fetal and neonatal anomalies. Meanwhile, medication of the mother during pregnancy should be avoided unless specific drug therapy is absolutely essential, especially with potentially harmful drugs during the first trimester. [265]

Undoubtedly, fetal exposure to maternal medications can cause many serious congenital problems in the neonate. Most drugs cross the placental barrier and most mothers

Table 8-3 Neonatal Goitrogenic Medications

Antiasthmatics (iodide)	Iothiouracil
Arthrital (alphidine)	Lithium carbonate
Blood "tonics" (iodide)	Methimazole
Caffedrine	Methylxanthines
Calcidrine syrup	Pefflan syrup
Chlorpromazine	Phenylbutazone
Chlorpropamide	Potassium iodide
Ephedrine compound elixir	Propylthiouracil
	Quadrinal
Felsol powders	Radioactive iodine
Hexylresorcinol	Sulfonamides
Iodides	Sulfonylureas

take many more medications during pregnancy than is generally realized. In one group of 67 consecutive private patients, each mother reported taking an average of 4.5 medications containing 8.7 drugs (vitamins were counted as one drug) during the last three to nine weeks of pregnancy. And 80% of these were taken without medical supervision or knowledge. These data did not include medications provided in the hospital prior to delivery. Two mothers took 23 different drugs. Most mothers took antacids (60%), aspirin (69%), and vitamins (86%). Dosages of up to 1.30 Gm. of aspirin daily in mothers during the last week of pregnancy were found to be responsible for platelet dysfunction (inhibition of collagen aggregation) and diminished factor XII (Hageman factor) activity in the neonate. In over 21% of the latter, hemorrhagic phenomena (bilateral periorbital purpura, cephalhematoma, and gastrointestinal bleeding) were noted at birth.[235,236,237]

In a notable case, ovarian hyperstimulation syndrome induced with the gonadotropic stimulator, clomiphene citrate, yielded a septuplet placenta with the pathological features, eccentric cord insertion and an amnion nodosum. Only three of the neonates survived.[273] By 1978 the drug, under the trade name Clomid, was being widely used. In properly selected patients, it produces ovulation in 85% of patients and pregnancy in up to 60%, with an incidence of multiple pregnancies of about 8% (3 to 5 times normal).[303]

The fetus is apparently more sensitive to the effects of some medications than the mother. Respiration may be abolished in the fetus at a level of analgesia that does not impair maternal respiration. Death of the fetus *in utero* may be caused by morphine and some other respiratory depressants. On the other hand, dihydrocodeinone and meperidine appear to have negligible effect on the fetal respiration in some studies.[225] Respiratory depressants like the volatile anesthetic

Table 8-4 Drugs That Cross the Placental Barrier of Animals and Whose Effects on the Human Fetus Require More Evaluation*

Acetazolamide (Diamox)	Cytosine arabinoside	Nitrogen mustard
ACTH	Dactinomycin	Penicillin
Adrenocorticoids	6-Diazo-5-norleucine	Phenothiazines
Alcohol	Digitoxin	Phenformin (DBI)
Alkaloids	Erythromycin (Erythrocin,	Phenytoin (Dilantin)
Amphetamine	Ilosone)	Pyrimethamine (Daraprim)
Anesthetic gases	Fluorides	Radioactive isotopes
Antihistamines	5-Fluorouracil (5-FU)	Salicylates (aspirin)
Atropine	Hydergine (ergot alkaloids)	Selenium and its salts
Azaserine	Imipramine	Streptomycin
Barbiturates	Insulin	Thallium and its salts
Bismuth and its salts	Lead and its salts	Thyroxin
Biguanide derivates	Lithium and its salts	Thio-tepa
Boric acid	LSD (lysergic acid diethylamide)	Thiamylal
Buclizine	Marihuana	Tranylcypromine (Parnate)
Busulfan (Myleran)	Meclizine (Bonine)	Triethylenemelamine (TEM)
Caffeine	Mepacrine (quinacrine)	Triparanol
Chlorcyclizine	Meprobamate	Urethan
Chlorpromazine (Thorazine)	6-Mercaptopurine (Purinethol)	Vinblastine (Velban)
Colchicine	Mercurials	Vincristine (Oncovin)
Cyclizine (Marezine)	Neostigmine (Prostigmin)	

* These drugs cross the placental barrier and some of them have been shown to damage the fetuses of animals (chicks, hamsters, mice, rabbits, rats). Further investigation may possibly reveal that they damage human fetuses also, but not necessarily.[225,238–242,246,248,250,255,262–265,272]

gases, barbiturates, chloral hydrate, and paraldehyde may reach concentrations in the fetal circulation equivalent to those in the maternal circulation, or even higher. Some fetal barbiturate levels reach equilibrium with maternal levels in 3 to 5 minutes after therapeutic doses. However, with maternal suicidal doses, the fetal barbiturate levels may be almost twice as high as the mother's because of less effective detoxication and elimination by the fetus.[225]

Severe hypoglycemia (20 mg. glucose per 100 ml. of blood at 4 hours of age) was observed in one neonate after the mother had been receiving chlorpropamide (Diabinese) throughout pregnancy. The level of glucose in the infant's serum dropped as low as 75 mcg./ml. even after intravenous glucose. It was necessary to give glucose subcutaneously, intravenously, and by gavage to save the child. Because of prompt treatment the child apparently sustained no brain damage and was normal in other respects at one year of age.[170]

Fetal death and intrauterine hemorrhage may occur when oral anticoagulants such as bishydroxycoumarin (Dicumarol) and sodium warfarin (Coumadin, Panwarfin, Prothromadin) are administered during pregnancy, even with accepted therapeutic dosages. Since these drugs cross the placental barrier,* close observation and laboratory control are mandatory.[114] Other drugs that are known to cause fetal and neonatal defects include antimicrobials (chloramphenicol, nitrofurantoin, novobiocin, streptomycin, sulfonamides, tetracyclines, etc.), antineoplastics (chlorambucil, methotrexate, etc.), antithyroid agents, barbiturates in excess, iodides, opiates, oral androgens, estrogens and progestogens, oral anticoagulants, radiopaque iodine diagnostic agents, and thalidomide.[275]

Excessive use of alcohol by women during pregnancy can result in a characteristic pattern of congenital abnormalities, termed the fetal alcohol syndrome. Both prenatal-onset and postnatal developmental and performance deficiencies are present. First recognized in this country in 1972, the syndrome consists of behavioral, craniofacial, limb, and neurological anomalies and, in nearly 50% of reported cases, cardiac septal defects, genital abnormalities, and hemangiomas.[1,2] Primary anomalies of the head and face include microcephaly, short fissures of the eyelids, midfacial defects, and a flattened elongated vertical groove in the upper lip. Malformations of the hands include abnormal palmar creases and joined, deviated, or permanently flexed fingers and toes. The IQs of affected individuals average 35-40 points below normal.[309]

Studies in animals corroborate observations that alcohol is a potent teratogen which also increases the incidence of stillbirths, resorptions, and spontaneous abortions. The latter observations in animals are particularly important because of the inherent difficulties of assessing risk factors related to spontaneous abortions in humans.

Some cholecystographic agents containing iodine, such as iophenoxic acid (Teridax) remain in the mother's blood for several decades (>30 years), enter the fetal blood during pregnancy, and create problems in the child. After a single oral 3 Gm. dose, the maternal PBI may range from 2,000 to 14,000 mcg. per 100 ml. One mother delivered three children, then received Teridax in 1958, and delivered three more children in 1961, 1963, and 1965. When the fourth child appeared to be retarded and showed signs of hypothyroidism, the PBI values were found to be 158, 125, 84 and 30 mcg. % respectively in the mother and the last three children, but normal in the first three children delivered before Teridax was administered to the mother. Prolonged retention appears to be due to enterohepatic circulation and protein binding.[212]

Iodide, present in antiasthmatics, antirheumatics, blood "tonics", and expectorant medications (25,000 to 350,000 mcg./dose) can cross the placental barrier and after about the twelfth week of gestation be taken up by the fetal thyroid and induce congenital goiter and hyperthyroidism. This was first reported in 1962 and it pertains to over-the-counter as well as prescription medications. By inhibiting the synthesis and release of hormone which leads to hypertrophy and hyperplasia of the thyroid gland, iodide induces goiters prenatally that are sometimes large enough to cause neonatal respiratory distress and occasionally asphyxia, and may interfere

---

*Heparin, which does not cross the placental barrier may be more safely used.

Table 8–5 Examples of Drugs Excreted in the Mother's Milk[266–268,305]

Acetaminophen (Tempra, etc.)
Alcohol
Allergic agents (allergens)
Aloe
Amantadine (Symmetrel)
Ambenonium chloride (Mytelase)
Aminophylline
p-Aminosalicylic acid (PAS)
Amitriptyline (Elavil)
Amphetamines (Benzedrine, etc.)
Ampicillin (Amcill, Omnipen, Penbritin, Polycillin, Principen, etc.)
Antibiotics
Antibodies (diphtheria, slight)
Anthraquinone cathartics (Dorbane, Dorbantyl)
Antihistamines
Aspirin
Atropine
Barbiturates
Bishydroxycoumarin (Dicumarol)
Bromides
Brompheniramine (Dimetane)
Caffeine
Calciferol (vitamin D)
Calomel
Carbenicillin disodium (Geopen, Pyopen)
Carbimazole (Neo-Mercazole)
Carisoprodol (Rela, Soma)
Carotene
Cascara
Cathartics and laxatives
Cephalexin (Keflex)
Cephalothin (Keflin)
Chloral hydrate (rectally)
Chloramphenicol (Chloromycetin)
Chlorazepate (Tramexene)
Chlordiazepoxide (Librium)
Chlormadione (Estalor-21)
Chloroform
Chloroquine (Aralen)
Chlorotrianisene (Tace)
Chlorpromazine (Thorazine)
Colchicine
Codeine
Corticotropin
Cortisone
Cyclamate
Cyclopenthiazide (Navidrix)
Cyclophosphamide (Cytoxan)
Cyclopropane
Cycloserine (Seromycin)
Danthron (Dorbane, etc.)
DDT
Demethylchlortetracycline (Declomycin, Demeclocycline)
Desipramine (Norpramin)
Dextroamphetamine (Dexedrine, etc.)

Dextrothyroxine (Choloxin)
Diazepam (Valium)
Dihydrotachysterol (Hytakerol)
Diphenhydramine (Benadryl)
Diphtheria antibodies
Emodin
Ephedrine
Ergot alkaloids
Erythromycin (Ilosone, E-mycin, Erythrocin)
Estrogens
Ether
Ethinamate (Valmid)
Ethisterone (Pranone)
Ethyl biscoumacetate (Tromexan)
Ferrous sulfate
Flufenamic acid (Arlef)
Fluorides
Fluoxymesterone (Halotestin, etc.)
Folic acid
Furosemide (Lasix)
Gallium-67
Guanethidine (Ismelin)
Heroin
Hexachlorobenzene
Hydrochlorothiazide (Esidrix, Hydrodiuril, etc.)
Hydroxyphenbutazone (Tandearil)
Hydroxypropylcarbamate (Robaxin)
Hydroxyzine (Atarax, Vistaril)
Imipramine (Tofranil)
Indomethacin (Indocin)
Iodine [131] (Iodides)
Iopanoic acid (Telepaque)
Iron (ferrous)
Iron-dextran (Feosol, Imferon)
Isoniazid (Nydrazid)
Kanamycin (Kantrex)
Lithium carbonate (Eskalith, Lithane, Lithonate)
Levopropoxyphene (Novrad)
Lincomycin (Lincocin)
Lindiol
Lynestrenol
Lyothyronine sodium (Cytomel)
Mandelic acid
Medroxyprogesterone (Provera)
Mefenamic acid (Ponstel)
Mepenzolate bromide (Cantil)
Meperidine (Demerol)
Meprobamate (Equanil, Miltown)
Mercury
Mesoridazine besylate (Serentil)
Mestranol
Metals, minerals, and salts
Methacycline (Rondomycin)
Methadone HCl (Dolophine)
Methdilazine (Tacaryl)
Methenamine (Hexamine, etc.)
Methimazole (Tapazole)

Methocarbamol (Robaxin)
Methyclothiazide & deserpidine (Enduronyl)
Methyldopa (Aldomet)
Metronidazole (Flagyl)
Morphine
Nalidixic acid (NegGram)
Narcotics
Neomycin sulfate (Mycifradin)
Nicotine
Nitrofurantoin (Furadantin)
Norethindrone (Norlutin)
Norethisterone ethanate
Norethynodrel (Enovid)
Novobiocin (Albamycin)
Oral contraceptives
Oxacillin (Prostaphlin)
Oxyphenbutazone (Tandearil)
Papaverine
Penethamate hydriodide (Neopenil, Leocillin)
Penicillins (G, benzathine, etc.)
Pentazocine (Talwin)
Pentothal
Phenacetin
Phenaglycodol (Ultran)
Phenformin (DBI, Meltrol)
Phenindione (Hedulin, Dindevan)
Phenolphthalein
Phenylbutazone (Butazolidin)
Phenytoin (Dilantin)
Piperacetazine (Quide)
Potassium iodide
Primidone (Mysoline)
Prochlorperazine (Compazine)
Propantheline (Pro-banthine)
Propoxyphene (Darvon)
Propranolol (Inderal)
Propylthiouracil
Pseudoephedrine
Pyrazolones (Isopyrine, etc.)
Pyrimethamine (Daraprim)
Quinidine
Quinine sulfate
Radioactive ions (gallium, iodine, sodium, etc.)
Reserpine (Serpasil, etc.)
Rh antibodies
Rhubarb
Ribonucleic acid (RNA)
Salicylates
Scopolamine
Senna (Senokot)
Sodium chloride (radioactive)
Sodium fusidate
Sodium salicylate
Spironolactone (Aldactone)
Streptomycin
Sulfamethoxazole (Gantanol)
Sulfadimethoxine (Madribon)
Sulfanilamide
Sulfapyridine
Sulfathiazole

Table 8-5   Examples of Drugs Excreted in the Mother's Milk [266-268,305]

Sulfisoxazole	Thiouracil	Trimeprazine (Temaril)
Tetracyclines	Thyroid	Tripelennamine (Pyrabenzamine)
Thiazides	Tolbutamide (Orinase)	Valproic acid (sodium valproate)
Thiopental sodium (Pentothal)	Tranylcypromine (Parnate)	Vitamins A, B, C, D, E, K
Thioridazine (Mellaril)	Trifluoperazine (Stelazine)	Warfarin sodium (Coumadin)

with delivery. Impaired growth and mental retardation may be sequelae. Steam inhalations and forcing of fluids for bronchitis during pregnancy are far safer alternatives to iodide therapy. Also, mothers who are breast feeding their infants must avoid medications containing therapeutic doses of iodides as they are excreted in the mother's milk. Vitamin-mineral supplements containing up to 150 mcg. of iodide per dose have not been implicated in goitrogenic problems either during lactation or pregnancy. But all medications containing goitrogenic doses of iodide should be available only on prescription. Other goitrogenic medications include antithyroid drugs (iothiouracil, methimazole, propylthiouracil), chlorpromazine, lithium carbonate (up to 8% incidence of neonatal goiter), phenylbutazone, radioactive iodine, sulfonamides, sulfonylureas, and some of the other drugs shown in Table 8-3. [20,58,92,112,133,276,277]

Cogoitrogens have been discovered. Marked synergism occurs between the methyl xanthines (theophylline>caffeine >theobromine which alone are strongly goitrogenic) and propylthiouracil. Iodide markedly enhances the antithyroid potency of sulfadiazine, and the combination of subgoitrogenic doses of iodide and phenazone have led to goiter. [276-277]

Nearly all drugs, if they are administered during pregnancy, appear in the mother's milk or influence secretion of the milk (see Table 8-5). For this reason, mothers who must take potent drugs like iothiouracil, methimazole, thiouracil or propylthiouracil should not breast feed their infants. Goiter and agranulocytosis may be caused by these drugs. [114] Diet is also an important factor. Alcohol must be taken in moderation. Symptoms appeared in an infant whose mother consumed 750 ml. of Port wine in a period of 24 hours. Allergic responses may be observed in the infant when the mother consumes al-

lergenic agents such as eggs, cottonseed, flaxseed, peanuts and wheat. Death of the infant has resulted from methylglyoxal excreted by thiamine deficient mothers. [266,267]

Increased bowel activity may result if the mother ingests anthraquinone derivatives (aloin, cascara, senna, Dorbane, Dorbantyl, etc.). Secretion of milk may be depressed by atropine and nicotine. Drowsiness and skin rash may appear in the newborn infant after maternal bromide intake. Death of an infant followed maternal DDT inhalation. Methemoglobinemia may occur, but rarely, with phenytoin. Ergotism in the neonate was induced by maternal ergot alkaloid intake. Lead from nipple shields containing lead appeared in the milk. [268]

Especially important is the initial neonatal drug addiction due to fetal intake of narcotics after ingestion or parenteral injection into the mother during pregnancy or labor. Heroin produces perinatal addiction in nine out of ten of the breast-fed infants exposed. This problem urgently needs investigation. In fact, much more investigation of the excretion of drugs and their metabolites in human milk is needed. No NDA should be approved until this type of information has been developed if the new medication will be taken by women who nurse their own children or supply milk for other infants.

The CNS Barriers. The extent, mechanism and rapidity of exchange of a drug between the plasma and the cerebrospinal fluid (blood-CSF barrier), the plasma and the extracellular fluid (ECF) of the brain (blood-brain barrier), or between the CSF and ECF may markedly influence patient response to medications. Some drugs like amphetamine and other phenylisopropylamines readily cross the blood-brain barriers while many drugs like bishydroxycoumarin and the catecholamines do not readily cross the barriers. This is particularly important to know when using a drug like methotrexate that does not cross the barrier, since meningeal leukemia is common and responds to the drug injected intrathecally.

The CSF acts as a buffer for the nervous system against complex physical and chemical insults. It is contained in the sac formed by two of the three membranes (meninges) enveloping the brain and spinal cord. The innermost, the *pia mater,* immediately invests and follows every contour of the brain and spinal cord. External to the pia mater is the subarachnoid cavity filled with the CSF and bounded externally by the *arachnoid.* External to the arachnoid is the subdural potential space and the *dura mater.* The cerebrospinal fluid is constantly elaborated (perhaps with the aid of carbonic anhydrase) in the vascular choroid plexuses, and possibly in the perivascular spaces and the ependymal cells of the ventricles and the spinal canal. It passes via the choroid villi into the ventricles of the brain, and via the foramina of Magendie and Luschka into the subarachnoid spaces. The fluid amounting to 150–220 ml. in the adult, therefore occupies the ventricles, the central canal of the spinal cord, the subarachnoid space (including the cisterna magna behind the cerebellum and between it and the medulla oblongata, the cisterna pontis ventral to the pons, and the cisterna basalis containing the circle of Willis), and the perivascular spaces of the central nervous system and their continuations. It thus communicates at the brain with the tissue spaces within the nerve sheaths (and via these with the lymphatics) and also with the tissue spaces around the blood vessels that penetrate the highly vascular pia mater. Through these channels drugs may pass between the ECF of the brain and the CSF. And the CSF communicates with the plasma via the cisterna magna and the choroid plexus cells of the fourth ventricle.[219]

But constant rapid secretion of CSF normally builds up pressures in the meningeal sac that are periodically higher than the venous pressure. When the pressure of the fluid is higher than the venous pressure, CFS flows out through the one-way valves of the arachnoidal villi into the venous sinuses or lacunae. These valves close whenever venous pressure is greater than that of the CSF. A drug must therefore enter the CSF at a rapid rate, mainly via the choroid plexuses, to attain any appreciable concentration in the face of the rapid bulk turnover (about 30% per hour). The hydrostatic pressure is a major factor in preventing accumulation of some drugs and in completely excluding others.[103] However, the direction of fluid transport across the membranes of choroid plexuses and parenchymal capillaries may be reversed in response to osmotic shifts in the blood.[224]

Protein does not readily enter either the CSF (15 mg. % in the lumbar region, 5 mg. % in the ventricles) or the brain ECF. But some drugs in the unbound form cross the blood-brain barrier (walls of the brain capillaries and the glial membranes that separate the plasma and the ECF of the brain) and the blood-CSF barrier (choroid plexuses that separate the plasma and the CSF) through simple diffusion or by active secretory mechanisms. They enter the CSF and ECF of the brain most readily if they have (1) high lipoid solubility, (2) low degree of ionization, and (3) low affinity for plasma proteins. The pH and various other gradients previously discussed then play their roles.

Weak organic acids diffuse to areas of higher pH and weak organic bases diffuse to areas of lower pH. Metabolic acidosis or alkalosis causes minimal changes in the normally more acid CSF because of the slow exchange of the bicarbonate ion between blood and CSF. But respiratory acidosis or alkalosis tends to shift the CSF and intracellular pH to that of the plasma. Blood pCO_2 strongly affects drug distribution. Thus hypercapnia produced in test animals by inhalation of relatively high concentrations of CO_2 causes more of the weak organic acids such as acetazolamide, phenobarbital, and salicylate to migrate to the brain or CSF from the plasma than normally. Hypocapnia produced by hyperventilation causes less of the phenobarbital and salicylate to enter but has no appreciable effect on acetazolamide. Possibly a change in the protein-binding of the drug caused by altered pH may offset the expected change in migration since the drug is very highly bound.

Drugs that alter the tonicity of the blood or its pressure may cause shifts of fluid from the blood to the CSF or the ECF of the brain or in the opposite direction, but the total volume of fluid in the central nervous system tends to remain constant. Hydrocephalus may develop if a tumor or inflammation blocks the passage of fluid via an aqueduct or foramen or many arachnoidal villi.

The transfer of drugs across CNS barriers may be significantly increased by certain pathologic conditions involving anoxia and inflammation or laceration of the brain. The permeability of the barriers to oxytetracycline, penicillin, and streptomycin is significantly increased during active tuberculous meningitis. The barrier is apparently lacking in the vascular supply to brain tumors and this permits their localization by injecting a radioactive tracer into the blood stream and observing with a scintillation counter.

Drugs that cross the CNS barriers and contact receptors bathed by the ECF and CSF often produce very different effects from those produced by the usual routes of drug intake. A small dose of atropine (1 ml. of 1% solution) injected directly into the CSF of test animals produces paralysis of the vagus in a few seconds. Curare injected intrathecally produces excitation, increases in reflex action, convulsions, and finally death from respiratory paralysis. Sodium thiocyanate by this route also produces strong excitation and convulsions. And epinephrine (0.5 ml. of 1% solution) does not elevate blood pressure.[104]

Drug Binding

Drugs may be bound (1) to specific proteins whereby they may in a few instances act as haptens, particularly with covalent binding, and initiate autoimmune (hypersensitivity) reactions, (2) to receptor sites whereby they initiate characteristic actions and produce corresponding effects in the body, or (3) to protein and other constituents of the body whereby they are inactivated and stored. The last two types of binding are of major importance in drug distribution and all three are of vital importance to patient response. Degree of binding is affected by pH, temperature, and inherent affinities as measured by association constants.

Drugs that enter the vascular fluids are reversibly bound with varying degrees of tenacity by means of ionic and covalent bonds and van der Waal's forces to proteins. They are usually bound first to albumin, and when this is saturated, to globulins and other frac-

tions.* Drugs also enter the other body fluids and are bound in the tissues. Binding in the circulatory fluids and the tissues destroys the ability of drugs to bind with and act at receptors, to enter the glomeruli, and to cross membranes freely. Therefore it influences onset, intensity, and duration of action by controlling amount and location of drug, and its time of retention in the body.

Delay in onset is caused by removal of the activity of some of the first doses of a drug through binding. This is one reason why a loading dose is sometimes necessary. All protein binding sites must be saturated as promptly as possible if onset of drug effects are to be achieved without undue delay. A desired intensity of effect can only be achieved when allowance for inactivation through binding is made in the dosage regimen. Since the reservoir of circulating, bound drug as well as bound drug in the tissues is in equilibrium with unbound drug, as the latter is eliminated bound drug is released to maintain active drug levels in the blood and tissue fluids and at receptor sites. This process of unbinding continues until all bound drug is released, metabolized, and excreted, or until more drug is received and the process repeated.

Both degree and tenacity of plasma protein binding vary widely. Bishydroxycoumarin is 99% bound to plasma proteins, phenylbutazone 98%, warfarin 97%, diazoxide 90%, sulfonamides up to 85%, thiopental 65%, riboflavin 60%, phenacetin 30%, acetaminophen and aspirin 25%, and antipyrine is essentially unbound. The rate of binding is influenced by the percentage of reactive chemical groups on drug molecules that approach the receptor sites at the correct angle for interaction. The percentage can be improved by two orders of magnitude through suitable physicochemical treatment, and as a result the response of the patient dramatically increased.[93]

Tenacity of drug binding is of vital importance to the patient. Drug safety and efficacy

---

* Thyroxine is bound first to α-globulins and when all the binding sites on these globulins are saturated it is then bound to albumin. The extent and nature of protein-binding is determined by analytical centrifugation, electrophoresis, equilibrium dialysis technique, gel filtration, preparative ultracentrifugation, or ultrafiltration. (*Lancet* 1:73-74 (Jan. 10) 1970).

may be affected by the impact of binding tenacity on drug storage and redistribution in fluids and tissues. In drug intoxication where drugs in high overdosage become strongly bound to serum proteins or firmly imbedded in the body lipids, measures such as hemodialysis may be unsuccessful. And in patient evaluation, competitive protein binding forms the basis for sensitive assays for 17β-estradiol, progesterone, testosterone, and other steroids in the plasma and urine.

Tissue Storage

During distribution in the circulating and extravascular fluids many drugs and chemicals are removed and selectively stored in various tissues of the body according to affinities created by binding, solution, and other storage mechanisms. Drugs and other chemicals are stored in (1) deposits of fat, (2) within cells, or (3) extracellularly within a given tissue. Since stored drug is in equilibrium with unbound drug in the body fluids, these three reservoirs therefore may provide drug to receptors and cause physiological effects long after medication has been discontinued. This situation may be particularly hazardous if a severe drug reaction occurs and cannot be arrested, especially in patients with impaired renal function.

For this reason long-acting sulfonamides may be very hazardous in patients who experience a severe reaction such as the Stevens-Johnson syndrome. Not only are these drugs slowly excreted, but they also are extensively bound to plasma protein and may not be completely released for protracted periods. Hypersensitivity reactions may thus continue to be exacerbated, and concomitant medication that increases rate of release from storage may make the situation even worse. The outcome may be irreversible and fatal. See Chapter 10 *Drug Interactions.*

The extent and location of storage of a drug in the various tissues of the body is governed by affinities arising from the specific physical and chemical properties of tissue constituents and of the drugs. Some drugs have an affinity for the strongly ionic groups of the mucopolysaccharides of the connective tissue. Some like lead, strontium, and tetracyclines become fixed in the matrices of bone. Others bind to the nucleoproteins of cell nuclei, phospholipids, and other constituents of the tissues. Some drugs accumulate in the hair, nails, and other tissues containing scleroprotein. And still others tend to accumulate in adipose tissue.

Fat Storage. Drugs and other chemicals that have a high lipid solubility tend to accumulate in body fat. In an obese patient, whose body content of fat may be as high as 50%, storage may be extensive. As high as 70% of a short acting, highly lipid-soluble barbiturate, considerable amounts of lipid-soluble drugs like dibenamine and phenoxybenzamine, appreciable quantities of chlorinated insecticides (aldrin, DDT, dieldrin, etc.), and other chemicals that are absorbed through environmental exposure, may be stored. A distinct improvement in obesity or even fasting by a normal individual may then cause mobilization of the stored chemicals. DDT, inactive when stored in the fat of a patient, passes from adipose tissue to plasma and becomes active during a weight reduction program. The quantities usually encountered are not toxic but a problem arises because DDT is an inducer of drug metabolizing enzymes. Therefore, the effects of chlordiazepoxide, meprobamate, methyprylon and other affected drugs that are being taken as the insecticide is activated are often diminished in intensity. The reverse situation is of course true. An individual who is becoming steadily more obese is able to absorb larger quantities of chlorinated hydrocarbons and other lipid-soluble drug inducing chemicals without experiencing any alteration in the efficacy of medications he may be taking.[28]

Cellular Storage. Some drugs are actively transported into the cells of a specific organ such as the brain or liver where they accumulate in high concentrations through reversible binding with intracellular nucleoproteins, phospholipids, or proteins. Acetazolamide localizes in the caudate nucleus, hippocampus, and hypothalamus. Barbiturates are bound to tissue proteins, particularly in the liver and kidney. Bilirubin localizes in the basal ganglia in kernicterus. Acridine antimalarials appear to be bound to intracellular components in the cell nucleus, such as nucleic acids.[104] Cellular concentrations of some drugs may reach very high levels. About 4 hours after a single dose of quinacrine, the liver level may be 2,000 times the plasma level, and after prolonged administration the ratio between the two levels may reach 22,000 to 1. These high concentrations probably result from strong binding to nucleoproteins in the cell nuclei. Nevertheless, though much higher levels of drug may be reached within the cell than in the extracellular fluid, as the drug is eliminated through metabolism and excretion it gradually passes out of the cell and is eventually completely removed from the body.[230]

Since the normal pH gradient between extracellular fluid (pH 7.4) and intracellular fluid (pH 7.0) is small, the cellular concentration of weak bases is only slightly higher and of weak acids only slightly lower than in the extracellular fluid. Acidosis tends to move acids into cells and bases out of cells. Alkalosis tends to do the reverse.

Drugs cross membranes covering cells by means of the same mechanisms previously discussed under Absorption and Transport. Nonelectrolytes are generally transported by pH and other gradients across the lipid portions of the membrane and small molecules like urea pass through the aqueous pores. The same mechanism of simple diffusion also holds for transport across membranes covering the cell nuclei, mitochondria, and possibly other cellular components.

Redistribution

When the quantity of active drug administered by repeated oral or parenteral dosage or constant hypodermoclysis or intravenous infusion just offsets the quantity removed by biotransformation, binding, storage, and excretion, the total amount of drug within the body may remain at a fairly constant level. But a drug may nevertheless be shifted by other drugs, dietary and environmental chemicals, and other factors to and from receptors and binding sites in the body fluids and tissues, and across membranes from one body of fluid to another. Such transport may affect drug activity. This is one reason why attending physicians must watch for drug interactions and carefully control both diet and environment.

A drug may become less active if it is displaced from receptor sites by other chemicals with higher affinity for those sites or if it be-

comes more extensively bound to plasma protein or tissue constituents. Or it may become more active if it is displaced from binding sites, or released from storage in fats by dieting, or from storage in organs, tissues, and cells by changes in acid-base balance, blood flow and pressure, and other homeostatic and physicochemical factors that alter membrane permeability and the forces of transport mechanisms. Significant shifts of a drug may occur into or out of blood plasma, lymph, intracellular fluid, or transcellular fluid depots such as the cerebrospinal fluid and extracellular fluid of the brain. Through these displacements from binding sites and shifts in localization patterns more drug may be made available for action at receptor sites.

Thus therapeutic efficacy, which depends on the amount of drug bound to the appropriate receptors, is basically dependent on levels of drug at those receptors, and levels at any particular population of sites depends on rates of intake, patterns of distribution and redistribution, and rates of metabolism and excretion.

DRUG METABOLISM

Adverse drug reactions can often be avoided if drug metabolism theory is applied by the prescribing physician. Unnecessary reactions are sometimes often caused by genetically induced abnormalities in the patient such as enzyme deficiencies, by immaturity of enzymes in infants, or by altered activity of normal enzymes (induction or inhibition). When any of these exist, it is impossible to prescribe rationally on the basis of a memorized schedule of dosages, contraindications, and other precautionary information. Variations in rates of metabolism among individuals may account in part for the 30-fold variation in plasma levels that has been observed with the same dose of a drug. Even the same dose given to the same patient at different times may achieve either a toxic, or a therapeutic, or an inadequate effect.[5]

A drug that is absorbed and distributed in the body is either excreted unchanged or as metabolites derived from the drug through one or several enzymatic processes. These processes may produce beneficial or adverse responses to medication depending on the circumstances. They are influenced by absorption rate, age, binding of the drug, disease, displacement from binding and receptor sites, enzyme induction or inhibition, excretion rate, hereditary constitution, hormonal balance, interactions with other drugs, lipoid solubility, molecular modification, nutritional status, pregnancy, sex, and many other factors. Because of the varying and complex relationships that exist between a given drug and the factors affecting its biological transformations, prediction of therapeutic results and adverse effects cannot be made with complete confidence at the present stage of our knowledge. [5, 15, 28, 44]

Much of the information on drug metabolism has been obtained in animals and tissue cultures and still remains to be evaluated clinically. Nevertheless enough data are now available to warrant application in a general way to improve human therapeutics and explain some types of drug interactions and other abnormal responses to medication. Extrapolations must be made cautiously, however, because abnormal responses that occur in animals through modification of biotransformation may not occur in man or may not take place as rapidly and intensely. And the reverse is also true. Animal enzyme systems and metabolic pathways often differ markedly from those in man.

Drug metabolism is apparently directed toward converting drugs into more readily eliminated gases, degradation fragments, and more polar compounds (less lipid-soluble). These metabolites are (1) less able to bind to circulating proteins of lymph and plasma and constituents of cells and tissues, and are thus more available for glomerular excretion, (2) less soluble in fats and therefore less able to be stored in adipose tissue, (3) less able to cross membranes and enter and be stored in cells and transcellular fluid reservoirs, and (4) less able to be reabsorbed by the urinary tubules and therefore more readily excreted.

Metabolic processes are protective against drug insults to the body. They are separate from the natural intermediary anabolic and catabolic processes within the body, and they continue until all administered drug is eliminated unchanged or as metabolites, or is permanently bound in some tissue. Specialized enzymes metabolize alkaloids, hydrocarbons, synthetic chemicals, and other foreign substances that are absorbed, ingested, or inhaled via the diet, environment, or medica-

tions. If some highly bound substances like chlorpromazine,* phenylbutazone, and thiopental were not converted to metabolites that are readily excreted, their physiologic effects would last a lifetime. [44]

The enzymes active in drug metabolism carry out *conjugation* (salicylic acid to salicyluric acid; sulfanilamide to *p*-acetylaminobenzenesulfonamide; phenols to sulfates and glucuronides), *deamination* (amphetamine to phenylacetone and ammonia), *demethylation* (chlorpromazine and other phenothiazines to tricyclic compounds resembling the imipramine type of antidepressant; meperidine to meperidinic acid, normeperidine and normeperidinic acid), *hydrolysis* (procaine to diethylaminoethanol and benzoate), *methylation* (niacin to N-methylnicotinamide), *oxidation* (acetanilid to acetaminophen; chlorpromazine to the 3,7 dihydroxy compound and sulfoxides; phenylbutazone to oxyphenbutazone and thus Butazolidin becomes Tandearil; alcohol to acetaldehyde), and *reduction* (nitrophenols to aminophenols). By means of these reactions, drugs are converted into metabolites that are less active, equally active, or more active, and perhaps at times more toxic than the unchanged form. Thus, nalidixic acid is partially converted to an equally active metabolite, hydroxynalidixic acid. Acetohexamide (Dymelor) is converted to an active metabolite, hydroxyhexamide. About 10% of a dose of codeine is converted to the narcotic morphine. Ephedrine is N-demethylated to form a metabolite with similar pharmacologic properties. Prontosil† had to be split to form the active metabolite sulfanilamide before it became effective. And the metabolically active form of vitamin D_3 appears to be 25-hydroxycholecalciferol. This metabolite must be produced in the liver before the vitamin can perform its functions in the intestine (calcium transport) or in the bone (calcification of bone with the aid of parathyroid hormone). [31]

---

*The number of metabolites produced may be large. Chlorpromazine yields about 24.

†Prontosil, chemically *p*-[(2,4-diaminophenyl)azo] benzenesulfonamide, is an azo dye that was first patented by Kearer and Mietzsch of IG Farbenindustrie and first used clinically against staphylococcal septicemia in a 10-year-old boy with dramatic curative response (1933). Domagk reported its protective value against streptococcal and other infections in mice (1935) and for his work received a Nobel Prize (1938).

The biotransformation of some drugs can proceed via more than one pathway. At times this may be hazardous. Chloramphenicol provides an illustration of one type of problem associated with multiple metabolic processes. In man, glucuronidation is the major route of metabolism of the drug and this can be stimulated by certain inducers (see below). However, reduction of its NO_2 group is another route and this yields a metabolite that may act as a hapten which couples with protein to form an antigen that stimulates the production of antibodies against the drug. If this occurs in a given patient, attempts to counteract with higher doses the lowered activity caused by the enzyme induction may intensify the hypersensitivity reactions caused by antibody formation. This problem may be insurmountable in some patients.[207]

Two other problems associated with chloramphenicol, although unrelated, appear to have metabolic origins. The first is a reversible bone marrow suppression characterized by arrested cell maturation, ferrokinetic changes indicative of suppressed erythropoiesis, normally cellular marrow, reticulocytopenia, and vacuolization in erythroid and myeloid cells. This appears to be caused by the inhibition of protein synthesis by the mitochondria of the bone marrow. The second, a rare but far more serious complication, is characterized by aplasia or hypoplasia of bone marrow, delayed onset of three to six weeks after the last dose, lack of a dose-effect relationship, pancytopenia, and usually death from hemorrhage or infection. This aplastic anemia appears to be caused by a genetically determined biochemical anomaly, and withdrawal of the drug upon the early appearance of bone marrow suppression will not necessarily prevent the development of the condition. And this serious complication cannot as yet be predicted.[207]

The rate of formation of metabolites and their characteristics are major factors governing intensity, type and duration of drug action in the body and therefore patient response. The index of drug duration that is usually employed is the half-life.

Half-Life

The half-life of a dose of a given drug has been variously defined as the time required (1) to eliminate one-half of the drug administered to the patient, (2) to eliminate one-half of the biologically available drug, (3) to lower the blood level of a drug to one-half of its initial peak level, (4) to eliminate one-half of the activity of the drug, and (5) to reduce to one-half the amount of unchanged drug in the body once equilibrium is established.

Half-life has been defined in many ways, according to the method of determination and the parameters selected. The third definition is usually used for several reasons, but by any method it is sometimes difficult to determine in any meaningful sense. Not all of a drug given orally may be absorbed. Not all of an absorbed or injected drug is distributed to its site of action. Drug binding, storage, transport and excretion that play significant roles in determining half-life may be altered by other chemicals and dietary and environmental influences. Drug concentration peaks may form rapidly and drop rapidly and thus become difficult to locate. They may bear no close relationship to the therapeutic activity of a drug. The drug may be eliminated by some combination of biliary, fecal, lacrimal, mammary, perspiratory, respiratory, salivary, and urinary excretion or almost entirely by one route. There are many reasons why the half-life must be interpreted with respect to other factors. However, the half-life does give some indication of metabolism and excretion rates relative to other drugs and forewarns about the possibility of accumulation or the need to alter the frequency of dosage.

The half-life and therefore the therapeutic activity of a drug depends on the net effect of several variables on bioavailability: (1) the rate at which the minimum effective concentration (MEC) of the drug and its active metabolites reach receptor sites, (2) the duration and extent of binding at those sites, (3) the rate at which the drug is biotransformed into metabolites that are more active than it is, (4) the rate at which the drug is converted into metabolites that are less active than it is, (5) the extent of inactivation through plasma binding and localization in certain tissues, (6) the extent of activation of bound or stored drug through displacement from binding sites and release from depots, and (7) the rate at which the drug and its active metabolites are excreted.

The net effect when factors 1, 2, 3, and 6

that tend to increase activity are balanced against the remaining factors that tend to decrease activity determines whether the effects of a drug in the body are increasing, decreasing, or remaining constant. The important considerations in medicating a patient with a given dosage are: (1) What is the initial peak blood level? (2) How soon is this level reached? (3) What is the minimum effective concentration (MEC) of the given drug? (4) How soon is the MEC reached? (5) How long is the MEC maintained by each dose?

Reduction in the amount of unchanged drug in the body or urinary elimination is seldom if ever a linear (1st order) reaction. The drug may be distributed unevenly among the body compartments and pass into and out of these compartments at different rates. The drug may be excreted by several routes at different rates and percentages. It may be metabolized by different enzymatic pathways. The metabolites may be less ac-

tive, equally active, or more active than the parent compound. For these and other reasons the decay of the activity of a drug in the body through storage, binding, metabolism, and excretion is a very complex process and the results of attempts to express the decline in activity mathematically are frequently frustrating.

Even working backwards from terminal plasma concentrations does not ensure a valid half-life because so many patient variables are involved and these change from one patient to another and in the same patient over a period of time. Rate of decay of activity is altered by the magnitude of the dose, substances that induce or inhibit drug-metabolizing enzymes, variations in body fluid volumes, and other factors.

The many pharmacodynamic factors concerned with attainment of therapeutically effective levels of a drug are discussed in earlier sections (pages 242 and 246). The duration of

Table 8-6 Examples of Diseases Caused by Enzyme Deficiencies [56,63,154,156,157,297]

Deficient Enzyme	Condition
Adenosine triphosphatase	Hemolytic anemia (congenital nonspherocytic)
Alkaline phosphatase	Hypophosphatasia
Amylo-(1,4-1,6)-transglucosidase	Glycogen storage disease (c)
Amylo-1,6-glucosidase	Glycogen storage disease (b)
Arginase	Argininemia
Catalase	Acatalasemia
Cystathionine cleavage enzyme	Cystathioninuria
α-Antitrypsin	Pulmonary emphysema
Dehalogenase	Goitrous cretinism
2,3-Diphosphoglycerate mutase	Hemolytic anemia (congenital nonspherocytic)
Galactose-1-phosphate uridyl transferase	Galactosemia
Glucose-6-phosphatase	Glycogen storage disease (a)
Glucose-6-phosphate dehydrogenase	Hemolytic anemia (Heinz body)
Glucose phosphate isomerase	Hemolytic anemia (congenital nonspherocytic)
Glucuronyl transferase	Congenital hyperbilirubinemia
Glutathione peroxidase	Hemolytic anemia (congenital nonspherocytic)
Glutathione reductase	Hemolytic anemia (drug sensitivity)
Glutathione synthetase	Hemolytic anemia (congenital nonspherocytic)
Hexokinase	Hemolytic anemia
Homogentisic acid oxidase	Alkaptonuria
Hypoxanthine-guanine phosphoribosyl-transferase	Gout (genetically distinct subtype)
Hypoxanthine-guanine phosphoribosyl-transferase	Lesch-Nyham syndrome
L-Phenylalanine hydroxylase	Phenylketonuria
Methemoglobin reductase (diaphorase I)	Methemoglobinemia (one type)
p-Hydroxyphenylpyruvic acid oxidase	Tyrosinosis
6-Phosphogluconate dehydrogenase	Hemolytic anemias (congenital and drug-induced)
Phosphoglycerate kinase	Hemolytic anemia (congenital nonspherocytic)
Pyruvate-kinase	Hemolytic nonspherocytic anemia
Triosephosphate isomerase	Hemolytic nonspherocytic anemia
2,3-Diphosphoglycerate mutase	Hemolytic nonspherocytic anemia
Tyrosinase	Albinism
Uroporphyrinogen-producing enzyme	Hemolytic anemia (drug sensitivity)

the MEC is governed by the amount of drug administered, frequency of dosage, rate of intake, distribution patterns, rate of metabolism, and rate of excretion. The rate of metabolism is governed by pH; solubility and concentration of drug; its molecular structure; rate of penetration into tissues, cells, and cell components; quantity, maturity, and activity of enzymes; and other factors that control enzymatic transformation of drugs. The factors that influence excretion rates are covered later in this chapter.

Among some of the most important pharmacogenetic considerations that influence the half-life, therapeutic activity, or toxicity of a drug and that are of major significance in predicting and achieving a desired patient response are (1) enzyme deficiencies, (2) enzyme induction, (3) enzyme inhibition, (4) autoimmune (immune response) phenomena, (5) rare metabolic anomalies, and (6) metabolic stresses.

Enzyme Deficiencies

Because the disposition of drugs in the body is mediated largely by enzymatic processes, the mechanisms and kinetics of drug distribution, utilization, or elimination and therefore patient responses to medication are modified by congenital enzyme anomalies or modifications of normal enzymes. These enzyme problems, named *inborn errors of metabolism* by Garrod in 1908, may have local or general, primary or secondary, highly specific or nonspecific and highly hazardous or innocuous consequences.[201]

An enzyme may be so specific in its activity that any anomaly or adverse effect of a drug on the enzyme may interfere with only one molecular structure. Thus the enzyme system that N-demethylates aminopyrine is different from the one that N-demethylates aminoazo dyes. But interference with various other enzymes may affect the metabolism of many compounds. Thus some hydrolytic enzymes will split a wide range of ester, peptide or other bonds. The gastric proteolytic enzyme pepsin converts many proteins of the diet into peptones and proteoses by breaking peptide bonds.[26]

In many pathologic conditions, altered morphology in the patient has usually been related first to a clinical disorder, then to a

biochemical defect, and finally to a genetic basis for the defect. Familial hypercholesterolemia (autosomal dominant), familial hyperlipemia (autosomal recessive), Wilson's disease (autosomal recessive), and dozens of other metabolic problems have been identified. Many of these genetically determined biochemical defects are enzyme deficiencies which are being identified in increasing numbers each year (see Table 8-6).* Now that we can synthesize enzymes, genes, lysosomes, and other cell components, we may eventually be able to exert genetic control, and eliminate drug reactions that occur as a consequence of genetic defects.† Cellular probing for genetic information will undoubtedly provide us with powerful therapeutic tools.[21, 63, 111, 202]

Genetically determined metabolic anomalies express themselves as a wide range of problems, including many hypersensitivities. So many of these enzymatic anomalies are constantly being detected and associated with drug reactions, it appears that practically all of these types of reactions may eventually be explained on the basis of an inherited problem that predisposes the patient to a hypersensitivity state. The term "idiosyncracy," has probably outlived its usefulness as a word. It could now be replaced by "rare phenotype," since more and more so-called idiosyncratic drug reactions can be explained by genetic mechanisms.[37] These types of hypersensitivity reactions, however, must not be confused with allergic drug reactions caused by immunological responses (see pages 279-281).

Enzyme deficiencies vary with the ethnic origins of a population. INH acetylase deficiency (in slow inactivators of isoniazid) is

---

†The first human genetic engineering was attempted in 1970 when Rogers of the Oak Ridge National Laboratory provided harmless Shope papilloma virus to Terheggen of the Cologne Kinderkrankenhaus for use in two German sisters with arginemia. The virus was introduced to provide missing genetic information in their DNA needed for making arginase.[228]

* The number of diseases caused by enzyme deficiencies is increasing very rapidly. The reader is referred to repeatedly updated textbooks such as: Stanbury J B, Wyngaarden J B, Fredrickson D S: *The Metabolic Basis of Inherited Disease.* McGraw-Hill, New York, 1978. Some of the most dramatic recent medical advances have been achieved through correction of newly identified enzyme deficiencies.

found less frequently in Eskimos and Japanese than in Caucasians and Negroes.[111] See Table 8-7 on page 276. The most thoroughly investigated enzyme deficiency, that of glucose-6-phosphate dehydrogenase, is found with the highest incidence in Mediterranean races and African tribes.

Glucose-6-phosphate Dehydrogenase Deficiency. The significance of a deficiency of glucose-6-phosphate dehydrogenase (G6PD) as an intrinsic erythrocyte defect that causes drug toxicity, particularly Heinz body hemolytic anemia was not revealed until 1956, although the problem was reported as early as 1926.[27] It is appreciated best by cutting across the disciplines of biochemistry and immunology.[1,2,10,11,19,22,118]

Acute hemolytic intoxication caused by an unknown mechanism was first observed among chemical workers in Germany in 1890 by Heinz. He noted brown-to-green blood, cyanosis, and the presence of spherical inclusion bodies (Heinz bodies) in the red cells of affected persons. The condition was induced by aromatic amino, nitro, and oxy compounds such as aniline, nitrobenzene, phenylhydrazine, and quinones, used as intermediates in the preparation of dyes, explosives, and photographic chemicals. It is now known to be induced also by certain anti-infectives (chloramphenicol, nitrofurans, sulfonamides, etc.), antimalarials (pamaquine, primaquine, and other 8-aminoquinolines), analgesics and antipyretics (acetanilid, aspirin, phenacetin, pyramidon, etc.), certain foods (fava beans and pollen), chlorates, nitrites, methylene blue, naphthalene, probenecid, sulfones, vitamin K, and a rapidly growing list of many other drugs and other chemicals. These act as catalysts in the sequential irreversible denaturation of hemoglobin by oxygen. Methemoglobinemia appears early and is followed by sulfhemoglobinemia and Heinz bodies. Heinz bodies may form in less than 15 minutes after a potent hemolytic chemical like aniline or hydroxylamine contacts red cells. Thus, the presence of these bodies and modified hemoglobin in red cells is an early warning sign of the specific type of hemolytic anemia provoked by various drugs in certain persons.[53,55,165]

Reports that diabetic acidosis, uremia, virus infections (infectious hepatitis, infectious mononucleosis, and viral respiratory infec-

tions), bacterial pneumonias, and septicemias (typhoid, etc.), including many infections that are arthropod-borne, also precipitate hemolytic anemia in susceptible subjects may have far-reaching significance. Possibly the African epidemics of jaundice associated with dark urine and occurring in its severest form in males, may indicate a relationship to a trait present in susceptible individuals.[2,59,60]

In 1956, Carson demonstrated that the Heinz body type of hemolytic anemia was caused by an inherited deficiency of glucose-6-phosphate dehydrogenase (G6PD), an enzyme required to catalyze the early stage of the only oxidative pathway available to erythrocytes, the pentose phosphate pathway.[19] This deficiency may be inherited as a sex-linked character with full expression in hemizygous males (with one X-chromosome carrying the mutant gene and one normal Y-chromosome) and in homozygous females (with two X-chromosomes carrying the mutant gene) and partial expression in heterozygous females (with one X-chromosome carrying the mutant gene and one normal X-chromosome).* It is found in up to 58% of Kurds, up to 65% of Arabians, some Mediterranean populations (Ashkenazic and Sephardic Jews, Greeks, Iranians, Persians, Sardinians, Serbs), up to 33% in some African tribes (Bondei, Digo, Ganda, Giriama, Kikuyu, Luo, Masai, Sambaa, Zibua), up to 33% of Thais, up to 16% in other Asiatic populations (Chinese, Filipinos, Indians-Parsees, Javanese, Micronesians), about 6 to 15% in American Negro males, and about 16% in some American Indians (Oyana males).[1,2,10,11,89,116] Negro troops stationed in Korea, Vietnam and elsewhere sustained allergic reactions to antimalarials because of this enzyme deficiency.[19,53,89]

A significant decline in the incidence of G6PD deficiency in young Negro males has been reported in the United States. This decline may be due to the fact that the deficiency is a hemizygous X-linked trait and that there is an increasing tendency for Negro outbreeding with whites and Indians

---

*The World Health Organization estimates that 100,000,000 individuals throughout the world have inherited this condition. It is one of the most prevalent of the hereditary enzymatic defects of clinical significance.[274]

having lower frequencies of G6PD deficiency.[116]

In several of the populations, the incidence of the trait approximately parallels that of the sickle-cell trait and tends to be found where malaria abounds.[116] These traits may exemplify balanced polymorphism, i.e., the deleterious consequences of possessing such genes are offset by certain advantages, particularly in heterozygotes in their own environment. But if they move they may lose the advantage. If an affected Greek, Iranian, or Sephardic Jew for example moves from a Mediterranean country where his enzyme deficiency protects him from falciparum malaria to another country like the United States where the hazard is essentially nonexistent, he then receives no advantage but only disadvantages such as hypersensitivity to certain medications.

Apparently the trait of G6PD deficiency is protective since malaria parasites, for two metabolic reasons, may multiply less rapidly in cells deficient in the enzyme.[2,116,147] G6PD deficient cells have a subnormal concentration of glutathione which is required in its reduced form for growth of plasmodia. Also the rate of metabolism by the hexose monophosphate-shunt pathway used by the malaria parasites is diminished in these enzyme deficient cells.[19]

G6PD deficiency leads to defective direct oxidation of glucose in erythrocytes because of a fall in reduced glutathione (GSSG), triphosphopyridine nucleotide (TPN) and diphosphopyridine nucleotide (DPN). Even cells with the deficiency, however, function normally until they come into contact with oxidative chemicals that accelerate the transfer of hydrogen from TPNH, GSSG, hemoglobin, free SH groups of proteins, and other donors. These chemicals apparently react with oxyhemoglobin to form hydrogen peroxide (H_2O_2), which is normally decomposed when adequate amounts of reduced glutathione and glutathione peroxidase are present. But when the enzyme deficiency exists, GSSG is not adequately regenerated through the TPN-TPNH cycle, the H_2O_2 is not destroyed, the normal equilibrium (R-SH$\rightleftharpoons$R-SS-R) is shifted toward the right with the formation of improper -SS- bridges, and the hemoglobin in the drug-sensitive red cells is oxidized and otherwise denatured, with for-

mation of characteristic intracellular spherical inclusion bodies (Heinz bodies) and hemolysis.

G6PD deficiency does not appear to be the result of the same mutation in all who are affected because the following vary from one population to another: (1) properties of the enzyme, (2) severity of the deficiency, and (3) susceptibility of affected individuals to hemolysis when they are exposed to various drugs. Several electrophoretic variants of the enzyme have been detected, as well as differences in substrate affinities and optimum pH for activity.[89] Most deficient Caucasians, predominantly male Greeks and Southern Italians, have significantly lower red cell G6PD activity than affected Negro males. The males of the Barbieri family of Northern Italy, however, have on the average only a 50% decrease in the G6PD enzyme. Affected Caucasian males also have a significantly decreased level in liver, saliva, skin and white cells whereas affected Negro males have normal or near normal levels in these tissues and cells. Among Greek, Italian and Malayan populations there is a significant incidence of neonatal jaundice and kernicterus in G6PD deficient infants whereas it is rare among American Negroes and Sephardic Jews.

Also all cases of chronic nonspherocytic hemolytic anemia associated with the deficiency have involved Caucasians only. And the hemolytic reaction induced by drugs is usually mild and self-limiting in deficient Negroes while it is often very severe and not self-limiting in deficient Caucasians. Among these Caucasians, in contrast to the Negroes, the G6PD level is not significantly higher in younger erythrocytes than in the older cells.[150,178]

The amount of drug administered may strongly influence the severity of the hemolysis in the presence of the enzyme deficiency. Deficient Negroes are not affected by aspirin until the dose reaches about 5 Gm. No instances of the blood dyscrasia were noted with doses under 4 Gm.

Any agent that stimulates the pentose phosphate pathway, i.e., the hexosemonophosphate (HMP) shunt pathway, may be potentially hemolytic for they can carry electrons from cellular components such as GSH and TPNH to molecular oxygen in the oxidation-reduction system. Typical examples are drugs with *ortho* and *para* hydroxyphenyl-amine, quinone-quinhydrone-hydroquinone, and other potential ketone-imine and quinone structures.

Some drugs such as aminoquinones, quinones, and certain dyes can short circuit the system by reacting with the TPNH and oxiding it back to TPN. [+] See Fig. 8-2.

All patients are sensitive to these oxidative structures. A high enough blood level, attained through high dosage, decreased excretion, decreased metabolism or other situations, is hazardous even for patients with normal amounts of G6PD. They are particularly hazardous for those deficient in the enzyme.

The lens of the eye, like the erythrocyte, is also concerned with maintaining specialized protein that is rich in sulfhydryl through generation of TPNH and preservation of GSH. Thus inhibition of G6PD with substances like galactose or the introduction of oxidants like beta-naphthol, dinitrophenol, or naphthalene, can cause cataracts. These cataractogenic agents (1) induce formation of quinones, (2) lower GSH levels, (3) oxidize protein sulfhydryl groups, (4) stimulate glucose consumption, (5) deplete organic phosphates, (6) cause cation changes and swelling of tissue, and (7) precipitate lens protein into inclusion bodies (cataracts).[53] The main cataractogenic effects may be produced by the metabolized quinones.

Any drug that causes Heinz body anemias or biochemical defects that predispose patients to these anemias may cause the formation of cataracts and other ocular anomalies. Even when there is no G6PD deficiency, some oxidative drugs, e.g., methylene blue can enter the cycle, as shown in Figure 8-2, and speed up the oxidative process to such an extent that a hemolytic crisis may occur.

A simple visual test for the G6PD deficiency is readily available. Reduction (decolorizing) of brilliant cresyl blue with a suitable buffer, red cell hemolysate, and stabilizer occurs when TPNH is formed by the following reaction:

$$\text{Glucose-6-phosphate} + \text{TPN} \xrightarrow{\text{G6PD}}$$
$$\text{6-Phosphogluconate} + \text{TPNH}$$

The TPNH reduces the dye to its colorless form. The rate at which the color of the dye disappears is proportionate to the enzyme content of the red cells. If the color does not disappear in 2 hours the cells are considered to be deficient. Commercially produced test kits are now becoming available for detecting various enzyme deficiencies.

It is therefore now possible to predict that a patient with the G6PD enzyme deficiency will react adversely to a specific molecular structure. And more is constantly being learned about the relationships between drugs and patients with this genetic problem. Yet most of the data remain buried in the literature and laboratory files. Because physicians usually prescribe by name only, without recognition of the molecular structure and its biochemical significance, they are not as a rule able to detect a compound that will react unfavorably in their abnormal patients.

It is well known that certain types of drugs can cause severe, sometimes fatal, hemolytic anemias when the enzyme deficiency exists. A variety of simple microscopic and spectrophotometric procedures are available for detecting incipient hemolytic problems. Nevertheless, many potent oxidant drugs have been marketed without data from any one of these tests having been included in research protocols and NDA applications. And most drugs are still prescribed, without a screening test and without adequate follow-up, for members of ethnic groups in which these problems often exist. Microscopic examination of erythrocytes for Heinz bodies and spectrophotometric detection of methemoglobin should be routine tests with such potentially

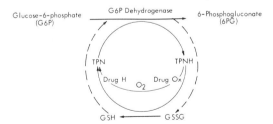

Fig. 8-2. Glucose-6-phosphate (G6P) oxidative conversion to 6-phosphogluconate (6PG) is catalyzed by the enzyme glucose-6-phosphate dehydrogenase (G6PD) in the presence of triphosphopyridine nucleotide (TPN) conversion to its reduced form (TPNH), and glutathione regeneration of TPN as it passes from the oxidized form (GSSG) to the reduced form (GSH).

hazardous investigational drugs. And careful screening of patients with pertinent ethnic origins is essential before these drugs are prescribed.

Enzyme deficiencies and their variants that induce hemolytic anemias are constantly being discovered as sensitive methods of detection become perfected. Apparently, any medications that affect the glycolytic pathways in erythrocytes may induce hemolytic responses. But effects are often difficult to predict. Thus the essential endogenous chemical, glucose, increases hemolysis under certain conditions, but it may diminish it under others. [297]

Hemolytic enzyme deficiencies that have been identified since the discovery of glucose-6-phosphate dehydrogenase deficiency are discussed below in alphabetical order.

Hexokinase Deficiency. A severe hereditary hemolytic anemia attributed to a hexokinase deficiency was described for the first time in 1967. The enzyme is probably active in a critical rate-limiting step in glycolysis via the Embden-Meyerhof pathway (not by the pentose phosphate pathway) in the young reticulocytes. When its activity is lowered through rapid decay because of an inherited abnormality, the erythrocytes age prematurely with consequent hemolysis. [154,157]

Pyruvate-kinase Deficiency. The existence of this inherited nonspherocytic anemia was first recorded in 1961, and more than 80 cases were reported during the first five years after it was noted. [66,156] This represented the first reported instance of an inborn metabolic error involving the main pathway of glycolysis in a human tissue whereby energy for the mature erythrocyte is derived from anaerobic conversion of glucose to lactate via the Embden-Meyerhof cycle. [156]

This enzyme deficiency disease is characterized by large discoidal erythrocytes that are often irregularly contracted, crenated, or spiculated, also by a deficiency of enzymes in the glycolytic pathway (not in the hexose-monophosphate shunt), as well as the other symptoms of dark urine, jaundice, splenomegaly, and high incidence of gallstones. Next to G6PD deficiency it is the most frequently encountered cause of congenital nonspherocytic hemolytic anemia. Hemolysis continues after splenectomy is performed because the liver is the "graveyard" for the deficient cells. The degree of hemolysis may be exacerbated by administration of glucose in disease caused by some variants of the deficiency.

Other related hemolytic nonspherocytic anemias are caused by deficiencies of *triose-phosphate isomerase, 2,3-diphosphoglycerate mutase,* and other enzymes listed in Table 8-6 on page 269.

Red cells become particularly sensitive to hemolysis with certain drugs and patients become highly susceptible to recurrent infections when there are deficiencies of *glutathione, glutathione reductase,* the *enzyme that converts porphobilinogen to uroporphyrinogen,* and related substances. Lack of glutathione (GSH) may result in oxidative destruction of hemoglobin, improper functioning of cellular enzymes, metabolic blockage through combination with functional sulfhydryl groups that are normally protected by GSH, and protein denaturation through biological chain reactions brought about by sulfhydryl-disulfide interchanges. [63]

Other Metabolic Anomalies

Since both drug metabolism and pharmacological responses to drugs ultimately depend on the activity of enzymes which are genetically controlled, atypical phenotypes (genetic variants) with enzyme anomalies are very likely to be revealed by potent drugs and overdosage. Characteristic adverse reactions are produced. But, because many of these reactions are extremely rare, they may not appear until after a drug has been very widely used. Even then they may not be immediately recognized in propositi as adverse drug-induced responses that are caused by genetic errors until several other patients of the same phenotype have also received the incriminated drug and reacted adversely. [37,111]

As more knowledge of rare inherited anomalies becomes available, as well as more sensitive tests to identify each specific type, we shall be able to predict more accurately when rare hypersensitivity reactions will occur and thereby reduce some of the hazards of drug therapy. Proper selection of alternative medications and suitable adjustment of dosage will enable physicians to circumvent such rare events.

The following representative problems, arranged in order of their discovery, illustrate the hazard faced by patients with enzyme anomalies who receive potent medications.

Hemoglobin Abnormalities. An abnormal and characteristic hemoglobin (Hb) is found in a number of hemolytic diseases, including sickle cell anemia (HbS), sickle cell hemoglobin C disease (HbC), congenital Heinz body anemias (Hb Köln, Hb Seattle, Hb St. Mary, Hb Zürich), and certain mild hemolytic anemias (HbD, HbE). The majority of inherited hemoglobin abnormalities are associated with anemias and they seem to result from amino substitution in the β polypeptide chain. However in thalassemia, the most common disease caused by hemoglobin abnormality, the error is depression of alpha chain synthesis. Instead of the four chains found in normal hemoglobins (2α and 2β in HbA; 2α and 2δ in HbA$_2$; 2α and 2γ in HbF; and 2α and 2ε in Gower-2) the hemoglobin is mainly HbF.

Hemoglobin S. In 1949, the first of the fourteen known abnormal hemoglobins was recognized as the biochemical determinant of sickle cell anemia, and it became known as hemoglobin S. The only difference between it and normal hemoglobin is replacement of glutamic acid by valine in the β chain. Anemia is always present in those that inherit this variant of hemoglobin. Hemolysis may be induced in these individuals during anesthesia or periods of anoxia, in severe pulmonary infection, or while traveling in unpressurized aircraft.[198]

Hemoglobin H. This inherited variant of hemoglobin (HbH) was reported in 1959 to consist of four β-polypeptide chains. It usually occurs in the hemolytic anemia, thalassemia, and is found most often among Chinese, Filipinos, and Thais, and sometimes among Greeks. Those who have HbH disease possess two nonallelic genes, one for thalassemia and one for HbH. The erythrocytes have a life span of only about 40 days, one third of the normal span, because of the tendency of HbH to form methemoglobin. HbH is readily denatured by drugs like acetanilid, aminophenol, amyl nitrite, methylene blue, nitroglycerin, phenacetin, sodium nitrite, sulfonamides, and other methemoglobin forming agents, with production of anemia.[199,200]

Hemoglobin Zürich. This mutant was discovered in 1960 in the members of a Swiss family who developed severe hemolytic anemia following sulfonamide (sulfadimethoxine and sulfamethoxypyridazine) therapy.[42] Their hemoglobins contained three unusual peptides created by replacement of histidine, the amino acid normally present in position 63 of the β chain, by arginine. Phenotypes with this metabolic error were prone to develop anemia and jaundice and their erythrocytes were readily lysed by primaquine and certain other drugs.[37,42]

Succinylcholine Sensitivity. Prolonged apnea produced by succinylcholine, first clinically observed and reported in 1952, led to the recognition of plasma *pseudocholinesterase* polymorphism. This becomes apparent as a sharply discontinuous variability of drug response. The genetically determined sensitivity to the drug is associated with its use in patients with abnormal serum cholinesterase activity. The genetic variants (phenotypes) with an atypical enzyme pseudocholinesterase can be clearly identified with the aid of "dibucaine numbers." These values are determined and plotted as percentages of inhibition by dibucaine of the hydrolysis of benzoylcholine used as the substrate for plasma pseudocholinesterase.[166,180,181]

Normally, succinylcholine is very rapidly converted into the relatively inactive metabolite succinylmonocholine in the blood. The usual 40 mg. dose is destroyed in less than a minute and the effects wear off in three or four minutes. But in a patient with atypical esterase, excessive amounts of the drug reach and depolarize the nerve endplate at the neuromuscular junctions. As a result he may not be able to breathe adequately for a prolonged period of time, e.g., 8 to 10 hours after receiving the drug by continuous infusion during prolonged anesthesia (1 Gm. or more per hour). The prolonged apnea does not occur in deficient patients when other muscle relaxants (decamethonium, tubocurarine, etc.) that are not destroyed by cholinesterases are administered.[63]

Brain damage from hypoxia is always a potential hazard with muscle relaxants. Adequate facilities for artificial respiration should always be available when these drugs are used, especially succinylcholine. In some mental institutions the use of this drug is prohibited because brain damage that results from its use during electroconvulsive therapy may not be recognized in mental patients.

Isoniazid Neuropathy. In 1953, and independently in 1954, patients were first found to inactivate the antituberculosis agent isoniazid through acetylation at different rates.[185,186] Subsequently, the hereditary nature of the variation became well established, and individuals were found to be either slow or rapid inactivators who yielded isoniazid half-lives of 140 to 200 minutes or 45 to 80 minutes respectively, depending on the amount of acetylase present. Ability to acetylate isoniazid is controlled by an autosomal dominant gene, and slow inactivators appear to be homozygous for a gene that fails to produce normal acetylating enzyme.[39]

Slow inactivators (deficient in acetylase) tend to build high blood levels of the drug which seems to interact with and deactivate pyridoxine (vitamin B_6). The resulting avitaminosis causes disturbances of the nervous system, including a peripheral neuropathy. The relative degree of hazard, that varies with ethnic origin, is shown in Table 8-7.

Refractory Rickets. An inherited lack of alkaline phosphatase causes a form of vitamin-D resistant refractory rickets, known as hypophosphatasia.[188] In this condition, first reported in 1957, treatment with vitamin D is ineffective.

Hypophosphatasia should not be confused with the deficiency, determined by a dominant sex-linked gene, on the X-chromosome, recognized since about 1937, and now categorized as Type I resistant rickets.[187] The latter is also known as endogenous rickets, ideopathic osteomalacia (adult), late rickets, Milkman's syndrome (adult), phosphate diabetes, primary vitamin-D refractory rickets,

Table 8-7   Ethnic Distribution of Slow and Rapid Isoniazid Inactivators [185,194-196]

Ethnic Group	Percentage of Rapid Inactivators	Percentage of Slow Inactivators
Eskimo	95.4	4.6
Japanese	86.7	13.3
American Indians	78.5	21.5
Latin Americans	67.2	32.8
American Negroes	47.5	52.5
White Americans and Canadians	44.9	55.1

rachitis tarda, raised resistance to vitamin D (RRD), and tubular rickets. In treating patients with this deficiency which causes a defect of renal tubular reabsorption of plasma phosphate, massive doses of vitamin D are administered. But prolonged doses near toxic levels (1.25 to 12.5 mg. daily) may cause calcifications in the tissues and possibly death from renal failure caused by calcium deposits.[63]

α_1-Antitrypsin Deficiency. A genetically determined deficiency of α_1-antitrypsin, the proteinase inhibitor that comprises about 90% of the α_1-globulin fraction of human serum, is associated with pulmonary emphysema. Since the discovery of this relationship in 1963, dozens of investigators have made electrophoretic, enzymatic, immunologic and other studies that have shown the familial nature of the condition. The deficiency can be readily detected.[213,214]

Anticoagulant Resistance. Exceptional inherited resistance to oral anticoagulant drugs (bishydroxycoumarin, phenylindandione, warfarin), was first described in 1964. The propositus for the anomaly was a 73-year-old man with a recently sustained myocardial infarct. Although anticoagulants were administered to him orally and intravenously in doses varying widely (e.g., from 40 to 1010 mg. of warfarin) and although absorption was complete, blood levels were proportionate to the dosage, and protein binding (97%) and urinary excretion of the metabolites were normal, the prothrombin response was much less than that for a normal person. Also the effect of vitamin K on the hypoprothrombinemia produced by the drugs was much greater in the propositus than in patients who responded normally. Six relatives displayed the same anomaly. The atypical response may be controlled either by a single autosomal or by an X-linked dominant gene, perhaps by an atypical regulator gene that produces an atypical repressor with decreased affinity for anticoagulants or increased affinity for vitamin K or both.[37,113]

Phenytoin Toxicity. In 1964, the relative inability of certain genetic phenotypes to parahydroxylate phenytoin was found to be the cause of toxic reactions. Ataxia, mental blunting, and nystagmus occurred early in otherwise healthy patients receiving normal doses of the drug, apparently because of a deficiency of the specific enzyme phenytoin parahydroxylase. This deficiency decreased the rate of urinary excretion and caused unchanged drug to accumulate in the plasma. One deficient patient who received a minimal dose of 300 mg. daily reached a plasma level of 70 mcg. per ml. of monohydroxylated phenytoin in two weeks. [37,77]

Hydralazine Sensitivity. In 1967, the sensitivity of certain patients (genetic variants) to hydralazine was related to a deficiency of acetylating enzyme. Those who are slow acetylators are more prone than rapid acetylators to develop antinuclear antibody when they receive the drug and to develop a condition that mimics systemic lupus erythematosus in every clinical feature. [37,182]

Phenacetin Hypersensitivity. A rare hypersensitivity to acetophenetidin (phenacetin) was first described in 1967. The propositus was a teenage patient with a profound methemoglobinemia caused by addiction to the drug. The youngster was found to be unable to de-ethylate the drug to form the usual metabolite (acetaminophen). Instead, other metabolic pathways produced more than the usual small amounts of hydroxyphenetidin and hydroxyphenacetin, potent methemoglobin-forming agents. A sister possessed the same genetic defect, but the rest of her family did not. [37,135]

Hypoxanthine Guanine Phosphoribosyltransferase (HGPRT) Deficiency. A deficiency of this enzyme whose activity is determined by a gene on the X-chromosome, presents problems when hyperuricemia and uric acid crystalluria are treated with allopurinol (Zyloprim). As first reported in 1970, this uricosuric agent in the presence of the enzyme deficiency may cause an increase in hypoxanthine and xanthine levels in the blood. [71]

HGPRT deficiency is responsible for the familial disease of male children first reported by Lesch and Nyhan in 1964. Features of the disease include aggressive behavior, choreoathetosis, gout, hyperuricosuria, mental retardation, motor handicaps, neurological dysfunction, obsessive self-mutilation, and spastic cerebral palsy. Most children die before they reach maturity from pneumonia, progressive inanition, or uremia. [30,76,100]

Allopurinol Hypersensitivity. A severe, allopurinol-induced hypersensitivity reaction (azotemia, eosinophilia, toxic epidermal necrolysis, oliguria), that ended in extensive intracutaneous infections, sepsis, pneumonia and death was reported in 1970. Drug-induced cutaneous eruptions of the type encountered are associated with a 30% mortality rate. Because such death is a rare event, the only one reported for the drug which is a potent enzyme inhibitor with side effects that are usually mild and self-limiting, perhaps the etiology is a genetically determined hypersensitivity that should be fully investigated. [37,64] Problems of this type, especially with newly marketed medications, are continually appearing in the clinical literature.

Miscellaneous Anomalies. The large variety of inherited metabolic anomalies may be illustrated by the following random list that involved drugs, foods, and environmental chemicals.

1. Ability or inability to taste certain chemicals, e.g., methimazole, methylthiouracil, phenylthiourea, propylthiouracil, etc. [63]

2. Lack of catalase in the blood (acatalasia). Catalase is involved in ethyl alcohol metabolism and its absence may sensitize an individual to alcohol. The enzyme also converts methyl alcohol to toxic formaldehyde. Acatalasia may thus tend to protect those who ingest methanol from possible blindness. [63,192]

3. Inability to smell certain chemicals, e.g., hydrocyanic acid. [63,191]

4. Hyperthermic reaction to general anesthetics, e.g., ether, halothane, etc. Of 24 relatives of the propositus receiving anesthetics, 10 died from sudden hyperpyrexia. [189]

5. Extrapyramidal reactions to phenothiazines (21% of patients develop akathisia, 15% parkinsonism, and 2% dyskinesia). These appear to occur where there is a hereditary predisposition and different ethnic groups respond differently. [63,190,215]

6. Flare reactions to intradermal injections of certain chemicals, e.g., chymotrypsin, histamine, xanthine, xanthosine, etc. [63,216]

7. Excretion of malodorous methyl mercaptan (methanethiol) after eating asparagus. In one test, 40% were excretors and 60% were nonexcretors of this chemical which is used as an indicator in natural gas and produces the odor of skunks. The excretor character is

determined by an autosomal dominant gene.[193]

8. Excretion of a red pigment (betanin) after eating beets. About 10% of some populations are excretors. The excretor character is determined by an autosomal recessive gene.[193]

9. Jaundice and drug toxicity from deficiency of glucuronidation.[63,197]

10. The Crigler-Najjar syndrome caused by failure of the ester type of glucuronidation of bilirubin.[220]

11. Nonhemolytic familial jaundice caused by dysfunction of the glucuronyl transferase system.[63] Kernicterus produced by acetaminophen, sulfonamides, vitamin K, etc.[197,221]

12. Gout and hyperuricemia produced by chlorothiazide, mecamylamine, mercurial diuretics, pempidine, pyrazinamide, and some other drugs in predisposed patients.[63,222]

13. Diabetes caused by chlorothiazide, dihydroflumethiazide, hydrochlorothiazide, and some other drugs in patients with an inherited predisposition.[63]

14. Insulin resistance in juvenile diabetics.[177]

Other conditions caused by inherited metabolic defects are constantly being discovered. And the true causes of older diseases, such as glaucoma,[184] insulin resistance in juvenile diabetes mellitus,[177] chloromycetin toxicity in infants (failure of glucuronidation),[197] familial dysautonomia,[184] diabetes insipidus,[184] maple syrup urine disease (branched-chain keto acid decarboxylases),[179] hyperrigidity with anesthetics,[184] and optic atrophy (G6PD Worcester) are being traced to enzyme anomalies.[178]

Even a cursory review of the above pharmacogenetic problems caused by inherited anomalies immediately suggests the possibility that (1) drugs may be used to reveal incipient diseases that can be controlled while still in the subclinical stage, (2) response to medications may be altered in the presence of inherited conditions such as diabetes, glaucoma (angle-closure), glycogen storage disease, gout, hemolytic diseases, hereditary methemoglobinemia (enzymatic form), jaundice (familial nonhemolytic), lack of glucuronyl transferase, mongolism, phenylketonuria, and prophyria, (3) many severe drug reactions with unknown etiologies may eventually be traced to enzyme deficiencies, atypical enzymes, abnormal carriers, and other genetically determined anomalies and genetic predispositions that alter drug metabolism, excretion, and action, and (4) every physician who prescribes medications for many patients must expect and cannot always avoid rare, severe and occasionally fatal drug reactions because of these pathogenetic problems.[6,37,38,56,101,184,203-206]

Enzyme Induction

In 1952, Richardson reported that 3-methylcholanthrene increased the activity of the hepatic microsomal enzymes so markedly in rats that potent liver carcinogens like certain dimethyl aminoazobenzene derivates added to the diet were metabolized so rapidly they did not produce hepatomas.[123] Subsequently, other investigators at the Medical School of the University of Wisconsin noted that methylated aminoazo dyes and coplanar polycyclic hydrocarbons stimulated the rate of their own metabolic biotransformation by increasing the activity of the same enzymes.[171,172] Other investigators since then have uncovered a wide variety of drugs and other chemicals that can stimulate their own metabolism or that of certain other lipid-soluble endogenous and exogenous substances.[4,65,86]

This phenomenon, whose discovery marked the beginning of a very important era in medical research, became known as *enzyme induction*.[173] It may have harmful or beneficial effects in the patient.[174-176] Since induction is more frequently encountered in therapeutics as a form of drug interaction, it is covered in more detail in Chapter 10.

Enzyme Inhibition

Inhibition of drug metabolizing enzymes by drugs was first noted in 1954 with the metabolite of SKF-525-A (diphenylpropylacetic acid). Microsomal enzyme inhibition produces effects opposite to those of enzyme induction. It usually increases the physiological activity of drugs whose biotransformation is inhibited, because their conversion into less active metabolites is retarded or prevented. If, however, the metabolites of a given drug happen to be equally or more potent that the drug itself, then enzyme inhibition either has no effect on patient response or it decreases the expected overall activity.[18] It may under certain circumstances cause serious adverse reactions,[45] or it may be beneficial.[68]

Since enzyme inhibition is frequently encountered in therapeutics as a form of drug interaction, it is covered in more detail in Chapter 10.

Immune Reaction Phenomena

Drug-induced "autoimmune" hemolytic anemia was first authenticated in 1954 in a patient during a course of stibophen injected for schistosomiasis. This was about ten years after a previous course of treatment in that patient with the same drug. When the patient's red cells were examined during the period of his acute, intravascular, hemolytic episode, an immunological mechanism was revealed and the drug itself was identified as the antigen. It induced the formation of an antibody which, in the presence of the drug, agglutinated normal red cells and sensitized them to the antiglobulin serum. When the drug was absent, the normal red cells were not affected by the serum of the patient. Destruction of the red cells *in vivo* was apparently a secondary effect of a drug-antidrug reaction.[55]

In 1964, ten years after this first reported immune reaction to a drug, a case of agranulocytosis caused by an antibody against aminopyrine (Pyramidon) was demonstrated *in vitro*. This antibody was highly cell-specific and active against drugs containing the phenazone moiety.[226]

Similar incidents of acute intravascular hemolysis, all of which are rare, have been reported with antazoline sulfate, *p*-aminosalicylic acid, chlorpromazine, dipyrone, insecticides, isonicotinic acid hydrazide, methyldopa, penicillin (large doses), phenacetin, pyramidon, quinidine, quinine, and sulfonamides. In each event, the drug itself must be present before antibodies can be demonstrated in the patient's serum.[81,87]

The basic requirements for many other drugs to elicit a toxic immunologic response is attachment through covalent linkage of a hapten (the drug or its metabolites) to a protein or other component of the blood or a tissue. By means of this coupling mechanism, a polyvalent drug or other hapten that is not in itself antigenic, forms an antigenic complex that can induce the formation of specific antibodies against the drug or the given tissue component. Thus, an immune reaction is produced within the body when the drug is again administered.

Drugs with immunogenic capacity include alkylators like carbon tetrachloride, chloramphenicol, dimethyl sulfate, nitrogen mustards and some antineoplastics. Other drugs that produce such hypersensitivity reactions are acylators. The classic example of immunogenesis is penicillin, but aromatic hydroxylamines, drugs under the influence of ultraviolet irradiation (free radicals), phthalimides, various carcinogenic and teratogenic agents, and many other drugs may combine with the amino groups of protein, especially with the amino groups of lysine in protein.

Possibly the teratogenic effects of some drugs may be caused by related reactions between the nucleoproteins of genetic material and an acylator like phthalimide (see Fig. 8-3).

Coupling of drugs to tissue proteins may elicit severe hypersensitivity reactions and blood dyscrasias. The types of structures (Fig. 8-4) should be suspect until proven otherwise because they tend to couple readily.

When coupling occurs, the immunological system that is established with erythrocytes, globulins, tissue proteins and other body components induces attachment of antibody. This can be hazardous for the patient. If attachment of antibody to erythrocytes is followed by complement fixation the cells are

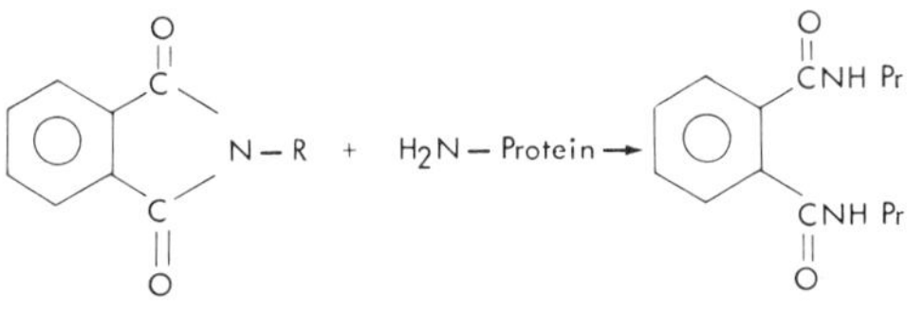

Fig. 8-3. Acylation of protein as a possible carcinogenic or teratogenic mechanism.

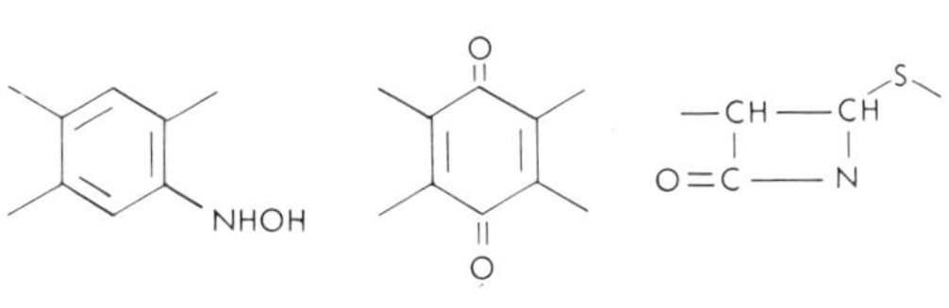

Fig. 8-4. Hapten structures that are potentially antigen-producing after coupling with protein.

lysed. Hemolysis induced by this mechanism may be very damaging, and possibly lethal.

A drug containing the quinone structure may cause hemolysis by two mechanisms. First, it may enter the G6PD cycle and cause hemolysis, particularly when the G6PD enzyme is deficient. Secondly, it may couple with protein and induce an autoimmune response in the manner described above. Any drug with this potential should be checked for irreversible coupling with protein by means of radioactive techniques.

These findings strongly suggest that simultaneous administration of a protein medication like gamma globulin and an acylating agent like penicillin should be avoided, for sensitization to both agents may be induced through linkage of the two. Also basic drugs like chloroquine, kanamycin, neomycin, polymycin, and streptomycin may form antigens through an affinity for chondroitin sulfate, DNA, nucleic acid, and high molecular weight drugs like heparin. However, drugs that bind loosely with protein in the blood apparently do not form antigens by this loose type of binding.

Immune reactions that are the basis for hemotoxic drug reactions can be detected and investigated by means of the Coombs antiglobulin test. This test is the principal *in vitro* one used for demonstrating the attachment of antibodies to erythrocytes. Some drugs mediate this attachment of antibodies or complement or both to the red cells. The mechanism of three different processes of immune injury with drugs to erythrocytes have been elucidated with this test: (1) the hapten type that results in antigamma reactions, (2) the type that results in anti-C' reactions, and (3) the α-methyldopa type that result in antigamma reactions which do not require the drug to be present in the test.[223]

Some drugs producing autoimmune hemolytic anemias generate several different autoantibodies. α-Methyldopa is a good example. Between 3 to 6 months after starting therapy with the drug, 10-30% develop red cell autoantibodies. The resulting anemia is severe enough to be overt in about 2% of the patients showing a positive antiglobulin test. The drug also develops an antinuclear factor.[169]

The severity of the hemolytic anemia produced by the above drugs is related to the amount of autoantibodies in the serum and on the red cells. A number of diseases can be attributed to this mechanism and thereby identified. However, diagnosis of various autoimmune and enzyme deficiency diseases including hypersensitivity to drugs is sometimes difficult to establish. Skin tests are often negative in spite of a definite clinical history of drug allergy, and fatal accidents occur too often. Attempts have therefore been made to develop an urgently needed *in vitro* test for drug allergy. A promising one is the lymphocytic transformation test (LTT). In immediate type allergies (anaphylactic shock, angioneurotic edema, asthma, coryza, spasmodic cough, and urticaria) as well as in delayed types, the test is nearly 100% accurate. It also agrees with patch tests in all cases of contact dermatitis.

LE Autoantibodies. The causative factor of systemic lupus erythematosus (SLE) is a group of antinuclear autoantibodies* that can be found associated with gamma globulin in blood plasma, exudates, transudates, and urine that contains protein. This is the first well documented example of antibodies to nuclear components. Diagnosis of the disease is made by finding uniquely characteristic LE cells (leukocytes with typical inclusions) in bone marrow and in the blood. The disease is demonstrated readily through the formation of LE cells when plasma from an infected person is added to a substrate of chicken or horse leukocytes (most susceptible) or dog or guinea pig leukocytes (highly susceptible). It induces a false positive test for syphilis. Some other diseases, various drug reactions, and certain fungi also induce the emergence of LE cells. Thus the LE cell phenomenon appears in individual cases of dermatitis herpetiformis, leukemia, multiple myeloma, pernicious anemia, primary amyloidosis, etc.

In addition, LE antibodies overlap those found in certain other diseases such as Hashimoto's disease, hepatitis, and rheumatoid arthritis. A DNA skin test that is reported to be highly specific has been developed, however, to differentiate between LE and rheumatoid arthritis. This test is sometimes used in

---

*The LE factor crosses the placental barrier and produces a transitory LE phenomenon in the neonate.

screening patients on drug therapy for induction of LE by medication.[80,88]

The manifestations of drug-induced LE are similar to those found in spontaneously occurring systemic lupus erythematosus. The following may occur in varying intensities: arthralgia, arthritis, connective tissue lesions in the dermis, synovial membranes and vascular system, hemolytic anemia, lymphadenopathy, muscular atrophy and weakness, pleurisy, prolonged fever, renal disease, typical erythematosus butterfly facial lesions, and ulcerations. Some of these may not occur and some may become chronic and progressive. Normal infections, severe emotional or physical stresses and sunlight may exacerbate or precipitate the disease.

A wide variety of chemically dissimilar drugs have activated the syndrome (see Table 9-9, Chapter 9). They have been divided into two classes: (1) those that precipitate a disease resembling SLE by virtue of their pharmacologic properties and (2) those that produce an allergic (immune reaction) response. In the second group are anticonvulsants, hydralazine, isoniazid, and procainamide. Some patients with hydralazine-induced LE still had clinical manifestations and a positive antinuclear factor up to 9 years after withdrawal of the drug. Between 8% and 13% of hereditarily predisposed patients are affected. Over 150 cases of hydralazine-induced LE have been reported in the literature.[217,232]

A positive antinuclear factor and LE cells have been found in 18 reported cases of LE during treatment of tuberculosis with isoniazid. Since both hydralazine and isoniazid and other drugs induced the disease most commonly in patients who are slow acetylators, there is a possibility that drug induced LE is produced only in patients who are genetically predisposed. Careful documentation of this type of drug response is essential in order to prove whether this relationship actually exists.[80,88,217,232-234]

Metabolic Stresses

Application of stresses to the body of the patient often reveals latent disease, e.g., exercise to disclose electrocardiographic evidence of myocardial ischemia, glucose loading to unmask diabetes, and stimulation of an adrenal cortex, ovary, thyroid, or other organ with its tropic hormone to pinpoint a primary deficiency or malfunction. At the molecular level, highly specific provocative tests have been devised. Thus, the lymphocyte-stimulating effect of phytohemagglutinins (PHA) is diagnostic for the carrier state of two rare genetic disorders characterized by deficiencies of specific lysosomal enzymes. In both heterozygous and homozygous carriers of the trait for Pompe's disease, a deficiency of lymphocyte lysosomal acid α-1,4-glucosidase is revealed when the enzyme levels do not rise with stimulation by PHA. This lack of response also holds true in heterozygous carriers of a new and yet unnamed genetic disease (bleeding, hypotonia, lethargy, vomiting, and death in infants) characterized by a deficiency of lysosomal acid phosphatase activity.[16]

Not only in diagnosis, but also in testing drugs, appropriate metabolic stresses must be applied. Since more stringent FDA regulations have been in effect massive overdoses must be applied to animals to determine whether the potential exists for carcinogenic, mutagenic, teratogenic, or other hazardous metabolic responses. Many drugs (and other chemicals) at doses far beyond therapeutic or normally tolerated levels will produce such deleterious effects. Nevertheless whenever such highly abnormal stresses signify that potentials for damaging effects exist, the drug cannot be marketed and drugs already on the market must be withdrawn.

Serious potential metabolic hazards exist with all physiologically active chemicals, but three questions remain unanswered. *Which animal models are suitable? Which results of chemical and physical stresses in specific animal models can be extrapolated to man? How great a stress is significant and reasonable in testing specific molecular structures?* See also Chapter 3. The significance of animal responses to severe metabolic stresses when they are extrapolated to man requires more study.[25]

Legal Implications of Anomalies

The foregoing sections briefly outline representative types of pharmacogenetic problems that require further analysis. Meanwhile, every prescribing physician will find it mandatory to consider these and similar situations in every plan of therapy. He must be aware that in any large number of patients, a few are genetically constituted so that they have a relative inability to detoxify certain drugs by means of biotransformation. Therefore, these unfortunate patients are much more likely to sustain serious adverse effects, some of which are life-threatening.

When a medication injures a patient and a lawsuit is brought against the physician, the hospital, the pharmacist, or the manufacturer, is it proper for an attorney to ask whether the patient has a rare anomaly and whether tests to detect it were made? If the patient does have an enzyme deficiency or other genetically determined anomaly that causes a sensitivity to the implicated drug, who is at fault? The patient, if he was aware of a previous drug interaction or of his inborn error of metabolism, but did not mention it to the physician? The physician, if he did not detect the inherited problem? The manufacturer, if he did not include warnings in the package circular against the known contraindications? The hospital, if the administrator did not adequately alert all the members of the staff to the problem? The resident, intern, or other member of the hospital medical staff, if he did not take the genetic defect into consideration? The hospital pharmacist, if he did not keep adequate patient medication records or check the patient's medication records for the hypersensitivity? The answers to these questions are not available. Ultimate responsibility will probably have to be determined on the merits of individual cases until enough precedents are established. Meanwhile, the legal significance of proper screening of the patient seems obvious, but in many instances adequate and reliable screening techniques are not available.

DRUG ACTION

The intensity of both beneficial and harmful effects of a drug in the patient are governed by (1) the formulation characteristics of the medication containing the drug, (2) the pharmacodynamics of the drug and the pharmacokinetics of its absorption, distribution, metabolism, and excretion, (3) the concentration of active drug at its site(s) of action, (4) the length of time the drug remains in contact with its "receptors," (5) the chemical structure and properties of the drug and their influence on the formation of the "drug-receptor complex" at the site of action, (6) the interactions of agonists, antagonists, enzyme inducers and inhibitors, and other chemicals at the same or different "receptor sites," and (7) factors that influence mechanisms of action.

The following classical mechanisms of drug action are largely based on hypothetical concepts deduced from experimental results.[230] Extensive investigation remains to be conducted to prove and improve these concepts.[164]

Mechanisms of Drug Action

Some drugs, like general anesthetics, produce their effects in the body by interacting at relatively high concentrations with tissues. But most drugs act at relatively low concentrations by selectively combining with and thereby modifying sensitive *receptors** (cell membranes, enzymes, or other cellular components) with specialized functions in intact cells. *Drug action* (modification of these cellular components) results in *drug effects* (biochemical and physiological changes) in the body that characterize the clinical utility of the drug. The intensity of the drug effects (patient response), which depends on the intensity of the drug action at the receptors, has been explained on the basis of percentage of receptors occupied, the rate of drug-receptor combination, and other mechanisms.[164] But only very dilute concentrations, usually a few mcg. per ml., are required.

Drug-receptor combinations, i.e., *drug-receptor complexes,* are formed by reversible interactions (bondings) of varying strengths between reactive groups on drug molecules and reactive chemical groups (amino, carboxyl, phosphate, sulfhydryl, etc.) known as *receptor groups* or *receptor sites* on the receptors. Only cell components that interact with drugs to produce drug effects are true *receptors.* Other groups that interact with drugs without initiating a drug reaction, such as

---

*Studies with various drugs have enabled investigators to arrive at an estimate of 1.6×10^5 receptor molecules per cell, covering about 1/5000 of the cell surface.

those that reversibly bind drugs to cell and plasma proteins and to enzymes involved in biotransformation and drug transport, are referred to as *acceptors, binding sites, secondary or silent receptors, storage sites, etc.* Binding may take place by means of firm covalent or coordinate bonds or ionic, hydrogen, or other weak bonds such as Van der Waal's forces, and possibly also through the formation of clathrates or inclusion complexes with no binding. The rate of binding and therefore intensity of effects is influenced by the percentage of reactive chemical groups on drug molecules that approach the receptor sites at the correct angle for binding. The percentage can be improved by two orders of magnitude through suitable physicochemical treatment. Dissociation constants for drugs and receptors are being determined as a means of evaluating drug action. Better models are constantly being evolved as tools useful to explain and predict drug potency, receptor selectivity, adverse effects, and efficacy. A kinetic theory of drug action has been thoroughly reviewed.[164] On the basis of rate of drug-receptor combination, the differences in rates of action and potency, and the fading response to drugs can be neatly explained.

The manner in which a drug arrives at its receptor sites has been considered with the aid of mathematical models that explain why access to the receptors is limited by diffusion and perfusion factors. The rise of concentration at receptors always lags behind that at the site of administration. But many other variables are encountered in analyzing the complex mechanisms of patient response. Flow of vascular fluids, cardiac output, volume of extracellular space, diffusion delay, uptake and inactivation by binding at silent receptor sites, and indirect modes of action are just a few of the important factors to be considered.[164]

Drugs that have affinity for and combine with receptors and thereby initiate drug actions which produce corresponding effects are termned *agonists.* They possess *efficacy* and may be fully active *(full agonists)* or somewhat less active *(partial agonists).* The effects of a full agonist and a partial agonist acting on the same effector may be additive or antagonistic. Drugs that combine with receptors more strongly than agonists, but do not initiate drug action and therefore do not have efficacy, are termed *competitive antagonists.* They enter into *competitive interactions* with other drugs through occlusion of receptor sites. The combinations with the receptors may be reversible or irreversible.

They types of receptors in the body are numerous but many of the most significant drug actions and competitive drug interactions occur at neuroeffectors.

Classification of Neuroeffectors

Neuroeffective receptors in the body may be classified as a working hypothesis according to the relative potencies of specific agonists and the effects or lack of effects of specific antagonists.

The variety and variants of the classical receptors may be large, as new ones are constantly being discovered in various species. However, for the purpose of explaining autonomic drug actions and interactions, the pertinent receptors may be subdivided on the basis of agonists and antagonists into muscarinic, nicotinic, α-adrenergic, and β-adrenergic receptors. Some investigators point out, however, that identification and nomenclature is much more natural in terms of the relevant antagonist (dibenamine, hexamethonium, hyoscine, phentolamine, propranolol, tubocurarine, etc.)

Muscarinic Receptors. These are cholinotropic receptors where acetylcholine (ACh) acts on smooth muscle, where parasympathomimetic drugs can mimic the effects of acetylcholine, and where agents like atropine can block the smooth muscle effects of cholinomimetics and ACh. Thus by blocking muscarinic responses, atropine prevents cardiac slowing and salivary secretion when cholinergic drugs stimulate the muscarinic receptors. Curare does not block the effects of ACh at these receptors.

Nicotinic Receptors. These are cholinotropic receptors where ACh acting on striated muscle mimics the effects of nicotine, and where blocking drugs like curare can block the striated muscle effects of ACh. The effects of ACh at these receptors are not blocked by atropine.

Nicotinic receptors are also present in the autonomic ganglia where ACh and related drugs initially stimulate and then block the impulses.

α-Adrenergic Receptors. These are adrenotropic receptors where epinephrine (most potent), phenylephrine, norepinephrine, and certain other catecholamines usually *excite* smooth muscle (intestinal muscle, however, is inhibited), and where α-adrenergic blocking agents such as the haloalkylamines and imidazolines (phenoxybenzamine, etc.) can block the excitation. The α-adrenergic receptors are usually excitatory. To date, the receptors identified in the salivary glands, skin and spleen are of the α variety only. But, along with β-receptors, they are found in the eye (radial muscle), blood vessels, stomach, intestines, bladder, and uterus.

β-Adrenergic Receptors. These are adrenotropic receptors where epinephrine, isoproterenol (most potent) and other catecholamines usually *inhibit* smooth muscle (the myocardium, however, is stimulated and cardiac output increased), and where β-adrenergic blocking agents like dichloroisoproterenol, pronethalol (Nethalide), and propranolol (Inderal) can block the inhibition. To date, the receptors identified in the heart and lungs are of the β variety only.

Both epinephrine and norepinephrine, the primary adrenergic neurohumoral transmitters in the body, affect both α and β adrenergic receptors. But epinephrine strongly affects the α whereas norepinephrine only weakly affects β receptors, except on cardiac β receptors. However, epinephrine relaxes the intestinal smooth muscle by acting on both types of adrenergic receptors and therefore both α- and β-adrenergic blocking agents must be used to inhibit the relaxant effect of epinephrine completely.

Additional types of receptors have been proposed, not only for the nervous system but also for metabolic actions. The following have been well established: (1) ACh is the neurohumoral transmitter of nerve impulses at all peripheral neural sites except at the terminals of most post-ganglionic sympathetic nerve fibers where norepinephrine functions, and (2) ACh and norepinephrine are the neurohumoral transmitters of cholinergic and adrenergic nerve impulses at some sites within the central nervous system. But some specific receptors in this system and the pertinent excitatory and inhibitory transmitters remain to be established.

Extremely sensitive and delicate balances exist among the neurohumors and their actions at the various effectors. Because of this, it is wise never to introduce any drug into the body unless the entire map of actions, reactions, and interactions has been clearly visualized and understood. The drug may induce effects in neurons that will make systems other than the target system vulnerable to adverse responses.

The response of patients to drugs in terms of chemical and physical reactions are poorly understood. Many *theories* have been propounded to explain drug effects, threshold response, agonist-antagonist interactions, desensitization, and other aspects of drug therapy. But we still do not know the chemical nature of receptors, precise affinity constants of agonist-receptor reactions, the stages between drug action at a receptor and the corresponding effect produced in the body, nor even the chemical structure of some drugs that are put into the body.

Until we can advance beyond empirical use of medications, beyond therapy whose action is largely based on as yet incompletely proved theories, we shall continue to treat patients many times without a truly rational basis.

DRUG EXCRETION

Both the activity and the toxicity of a drug are strongly influenced by the rate at which it and its active metabolites are excreted. In general, the more slowly they are excreted from the body, the higher the drug blood levels attained, the greater the amount of active chemical made available for receptors, and the greater the activity and toxicity induced, and vice versa. Since most unmetabolized drugs and their active metabolites are excreted in the urine, the urinary route is of major importance in determining efficacy and safety of medications. The biliary, fecal, lacrimal, mammary, perspiratory, respiratory, and salivary routes of excretion, as well as slow removal in trimmed hair and nails, shed epidermis and extracted teeth also play additional but usually minor roles. However, drugs may be extensively excreted in the feces if they are not well reabsorbed after biliary excretiion or they are not completely absorbed from oral dosage forms after ingestion.

Drugs and metabolites excreted in the bile may be largely reabsorbed in the intestines and enter into an enterohepatic cycle. Also drugs excreted in the saliva and tears are largely swallowed and thus small amounts of drug may theoretically enter into an enterosalivary or enterolacrimal cycle. Part of a drug and its metabolites may therefore be partially excreted and returned to the plasma by these cycles and gradually eliminated in the urine.

Gaseous drugs such as the general anesthetic gases and gaseous end products of metabolism such as CO_2 are eliminated via the respiratory route. The rate of elimination of volatile drugs and gaseous metabolites is governed largely by (1) the relative tensions (partial pressures) of the gas in the inspired air, in the alveoli, and in the blood flowing through the capillaries in the lungs, (2) the solubility of the drug in the blood and the tissue fluids, (3) the rate of blood flow in the alveoli and tissues, and (4) the presence of other gases.

Drugs excreted in the milk of nursing mothers can cause undesirable pharmacological effects and possibly intoxication of the neonate. Women who are receiving antidiabetic, anti-infective, antithyroid, and other potent medication that cannot be handled by immature enzyme systems, should not nurse infants. Until proven otherwise, any drug that crosses the placental barrier and is contraindicated in pregnancy should probably be suspected of being eliminated in the milk (see page 261). Specific examples include sulfonamides, analgesics, and narcotics.

Urinary excretion of drugs produces essentially the opposite effects of drug absorption from the gastrointestinal tract. Whereas increased rate of intake within therapeutic limits, tends to increase blood levels, physiological action and efficacy, increased rate of excretion tends to do the opposite. Formulation factors have an important influence on rate and extent of absorption, whereas these generally have little effect on excretion once the drug is distributed in the body.

On the other hand, the mechanisms of absorption and the many factors that control absorption are the same ones that govern excretion. Thus, electrochemical, hydrostatic, and osmotic gradients, lipid-water partition coefficients, flow rate and pressure of vascular fluids, active transport mechanisms, and other transport factors discussed on pages 250-256 control the transport of drug out of the body into the urine in much the same manner that they control the passage of drugs into the body from the gastrointestinal tract. Many of the pharmacokinetic considerations are similar. Excretion may be enhanced or decreased by suitable control of pH, blood pressure and flow, carriers, chelation, secretion, and various other factors.

Overall, four aspects of excretion must be considered: (1) glomerular filtration, (2) tubular secretion, (3) active tubular reabsorption, and (4) passive tubular reabsorption. The first two act to remove drugs and their metabolites and eliminate them in the urine. The last two tend to counteract elimination by transporting some of the excreted substances back into the body. The actual rate and extent of excretion is the net effect of these factors. [219,230,231]

Glomerular Filtration

Glomerular filtration is a physical function of the quarter billion nephrons in the kidney cortices. It involves the transport of large volumes of extracellular fluid (total ECF of 12.5 liters every 10 minutes) containing electrolytes, nutrients, and other filterable constituents including waste products from the blood into the glomerular filtrate. The filtered substances cross the lipid-containing membrane that separates the fine vasculature from the glomerular filtrate. Most of the filtered substances are readily reabsorbed from the renal tubules by passive and active transport mechanisms to maintain homeostasis of the ECF but about 1 ml. per minute of urine is not reabsorbed and is excreted.

The rate of glomerular filtration of a drug is altered by any changes in: (1) number of functioning glomeruli, (2) hydrostatic pressure within the glomerular vasculature, (3) osmotic pressure created by the nondiffusible constituents of the vascular fluid, (4) renal blood flow, (5) extent of plasma binding, and (6) back pressure from the tubules, ureters, and bladder. Thus common causes of a reduced rate of glomerular filtration are pathologic changes in the renal vascular bed, and changes in renal plasma pressure and flow induced by cardiac failure, antihypertensives, pressor agents, diuretics, etc., and various other drugs. Also drugs bound to protein do not gain access to the glomerular capsule and cannot be filtered into the urine.

Tubular Secretion

Secretion of drugs and certain other substances takes place in the proximal tubules with the aid of several active carrier-mediated processes. One major system transports acids (acetylated sulfonamides, glucuronides, penicillin, salicylic acid, thiazides, uric acid, etc.) and another transports bases (choline, histamine, quinine, tetraethylammonium, tolazoline, etc.). Other specialized systems transport amino acids, glucose, vitamins, and other drugs.

Tubular Reabsorption

Reabsorption of 99% of the glomerular filtrate by the proximal and distal tubules and Henle's loop is a passive process that maintains homeostasis (acid-base balance, volume, and composition) of the extracellular fluid. The rate of reabsorption of drugs is governed by the concentration, hydrostatic, osmotic, and pH gradients at the membrane, drug solubility, tubular fluid volume, and other active and passive transport factors.[219]

The mechanisms of excretion via the urinary system are in many respects the same as those governing absorption from the gastrointestinal tract; many of the same factors influence both the glomerular filtration and reabsorption processes. For instance, a drug in the nonionized, lipid-soluble state tends to be more rapidly reabsorbed and therefore more slowly excreted than a drug in its highly ionized, water-soluble state. Therefore, weak acids like barbiturates, phenylbutazone, salicylic acid, and sulfonamides tend to be more rapidly excreted as the urine is made more alkaline, and vice versa. Also weak bases like amphetamines, ephedrine, meperidine, and quinine tend to be more rapidly excreted as the urine is made more acid, and vice versa.[43,168]

Like gastrointestinal absorption rates, urinary excretion rates vary with the pK_a values of the drugs. The urinary excretion of strongly basic drugs like mecamylamine, tol-azoline, and the tricyclic antidepressants (Aventyl, Elavil, Pertofrane, and Tofranil) with a pK_a above 9 are not significantly decreased by alkalinizing the urine because of pH of 8 is about the maximum attainable through physiological processes. And even at pH 8 these strong bases are still ionized and readily excreted. A weaker base like meperidine with a pK_a of 8.7 is practically completely ionized only if the pH is below 6; essentially no drug is then reabsorbed and all drug filtered by the glomeruli is eliminated in the urine. On the other hand, a weak acid like sulfadiazine with a pK_a of 6.5 is less than 1% ionized at pH 1, about 24% at pH 6, and nearly all ionized at pH 8. Thus, the urine should be made definitely alkaline to facilitate excretion of the weakly acidic sulfonamides.[15,35,43,161-163]

Products being excreted in the urine must remain in solution in order to be eliminated from the body. Since pH exerts such a significant influence on solubility and rate of urinary excretion, it should be carefully controlled to avoid insoluble deposits (crystalluria) and toxic blood levels.

A sudden shift in a homeostatic indicator may create excretion problems. A severely hypertensive patient whose blood pressure is reduced with potent hypotensives may manifest a high BUN. The glomeruli that maintained a normal excretion of urea by gradually increasing pressure may not function as effectively under the reduced pressure until they adjust once again to the altered situation.

If the pH of the urine is raised too high with sodium bicarbonate, e.g., when preventing decreased urinary citrate excretion due to metabolic acidosis with a carbonic anhydrase inhibitor like acetazolamide, nephrocalocosis may occur. Precipitation of calcium phosphate is favored both by the high pH and the decreased binding of calcium in soluble citrate complexes. Hypercalciuria should be noted if present and the risk of precipitating renal calculi carefully weighed in patients receiving such therapy. When administering some drugs, factors influencing metabolic and excretory mechanisms may require carefully balancing in order to avoid undesirable complications.

Table 8-8 Medication Warnings

1. **Avoid the use of alcoholic beverages while taking this medication**—For sedatives, hypnotics, and other CNS depressant drug products such as barbiturates, certain antihistamines, and tranquilizers that are potentiated by alcohol, as well as aspirin and other drugs that produce adverse drug interactions with alcohol.

2. **Swallow these tablets whole. Do not chew them**—For tablets with enteric coatings, or those containing an irritant, dye, or other substance that should not remain in contact with the teeth and oral tissues.

3. **Do not drive a car or operate machinery if this medication makes you drowsy**—For certain analgesics, antihistamines, hypnotics, narcotics, psychochemicals, and other drugs with drowsiness as a side effect.

4. **Do not take the following while taking this medication**—For the prevention of serious drug interactions. Alcoholic beverages, aspirin, other OTC drugs, and certain foods appear frequently on these lists.

5. **Do not allow this medication to contact the skin, eyes, or clothing**—For all drugs that irritate, stain, or otherwise cause impairment or damage to dermatomucosal surfaces and the clothes.

6. **Take this medication on an empty stomach**—For certain antimicrobials and other drugs that are inhibited by, and for MAO inhibitors and other drugs that are potentiated by, certain food constituents.

7. **Do not take this medication with fruit juice**—For certain antimicrobials and other drugs that tend to be destroyed by the constituents of fruit juices.

8. **Take this medication X hour(s) before meals**—For drugs like atropine, belladonna, methylphenidate, and propantheline that require precise timing before intake of food to obtain the desired gastrointestinal effects, or for the drugs mentioned in paragraph 6 that require a specific minimum time for them to be absorbed before food can interfere.

9. **Do not take this medication with milk or milk products, but take with water or juice**—For drugs like tetracycline that are inactivated by calcium or other constituents of dairy products.

10. **Take this medication with plenty of water**—For uricosuric drugs like allopurinol to prevent formation of xanthine calculi and precipitation of urates, and for slightly soluble drugs like certain sulfonamides to prevent crystalluria.

11. **Take this medication immediately before, with, or immediately after meals**—For nauseating or irritating medications such as PAS, APC, aspirin, indomethacin, isoniazid, etc.

12. **This medication may color the urine**—For drugs like phenazopyridine that colors the urine red (suggesting bleeding) and methylene blue that colors the urine blue.

13. **Do not take this medication with antacids**—For drugs like ferrous gluconate and ferrous sulfate which form insoluble iron compounds that are poorly absorbed in the presence of alkalies.

14. **Do not take aspirin with this medication**—For drugs like coumarin anticoagulants, phenylbutazone, probenecid, and spironolactone that are known to interact adversely.

15. **Do not take mineral oil with this medication**—For drugs like dioctyl sodium sulfosuccinate and oil-soluble vitamins.

16. **Take orange juice, bananas, and other foods high in potassium while taking this medication**—For diuretics like ethacrynic acid, furosemide, and hydrochlorothiazide, and steroids like aldosterone and desoxycorticosterone that tend to cause hypokalemia.

VARIABILITY OF PATIENT RESPONSE

Even a cursory review of this chapter makes it quite clear that variability of patient response is the ultimate hazard. To some it might seem that the multiplicity of hazards cited are so overwhelming that only a fool or a foolhardy individual would ever prescribe a medication. This, of course, is not true. The prescribing of oxygen, salt, water, or certain foods may be hazardous under certain patient conditions. Oxygen can cause lung damage if it is administered in large amounts over long periods of time, and retrolental fibroplasia followed by permanent impairment of vision in premature infants if it is kept at high levels in the incubator. Salt ingestion can be very hazardous to patients with congestive heart failure and certain other conditions. Water balance is also extremely important. But no wise man could condemn their proper use. Fundamentally, each prescription is an exercise of judgment on the part of the physician based on his long training, experience, and acuminous knowledge. Every cure is a triumph of therapy; every failure a stimulus to seek further needed therapeutic modalities.

Errors Made by the Patient

When a serious adverse reaction or death is surprisingly associated with a drug that has been used safely and effectively for a relatively long period of time, detection of the exact cause may be very difficult. The possible cause may be: (1) toxicity developed through improper storage and handling, (2) adverse interaction with other medications, (3) improper selection or administration of the drug, (4) rare hypersensitivity, or (5) failure of the patient to follow directions properly.

In some studies more than half of all the patients surveyed did not comply with recommendations and directions given them by their physician. They frequently ignored or forgot instructions and thereby caused the medication to be ineffective or to create hazards for themselves. It is therefore often desirable for the patient to receive specific written instructions to reinforce the verbal ones.

The warnings in Table 8-8 with pertinent lists of foods, drugs, and other chemicals, must be heeded when they are called for in the plan of therapy. They can be printed on separate slips of paper and handed to the patient as necessary. With some medications patients should be given more than one of these warnings.

The physician often finds it necessary to determine why his patient is not responding satisfactorily to medication that has always been safe and effective in similar conditions in many other patients. He can usually rule out deficiency of the drug product itself, but he must keep the possibility in mind. Some of the reasons why the patient may respond unfavorably to sound therapy are:

1. Failure to obtain the drug prescribed (error, counterfeit product, substitution, etc.).
2. Failure to follow the dosage schedule ordered by the physician.
3. Failure to avoid interacting medications, including OTC drug products.
4. Failure to avoid interacting foods and environmental chemicals.
5. Failure to follow one or more of the other medication warnings given above.
6. Failure to take the correct amount of fluids.
7. Failure to report response to the medication completely and truthfully.
8. Failure to undertake supplementary measures as directed.
9. Placebo response.

In every plan for therapy the patient has certain inescapable responsibilities. He must carefully read the directions on the label and if he does not understand them, ask for clarification. He must follow all instructions precisely and must not omit a dose, or take too much, or too little, or take the medication too often or for longer than necessary. The patient must collect specimens of sputum, urine, etc., exactly as specified at the exact times and under the precise periods requested so that his physician can follow his progress properly. He must fast or restrict his diet as necessary and follow all other instructions meticulously.

Hazardous Responses

The information on patient response presented in this chapter demonstrates that serious adverse reactions to both prescription and nonprescription medications can be associated with virtually every organ and function of the body. Posterior subcapsular cataracts in steroid treated children,[14] blindness from betamethasone eye drops,[29] poisoning with boric acid,[46,73,139] red cell aplasia resulting from antituberculosis therapy,[48] intracranial hemorrhage with amphetamine,[49] liver injury from halothane,[52] fatal hepatitis due to indomethacin,[51,67] severe reaction from anticholinesterase eye drops,[69] hepatotoxicity and fatalities after methoxyflurane anesthesia,[70,278] hyperglycemia from trioxazine,[75] lung disease caused by various drugs,[85] teratogenic effects from various drugs,[95,96] intestinal ulceration with mefenamic acid,[97,110] fatal nephritis with phenacetin,[107] permanent deafness with ethacrynic acid,[117] allergic reactions with antimicrobials,[120,126,142,145] visual impairment with an antimalarial,[125] thrombophlebitis with oral contraceptives,[140] physical and phychological dependence with methamphetamine[141] and delayed, severe, prolonged and fatal effects from radiopaque diagnostic drugs[155] are representative examples which indicate the variety of problems with which the physician must contend. They were selected at random from current medical journals. Some of these and many other iatrogenic problems were unpredictable at the time they were first associated with a drug. This is why this type of information should be avidly sought by every physician who prescribes medications and should be widely and thoroughly disseminated as promptly as possible.

Reports on Suspected Adverse Reactions to Drugs, published on file cards by the FDA,[41] *Side Effects of Drugs*, a comprehensive review of adverse drug effects published every few years by the Excerpta Medica Foundation,[99] *Clin-Alert*, *Medical Letter*, *Drug Intelligence*, *International Pharmaceutical Abstracts*, *Clinical Abstracts* in the *American Journal of Hospital Pharmacy*, and other publications (see pages 111 to 114, are useful sources for keeping abreast of hazardous responses.

The difficult task of keeping adequately abreast of the literature on adverse reactions, however, is only one problem facing the physician who prescribes medications. He must also cope with other serious problems in controlling patient responses, such as the error made in administering medications to the patient (often beyond his control),[9,90,91,131] drug abuse and misuse,[36,72,102,149,244] and undesirable effects due to multiple drug therapy.[148,158,159] These subjects, including the impact of diet,[13,17,78,129] environmental chemicals,[83,94,98,138] adverse drug reactions and interactions, are discussed in the next two chapters under *Adverse Drug Reactions* and *Drug Interactions*.

SELECTED REFERENCES

1. Allison AC: Glucose-6-phosphate dehydrogenase deficiency in red blood cells of East Africans. *Nature* 186: 531-532 (May 14) 1960.
2. Allison AC, Clyde DF: Malaria in African children with deficient erythrocyte glucose-6-phosphate dehydrogenase. *Br Med J* 1:1346-1349 (May 13) 1961.
3. American Association of Blood Banks: Standards for a blood transfusion service. Chicago, 1966; *Med Let* 12:12 (Feb 6) 1970.
4. Anon: Drugs and light for the prevention and treatment of neo-natal jaundice. *Drug Ther Bull* 8:25-27 (Mar 27) 1970.
5. Azarnoff DL: Application of metabolic data to the evaluation of drugs. *JAMA,* 211:1691 (Mar 9) 1970.
6. Baker SBdeC, Tripod J: *Sensitization to drugs.* Proceedings of the European Society for the Study of Drug Toxicity, vol X, Amsterdam, Excerpta Medica, 1969.
7. Ballard BE: Biopharmaceutical considerations in subcutaneous and intramuscular drug administration. *J Pharm Sci* 57:357-78 (Mar) 1968.
8. Moser RH: Iatrogenic disorders. *Mil Med* 135:619-629 (Aug) 1970.
9. Barker KN: The effects of an experimental medication system on medication errors and costs. *Am J Hosp Pharm* 26:324-333 (June) 1969.
10. Berry DH: Erythrocyte enzyme deficiency anemias in children: a review. *Lancet* 86:144-8 (Mar) 1966.
11. Beutler E: Glucose-6-phosphate dehydrogenase deficiency. *Br J Haemat* 18:117-121 (Feb) 1970; *Blood* 14:103-139, 1959.
12. Beware the catheter in accident patients. *Med News-Trib* (June 5) 1970.
13. Boyd EM: Diet and drug toxicity. *Clin Toxicol* 2:423, 1969.
14. Braver DA, Richards RD, Good TA: Posterior subcapsular cataracts in steroid treated children. *Arch Opthal* 77:161-162 (Feb) 1967.
15. Brodie BB: Kinetics of absorption, distribution, excretion, and metabolism of drugs in *Pharmacologic Techniques in Drug Evaluation,* (ed.: Nodine and Siegler), Chicago, Year Book Medical Publishers, pp. 69-88, 1964.
16. Brodie BB, Hogben CAM: Some physico-chemical factors in drug action. *J Pharm Pharmacol* 9:345-380, 1957.
17. Buchner LA, Carbone G, Reisberg C, et al: Chinese restaurant syndrome. *Morbidity & Mortality Weekly Report* 19:272 (July 18) 1970.
18. Burns JJ, Conney AH: Enzyme stimulation and inhibition in the metabolism of drugs. *Proc Roy Soc Med* 58:955-960 (Nov) 1965.
19. Carson PE, et al: Enzymatic deficiency in primaquine sensitive erythrocytes. *Science* 124:484-485, 1956; Glucose-6-phosphate dehydrogenase deficiency and related disorders of the pentose phosphate pathway. *Am J Med* 41:744-761 (Nov) 1966.
20. Carswell F, Kerr MM, Hutchinson JH: Congenital goitre and hypothyroidism produced by maternal ingestion of iodides. *Lancet* 1:1241-1243 (June 13) 1970.
21. Cellular probing for genetic information. *JAMA* 213:289-290 (July 13) 1970.
22. Childs B, Zinkham WH: The genetics of primaquine sensitivity of the erythrocytes in *Biochemistry of Human Genetics* (ed., Wolstenholme GEW, O'Connor CM). New York, Little Brown, 1959.
23. Coldwell BB, Solomonraj G, Boyd EM, et al: The effect of dosage form and route of administration on the absorption and excretion of acetysalicylic acid in man. *Clin Toxicol* 2:111-126 (Mar) 1969.
24. Colwell JA, Kravitz A, Homi J, et al: The acidity of intravenous dextrose solutions. *Hosp Form Manag* 4:24-26 (Aug) 1969.
25. Comides GJ: Special problems of safety in long-term chemotherapeutics. *Safer and More Effective Drugs.* Washington, American Pharmaceutical Association, Academy of Pharmaceutical Sciences, 1968.
26. Cooney AH, Burns JJ: Factors influencing drug metabolism, *Adv Pharmacol* 1:31-58, 1962.
27. Cordes W: Experience with plasmochin in malaria. *15th Annual Report,* United Fruit Company Medical Department, pp 66-71, 1926.
28. Crawford JS, Rudofsky S: Some alterations in the pattern of drug metabolism associated with pregnancy, oral contraceptives, and the newly born. *Br J Anaesth* 38:446-454, 1966.
29. Crompton DD: Blindness from betamethasone eye drops. *Med J Australia* 2:963-964 (Nov 12) 1966.

30. Lesch M, Nyhan WL: A familial disorder of uric acid metabolism and central nervous system function. *Am J Med* 36:561-570 (Apr) 1964.

31. deLuca HF: 25-Hydroxycholecalciferol; the probable metabolically active form of vitamin D₃ *Arch Int Med* 124:442-450 (Oct) 1969.

32. Done AK: Perinatal drug hazards. *Symposium on Factors Related to the Development of Safer and More Effective Drugs,* Washington, American Pharmaceutical Association, Academy of Pharmaceutical Sciences, 1968.

33. Dreisbach RH: *Handbook of Poisoning.* Los Altos, Ca, Lange, 1974.

34. Dunlop E: Ten year review of psychotropic drugs in psychiatric practice. *Sensitization to Drugs.* Amsterdam, Excerpta Medica Foundation, 1969.

35. Effect of pH of the urine on antimicrobial therapy of urinary tract infections. *Med Let* 9:47-48 (June 16) 1967.

36. Epidemiology of drug abuse, *Lancet* 2:1114-1115 (Nov 22) 1969.

37. Evans DAP: Genetically controlled idiosyncratic reaction to drugs. *Sensitization to Drugs.* Amsterdam, Excerpta Medica Foundation, 1969.

38. Evans DAP, Clarke CA: Pharmacogenetics. *Br Med Bull* 17:234-240 (Mar) 1961.

39. Evans DAP, Manley KA, McKusick VA: Genetic control of isoniazid metabolism in man. *Br Med J* 2:485-491 (Aug 13) 1960.

40. Fincher JH: Particle size of drugs and its relationship to absorption and activity, *J Pharm Sci* 57:1825-1835 (Nov) 1968.

41. Food and Drug Administration: *Reports on Suspected Adverse Reactions to Drugs,* vol. 66-70. Washington, D.C., U.S. Department of Health, Education and Welfare, 1966-1970.

42. Frick PG, Hitzig WH, Betke K: Hemoglobin Zurick I. A new hemoglobin anomaly associated with acute hemolytic episodes with inclusion bodies after sulfonamide therapy. *Blood* 20:261-271 (Sep) 1962.

43. Garrett ER: Drug systems affecting availability and reliability of response. *J Am Pharm Assoc* NS9:110-112 (Mar) 1969.

44. Gilette JR: Biochemistry of drug oxidation and reduction of enzymes in hepatic endoplasmic reticulum. In Siegler PE, Moyer JH III: *Animal and Clinical Pharmacologic Techniques in Drug Evaluation,* Chicago, Year Book, p. 48-66, 1967.

45. Goldberg LI: Monoamine oxidase inhibitors; adverse reactions and possible mechanisms. *JAMA* 190:456-462, 1964.

46. Goldbloom RB, Goldbloom A: Boric-acid poisoning. *J Pediat* 43:631-643 (Dec) 1953.

47. Goldstein SW (editor): *Symposium on Factors Related to the Development of Safer and More Effective Drugs.* Washington, American Pharmaceutical Association, Academy of Pharmaceutical Sciences, 1968.

48. Goodman SB, Block MH: A case of red cell aplasia occurring as a result of antituberculous therapy. *Blood* 24:616-623 (Nov) 1964.

49. Goodman SJ, Becker DP: Intracranial hemorrhage associated with amphetamine abuse. *JAMA* 122:480 (Apr 20) 1970.

50. Green BA: Clinical anesthesia conference. *NYS J Med* 56:104-107 to 57:4039-4041 (Dec) 1957.

51. Guerra M: Toxicity of indomethacin. *JAMA* 200:552 (May 8) 1967.

52. Halothane and liver injury. *Med Let* 10:7-8 (Jan 26) 1968.

53. Harley JD, Mauer AM: Studies on the formation of Heinz bodies. I. Methemoglobin production and oxyhemoglobin destruction. *Blood* 16:1722-1735, 1960; II. The nature and significance of Heinz bodies. *Blood* 17:418-433, 1961.

54. Harold LC, Baldwin RA: Ecologic effects of antibiotics. *FDA Papers* 1:20-24 (Feb) 1967.

55. Harris JW: Studies on the mechanism of drug-induced hemolytic anemia. *J Lab Clin Med* 44:809-810, 1954.

56. Harris H: *Human Biochemical Genetics,* London, Cambridge University Press, 1959.

57. Harvey PW, Purnell GV, et al: Fatal case of gas gangrene associated with intramuscular injections. *Br Med J* 1:744-746 (Mar 23) 1968; intramuscular injections and gas gangrene. *Br Med J* 2:241-242 (Apr 27) 1968.

58. Hassan A, Aref GH, Kassem AS: Congenital iodide-induced goitre with hypothyroidism. *Arch Dis Child* 43:702-704 (Dec) 1968.

59. Jandl JH: The Heinz body hemolytic anemias. *Ann Intern Med* 58:702-709 (Apr) 1963.

60. Jandl JH, Hoffman JF, Weed RL, et al: Symposium on disorders of the red cell. *Am J Med* 41:657-830 (Nov) 1966.

61. Jetter WW, Hunter FT: Death from attempted abortion with a potassium permanganate douche. *N Engl J Med* 240:794-798 (May 19) 1949.

62. Jick H, Slone D, Shapiro S, Lewis GP: Clinical effects of hypnotics. *JAMA* 209:2013-2015 (Sep 29) 1969.

63. Kalow W: *Pharmacogenetics.* Philadelphia, Saunders 1962.

64. Kantor GL: Toxic epidermal necrolysis, azotemia, and death after allopurinol therapy. *JAMA* 212:478-479 (Apr 20) 1970.

65. Kater RMH, Tobon F, Iber FL: Increased rate of tolbutamide metabolism in alcoholic patients. *JAMA* 207:363-365 (Jan 13) 1969.

66. Keitt AS: Pyruvate kinase deficiency and related disorders of red cell glycolysis. *Am J Med* 41:762-785 (Nov) 1966.

67. Kelsey WM, Scaryj M: Fatal hepatitis probably due to indomethacin. *JAMA* 199:586-587 (Feb 20) 1967.

68. Kettel LJ, Hasegawa J, Kwaan HC, et al: Report of the Committee on Therapeutic Agents on the use of methotrexate in leukemia, trophoblastic neoplasms and psoriasis. *Hosp Form Manag* 3:19-22 (Jan) 1968.

69. Kinyon GE: Anticholinesterase eye drops—need for caution. *N Engl J Med* 280:53 (Jan 2) 1969.

70. Klein NC, Jeffries GH: Hepatotoxicity after methoxyflurane administration. *JAMA* 197:1037-1039 (Sep 19) 1966.

71. Kogut MD, Donnell GN, Nyhan WL, et al: Disorder of purine metabolism due to partial deficiency of hypoxanthine-guanine phosphoribosyl-transferase. *Am J Med* 48:148-161, 1970.

72. Kramer JC, Fischman VS, Littlefield, DC: Amphetamine abuse: Pattern and effects of high doses taken intravenously. *JAMA* 201:305-309 (July 31) 1967.

73. Krantz JC, Carr CJ: *The Pharmacologic Principles of Medical Practice.* ed 7, p 244. Baltimore, Williams and Wilkins, 1969.

74. Kruger-Thiemer E, Bunger P: The role of the therapeutic regime in dosage design. *Chemotherapia* 10:61-73, 129-144, 1965-66.

75. Krumholz WV, Chipps HI, Merlis S: Clinical effects of trioxazine, with a case report of hyperglycemia as a side effect. *J Clin Pharmacol* 7:108-110 (Mar-Apr) 1967.

76. Seegmiller JE, Rosenblum FM, Kelley WN: Enzyme defect associated with a sex-linked human neurological disorder and excessive purine synthesis. *Science* 155:1682-1684 (Mar) 1967.

77. Kutt H, Wolk M, Scherman R, *et al:* Insufficient parahydroxylation as a cause of diphenylhydantoin toxicity. *Neurol* 14:542-548, 1964.

78. Kwok RHM: Chinese restaurant syndrome. *N Eng J Med* 278:796 (Apr 4) 1968.

79. Lane JM, Ruben FL, Abrutyn E, Millar JD: Deaths attributable to smallpox vaccination 1959 to 1966, and 1968. *JAMA* 212:441-444 (Apr 20) 1970.

80. Lee SL, Rivero I, Siegel M: Activation of systemic lupus erythematosus by drugs. *Arch Int Med* 117:620-626, 1966.

81. Parker CW: Drug reactions in *Immunological Diseases* (eds., Santer M, Alexander HL), Boston, Little Brown, 1965.

82. Levine RR: Factors affecting gastrointestinal absorption of drugs. *Am J Dig Dis* 15:171-188 (Feb) 1970.

83. Lijinsky W, Epstein SS: Nitrosamines as environmental carcinogens. *Nature* 225:21-23 (Jan 3) 1970.

84. Lithium for manic-depressive states. *Med Let* 12:10-12 (Feb 6) 1970.

85. Lung disease caused by drugs. *Br Med J* 3:729-730 (Sep 27) 1969.

86. MacDonald MG, Robinson DS, Sylwester D, Jaffe JJ: The effects of phenobarbital, chloral betaine, and glutethimide administration on warfarin plasma levels and hypoprothrombinemic responses in man. *Clin Pharm Therap* 10:80-84 (Jan Feb) 1969.

87. MacGibbon BH, Longbridge LW, Howihane DO, *et al:* Autoimmune hemolytic anemia with acute renal failure due to phenacetin and *p*-aminosalicylic acid. *Lancet* 1:7-10 (Jan 2) 1970.

88. Mackay IR, Cowling DC, Hurley TH: Drug-induced autoimmune disease: hemolytic anemia and lupus cells after treatment with methyldopa. *Med J Austral* 2:1047 (Dec 7) 1968.

89. Marks PA, Banks J: Drug-induced hemolytic anemias associated with glucose-6-phosphate dehydrogenase deficiency: a genetically heterogenous trait. *Ann NY Acad Sci* 123:198-206 (Mar 12) 1965.

90. Martin EW: *Dispensing of Medication.* Easton, Pa. Mack Publishing, 1971.

91. ———: *Techniques of Medication.* Philadelphia, Lippincott, 1969.

92. Martin MM, Rento RD: Iodide goiter with hypothyroidism in 2 newborn infants. *J Pediat* 61:94-99 (Jan) 1962.

93. McArthur JN, Smith MJH: The determination of the binding of salicylate to serum proteins. *J Pharm Pharmacol* 21:589-594, 1969.

94. McCutcheon RS: Poisoning. *Pharm. Index* 11:4-8 (Nov) 1969.

95. ———: Teratogenic drugs. *Pharm Index* 11:5-8 (Sep) 1969.

96. Meadow SR: Anticonvulsant drugs and congenital abnormalities. Lancet 2:1296 (Dec 14) 1968.

97. Mefenamic acid (Ponstel). *Med Let* 9:77-78 (Oct 6) 1967.

98. Meier H: Effects of carbon tetrachloride on microsomal enzymes. *Experimental Pharmacogenetics.* New York, Academic Press, 1963.

99. Meyler L, Excerpta Medica Foundation, *et al: Side Effects of Drugs.* vol 1 to 5, The Hague, Mouton and Co., 1966.

100. Proceedings of the seminars on the Lesch-Nyhan syndrome. *Fed Proc* 27:1019-1112 (July-Aug) 1968.

101. Miller SE: *A Textbook of Clinical Pathology.* Baltimore, Williams and Wilkins, 1966.

102. Milman DH: Marihuana psychosis. *JAMA* 210:2397-2398 (Dec 29) 1969.

103. Milne MD: Influence of acid-base balance on efficacy and toxicity of drugs. *Proc Roy Soc Med* 58:961-963.

104. Mitchison DA: Estimating drug-dosage regimens. *Lancet* 2:1069-1070 (Nov 15) 1969.

105. Modell W: Hazards of new drugs. *Science* 139:1180-1185 (Mar 22) 1963.

106. Montserrat-Eteve S: The importance of drug-patient relation in prediction of therapeutic response. *The Present Status of Psychotropic Drugs.* Amsterdam, Excerpta Medica Foundation, 1969.

107. Moolten, SE, Smith LB: Fatal nephritis in chronic phenacetin poisoning. *Am J Med* 28:127:134 (Jan) 1960.

108. Morgan NR, Waugh TR, Boback MD: Volkmann's ischemic contracture after intra-arterial injection of secobarbital. *JAMA* 212:476-478 (Apr 20) 1970.

109. Morris RW: Coagulants and anticoagulants. *Pharm Index* 12:5-8 (Jan) 1970.

110. ———: Trends in centrally acting drugs. *Pharm Index* 11:5-12 (May), 4-8 (June), 4-7 (July) 1969.

111. Motulsky AG: The genetics of abnormal drug responses. *Ann NY Acad Sci* 123:167-177 (Mar 12) 1965.

112. Murray IPC, Stewart RDH: Iodide goitre. *Lancet* 1:922-926 (Apr 29) 1967.

113. O'Rielly RA, Aggeler PM, Hoag MS, *et al:* Hereditary transmission of exceptional resistance to coumarin anticoagulant drugs: the first reported kindred. *N Eng J Med* 27:809, 1964.

114. Package insert (official brochure).

115. Pellissier NA, Burgee SL: Guide to Incompatibilities. *Hosp Pharm* 3:15-32 (Jan) 1968.

116. Petrakis NL, Wiesenfeld SL, Sams BJ, *et al:* Prevalence of sickle-cell trait and glucose-6-phosphate dehydrogenase deficiency. *N Engl J Med* 282:767-770 (Apr 2) 1970.

117. Pillay VKG, Schwartz FD, Aimi K, *et al:* Transient and permanent deafness following treatment with ethacrynic acid in renal failure. *Lancet* 1:77–79 (Jan 11) 1969.

118. Prankard TAJ: Hemolytic effects of drugs and chemical agents. *Clin Pharmacol Ther* 4:334–350, 1963.

119. Prescott LF: Pharmacokinetic drug interactions. *Lancet* 2:1239–1243 (Dec 6) 1969.

120. Principal toxic, allergic, and other adverse effects of antimicrobial drugs. *Med Let* 10:73–76 (Sep 20) 1968.

121. Brodie BB, Erdos EG (eds): Proceedings of the First International Pharmacological Meeting. vol 6. *Metabolic Factors Controlling Duration of Drug Action.* 1962.

122. Rall DP, Zubrod CG: Mechanisms of drug absorption and excretion. *Ann Rev Pharmacol* 2:109–128, 1962.

123. Richarson HL, Stier AR, Boreva-Nachtnebel E: Liver tumor inhibition and adrenal histologic responses in rats to which 3'-methyl-4-dimethylaminoazobenzene and 20-methylcholanthrene were simultaneously administered. *Cancer Res* 12:356–361, 1952.

124. Rosenstein S, Lamy PP: Some aspects of polymorphism. *Am J Hosp Pharm* 26:598–601 (Oct) 1969.

125. Rothermich NO: Visual impairment from antimalarial drug. (Comments by Lazarus RJ). *N Engl J Med* 275:1383 (Dec 15) 1966.

126. Sanders DY: Rash associated with ampicillin in infectious mononucleosis. *Clin Pediat* 8:47–48 (Jan) 1969.

127. Schanker LS: Mechanisms of drug absorption and distribution. *Ann Rev Pharmacol* 1:29–44, 1961.

128. ———: Passage of drugs across body membranes. *Pharmacol Rev* 14:501–530, 1962.

129. Schaumberg HH, Byck R, Gerstl R, *et al:* Monosodium L-glutamate; its pharmacology and role in the chinese restaurant syndrome. *Science* 163:826–828 (Feb 21) 1969.

130. Scheindlin S: Aspects of current parenteral formulation. *Bull Parent Drug Assoc* 24:31–39 (Jan–Feb) 1970.

131. Schimmel EM: The hazards of hospitalization. *Ann Intern Med* 60:100–110, 1964.

132. Schou J: Absorption of drugs from subcutaneous connective tissue. *Pharmacol Rev* 13:441–464, 1961.

133. Schou M, Amdisen A, Jensen SE, *et al:* Occurrence of goiter during lithium treatment. *Br Med J* 3:710–713 (Sep 21) 1968.

134. Sellers EM, Koch-Weser J: Protein binding and vascular activity of diazoxide. *N Engl J Med* 281:1141–1145 (Nov 20) 1969.

135. Shahidi NT: Acetophenetidin sensitivity. *Am J Dis Child* 113:81–82 (Jan) 1967.

136. Shapiro S, Glon D, Lewis GP, *et al:* Clinical effects of hypnotics. *JAMA* 209:2016–2020 (Sep 29) 1969.

137. Shirkey HC: Therapeutic reliability of variously manufactured drugs: generic-therapeutic equivalence. *J Pediat* 76:774–776 (May) 1970.

138. Shults WT, Fountain EN: Methanethiol poisoning. *JAMA* 211:2153–2154 (Mar 30) 1970.

139. Skipworth GB, Goldstein N, McBride WP: Boric acid intoxication from "medicated talcum powder." *Arch Derm* 95:83–86 (Jan) 1967.

140. Slugglet J, Lawson JP: Side effects of oral contraceptives. *Lancet* 2:612 (Sep 16) 1965.

141. Smith DE: Physical vs. psychological dependence and tolerance in high-dose methamphetamine abuse. *Clin Toxicol* 2:99–103 (Mar) 1969.

142. Smith JW, Johnson JE, III, Cluff LE: Studies on the epidemiology of adverse drug reactions: II. An evaluation of penicillin allergy. *N Engl J Med* 274:998–1002 (May 5) 1966.

143. Smith JW, Seidl LG, Cluff LE: Studies on the epidemiology of adverse drug reactions: V. Clinical factors influencing susceptibility. *Ann Int Med* 65:629–640, 1966.

144. Sollmann T: *Pharmacology,* p. 366. Philadelphia, Saunders, 1957.

145. Stewart GT: Allergenic residues in penicillins. *Lancet* 1:1177–1183 (June 3) 1967.

146. Stewart WC, Madill HD, Dyer AM: Night vision in the miotic eye. *Can Med Assoc J* 99:1145 (Dec 14) 1968.

147. Stuckey WJ, Jr: Hemolytic anemia and erythrocyte glucose-6-phosphate dehydrogenase deficiency. *Am J Med Sci* 251:104–115 (Jan) 1966.

148. Symposium on iatrogeny. *J Einstein Med Cent* 7:229–300 (Oct) 1959.

149. Talbott JA, Teague JW: Marihuana psychosis. *JAMA* 210:299–302 (Oct 13) 1969.

150. Tarlov AR, Brewer GJ, Carson PE, *et al:* Primaquine sensitivity. Glucose-6-phosphate dehydrogenase deficiency: an inborn error of metabolism of medical and biological significance. *Arch Int Med* 109:209–234, 1962.

151. Teorell T: General physico-chemical aspects of drug distribution. In Raspé G (ed): *Schering Workshop on Pharmacokinetics,* Berlin (May 8–9, 1969), Advances in Biosciences 5, Braunschweig, Germany, Vieweg & Sohn, 1970.

152. The choice of therapy in the treatment of cancer. *Med Let* 12:13–20 (Feb 20) 1970.

153. Thiabendazole (mintezol)—a new anthelmintic. *Med Let* 9:99–100 (Dec 15) 1967.

154. Thompson RHS, Wooton IDP: *Biochemical Disorders in Human Disease.* New York, Academic Press, 1970.

155. Thorotrast. *Clin-Alert* No 54 and 77, 1963; 59 and 181, 1964; 257, 1965; 160 and 188, 1966; 58, 1967; 146 and 173, 1968.

156. Valentine WN, Franaka KR, Miwa S: A specific erythrocyte glycolytic enzyme defect (pyruvate-kinase) in three subjects with congenital nonspherocytic hemolytic anemia. *Fr A Am Physicians* 74:100, 1961.

157. Valentine WN, Oski FA, Paglia DE, *et al:* Hereditary hemolytic anemia with hexokinase deficiency. *N Engl J Med* 276:1–11 (Jan 5) 1967.

158. van Dam EE, Overkamp M, Haanen C: The interaction of drugs. *Lancet* 2:1027 (Nov 5) 1966.

159. Vere DW: Errors of complex prescribing. *Lancet* 1:37–373 (Feb 13) 1965.

160. Vogler WR, Huguley CM, Jr, Kerr W: Toxicity and antitumor effect of divided doses of methotrexate. *Arch Int Med* 115:285–293 (Mar) 1965.

161. Wagner JG: Biopharmaceutics: absorption aspects. *J Pharm Sci* 50:359–386 (May) 1961.

162. Wagner JG: *Biopharmaceutics & Relevant Pharma-*

cokinetics. Drug Intelligence Publications, Hamilton, IL, 1971.

163. Wagner JG: *Fundamentals of Clinical Pharmacokinetics.* Drug Intelligence Publications, Hamilton, IL, 1975.

164. Waud DR: Pharmacological receptors. *Pharmacol Rev* 20:49-88, 1968.

165. Webster SH, Liljegren EJ, Zimmer DJ: Heinz body formation by certain chemical agents. *J Pharmacol Exp Ther* 95:201-211, 1949.

166. Whittaker M: Genetic aspects of succinycholine sensitivity. *Anesthesiol* 32:143-150 (Feb) 1970.

167. Winterstein H: The actions of substances introduced into the cerebrospinal fluid and the problem of intracranial chemoreceptors. *Pharmacol Rev* 13:71-107, 1961.

168. Worden AN, Harper KH: Oral toxicity as influenced by method of administration. In *Some Factors Influencing Drug Toxicity.* Amsterdam, Excerpta Medica Foundation, 1964.

169. Worllege SM: Drug-induced hemolytic anemia with an immunological mechanism. In *Sensitization to Drugs,* pp. 19-26. Amsterdam, Excerpta Medica Foundation, 1969.

170. Zucker P, Simon G: Prolonged symptomatic neonatal hypoglycemia associated with maternal chlorpropamide therapy. *Pediat* 42:824 (Nov) 1968.

171. Brown RR, Miller JA, Miller EC: The metabolism of methylated aminoazo dyes. *J Biol Chem* 209:211-222, 1954.

172. Conney AH, Miller EC, Miller JA: The metabolism of methylated aminoazo dyes. *Cancer Res* 16:450-459, 1956.

173. Conney AH: Pharmacological implications of microsomal enzyme induction. *Pharmacol Rev* 19:317-366, 1967.

174. Crigler JF, Gold NI: Sodium phenobarbital-induced decrease in serum bilirubin in an infant with congenital nonhemolytic jaundice and kernicterus. *J Clin Invest* 45:998-999, 1966.

175. Bledsoe T, Island DP, Ney RL, *et al:* An effect of o,p'-DDD on the extraadrenal metabolism of cortisol in man. *J Clin Endocrinol* 24:1303-1311 (Dec) 1964.

176. Kupfer D: Enzyme induction by drugs. *Bio Science* 20:705-709 (June 15) 1970.

177. Faulk W P, Tomsovic EJ, Fudenberg HH: Insulin resistance in juvenile diabetes mellitus. *Am J Med* 49:133-139 (July) 1970.

178. Snyder LM, Necheles TF, Reddy W J, *et al:* G-6-PD Worcester; a new variant, associated with X-linked optic atrophy. *Am J Med* 49:125-132 (July) 1970.

179. Schulman JD, Lustberg TJ, Kennedy JL, *et al:* A new variant of maple syrup urine disease (branched chain ketoaciduria). *Am J Med* 49: 118-124 (July) 1970.

180. Bourne JG, Collier HOJ, Somers, GF, *et al:* Succinyl-choline (succinylcholine). Muscle relaxant of short action. *Lancet* 1:1225-1229 (June 21) 1952.

181. Kalow W, Genest K: A method for the detection of atypical forms of human serum cholinesterase. Determination of dibucaine numbers. *Can J Biochem* 35:339-346, 1957.

182. Perry HM, Sakamoto A, a Tan, EM: Relationship of acetylating enzyme to hydralazine toxicity. *Proc Centr Soc Clin Res* 40:81, 1967.

183. Knox WE, Auerbach VH, Lin ECC: Metabolic adaptations. *Physiol Rev* 36:225-227 (Apr) 1956.

184. La Du BN, Kalow W (ed): Pharmacogenetics. *Ann NY Acad Sci* 155:2, 691-1001 (July 31) 1968.

185. Hughes HB, Biehl JP, *et al:* Metabolism of isoniazid in man as related to the occurrence of peripheral neuritis. *Am Rev Tuberc* 70:266-273, 1954.

186. Bönicke R, Reif W: Enzymatische inaktivierung von isonikotinsäurehydrazid im menschlichen und tierischen organismus. *Arch Exp Path Pharmakol* 220:321, 1953.

187. Albright F, Butler AM, Bloomberg E: Rickets resistant to vitamin D therapy. *Am J Dis Child* 54:529-547, 1937.

188. Fraser D: Hypophosphatasia. *Am J Med* 22:730-746, 1957.

189. Denborough MA, Lovell RRH: Anaesthetic deaths in a family. *Lancet* 2:45 (July 2) 1960.

190. World Health Organization: Some differences in the effects of and needs for psychotropic drugs in different cultures. *Tech Rep Ser* 152:46-48, 1958.

191. Kalmus H, Hubbard SJ: *The Chemical Senses in Health and Disease.* Springfield, Ill, Charles C Thomas, 1960, p. 61.

192. Stanbury JB, Wyngaarden JB, Frederickson DS: Acatalasia. In Wyngaarden JB, Frederickson DS (ed.): *The Metabolic Basis of Inherited Disease* New York, McGraw-Hill 1966, pp. 1343, 1355.

193. Allison AC, McWhirter KG: Two unifactorial characters for which man is polymorphic. *Nature* 178:748-749 (Oct 6) 1956.

194. Armstrong AR, Peart HE: A comparison between the behavior of Eskimos and non-Eskimos to the administration of isoniazed. *Am Rev Resp Dis* 81:588-594, 1960.

195. Harris HW, Knight RA, Selin MJ: Comparison of isoniazid concentrations in the blood of people of Japanese and European descent. *Am Rev Tuberc* 78:944-1438, 1958.

196. Mitchell RS, Bell JC, Riemensnider DK: Further observations with isoniazid inactivation tests. Washington D.C., Veterans Administration, 19th Conference. *Chemother Tuberc Trans* 19:62, 1960.

197. Weiss CF, Glazko J, Weston JK: Chloramphenicol in the newborn infant: a physiologic explanation of its toxicity when given in excessive doses. *N Engl J Med* 262:787-794 (Apr 21) 1960.

198. Pauling L, Itano HA, Singer SJ, Wells IC: Sickle cell anemia, a molecular disease. *Science* 110:543-548 (Nov 25) 1949.

199. Rigas DA, Koler RD, Osgood EE: Hemoglobin H. *J Lab Clin Med* 47:51-64 (Jan) 1956.

200. Jones RT, Schroeder WA, Balog JE, *et al:* Gross structure of hemoglobin H. *J Am Chem Soc* 81:3161 (June 20) 1959.

201. Garrod AE: The Croonian lectures on inborn errors of metabolism. *Lancet* 2:1, 73, 142, 214, 1908.

202. McKusick VA: Mechanisms in the genetic diseases of man. *Am J Med* 22:676-686 (May) 1957.

203. Knox WE, Hsia Dy-y: Pathogenetic problems in phenylketonuria. *Am J Med* 22:687-702 (May) 1957.

204. Holzel A, Komrower GM, Schwarz V: Galactosemia. *Am J Med* 22:703-711 (May) 1957.
205. Stanbury JB, McGirr EM: Sporadic or non-endemic familial cretinism with goiter. *Am J Med* 22:712-723 (May) 1957.
206. Prankerd TAJ: Inborn errors of metabolism of red cells of congenital hemolytic anemias. *Am J Med* 22:724-729 (May) 1957.
207. Chloramphenicol-induced bone marrow suppression. *JAMA* 213:1183-1184 (Aug 17) 1970.
208. Editorial: Intravenous additives, polypharmacy and patient safety. *Drug Intell* 2:143 (June) 1968.
209. Autian, J: Interaction between medicaments and plastics. *J Mondial Pharm* pp. 316-341 (Oct-Dec) 1966.
210. Physician's liability for drug reactions. *JAMA* 213:2143-2144 (Sep 21) 1970.
211. Dunworth RD, Kenna FR: Incompatibility of medications in intravenous solutions. *Am J Hosp Pharm* 22:190-191 (Apr) 1965.
212. Jankowski JJ, Feingold M, Gellis SS: Effect of maternal ingestion of iophenoxic acid (Teridax) on protein-bound iodine: report of a family. *J Pediat* 70:436-438 (Mar) 1967.
213. Laurell CB, Eriksson S: Electrophoretic α-globulin pattern of serum in α_1-antitrypsin deficiency. *J Clin Lab Invest* 15:132-140, 1963.
214. Townley RG, Tyning F, Lynch H, *et al:* Obstructive lung disease in hereditary α-antitrypsin deficiency *JAMA* 214:325-331 (Oct 21) 1970.
215. Ayd FJ: A survey of drug-induced extrapyramidal reactions. *JAMA* 175:1054-1060 (Mar 25) 1961.
216. Kalmus H, Willoughby DA: Flare reactions to intradermal injections of xanthosine and chymotrypsin. *Heredity* 14:227, 1960.
217. Alarc-Segovia D: Drug-induced lupus syndromes. *Mayo Clin Proc* 44:664-681 (Sep) 1969.
218. Dost FH: Opening. *In Schering Workshop on Pharmacokinetics, Berlin 1969.* Advances in the Biosciences 5. Braunschweig, Germany, Vieweg & Sohn 1970.
219. Best CH, Taylor NB: *The Physiological Basis of Medical Practice,* ed. 7 Baltimore, Williams & Wilkins, 1961.
220. Childs B, Sidbury JB, Migeon CJ: Glucuronic acid conjugation by patients with familial nonhemolytic jaundice and their relatives. *Pediat* 23:903-913 (May) 1959.
221. Brown AK, Zuelzer WW: Studies on the neonatal development of the glucuronide conjugating system. *J Clin Invest* 37:332-340 (Mar)
222. Ogryzlo MA: The renal factor in the etiology of primary gout. *Can Med Assoc J* 83:1326-1327 (Dec 17) 1960.
223. Croft JD, Swisher SN, Gilliland BC, *et al:* Coombs'-test positivity induced by drugs. *Ann Int Med* 68:176-187 (Jan) 1968.
224. Ruch TC, Fulton JF: *Medical Physiology and Biophysics* ed. 18 Philadelphia, Saunders, 1960, pp. 899-902.
225. Sapeika BA: The passage of drugs across the placenta. *S Afric Med J* 34:49-55 (Jan) 1960.
226. Theirfelder von S, Magis C, Saint-Paul M, *et al:* Die Pyramidon-Agranulozytose. *Dtsch Med Wschr* 89:506 (Mar 13) 1964.
227. Ferholt JB, Stone WN: Severe delirium after abrupt withdrawal of thiothixene in a chronic schizophrenic inpatient. *J Nerv Ment Dis* 150:400-403 (May) 1970.
228. Two sisters given first therapy by genetic engineering. *Med News-Trib* 2 (No 36):1 (Sep 4) 1970.
229. Cephaloglycin (Kafocin). *Med Let* 12:81-82 (Oct 2) 1970.
230. Goodman LS, Gilman A: *The Pharmacological Basis of Therapeutics,* New York, Macmillan 1970.
231. Gladtke E: The systematic influence of elimination. *In Schering Workshop on Pharmacokinetics, Berlin 1969.* Advances in Biosciences 5. Braunschweig, Germany Vieweg & Sohn, 1970.
232. Drug-induced lupus syndromes. *Br Med J* 1:192-193 (Apr 25) 1970.
233. Hargraves MM, Richmond H, Morton R: Presentation of two bone marrow elements: the "tart" cell and the "L.E." cell. *Proc Staff Mtg Mayo Clin* 23:25-28 (Jan 2) 1948.
234. Alarcon-Segovia D, Wakim KG, Worthington JW, *et al:* Clinical and experimental studies on the hydralazine syndrome and its relationship to systemic lupus erythematosus. *Medicine* 46:1-33 (Jan) 1967.
235. Moya F, Thorndike V: Passage of drugs across the placental barrier. *Am J Obstet Gynec* 84:1779-1798 (Dec 1) 1962.
236. Bleyer WA, Au WYW, Lange WA, Sr, *et al:* Studies on the detection of adverse drug reactions in the newborn I. Fetal exposure to maternal medication. *JAMA* 213:2046-2048 (Sep 21) 1970.
237. Bleyer WA, Breckenridge RT: Studies on the detection of adverse drug reactions in the newborn II. The effects of prenatal aspirin on newborn hemostasis. *JAMA* 213:2048-2053 (Sep 21) 1970.
238. Stuart DM: Teratogenicity and teratogenic drugs, *Pharm Index* 8 (Aug) 1966.
239. Apgar V: Drugs in pregnancy. *JAMA* 190:840-841 (Nov 30) 1964.
240. Cohlan SQ: Fetal and neonatal hazards from drugs administered during pregnancy, *NY State J Med* 64:493-499 (Feb 15) 1964.
241. Skirkey HC: The innocent child. *JAMA* 196:418-421 (May 2) 1966.
242. Smart RG, Bateman K: The chromosomal and teratogenic effects of lysergic acid diethylamide. *Can Med Assoc J* 99:805-810 (Oct 26) 1968.
243. Beckman H: Drugs in the developing fetus. In *Dilemmas in Drug Therapy,* p. 140-144 Philadelphia, Saunders, 1967.
244. Nora JA, Trasler DG, Fraser FC: Malformations in mice induced by dextroamphetamine sulfate. *Lancet* 2:1021-1022 (Nov 13) 1965.
245. Gordon HR: Fetal bradycardia after paracervical block. *N Engl J Med* 279:910-914 (Oct 24) 1968.
246. Toxoplasmosis-treatment with pyrimethamine (Daraprim). *Med Let* 10:107-108 (Dec 27) 1968.
247. Weinstein L, Dalton D: Host determinants of response to antimicrobial agents. *N Engl J Med* 279:526-528 (Sep 5) 1968.
248. Grumback MM, Ducharne JR: The effects of androgens on fetal sexual development. *Fert Steril* 11:157-180 (Feb) 1960.
249. Nora JA *et al:* Dextroamphetamine teratogenicity. *Lancet* 2:1021 (Nov 13) 1965; *Clin-Alert* No. 9 (Jan 5) 1966.

250. Goldstein A, Aronson L, Kalman L: Chemical teratogensis. In *Principles of Drug Action,* pp 711-735. New York, Harper & Row, 1968.

251. Adamson K, Joelson I: The effects of pharmacological agents upon the fetus and newborn, *Am J Obstet Gynec* 96:437-460 (Oct 1) 1966.

252. Lenz W: Malformations caused by drugs in pregnancy, *Am J Dis Child* 112: (Aug) 1966.

253. Sutherland JM: Fatal cardiovascular collapse of infants receiving large amounts of chloramphenicol, *Am J Dis Child* 97:761-767 (June) 1959.

254. Weinstein L, Dalton C: Host determinants of response to antimicrobial agents, *N Engl J Med* 279:467-473 (Aug 29) 1968.

255. Warkany J, Shirkey HC: *Drugs and teratology in pediatric therapy,* pp. 148-150 St. Louis, Mosby, 1968; Warkany J: *Congenital Malformations.* Year Book, Chicago, 1971.

256. Wilkins L: Masculinization of female fetus due to orally given progestins. *JAMA* 172:1028-1032 (Mar 5) 1960.

257. Monnet P, Kalb JC, Pujol M: Toxic influence of isoniazid on fetus. *Lyon Med* 218:431-455, 1967.

258. Galina MP, Avnet ML, and Einhorn A: Iodides during pregnancy: apparent cause of neonatal death. *N Engl J Med* 267:1124-1127 (Nov 29) 1962.

259. Aaron HH, Schneirson SJ, Siegel E: Goiter in newborn infant due to mother's ingestion of propylthiouracil. *JAMA* 159:848-850 (Oct 29) 1955.

260. Rodriguez SU, Leikin SL, Hiller MC: Neonatal thrombocytopenia associated with ante-partum administration of thiazide drugs. *N Engl J Med* 270:881-884 (Apr 23) 1964.

261. Larsson Y, Sterky G: Possible teratogenic effect of tolbutamide in a pregnant prediabetic. *Lancet* 2:1424-1425 (Dec 31) 1960.

262. Cohlan SQ: Excessive intake of vitamin A as a cause of congenital anomalies in rats. *Science* 117:535-536 (May 15) 1953.

263. Cohlan SQ: Congenital anomalies in rats induced by excessive intake of vitamin A during pregnancy. *Pediatrics* 13:556-567, 1964.

264. Lucey JF, Dolan RC: Hyperbilirubinemia of newborn infants associated with parenteral administration of vitamin K analogues to mothers. *Pediatrics* 23:553-560 (March) 1959.

265. Apgar V, Cohlan SQ, Fish SA, *et al:* Should you give her that drug during pregnancy? *Patient Care* 3:84-92 (July) 1969.

266. Bartig D, Cohon MS: Excretion of drugs in human milk. *Hosp Form Manag* 4:26-27 (Apr) 1969.

267. Knowles JA: Excretion of drugs in milk—a review. *J Pediat* 66:1068-1082, 1965.

268. ———: *Pediatric Therapy,* ed. 3, pp. 175-177. St. Louis, Mosby 1968-1969.

269. Apgar V: Comparison of regional and general anesthesia in obstetrics with special reference to transmission of cyclopropane across the placenta. *JAMA* 165:2155, 1957.

270. Hapke FB, a Barnes AC: The obstetric use and effect of fetal respiration of Nisentil. *Am J Obstet Gyn* 58:799-801 (Oct) 1949.

271. Smith EJ, Nagyfy SF: A report on the comparative study of newer drugs used for obstetrical anesthesia. *Am J Obst Gyn* 58:695-702 (Oct) 1949.

272. Halasey TG, and Dille JM: Observations of 3-hydroxy-*N*-methylmorphinan hydrobromide (Dromoran) on fetal respiratory movements of the rabbit. *Proc Soc Exp Biol Med* 78:808-810, 1951.

273. Aiken RA: An account of the Birmingham "sextuplets." *J Obstet Gynaec Br Cwlth* 76:684-691 (Aug) 1969. Cameron, AH, *et al:* Septuplet conception: placental and zygosity studies. *Ibid* 76:692-698 (Aug) 1969.

274. World Health Organization: Standardization of procedures for the study of glucose-6-phosphate dehydrogenase. *Tech Rep Ser* 366:5-35, 1967.

275. Mellin GW, Katzenstein M: The saga of thalidomide. Neuropathy to embryopathy with case reports of congenital anomalies. *N Engl J Med* 267:1184-1193 (Dec 6) 1962.

276. Pasternak DP, Socolow EL, Ingbar SH: Synergistic interaction of phenazone and iodide on thyroid hormone biosynthesis in the rat. *Endocrinol* 84:769-777 (Apr) 1969.

277. Wolff J, Varrone S: The methyl xanthines—a new class of goitrogens. *Endocrinol* 85:410-414 (Sep) 1969.

278. Panner BJ, Freeman RB, Roth-Moyo LA, *et al:* Toxicity following methoxyflurane anesthesia. I. Clinical and pathological observations in two fatal cases. *JAMA* 214:86-90 (Oct 5) 1970.

279. Ravin RL: An I.V. additive program-suggested procedures. *Hosp Form Manag* 3:35-38 (Oct) 1968.

280. Williams JT, Moravec DF: Intravenous therapy. *Hosp Form Manag* 1:44 (Aug) 1966, and subsequent papers compiled into *Intravenous Therapy.* Chicago, Clissold Books, 1967.

281. Mixing drugs with intravenous infusions. *Drug Ther Bull* 8:53-56 (July 3) 1970.

282. Adding drugs to intravenous infusions. *Lancet* 2:556-557 (Sep 12) 1970.

283. Workshop on parenteral incompatibilities. *Am J Hosp Pharm* 23:596-603 (Nov) 1966.

284. Patel JA, Phillips GL: A guide to physical compatibility of intravenous drug mixtures. *Am J Hosp Pharm* 23:409-411 (Aug) 1966.

285. Meisler JM, Skolaut MW: Extemporaneous sterile compounding of intravenous additives. *Am J Hosp Pharm* 23:557-563 (Oct) 1966.

286. Gallelli JF: Stability studies of drugs used in intravenous solutions. Part 1. *Am J Hosp Pharm* 24:425-433 (Aug) 1967.

287. Parker EA: Solution additive chemical incompatibility study. *Am J Hosp Pharm* 24:434-439 (Aug) 1967.

288. Sister Mary Edward: pH—an important factor in the compatibility of additives in intravenous therapy. *Am J Hosp Pharm* 24:440-449 (Aug) 1967.

289. Fowler TJ: Some incompatibilities of intravenous admixtures. *Am J Hosp Pharm* 24:450-457 (Aug) 1967.

290. Donn R: Intravenous solution manual & incompatibility file—its use in a community hospital. *Am J Hosp Pharm* 24:459-461 (Aug) 1967.

291. Webb JW: A pH pattern for I.V. additives. *Am J Hosp Pharm* 26:31-35 (Jan); 197 (Apr); 249 (May); 23 (June); 24 (June) 1969.

292. Patterson TR, Nordstrom KA: An analysis of intravenous additive procedures on nursing units. *Am J Hosp Pharm* 25:134-137 (Mar) 1968.

293. Compatibility digest. *Am J Hosp Pharm* 26:412-413 (July); 543-544 (Sep); 653-655 (Nov) 1969; etc.

294. Burton D, Garrison T: A pharmacy admixture program for anesthesiology. *Am J Hosp Pharm* 26:588-591 (Oct) 1969.

295. Gallelli JF, MacLowery JD, Skolaut MW: Stability of antibiotics in parenteral solutions. *Am J Hosp Pharm* 26:630-635 (Nov) 1969.

296. David NM, Turco S, Sively E: A study of particulate matter in I.V. infusion fluids. *Am J Hosp Pharm* 27:822-826 (Oct) 1970.

297. Fairbanks VF, Fernandez MN: The identification of metabolic errors associated with hemolytic anemia. *JAMA* 208:316-320 (Apr 14) 1969.

298. Prescott LF, Steel RF, and Ferrier WR: The effect of particle size on the absorption of phenacetin in man. *Clin Pharmacol Ther* 11:496-504 (July-Aug) 1970.

299. Jacob JT, Plein EM: Factors affecting the dissolution rate of medicaments from tablets. *J Pharm Sci* 57:798-801 (May) 1968.

300. Marshall TR, Ling JT, Follis G, Russell M: Pharmacological incompatibility of contrast media with various drugs and agents. *Radiology* 84:536-9, 1965.

301. David TJ. Nature and etiology of the Poland anomaly. *N Engl J Med* 287:487-9 (Sep 7) 1972.

302. Carakushansky G, Neu RL, Gardner LI: Lysergide and cannabis as possible teratogens in man. *Lancet* 1:150-1 (Jan 18) 1969.

303. Hecht F, Beals RK, Lees MH, et al: Lysergic-acid-diethylamide and cannabis as possible teratogens in man. *Lancet* 2:1087 (Nov 16) 1968.

304. AMA Department of Drugs: *AMA Drug Evaluations.* Publishing Sciences Group, Inc., Littleton, MA, 1977.

305. O'Brien TE: Excretion of drugs in human milk. *Am J Hosp Pharm* 31:844-54 (Sep) 1974.

306. FDA/HEW: Sudden withdrawal of propranolol dangerous. *FDA Drug Bull* 5:6 (Apr-Jun) 1975.

307. King JC: *Guide to Parenteral Admixtures.* Cutter Laboratories Inc, St. Louis, MO, 1978.

308. FDA/HEW: Fibrinogen withdrawn from the market. *FDA Drug Bull* 8:15 (Mar-Apr) 1978.

309. FDA/HEW: Fetal alcohol syndrone. *FDA Drug Bull* 7:18 (Sep-Oct) 1977.

9 Adverse Drug Reactions

Severe, sometimes irreparable damage to the body is too often caused by both over-the-counter and prescription medications. Because of serious reactions to one or more drugs in these medications, some 8,500,000 patients were admitted to hospitals during the 1960's in the United States (on an average, 1 for every 24 individuals).* Many of these reactions persisted as incapacitating conditions or terminated fatally. Many of the patients who developed aplastic anemia, suffered from anaphylactic shock, underwent a hypertensive crisis, or otherwise reacted so adversely to a drug that they did not survive, would have lived if they had received no drug therapy.[38] A much more cautious, more sophisticated, and more thoughtful approach to medication of the patient is urgently needed to decrease the alarming incidence of iatrogenic disease that was first fully uncovered by investigators between 1964 and 1970.[3,8, 13-17,39,58,72,74,90,91]

The most serious of the drug-induced diseases cause severe handicaps, incapacitation, or death. Some, like allergic reactions, e.g., anaphylactic shock, may be practically instantaneous.[73] Others, like blood dyscrasias and nephrotoxic effects, may develop more slowly. The effects may be of short duration or prolonged, and reversible or irreversible. They may occur only after a lag period which is sometimes characteristic of the drug. The radiation effects of some drugs, for example, may be delayed for years (see page 28). Also, redistribution of certain drugs in the body may cause problems long after their withdrawal. Thus, sensitivity to respository penicillins presents a special problem.[106] Also, gradual release of a drug into the blood stream from the liver where it is stored sometimes causes problems in other organs of the body. This mechanism accounts for the delayed retinopathy that sometimes occurs with chloroquine, perhaps years after the drug has been discontinued.[87] Obviously, it is imperative that long-term, intensive coordinated studies of each type of drug-induced disease be undertaken.

Malpractice lawsuits based on severe drug reactions (ADRs, drug adverse reactions, DARs, adverse drug experiences, ADEs) due to allegedly improper prescribing and administration of medications have steadily increased in recent years. But, because no general agreement on the meaning of drug reaction terminology has been reached, legal arguments become bogged down in semantic problems and physicians and medications are often incorrectly condemned. Both medical and pharmaceutical terminology require clarification, standardization, and continual updating in order to improve legal and professional communication and thereby remove some of the iatrogenic hazards to patients and legal hazards to practitioners.

Complications in Diagnosing ADRs

Adverse drug reactions are the most difficult diagnoses that a physician makes. Most

---

*See the introduction to Chapter 1. ADR data to date are so incomplete and unrepresentative that the nature and scope of the drug experience problem still cannot be delineated with scientific accuracy. Some of the most accurate evaluations have been conducted by Nelson S. Irey, director of the Registry of Tissue Reactions to Drugs, Armed Forces Institute of Pathology, Washington, DC 20305.[326,329-31]

of the ADRs reported in the literature are really *suspected,* not proved. As the adjective implies these are working, often tentative diagnoses. Obviously, faulty statistics can therefore readily be drawn from the literature.

Another very serious complication is use of the term "drug." It is commonly applied to either a drug product or an active ingredient. But the literature attributes all ADRs that occur with a product to the "active ingredient" only. Thus, until the data published in the literature are presented in terms of both active and inactive ingredients as well as the product name this situation will always be a major complication in the epidemiology of adverse drug experiences.*

When such complications as unreliable ADR diagnosis and inconsistency of ADR terminology are added to placebo effect, inadequate ADR reporting, and poor communication no one should be surprised that adverse drug reactions and interactions are confusing and poorly understood by many practitioners. More emphasis on proper use of medications in the medical curricula is sorely needed.

In this era of chemotherapy physicians should prescribe drugs with at least the same care and criteria they use in recommending elective, necessary, or emergency surgery for a patient. They should carefully consider the benefits and hazards of taking the drug(s) and whether in the patient's particular situation it is advisable to have "chemical surgery." Only then will the problem of adverse drug reactions fall into proper focus. [324-5]

Definition of Drug Reaction

A drug reaction may be perceived through signs and symptoms or through abnormal clinical laboratory test results, and it may manifest itself as a disease or syndrome.

When a drug is administered to a human being, two types of drug actions may or may not occur: (1) *desired drug actions* which are

---

*Hidden agents (in foods, beverages, and drugs) that cause reactions have been described and lists of products containing specific drugs that produce allergic reactions are available from such sources as The Allergy Foundation of Lancaster County, Lancaster, PA 17604. [333-7] FDA's efforts in this area have been inadequate in the opinion of allergists.

the preventive, diagnostic, prognostic, or therapeutic effects primarily sought, or (2) *undesirable drug reactions* which are the effects not primarily sought. Of course, neither would result from *no action* which may be most desirable.

No drug is so precisely specific for receptors and properly potent in its effects that it is effective in exactly the desired manner in each patient to whom it is given. No drug is absolutely free of some capacity to produce unsought reactions in a certain percentage of patients. These unsought reactions may be harmful or harmless. They may even be beneficial The harmful effects (serious adverse reactions), however, are the ones that cause concern—anxiety for the patient's welfare, and apprehension lest the prescriber be involved in litigation.

Optimum medication of humans requires every physician to balance therapeutic effectiveness against possible undesirable reactions. Thus, the judgment of the physician is continually needed as he evaluates his patient on the one hand and the drug actions and reactions on the other. The most critical decision that he may be called upon to make is whether a given "reaction" is actually caused by the medication or by something else.

In attempting to cope with semantic problems arising from the term "adverse drug reactions," the Food and Drug Administration coined the term *adverse drug experiences* for *all* adverse reactions associated with any given drug therapy, i.e., those occurring during or subsequent to the administration of the given medication. Thus, all reactions that occur in a patient while he is receiving a drug, or within a certain period of time after he has stopped taking the drug, are grouped under this heading, whether they are *adverse experiences definitely caused by a drug* or *adverse experiences not definitely caused by a drug.* Mere *association* of an adverse effect with a drug does not establish a cause and effect relationship. It does not automatically justify classification of the effect as an adverse reaction induced by the drug.

Classification of Drug Reactions

Only when adverse experiences are definitely shown to be caused by a drug can they correctly be called *drug reactions*. Otherwise, they are simply adverse experiences which may be coincidental with drug therapy but not necessarily caused by it. Even if a reaction is definitely shown to be a drug reaction, it should not necessarily be called a *serious* drug reaction. This term should be reserved only for those reactions which are definitely harmful to the patient, possibly life threatening (Table 9-1); otherwise they should be called *minor* drug reactions (Table 9-2). Every drug reaction, serious or minor, can be classified as a (1) *side effect,* (2) *extension effect,* or (3) *drug interaction effect.* It may be localized or systemic.

A side effect is different pharmacodynamically from that effect primarily sought. Different pharmacologic mechanisms may be involved or different organs may be affected by the same pharmacologic mechanism. For example, an antibiotic may produce diarrhea as a secondary effect, although its primary effect is antimicrobial. The diarrhea is usually the result of a direct local irritation of the mucosa. Additional side effects such as nausea and vomiting may also be produced concurrently by the irritation. Another example is that of an anticholinergic agent administered to relieve the pain of peptic ulcer or spastic conditions of the gastrointestinal tract by means of its parasympatholytic activity. Other secondary autonomic effects such as blurring of vision, dryness of mouth, dumping

syndrome, and ataxia often cannot be avoided. Immunologic reactions (hypersensitivity) and idiosyncrasy may also be the cause of side effects of varying degrees of severity. Classification of such effects has been published by an allergist.[332]

Side effects usually occur when a drug has more than one pharmacologic action. It then may influence more than one body system, perhaps have multiple neurologic or muscular activities. Thus dextroamphetamine, used primarily as an antihyperkinetic or anorexigenic to control appetite because of its CNS stimulant properties, may cause the following

Table 9-2 Examples of Minor Drug Reactions[a]

Acidosis	Hiccup
Anorexia	Nausea
Chromatopsia	Paresthesias, mild
Cramps	Pharingitis
Diarrhea, mild	Proctitis
Dizziness	Pruritus ani
Drowsiness	Skin rash, mild
Euphoria	Stomatitis
Fatigue	Vaginitis
Fever, low grade	Vertigo
Glossitis	Vomiting
Headache	Weakness

[a] Some of these reactions may become serious adverse drug reactions if they are sufficiently intensified. A patient may be incapacitated by a very severe acidosis, emesis, headache, etc.

Table 9-1 Examples of Major Adverse Drug Reactions

Addiction (physical or psychological dependence)	Libido reduction (severe)
Allergic reactions (hypersensitivity)	Libido enhancement (severe)
Anaphylactic shock	Liver dysfunction
Atrophy of any organ or tissue	Mental depression (severe)
Blood dyscrasias (agranulocytosis, aplastic anemia, bone marrow depression, thrombocytopenia, etc.)	Mutation
	Ocular damage (blindness, etc.)
	Pancreatitis
Blood pressure changes (severe)	Paralysis
Blood sugar changes (severe)	Peripheral vascular collapse
Cancer (neoplastic disease)	Photosensitivity (severe)
Cardiopathy (arrhythmias, decompensation, etc.)	Psychoses
Coma	Resistant organisms
Convulsions	Respiratory depression
Death	Skin reactions, severe (see Table 9-10)
Encephalopathy (severe CNS involvement)	Superinfections
Exacerbation (peptic ulcer, infections, etc.)	Teratism
Hearing impairment (deafness, etc.)	Thyroid depression
Hemorrhage (severe)	Tolerance
Impairment of psychomotor activity	Ulceration
Iodism, bromism, etc.	Withdrawal symptoms (severe)
Kidney dysfunction	

Table 9-3   Categories of Adverse Drug Experiences

Adverse Experiences Caused by the Drug
  Major Adverse Drug Reactions
    Drug Interactions
    Extension Effects
      Accumulation
      Overdosage
    Side Effects
      Hypersensitivity (Allergy)
      Idiosyncrasy (Phenotype)
  Minor Adverse Drug Reactions
    Drug Interactions
    Extension Effects
      Accumulation
      Overdosage
    Side Effects
      Hypersensitivity (Allergy)
      Idiosyncrasy (Phenotype)
Adverse Experiences Not Caused by the Drug
  Effects of Concurrent Diseases
  Effects of Concomitant Medication
  Effects of Misuse of Medications
  Effects of Diet
  Effects of Incompatibilities
  Effects of Environmental Factors
  Effects of Life Style
  Faults of the Patient
  Psychogenic Effects

unwanted reactions: blood pressure elevation, diarrhea, gastrointestinal disturbances, headache, impotence, insomnia, overstimulation, restlessness, sweating, tachycardia, and tremor.

In contrast to side effect, an extension effect is the same pharmacodynamically as that effect primarily sought, but it differs in the extent of the effect produced. For example, a given dose of insulin may lower an elevated blood sugar level just enough to produce a normal level in one patient whereas the same dose in another patient with the same degree of elevation may produce severe hypoglycemia and even coma. Thus a side effect differs in the *type* of effect and an extension effect in the *degree* of effect produced.

The third type of drug reaction, drug interaction, is discussed fully in Chapter 10. Potentiation, antagonism and other modifications of activity may be involved.

Dangerous effects may result from *idiosyncrasy* (a susceptibility peculiar to a rare phenotype), *hypersensitivity* (hyper-reactivity, often antigenic), *overdosage* (too large a dose given or taken intentionally for homicidal or suicidal purposes, or given or taken in error),

or from *accumulation* in the body (prolonged half-life) because of renal failure, affinity for certain tissues, or some other reason. Table 9-3 summarizes the categories of adverse drug experiences that can occur.

Adverse experiences not caused by the primary drug being given, but sometimes attributed to it are listed in Table 9-3. One of these, misuse of medications, is creating very serious problems that are causing worldwide concern among knowledgeable health professionals. Suboptimal use of antimicrobial agents has changed the patterns of pathogenic organisms encountered in hospitals and caused the emergence of many types of resistant organisms responsible for bacillary dysentery, gonorrhea, influenza, leprosy, meningitis, septicemia, travelers' diarrhea, typhoid, and various other life-threatening diseases. This is particularly disquieting since resistance as well as virulence can be transmitted from one bacterium to another through conjugation and bacteriophages. The author of this volume has reviewed the problem of antibiotic misuse for FDA.[338-57]

Other adverse drug effects not classifiable as drug experiences are caused by the serious national problem of overuse of medications, especially of psychoactive agents. During the 1960s use of prescription drugs increased more than 50 percent and during the 1970s about 200 million prescriptions for tranquilizers alone are being dispensed each year. Many people have developed the habit of depending on these drugs instead of resolving the underlying problems. Thus 10 percent of the adult population are using the two most commonly prescribed antianxiety drugs, diazepam (Valium) and chlordiazepoxide (Librium). And 20 percent of all 2 billion prescriptions dispensed call for medications that alter behavior by affecting mental processes including, in addition to antianxiety drugs, the antidepressants, antipsychotics, and hypnotics and sedatives. These drugs have been involved in accidents with automobiles and dangerous machinery, homicides, suicides, and a long list of serious adverse drug reactions.[327-8,342]

Significance of Drug Reactions

Drug reactions (side effects, extension effects, and the effects of drug interactions) vary in significance according to their nature and the circumstances. They may be: (1) *adverse* (euphoria and sedation in taxi drivers) or *beneficial* (euphoria and sedation in cancer patients), (2) *significant* (agranulocytosis) or *insignificant* (slight drowsiness), (3) *apparent* (generalized urticaria) or *hidden* (leukopenia), (4) *severe* (coma) or *mild* (slight somnolence), (5) *acute* (acute hepatitis) or *chronic* (chronic dermatitis), (6) *immediate* (anaphylactic shock) or *delayed* (cirrhosis of the liver). These are a few examples of antonymous implications. Others can be found.

Obviously, the term "adverse" is only one of many qualifying adjectives for drug reactions. In fact, the same reaction may be either beneficial or adverse, depending on the circumstances. Nevertheless, there has been a tendency to classify all drug reactions as adverse. This approach creates unnecessary medicolegal problems and beclouds information for the physician. He needs to know which drug reactions require his special attention. If every possible drug reaction reported for each drug is listed as adverse, he is not aided very much in making professional judgments. In fact, prescribers often depend upon certain drug reactions, such as dryness of the mouth, to serve as an indicator of adequate dosage.

Minor drug reactions may serve a useful purpose by alerting the physician to the possibility of more serious impending toxicities. Thus penicillin skin rashes and urticaria have been followed by anaphylaxis, thalidomide neuritis by phocomelia, and triparanol alopecia by cataracts.

The physician should be given as much guidance as possible by up-to-date reference material as he constantly does the following: (1) balances the seriousness of possible reactions against the beneficial effects for each drug he considers, (2) compares the relative efficacy and safety of each of the available competitive medications that appear to be worthy of consideration for his patient, (3) evaluates the seriousness of the condition being treated, and (4) critically reviews the total condition of the patient. He may actually decide, for example, to have his patient face the possibility of a serious adverse reaction with a given drug if it is the only medication available for treating a life-threatening condition.

The prescribing physician realizes that he must not only understand drug reaction theory; he must also have an acute awareness of all possible effects of the medications he prescribes, and their significance. He must know how to deal with rare situations which occur perhaps once in many thousands or even millions of doses. He is then in a strong position to serve his patients as well as to forestall any lawsuits he otherwise might incur and to know his legal status. Typical examples, which show what the physician faces, include: anaphylactic death in a 24-year-old man after one throat lozenge containing benzocaine; severe hemorrhagic cardiac lesions from a therapeutic dose of Adrenalin; death due to irreversible ventricular fibrillation caused by an injection of calcium in digitalis intoxication; severe fall in blood pressure and sudden death through potentiation of a hypotensive drug with an anesthetic; and permanent severe blood dyscrasia with PAS. These are rare occurrences, but nevertheless the physician must be instantly ready to take counteractive measures against these and thousands more that are seldom seen if patients with such rare idiosyncrasies and hypersensitivities are to survive.

Criteria for Drug Reactions

The criteria which must be examined in order to establish that a drug reaction has occurred may be grouped under the headings: (1) problems of the physician, (2) environmental problems, and (3) problems with the patient.

Problems of the Physician. These are largely concerned with proper precautions and observation.

1. *Did the physician take all reasonable precautions?* Did he inquire and test the patient to determine whether he was sensitive to the drug? Did he withdraw all other medication that might interact adversely with the one he wishes to prescribe? Did he allow time for elimination of long-acting interfering medications? Did he warn the patient about taking over-the-counter medications concurrently? Did he check the diet for possible interactions—for example, cheese and beer—if he is using certain monoamine oxidase inhibitors for a depressive state? Did he carefully avoid all physical, chemical, and thera-

peutic incompatibilities? The list of such questions is very long indeed.

2. *Did the physician personally observe the adverse reactions?* Can he state, without reservation, that he personally observed the adverse drug reaction take place after he administered the implicated drug so that a definite cause-and-effect relationship was clearly established? Physicians have injected penicillin into patients who immediately suffered anaphylactic shock and died. In a case with such an instantaneous response, there can be little doubt that the drug caused the reaction. On the other hand, physicians have occasionally reversed their conclusion that a given drug had caused a certain reaction when more information became available.

3. *Did the "drug reaction" pose an immediate or potentially serious hazard?* Circumstances alter the significance of situations. For example, deep sedation as a side effect of an antihistamine used to treat an allergy in the driver of a taxicab may create a hazard for the driver and his passengers, whereas the same side effect when the drug is used to treat an allergy in a dangerous psychotic may temporarily remove a hazard for the psychotic's neighbors. In the first instance the reaction is truly an adverse one, whereas in the second situation the same reaction is actually beneficial. On the other hand, the situation may be completely reversed with lower dosage. The taxi driver may then function better under the pressure of city driving and the psychotic may go out of control and commit a crime.

Environmental Problems. These are concerned with environmental factors affecting both the patient and the drug.

1. *Are factors in the environment responsible?* Hazardous substances which come into contact with the patient can greatly alter his reaction to drug therapy. Solvent vapors, industrial fumes, and other toxic pollutants in the inhaled air or constituents of his food or items he touches can affect enzyme systems, drug receptors, or kidney, liver, and lung tissues. Unusual drug reactions (interactions) may occur as a result of simultaneous exposure to such chemicals.

2. *Was the drug properly stored?* Was it affected by exposure to sunlight or to temperatures and humidity above normal after leav-

ing the production line, perhaps during transportation, or in the pharmacy, or in the physician's office, or in the patient's home? Highly toxic products can be formed when some drugs deteriorate because of improper or prolonged storage beyond the expiration date. Perhaps the prescription was left near a heating unit or exposed to sunlight on a windowsill? Should the drug or improper storage then be blamed for the resulting adverse effects?

Problems of the Patient. These are concerned with the interaction of the patient and the drug, and with the characteristics of the patient.

1. *Did the patient receive the drug prescribed?* Substitution is always a possibility and may be permitted under certain specified circumstances. A substitute drug (another brand or a different drug entirely) may be the cause of an adverse reaction, whereas the drug originally prescribed may be blamed for the reaction. Also, medication errors occur too frequently. See page 121.

2. *Did the patient take the drug?* Serious side effects have been reported for a drug and then later it was discovered that the patient did not even take the drug being condemned. This is one reason why pharmaceutical laboratories are now developing quick tests for body fluid (urine, etc.) levels of drugs to verify that the correct drug was taken in the correct amount.

3. *Did the patient receive the proper dose?* The prescribing physician must constantly consider patient differences in absorption, distribution, metabolism, and excretion rates. Physiological mechanisms, including metabolizing enzyme systems vary with age, sex, race, and other inherent characteristics; with various temporary conditions such as diarrhea, lactation, menstruation, nausea, pregnancy, and vomiting; and with various chronic conditions such as asthma, diabetes, hypertension, kidney disease, and peptic ulcer. The physician must always consider the particular characteristics of the individual patient in prescribing the correct dose. See page 102.

4. *Did the patient receive other medication at about the same time?* Did the patient simultaneously take over-the-counter self-medication? Did the patient take medication pre-

scribed for another patient, on a layman's recommendation, or medication prescribed by another physician? Sometimes an outpatient does not reveal that several physicians are seeing him and prescribing drugs for him. In some hospitals, patients may receive an average of 14 different drugs during their stay, and some receive more than twice this number, sometimes simultaneously from different physicians. The frequency of reactions in several studies is proportional to the number of drugs administered. See page 356. When large numbers of drugs are taken, the chances of drug interactions and drug incompatibilities, particularly therapeutic incompatibilities, occurring are very high. Additive, synergistic, or potentiating effects can occur. Also various antagonizing effects can occur. See Drug Interactions, page 351. Finally, long acting medication may be carried in the body for several days and create problems with subsequent medication.

5. *Was the adverse experience a symptom of a disease?* Signs and symptoms of diseases often resemble drug reactions. Is another disease present in addition to the one being treated? If a disease is present, does it induce alterations in the action and effects of the prescribed medication?

6. *What is the sex of the patient?* Special precautions must be taken when administering drugs to females. See page 104.

7. *What is the history of the patient?* Hereditary traits may adversely affect the patient. See pages 104 and 203.

8. *What is the age of the patient?* Young children and geriatric patients tend to be more reactive than younger adults to medications. See page 102.

9. *What is the weight of the patient?* In general, the heavier the patient the larger is the dose that he can tolerate but there are exceptions to this rule. See page 104.

10. *What is the temperament of the patient?* Patients with different temperaments respond differently. See page 104.

11. *What is the race of the patient?* Different ethnic groups are known to react differently to medication. See page 104.

12. *What is the effect of heat and cold?* Some drugs may cause different responses in patients subjected to severe environmental stresses. See page 103.

13. *Did the patient have a placebo effect?* Many patients react psychosomatically to any substance taken, even if it is pharmacologically inert.

14. *Was the patient overdosed?* The adverse effects that occur when a drug is ingested or injected in large quantities by accident or with suicidal or homicidal intent cannot be truly termed an adverse drug reaction. Human error or attitude should not be a basis for condemning a drug.

Obviously, a physician thoroughly trained in clinical drug toxicology should evaluate any adverse drug reaction. Usually it is necessary to study the patient in depth, considering total drug usage, rationale for use of the medication, and overall efficacy.[8] In reporting drug reactions, physicians should simply report signs, symptoms, abnormal clinical laboratory test results, syndromes, and diseases occurring without prejudgments for the information of FDA and drug manufacturers.

Adverse Drug Reaction Information

The following two monographs provide examples of the types of information the physician requires at his finger tips. The two classes of drugs covered are widely used in the United States and they present special hazards. Unfortunately, no single reference source is available to provide the physician with complete information on all contraindications, warnings, precautions, and adverse effects of all drugs now in use. To develop such a source may be beyond the capabilities and motivation of any segment of our economy except a government agency such as FDA or a large foundation or institution with funds available for such a purpose. For this reason, the task of compiling a *United States Prescription Drug Compendium* by FDA itself or in collaboration with other suitable sponsors has encountered economic and political obstacles that have not as yet been surmounted.[55]

Barbiturates

(Amobarbital, aprobarbital, barbital, butabarbital, cyclobarbital, heptabarbital, mephobarbital, metharbital, pentobarbital, probarbital, phenobarbital, secobarbital, thiopental, vinbarbital, etc.)

Warnings—Warn patients against the operation of automobiles or machinery after receiving barbiturates parenterally (as in office procedures) or orally in doses large enough to impair reaction time and judgment.

Contraindications—Do not use in patients with known allergy or hypersensitivity to barbiturates, with a history of latent or manifest porphyria, with known previous addiction to drugs of the sedative-hypnotic group, or with severe respiratory embarrassment (status asthmaticus). Do not inject any barbiturate intravenously where there is complete absence of suitable veins.

Precautions—Barbiturates stimulate microsomal enzyme induction and thereby increase the rate of metabolism of many drugs and decrease their efficacy, e.g., decrease the anticoagulant effects of coumarin derivatives. Since barbiturates are primarily detoxified in the liver, use with caution in patients with hepatic impairment. Guard against the development of psychological dependence. Abrupt discontinuance after such dependence has been established may precipitate withdrawal symptoms, including convulsions. Withdraw gradually after prolonged or excessive use. Use barbiturates cautiously in the presence of a moderate degree of hypotension from any cause, in conditions in which the hypnotic effect may be prolonged (excessive premedication, patients with asthma, severe cardiovascular disease including peripheral circulatory failure, increased intracranial pressure, or myasthenia gravis).

Because respiratory depression and laryngospasm may develop when an overdose of a barbiturate is injected intravenously or rectally or the patient over-responds, do not administer without the ready availability of resuscitative equipment, including provision for endotracheal intubation and support of circulation. Take special care when administering barbiturates to patients with any degree of respiratory embarrassment or obstruction. Sodium thiopental injection, for example, is considered to have the same potential as an inhalation anesthetic. Therefore protect the patency of the airway at all times.

Do not use barbiturates rectally in patients who are to undergo rectal surgery or in the presence of bleeding, inflammatory, neoplastic, or ulcerative lesions of the lower bowel. A person competent in anesthetic management should be in constant attendance when barbiturates are administered rectally, because surgical anesthesia may ensue when doses ordinarily sedative are given to sensitive patients. Rectal irritation may follow rectal administration. If a rectally administered dose is evacuated, assess the effects of any retained portion before repeating the dose.

Adverse Reactions—*Habit forming. Idiosyncratic reactions* (excitement, hangover, pain) and *allergic reactions* (particularly in persons subject to angioedema, asthma, urticaria or similar conditions). *Psychological dependence. Respiratory depression. Skin rash.*

The high potential for abuse, adverse reactions, and fatalities with barbiturates when suitable substitutes are available has raised the question of their need except perhaps in epilepsy.

Coumarin Anticoagulants

(Acenocoumarin, acenocoumarol, bishydroxycoumarin, ethyl biscoumacetate, sodium warfarin)

Warnings—The anticoagulant effects of these potent drugs tend to be cumulative and prolonged. Examine the patient frequently for adverse effects and withdraw the medication immediately at the earliest sign of bleeding. Any type of bleeding episode indicates the need for critical evaluation of the patient's condition. *Treat each patient individually!* Control dosage very carefully with the aid of periodic prothrombin time determination. Clotting and bleeding times are *not* suitable guides for adjusting dosage. When giving heparin with coumarin anticoagulants bear in mind that heparin prolongs the one-stage prothrombin time. Wait for 3 to 4 hours after the last dose of heparin so that a valid prothrombin time may be obtained.

Because coumarin anticoagulants pass through the placental barrier, both mother and fetus are subject to the hazards of this type of anticoagulant therapy; fetal or neonatal hemorrhage and intrauterine death have occurred. Carefully evaluate pregnant women who are candidates for anticoagulant therapy and critically review the indications. Weigh the risk of withholding the drug (embolization, postoperative thrombophlebitis, thrombosis) against the possible hazards entailed in administering it. Since the drug appears in the mother's milk, observe the nursing infant for evidence of hypoprothrombinemia and unexpected bleeding. The newborn are particularly sensitive to anticoagulants because of vitamin K deficiency.

Exercise great caution in patients with impaired liver function, particularly those with cirrhosis or hepatitis; the return to normal prothrombin times is much delayed in such patients after discontinuance of the anticoagulant. Use these medications extremely carefully in patients with nephritis (avoid altogether in acute nephritis, particularly if there are red blood cells in the urine); with sabacute bacterial endocarditis, severe to moderate hypertension, allergic and anaphylactic disorders, menometrorrhagia, polycythemia vera, vasculitis, ulcerating or granulomatous lesions, or toxic-infectious syndromes, in debilitated or seriously ill patients, and in menstruating or pregnant women.

In hemorrhagic emergencies withdraw the anticoagulant medication, and if necessary, rapidly restore prothrombin levels by transfusing whole blood. If the prothrombin activity falls below 15% of normal, administer vitamin K as indicated. Do not use this vitamin (phytonadione, etc.) unless necessary as it complicates further anticoagulant therapy.

Contraindications—Do not use in the presence of: Blood dyscrasias (hemophilia, hypoprothrombinemia, thrombocytopenia, etc.); recent or contemplated surgery of the brain, eye, or spinal cord or where large open surfaces are produced by surgery, trauma, or ulceration; bleeding; hemorrhagic tendencies, particularly when associated with inaccessible ulcerations, active ulceration, or trauma of the gastrointestinal, genitourinary, or respiratory tracts; capillary permeability; cerebrovascular hemorrhage; aneurysms (cerebral, dissecting aorta); pericardial effusions; sabacute bacterial endocarditis; eclampsia, preeclampsia, or threatened abortion; lumbar and regional block anesthesia; polyarthritis; vitamin C or K deficiency; colitis; continuous tube drainage of stomach or intestines; diverticulitis; severe hepatic or renal disease; acute nephritis; suspected intracranial hemorrhage; visceral carcinoma; or severe hypertensions. Do not use when there is lack of patient cooperation or where laboratory facilities are inadequate.

Precautions—Prescribe with great care and have suitable laboratory facilities available for proper evaluation and control of dosage. Take care in selecting patients to insure that they will be cooperative; very carefully evaluate alcoholics and those who are emotionally unstable, psychotic, or senile.

Use with caution in debilitated and cachectic patients and in those with active tuberculosis, liver or kidney impairment or disease, moderate hypertension, severe diabetes, or a history of ulcerative diseases of the gastrointestinal tract, in those with indwelling catheters, and in those who have occupations that carry a hazard of significant physical injury. Also use with caution during menstruation and the postpartum period. Reduce the dose when necessary in patients with congestive heart failure; they often become more sensitive to the coumarin anticoagulants.

The intensity and duration of action and the probability of hemorrhage are increased by lowering the intake of vitamin K (by dieting, lowered bile output to the intestines, suppressing the vitamin K producing flora of the intestines with antimicrobials, or increasing the intake of dietary fat), since these anticoagulants act by antagonism of this vitamin; by the effects of alcoholism, fever, renal insufficiency, scurvy, and X-ray exposure; by drugs that displace the anticoagulants from protein-binding sites in the plasma (diphenylhydantoin, indomethacin, phenylbutazone, oxyphenbutazone, etc.), and by drugs that depress prothrombin formation in the liver (quinidine, quinine, salicylates, etc.). The anticoagulant action and the hemorrhagic hazard are decreased by diarrhea (reduced absorption and loss of drug in the stool), by increased intake of vitamin K, and by drugs that stimulate metabolic degradation of the anticoagulants through enhanced microsomal enzyme activity (barbiturates, phenytoin, glutethimide, griseofulvin, meprobamate, etc.). When administering or withdrawing interacting drugs adjust the dosage of the anticoagulant medication accordingly. See *Drug Interactions* (page 351).

Bleeding following oral coumarin anticoagulant therapy does not always correspond with prothrombin activity. Significant gastrointestinal or urinary tract bleeding may indicate the presence of an underlying occult lesion. Patients with congestive heart failure frequently become more sensitive to the medication. In such cases reduce the dosage appropriately.

Adverse Reactions—Deaths from drug interactions which affect metabolic enzymes or binding to plasma proteins, and from fetal hemorrhage. Hemorrhages from mucous membranes, ulcerative lesions, and wounds, hematuria, hemorrhagic necrosis of the female breast and other areas; intestinal obstruction and paralytic ileus from intramural or submucosal hemorrhage; petechial and purpuric hemorrhages, excessive uterine bleeding (menstrual flow is usually normal). Minor side effects (abdominal cramps, alopecia, diarrhea, fever, and skin rash).

Epidemiology of Adverse Drug Reactions

Several definitive epidemiologic studies of adverse drug reactions have been made in a number of hospitals. [13,15,16,39,58,74,92,93,98,121,128] In the study by Meleney and Fraser [58] at the *outpatient* clinic of the University of Florida Teaching Hospital, data were collected from 749 consecutive patients and computerized for analysis. The findings were typical. The patient population ranged in age from 16 to 78, with over half aged 50 or older and the largest number aged 60 to 69. There were 15% more women than men, and the average age of the men was slightly higher than that of the women. During the two months preceding their visit to the clinic, the patients had taken 2,730 drugs in 540 different formulations. This was an average of 3.6 drugs per patient. The number ranged up to 16, but 71 patients had taken no drugs. The number of drugs taken tended to increase with age and was higher for women (average 4.1) than for men (average 3.1). *One-third of all drugs taken were not prescribed by physicians.* [58]

The categories of drugs most frequently implicated are shown in Table 9-4. Aspirin, in the first category (CNS) accounted for nearly 19% of total drug usage. The next most frequently used, in descending order, are listed in the Table.

Of the total number of patients, 268 (36%) had experienced at least one adverse reaction from 375 of the medications taken (126 different drugs). The categories of the drugs that caused the highest percentage of adverse reactions in descending order, were anti-infectives (41.3%), central nervous system drugs (29.1%), hormones (8.3%), biologicals (4.8%), autonomics (3.5%), antihistamines (2.7%), cardiovasculars (2.4%), and electrolytic, caloric, and water balance agents (2.1%). Penicillin, in the anti-infective category, the one most frequently implicated, [73] caused by far the largest number (28%) of the adverse reactions. Next worst offenders were sulfonamides (13%), codeine (6.5%), tetanus antitoxin (5%), aspirin (3.5%), and morphine (3.5%). See Table 9-4. The true incidence of abnormalities resulting from the intensive use of immunizing biologicals still remains to be determined. [77]

The body systems most frequently affected by adverse drug reactions, according to

Table 9-4   Summary of Medication Used by Outpatients [58]

Drug Categories Used Most Frequently (% of All Drugs)	Drugs Used Most Frequently by Outpatients	ADR Drug Categories Used Most Frequently (% of Usage)*	Drugs With Highest ADR Frequencies (% of All Reactions)
CNS drugs (40.1%)	Aspirin (19%)	Anti-infectives (41.3%)	Penicillin (28%)
Gastrointestinal drugs (12.9%)	Librium	CNS drugs (29.1%)	Sulfonamides (13%)
Hormones (8.0%)	Milk of magnesia	Hormones (8.3%)	Codeine (6.5%)
Anti-infectives (7.2%)	Valium	Biologicals (4.8%)	Tetanus antitoxin (5.0%)
Antihistamines (6.3%)	Maalox	Autonomics (3.5%)	Aspirin (3.5%)
Cardiovasculars (5.1%)	Indocin	Antihistamines (2.7%)	Morphine (3.5%)
Electrolytic, caloric, water balance agents (4.4%)	Penicillin G	Cardiovasculars (2.4%)	
Vitamins (4.0%)	Phenobarbital	Electrolytic, caloric, water balance agents (2.1%)	
Autonomics (3.0%)	Tetracycline HCl	Diagnostics (1.1%)	
Others (9.0%)	Vitamin B_{12}	Others (4.7%)	

* ADR—adverse drug reaction.

Cluff's study of 714 *hospitalized patients* over a three-month period at Johns Hopkins Hospital, were the gastrointestinal (35.6%), neuromuscular (15.8%), metabolic (13%), cardiovascular (11.6%), cutaneous (10.3%), hematologic (4.8%), renal (3.4%), pulmonary (1.4%) and remaining systems (1.4%). Several systems were involved in 2.7%. About 7% of all the reactions observed were life-threatening. Cluff and his colleagues found that the categories most frequently implicated were antimicrobials and cardiovasculars (21.2%), hypnotics and sedatives (13.0%), insulin (8.9%), and antihypertensives (8.2%). The order of the drug categories undoubtedly varies from one ward, or service, or institution to another because of type of patient load, prescribing practices, and other factors.

The relative degree of hazard for nine major categories of medications in terms of frequency of fatal and nonfatal adverse effects reported per million prescriptions are shown in Table 9-5. The ratio of the fatal to the nonfatal is about 1:7.

These data, as reported to the British Committee on Safety of Drugs in 1968, provide some indication of relative hazard. But they do not indicate the actual degree of hazard because reporting of adverse drug effects is notoriously poor. Probably no more than 25% of fatal reactions and a far smaller percentage of nonfatal ones were reported to the Committee.[292] In Denmark only about 2% of adverse drug experiences are reported. A low level of reporting also appears to exist in the United States. In a recent Yale study only slightly more than 1% of ADRs were reported spontaneously.

Table 9-5   Adverse Reactions per Million Rx for Major Drug Categories[292]

Drug Categories	Fatal	Nonfatal
MAO inhibitors	10.0	67.5
Phenothiazine tranquilizers	3.4	20.7
Tricyclic antidepressants	2.4	26.0
Thiazides	1.8	8.8
Benzodiazepines	0.9	9.8
Penicillins	0.4	4.2
Antihistamines	0.3	4.9
Corticosteroids	0.3	2.2
Barbiturates	0.2	1.5

Multiple drug therapy can induce multiple medication reactions. In a Negro soldier who received a chloroquine-primaquine tablet, two types of drug reactions proceeded simultaneously. He experienced an immediate, severe hypersensitivity reaction (angioneurotic edema and urticaria) and also developed hemolytic anemia.[114]

Adverse reactions occur more frequently in whites than in blacks, in women than in men, and in persons over 50 years of age than in younger age groups. The incidence increases with an increase in the number of medications administered and in the length of time they are administered.[121] See Table 10-1.

But signs and symptoms resembling adverse drug effects are often reported by patients who are neither suffering from a clinically detectable disease nor receiving medication.[115,116] Reidenberg pointed out that if the baseline incidence of symptoms in an untreated population is not subtracted from the incidence of symptoms in the treated population, the values for incidence of side effects and drug toxicity will be too high. This error of ADR exaggeration is just as important as the opposite error of ADR understating because of missed cases.

Critical analysis by Meleney of his group of 749 out-patient records revealed that 78% of the reported adverse reactions were probably authentic but 22% were doubtful. Incidentally, only 10 of the 749 out-patients manifested an adverse drug reaction at the time of examination.[58] Also, Irey and his colleagues at the Registry of Tissue Reactions to Drugs, using rigid criteria for their first 1,200 adverse drug reaction cases, have reported that only 8% of the cases could definitely be classified as causative, 30% probable, 40% possible, 19% coincidental, and 3% not related.[118] From surveillance of adverse drug reactions during a one-year period (March 1, 1967 to Feb. 28, 1968) at the Wood Veterans Administration Center, Marquette School of Medicine, Milwaukee, Wisconsin, the investigators, using strict criteria for determining what constitutes an adverse reaction, found an incidence rate of only 1.54% (128 of 8,291 patients).[231]

Sometimes patients must tolerate severe side effects to receive the benefit of specific therapy. With thiabendazole (Mintezol), an advance in anthelmintic therapy for *Strongyloides stercoralis, Ascaris lumbricoides,* etc., 54% of the patients receiving the drug may be incapacitated for as long as 24 hours following doses of 50 mg. kg. Activities requiring mental alertness must be prohibited during such therapy.[117] The price paid by patients for drug therapy in terms of discomfort and incapacitation is sometimes high.[62,67] It can be too high and inexcusable if the therapy is excessive or irrational (see page 26).

Long-term therapy, or sometimes short-term therapy, with a toxic medication used to treat a specific disease may cause another disease. The given disease-producing medication may affect a healthy organ, but it is much more likely to injure a diseased organ or throw a subclinical or controlled state into a full blown case. Long-term systemic (and in some cases even topical) corticosteroid therapy can cause severe problems. In patients with leukemia or lymphoma it is likely to cause systemic fungus infections. It may also accelerate bone demineralization (osteoporosis) through its antianabolic effects and in prolonged high doses form subcapsular cataracts.[132] Extended broad spectrum antibiotic therapy is likely to induce candidiasis due to disruption of the normal ecologic balance of the intestinal flora.[48] Subclinical hepatic disease may be exacerbated by agents such as chlorpromazine, chlorothiazide, halothane, PAS, phenacetin, phenylbutazone, and the other drugs listed in Table 9-20, and subclinical renal disease may be exacerbated by the agents listed in Table 9-21.

Persistent use of many medications that affect the nervous systems may cause irritability and other personality changes and thereby have profound impact on the patient, his family, and his associates. Reserpine is an important cause of depression, an adverse reaction that should be promptly recognized. Anorexigenic agents, nasal decongestants, and other common medications when used in high or prolonged dosages may be the source of uncontrollable conflicts among individuals. The implications of this potential are obvious and may engender hazards that may reach far beyond the individual immediately involved.[47,129]

Types of Hazardous Drug Reactions and Their Etiologies

Drug-induced diseases include the entire spectrum of undesirable conditions that have been reported in man. They may affect any cell, tissue, organ or body system and any pharmacodynamic mechanism concerned with absorption, distribution, metabolism, pharmacologic action, or excretion of drugs. Usually they are predictable because frequently they are extensions of the known pharmacologic actions of the drug. Some are related dirctly to size and duration of dosage, whereas others are not dose-related and result from hypersensitivities and phenotypical predispositions. They are at times bizarre, and may have unexpected repercussions.[122] Possibly the characteristics of the human race, in adapting to potent drug therapy, may have been modified through alteration of genetic material. But, even though side effects may not be harmful biologically, still, cosmetic effects such as achromotrichia, pigmentation of the skin or teeth, or depigmentation of areas of the skin, may be psychologically damaging.

Drugs can be lethal when improperly used. Even when properly used, many drugs have a low but definite mortality incidence or very severe sequelae. Examples can be found throughout the literature. A mortality rate of 1 in 25,000 is found with intravenous pyelography, which is considered to be a safe procedure.[244] Amputations of segments of gangrenous limbs have been necessary subsequent to intra-arterial injection of thiopental.[244] One in 5,000 to 1 in 100,000.[323] patients receiving halothane anesthesia, depending on the type of operation, die from massive hepatic necrosis. Since this anesthetic may be a sensitizing agent or hepatotoxin in some patients, any one experiencing an unexplained sudden temperature elevation in the immediate post-operative period should not receive the drug again.[229,323]

Adverse drug reactions frequently mimic respiratory, dermatologic, and other diseases. *Thus a "disease" may be diagnosed and treated with medications without recognizing the fact that the disease was drug-induced and that instead of giving more drugs it was only necessary to withdraw all medications and per-*

mit the body to reverse the pathologic condition.

The most hazardous adverse effects of medications are briefly discussed below in alphabetical order: addiction, blood dyscrasias, carcinogenicity, cardiovascular toxicity, congenital anomalies, dermatomucosal toxicity, diabetogenicity, gastrointestinal toxicity, hepatotoxicity, nephrotoxicity, neurotoxicity including oculotoxicity and ototoxicity, and finally pulmonary toxicity. In any attempt to classify adverse effects there is always considerable overlap because few drugs affect any single body system. This is evident in the following categories.

Addiction. Patients may become more or less strongly habituated to a wide variety of drugs. The abuse of alcohol, amphetamines, barbiturates, narcotics, and psychochemicals is widely recognized.[66,159,160] In the United States there are more than 400,000 known heroin addicts, half of them in New York City, and as many as 80 million Americans have tried marijuana, according to 1977 estimates. During 1970 in New York alone, more than 1,100 persons died from narcotic-related causes, a large percentage under 20 years of age, and 5 of these were only 14 years old. Deaths from drug use have been reported for children much younger even than the teens. In all ages, females outnumber the males. Half of the addicts started drug-taking with stimulants, 25% with marijuana, and 10% with sedatives. Alcohol may also play a role.[152] Although only a very small proportion of drug-dependent Australian women were found to be dependent on alcohol, 55% of drug-dependent men were also alcohol-dependent.[218]

All over the world, drug abuse has long presented many medical problems, but their full effects on the addict have not yet been thoroughly investigated and evaluated. Known complications include a wide range of emotional and physical problems including cerebral atrophy,[153] chromosome breakage,[149] and hepatitis.[151,157] Ganja (cannabis), LSD and mescaline have been shown to have a teratogenic potential.[289] Perhaps the most difficult problem of all is how to help the addict to break his habit. The criteria for recovery from drug dependence have been clearly defined, but they are very difficult to meet, particularly with those addicted to "hard" drugs like heroin, and substitution of a less harmful narcotic may be the only recourse.[158]

Even common analgesics like acetanilid, aspirin, and phenacetin and even "safe" sedatives like bromides have some potential for addiction, at least a potential for psychological dependence, if taken continually for prolonged periods.* In fact, all central nervous system depressant or stimulant drugs appear to have this potential. Their repeated euphoric or other effects that alter the level of consciousness may create a compulsion, a desire that may at times be overwhelming. Such addiction may be characterized by a tendency to increase dosage, either to maintain the given level of needed effect as tolerance develops, to intensify the effect that is so strongly desired, or to cope with the after effects of abuse or misuse. Psychological dependence or physical dependence or both may occur with deleterious effects on both the mental and somatic processes.[4,18,69,122]

Despite the hazards, however, a large number of proprietary medications containing hallucinogenic drugs are sold without a

Table 9–6   Hallucinogenic Medications*

Alophen	Neo-Nyte
Asthamdor	Nytol
At-Eaze	Quietabs
Compoz	Relax
Contac	San-Man
Devarex	Serene
Donnagel	Sleep-eze
Donnagel-PG	Sleep-tite
Dormeez	Sominex capsules
Doze-Off	Sominex tablets
Endotussin-C	Super-Sleep
Endotussin-NN	Sure-Sleep
Femicin	Trangest
Lullaby	Tranquil
Mr. Sleep	Travel-eze

* These OTC (over-the-counter, nonprescription, proprietary) potentially hallucinogenic medications contain ingredients such as antihistamines (e.g., chlorpheniramine maleate, methapyrilene HCl, or pyrilamine maleate), belladonna or stramonium alkaloids (e.g., homatropine, hyoscyamine, or scopolamine), and various other ingredients such as phenylpropanolamine, salicylamide, etc.

*The frequency of significant analgesic abuse in women with reactive depression, chronic neurosis or inadequate personality may be as high as 1 in 3. Psychological dependence was uncovered in one patient who consumed more than 1 kg. of an analgesic agent over a 6 month period; "to calm me down" and "to get my strength back" are typical excuses.[70]

prescription. Table 9-6 lists a number that are readily available and virtually free of government control. They contain belladonna or other solanaceous alkaloids such as scopolamine in combination with antihistamines such as pethapyrilene, and sometimes aspirin, potassium bromide, and other ingredients. Confusion, delirium, disorientation, hallucinations (auditory and visual), and psychotic behavior are typical symptoms of intoxication with any one of some 130 sedatives, sleep aids, and other easily purchased over-the-counter remedies containing ingredients that affect the mind. These drug products, usually regarded as "safe," may uncover schizophrenic pathology and induce other personality problems, including attempts at suicide. In 1968, Leff and Bernstein described with unsurpassed clarity the signs and symptoms of the dose-related intoxication produced by belladonna alkaloids: [123]

"Among the initial symptoms are slight bradycardia, and dryness and burning of the oral mucosa, with thirst and difficulty in swallowing also being present. Shortly after this phase, there may follow a slight tachycardia, as well as dilation of the pupils and cycloplegia causing blurred vision and photophobia. The skin becomes hot, dry, and flushed, due to the peripheral vasodilation and the inhibition of sweating. Due to the latter effect, the body temperature may rise and, especially in the very young, may become quite alarming. Although there may be a weak, rapid pulse, this effect may not be noticeable in infants or old people. Palpitation, urinary urgency with difficulty in micturition, and abdominal distention may occur.

"With more severe intoxication the patient may show slurred speech, ataxia, confusion, disorientation, muscular weakness and incoordination, agitation and other evidence of manic-like symptoms, such as excitement and giddiness. Nausea and vomiting may also be present at this time. Manifestations of an acute organic psychosis are seen, such as decreased memory with possible amnesia for the toxic episode, disorientation, hallucinations, usually visual, along with the confusion, disorientation and agitated excitement mentioned earlier. This syndrome reaches its peak within several hours of the ingestion and usually disappears within several days. However, we have observed that intoxication with between 3 and 8 mg. of scopolamine has persisted for between 24 to 36 hours. We have also seen that evidence of psychotic thinking has persisted for many months after the initial ingestion. This may be due to either the mental state which caused the ingestion, an un-masking of underlying psychopathology by the drug or long term effects of the intoxication itself. Because of the fairly wide margin of safety, even with scopolamine, most cases do not progress to death. However, in severe intoxication, death may occur, due to a decrease in blood pressure, circulatory collapse, diminished respirations, with death ultimately resulting from respiratory insufficiency after paralysis and coma."

The Bureau of Narcotics and Dangerous Drugs maintains rigid control over the distribution of central nervous system depressants and stimulants (see page 96). Hallucinogens such as diethyltryptamine (DET), dimethyltryptamine (DMT), lysergic acid diethylamide (LSD), mescaline, marijuana, peyote, psilocybin, 2,5-dimethoxy-4-ethylamphetamine (DOET), and 2,5-dimethoxy-4-methylamphetamine (DOM or STP) cannot be sold legally in the United States, and permission for experimental use of these substances, except for use of peyote in certain tribal religious rites in the Native American Church, must be obtained from the FDA. Legitimate sources of supply are severely limited. Thus LSD and psilocybin are obtainable legally only through the National Institutes of Mental Health.

LSD. The dangers of LSD and other hallucinogenic drugs to borderline psychotics and depressed individuals are universally recognized. Only 100 mcg. of LSD can cause hallucinations and uncontrolled behavior. Yet the black market flourishes and provides these drugs diluted in powders, capsules, sugar cubes, and other dosage forms for their psychedelic effects (unpredictable mood changes, sometimes tending towards euphoria, at other times towards deep depression, depersonalization, hallucinations, sensory distortion, and vivid fantasies). The affected individual and those around him are subjected to the hazards of impaired judgment and panic that on occasion lead to attempts to fly, dangerous driving, hostility, and loss of inhibitions. Bodily injury and occasionally death, intentional or accidental, often ensue and psychic dependence may destroy the capacity of the individual to function normally.

Marijuana. Marijuana (marihuana) is claimed by its advocates to be no more harmful than cigarettes and alcohol and during 1970 the standardized drug supplied by Federal government agencies began to be used in terminal cases of cancer in an attempt to eliminate the need for potent antidepressants and analgesics.[119] Nevertheless, the drug can produce serious emotional disturbances and personality changes. Patients have required intensive psychiatric care after consecutively smoking 12 or 15 marijuana cigarettes, and some have been institutionalized. Aggressive, impulsive, and paranoid behavior, depersonalization, depression, delusions, hallucinations, indolence, memory loss, neglect of personal hygiene, and severe mental confusion have all been observed and are intensified when the drug is combined with other agents such as alcohol and amphetamines.[151,154]

The effects of large doses of marijuana are very similar to the effects of LSD described above. It induces the following physical effects: appetite increase, conjunctival congestion (red eye), diarrhea, dryness of the mouth, hypoglycemia, hypothermia, muscular incoordination, mydriasis, nausea, photophobia, postural hypotension, respiratory depression, spasms, and urinary frequency.[83, 125, 127]

Those who advocate legalization of the use of marijuana may not be aware of its truly great potential for harm and may be misled and make poor judgments because of the fact that much of the drug found in the United States is of inferior potency. Escalation from marijuana to "hard" drugs like heroin is a major hazard. Also, with prolonged heavy use, carcinoma of the lung, fetal effects, brain damage, are possibilities which require investigation. On the other hand, occasional use of small amounts is often harmless and may be therapeutic in some conditions such as glaucoma. FDA had over 80 INDs for the drug in 1977.

Amphetamines. Amphetamine (Benzedrine), the first member of its class of sympathomimetic amines with CNS stimulant activity, was introduced into medicine as an analeptic and euphoric in the middle 1930's and through the following decades the dependency-producing property of this drug and its congeners became even more psychologically destructive than heroin. Too freely available, too freely prescribed, and probably more treacherous than any other addicting substance, amphetamines have damaged in-

dividuals much more than they have helped them. Their usefulness in medicine has been repeatedly questioned. They most certainly no longer have a valid place in the treatment of depression, dysmenorrhea, fatigue, hypotension, migraine, narcotic intoxication, nocturnal enuresis, and premenstrual tension.

These CNS stimulants, nevertheless, have been effectively used in minimal brain dysfunction (hyperkinetic behavior disorders) in children, in narcolepsy, in obesity, and in certain types of epilepsy. However, because they have a significant potential for abuse and tolerance, they should be restricted to short term use. They should also be used cautiously in combination because they enter into many adverse interactions, some of which are life-threatening, e.g., hypertensive crisis with monoamine oxidase inhibitors. The following warnings were compiled by the FDA during 1970:

Warnings for Amphetamines

"Tolerance—Tolerance to the anorectic effect usually develops within a few weeks. When this occurs, the recommended dose should not be exceeded in an attempt to increase the effect; rather, the drug should be discontinued. Amphetamines may impair the ability of the patient to engage in potentially hazardous activities such as operating machinery or driving a motor vehicle; the patient should therefore be cautioned accordingly.

Drug Dependence—Amphetamines have a significant potential for abuse. Tolerance and extreme psychological dependence have occurred. There are reports of patients who have increased the dosage to many times that recommended. Abrupt cessation following prolonged high dosage administration results in extreme fatigue and mental depression; changes are also noted on the sleep EEG. Manifestations of chronic intoxication with amphetamines include severe dermatoses, marked insomnia, irritability, hyperactivity, and personality changes. The most severe manifestation of chronic intoxication is psychosis, often clinically indistinguishable from schizophrenia.

Usage in Pregnancy—Safe use in pregnancy has not been established. Reproduction studies in mammals at high multiples of the human dose have suggested both an embryotoxic and a teratogenic potential. Therefore, use of amphetamines by women who are or who may become pregnant, and especially those in the first trimester of pregnancy, requires that the potential benefit be weighed against the possible hazard to mother and infant.

Usage in Children—Amphetamines are not recommended for use as anorectic agents in children under 12 years of age."

According to D. E. Smith,[97] the use of high doses of methamphetamine ("speed") was the major adolescent problem in the Haight-Ashbury district in San Francisco, as in Japan, Greenwich Village in New York City, and other areas supporting the drug subculture. The abuse of this drug (*"speed binge"*) is divided into two phases. During the *action phase,* the user (*"speed freak"* or *"meth head"*) injects 1 to 10 doses IV daily and with each injection experiences a *"flash"* or *"full body orgasm."* Between injections he is euphoric, hyperactive and hyperexcitable. This phase may be prolonged for many days without sleep and with little food. The *reaction phase* follows when he runs out of drug or ceases his injections because of confusion, fatigue, panic, paranoia, or some other reason. He may sleep for as long as two days from sheer exhaustion, then awaken very hungry, eat ravenously, and finally enter a state of severe psychological depression that may become so intolerable that he begins injecting the drug again.

Prolonged IV injections of high doses of methamphetamine lead to acute psychiatric problems, hepatitis, malnutrition, and various dermatologic conditions including skin abscesses. Smith subdivides the psychiatric problems into (1) acute anxiety, (2) psychosis, (3) exhaustion, and (4) withdrawal reactions. The psychotic type of reaction, with auditory and visual hallucinations and paranoia, is the most dramatic and difficult to manage. Submerged in fear, the "speed freak" may compound his problems by medicating himself IV with barbiturates and heroin, and thereby acquire secondary dependencies.

Tolerance produces tremendous variability in the amount of drug that can be taken and in the nature and response to the drug by the body and mind. Death has been reported from 120 mg. rapidly injected IV and some addicts have lived after injecting as much as 100 grams during one "run" or "speed binge" (e.g., after "shooting" one "spoon" or about 1 gram of "speed" every few hours for 12 days). Such large doses may at times be tolerated partly because inferior black market drug is used. Addicts consider 100 mg. (a "dime bag") a small dose and yet after a long interval without injections, they may become "over-amped" with this quantity and require medical attention. In one teenage neophyte, who did not survive following ingestion of two packets of methamphetamine during a chase by the police, a temperature of 108°, a blood level of 2.2 mg./100 ml., and a urine level of 55 mg./100 ml. were recorded during attempts to resuscitate him after he had been convulsing and brought to the hospital apneic, cyanotic, fasciculating, and unconscious.[47,97]

Bartholomew[4] has reviewed various reasons given for taking amphetamines. Patients seen by a number of physicians admitted taking these drugs to cope with (1) physical, (2) personality, and (3) sexual problems. Specific problems are cited below. Obviously, ignorance, superstition and other factors contributed to faulty use.

Physical problems include obesity, fatigue, the need to stay awake, to offset lethargy or sleepiness induced by barbiturate, marijuana, or other drugs and to overcome the onset of drunkenness. Individuals who work throughout the night, interstate truck drivers, party goers, and students cramming for examinations were frequenty involved. Typical statements were:

"I started taking them to keep awake."
"It peps you up." "Makes you feel awake." "Gives you vitality." "You can stay awake all weekend." "You don't need to go home on Saturday night."

Personality problems included anxiety, depression, and feelings of inferiority. Other psychological factors were hedonism, sensitivity, and uncontrollable desires to belong to a group, to achieve satisfaction, and an unrealistic sense of being superhuman. Typical statements were:

"I can't dance with girls without it."
"You enjoy things better, get a better effect." "You don't care what is said about you." "They give me confidence and a feeling of exhilaration." "Usually I feel insecure and have no confidence in myself, but on drugs I feel full of confidence and I am more creative; I like to live 24 hours a day, I want to be a poet and my mind is much more clearer with amphetamines." "I felt I was a genius." "I felt I could do anything I could turn my

hand to." "All my friends were taking them and when I was offered some pills, I felt I had to take them to be in with the crowd." "Everybody does it so you do." "You just take them to be with it." "They were all the rage." "They make me feel intelligently alive." "They take all the tension out of my body." "My boyfriend gave me some amphetamines to make me more lively." "I came to Sidney looking for excitement, and that means taking drugs."

Sexual problems included impotence and the influence of homosexuality. Typical statements were:

"I took the drug to delay ejaculation." "I came because I am homosexual and the homosexuals I met here were taking drugs."

Withdrawal. Abrupt discontinuance of some addicting drugs may create severe withdrawal symptoms. When certain analgesics, sedatives, hypnotics, and other CNS depressant drugs are suddenly discontinued subsequent to intensive or long-term therapy or drug abuse, excessive stimulation and even grand mal epileptic seizures and death may occur. Barbiturates and narcotics are notorious in this regard.

Management of opiate addiction with methadone[59] and also the longer acting methadol appears to be of value, but FDA requirements for their use are stringent.

Identifying and Managing Drug Abuse. Physicians face major problems in identifying and managing adverse reactions to commonly abused drugs like the *amphetamines* (benzedrine, or "bennies," methamphetamine or "speed," methylphenidate, phenmetrazine, etc.), *anticholinergics* (atropine, belladonna, scopolamine, etc.), *CNS depressants* (barbiturates or "goof balls," chlordiazepoxide, diazepam, ethchlorvynol, glutethimide, meprobamate, etc.) *hallucinogens* (cannabis products like hashish, tetrahydrocannabinol or THC; marijuana or "pot"; dimethyltryptamine or DMT; lysergic acid diethylamide or LSD or "acid"; mescaline or peyote; psilocybin, STP, etc.), and narcotics (cocaine or "big C," heroin or H or "horse," hydromorphone, meperidine, methadone, morphine, opium, etc.).* Emergency treatment is often

---

* A glossary of some of the slang terms used by addicts appears in *The Drug Scene* (New York, McGraw-Hill Book Co., 1968), by Donald B. Louria, and other works.[53,108]

necessary before the results of laboratory tests can be obtained and rapid reliable tests for the identity of some drugs like LSD or cannabis in the body are not readily available. Treatment must usually be based strictly on clinical findings. See Table 9-7.[21-23,150]

In an all-out effort to stem the vast and increasing abuse of hallucinogens, marijuana, narcotics, sedatives, stimulants, and other dangerous drugs, the U.S. government is taking the following steps: (1) increasing prevention, rehabilitation, and treatment through HEW backed efforts by communities and the Public Health Service, (2) tightening control and enforcement by the Justice Department through registration at all levels of distribution including physicians, (3) reducing criminal penalties for possession, eliminating mandatory sentences, and expunging references to illegal acts from official records under certain circumstances, (4) authorizing research and education relating to Justice Department cooperation with states and localities, forfeitures, inspections, law enforcement, and searches including "no knock" provisions, (5) financing for community health centers, drug abuse education, enforcement personnel, and special projects, (6) limiting use of amphetamines by restricting recommended medical uses and production. Production quotas are established annually.

The United States Department of Health, Education, and Welfare (HEW) has compiled a bibliography of about 3,000 citations on drug dependence and abuse.[103] It is available from the National Clearinghouse for Mental Health Information. HEW has also prepared a number of other useful brochures which are available from the Government Printing Office, including *Answers to the Most Frequently Asked Questions About Drug Abuse.*

Drug abuse in the United States is not primarily a medical problem, but a much broader problem of society. This serious hazard can only be controlled within the framework of our national economic, political and social goals by more effective coordination at Federal, state, and local levels of all efforts directed toward strengthening family structure and community discipline. Problems of

Table 9-7   Table of Drug Abuse Reactions [21-23]

Drug	Clinical Findings*
Amphetamines	Activity stereotyped; aggressiveness, blood pressure elevated; cardiac arrhythmia; circulatory collapse, confusion, high fever; mouth dry; paranoid ideation; respiration shallow; tendon reflexes hyperactive; and sweating. Withdrawal symptoms may include aching muscles, apathy, depression, somnolence, and ravenous hunger.
Anticholinergics	Amnesia, answers nonsensical; disorientation; distorted body image, mucosae and skin dry and flushed; pupils dilated; sensorium cloudy; visual hallucinations without distortion of perception; and urinary retention. No specific withdrawal syndrome.
CNS depressants	Ataxia; blood pressure depressed; coma; confusion; nystagmus on lateral gaze; respiration depressed; shock; slurred speech; and tendon reflexes depressed. Withdrawal symptoms may include agitation, cardiovascular collapse, chronic blink reflex, convulsive seizures, delirium, high fever, insomnia, psychosis, and tremulousness.
Hallucinogens (Cannabis products)	Distorted body image and perception but sensorium often clear; conjunctivae red, hallucinations rare, postural hypotension; pupils normal; and tachycardia. No specific withdrawal syndrome.
Hallucinogens (LSD type)	Anxiety; blood pressure elevated; delusions; distorted perception and body image but sensorium often clear; pupils dilated but reactive to light; skin papillae erectile (gooseflesh); sweating; tendon reflexes hyperactive; and visual hallucinations kaleidoscopic. No specific withdrawal syndrome.
Narcotics	Blood pressure depressed; coma; pulmonary edema; pupils pinpoint, fixed; respiration depressed; sensorium depressed but patient may appear alert and normal; and shock. Withdrawal symptoms include aching muscles, chills, dehydration, diarrhea, elevated blood pressure, pulse rate, respiratory rate and temperature, erectile skin papillae, lacrimation, nausea, restlessness followed by sleep, rhinorrhea, twitching, vomiting, weakness, and yawning.

* Depending on the severity of the reaction, all of these findings may or may not be present and some may occur in varying degrees of intensity.

such magnitude have been solved in other societies with drastic means such as capital punishment and sterilization. Drug abuse can be solved in the United States with the instruments it has available if the will to do so is properly mobilized.

Blood Dyscrasias. Some pathological conditions of the blood and the hematopoietic system are caused most often by medications or other chemicals. Patients with certain inborn or acquired characteristics (see page 269) may be particularly susceptible to such adverse hematic reactions. Therefore, drugs that have the potential to induce these conditions are contraindicated in such patients. Also concurrent therapy, with two or more drugs that are known to cause severe dyscrasias such as those resulting from bone marrow depression (bone marrow aplasia, depressed hematopoiesis) is contraindicated in *all* patients. [232]

The categories of drug-induced blood dyscrasias that have been used for reporting adverse drug reactions include (1) agranulocytosis (granulocytopenia) or leukopenia, (2) aplastic (hypoplastic) anemia, (3) hemolytic anemia, (4) megaloblastic anemia, (5) pancytopenia, and (6) thrombocytopenia. The Registry on Blood Dyscrasias which was permanently established in 1957 by the American Medical Association included the category of Erythroid Hypoplasia without Pancytopenia. [6,37,81]

Agranulocytosis, although rare, is the most frequently observed blood dyscrasia. It is caused by drugs in most cases, often through an immune mechanism, but also by inducing marrow hypofunction or interfering with other hematopoietic mechanisms. Typical clinical signs and symptoms associated with this acute, grave adverse drug reaction usually appear explosively, often precipitated by a secondary bacterial invasion. The mortality

Table 9-8   Drugs Which Can Induce Blood Dyscrasias[a]

Drug	Agranulocytosis (Leukopenia)	Aplastic Anemia	Hemolytic Anemia	Megaloblastic Anemia	Pancytopenia	Thrombocytopenia
Acetanilid			*			
Acetazolamide (Diamox)		*			*	*
Acetophenetidin		*	*		*	*
Acetylphenylhydrazine			*			
Acetylsalicylic acid (Aspirin)	*	*	*		*	*
Allyl-isopropyl-acetylcarbamide (Sedormid)						*
Aminopyrine (Pyramidon)	*	*	*			
Amodiaquine (Camoquin)		*				
Antihistamines		*				
Antineoplastics		*				
Antipyrine (Phenazone)			*			
Arabinoside				*		
Arsenicals (Organic)		*				
Arsenobenzenes						*
Azathioprine (Imuran)	*			*		*
Barbiturates		*		*	*	*
Busulfan (Myleran)					*	*
Butazolidin	*	*			*	*
Carbamazepine (Tegretol)	*	*				*
Carbimazole		*				
Carbutamide		*				
Cephalothin Sodium (Keflin)				*		*
Chloramphenicol (Chloromycetin)	*	*	*		*	*
Chlordiazepoxide (Librium)	*	*				
Chlorothiazide (Diuril)	*	*			*	*
Chlorpromazine (Thorazine)	*		*			
Chlorpropamide (Diabinese)		*			*	*
Cinchophen	*					
Clofibrate (Atromid-S)	*	*				
Colchicine	*	*				*
Cyclophosphamide (Cytoxan)	*	*				*
Cytarabine (Cytosar)	*			*		*
Cytosine (Cytarabine)	*			*		*
Diaminophenylsulfone			*			
Digitalis glycosides	*	*			*	*
Dimercaprol (BAL)			*			
Diphenylhydantoin (Dilantin)				*		
Dipyrone	*	*				*
Ethchlorvynol (Placidyl)			*			*
Ethosuximide (Zarontin)	*	*				
5-Fluorouracil				*		
Furaltadone			*			
Furazolidone (Furoxone)			*			
Gold compounds		*			*	*
Hydantoins		*				*
Hydrochlorothiazide (Hydrodiuril)						*
Hydroxyurea (Hydrea, Hydroxycarbamide)	*			*		*
Hydroflumethiazide (Diucardin, Saluron)	*	*				*
Imipramine (Tofranil)	*					
Indomethacin (Indocin)	*	*	*			*

[a]The sources used to compile this table were selected on the basis of apparent reliability of authorship.[1,7,10,12,17,19,24,30,35,42–44,54,61,63,68,79,85,89,94,100,109,110,113,132,232,306,307]

Table 9-8　Drugs Which Can Induce Blood Dyscrasias *(Continued)*

Drug	Agranulocytosis (Leukopenia)	Aplastic Anemia	Hemolytic Anemia	Megaloblastic Anemia	Pancytopenia	Thrombocytopenia
Iothiouracil (Itrumil)	*					
Irradiation (radioactive drugs)		*				
Isoniazid			*			
Melphalan (Alkeran)		*				*
Mepazine (Pacatal)	*	*			*	
Mephenytoin (Mesantoin)	*	*	*	*	*	*
Meprobamate (Equanil, Miltown)	*	*			*	*
6-Mercaptopurine (Purinethol)	*			*		*
Mesoridazine (Serentil)	*	?	?		?	?
Methicillin (Staphcillin)	*		*			*
Methimazole (Tapazole)	*	*			*	*
Methophenobarbital				*		
Methyldopa (Aldomet)	*	*			*	*
Methylene blue			*			
Methyl-phenyl-ethyl-hydantoin	See *Mephenytoin* above					
Methylthiouracil		*				
Nitrofurantoin (Furandantin)			*			
Nitrofurazone (Furacin)			*			
Novobiocin						*
Oxyphenbutazone (Tandearil)	*	*				
Pamaquine			*			
Para-aminosalicylic acid			*			
Paradione	*	*			*	*
Penicillin	*	*	*		*	*
Pentaquine			*			
Pentazocine (Talwin)	*					
Phenacemide (Phenurone)		*				
Phenantoin (Mesantoin)		*	*		*	
Phenindione	*					
Phenothiazines	*	*	*	*	*	*
Phenylbutazone (Butazolidin)	*	*			*	*
Phenylhydrazine			*			
Phenytoin sodium				*		
Plasmoquine			*			
Potassium perchlorate		*				
Primaquine			*			
Primidone (Mysoline)		*		*		
Probenecid (Benemid)			*			
Procainamide (Pronestyl)	*	*				
Procarbazine (Matulane)	*	*				*
Prochlorperazine (Compazine)	*					
Promazine (Sparine)	*					
Propylthiouracil	*					*
Pyrazolones (See Aminopyrine, Antipyrine)	*	*	*			*
Pyrimethamine (Daraprim)	*			*	*	*
Quinacrine (Atabrine)		*	*			*
Quinidine	*	*	*		*	*
Quinine			*			*
Rifampin (Rifadin, etc.)	*		*			*
Streptomycin	*	*	*		*	*
Stibophen (Fuadin)			*			*
Sulfonamides	*	*	*		*	*
Sulfasalazine (Azulfidine)			*			

A question mark (?) indicates an early indication or a definite possibility of occurrence with a new drug. A few drugs in this table are no longer marketed but are retained because of similarity in structure to drugs that are prescribed.

Table 9-8 Drugs Which Can Induce Blood Dyscrasias *(Continued)*

Drug	Agranulo-cytosis (Leukopenia)	Aplastic Anemia	Hemolytic Anemia	Megalo-blastic Anemia	Pancyto-penia	Thrombo-cytopenia
Sulfacytine (Renoquid)	?	?	?		?	?
Sulfadiazine	*		*			
Sulfamethizole	*	*			*	
Sulfamethoxazole (Gantanol)	*	*	*			*
Sulfisoxazole (Gantrisin)		*	*		*	*
Sulfoxone			*			
Tetracycline	*		*		*	*
Thiacetazone (Seroden, etc.)		*	*			
Thiazolsulfone (Promizole)			*			
Thiocyanates		*				
Thioguanine	*			*		*
Thioridazine (Mellaril)	*					
Thiouracil	*					*
Tolbutamide (Orinase)	*	*			*	*
Triamterene (Dyrenium)		*		*		
Trimethadione (Tridione)	*	*			*	*
Tripelennamine (Pyribenzamine)	*					
Vincristine	*	*				
Vitamin K water-soluble analogues			*			

rate may reach 50%. Agranulocytosis must be differentiated from acute aleukemia and aplastic anemia. [30,42-44,63,130]

Aplastic anemia (aregenerative anemia, bone marrow failure, hypoplastic anemia, primary refractory anemia), first named by Ehrlich in 1888, is the most serious of the drug-induced blood dyscrasias. The mortality rate may reach 80-100% if the causative agent is not identified and withdrawn rapidly, and appropriate therapy initiated.

In pure aplastic anemia, there is complete absence of all types of hematopoiesis in the marrow. Other types of aplastic anemia may affect the production of only one or two of the elements of the blood, and result in various combinations of anemia, leukopenia, and thrombocytopenia. The clinical symptoms of aplastic anemia may appear rapidly, particularly with antineoplastics and ionizing irradiation. But with most chemicals the onset is insidious and delayed, often not manifesting itself until some time after the offending agent has been removed.

In the past, many cases of aplastic anemia have been designated idiopathic (chloramphenicol in 50% of all cases). As the mechanisms of adverse drug reactions become better understood, the condition may often be explained on the basis of bone marrow toxicity resulting from inherited sensitivities to drugs and from the actions of environmental chemicals such as benzene, carbon tetrachloride, hair dyes, insecticides (DDT, lindane), plant sprays, solvents, TNT, and trichloroethylene. Other etiologic agents include congenital conditions (e.g., the Fanconi syndrome) and ionizing irradiation. It is sometimes associated with tumors of the thymus. [131]

Hemolytic anemia is discussed in Chapter 8 in connection with hypersensitivity and pharmacogenetic influences. Table 9-8 lists many medications that have been implicated in this and the other blood dyscrasias.

Carcinogenicity. Cancer, the second leading cause of death by disease, is undoubtedly the most complex health problem urgently requiring solution. The International Cancer Congresses and other groups repeatedly review the most recent medical knowledge concerning the 200 or more malignant diseases which physicians must identify and attempt to treat. Yet, in spite of good communication, progress is painfully slow. Many malignant neoplastic disease entities are not easy to pinpoint and for practically all of them no cures are available, only palliatives.* The major difficulty lies in the fact that they are almost certainly composite processes—biochemical and immunological as well as viral. This makes the development of prognostic indicators as well as identification very difficult. But metabolic studies of *in vitro* cultures of malignant cells, identification of cancer-producing viruses, synthesis of DNA, and other techniques are improving insight. Also, with more accurate characterization of the proteins involved, classification of neoplasms is becoming more precise. The cancerous disorders are now frequently designated by means of the protein products of neoplastic cells, disorders of immunoglobulin synthesis (alpha, gamma, and mu chain diseases), or other specific biochemical terminology.[2]

So many chemicals and other agents (disease, faulty nutrition, genetic influences, immunologic deficits, implants, parasites, radiation, tobacco, trauma, viruses, etc.) appear to induce cancer or predispose patients to the disease that it is difficult to define the causative agent. While much human cancer is induced by chemicals, certain microorganisms are undoubtedly involved. Polyoma virus is a known potent oral tumorigenic agent.[137] Breast cancer, Burkitt's lymphoma, cervical cancer, leukemia, postnasal cancer and sarcoma are all strongly suspected of being caused by viruses. These and other carcinogens are found in the air, food, water, or the environmental substances contacting man.

In the environments of large metropolitan areas, some known carcinogens like 3,4-benzopyrene are ubiquitous. So also are industrial pollutants, pesticides, solvents, and various vapors and suspended particulate substances that have been implicated as carcinogens. In these congested areas, such a vast array of potential carcinogens is present that it is exceedingly difficult to decide definitely that any given drug or other chemical is the carcinogenic culprit in a specific patient. Table 9-9 lists some typical agents.

Table 9-9   Typical Carcinogenic Agents

Aflatoxins	Hair dyes
o-Aminoazotoluene	(phenylenediamines)
2-Aminofluorene	Herbicides
Androgens	Implants (metal, plastic)
Antineoplastics	Maleic hydrazide (liver
(alkylating)	tumors, mice)
Antivitamins	3-Methylcholanthrene
Asbestos	Naphthylamines
Benzene	Nitrites
Biphenylamines	Nitrofurans
3,4-Benzopyrene	Nitrosamines
Busulfan	N-Nitrosodialkylamines
Carbon tetrachloride	Norethindrone c
Chloroform	mestranol?
Corticosteroids	Oral contraceptives?
Cyclamates	Pesticides*
Cytotoxic antineoplastics	Pronethalol (Alderlin)
4-Dimethylamino-	Radiation
azobenzene	Thioacetamide
Dimethylbenzanthracene	Tobacco smoke
Dioxane	TRIS (flame retardant)
Epinephrine	Trypan blue
Estrogens	Viruses
Food Additives (some)	Vitamins (deficiency or
Freons (liver tumors,	excess)
mice)*	
Griseofulvin (liver	
tumors, mice)	

* For example, when Freons used as propellants are combined with piperonyl butoxide, a pyrethrin pesticide synergist.[134]

Aflatoxins, produced by *Aspergillus flavus,* a pathogenic mold that may be present in certain nuts, cereals, and other items used as food, are potent carcinogens. In 1960, poultry feed containing contaminated peanut meal induced the mysterious turkey X disease that killed more than 50% of the British turkeys. The nitrosamines also are potent carcinogens in a wide range of organs of various species. These may be formed during cooking when ingested nitrites† react chemically with secondary amines present in the food.[52] Those who contact certain chemicals in laboratories or in industrial chemical plants may be particularly vulnerable.[51] Benzidine, used to detect occult blood, and other aromatic amines have been implicated in cancer of the urinary bladder and of the pan-

---

*Complete remissions have been achieved at the National Cancer Institute in six types of fast growing cancers: acute leukemia, Burkitt's lymphoma, certain childhood solid tumors, choriocarcinoma, Hodgkin's disease, and testicular tumors.

---

† During 1971 the FDA took steps to lower the present limit of 100 ppm permitted in foods to perhaps a tenth of that concentration because of its carcinogenic potential.

creas. Mustard gas creates the occupational hazard of oral and upper respiratory tract neoplasms in workers who produce this chemical. N-methyl-N-nitrosourea is a potent carcinogen in dental tissue. Other well known carcinogenic chemicals include *o*-aminoazotoluene, biphenylamines, 4-dimethylaminoazobenzene or butter yellow, the insecticide 2-aminofluorene and its amide, the solvents N-nitrodimethylamine, carbon tetrachloride and dioxane, thioacetamide used to generate H_2S in the analytical laboratory, 3-methylcholanthrene of coal tar, and several dyes including Trypan blue. [135,137]

At a symposium in 1970, the herbicide maleic anhydride and the pesticide 1-(1-naphthyl)-2-thiourea (ANTU) were reported to be carcinogens in test animals. The commercial grade of the herbicide contains 2-naphthylamine, a known bladder carcinogen in man and the dog but not in the mouse or rat. [133]

A genetic element is present in the development of some malignancies, e.g., a familial polyposis exhibits dominant inheritance, xeroderma pigmentosa is inherited by a recessive gene, and possibly a predisposition to carcinoma of the breast is inherited. [133] When a predisposition to develop a malignant neoplastic disease is genetically acquired, no more than two or three viral genes may be responsible for carcinogenesis. [135]

Regulatory scrutiny of the carcinogenic potential of foods, drugs and cosmetics by the FDA has properly become very intensive and regulatory action is often prompt and rigid, partially because of the insertion of the Delaney clause in the Federal Food, Drug, and Cosmetic Act. [31] This clause states that:

"No additive shall be deemed to be safe if it is found to induce cancer when ingested by man or animal, or if it is found after tests which are appropriate for the evaluation of the safety of food additives, to induce cancer in man or animal. . ." [31]

The above statement has led to the removal of products like cyclamates that were used in dietary beverages, drug products, and foods for as long as 25 years. It has also led to re-examination of products generally regarded as safe (the GRAS list). Saccharin, monosodium glutamate, and many others will undoubtedly be restricted as to their use and some will be removed from the market.

Action must now be taken by the government immediately cancer has been produced, even when extremely high doses of a drug, food additive, herbicide, pesticide, or other chemical have been used to challenge the cancer-producing mechanisms of a test animal. The crux of this facet of the problem of carcinogenicity may reside in the development of a new and more meaningful definition of "tests which are appropriate for the evaluation . . ."

Occasionally, some medications have been found to be carcinogenic, usually only in very high dosages, but unfortunately, not always before they are administered to patients. Sometimes the carcinogenic activity of a drug in animals is not discovered until after the drug has been used in clinical trials or rarely even long after they have been marketed. With investigational drugs, trials are immediately halted, and the patients who have taken the drugs are monitored for at least five years.* With drugs already on the market, however, the problem is not so easy. A decision to withdraw the drug from human use, based only on animal data, may be necessary. This always raises the problem of how valid this type of extrapolation to man really is. When widely used drugs, such as the nitrofurans, produce tumerogenic evidence in test animals (Aug., 1970), FDA ad hoc and advisory committees are placed under tremendous pressure. The hazard to the patient may or may not be real whenever these situations arise.

The fact that some antineoplastic drugs may themselves be carcinogenic under certain circumstances is startling. Busulfan (Myleran) produces dysplasia in multiple organ systems and abnormal cellular changes in exfoliated cells of the oral mucosa. Methotrexate enhances the carcinogenic effect of dimethylbenzathracene (buccal pouch of the hamster). Further investigation is needed to determine the prognosis when patients with

---

*At the beginning of the 1970's several pharmaceutical companies including Lederle, Merck and Ortho were conducting follow-ups on such patients. Drug-induced cancers associated with such common drugs as the sex hormones are being ever more intensively studied and the risks evaluated by means of epidemiologic case-control methods.

occult dysplastic lesions are simultaneously exposed to environmental carcinogens and subjected to certain types of antineoplastic therapy. [137]

Also, antineoplastic therapy tends to be immunosuppressive. This may provide a rational form of therapy for some types of cancer. It may not be a good treatment modality where immunity is an important consideration in overcoming other types of the disease.

Cardiovascular Toxicity. Medications have induced serious cardiac and vascular problems, ranging from various types of arrhythmias to hypertensive crises and cerebrovascular accidents. Practically all drugs have the potential to produce toxic effects on the heart or blood vessels and this potential may be considerably magnified in the presence of cardiovascular disease. Unfortunately, certain drugs have been widely used for prolonged periods before their cardiovascular toxicities were revealed.

Phenothiazines, beginning with chlorpromazine (Thorazine) and later many other related psychotropic drugs were used "safely" in psychiatry for many years. Then reports of cardiac dysrhythmias, conduction disturbances, electrocardiographic changes suggestive of infarction, and sudden death* began to appear about 1963. [220-223] Similar reports also appeared for the tricyclic antidepressants (dibenzazepines, dibenzocycloheptenes), a group that includes amitriptyline (Elavil), desipramine (Pertofrane), imipramine (Tofranil), nortriptyline (Aventyl), protriptyline (Vivactil), and trimipramine (Surmontil). Both the phenothiazines and tricyclics, in addition to their psychotropic effects resulting from central nervous system action, also produce adrenolytic, atropine-like, and hypotensive effects. [224-227]

Apparently, through competition at receptor binding sites, these drugs inhibit uptake of norepinephrine and high concentrations of the catecholamine occur in the blood and urine, comparable to those found in pheo-

chromocytoma. Their cardiotoxicity may be due to the elevated plasma catecholamine levels plus the depletion of myocardial catecholamine that follows prolonged administration. Also alterations in the myocardial mitochondria and deposits of mucopolysaccharides in the arterioles of the subendocardium have been found on autopsy in patients who have died after receiving phenothiazines for many years. The antidotes used in adverse reactions, overdosage, and suicidal attempts with these agents have logically included cholinergic drugs like neostigmine. Beta-adrenergic blocking agents have also been used. [225,237,291]

Very few, if any, medications can be given for long periods without increasing the potential for cardiovascular damage. When careful follow-up reveals EKG changes or dysrhythmias or other evidence of toxicity, the patient should be switched to another group of agents with similar pharmacological effects but different molecular structure. [237] Physicians everywhere have been alerted to the possible long-range effects of the oral contraceptives such as cerebrovascular disorders, pulmonary embolism, retinal thrombosis, and thrombophlebitis.

Cardiac glycosides (digitoxin, digoxin, etc.) sympathomimetics (epinephrine, levarterenol, etc.) xanthine derivatives (aminophylline, caffeine, etc.), and other myocardial stimulants may produce arrhythmias under certain conditions. In the presence of hypertrophic subaortic stenosis, these inotropic drugs paradoxically impede left ventricular outflow. The hazards of digitalis toxicity are enhanced in the presence of diuretics if they cause hypokalemia and also in the presence of reserpine. The sympathomimetics, even in small doses, may produce arrhythmias when used with certain anesthetics like cyclopropane and halothane, and in excessive doses, they can cause anatomic myocardial damage as well as arrhythmias. In the presence of coronary insufficiency, drugs like aminophylline and the sympathomimetics that increase oxygen consumption through myocardial stimulation may induce myocardial ischemia. [236]

Anesthetics (general and local), barbiturates, parasympathomimetics, procainamide, quinidine, and certain other drugs are not

---

*In one study, 12 out of 87 autopsied neuropsychiatric patients who had received phenothiazine tranquilizers had sudden, unexpected deaths and no anatomic cause of death was found other than cardiac abnormalities.

only direct myocardial depressants, but some of them may also induce paradoxical effects. Thus, the antiarrhythmic drugs, procainamide and quinidine, may produce severe arrhythmias, particularly in the presence of cardiac disease.

Myocardial damage may be caused by the direct toxic effects of drugs like antimony, arsenicals, emetine, ethyl alcohol, and lead. *Antimony* has caused arrhythmias and conduction abnormalities. Although the toxic effects occur rarely, the prognosis is gloomy and sudden death is not uncommon. *Arsenicals* have caused interstitial myocarditis with fibrosis, edema, and eosinophilic and mononuclear infiltration of the myocardium. *Emetine,* with its narrow margin of safety, may cause degeneration and necrosis of myocardial fibers. *Doxorubicin* (Adriamycin), an antineoplastic agent, may produce dose-related myocardial necrosis. Vitamin E and tamoxifen are being investigated as protectives. *Ethyl alcohol* may cause arrhythmias and conduction disturbances in association with focal myocardial fibrosis and necrosis compensated by myofiber hypertrophy. Terminal chronic *lead* poisoning cases have evidenced myocarditis associated with interstitial fibrosis and a serous exudate.[236]

Some medications may cause myocardial damage as a result of hypersensitivity reactions. Carbutamide, chlorpromazine, chlortetracycline, penicillin, phenylbutazone, streptomycin, and sulfonamides are a few of the drugs reported to produce systemic hypersensitivity reactions. Interstitial myocarditis and less frequently granulomatous myocarditis have been described in patients suffering from such reactions.

Still other medications may damage the myocardium as a result of overdosage or drug interaction by indirect action. Anesthetics (decrease sympathetic activity), anticholinergics like atropine (blocks parasympathetic receptors), reserpine and other drugs that release catecholamine, CNS stimulants like pentylenetetrazol (increase sympathetic activity), ganglionic blocking agents like hexamethonium (interrupt transmission in sympathetic ganglia), vasodilators such as hydralazine and nitroglycerin (produce reflex increase in contractility and rate of the heart), vasoconstrictors such as angiotensin

or methoxamine (produce reflex bradycardia), and beta adrenergic agents such as isoproterenol (cause cardiac overwork and in large doses myocardial necrosis) are examples of drugs that are prone to produce adverse effects in the presence of latent congestive heart failure or myocardial ischemia. Arrhythmias and heart failure have occurred during surgery in patients who have received reserpine treatment over a long period of time, also angina pectoris and myocardial infarction may occur during hydralazine therapy.[132,236]

Damage to the blood vessels may result from excessive vasoconstriction or vasodilation or it may result from hypersensitivity. Extreme vasoconstriction due to excessive administration of ergot alkaloids or sympathomimetics may produce necrosis. It may also elevate the blood pressure and cause acute pulmonary edema, cerebrovascular accidents, or myocardial infarction. Extreme vasodilation produced by combinations of drugs such as nitrites, alpha-adrenergic blocking agents, catecholamine depletors, ganglionic blocking agents, histamine releasing agents, and spinal anesthetics results in severe hypotension and occasionally coma and death. Hypersensitivity reactions may produce peripheral vascular collapse with severe hypotension and death. Also polyarteritis and blood vessel damage may be seen with adverse reactions to penicillin, sulfonamides, and certain other drugs.[132,236]

Various drug interactions which induce hazardous cardiovascular crises such as the effect of imipraminelike drugs and monoamine oxidase inhibitors in potentiating the pressor response to exogenous epinephrine and other sympathomimetics are covered in Chapter 10.

Congenital Abnormalities. The adverse effects of drugs on the fetus, neonate, and nursing infant are discussed on pages 256 to 262. The tables presented there are indicative of the complexity and seriousness of the problem. Anticonvulsants, antineoplastics, and other categories of the potent drugs available may be teratogenic, particularly if used during the first trimester of pregnancy.[57] Even medication of the male must be considered. Antineoplastics and immunosuppressives given either to a female *or her consort* just prior to conception could conceivably be teratogenic. This needs investigation.

Most drugs now on the market have not been shown to be safe for use during pregnancy, at term, and during labor. Therefore, most drugs carry the following types of statements in the labeling:

"The effects of this drug on the fetus and the extent of transplacental passage of this drug are unknown. Therefore, its use during the first and second trimester should be confined to instances where need outweighs possible hazards."

"Since thiazides appear in breast milk, this drug is contraindicated in nursing mothers. If use of the drug is deemed essential, the patient should stop nursing. Meprobamate and thiazides cross the placental barrier and appear in cord blood. When this drug is used in women of child-bearing age, its potential benefits should be weighed against its possible hazards to the fetus. These hazards include fetal or neonatal jaundice, thrombocytopenia, and possibly other adverse reactions which have occurred in the adult."

"The safety of this drug in pregnancy has not been established; hence it should be given only when the anticipated benefits to be derived from treatment exceed the possible risks to mother and fetus."

Teratogenesis, the production of physical defects in the fetus during its development, must be differentiated from mutagenesis, the production of genetic mutations. [9,27,45,49,50,75] Teratogenic effects produced with large doses in test animals are extrapolated to man with much less certainty than carcinogenic effects.

Dermatomucosal Toxicity. It is often very difficult to show a definite cause and effect relationship between a drug and a skin eruption. Because many cases are idiopathic in origin and many etiologic agents surround the patient, the only way to obtain proof that the condition is definitely induced by a specific drug, is to withdraw the medication, wait until the reaction subsides, and then rechallenge the patient with the same medication. However, *a second challenge to the patient may be extremely hazardous,* and should not be attempted in most instances. Serologic procedures, such as the basophil degranulation test, may eventually be developed and provide much safer modes of etiologic identification. [201]

Meanwhile, the physician is occasionally faced with very severe drug-induced eruptions that are life-threatening. Those that have definitely been caused by drugs include exfoliative dermatitis, Stevens-Johnson syndrome (erythema multiforme exudativum), a syndrome resembling systemic lupus erythematosus (SLE), and toxic epidermal necrolysis. The very severe cases may permanently handicap the patient or cause his death. Out of a total of 57 cases of these drug-induced conditions collected from the literature by Rostenberg and Fagelson (see Table 9-10) over one 5-year period, 21 (37%) were caused by sulfonamides, and 14 deaths occurred, 5 (36%) of which were caused by sulfonamides. [201,233] When these very rare conditions occur, they must be promptly identified and the etiologic agent immediately withdrawn.

Exfoliative dermatitis is characterized by scaling and erythema with induration or thickening of the skin. This skin eruption is associated with exfoliative forms of psoriasis, pityriasis rubra pilaris, and other usually benign skin conditions. However, 2 (33%) of the 6 cases of the drug-induced eruptions tabulated by Rostenberg and Fagelson terminated in death. [201]

Stevens-Johnson syndrome, a variant of erythema multiforme bullosum may be caused by hypersensitivity or immune reaction. It is the most common of the severe drug-induced skin eruptions. High fever and severe headache precede balanitis, conjunctivitis, rhinitis, stomatitis, and urethritis which are usually followed in a few days by the appearance of succulent, erythematous papules with a hemorrhagic central iris or bull's eye consisting of concentric red circles. Bullae and vesicles resembling pemphigus may also be present. If this very severe drug reaction progresses, the patient becomes extremely ill and manifests many signs of toxicity—headache, joint pains, malaise, prostration, rapid weak pulse, weakness, and a purulent ocular exudate indicating serious ocular involvement that may eventuate in partial or total blindness. Erosions on the mouth and lips have a red base and are covered with a grayish-white pseudomembranous exudate. The lips and tongue may be swollen. Necrolysis of various tissues may occur in advanced stages. Recovery, if it takes place, is very slow. [201,203]

Table 9-10   Life-Threatening Drug-Induced Skin Eruptions [132,164-204,233,245,310,321]

Drug Eruptions	Drugs Involved	Reported Sequelae
Exofoliative dermatitis	Aminosalicylic acid (PAS)	Hepatitis, hemolytic anemia
	Antidiabetics, oral	
	Arsenicals	
	Barbiturates	
	Carbamazepine (Tegretol)	
	Demeclocycline (Declomycin)	
	Diphenylhydantoin (Dilantin)	Atypical lymphocytes, hypoproteinemia, hepatosplenomegaly
	Diphtheria and tetanus toxoids and pertussis vaccine, absorbed and Salk poliomyelitis vaccine.	Death; probably due to penicillin in the poliovirus vaccine.
	Furosemide (Lasix)	
	Gold	
	Griseofulvin (Grifulvin)	Lymphadenopathy
	Hydroflumethiazide (Saluron)	
	Isorbide (Isordil)	
	Measles virus vaccine	
	Mercury	
	Methotrimeprazine (Levoprome)	
	Nitrofurans	
	Nitroglycerin	
	Oral antidiabetics	
	Oxyphenbutazone (Tandearil)	
	Penicillin	
	Phenindione (Hedulin)	Hepatitis, nephritis
	Phenothiazines	
	Phenylbutazone (Butazolidin)	
	Phenytoin (Dilantin)	
	Streptomycin	
	Sulfamethoxypyridazine (Midicel)	Death
	Sulfasalazine (Azulfidine)	
	Sulfisomide (Elkosin)	
	Sulfonamides	
	Tetracyclines	
Stevens-Johnson syndrome (Erythema multiforme)	Aminophenazone	
	Ampicillin	
	Antipyrine	
	Arsenicals	
	Barbiturates	
	Carbamazepine (Tegretol)	
	Chloramphenicol	
	Chlorpropamide (Diabinese)	
	Clindamycin	
	Codeine	
	Cold preparation 666	
	Diphenylhydantoin (Dilantin)	Death
	Diphenylhydantoin and trimethadione	Lupus erythematosus occurred simultaneously.
	Mephenytoin, (Mesantoin)	
	Novobiocin	
	Oxyphenbutazone (Tandearil)	
	Paramethadione	
	Penicillin	
	Phenolphthalein	
	Phenylbutazone (Butazolidin)	
	Rifampin (Rifadin, Rimactane, etc.) [322]	
	Salicylates	
	Salizopyrine	
	Sulfadimethoxine (Madribon)	
	Sulfamethoxypyridazine (Kynex, Midicel)	Death; 2 out of 14 cases

Table 9-10   Life-Threatening Drug-Induced Skin Eruptions *(Continued)*

Drug Eruptions	Drugs Involved	Reported Sequelae
	Sulfasalazine (Azulfidine)	
	Sulfisomidine (Elkosin)	
	Thiacetazone (Amithiozone)	Death
	Thiazides	
	Thiouracil	
	Trimethadione (Tridione) and phenobarbital	Lupus erythematosus with subsequent medication
	Triple sulfas (Sulphatriad)	
	Tetracycline	
Toxic epidermal necrolysis (Lyell's Syndrome)	Acetazolamide (Diamox)	
	Antihistamines	
	Antipyrine	
	Barbiturates	
	Chenopodium oil	Death
	Dapsone	
	Diallylbarbituric acid	
	Diphenylhydantoin (Dilantin)	Death
	Diphtheria	
	Ethylmorphine HCl (Didial)	
	Gold salts	
	Ipecac	
	Methyl salicylate	
	Neomycin sulfate	
	Nitrofurantoin (Furadantin)	Death; etiology questionable
	Opium powder	
	Oxyphenbutazone (Tandearil)	
	Penicillin	
	Pentazocine (Talwin)	
	Phenobarbital	
	Phenolphthalein	
	Phenylbutazone (Butazolidin)	Death; one out of four
	Procaine penicillin, aqueous injection, and oral mixed sulfonamide preparation	
	Sulfadimethoxine (Madribon)	Death; leukopenia
	Sulfamethoxypyridazine (Kynex, Midicel)	
	Sulfasalazine (Azulfidine)	
	Sulfathiazole	Death
	Sulfisomidine (Elkosin)	
	Sulfonamides	
	Tetracycline	
Lupus erythematosus	Aminosalicylic acid	
	Chlorpromazine (Thorazine)	
	Chlortetracycline (Aureomycin)	
	Corticosteroid withdrawal	
	Digitalis (long term)	
	Diphenylhydantoin (Dilantin)	
	Ethosuximide (Zarontin)	
	Gold compounds (long term)	
	Griseofulvin	
	Guanoxan	
	Hydantoin anticonvulsants	
	Hydralazine (Apresoline)	
	Isoniazid (Nydrazid)	
	Isoquinazepon	
	Mephenytoin (Mesantoin)	
	Methyldopa (Aldomet)	
	Methysergide	
	Methylthiouracil	
	Oral contraceptives (mestranol?)	

Table 9–10   Life-Threatening Drug-Induced Skin Eruptions *(Continued)*

Drug Eruptions	Drugs Involved	Reported Sequelae
	Oxyphenbutazone (Tandearil)	
	Para-aminosalicylic acid (PAS)	
	Penicillamine	
	Penicillin	
	Phenobarbital (long term)	
	Phenylbutazone (Butazolidin)	
	Practolol	
	Primidone (Mysoline)	
	Procainamide (Pronestyl)	
	Propylthiouracil	
	Reserpine (long term)	
	Rifampin (Rifadin, Rimactane, rifampicin)	
	Streptomycin	
	Sulfadiazine	
	Sulfadimethoxine	
	Sulfamethoxypyridazine (Kynex)	
	Sulfasalazine (Azulfidine)	
	Sulfonamides (long acting)	
	Tetracycline	
	Thiazides (long term)	
	Trimethadione (Tridione, troxidone)	

Lupus erythematosuslike drug-induced syndrome resembles SLE. It develops in about 10% of patients receiving hydralazine therapy for long periods (see page 277), and may be due to coupling of a drug acting as a hapten, with body protein. It is also a frequent complication of procainamide (Pronestyl) therapy. The drug-induced disease may also sometimes be the result of exacerbation of a latent SLE. It is difficult to diagnose by means of the LE phenomenon because LE cells are found in acquired hemolytic anemia, chronic hepatitis, dermatitis herpetiformis, dermatomyositis, leukemia, miliary tuberculosis, moniliasis, multiple myeloma, pernicious anemia in relapse, polyarteritis nodosa, rheumatoid arthritis, scleroderma, and perhaps other conditions. Also the cells are not always found when SLE is present. [201,202]

Toxic epidermal necrolysis was first described by Lyell in 1956 as a condition resembling "scalding of the skin." Characterized by erythema and tenderness, followed by loosening and peeling of large areas of the skin, this eruption predominates in females. Symptoms include confusion, fever and swelling of the eyes with easy removal of the superficial layers of the skin by gentle rubbing. Many drugs have been implicated in this condition (see Table 9–10) and 5 out of 13 cases tabulated by Rostenberg and Fagelson terminated in death. However, in many cases reported in the literature, no drugs were implicated. [201-204]

In addition to the terms used to describe these four life-threatening categories, the following adjectives and nouns have been used to categorize other dermatomucosal drug reactions: achromotrichia, acneform, alopecia, angioneurotic edema, atrophy, bullous, depigmented, ecchymotic, eczematoid, erythematous, erythema nodosum, exanthematic, fixed, furunculoid, hirsutism, hyperpigmented, ichthyosislike, lichenoid, lichenplanuslike, macular, maculopapular, morbilliform, monilial, nail changes, necrotic, papular, petechial rash, photosensitization, porphyria, pruritus, purpura, scarlatiniform, striae, tumorlike, urticarial, and vesicular. A large number of medications have been implicated; they mimic practically every known cutaneous disease. One of the most frequently encountered types of adverse drug reactions is the cutaneous. [5,132,207,233]

Some of the above dermatologic conditions, e.g., angioneurotic edema, appear to have a strong familial tendency and some may be forerunners of impending serious adverse reactions. Any of these benign eruptions, if sufficiently exacerbated, may become a serious threat to the patient. The number of drugs and other agents that cause some of these skin eruptions appears to be large.

Cairins has listed 31 causes for pruritus. Nevertheless, very few biochemical mechanisms for rash production have been elucidated. Of the many causes given for pruritus, only *serotonin* in carcinoid syndrome, *calcium* in hyperthyroidism, and *bile acids and salts* in jaundice and pruritus gravidarum appear to be definitely incriminated. Even with these three etiologic agents, more proof is needed. [162,206]

Some drugs cause a wide variety of skin rashes and eruptions, depending on the severity of the reactions, but fortunately the skin reactions are usually rare. With allopurinol (Zyloprim), for example, the most common rash is maculopapular, but exfoliative, purpuric and urticarial lesions have also occurred. Sodium warfarin (Coumadin) has caused alopecia, dermatitis, urticaria, and even necrolysis of the skin. The penicillins, although noted for their low order of toxicity, are potent sensitizing agents. The most common types of allergic responses are skin eruptions varying widely in character, distribution, and intensity. They range from morbilliform, erythema nodosumlike, purpuric and urticarial eruptions to life-threatening erythema multiforme (Stevens-Johnson) and exfoliative dermatitis. Pyrazolon derivatives like antipyrine, aminopyrine, oxyphenbutazone and phenylbutazone must sometimes be rapidly and permanently withdrawn because of marked sensitivity manifested by exfoliative dermatitis, Stevens-Johnson syndrome, or toxic epidermal necrolysis. Older drugs that cause a variety of cutaneous reactions include aloin, arsenicals, bromides, iodides, mercurials, phenolphthalein, and salicylates. Notorious inducers of adverse dermatologic reactions include the drugs listed in Tables 9-10 to 9-19.

Photosensitization, or susceptibility to dermatitis caused by exposure to sunlight, is being associated more frequently with a wide variety of drugs and other agents (see Table 9-11). This phenomenon is of three types: photoallergy, phototoxicity and photoaugmentation. A *photoallergic reaction* occurs when (1) the photosensitizing chemical forms a hapten through absorption of light rays, then (2) the hapten forms an antigen by combination with a skin protein, and finally (3) an antigen-antibody reaction occurs in the skin when it is rechallenged with the offending agent. A delayed eczematoid or polymorphic dematitis is elicited by ultraviolet light above 3200 Å (through window glass). A *phototoxic reaction* occurs when (1) the photosensitizing chemical absorbs ultraviolet energy, then (2) the photoactivated chemical transfers this energy to vulnerable cellular constituents, and (3) the cells sustain damage, manifested as a more or less severe sunburn. The dermatitis appears after the first exposure to ultraviolet light of the wavelengths (2900-3000 Å) that normally cause sunburn. A *photoaugmentation reaction* occurs when ultraviolet light potentiates the reactivity of the skin by means of a direct effect on cellular components that make them more vulnerable to contact dermatitis. Some photosensitivity reactions are paradoxical. For instance, several sunscreen agents that have been used to prevent sunburn may themselves photosensitize an individual.

Diabetogenicity. A number of drugs produce reversible glucosuria, but some induce chronic or permanent diabetes mellitus through a necrotic action on the β-cells of the islets of Langerhans. The long-term administration of glucose, growth hormone and certain other drugs may induce hyperglycemia, but this may be prevented by simultaneous treatment with insulin. On the other hand, the β-cytotoxins including alloxan, a few of its N-substituted derivatives, certain ascorbic acid and quinoline derivatives, and streptozotocin are rapidly destructive of β-cells and induce a chronic and sometimes a life-long diabetes mellitus. Drugs that are closely related structurally to any of these chemicals must be carefully studied for diabetogenic effects before they are approved for medical use.

Commonly used drugs that are diabetogenic in some patients under some conditions include ACTH, ethacrynic acid (Edecrin), glucocorticoids, nicotinic acid, sulfonamides like chlorthalidone (Hygroton), clorexolone (Nefrolan), and furosemide (Lasix), and thiazides such as chlorothiazide (Diuril), diazoxide (Hyperstat), hydrochlorothiazide (Hydrodiuril), and polythiazide (Renese). [33,60,132,293]

Gastrointestinal Toxicity. Gastrointestinal reactions to medications are the ones most frequently observed and fortunately they are usually the least hazardous. Many of them (diarrhea, nausea, vomiting, etc.) appear in

Table 9-11 Photosensitizers [132,163,205,206,208-217,233,308]

Acetohexamide (Dymelor)
Acridine preparations (slight)
Agave lechuguilla (amaryllis)
Agrimony
9-Aminoacridine
Aminobenzoic acid
Amitriptyline (Elavil, etc.)
Anesthetics (procaine group)
Angelica
Anthracene
Antimalarials
Arsenicals

Barbiturates
Bavachi (corylifolia)
Benzene
Benzopyrine
Bergamot (perfume)
Bithionol (Actamer, Lorothidol)
Blankophores (sulfa derivatives)
Bulosemide (Jadit)
Bromchlorsalicylanilid
4-Butyl-4-chlorosalicylanilide

Carbamazepine (Tegretol)
Carbinoxamine d-form (Twiston R-A)
Carbutamide (Nadisan)
Carrots, wild
Cedar oil
Celery
Chlorophyll
Chlorothiazide (Diuril)
Chlorpromazine (Thorazine)
Chlorpropamide (Diabinese)
Chlortetracycline (Aureomycin)
Citron oil
Citrus fruits
Clover
Coal tar
Contraceptives, oral

Demeclocycline (Declomycin, demethylchlortetracycline)
Desipramine (Norpramin, Pertofrane)
Dibenzopyran derivatives
Dicyanine-A
Diethylstilbestrol
Digalloyl trioleate (sunscreen)
Dill
Diphenhydramine hydrochloride (Benadryl)
Diphenylhydantoin (Dilantin)

Eosin (slight)
Estrone

Fennel
Fluorescein dyes

5-Fluorouracil
Furocoumarins (bergamot oil)

Glyceryl p-aminobenzoate (sunscreen)
Gold salts
Grass (meadow)
Griseofulvin (Fulvicin)

Hematoporphyrin
Hexachlorophene (rare)
Hydrochlorothiazide (Esidrix, HydroDiuril)

Imipramine HCl (Tofranil)
Isothipendyl (Theruhistin)

Lady's thumb (tea)
Lantinin
Lavender oil
Lime oil

Meclothiazide (Enduron)
Mepazine (Pacatal)
9-Mercaptopurine
Methotrimeprazine (Levoprome)
Methoxsalen (Meloxine, Oxsoralen)
5-Methoxypsoralen
8-Methoxypsoralen
Monoglycerol para-aminobenzoate
Mustards

Nalidixic acid (NegGram)
Naphthalene
Nortriptyline (Aventyl)

Oxytetracycline (Terramycin)

Para-dimethylaminoazobenzene
Paraphenylenediamine
Parsley
Parsnips
Penicillin derivates (Griseofulvin)
Perloline
Perphenazine (Trilafon)
Phenanthrene
Phenazine dyes
Phenolic compounds
Phenothiazines (dyes [methylene blue, toluidine blue], etc.)
Phenoxazines
Phenylbutazone (Butazolidin)
Pitch and pitch fumes
Porphyrins
Prochlorperazine (Compazine)
Promazine hydrochloride (Sparine)
Protriptyline (Vivactil)

Promethazine hydrochloride (Phenergan)
Psoralens (perfume)
Pyrathiazine hydrochloride (Pyrrolazote)
Pyridine

Quinethazone (Hydromox)
Quinine

Rose Bengal perfume (slight)
Rue

Salicylanilides
Salicylates
Sandalwood oil (perfume)
Silver salts
Smartweed (tea)
Stilbamidine isethionate
Sulfacetamide
Sulfadiazine
Sulfadimethoxine
Sulfaguanidine
Sulfanilamide (slight)
Sulfamerazine
Sulfamethazine
Sulfapyridine
Sulfathiazole
Sulfonamides
Sulfisomidine (Elkosin)
Sulfonylureas (antidiabetics)

Tetrachlorsalicylanilide (TCSA)
Tetracyclines
Thiazides (Diuril, HydroDiuril, etc.)
Thiophene
Thiopropazate dihydrochloride (Dartal)
Tolbutamide (Orinase)
Toluene
Tribromosalicylanilide (TBS), (deodorant soaps)
Trichlormethiazide (Metahydrin)
Tridione
Triethylene melamine (TEM)
Triflupromazine hydrochloride (Vesprin)
Trimeprazine tartrate (Temaril)
Trimethadione (Tridione)
Tripyrathiazine
Trypaflavine
Trypan blue

Vanillin oils

Water ash

Xylene

Yarrow

Table 9-2 that lists minor drug reactions. Nevertheless, if these minor reactions are sufficiently exacerbated, they can readily incapacitate and sometimes seriously harm a patient. Such minor reactions may also be indicators of more serious reactions that are developing or have developed.

Gastrointestinal hemorrhaging of any degree should never be regarded lightly. But it is a common occurrence with the most widely used drug, namely aspirin. The bleeding induced by this drug may be occult or overt. Occult loss of blood occurs in 70% of patients who repeatedly ingest aspirin either from local irritation or from prolongation of the bleeding time by reduction of platelet stickiness. Overt loss of blood occurs when aspirin is taken in the presence of underlying lesions such as atrophic gastritis, esophagitis and peptic ulcer. Vasirub pointed out, "An uncommon effect of a common drug, gross gastric hemorrhage, may thus become an unmasker of unsuspected pathologic lesions." [219]

Gastrointestinal hemorrhaging with anticoagulant therapy has been critically reviewed by Babb *et al.* [230] They point out that melena, hematemesis and hematochezia may be harbingers of serious underlying disease. In their review they subdivide the gastroenterologic complications of anticoagulant therapy into (1) hemorrhage into the intestinal lumen, (2) intramural hemorrhage with secondary ileus, (3) retroperitoneal hemorrhage, (4) hemorrhage into the intraabdominal organs, (5) rectus abdominis hematoma, and (6) reactions to phenindione, i.e., diarrhea and hepatitis. In a total of 4615 patients in 8 series who received anticoagulants, the incidence of overall hemorrhage ranged from 5 to 48%, of major hemorrhage from 0.8 to 12%, and of gastrointestinal hemorrhage

Table 9-12   Drugs Causing an Acneform Reaction [132,233]

ACTH
Androgenic hormones
Bromides
Corticosteroids
Cyanocobalamin
Hydantoins
Iodides
Methandrostenolone (Dianabol)
Methyltestosterone (Metandren, etc.)
Oral contraceptives

Table 9-13   Drugs Causing Alopecia [132,233,299,309]

Alkylating agents
Anticoagulants
Antimetabolites
Bleomycin (Blenoxane)
Mepesulfate
Mephenytoin (Mesantoin)
Methimazole
Methotrexate
Norethindrone acetate
   (Norinyl, Norlestrin, Ortho-Novum)
Quinacrine
Oral contraceptives
Sodium warfarin (Coumadin)
Trimethadione (Tridione)
Triparanol (Mer-29)

from 3 to 4%. In patients with major hemorrhagic episodes 33 to 53% had serious bleeding in the gastrointestinal tract. In another survey 228 medical specialists reported that they had observed serious hemorrhage following anticoagulant therapy for myocardial infarction with 30 deaths due to exsanguination after gastrointestinal bleeding. The most common underlying lesion was peptic ulcer; other conditions included cancer, diaphragmatic hernia, diverticula, and hemorrhoids.

Other drugs that have been implicated in gastrointestinal bleeding include ethacrynic acid (Edecrin), ibufemac, indomethacin (Indocin), phenacetin, and pyrazolone derivatives such as phenylbutazone (Butazolidin). Death may result from peritonitis due to perforation of gastric ulcers following ethacrynic acid (Edecrin) therapy. After seven weeks on this drug, one patient on autopsy was found to have both gastric and duodenal ulcers. [238] Gastric ulcerations complicated by massive gastrointestinal hemorrhage and perforation have been repeatedly associated with indomethacin (Indocin) therapy. [239] Gastroduodenal ulcerations with perforations and occult blood loss have been reported with phenylbutazone (Butazolidin). [60] Other drugs associated with gastrointestinal ulcerations include the salicylates, corticosteroids, flufenamic acid, and potassium chloride.

Colitis, esophagitis, pharingitis, proctitis, stomatitis, and other conditions that result from irritant effects may be induced by a number of drugs. Stomatitis has been associated with cytostatic drugs such as certain alkaloids (trimethylcolchicinic acid, and vincristine), alkylating agents (thiotepa), antimetabolites (duazomycin, fluorodeoxyuridine, 5-fluorouracil, hydroxyurea, and methotrexate), as well as calomel, indandiones, and mercurial diuretics.

The undesirable effects of mineral oil such as its tendency to prevent gastrointestinal absorption of lipid-soluble vitamins and other drugs were discussed previously. Also the necrotizing effects of potassium chloride in the intestines were covered previously. The list of drugs that adversely affect the gastrointestinal tract has been growing constantly and rapidly.

Hepatotoxicity. Many drugs are capable of damaging the liver under certain circumstances. Hepatotoxic medications may alter hepatic function and induce hepatocellular changes including necrosis, as well as hepatomegaly and jaundice. These medications may possibly modify any of the hepatic functions such as *detoxication* of drugs, hormones, intestinal putrefactive products, and other endogenous and exogenous substances, *excretion* of bile (bile salts, bilirubin, etc.), *formation* of heat and vitamin A, *gluconeogenesis, glycogenolysis, liberation* of depressor principle, *metabolism* of drugs, carbohydrates, proteins and fats, *production* of bile acids, cholesterol, fibrinogen, heparin, hormones, and prothrombin and *reticuloendothelial activity.* Damage to the liver that alters any of its functions or produces significant hepatic insufficiency may have far-reaching effects on the brain (hepatic encephalopathy), endocrine glands, skin (pruritus), and other parts of the body.

Damage to the drug metabolizing microsomal enzymes of the liver may significantly decrease its capacity to conjugate and otherwise detoxicate drugs, i.e., decrease the rate of formation of metabolites and therby reduce the rate of urinary excretion of medications. The insufficiency may cause drug concentrations in the blood and tissues to rise to highly toxic levels. Severe, inadequately corrected cases can be fatal. Many hepatotoxic drugs are therefore contraindicated in patients with hepatic insufficiency whether it results from disease or some other cause; also in the very young or elderly, as they cannot cope with these toxic drugs because of their immature or impaired microsomal enzyme systems. If potentially hepatotoxic drugs must be administered, the patient must always be monitored closely and blood levels checked frequently. Hepatic tolerance to a drug may vary greatly from one individual to another.

Table 9-14　Drugs Causing Contact Dermatitis [41,132,233,298,300,311]

Acriflavine	Cyclomethycaine	Para-aminosalicylic acid
Amethocaine		Parabens
Antazoline	Diphenhydramine	Penicillin
Antazoline and phenocide	Domiphen	Peru balsam
Antazoline and pyribenzamine		Phenindamine
Antihistamine	Ephedrine	Phenocide and antazoline
Arsphenamine		Phenol
Atabrine	Formaldehyde	Potassium hydroxyquinoline
		sulfate
Bacitracin (occupational)	Halogenated phenolic	Procaine and other anesthetics
Benzocaine	compounds	Promethazine
Benzoyl peroxide and	Hedaquinium chloride	Propamidine
chlorhydroxyquinoline		Pyribenzamine and antazoline
Bleomycin (Blenoxane)	Iodine	
	Iodochlorhydroxyquinoline	Quinacrine (Atabrine)
Cetrimide	Isoniazid (occupational)	Quinine
Chloramphenicol		
Chlorcyclizine	Lanolin	Resorcin
Chlorhexidine		
Chlorhydroxyquinoline and	Meprobamate	Spiramycin (occupational)
benzoyl peroxide	Mepyramine (Pyrilamine)	Streptomycin
Chloroxylenol	Mercurials	Sulfonamides
Chlorphenesin	Mercury	Sulfur and salicylic acid ointment
Chlorpromazine		Tetracyclines
Colophony	Neomycin	Thiamine
Crotamiton	Nitrofurazone	Thimerosal (Merthiolate)
	Novobiocin	

Liver changes induced by drugs given alone or in certain combinations may occur immediately or they may be delayed for months after withdrawal of the medication. The changes may have a familial component and not be dose-related or they may be dose-related and reversible upon cessation or reduction of therapy. Some conditions like hepatocellular or hepatocanalicular jaundice may progress until they are irreversible, and may then persist for years as a chronic disease that may eventually terminate in death. See also Enzyme Induction, Enzyme Inhibition, and Other Metabolic Anomalies (pages 274 to 279).

Drug-induced liver damage may also be the result of hypersensitivity. Paraminosalicylic acid, chlorpromazine, and certain other drugs can produce severe allergic reactions through the formation of erythrocytic antigens. Subsequent administration of these

Table 9–16 Drugs Causing Lichenoid Reactions [132,233,295]

Amiphenazole (Daptazole)
Chloroquine
Gold salts compounds
Organic arsenicals
Para-aminosalicylic acid
Quinacrine (Atabrine, mepacrine)
Quinidine
Thiazides

drugs after they have been withdrawn for a period of time may initiate an antigen-antibody type of reaction with the development of blood dyscrasias, eosinophil invasion of liver secretions, fever, hypertrophy of lymph nodes, jaundice, rash, and urticaria.

Jaundice is the most frequently observed manifestation of iatrogenic hepatotoxicity. The syndrome, characterized by hyperbilirubinemia and depositions of bile pigments in

Table 9–15 Drugs Causing Fixed Eruptions [132,202,233,295,297]

Acetanilid	Disulfiram and alcohol	Pyrimidine derivatives
Acetarsone	Eosin	Quinacrine
Acetophenetidin	Ephedrine	Quinidine
Acetylsalicylic acid	Epinephrine	Quinine
Aconite	Ergot alkaloids	Reserpine
Acriflavine	Erythrosin	Salicylates
Aminopyrine	Eucalyptus oil	Santonin
Amobarbital	Formalin	Saccharin
Amodiaquine	Frangula	Scopolamine
Amphetamine sulfate	Gold compounds	Sodium salicylate
Anthralin	Griseofulvin (Grifulvin)	Sterculia gum
Antimony potassium tartrate	Iodine	Stramonium
Antipyrine	Ipecac	Streptomycin
Arsphenamine	Ipomea	Strychnine
Barbital	2-Isopropyl-4-pentenoyl urea	Sulfadiazine
Barbiturates	(Sedormid)	Sulfaguanidine
Belladonna	Karaya gum	Sulfamerazine
Bismuth salts	Magnesium hydroxide	Sulfamethazine
Bromides	Meprobamate	Sulfamethoxypyridazine (Kynex)
Chloral hydrate	Mercury salts	Sulfapyridine
Chlorguanide	Methenamine	Sulfarsphenamine
Chloroquine	Neoarsphenamine	Sulfathiazole
Chlorothiazide and sun	Opium alkaloids	Sulfisoxazole (Gantrisin)
Chlorpromazine	Oxophenarsine	Sulfobromophthalein sodium
Chlortetracycline	Oxytetracycline (Terramycin)	Sulfonamides
Cinchophen	Para-aminosalicylic acid	Tetracyclines
Copaiba	Penicillin	Thiambutosine
Dextroamphetamine	Phenacetin	Thiram and alcohol
Diacetyldiphenolisatin	Phenazone	Thonzylamine HCl (Neohetramine)
Diallybarbituric acid	Phenobarbital	Tripelennamine (Pyribenzamine)
Diethylstilbestrol	Phenolphthalein	Trisodium arsphenamine sulfate
Digilanid	Phenylbutazone (Butazolidin)	Tryparsamide
Digitalis	5-Phenylethylhydantoin	Urease
Dimenhydrinate (Dramamine)	Phenylhydantoin	Urginin
Dimethylamine acetarsone	Phenytoin	Vaccines and immunizing agents
Diphenhydramine (Benadryl)	Phosphorus	
Diphenylhydantoin (Dilantin)	Potassium chlorate	

Table 9-17   Drugs Causing Morbilliform Reactions [132,233]

p-Aminosalicylic acid (PAS)	Mercurials
Anticonvulsants	Methaminodiazepoxide
Anticholinergics	Novobiocin
Antihistamines	Organic extracts
Barbiturates	Para-aminosalicylic
Chloral hydrate	acid
Chlordiazepoxide	Penicillin
(Librium)	Phenothiazines
Chlorothiazide (Diuril)	Phenylbutazone
Chlorpromazine	(Butazolidin)
(Thorazine)	Quinacrine (Atabrine)
Gold salts	Salicylates
Griseofulvin (Grifulvin)	Serums
Hydantoins (Dilantin,	Streptomycin
etc.)	Sulfonamides
Insulin	Sulfones
Meprobamate	Tetracyclines
	Thiouracil

Table 9-19   Drugs Causing Urticaria [132,233]

ACTH	Mercurials
Amitriptyline	Nitrofurantoin
Barbiturates	(Furadantin)
Bromides	Novobiocin
Chloramphenicol	Opiates
(Chloromycetin)	Penicillin
Dextran	Penicillinase
Enzymes	Pentazocine (Talwin)
Erythromycin	Phenolphthalein
(Erythrocin, Ilotycin)	Phenothiazines
Griseofulvin (Grifulvin)	Propoxyphene (Darvon)
Hydantoins (Dilantin,	Rifampin (Rifadin,
etc.)	Rimactane,
Insulin	rifampicin)
Iodides	Salicylates
Iodopyracet (Diodrast)	Serums
Meprobamate (Equanil,	Streptomycin
Miltown)	Sulfonamides
Meperidine (Demerol)	Tetracyclines
Meprobamate	Thiouracil

the dermatomucosal membrances with resulting yellow appearance, has been classified by Schaffner, according to the abnormal processes involved, into three main types: (1) *cholestatic* (hepatocanalicular), (2) *hepatocellular* (necrotic), and (3) *hemolytic*. The latter is not induced through a hepatotoxic mechanism. Other authors add a fourth class: *mixed.* Table 9-20 lists drugs that have been implicated under these four headings. [86,88]

Cholestatic jaundice, which may or may not be accompanied by portal inflammation (cholangiolitis) occurs when drugs modify hepatic excretion or secretion through alteration of the canaliculi. All of the drugs listed in the first column of Table 9-20, except the steroids, may produce cholangeolitic chole-

Table 9-18   Drugs Causing Purpura [132,233,312]

ACTH	Griseofulvin (Grifulvin)
Allopurinol (Zyloprim)	Iodides
Amitriptyline (Elavil,	Mepesulfate
Endep, etc.)	Meprobamate
Anticoagulants	Oxyphenbutazone
Barbiturates	(Tandearil)
Carbamides	Penicillin
Chloral hydrate	Phenylbutazone
Chlorothiazide (Diuril)	(Butazolidin)
Chlorpropamide	Quinidine
(Diabinese)	Rifampin (Rifadin,
Chlorpromazine	Rimactane,
(Thorazine)	rifampicin)
Corticosteroids	Sulfonamides
Digitalis	Thiazides
Fluoxymesterone	Trifluoperazine
Gold salts	

static jaundice. This may be characterized by obstructive jaundice, possibly with blood dyscrasia, eosinophilia, fever, or rash. The steroid-induced syndrome does not include inflammation or sensitization of the patient. Hepatocellular or necrotic jaundice resembles severe viral hepatitis. Drugs inducing this type of liver damage may produce a mortality as high as 50%. Hemolytic jaundice may be caused by a hypersensitivity reaction as noted above, or by direct toxic action on the erythrocytes or by depletion of glutathione or interference with the pathways of glucose metabolism in the erythrocytes. See page 273.

Nephrotoxicity. Kidney damage is one of the most perilous hazards of medication. Nephrotoxic drugs and other agents (see Table 9-21) may damage enough nephrons directly or indirectly to alter signficantly the urinary excretion rate of the drugs themselves as well as other constituents of the extracellular fluid (ECF). The resulting renal insufficiency, or even possibly renal failure, can cause elevated highly toxic blood and tissue levels of these constituents. The characteristic signs and symptoms of uremia, may develop. Nephrotoxic medications are therefore usually contraindicated in patients with renal insufficiency, regardless of the cause. However, if a decision is made to administer a drug known to have a nephrotoxic potential to a patient with decreased renal function, he must always be monitored closely

Table 9-20 Drugs That May Induce Liver Disease[a]

Drug	Cholestatic Jaundice	Hemolytic Jaundice	Hepatocellular Jaundice	Mixed Jaundice
Acetaminophen (Tylenol)			*	
Acetanilid		*		
Acetohexamide (Dymelor)				*
Actinomycin			*	
Amitriptyline (Elavil, etc.)	*			
Amphetamine		*		
Arsenicals	*		*	
Arsphenamine	*			
ASA			*	
Beta-phenylisopropylhydrazine (Catron)			*	
Carbamazepine (Tegretol)	*		*	
Carbamazine	*			
Carbarsone	*			
Carbutamide				*
Chlorambucil (Leukeran)			*	*
Chloramphenicol (Chloromycetin)	*			*
Chlordiazepoxide (Librium)	*		*	
Chloroform			*	
Chlorothiazide (Diuril)	*			
Chlorpromazine (Thorazine)	*			
Chlorpropamide (Diabinese)	*			*
Chlorprothixene (Taractan)	*			
Chlortetracycline (Aureomycin)			*	
Cinchophen				b
Colchicine			*	
Diazepam (Valium)	*			
Diethylstilbestrol	*			*
Dinitrophenol	*			*
Ectylurea	*			
Erythromycin estolate (Ilosone)				*
Ethacrynic acid (Edecrin)				b
Ethionamide (Trecator)			*	
Ethyl carbamate			*	
Gold salts				*
Glucosulfone sodium (Promin)		*		
Griseofulvin	*			
Halothane			*	
Indomethacin			*	
Imipramine			*	
Iopanoic acid			*	
Iproniazid (Marsilid)			*	
Isocarboxide (Marplan)			*	
Isoniazid			*	*
MAO inhibitors			*	
Mepazine (Pacatal)	*			
Mepharsen				*
Meprobamate	*			
6-Mercaptopurine (Purinethol)				*
Metahexamide			*	
Methandrostenolone (Dianabol)	*			
Methimazole (Tapazole)	*			
Methotrexate			*	
Methoxyflurane			*	
Methyldopa (Aldomet)				b
Methylestrenolone (Normethandrone)	*			
Methyltestosterone	*			
Mitomycin			*	
Neoarsphenamine		*		

[a] These hepatotoxicities have all been reported in the literature.[11,20,25,26,32,34,36,40,46,56,64,71,76,78,80,82,84,88,95,99,100–102,105,107,111,112,136,313–316]

[b] Potentially fatal complications. Read labeling carefully.[120]

Table 9-20 Drugs That May Induce Liver Disease *(Continued)*

Drug	Cholestatic Jaundice	Hemolytic Jaundice	Hepatocellular Jaundice	Mixed Jaundice
Nicotinic acid	*			
Norethandrolone (Nilevar)	*			
Norethindrone (Norlutin)	*			
Norethisterone (Norethindrone)	*			
Norethynodrel (Enovid)	*			
Novobiocin			*	
Oxyphenbutazone (Tandearil)			*	
Oxytetracycline				*
Paracetamol			*	
Para-aminobenzyl caffeine	*			
Para-aminosalicylic acid (PAS)	*	*	*	*
Penicillin			*	
Perphenazine (Trilafon)	*		*	
Phenacemide (Phenurone)		*	*	
Phenacetin			*	
Phenazopyridine	*			
Phenelzine (Nardil)		*		
Phenantoin (Mesantoin)		*		
Phenindione (Danilone)				*
Pheniprazine (Cavodil)			*	
Phenobarbital				*
Phenothiazine	*			
Phenoxypropazine			*	
Phenylbutazone (Butazolidin)		*		
Phenylhydrazine				*
Phenytoin (Dilantin)			*	*
Polythiazide (Renese)		*		
Primaquine				*
Probenecid (Benemid)	*			
Prochlorperazine (Compazine)	*			
Promazine (Sparine)				*
Propoxyphene (Darvon)	*			
Propylthiouracil				*
Pyrazinamide (Aldinamide)			*	
Quinacrine (Atrobrine)				*
Quinethazone (Aquamox, Hydromox)			*	
Quinine		*		
Rifampin				*
Sulfadiazine	*			*
Streptomycin			*	
Sulfanilamide	*			
Sulfonamides				*
Sulfones	*			
Sulfonylureas	*			
Tannic acid			*	*
Tetracycline (Achromycin, Tetracyn, etc.)			*	
Thiouracil	*		*	
Tolbutamide	*			
Tranylcypromine (Parnate)				*
Triacetyloleandomycin (Cyclamycin, TAO)			*	*
Trichloroethylene			*	
Trimethadione (Tridione)			*	*
Urethane			*	
Zoxazolamine (Flexin)			*	

Table 9-21   Agents That May Induce or Exacerbate Kidney Disease [132,138-148,235,242,312,317,318]

Acetazolamide (Diamox)	Diuretics	Para-aminosalicylic acid (PAS)
Allopurinol	Diurgin (mercurial diuretic)	Paradione
Aminonucleotides	Electroshock	Paramethadione (Paradione)
Amitriptyline (Elavil)	Ethacrynic acid (Edecrin)	Penicillamine
Amphotericin B (Fungizone)	Ether	Penicillin
Aniline	Ethylene dichloride	Pentamide
Antimony compounds	Ethylene glycol	Phenacetin
Antineoplastics	Ethylene glycol dinitrite	Phenazopyridine (Pyridium)
Arsine and arsenic	Furosemide (Lasix)	Phenindione (Danilone, Hedulin)
Bacitracin	Gentamicin	Phenobarbital hemolysis
Bee stings	Gold compounds	Phenylbutazone (Butazolidin)
Benzene	Heat stroke	Poison oak
Beryllium	Homolysins	Polymyxin B (Aerosporin)
Biphenyl (chlorinated	Hydralazine HCl (Apresoline)	Probenecid (Benemid)
compounds)	Hydrochlorthiazide (Hydrodiuril)	Propylene glycol
Bismuth compounds	Hypercalcemia	Puromycin
Bleomycin (Blenoxane)	Hyperkalemia	Radiation
Cadmium compounds	Hyperuricemia	Rifampin
Cantharides (Spanish fly)	Iron salts	Rotenone
Carbonic anhydrase inhibitors	Kanamycin (Kantrex) sulfate	Salicylates
Carbon monoxide	Lead compounds	Silver compounds
Carbon tetrachloride	Mannitol	Snake venom
Cellosolve (2-ethoxyethane)	Meralluride (Mercuhydrin)	Spider venom
Cephaloridine	Mercaptomerin (Thiomerin)	Spironolactone (Aldactone)
Cephalothin	sodium	Streptomycin
Cephalosporins	Mercurophylline (Mercupurin)	Sucrose
Chlorinated hydrocarbons	sodium	Sulfamethoxazole-trimethoprim
(insecticides)	Mercury (organic and inorganic)	Sulfonamides
Chlormerodrin (Neohydrin)	Mersalyl (Salyrgan)	Tetrachloroethylene
Chlorothiazide (Diuril)	Methemoglobin producers	Tetracyclines
Colchicine	Methicillin	Thallium compounds
Colistimethate	Methotrexate	Thiazides
Colistin (Coly-Mycin)	Methoxyflurane (Penthrane)	Thyroid preparations
Contrast agents (high	Methyl alcohol	Triamterene (Dyrenium)
concentration)	Methyl cellusolve	Tridione
Copper compounds	Mushroom poison	Trimethadione (Tridione)
Corticosteriods	Narcotics	Uranium compounds
Cresol	Neomycin	Vancomycin (Vancocin) HCl
Diallylacetic acid	Nephroallergens	Vasoconstrictors
Diatrizoate	Nitrofurans	Vasopressors
Diethylene glycol	Nitrofurantoin (Furandantin)	Zoxazolamine (Flexin)

and his blood levels must be checked frequently.

Severe nephrotoxicity may result from (1) direct damage to the structure or the function of the nephrons with a toxic chemical like carbon tetrachloride or mercuric chloride, (2) immune reaction to a compound like aminonucleotide that causes a condition resembling nephritis or the nephrotic syndrome, (3) hypersensitivity to substances like the sulfonamides that may cause angiitis within the kidney, (4) chronic poisoning with lead or other heavy metals, or (5) exacerbation of existing renal disease with cathartics, diuretics, and certain other drugs. Thus, uremia can be exacerbated with antineoplastics,

corticosteroids, diuretics, nitrofurans, narcotics, tetracyclines, thyroid preparations, vasoconstrictors and vasopressors.

Drug-induced kidney dysfunction may arise directly not only from damage to the glomerular filtration apparatus, but also from damage to enzymes, cells, membranes and other components involved in the active and passive tubular secretion and reabsorption of endogenous and exogenous substances. Dysfunction may also arise as a secondary effect. Thus, a severe hypokalemia caused by a drug may induce hypokalemic nephropathy. Serious problems may arise in a patient when, because of renal damage, (1) the volume (50-60% of body weight) and composition of the extracellular fluid are shifted outside their normal narrow limits, and (2) the electroneutrality of the excreted, secreted, or reabsorbed fluids is disturbed. Nephrotoxicity is closely related to disturbances of fluid and electrolyte balance.

Disturbances of Fluid and Electrolyte Balance. Hypovolemia, either from simple dehydration or combined sodium and water depletion, may result from excessive drug-induced diuresis, vomiting or diarrhea, or tubular necrosis. Dry tongue, nausea, postural hypotension, rapid pulse, reduced turgor of the skin, thirst, weakness, and possibly shock, are typical findings.

Drug-induced shifts in concentrations of electrolyte (bicarbonate, chloride, potassium, sodium, and certain organic anions) in the ECF may cause serious problems. *Hyponatremia,* with the signs and symptoms of water intoxication, causes ECF fluid to move into the cells. CNS effects may occur, including confusion, irritability, lethargy, possibly progressing to convulsions, coma, and death. *Hypernatremia,* accompanied by dehydration, hypertoxicity, and water loss, may be encountered in patients unable to drink adequate quantities of water because they are stuporous or comatose; drug toxicity may possibly induce these states.

Shifts in the potassium equilibrium may produce a wide range of clinical disorders because the element has a powerful effect on the excitability of cardiac and skeletal muscles and on kidney function. It is also an essential activator of certain enzyme reactions. *Hypokalemia,* (serum K level below 2 mEq./L.) induces neuromuscular effects (weakness, paralysis, and possibly death from respiratory insufficiency), serious cardiac arrhythmias especially in digitalized patients, renal tubular damage (multiple epithelial vacuoles, inability to concentrate the urine, and sometimes nocturia, polydipsia, and polyuria), gastrointestinal dysfunction (paralytic ileus), and metabolic acidosis. Implicated drugs include corticosteroids, diuretics including carbonic anhydrase inhibitors, ethacrynic acid, furosemide, mercurials, thiazides, and outdated tetracycline (epianhydrotetracycline). *Hyperkalemia,* potassium intoxication (serum K level above 7 mEq./L.), causes serious cardiac abnormalities (atrial asystole, intraventricular block and ultimately ventricular

standstill), neuromuscular effects (flaccid paralysis, weakness, and ultimately death). Implicated drugs include intravenous KCl therapy (especially if renal function is impaired), the aldosterone antagonist, spironolactone impairs ability of kidney to handle a K load and should not be given with K supplements) and traimterene (impairs tubular exchange of Na for K).

Acid base imbalance (pH below 7.35 or above 7.45) caused by metabolic, respiratory, or renal drug induced disturbances may seriously affect major vital organ systems. Death usually occurs below pH 6.8 or above 7.8. *Metabolic acidosis* occurs when the bicarbonate ion concentration is reduced as a result of excessive loss of alkali from the body or overload of acid or impaired renal function that prevents normal excretion of excess acid.

Drugs that have been implicated in metabolic acidosis include ammonium chloride, carbonic anhydrase, paraldehyde, and salicylates. Drugs that may cause metabolic alkalosis include corticosteroids, ethacrynic acid, furosemide, mercurial diuretics, and thiazides. Respiratory alkalosis results from salicylate intoxication, and respiratory acidosis may be caused by anesthetics. *Metabolic alkalosis* occurs when the bicarbonate ion concentration is elevated as a result of excessive loss of acid or overload of alkali or imparied renal function that prevents normal excretion of excess alkali. *Respiratory acidosis* occurs when elevated pCO_2 results from hypoventilation which may be caused by anesthetics and drugs that have effects on the neuromuscular and central nervous systems. Respiratory alkalosis occurs when reduced pCO_2 results from hyperventilation which may be induced by drugs that cause central nervous system injury involving the respiratory center.[148]

Neurotoxicity. Neurotoxic reactions, attributable to drugs, may occur in both the central and peripheral nervous systems, and may affect a wide range of organs and tissues, including the heart, sensory organs such as the ear and the eye, muscles, and the vasculature. Medications which adversely affect neurohumoral transmission of nerve impulses in the autonomic and central nervous systems, or which injure neurons through direct or allergic effects should be withdrawn promptly.

Nervous system toxicities manifest themselves mainly as adverse cerebrovascular conditions, CNS depression, convulsive states, encephalopathy, extrapyramidal syndromes, myelopathy, oculotoxicities, ototoxicities, peripheral neuropathy, or adverse behavior.

Adverse cerebrovascular conditions include four that are very hazardous.[234] (1) Cerebral infarcts may occur if drugs with antihypertensive effects cause cerebral ischemia and a sudden fall in blood pressure. Chlorisondamine, hexamethonium, and pentolinium are examples of drugs that have been implicated. (2) Hypertensive crises complicated by intracerebral or subarachnoid hemorrhage, and sometimes terminating in death may follow the administration of monoamine oxidase (MAO) inhibitors used either as antidepressants or antihypertensives when these drugs are given concomitantly with foods and drugs containing pressor principles (*Tyramine-rich Foods,* and *Sympathomimetics,* Table of Drug Interactions). (3) Intracerebral or subarachnoid hemorrhages may also occur when pressor amines (epinephrine, levarterenol, tyramine, and other sympathomimetic amines) unduly increase the intracranial blood pressure in the presence of berry aneurysms or clotting defects. These hemorrhages may also occur when anticoagulant drug therapy is poorly controlled. (4) Strokelike syndromes may be produced by sudden reductions of blood glucose with hypoglycemics, either oral or parenteral. These syndromes may be manifested by symptoms such as hemiparesis or toal hemiplegia after administration of anticonvulsants such as phenytoin.

CNS depression induced by drugs may occasionally be very severe and sometimes unexpected. The fatal synergism occurring with alcohol and barbiturates is discussed in the next chapter. The sedation and other depressant effects of analgesics, antihistamines, general anesthetics, hypnotics, narcotics, psychotropics, sedatives, and various other CNS depressants are well known. Combinations of such drugs may cause serious problems in some patients, including respiratory depression, coma, and possibly death. Some CNS depressant effects may be paradoxical. Thus, the sympathomimetic naphazoline, a nasal decongestant, may cause coma and lowered body temperature as the result of CNS depression, and therefore should not be used in children.

Convulsive states have been induced by (1) analeptics and CNS stimulants, e.g., amphetamines, bemegride, methylphenidate, pentylenetetrazol, and pictrotoxin, (2) anesthetics applied locally, e.g., lidocaine, procaine, and tetracaine in excessive mucosal concentrations or inadvertently injected IV, (3) antidepressants, e.g., the MAO inhibitors and the tricyclic antidepressants, (4) antifungals, e.g., diamthazole, (5) antihistamines, e.g., tripelennamine, (6) antimycobacterials, e.g., cycloserine and isoniazid, and (7) antipsychotics, e.g., phenothiazines and Rauwolfia alkaloids in high doses and in the presence of brain damage or epilepsy.

Encelphalopathy and myelopathy (encephalomyelitis, cerebellar syndromes, etc.), consisting of hemorrhagic lesions that result from direct drug toxicity or demyelinating lesions that result from allergic drug reactions, may be accompanied by seizures and other neurological disturbances. These conditions are rare but they have a high fatality rate. Drugs that have been implicated include: (1) antibacterials, e.g., iproniazid, isoniazid, penicillin, streptomycin, and sulfonamides, (2) anticonvulsants, e.g., chlordiazepoxide, chlorpromazine, hydantoins, meprobamate, phenobarbital, phenothiazines, primidone, reserpine, and other psychotropic drugs, (3) antidepressants, particularly combinations of MAO inhibitors and tricyclic antidepressants, whereby the former increase the serotonin and catecholamine content of the brain while the latter enhance adrenergic sensitivity centrally, (4) gold compounds used in rheumatoid arthritis, and (5) mercurial compounds.

Extrapyramidal syndromes such as akathisia, dystonia, and parkinsonism are characteristic adverse effects of phenothiazine tranquilizers and may occur with all psychotropics including the butyrophenones, benzoquinolizines, phenylpiperazines, and thioxanthines. The phenothiazines in particular, have so many adverse reactions associated with them that it is very difficult to summarize them briefly. See Addiction, Blood Dyscrasias, Cardiovascular Toxicity. Hepatotoxicity, and other hazardous drug reactions discussed in the previous sections of this chapter.

In addition to type of drug and level of dosage, the age and sex of the patient appear to affect the incidence of extrapyramidal symptoms. Women are more susceptible than men and older patients more than younger ones. Also some individuals are inherently more susceptible than others and a genetic influence may exist. These undesirable adverse effects appear to be induced in general by any drug that depletes or blocks catecholamines and serotonin (e.g., antipsychotics and methyldopa) and these drugs may be treated beneficially with drugs that antagonize the opposing neurohumoral agents acetylcholine and histamine (e.g., anticholinergics and antihistamines).

Dystonia or dyskinesia, manifested by myoclonic or tonic twitching of shoulder muscles, oculogyric crisis, spasms of the face, jaw, and tongue, and spastic retrocollis or torticollis, appears to be caused most frequently by piperazine phenothiazines. Examples of these drugs are acetophenazine (Tindal), fluphenazine (Prolixin), perphenazine (Trilafon), prochlorperazine (Compazine), and trifluoperazine (Stelazine). Patients receiving these drugs should be closely monitored. Occasionally chlorpromazine and most of the other psychotropic drugs* may induce the same condition, especially after parenteral administration. Fortunately it is rarely fatal and usually reversible with antiparkinsonism drugs, barbiturates, or caffeine, but it is often diagnosed incorrectly as encephalitis, hysteria, tetanus or some other acute CNS disorder. Its incidence ranges from essentially 0% with thioridazine to 3% or higher with halogenated piperazines such as fluphenazine. Parkinsonism occurs in 15 to 45% of the patients treated with psychotropic drugs.

Peripheral neuropathy resulting from medications is usually manifested as bilateral or unilateral palsies, paresthesias such as numbness, formication, or tingling of the extremities and the tongue, and a variety of other neurologic side effects such as fasciculations, muscle twitchings, tremors, unsteadiness of gait, and weakness of various muscles. The *antibacterials* chloramphenicol, nitrofurantoin, penicillins and sulfonamides have been most frequently implicated, often

with an associated optic neuritis. The *antituberculars* ethionamide, isoniazid, and streptomycin have also been implicated. Isonizid, particularly in slow metabolizers of the drug, causes neuropathy through increased pyridoxine excretion. The *antidepressants,* both the MAO inhibitors such as the hydrazides and tricylcics such as amitriptylene and imipramine, have produced peripheral neuropathy. A wide variety of other drugs have also been implicated, including arsenicals, chloroquine (prolonged use), disulfiram (in some alcoholics), ethacrynic acid (Edecrin), methimazole, perhexiline, polymyxin, sodium colistimethate (Coly-Mycin), and stilbamidine. [234]

Ocular Toxicity. Careful follow-up of patients receiving a drug that is known to affect sight adversely is essential so that if symptoms of ocular toxicity appear the drug can be withdrawn promptly and the adverse effects reversed if possible. Some oculotoxic drugs that are useful in treating serious conditions may be reinstituted at a lower dose after a rest period if the eyes return to near normal. This is frequently the case with certain antituberculosis drugs such as ethambutol (Myambutol), but if there is a genetically induced sensitivity to a drug, use of a succedaneum may be necessary.

Some drugs, although widely and safely used for various purposes, must be prescribed with great caution for ophthalmic use. The topical anesthetics dibucaine, dyclonine and tetracaine, although said to be less damaging than cocaine, when applied repeatedly in the eye have been associated with corneal opacification and loss of vision.

Cholinergic drugs which produce miotic effects include acetylcholine chloride (Miochol), bethanechol (Urecholine), carbachol (Carcholin, Doryl), demecarium (Humorsol), isoflurophate (DFP, Floropryl), methacholine (Mecholyl), neostigmine (Prostigmin), pholine (Echothiopate) iodide, physostigmine (Eserine) salicylate or sulfate, and pilocarpine HCl or nitrate. Such drugs may also produce ciliary spasm, as well as asthma due to constriction of the bronchi, and other parasympathomimetic effects.

Cholinergic blocking drugs which produce mydriatic effects include atropine sulfate, cyclopentolate (Cyclogyl) HCl, eucatropine HCl, homatropine HBr, hydroxyampheta-

---

* Notably the butyrophenones (haloperiodol, etc.).

mine (Paredrine) HBr, scopolamine HBr, and tropicamide (bis-Tropamide, Mydriacyl). Such drugs may also produce increased intraocular pressure and restlessness, as well as ataxia, disorientation, failure to recognize people, fever, flushing of the face, hallucinations, and incoherency, and particularly in young children if the dosage is excessive. *Acute glaucoma* may be precipitated by anticholinergics, and also by antidepressants such as amitriptylene and imipramine, antiparkinsonism drugs such as benztropine and procyclidine, and antipsychotics such as mepazine.

Sympathomimetics with mydriatic effects like epinephrine and phenylephrine (Neo-Synephrine) HCl, may also induce hypertension and cardiac arrhythmias. Caution must be observed with predisposed patients such as those with arteriosclerosis, bradycardia, hyperthyroidism, myocardial disease, and partial heart block.

Other drug-induced ocular disorders include *subcapsular cataracts* with corticosteroids such as betamethasone.[240] This drug can also cause *blindness* through faulty prescribing. A patient with chronic simple glaucoma may loose his sight if a physician prescribes betamethasone eye drops in the belief that he is prescribing a steroid for conjunctivitis.[241] *Blurred vision* may be induced with a number of antibiotics, including chloramphenicol (Chloromycetin), chlortetracycline (Aureomycin), demethylchlortetracycline (Declomycin), dihydrostreptomycin, streptomycin, and virgimycin (Rovamycin), with parasympatholytics including anticholinergics such as the belladonna alkaloids, with certain antihistamines, and other drugs. *Diplopia* may occur with drugs like aceptophenazine. *Optic neuritis* has been produced by chloramphenicol, isoniazid, *dl*-penicillamine, streptomycin and sulfonamides. *Retinopathy* associated with pigmentation has occured with 4-aminoquinoline antimalarials such as chloroquine and hydroxychloroquine, and with phenothiazines like chlorpromazine, prochlorperazine and trifluoperazine. Heavy metals such as gold and silver from drugs containing them may be deposited in the cornea and fine granular deposits of phenothiazines in both the cornea and lens have followed their long-term use. *Myopia* has been associated following therapy with acetazola-mide (Diamox), corticotropin, ethoxzolamide (Cardrase), hexamethonium, hydralazine (Apresoline), hydrochlorothiazide (Hydrodiuril), sulfonamides, and tetracycline. *Toxic amblyopia* has been reported with chlorpropamide and with high doses of nicotinic acid. Some widely used drugs induce many oculotoxicities, including the amblyopia, blurred, colored and flickering vision, and scotomata that have occurred with digitalis glycosides,[234] and the diplopia, loss of vision, proptosis, and retinal thrombosis with oral contraceptives.[132]

Otic Toxicity. Serious ototoxic complications resulting from drug therapy include deafness and vestibular damage. Hearing loss may be caused by several antibiotics, including dihydrostreptomycin (1% of patients), gentamycin (Garamycin), kanamycin (Kantrex), neomycin) Mycifradin), sodium colistimethate (Coly-Mycin given concurrently with an ototoxic agent), and streptomycin. It is also caused by phenylbutazone (Butazolidin), quinine, and salicylates.

Ethacrynic acid (Edecrin) has caused hearing loss within 20 minutes after administration and permanent deafness due to outer hair cell loss in the cochlea. When combined with one of the above ototoxic drugs rapid and permanent deafness occurs in a high percentage of patients receiving the combination.[132,243] Vestibular damage has been reported with several drugs, including streptomycin.

Adverse Behavior. Many drugs that affect the nervous systems have been responsible for various depressive reactions, deliria, psychoses, and withdrawal reactions. The worst offenders in producing depression are members of the reserpine type of alkaloids which release norepinephrine and reserpine from cerebral binding sites. Hypertensive patients receiving these Rauwolfia alkaloids are most likely to become highly depressed, even to the point of suicide. Other hypotensive agents that have apparently caused serious depression include hydralazine, guanethidine and methyldopa.

The anticholinergics such as benztropine, biperidin, and procyclidine, particularly in high dosage, have a potential to produce delirium, also tricyclic antidepressants with anticholinergic activity such as amitriptyline and imipramine. Even instillation into the eye of mydriatics such as cyclopentolate or homatropine 1% has produced delirium. In susceptible patients, excitement may be produced by barbiturates, bemegride, cycloserine, isonaizid, opiates, procaine IV, and a number of other drugs. Agitation, auditory, gustatory, tactile and visual hallucinations, and sometimes disorientation have occurred with penicillin (procaine penicillin IV), and impaired intellect and memory loss as sequelae to an anaphylactic reaction to the drug. Other related adverse behavioral reactions have occurred with many drugs including alkylating antineoplastics, antihistamines, atabrine, digitalis, disulfiram, and sulfonamides.

Psychoses or neuroses have been caused by a variety of drugs. The psychotic effects of high doses of stimulants like the amphetamines, especially methamphetamine are mentioned under Addiction above. Manifestations commonly observed are delusions, paranoid behavior and various kinds of hallucinations. These closely resemble the symptoms of schizophrenia. Other drugs such as methylphenidate and phemetrazine may have similar effects. Corticosteroids and phenurone not only have these effects but at times they may produce depression, euphoria, or neurotic conditions, depending on the patient and circumstances.

Withdrawal has been briefly mentioned in association with barbiturates, narcotics and other sedative drugs. When these drugs are taken by an individual at high doses or for prolonged periods of time, he cannot simply stop taking them without suffering characteristic withdrawal symptoms. He becomes agitated, anxious, confused, emotionally disturbed, and nauseous. He vomits, perspires from hyperthermia, trembles, and suffers with insomnia. If the withdrawal is sudden after excessive use he may have grand mal seizures, possibly status epilepticus, and delirium with persecutory visual hallucinations. If the agitation and hypothermia are sufficiently exhausting, cardiovascular collapse and death may ensue.[97,132,243] See the problems with Addiction (page 308).

Pulmonary Toxicity. Many adverse reactions to drugs closely resembles respiratory disease and therefore the true cause of such drug-induced conditions may be overlooked. In these cases, the attending physician may prescribe unnecessary medication rather than withdraw the offending agent.

Pulmonary disease may be induced directly as the result of (1) an allergic reaction, (2) an idiosyncratic reaction, or (3) a toxic reaction to a drug, or some combination of these. An adverse pulmonary effect may also be induced indirectly as the result of a generalized reaction to a drug. More than one such adverse effect may be caused simultaneously by some drugs. But, whether the pulmonary toxicities are induced directly or indirectly they are often reversible when the offending drug is withdrawn.

Asthma is the most common drug-induced respiratory disease and aspirin is the most common inducer of this disease. Asthmatic attacks may occur within 20 minutes after this drug is taken by patients with a history of asthma or nasal polyps and such attacks may be severe, prolonged, and occasionally fatal. Asthma may also be caused by the other drugs listed in Table 9-22. Of those listed, acetylcysteine, histamine, metacholine chloride, parasympathomimetics, and propranolol may exacerbate airway obstruction in asthmatics.

Systemic lupus erythematosus induced by drugs may cause respiratory disease associated with effusion, pleurisy, pneumonia, pulmonary edema, shrinking lungs, or other conditions resulting from alveolar atelectasis. Implicated drugs include many that are widely used, such as griseofulvin, hydralazine, isoniazid, methyldopa, PAS, penicillin, procainamide, sulfonamides, and tetracycline. See Table 9-22.

Polyarteritis or *periarteritis nodosa* induced by drugs may be accompanied by respiratory disease such as asthma, lung abscesses, and pneumonia. Implicated agents include DDT, hydantoins, iodides, penicillin, phenothiazines, and sulfonamides. See Table 9-22.

Pulmonary eosinophilic infiltrates as a result of an adverse drug reaction is more often observed after nitrofurantoin than any other drug. However, the condition with its characteristic symptoms of cough, dyspnea and fever with audible crepitations that are sometimes widespread, but without tachypnea, wheezing, or prolongation of expiration, may also be caused by imipramine, mephenesin

Table 9-22 Lung Diseases That May be Induced by Drugs [28, 161, 319, 358]

Disease	Drug
Asthma	Acetyl cysteine
	Allergenic extracts
	Anesthetics, local
	Antisera
	Aspirin
	Bromsulphalein
	Cephaloridine (Keflin, Loridine)
	Erythromycin (Erythrocin, Ilotycin)
	Ethionamide
	Griseofulvin (Grifulvin)
	Histamine
	Iron dextran (Imferon)
	Mercurials
	Methacholine chloride (Mecholyl)
	Monoamine oxidase inhibitors
	Neomycin
	Parasympathomimetics
	Penicillin
	Pentazocine (Talwin)
	Pituitary snuff
	Propranolol
	Pyrazolons
	Radiopaque organic iodides
	Sodium dehydrocholate
	Streptomycin
	Suxamethonium (Succinylcholine) chloride
	Tetracycine
	Vaccines
	Vitamin K
Intra-alveolar fibrinous edema	Bleomycin (Blenoxane)— deaths 1 per 100 patients
	Busulfan (Myleran)
	Cyclophosphamide (Cytoxan)
	Hexamethonium (Vegolysen)
	Mecamylamine (Inversine)
	Methysergide (Sansert)
	Pentolinium (Ansolysen)
Iodism	Iodine-containing compounds
Polyarteritis nodosa	Arsenicals (organic)
	Busulfan (Myleran)
	Gold salts
	Hydantoins (Dilantin, etc.)
	Iodides
	Mercurials
	Penicillin
	Phenothiazines
	Sulfonamides
	Thiouracils
Pulmonary embolism	Oily contrast media
	Oral contraceptives
Pulmonary eosinophilic infiltrates	Chlorpropamide
	Cromoglycate, disodium
	Hytrast (Iopydol, Iopidone)
	Imipramine (Tofranil)
	Mephenesin
	Methotrexate

Disease	Drug
	Nitrofurantoin (Furadantin)
	Para-aminosalicylic acid (PAS)
	Penicillin
	Sulfonamides

and the other drugs listed under pulmonary eosinophilia in Table 9-22.

In general, the lungs tend to be highly sensitive to other drugs and chemicals, even oxygen. Prolonged ventilation with high concentrations of this essential gas is very damaging to the lungs; it produces congestion, edema, fibrin exudate, hemorrhage, and finally fibrosis and hyperplasia of the alveolar linings. A number of drugs including lidocaine may cause respiratory depression and arrest.[246] Oil-containing medications, including cod liver oil and mineral oil may induce lipoid pneumonia. Iodized vegetable oils used for bronchography may induce granulomata that may be mistaken for carcinoma. Iodized oils injected inadvertently into a vein druing hysterosalpingography, myelography, or urethrography may cause oil emboli in the lungs. Pulmonary embolism is inevitable when these oils are injected. Deaths have been reported in a number of the above situations.[28, 161]

Other diseases may be secondary to drug-induced pulmonary disease. Thus, cor pulmonale may develop in drug addicts following pulmonary vascular obstruction caused by repeated IV injection of particles of heroin and other narcotics. Generalized enlargement of lymph nodes may result from the mediastinal effects of hydantoins, para-aminosalicylic acid or phenylbutazone. See also the effects of drug-altered respiration in the preceding section on Disturbances of Fluid and Electrolyte Balance.

What Is a Safe Drug?

Under the concept of "statistical morality" a drug that produced one fatality a year in each million patients who received it could be considered "safe" around 1900. But in the 1970's with infinitely more rapid distribution of drugs and practically instantaneous communication of drug information internationally, the entire world population of over three billion people may quickly become involved with a widely used medication. The potential then becomes 3,000 fatalities a year. This is unacceptable for most medications. The only possible exceptions are those used in life-threatening diseases associated with very high mortality. [120]

The risks with a common preventive agent like smallpox vaccine were discussed on page 108. Other situations have also been pointed out throughout the preceding chapters. But the safe use of any medication depends in the final analysis, on the knowledge and experience of the individual physician. He should be adequately familiar with the chemistry and pharmacology of the drugs he uses. Not only should he be able merely to associate generic or chemical names with brand names, but he should also be particularly interested in the physical, chemical, and biopharmaceutic properties, the metabolic fate, and other pharmacodynamic characteristics of every drug he prescribes. To abide fully by the old motto: "Primum non nocere," he now finds it essential to have much greater knowledge of pharmacology in depth so that "above all he does no harm." [120]

It is impossible to give an absolute definition for "safe drug" because safety of medications is a relative matter. It can only be measured in relationship to the potency, specificity and other characteristics of the drug, the characteristics of the patient, and

Table 9-23 Drugs That May Cause Gynecomastia [320]

Adrenocortical hormones [268]	HCG (human chorionic gonadotropin) [268]
Amitriphyline (Elavil, Endep, etc.)	Heroin [261]
Androgens [268]	Hormones [262,263]
Busulfan (Myleran) [132]	Isoniazid [264-267]
Cardiac glycosides [268]	Methyldopa [132]
Chlortetracycline (Aureomycin) [247]	Methyltestosterone [268]
Contraceptives, oral ("Ovosiston") [248]	Phenaglycodol (Ultran) [269-271]
Diethylstilbestrol [285,286]	Phenelzine (Nardil) [272]
Digitalis [249-254]	Phenothiazines [273,274]
Digitoxin [255]	Reserpine [275-277]
Estrogens [268]	Spironolactone (Aldactone) [278-284]
Ethionamide [256]	Steroids [268]
Griseofulvin (Grifulvin) [257-259]	Stilbestrol [285,286]
Haloperidol (Haldol) [260]	Vincristine (Oncovin) [287]
	Vitamin D_2 [288]

the hazards of the disease. [126] One oral tablet of penicillin can be almost immediately lethal in a patient who is highly sensitive to the drug. Certain drugs (see Table 9-23) cause gynecomastia which may be prodromal for malignant neoplastic disease. Antineoplastics have a very narrow margin between the therapeutic and toxic doses. In some instances, the therapeutic and toxic dose ranges overlap and highly toxic effects must be endured in order to achieve a therapeutic effect. Yet these and other potentially hazardous medications may be highly valuable when they are carefully used and the patients receiving them are closely monitored.

Large doses of some drugs can be taken without apparent harm. A 15-year-old boy took 49 capsules of clofibrate (Atromid-S) in attempted suicide. He became drowsy, developed pain in his arms and experienced difficulty in walking, but after five days there was no clinical or laboratory evidence of harm. [124] Patients who have tried to commit suicide with certain CNS depressants, e.g., thalidomide, have been unsuccessful. Death has been reported with as little as 12 Gm. (30 of the 400 mg. tablets) of meprobamate and survival with as much as 40 Gm. (100 of the 400 mg. tablets). The outcome is largely dependent on individual susceptibility and the length of time between ingestion and treatment. [132]

One aspect of drug safety that is extremely important, however, was mentioned previously with regard to prescribing. Overconcern with safety on the part of the physician may deny the patient fundamentally beneficial drug therapies.

Avoiding Adverse Effects

Some research workers (at Alza, Lilly, Merck, Schering, Upjohn and Wyeth) believe that new drug delivery systems that bypass both the liver and the gastrointestinal tract and approach target organs directly by more natural means may medicate patients more effectively. Many investigators believe that far fewer side effects would be encountered if each drug of suitable molecular structure compatible with topical tissues could be administered through these tissues by steady controlled release, over a specific time span, at the most suitable rate and adjusted to the body's circadian rhythm for that drug if it happens to be a hormone or other substance with diurnal blood level fluctuations.

Investigators are attempting to achieve such controlled release of drugs into the body by incorporating them into (1) plastic membranes for insertion into the conjunctival sac (antiglaucoma agents), (2) silicone rubber rings for insertion into the vagina (contraceptive agents), (3) polymeric membranes for insertion next to the buccal mucosa and the skin (cortisol, insulin, and prostaglandins) and other devices for topical sites.

If the numerous variables discussed in previous chapters can be circumvented by these means many adverse reactions will undoubtedly be prevented. Undesirable blood level peaks and valleys will be eliminated because absorption will be at a constant desired rate. pH and other factors in the gut will no longer influence the amount of drug absorbed and the rate at which it enters the blood stream. Large doses of the drug will not be necessary in order to overcome prompt metabolism because of immediate entry into the splanchnic circulation.

Until such delivery systems are developed, however, the physician must attempt to approach the ideal as closely as he can by suitable prescribing. Adverse reactions to medications may be avoided or at least decreased in frequency and intensity by a number of techniques of administration: (1) descreasing the rate of administration of parenterals, (2) decreasing the frequency of administration by the use of prolonged action, (3) buffering to the optimum pH before ingesting, injecting, or applying topically to sensitive surfaces, (4) adjusting the tonicity to that of the appropriate body fluid, (5) achieving appropriate rates of dissolution and absorption of drugs administered orally in solid dosage forms, (6) administering the minimum effective dose for the shortest possible period of time, and (7) monitoring closely the blood levels of toxic drugs, particularly those that are hepatotoxic or nephrotoxic.

Medications for which the risk-to-benefit ratio is so unsatisfactory that their use cannot be justified should be removed from the market promptly. But removal of a drug or even a hazardous chemical from distribution channels has not always been readily accomplished. Carbon tetrachloride (CCl_4) affords a particularly good example of the considerable length of time that is required sometimes to protect the public from a dangerous drug or toxic chemical. This chlorinated hydrocarbon, first discovered by a French physician in 1839 was available for more than 130 years. At various times it was used medically as an analgesic, anesthetic, and anthelmintic; cosmetically as a "dry shampoo"; commercially as a dry cleaning agent, fire extinguisher, and fumigant; and industrially as a chemical intermediate in the manufacture of chloroform, dyes, inks, insecticides, plastics, refrigerants, soaps, and other products.

Repeatedly, after each new use for this highly toxic, rapidly absorbed liquid was introduced, people were disabled or killed as a result of inhalation of vapors, percutaneous absorption, or ingestion, and such use was then discontinued.

A half pint of cleaning fluid containing CCl_4, spilled in an unventilated bathroom, produces lethal vapor concentration of 4420 ppm, or 442 times the maximum safe concentration. When sprayed on a fire from an extinguisher, the chemical is converted to the lethal World War II gas, phosgene, and other toxic decomposition products. It is extremely hazardous to man. [242]

Alcoholics, the obese, those contaminated with certain pesticides, and those who have taken certain drugs are highly susceptible to carbon tetrachloride intoxication. Phenobarbital causes test animals to be 100 times more sensitive than untreated animals. Susceptibility is also increased by cardiac disease, diabetes, hypersensitivity to halogenated hydrocarbons, increasing age, kidney or liver dysfunction, malnutrition, peptic ulcer, and pulmonary disease. The chemical causes heart, kidney, liver, and lung damage and is toxic to all cells of the body. Symptoms of intoxication mimic a wide variety of other conditions, thus making diagnosis difficult. There is no known antidote or specific treatment.

This highly dangerous chemical has caused death after an individual cleaned his necktie in the kitchen, a 7-year-old cleaned something from a rug in his bedroom, a 17-year-old cleaned the hot engine of his automobile, and other persons used the CCl_4 in some similar manner. A strong warning label was required under the Hazardous Substances

Act, beginning in 1961, but this was insufficient to prevent fatalities. Finally in the February 16, 1968 *Federal Register,* the FDA published a notice of its proposal to ban the chemical completely. Hearings began in May, 1969 and finally on August 19, 1970, after the government and industry had presented their cases, an FDA order banning CCl_4 for use in American households became final in November, 1970.[242]

Other drugs have long been injurious to patients and destructive of human life. Nevertheless, they remain readily available to the lay public, with inadequate warning labels. Boric acid, introduced in 1700 and the cause of 172 poisonings (83 fatal) reported from 1881 to 1960, is still widely used, although its use is banned in many hospitals. [96, 104] Many hazardous over-the-counter medications contain hallucinogens and other potent drugs (see Table 9-6). Phenacetin, freely sold in the analgesic PAC (phenacetin, aspirin, and caffeine) tablets is a known cause of fatal nephritis.[65] Over 2,000 cases of renal disease resulting from excessive use of analgesics have been reported in the world literature. Most of the analgesics contained phenacetin and most cases of analgesic-induced nephrotoxicity were reported in Scandinavia and Switzerland.

Timing may be very important in avoiding drug reactions. Some medications given concomitantly should be spaced as far apart as possible in the dosage schedule to prevent undesirable interactions. Timing with respect to food, time of day, etc. may also be important. But perhaps the most crucial precaution of all is to avoid taking drugs during pregnancy, unless the serious risks of congenital anomalies is more than offset by the need of the pregnant patient for medication. Too little attention is paid to this precaution. In a recent study of 168 obstetrical patients, all had received at least two drugs during the prenatal period, 93.4% had received five or more, and one took 32 different medications.[359]

A thorough study of all medications, not only prescription but also OTC drug products, consumed not only by the American public but by all peoples of the world should be completed as soon as possible. FDA has made a start with its DESI and OTC Review. Such studies, when concluded, should be followed by the development of appropriate consumer educational programs to delineate the hazards for the uninitiated.

SELECTED REFERENCES

1. Ball P: Thrombocytopenia and purpura in patients receiving chlorothiazide and hydrochlorothiazide. *JAMA* 173:663-665 (June) 1960.
2. Ballard HS, Hamilton LM, Marcus AJ, *et al,*: A new variant of heavy-chain disease (μ-chain disease). *N Engl J Med* 282:1060-1062 (May 7) 1970.
3. Barr DP: Hazards of modern diagnosis and therapy—The price we pay. *JAMA* 159:1452, 1955.
4. Bartholomew AA: Amphetamine addiction. *Med J Aust* 57:1209-1214 (June 13) 1970.
5. Beerman H, Kirsbaum RA, Criep LH: Adverse drug reactions. *Dermatologic Allergy,* Philadelphia, Saunders, 1967.
6. Best WR: Drug-associated blood dyscrasias. *JAMA* 185:286-290 (July 27) 1963.
7. Bigelow FS, Desforges JF: Platelet agglutination by an abnormal plasma factor in thrombocytopenic purpura associated with quinidine ingestion, *Am J Med Sci* 224:274-280, 1952.
8. Borda IT, Slone D, Jick H: Assessment of adverse reactions within a drug surveillance program. *JAMA* 205:645-647 (Aug 26) 1968.
9. Browne D: A mechanistic interpretation of certain malformations. In *Advances in Teratology* vol. 2, New York, Academic Press, 1967.
10. Calvert RJ, Hurworth E, MacBean AL: Megaloblastic anemia from methophenobarbital. *Blood* 13:894-898, 1958.
11. Carr AA: Colchicine toxicity. *Arch Int Med* 115:29-33 (Jan) 1965.
12. Casey TP: Drug-induced blood dyscrasias. *N Zealand Med J* 67:599, 1968.
13. Cluff LE: Adverse Reactions to Drugs: Methods of Study. In *International Encyclopedia of Pharmacology and Therapeutics,* sec 6, vol II, New York, Pergamon Press, pp 665-667, 1966.
14. Cluff LE, Johnson JE, III: Drug Fever. *Prog. Allerg.* 8:149-194, 1964.
15. Cluff LE, Thornton GF, Seidl LF: Studies on the epidemiology of adverse drug reactions. *JAMA* 188:976-983 (June 5) 1964.
16. Cluff LE, Thornton GF, Seidl LD, *et al:* Epidemiologic study of adverse drug reactions. *Trans Assoc Am Physicians* 78:255-266, 1965.
17. Collins IS: Hazards of drug therapy. *Med J Aust* 1:222-230 (Feb 15) 1964.
18. Committee on Problems of Drug Dependence: *Bulletin on Drug Addiction and Narcotics* and *Addenda* to the minutes of the Committee, Washington, D.C., Division of Medical Sciences, National Academy of Sciences—National Research Council, 1947 to date.
19. Crosby WH, Kaufman RM: Drug-induced blood dyscrasias. *JAMA* 189:417-418 (Aug 10) 1964.

20. Datey KK, Deshmukh SN, Dalvi SP, *et al:* Hepatocellular damage with ethacrynic acid. *Br Med J* 3:152-153 (July 15) 1967.

21. Diagnosis and management of reactions to drug abuse. *Med Let* 12:65-68 (Aug 7) 1970.

22. Dole VP, Kim WK, Eglitis I: Detection of narcotic drugs, tranquilizers, amphetamines, and barbiturates in urine. *JAMA* 198:349-352 (Oct 24) 1966.

23. Dole VP, Nyswander ME, Warner A: Successful treatment of 750 criminal addicts. *JAMA* 206:2708-2711 (Dec 16) 1968.

24. Donald D, Wunsch RE: Acute hemolytic anemia with toxic hepatitis caused by sulfadiazine; report of a case. *Ann Int Med* 21:709-711 (Oct) 1944.

25. Dowling HF, Lepper MH: Hepatic reactions to tetracycline. *JAMA* 188:307-309 (Apr 20) 1964.

26. Dubin HV, Harrell ER: Liver disease associated with methotrexate treatment of psoriatic patients. *Arch Derm* 102:498-503 (Nov) 1970.

27. Editorial: The difference between mutagenesis and teratogenesis, or how to tell the players from the spectacles. *Teratol.* 3:221-222 (Aug) 1970.

28. ———: Lung disease caused by drugs. *Br Med J* 3:729-730 (Sep 27) 1969.

29. ———: Psoriasis, methotrexate and cirrhosis. *JAMA* 212:314-315 (Apr 13) 1970.

30. Erslev AJ: Drug-induced blood dyscrasias; I. Aplastic anemia. *JAMA* 188:531-532 (May 11) 1964; Erslev AJ, Wintrobe MM: Detection and prevention of drug-induced blood dyscrasias. *JAMA* 181:114-119 (July 14) 1962.

31. Food and Drug Administration, U.S. Dept. Health, Education and Welfare: *Federal Food, Drug and Cosmetic Act* including Drug Amendments of 1962 with Explanations. Chicago, Commerce Clearing House, Inc., 1962.

32. Garvin CF: Toxic hepatitis due to sulfanilamide. *JAMA* 111:2283-2285 (Dec 17) 1938.

33. Goodman L, Gilman A: *The Pharmacological Basis of Therapeutics,* ed 4 New York, Macmillan, 1970.

34. Gutman AB: Drug reactions characterized by cholestasis associated with intrahepatic biliary tract obstruction. *Am J Med* 23:841-845 (Dec) 1957.

35. Hallwright GP: Agranulocytosis caused by methyldopa (Aldomet). *N Zealand Med J* 60:567, 1961.

36. Hanger FM, Jr., Gutman AB: Postarsphenamine jaundice apparently due to obstruction of the intrahepatic biliary tract. *JAMA* 115:263-271 (July 27) 1940.

37. Harris HW, *et al:* Registry of Adverse Drug Reactions. JAMA 203:31-34 (Jan 1) 1968.

38. Havard CWH: Drug-induced disease. In *Fundamentals of Current Medical Treatment,* London, Staples Press, 1965.

39. Hoddinott BC, Gowdey CW, Coulter WK, *et al:* Drug reactions and errors in administration on a medical ward. *Can Med Assoc J* 97:1001-1006 (Oct 21) 1967.

40. Holdsworth CD, Atkinson M, and Goldie W: Hepatitis caused by the newer amine-oxidase-inhibiting drugs. *Lancet* 2:621-623 (Sep 16) 1961.

41. Holt LE, Jr., McIntosh R, Barnett HL: *Pediatrics.* New York, Appelton-Century-Crofts, pp 889-890, 1962.

42. Huguley CM, Jr.: Drug-induced blood dyscrasias. DM: (Oct) pp 1-52 1963.

43. ———: Drug-induced blood dyscrasias II. Agranulocytosis. *JAMA* 188:817-818 (June 1) 1964.

44. ———: Hematological reactions. *JAMA* 196:408-410 (May 2) 1963.

45. Ingalls TH, Curley FJ: Principles governing the genesis of congenital malformations induced in mice by hypoxia. *N Engl J Med* 257:1121-1127 (Dec 5) 1957.

46. Kohn NN, Myerson RM: Xanthomatous biliary cirrhosis following chlorpromazine. *Am J Med* 31:665-670 (Oct) 1961.

47. Kramer JC, Fischman VS, Littlefield DC: Amphetamine abuse: pattern and effects of high dose taken intravenously. *JAMA* 201:305-309 (July 31) 1967.

48. Harold LC, Baldwin RA: Ecologic effects of antibiotics. *FDA Papers* 1:20-24 (Feb) 1967.

49. Legator MS, Jacobson CB: Chemical mutagens as a genetic hazard. *Clin Proc Child Hosp DC* 24:184-189 (May) 1968.

50. Lenz W: Epidemiology of congenital malformations. *Ann NY Acad Sci,* vol 123, 228-236, 1965.

51. Li FP, Fraumeni JF, Jr *et al:* Cancer mortaility among chemists. *J Nat Cancer Inst* 43:1159-1164 (Nov) 1969.

52. Lijinsky W, Epstein SS: Nitrosamines as environmental carcinogens. *Nature* 225:21-23 (Jan 3) 1970.

53. Louria DB: *The Drug Scene.* New York, McGraw-Hill, 1968.

54. MacGibbon BH, Loughride LW, Hourihane DO, *et al:* Autoimmune hemolytic anemia with acute renal failure due to phenacetin and *p*-aminosalicyclic acid. *Lancet* 1:7-10 (Jan 2) 1960.

55. Martin EW: United States Compendium of Drugs. *Lex et Scientia* 6:49-53 (Jan-Mar) 1969.

56. Masel MA: Erythromycin hepatosensitivity; a preliminary report of 2 cases. *Med J Aust* 49:560-562, (Apr 14) 1962.

57. Meadow SR: Anticonvulsant drugs and congential abnormalities. *Lancet* 2:1296 (Dec 14) 1968.

58. Meleney HE, Fraser ML: A retrospective study of drug usage and adverse drug reactions in hospital outpatients. *Drug Info Bull* 3:124-127 (July-Dec) 1969.

59. Methadone in the management of opiate addiction. *Med Let* 11:97-99 (Nov 28) 1969.

60. Meyer L: Side effects of drugs as reported in the medical literature of the world, vol I, II, III, IV, V, and VI, *Excerpta Medica,* New York, Excerpta Medica Foundation, 1957-1966.

61. Meyer LM, Heeve WL, Bertscher RW: Aplastic anemia after meprobamate (2-methyl-2-N-propyl-1, 3-propranediol dicarbamate) therapy. *N Engl J Med* 256:1232-1233 (June 27) 1957.

62. Meyler L, Peck HM: *Drug-Induced Diseases.* Amsterdam, Excerpta Medica Foundation, 1965.

63. Moeschlin S, Wagner K: Agranulocytosis due to occurrence of leukocyt-aglutinins. *Acta Hematol* 8:29, 1952.

64. Montes LF, Middleton JW, Fisher A: Hepatic dysfunction and fixed-drug eruption due to triacetyl-ole-andomycin. *Lancet* 1:662-663 (Mar 21) 1964.

65. Moolten SE, Smith IB: Fatal nephritis in chronic phenacetin poisoning. *Am J Med* 28:127-134 (Jan) 1960.

66. Morris RW: Trends in centrally acting drugs. Part 1—Depressants. *Pharm Index* 11:5-12 (May) 1969; Part 2—Stimulants. 11:4-8 (June) 1969; Part 3—Abuse and Misuse 11:4-7 (July) 1969.

67. Moser RH: Diseases of medical progress. *N Engl J Med* 255:606-614 (Sep 27) 1956; *Clin Pharmacol Ther* 2:446-522 (Apr) 1961.

68. Murad F: Immunohemolytic anemia during therapy with methyldopa. *JAMA* 203:149-151 (Jan 8) 1968.

69. Mowbrony RM: Hallucinogens. *Med J Aust* 57:1215-1220 (June 13) 1970.

70. Murray RM, Timbury GC, Linton AL: Analgesic abuse in psychiatric patients. *Lancet* 1:1303-1305 (June 30) 1970.

71. Nelson RS: Hepatitis due to carbarsone. *JAMA* 160:764-766 (Mar 3) 1956.

72. Norman PS, Cluff LE: Adverse drug reactions and alternative drugs of choice. In Modell W.: *Drugs of Choice,* St. Louis Mosby, pp. 30-47, 1966.

73. Northington JM: Penicillin hypersensitivity. *Clin Med* 71:803-805 (May) 1964.

74. Ogilvie RI, Ruedy J: Adverse drug reactions during hospitalization. *Can Med Assoc J* 97:1450-1457 (Dec 9) 1967.

75. Orgel LE: The chemical basis of mutation. *Adv Enzymol* 27:289-346, 1965.

76. Paine D: Fatal hepatic necrosis associated with aminosalicylic acid; review of the literature and report of a case. *JAMA* 167:285-289 (May 17) 1958.

77. Peeler RN, Kadull PJ, Cluff LE: Intensive immunization of man: evaluation of possible adverse consequences. *Ann Int Med* 63:44-57 (July) 1965.

78. Pflug GE: Toxicities associated with tetracycline therapy. *Am J Pharm* 135:438-450 (Dec) 1963.

79. Prout BJ, Edwards EA: Agranulocytosis during administration of "Atromid." *Br Med J* 2:543-544 (Aug 31) 1963.

80. Radke R, Baroody WG: Carbarsone toxicity; a review of the literature and report of 45 cases. *Ann Int Med* 47:418-427 (Sep) 1957.

81. Registry of Adverse Drug Reactions, Report of the Drug Reaction Registry Subcommittee of the Greater Philadelphia Committee for Medical-Pharmaceutical Sciences. *JAMA* 203:31-34 (Jan 1) 1968.

82. Robinson MJ, Rywlin AM: Tetracycline associated fatty liver in the male: report of an autopsied case. *Am J Dig Dis* 15:857-862, 1970.

83. Rodin EA, Domino EF, Prozak JP: The marihuana-induced "social high." *JAMA* 213:1300-1302 (Aug 24) 1970.

84. Rosenblum LE, Korn RJ, Zimmerman HJ: Hepatocellular jaundice as a complication of iproniazid therapy. *Arch Int Med* 105:583-593 (Apr) 1960.

85. Rosenstein BS, Lamy PP: Drug-induced disease: blood dyscrasias. *Hosp Form Manag* 5:13-17 (July) 1970.

86. Rosenstein S, Lamy PP: Drug-induced disease: the liver. *Hosp Form Manag* 5:17 (June) 1970.

87. Rothermich NO: Visual impairment from antimalarial drug. *N Engl J Med* 275:1383 (Dec 15) 1966.

88. Schaffner F: Iatrogenic jaundice. *JAMA* 174:1690-1695 (Nov 26) 1960.

89. Shaw RK, Raitt JW, Glazener FS: Agranulocytosis associated with thioridazine administration. *JAMA* 187:614-615 (Feb 22) 1964.

90. Schimmel EM: The physician as a pathogen *J Chron Dis* 16:1-4 (Jan) 1963.

91. ———: The hazards of hospitalization. *Ann Int Med* 60:100-110 (Jan) 1964.

92. Seidl LG, Thornton GF, Cluff LE: Epidemiological studies of adverse drug reactions, *Am J Pub Health* 55:1170-1175 (Aug) 1965.

93. Seidl LG, Thornton GF, Smith JW, *et al:* Studies on the epidemiology of adverse drug reactions III. Reactions in patients on a General Medical Service, *Bull John Hopkins Hosp.* 119:99-135, 1966.

94. Sheiman L, Speilvogel AR, and Horowitz HI: Thrombocytopenia caused by cephalothin sodium; occurrence in a penicillin-sensitive individual. *JAMA* 203:601-603 (Feb 19) 1968.

95. Sherlock S: Hepatic reactions to therapeutic agents. *Ann Rev Pharmacol* 5:429-446, 1965.

96. Skipworth GB, Goldstein N, McBride WP: Boric acid intoxication from "medicated talcum powder." *Arch Dermatol* 95:83-86 (Jan) 1967.

97. Smith DE: Physical vs. psychological dependence and tolerance in high-dose methamphetamine abuse. *Clin Toxicol* 2:99-103 (Mar) 1969.

98. Smith JW, Johnson JE, III, Cluff LE: Studies on the epidemiology of adverse drug reactions: II. An evaluation of penicillin allergy, *N Engl J Med* 274:998-1002 (May 5) 1966.

99. Steigmann F: The early recognition of drug-induced liver disease. *Med Clin N Am* 44:183-192, 1960.

100. Sternlieb P, Eisman SH: Toxic hepatitis and agranulocytosis due to cinchophen. *Ann Int Med* 47:826-834 (Oct) 1957.

101. Tornetta FJ, Tamaki HT: Halothane jaundice and hepatotoxicity. *JAMA* 184:658-660 (May 25) 1963.

102. Tyler MW, King EQ: Phenacemide in treatment of epilepsy. *JAMA* 147:17-21 (Sep 1) 1951.

103. U.S. Department of Health, Education, and Welfare: *Bibliography on Drug Dependence and Abuse.* Chevy Chase, Md., National Clearinghouse for Mental Health Information, 1966.

104. Valdes-Dapena MA Arey JB: Boric acid poisoning. Three fatal cases with pancreatic inclusions and a review of the literature. *J Pediat* 61:531-546, 1962.

105. Whitfield AGW: Chlorpromazine jaundice. *Br Med J* 1:784-785 (Mar 26) 1955.

106. Willcox, RR, Fryers GR: Sensitivity to repository penicillins. *Br J Vener Dis* 33:209-216, 1957.

107. Wilson GM: Toxicity of hypotensive drugs. *Practitioner* 194:51-55 (Jan) 1965.

108. Winn M, *et al: Drug Abuse: Escape to Nowhere.* Philadelphia, Smith, Kline and French Laboratories and National Education Association, 1967.

109. Wintrobe MM: The problems of drug toxicity in man; a view from the hematopoietic system. *Ann NY Acad Sci* 123:316-325 (Mar 12) 1965.

110. Ziegler HR, Patterson JN, Johnson WA: Death from sulfadiazine with agranulocytosis, jaundice and hepatosis, report of a case. *N Engl J Med* 233:59-61 (July 19) 1945.

111. Zimmerman HJ: Drugs and the liver. *DM* (May) p 1 1963.

112. ————: Toxic hepatopathy. *GP* 35:115-127 (Feb) 1967.

113. Zuckerman AJ, Chazan AA: Agranulocytosis with thrombocytopenia following chlorothiazide therapy. *Br Med J* 2:1338 (Nov 29) 1958.

114. Stevenson DD, McGerity JL: Simultaneous drug reactions in the same patient; Chloroquine-primaquine sensitivity. *JAMA* 212:624-626 (Apr 27) 1970.

115. Sluglett J, Lawson JP: Side-effects of oral contraceptives. *Lancet* 2:612 (Sep 16) 1967.

116. Reidenberg MM: Adverse drug reactions without drugs. *Lancet* 2:892 (Oct 21) 1967.

117. Salunkhe DS, Gaitonde BB, Vakil BJ: Clinical evaluation of a new antihelmintic—thiabendazole [2-(4'-thiazolyl) -benzimidazole]. *Am J Trop Med* 13:412-416 (May) 1964.

118. Irey N: Diagnoses on drug reactions: the first 1200 cases, *Registry of Tissue Reactions to Drugs,* Parts I-III, 1968.

119. First modern medical use for marihuana, *Drug Res Rep* 13:RN8 (Nov 11) 1970.

120. Samter M: Reaction to drugs. *Ill Med J* 136:159-166 (Aug) 1969.

121. Smith JW, Seidl LG, Cluff LE: Studies on the epidemiology of adverse drug reactions. *Ann Int Med* 65:629-640 (Oct) 1966.

122. Dunlap E: Ten year review of psychotropic drugs in psychiatric practice. In *Sensitization to Drugs,* Amsterdam, Excerpta Medica Foundation, 1969.

123. Leff R, Bernstein S: Proprietary hallucinogens. *Dis. Nerv Syst* 29:621-626 (Sep) 1968.

124. Greenhouse AH: Attempted suicide with clofibrate. *JAMA* 204:402-403 (Apr 29) 1968.

125. Marijuana, *Med Let* 12:33-35 (Apr 17) 1970.

126. Canada AT: Adverse drug reactions—some problems of definition, interpretation, and reporting. *Drug Intell* 1:372-377 (Dec) 1967.

127. Keeler MH: Marihuana induced hallucinations. *Dis Nerv Syst* 29:314-315 (May) 1968.

128. Simmons M, Parker JM, Gowdy CW, *et al:* Adverse drug reactions during hospitalization. *Can Med Assoc J* 98:175 (Jan 20) 1968.

129. Goodman SJ, Becker DP: Intracranial hemorrhage associated with amphetamine abuse. *JAMA* 212:480 (Apr 20) 1970.

130. Valentine WN: The leukopenic state and agranulocytosis. In Beeson PB, McDermott W, ed: *Cecil-Loeb Textbook of Medicine* Philadelphia, Saunders, 1967.

131. Moore CV: Normocytic normochromic anemias. In Beeson PB, McDermott W, ed: *Cecil-Loeb Textbook of Medicine,* Philadelphia, Saunders, p 1018, 1967.

132. Package inserts (official brochures) and other labeling.

133. Bonser G: Presentation at the Symposium on the Prevention of Cancer, Royal College of Surgeons, June, 1970.

134. Epstein SS: Biological approaches to estimation of environmental hazards. *Drug Info Bull* 3:150-152 (July/Dec) 1969.

135. Stanley W: Presentation to the Tenth International Cancer Congress, Houston, Texas, 1970.

136. Popper H, Rubin E, Gardiol D, *et al:* Drug-induced liver disease. *Arch Int Med* 115:128-136, 1965.

137. Dunlap CL, Robinson HBG: Current cancer concepts. Practical application of experimental cancer research. *JAMA* 215:457-458 (Jan 18) 1971.

138. Crandall WB, Macdonald A: Nephropathy associated with methoxyflurane anesthesia: A follow up report. *JAMA* 205:798-799, 1968.

139. Freeman RB, Maher JF, Schreiner GE, *et al:* Renal tubular necrosis due to nephrotoxicity of organic mercurial diuretics. *Ann Int Med* 57:34, 1962.

140. Glushien AS, Fisher ER: Renal lesions of sulfonamide type after treatment with acetazolamide (Diamox). *JAMA* 160:204-206, 1956.

141. Healy LA, Magid GJ, Decker JL: Uric acid retention due to hydrochlorothiazide. *N Engl J Med* 261:1358-1362, 1959.

142. Isaacs AD, Carlish S: Peripheral neuropathy after amitriptyline. *Br Med J* 1:1739, 1963.

143. Rosenstein S, Lamy PP: Drug-induced disease; the kidney. *Hosp Form Manag* 5:34-35 (Sep) 1970.

144. Rubenstein CJ: Peripheral polyneuropathy caused by nitrofurantoin. *JAMA* 187:647, 1964.

145. Schreiner GE: Toxic nephropathy. *JAMA* 191:849, 1965.

146. Schreiner GE, Maher JF: Drugs and the kidney. *Ann NY Acad Sci* 123:326, 1965.

147. Zumoff B, Hellman L: Reversal of chlorothiazide-induced hyperuricemia by potassium. *Clin Res* 8:35, 1960.

148. Beeson PB, McDermott W: *Cecil-Loeb Textbook of Medicine.* Philadelphia, Saunders, 1967.

149. Hoey J: LSD and chromosome damage. *JAMA* 212:1707 (June 8) 1970.

150. Taylor RL, *et al:* Management of "bad trips" in an evolving drug scene. *JAMA* 213:422-425 (July 20) 1970.

151. Kurtzman RS: Complications of narcotic addiction. *Radiology* 96:23-30 (July) 1970.

152. Finer MJ: Habituation to chlordiazepoxide in an alcoholic population. *JAMA* 213:1342 (Aug 24) 1970.

153. Von Zerssen, D: Cerebral atrophy in drug addicts. *Lancet* 2:313 (Aug 8) 1970.

154. Brill NQ: The marijuana problem. *Ann Int Med* 73:449-465 (Sep) 1970.

155. Lundberg GD: Drug abuse in the western world. *JAMA* 213:2082 (Sep 21) 1970.

156. Perman ES: Speed in Sweden. *N Engl J Med* 283:760-761 (Oct 1) 1970.

157. Davis LE: Hepatitis associated with illicit use of methamphetamine. *Pub Health Rep* 85:809-813 (Sep) 1970.

158. AMA Committee on Alcoholism and Drug Dependence: Recovery from drug dependence. *JAMA* 214:579 (Oct 19) 1970.

159. Kales A: Drug dependency. Investigations of stimulants and depressants. *Ann Int Med* 70:591-614 (Mar) 1969.

160. Schuster CR: Self administration of and behavioral dependence on drugs. *Ann Rev Pharmacol* 9:483-502, 1969.

161. Davies PDB: Drug-induced lung disease. *Br J Dis Chest* 63:57-70 (Apr) 1969.

162. Burrows D, Shanks RG, Stevenson CJ: Adverse reactions to drugs in a dermatology ward. *Br J Derm* 81:391 (May) 1969.

163. Bergfeld WF, et al: Photosensitivity to drugs and soaps. *Geriatrics* 24:130-138 (Apr) 1969.

164. Watts JC: Fatal case of erythema multiforme exudativum (Stevens-Johnson syndrome) following therapy with dilantin. *Pediatrics* 30:592-594 (Oct) 1962.

165. Bailey G, Rosenbaum JM, Anderson B: Toxic epidermal necrolysis. *JAMA* 191:979-982 (Mar 22) 1965.

166. Yaffee HS: Stevens-Johnson syndrome caused by chlorpropamide: Report a case. *Arch Derm* 82:636-637 (Oct) 1960.

167. Rallison ML, et al: Lupus erythematosus and Stevens-Johnson syndrome: Occurrence as reactions to anticonvulsant medication. *Am J Dis Child* 101:725-738 (June) 1961.

168. Betson JR, Jr, Alford CD: Stevens-Johnson syndrome secondary to phenobarbital administration in treatment of toxemia of pregnancy. *Obstet Gynec* 18:195-199 (Aug) 1961.

169. Rallison ML, O'Brien J, Good RA: Severe reactions to long-acting sulfonamides: Erythema multiforme exudativum and lupus erythematosus following administration of sulfamethoxypyridazine and sulfadimethoxine. *Pediatrics* 28:908-917 (Dec) 1961.

170. Melvin KEW, Howie RN: Fatal case of Stevens-Johnson syndrome after sulfamethoxypyridazine treatment. *Br Med J* 2:869-870 (Sep 30) 1961.

171. Ergas MS: Stevens-Johnson syndrome following treatment with sulfamethoxypyridazine. *Helv Paediat Acta* 16:374-377 (Sep) 1961.

172. Yaffee HS: Stevens-Johnson syndrome following sulfamethoxypyridazine (Kynex), treated successfully with triamcinolone. *US Armed Forces Med J* 10:1468-1472 (Dec) 1959.

173. Cohlan SQ: Erythema multiforme exudativum associated with use of sulfamethoxypyridazine. *JAMA* 173:799-800 (June 18) 1960.

174. Garner RC: Erythema multiforme associated with sulfamethoxypyridazine administration. *N Engl J Med* 261:1173-1175 (Dec 3) 1959.

175. Williams JD: Stevens-Johnson syndrome following administration of "sulphatriad." *Practitioner* 190:249-250 (Feb) 1963.

176. Harland RD: Stevens-Johnson syndrome with unusual skin features occurring in two patients undergoing treatment for pulmonary tuberculosis with thiacetazone. *Tubercle* 43:189-191 (June) 1962.

177. Browne SG, Ridge E: Toxic epidermal necrolysis. *Br Med J* 1:550-553 (Feb 25) 1961.

178. Oswald FH: Toxische epidermale necrolyse (Lyell). *Nederl T Geneesk* 107:999-1002 (June 1) 1963.

179. Coricciati L, Friggeri L: Epidermolisi necrosante acuta di allergia penicillinica (Sindrome di Lyell). *Minerva Derm* 37:150-152 (Apr) 1962; abstracted *Ital Gen Rev Derm* 4:28, 1963.

180. Vas CJ: Unusual complication of phenylbutazone therapy—toxic epidermal necrolysis. *Postgrad Med J* 39:94-95 (Feb) 1963.

181. Overton J: Toxic epidermal necrolysis associated with phenylbutazone therapy. *Br J Derm* 74:100-102 (Mar) 1962.

182. Grimmer H: Toxic epidermal necrolysis (Lyell). *Z Haut Geschlechtskr* 28:ix-xii (Feb 1) 1960.

183. Potter, B, Auerbach R, Lorincz AL: Toxic epidermal necrolysis: acute pemphigus. *Arch Derm* 82:903-907 (Dec) 1960.

184. Jarkowski TL, Martmer EE: Fatal reaction to sulfadimethoxine (Madribon): Case showing toxic epidermal necrolysis and leukopenia. *Am J Dis Child* 104:669-674 (Dec) 1962.

185. Maher-Loughnan GP, Tullis DC: Severe hypersensitivity to sulfamethoxypyridazine. *Lancet* 1:202 (Jan 23) 1960.

186. Faninger A: Beitrag zur Kenntnis der Etiologie der "Toxic epidermal necrolysis Lyell." *Hautarzt* 12:554-555 (Dec) 1961.

187. Holley HL: Drug therapy and etiology of systemic lupus erythematosus. *Ann Intern Med* 55:1036-1039 (Dec) 1961.

188. Alexander S: Lupus erythematosus in two patients after griseofulvin treatment of trichophyton rubrum infection. *Br J Derm* 74:72-74 (Feb) 1962.

189. Steagall RW, Jr: Severe reaction to griseofulvin. *Arch Derm* 88:218-219 (Aug) 1963.

190. Hahn AL: Systemic lupus erythematosus associated with procainamide therapy. *Missouri Med* 61:19-20, 23 (Jan) 1964.

191. Ladd AT: Procainamide-induced lupus erythematosus. *N Engl J Med* 267:1357-1358 (Dec 27) 1962.

192. Kaplan JM, et al: Lupus-like illness precipitated by procainamide hydrochloride. *JAMA* 192:444-447 (May 10) 1965.

193. Sulkowski SR, Haserick JR: Simulated systemic lupus erythematosus from degraded tetracycline. *JAMA* 189:152-154 (July 13) 1964.

194. Benton JW, et al: Systemic lupus erythematosus occurring during anticonvulsive drug therapy. *JAMA* 180:115-118 (Apr 14) 1962.

195. Bower G: Skin rash, hepatitis, and hemolytic anemia caused by para-aminosalicylic acid. *Am Rev Resp Dis* 89:440-443 (Mar) 1964.

196. Rantakallio P, Furuhjelm U: Diphenylhydantoin sensitivity: case with exfoliative dermatitis and atypical lymphocytes in peripheral blood. *Ann Paediat Fenn* 8:146-151, 1962.

197. Iams AM: Fatal exfoliative dermatitis following injection of triple antigen and Salk vaccine. *Am J Dis Child* 100:282-285 (Aug) 1960.

198. Reaves LE, III: Exfoliative dermatitis occurring in a patient treated with griseofulvin. *J Am Geriat Soc* 12:889-892 (Sep) 1964.

199. Brooks RH, Calleja HB: Dermatitis, hepatitis and nephritis due to phenindione (phenylindandione). *Ann Intern Med* 52:706-710 (Mar) 1960.

200. Strouse CD: Fatal exfoliative dermatitis after sulfamethoxypyridazine. *N Engl J Med* 264:39-40 (Jan 5) 1961.

201. Rostenberg A, Jr, Fagelson, HJ: Life-threatening drug eruptions. *JAMA* 194:660-662 (Nov 8) 1965.

202. Montgomery H: Dermatopathology, vol 1 and 2. New York, Hoeber, 1967.

203. Lyell A: Toxic epidermal necrolysis: an eruption resembling scalding of the skin. *Br J Derm* 68:355-361 (Nov) 1956.

204. Beare M: Toxic epidermal necrolysis. *Arch Derm* 86:638-653 (Nov) 1962.

205. Idson B: Topical toxicity and testing. *J Pharm Sci* 57:1-11 (Jan) 1968.

206. Cairns RJ: in Rook AJ, Wilkinson DS, Ebling JG, ed: *Textbook of Dermatology,* vol 2, Oxford, Blackwell, 1968.

207. Fellner MJ, Baer RL: Cutaneous reactions to drugs. *Med Clin N Am* 49:709-724 (May) 1965.

208. Harber LC, *et al:* Berloque dermatitis. *Arch Derm* 90:572-576 (Dec) 1964.

209. Sams WM: Contact photodermatitis. *Arch Derm* 73:142-148 (Feb) 1956.

210. Starke JC: Photoallergy to sandalwood oil. *Arch Derm 96:62-63 (July) 1967.*

211. Burry JN: Cross sensitivity between fenticlor and bithionol. *Arch Derm* 97:497-502 (May) 1968.

212. Epstein S: Chlorpromazine photosensitivity. *Arch Derm* 98:354-363 (Oct) 1968.

213. Fulton JE, Willis I: Photoallergy to methoxsalen. *Arch Derm* 98:445-450 (Nov) 1968.

214. Goldman GC, Epstein E: Contact photosensitivity dermatitis from sun-protective agent. *Arch Derm* 100:447-449 (Oct) 1969.

215. Burry JN: Persistent light reactions to buclosamide. *Arch Derm* 101:95-97 (Jan) 1970.

216. Luscombe HA: Photosensitivity reaction to nalidixic acid. *Arch Derm* 101:122-123 (Jan) 1970.

217. Bergfeld WF, Roenigk HHJ: Photosensitivity to drugs and soaps. *Geriatrics* 24:130-138 (Apr) 1969.

218. Rankin JG: Epidemiology of alcohol abuse. *Med J Aust* 57:1218-1220 (June 13) 1970.

219. Editorial: Aspirin and gastric hemorrhage. *JAMA* 215:790 (Feb 1) 1971.

220. Kelly HG, Fay JE, and Laverty SG: Thioridazine hydrochloride (Mellaril): its effect on the electrocardiogram and a report of two fatalities with electrocardiographic abnormalities. *Can Med Assoc J* 89:546-554 (Sep 14) 1963.

221. Schou M: Electrocardiographic changes during treatment with lithium and with drugs of the imipraminetype. *Acta Psychiat Scand* 39 (Suppl. 169): 258-259, 1963.

222. Desautels S, Filteau C, St.-Jean A: Ventricular tachycardia associated with administration of thioridazine hydrochloride (Mellaril): report of a case with a favorable outcome. *Can Med Assoc J* 90:1030-1031 (Apr 25) 1964.

223. Leestma JE, Koenig KE: Sudden death and the phenothiazines. *Arch Gen Psychiat* 18:137-148 (Feb) 1968.

224. Alexander CS, Nino A: Cardiovascular complications in young patients taking psychotropic drugs. *Am Heart J* 78:757-769 (Dec) 1969.

225. Stone CA, Porter CC, Stavorski JM, *et al:* Antagonism of certain effects of catecholamine-depleting agents by antidepressant and related drugs. *J Pharmacol Exp Ther* 144:196-204, 1964.

226. Cairncross KD: On the peripheral pharmacology of amitriptyline. *Arch Int Pharmacodyn Ther* 154:438-448 (Feb) 1965.

227. Carlsson, C, Dencker SJ, Grimby G, *et al:* Noradrenaline in blood-plasma and urine during chlorpromazine treatment. *Lancet* 1:1208 (May 28) 1966.

228. Local anesthetics for physicians and dentists. *Med Let* 13:5-7 (Jan 22) 1971.

229. Aach R: Halothane and liver failure. *JAMA* 211:2145-2147 (Mar 30) 1970.

230. Babb RR, Spittell JA, Bartholomew LG: Gastroenterologic complications of anticoagulant therapy, *Mayo Clin Proc* 43:738-751 (Oct) 1968.

231. Wang RIH, Terry LC: Adverse drug reactions in a veterans administration hospital. *J Clin Pharm New Drugs* 11:14-18 (Jan-Feb) 1971.

232. Wintrobe MM: The problems of drug toxicity in man—a view from the hematopoietic system. *Ann NY Acad Sci* 123:316-325 (Mar 12) 1965.

233. Baer RL: Cutaneous aspects of drug toxicity. *Ann NY Acad Sci* 123:354-365 (Mar 12) 1965.

234. Hollister LE: Nervous system reactions to drugs. *Ann NY Acad Sci* 123:342-353 (Mar 12) 1965.

235. Schreiner GE, Maher JF: Drugs and the kidney. *Ann NY Acad Sci* 123:326-332 (Mar 12) 1965.

236. Goldberg LI, Wenger NK: Cardiovascular toxicity. *Ann NY Acad Sci* 123:333-341 (Mar 12) 1965.

237. Cardiovascular complications from psychotropic drugs. *Br Med J* 1:3 (Jan 2) 1971.

238. Pain AK: Acute gastric ulceration association with drug therapy. *Br Med J* 1:634 (Mar 11) 1967.

239. Rothermich NO: An extended study of indomethacin. *JAMA* 195:531-536 (Feb 14) 1966.

240. Braver DA, Richards RD, Good TA: Posterior subcapsular cataracts in steroid treated children. *Arch Ophthalmol* 77:161-162 (Feb) 1967.

241. Crompton DO: Blindness from betamethasone eye drops. *Med J Aust* 2:963-964 (Nov 12) 1966.

242. Miller DC: The unmourned demise of an insidious killer. *FDA Papers* 4:4-8 (Dec-Jan) 1968.

243. Pillay VKG, Schwartz FD, Aimi K, *et al:* Transient and permanent deafness following treatment with ethacrynic acid in renal failure. *Lancet* 1:77-79 (Jan 11) 1969.

244. Cohen SM: Accidental intra-arterial injection of drugs. *Lancet* 2:361-371 (Sep 4) 1948.

245. Baer RL, Harris H: Types of cutaneous reactions to drugs. *JAMA* 202:710-713 (Nov 20) 1967.

246. Lidocaine (Xylocaine) as an anti-arrhythmic agent. *Med Let* 13:1-2 (Jan 8) 1971.

247. Hubble D: Aureomycin, improved nutrition, and gynecomastia. *Lancet* 2:1246:1247, 1955.

248. Beetz D, Schiller F: Andrologic changes in workers engaged in the production of oral contraceptives. *Z Ges Hyg* 15:924-927, 1969. Abst. by *Excerpta Med* III 24:5790, 1970.

249. Dall JLC: Digitalis intoxication in elderly patients. *Lancet* 1:194-195, 1965.

250. Labram CL: Gynecomastia and galactorrhea caused by drugs. *Concours Med* 87:6639, 1965. Cited by Meyler L, Herxheimer A: *Side Effects of Drugs. A Survey of Unwanted Effects of Drugs Reported in 1965-1967,* Baltimore, Williams & Wilkins C, vol 6, 1968, p 193.

251. LeWinn EB: Gynecomastia during digitalis therapy. *Clin Proc Jewish Hosp (Phila)* 4:123, 1950.

252. ———: Gynecomastia during digitalis therapy; report of eight additional cases with liver-function studies. *N Engl J Med* 248:316-320, 1953.

253. Rodstein M: Gynecomastia—an unusual manifestation of digitalis toxicity. *GP* 26:95-96 (Aug) 1962.

254. Singer EP: Gynecomastia following digitalis administration. *J Med Soc NJ* 64:557-559, 1967.

255. Squibb ER, & Sons: Digitoxin tablets USP. *Physicians' Desk Reference,* Oradell, N.J., Medical Economics, ed. 25, p. 1267, 1971.

256. Gernez-Rieuv CH, *et al:* Perfusions with ethionamide in the treatment of pulmonary tuberculosis. *G Ital Chemioter* 10:87-98, 1963. Cited by Meyler L: *Side Effects of Drugs. Adverse Reactions as Reported in the Medical Literature of the World 1963-1965,* New York, Excerpta Medica Foundation, vol 5, p 282, 1966.

257. Durand P, Borrone C, Scarabicchi S, *et al:* Hyperpigmentation and gynecomastia following griseofulvin treatment. *Minerva Med* 55:2422-2425, 1964.

258. Sheinlukht LA, *et al:* Side effects during griseofulvin treatment, and methods of their prevention. *Vestn Derm Vener* 10:39, 1965. Cited by Meyler L, Herxheimer A: *Side Effects of Drugs. A Survey of Unwanted Effects of Drugs Reported in 1965-1967,* Baltimore, Williams & Wilkins, vol 6, p 317.

259. Vollum DI: Oestrogenic effects of griseofulvin. *Trans St John Hosp Derm Soc* 54:204-206, 1968. Abst by *Excerpta Med* [III] 24:1333, 1970.

260. McNeil Laboratories Inc: Haldol.® *Physicians' Desk Reference,* Oradell, NJ, Medical Economics, ed 25, p 894, 1971.

261. Camiel MR, Alexander LL, Benninghoff DL: Drug addiction and gynecomastia. *NY J Med* 67:2494-2495, 1967.

262. Ayerst Laboratories: Premarin.® *Physicians' Desk Reference,* Oradell, NJ, Medical Economics, ed 25, p 572, 1971.

263. Levy DM, Erich JB, Hayles AB: Gynecomastia. *Postgrad Med* 36:234-241, 1964.

264. Borsella C, Merelli B: Appearance of gynecomastia in pulmonary tuberculosis patients during isoniazid therapy. *Gior Clin Med* 38:1744-1758, 1957.

265. Bottero A, Bassoli B, Romeo G: Several cases of gynecomastia in pulmonary tuberculosis patients treated with isoniazid. *Giron Ital Tuberc* 10:280-284, 1956.

266. Guinet P, Garin JP, Morneix A: Gynecomastia in a grave case of pulmonary tuberculosis during isonicotinic hydrazide therapy. *Lyon Med* 188:281-284, 1953.

267. Labram CL: Gynecomastia and galactorrhea caused by drugs. *Concours Med* 87:6639, 1965. Cited by Meyler L, Herxheimer A: *Side Effects of Drugs. A Survey of Unwanted Effects of Drugs Reported in 1965-1967,* Baltimore, Williams & Wilkins, vol 6, 1968, p 193.

268. Modell W: *Drugs of Choice.* St. Louis, Mosby, 1970.

269. Kurtz PL: The current status of the tranquillizing drugs. *Can Med Assoc J* 78:209-215, 1958.

270. Lilly and Company, Eli: Darvo-Tran.® *Physicians' Desk Reference,* Oradell, NJ, Medical Economics, ed 25, p 836, 1971.

271. Randall RV, Mattox VR: Gynecomastia and increased urinary steroids during treatment with phenaglycodol (Ultran): report of a case and observations in a normal subject. *Metabolism* 16:748-751, 1967.

272. Arroyo H: Gynecomastia induced by a monoamineoxidase inhibitor. *Presse Med* 74:1764, 1966.

273. Margolis IB, Gross CG: Gynecomastia during phenothiazine therapy. *JAMA* 199:942-944, 1967.

274. Smith, Kline & French Laboratories: Thorazine.® *Physicians' Desk Reference,* Oradell, NJ, Medical Economics, ed 25, p 1243, 1971.

275. Arnold OH: Modern management of arterial hypertension. *Wien Med Wschr* 106:913-916, 1956. Cited by Meyler L: *Side Effects of Drugs. Untoward Effects of Drugs as Reported in the Medical Literature of the World During the Period 1956-1957.* Amsterdam-New York, Excerpta Medica Foundation, ed 2, p 45, 1958.

276. Kurtz PL: The current status of the tranquillizing drugs. *Can Med Assoc J* 78:209-215, 1958.

277. Robinson B: Breast changes in the male and female with chlorpromazine or reserpine therapy. *Med J Aust* 2:239-241, 1957.

278. Clark E: Spironolactone therapy and gynecomastia. *JAMA* 193:163-164, 1965.

279. Mann NM: Gynecomastia during therapy with spironolactone. *JAMA* 184:778-780, 1963.

280. Restifo RA, Farmer TA: Spironolactone and gynecomastia. *Lancet* 2:1280, 1962.

281. Searle GD: Aldactone.® *Physicians' Desk Reference,* Oradell, NJ, Medical Economics, ed 25, p 1201, 1971.

282. Smith WG: Spironolactone and gynecomastia. *Lancet* 2:886, 1962.

283. Sussman RM: Spironolactone and gynecomastia. *Lancet* 1:58, 1963.

284. Williams E: Spironolactone and gynecomastia. *Lancet* 2:1113, 1962.

285. Dunn CW: Stilbestrol induced testicular degeneration in hypersexual males. *J Clin Endocrinol* 1:643-648, 1941.

286. Hendrickson DA, Anderson WR: Diethylstilbestrol therapy gynecomastia. *JAMA* 213:468, 1970.

287. Smith RH, Barrett O, Jr: Gynecomastia associated with vincristine therapy. *Calif Med* 107:347-349, 1967.

288. Ferrari AV: Gynecomastia during treatment with massive doses of vitamin D_2. *Minerva Med* (Torino) 2:541-542, 1950. Abst. by *Excerpta Med.* [III] 5:806, 1951.

289. Robson JM: Testing drugs for teratogenicity and their effects on fertility. *Br Med Bull* 26:212-216 (Sep) 1970.

290. Dunlop D: Abuse of drugs by the public and by doctors. *Br Med Bull* 26:236-239 (Sep) 1970.

291. Richardson HL, Graupner KL, Richardson ME: Intramyocardial lesions in patients dying suddenly and unexpectedly. *JAMA* 195:254-260 (Jan 24) 1966.

292. Wade OL: Pattern of drug-induced disease in the community. *Br Med Bull* 26:240-244 (Sep) 1970.

293. Rerup CC: Drugs producing diabetes through damage of the insulin secreting cells. *Pharmacol Rev* 22:485-518 (Dec) 1970.

294. Shelley JH: Phenacetin, through the looking glass. *Clin Pharmacol Ther* 8:427-471 (Mar) 1967.

295. Sneddon I: Drug toxicity and the dermatologist, *Practitioner* 194:90, 1965.

296. Baer RL, Harber LC: Photosensitivity induced by drugs, *JAMA* 192:989, 1965.

297. Welsh AL, Ede M: The fixed eruption: a possible hazard of modern drug therapy, *Arch Dermatol* 84:1004, 1961.

298. Stritzler C, Kopf AW: Fixed drug eruption caused by 8-chlortheophylline in Dramamine with clinical and histologic studies, *J Invest Dermatol* 34:319, 1960.

299. Cormia FE: Alopecia from oral contraceptives, *JAMA* 201:635, 1967.

300. Calnan CD: Contact dermatitis from drugs, *Proc Roy Soc Med* 55:39, 1962.

301. Leard SE, Greer WER, Kaufman IC: Hepatitis, exfoliative dermatitis and abnormal bone marrow during tridione therapy; report of a case with recovery, *N Engl J Med* 240:962, 1949.

302. Kolman RW, Sturgill BC: Lupus-like syndrome induced by procaine amide, *Arch Intern Med* 115:214, 1965.

303. Serpe SJ, Norins AL: Allergic purpura after administration of trifluoperazine, *NY State J Med* 61:3517-3518, 1961.

304. National Academy of Sciences: *Adverse Reactions Reporting Systems.* Report of the International Conference, Oct 22-23, 1970. Washington, DC, 1971.

305. Mielke CH, Britten AFH: Aspirin: a new nightmare for blood bankers. *N Engl J Med* 286:268-269 (Feb 3), 1972.

306. Maudlin RK: Drug-induced diseases. *J AM Pharm Assoc* NS13:316-22 (June) 1973.

307. Miller RR: Hospital admissions due to adverse drug reactions. *Ann Intern Med* 219-223 (Aug) 1974.

308. Stempel E, Stempel R: Drug-induced photosensitivity. *J Am Pharm Assoc* NS13:200-4 (Apr) 1973.

309. Rees RB: Cutaneous drug reactions. *Texas Med* 66:92-3 (Feb) 1970.

310. Harpey JP: Lupus-like syndromes induced by drugs. *Ann Allergy* 33:256-61 (Nov) 1974.

311. Breit R, Bandmann HJ: Dermatitis from lanolin. *Br J Dermatol* 88:414-6 (Apr) 1973.

312. Nessi R, Domenichini E, Fowst G: "Allergic" reactions during rifampicin treatment: a review of published cases. *Scand J Resp Dis* [Suppl] 84:15-9, 1973.

313. Sameshima Y, Shiozaki Y, Mizuno T, *et al:* Clinical statistics on drug-induced liver injuries. Drug-induced liver injuries in Japan in the past 30 years. *Japan J Gastroenterol* 71:799-807 (Aug) 1974.

314. Zimmerman HJ: Liver disease caused by medicinal agents. *Med Clin NA* 59(4): 897-907 (Jul) 1975.

315. Schaffner F: Hepatic drug metabolism with adverse hepatic reactions. *Vet Pathol* 12:145-56, 1975. Iatrogenic disease; nephrototoxic and hepatotoxic drugs.

316. Mann JL: *Can J Hosp Pharm* 28:127-130 (Jul-Aug) 1975

317. Leblanc A, Vernet A: La néphrotoxicité des médicaments II. Étude systématique des principaux médicaments nephrotoxique. *Praxis* 62:59-63 (Jan 16) 1973.

318. Bennett WM, Singer I, Coggins CJ: A guide to drug therapy in renal failure. *JAMA* 230:1544-53 (Dec) 1974.

319. Heinzer F, Favez G: Iatrogenic respiratory diseases. *Ther Umsch* 32:248-53 (Apr) 1975

320. Levantine A, Almeyda J: Drug reactions XXIV. Cutaneous reactions to cytostatic agents. *Br J Dermatol* 90:239-42 (Feb) 1974.

321. Griffiths ID, Kane SP: Sulphasalazine-induced lupus syndrome in ulcerative colitis. *Br Med J* 2:1188-9 (Nov 5) 1977.

322. Nyirenda R, Gill GV: Stevens-Johnson syndrome due to rifampin. *Br Med J* 2:1189 (Nov 5) 1977.

323. Bunker JP, Forrest WH, Jr, Mosteller F, *et al:* The *National Halothane Study.* Washington, DC, National Institute of General Medical Sciences, 1969.

324. Napke E: The Canadian drug adverse reaction reporting program. *Drug Info J* 9:224-32 (May-Sep) 1975.

325. ———: Gap to fill—human toxicology. *Can Fam Phys* 13:91-94 (Apr) 1969.

326. Karch FE, Lasagna L: Adverse drug reactions. *JAMA* 234:1236-41 (Dec 22) 1975.

327. Balter MB, Levine J, Manheimer DI: Cross-national study of the extent of anti-anxiety/sedative drug use. *N Engl J Med* 290:769-74 (Apr 4) 1974.

328. Waldron I: Increased prescribing of Valium, Librium, and other drugs—an example of the influence of economic and social factors on the practice of medicine. *Int J Health Serv* 7:37-62 (Jan) 1977.

329. Irey NS: Diagnostic problems in drug-induced diseases. *Drug-Induced Diseases,* vol 4, Excerpta Medica, Amsterdam, 1972.

330. ———: Adverse drug reactions and death. *JAMA* 236:575-8 (Aug 9) 1976.

331. ———: Tissue reactions to drugs. Reprinted from the Teaching Monograph Series published in *The American Journal of Pathology.* The Armed Forces Institute of Pathology, Washington, DC.

332. Lockey SD: Adverse reactions to drugs. *Pa Med J* 67:45-51 (Aug) 1964.

333. ———: Allergic reactions due to F D & C yellow No. 5 tartrazine, an aniline dye used as a coloring and identifying agent in various steroids. *Ann Allergy* 17:719-21 (Sep-Oct) 1959.

334. ———: Reactions to hidden agents in foods, beverages and drugs. *Ann Allergy* 29:461-6 (Sep) 1971.

335. ———: Sensitizing properties of food additives and other commercial products. *Ann Allergy* 30:638-41 (Nov) 1972.

336. ———: Drug reactions and sublingual testing with certified food colors. *Ann Allergy* 31:423-9 (Sep) 1973.

337. ———: *List of Drugs Manufactured by American Pharmaceutical Firms Containing Tartrazine.* The Allergy Foundation of Lancaster County, Pennsylvania, 1978.

338. Finland M, Jones WF, Jr: Occurrence of serious bacterial infections since introduction of antibacterial agents. *JAMA* 170:2188-97 (Aug 29) 1959.

339. Finland M: Antibacterial agents: uses and abuses in treatment and prophylaxis. *RI Med J* 43:499-504, 513-4, 520 (Aug) 1960.

340. Novitch M: Overmedication: international perspectives. Presented at AAAS Annual Meeting, Symposium on The Overmedicated Society, Dec 28, 1971.

341. Nelson G: Effect of promotion and advertising of over-the-counter drugs on competition, small business, and the health and welfare of the public. Hearings before Subcommittee on Monopoly, Senate Select Committee on Small Business, Dec 5, 6, 7, 8, 13, and 14, 1972.

342. Silverman M, Lee PR: *Pills, Profits and Politics.* University of California Press, Berkeley, 1974.

343. Achong MR, Hauser BA, Krusky JL: Rational and irrational use of antibiotics in a Canadian teaching hospital. *Canad Med Assoc J* 116:256-9 (Feb 5) 1977.

344. Percival A, Rowlands J, Corkill JE, *et al*: Penicillinase-producing gonococci in Liverpool. *Lancet* 2:1379-82 (Dec 25) 1976.

345. Blog FB, Chang A, De Koning GAJ, *et al*: Penicillinase-producing strains of *Neisseria gonorrhoeae* isolated in Rotterdam. *Br J Vener Dis* 53:98-100, 1977.

346. Ashford WA, Golash RG, Hemming VG, *et al*: Penicillinase-producing *Neisseria gonorrhoeae. Lancet* 2:657-8 (Sep 25) 1976; Penicillinase-producing *Neisseria gonorrhoeae.* MMWR 25:262 (Aug 27) 1976; (Oct 1) 1976; 26:29-30 (Feb 4) 1977; 26:153-4 (May 13) 1977.

347. Piot P: Resistant gonococcus from the Ivory Coast. *Lancet* 1:857 (Apr 16) 1977.

348. Spence MR, Stutz DR, Srimunta C, *et al*: Changing penicillin resistance of the gonococcus in Thailand. *J Am Vener Dis Assoc* 8:32-4 (Sep) 1976.

349. Center for Disease Control: Penicillinase (B-lactamase)-producing *Neisseria gonorrhoeae*—worldwide. *MMWR* 27:10, 15 (Jan 13) 1978.

350. Sampson CC: Penicillin-resistant gonococci in perspective. *J Nat Med Assoc* 69:139 (Mar) 1977.

351. Schwartz R, Rodriguez W, Khan W, *et al*: The increasing incidence of ampicillin-resistant *Haemophilus influenzae.* A cause of otitis media. *JAMA* 239:320-3 (Jan 23) 1978.

352. Turano A, Peretti P: Pyocine typing and drug resistance of *Pseudomonas aeruginosa. J Antimicrob Chemother* 3 (Suppl C):43-5 (Nov) 1977.

353. Sabath LD: Chemical and physical factors influencing methicillin resistance of *Staphylococcus aureus* and *Staphyloccus epidermidis. J Antimicrob Chemother* 3 (Suppl C):47-51 (Nov) 1977.

354. McCabe WR: Gram-negative bacteremia. *Disease-a-Month,* Year Book, Chicago, 1973.

355. Koornhof HJ, Jacobs M, Isaacson M, *et al*: Follow-up on multiple-antibiotic-resistant pneumococci—South Africa. *MMWR* 27:1, 2, 7 (Jan 6) 1978.

356. Finland M: Introduction. *Contemporary Standards for Antimicrobial Usage* (Eds: McCabe WR, Finland M). Vol XII in a series of monographs on Principles and Techniques of Human Research and Therapeutics (Ed: McMahon GF). Futura Publishing Co, Mount Kisco, NY, 1977.

357. Martin EW: Misuse of antibiotics—a 20-year literature review (1959-1978). Prepared for the Commissioner of Food and Drugs, 1978.

358. Parker MA: Possible pulmonary reaction to chlorpropamide. *N Engl J Med* 296:945-6 (Apr 21) 1977.

359. Doering PL, Stewart RB: The extent and character of drug consumption during pregnancy. *JAMA* 239:843-6 (Feb 27) 1978.

10 Drug Interactions

A drug interaction occurs whenever the diagnostic, preventive or therapeutic action of a drug is modified *in or on the body* by another exogenous chemical (interactant). The interactant may be another drug, or it may be some other substance in the diet or in the environment that has contacted the body. Modification of the action may produce beneficial, planned and expected, or adverse, unplanned and unexpected effects. The impact of an interaction on patient response may be medically significant or not, depending on the nature and intensity of the interaction. The effects of an *adverse* drug interaction may be reversible and leave no serious after-effects or irreversible and leave permanent damage, and these effects may be dose-dependent or related to individual susceptibility.

As broadly defined by some authors, a drug interaction is any reaction between a drug and any other chemical, whether that reaction occurs in contact with the body or completely outside the body during compounding, storage, testing, and other processing of medications. This concept defeats the main purpose of compiling drug interaction data, which is to provide the physician with specific information about *in vivo* responses of patients to medications when *exogenous* agents interfere. Therefore, *in vitro* chemical and physical incompatibilities, and the effects of drugs on naturally occurring body chemicals are not included among the drug interactions discussed in this chapter. Neither are *in vitro* clinical laboratory interferences.

Depression of tuberculin skin test sensitivity by oral contraceptives[24] is a diagnostic drug interaction. But the depression of aldosterone secretion by heparin,[300] production of a positive direct Coombs test by cephalothin,[138,328] elevation of 17-ketosteroid secretion by penicillin[51] and inhibition of insulin secretion by adrenergic drugs,[1992] although they may lead to false diagnoses and clinical problems, are the effects resulting from the *actions of single agents* in the body and are not drug interactions. Because diurnal and seasonal fluctuations, exercise, faulty technique, and other factors not directly associated with patient response to medications also cause errors during clinical testing, the problems associated with clinical laboratory interferences are discussed in Chapter 7, separately from the problems of patient response and drug interactions.

A true drug interaction may enhance, modify, diminish, or eliminate expected drug actions and effects or produce new ones. The risk of such an interaction occurring may exist in as many as 8 prescriptions out of every 100 prescribed, according to a computerized study of the medication histories of a group of 42,000 patients.[1376]

Attempts to predict drug interactions in man by using animals as subjects are often unsuccessful. Because of variations in enzyme systems, organs and tissues, extropolations are occasionally faulty. In rats, barbiturates inhibit metabolism of phenytoin whereas the reverse is true in man.[1557] Amphetamines produce no significant change in blood glucose levels in humans, but they do in animals.[1586] Vitamin C does not stimulate metabolism of antipyrine in man (nondeficient), but it does in guinea pigs.

Moreover, humans themselves do not react consistently to some drug interactions. Racial (genetic) differences may be important. Thus, in some Africans phenylbutazone tends to antagonize the hypoglycemic effect of oral antidiabetics whereas in most US patients the anti-inflammatory agent tends to enhance the hypoglycemic effect.[1689]

Unfortunately the probable incidence of adverse drug interactions, like those resulting from drug allergy, idiosyncrasy, and other types of intolerance to medications often cannot be determined accurately by premarketing animal studies and clinical investigations. Only after a medication has been in general use for several years can its adverse effects be fully identified, evaluated, and classified.

CLASSIFICATION AND SCOPE OF DRUG INTERACTIONS

Useful terms for describing drug effects include *homergic* which refers to two drugs producing the same overt effect, *heterergic* which refers to two drugs when only one of them produces a given effect, *homodynamic* which refers to drugs producing a given effect by means of the same mechanism of action* (agonists of the same receptors), and *heterodynamic* which refers to drugs producing the same effect† by a different action. Thus, the same pair of drugs can be homergic with respect to one effect and heterergic with respect to others, and the common effect of homergic drugs can be the result of homodynamic or heterodynamic action, depending on the specific situation. But no drug is so sharply focused pharmacologically that it has only one action and produces only one effect.

Major Categories

With the aid of the above terms, combined drug actions may be categorized into three broad types: addition, inhibition, and potentiation:[143]

---

* Drug *action* occurs when a drug combines with enzymes, cell membranes, or other specialized components of cells to initiate biochemical and physiological changes that are characteristic of the pharmacological properties of the drug.

† A drug effect is the result of drug action. Through actions on specific cells, the body systems, organs and tissues are affected (temperature change, pain relieved, diuresis, neuromuscular block, cardiac acceleration, sedation, and a vast number of other effects).

1. Addition of Effects. An *additive effect* occurs when the combined common effect of two or more homergic homodynamic drugs given concomitantly is greater than that expected for one of the drugs acting alone. The result of addition of the common effect produced by the drugs may be less than (*infra-addition*), equal to *(simple addition),* or more than *(supra-addition)* that produced by simple summation of that effect. *Summation* of effects occurs when all the effects of two or more drugs (homergic, heterergic, homodynamic, or heterodynamic) are exactly equal to the sum of the individual effects that are produced when the drugs are administered alone. This occurs when several drugs administered simultaneously exert their individual effects independently without any interactions or alteration of each other's intensity of effect. Drug interaction is not present in simple addition or summation but may be present in infra-addition (see inhibition) and supra-addition (see potentiation).

Simple addition is exemplified by trisulfapyrimidines, the official mixture of three sulfonamides (sulfadiazine, sulfamerazine and sulfamethazine) used orally. The blood levels and antimicrobial effects are about the same as those obtained with the same total dose of one of the sulfonamides. The mixture, however, has the advantages of not causing crystalluria and of decreasing some untoward renal reactions.

2. Inhibition of Effects. This term is sometimes very broad in its meaning. It may include antagonism, infra-addition, and any other term that connotes decreased drug effects. It can refer to any type of drug interaction that occurs when a substance given previously concurrently, or subsequently, partially or completely prevents a drug from exerting its action and producing its full effects in a patient. Various mechanisms may be involved. Thus, barbiturates inhibit the action of antihistamines and many other drugs through enzyme induction (see page 371) if the metabolites are less active than the original drug. If the metabolites are more active, e.g., when cyclophosphamide is converted to its three cytotoxic metabolites, then induction of the microsomal enzymes enhances the action of the drug. Sometimes drugs used for the same purpose inhibit each other, e.g., tetracycline inhibits the antibacterial activity of penicillin. The exact mechanisms of such inhibitory actions are not always known, but they will probably be identified eventually as biopharmaceutic or pharmacodynamic.

Antagonism, the result of a reversible or irreversible chemical or biological interaction that decreases drug effects, occurs when a drug with a given activity *(agonist)* is blocked by a drug with a nullifying action *(antagonist)*. Antagonistic drugs tend to cancel or oppose the effects of one another. Frequently encountered combinations of such drugs are: (1) A central nervous system (CNS) stimulant (amphetamine, caffeine, methamphetamine, picrotoxin) plus a CNS depressant (barbiturate, chloral hydrate, paraldehyde), (2) an antimuscarinic (homatropine) plus a parasympathomimetic (pilocarpine), (3) a sympathomimetic (ephedrine) plus an adrenergic blocking agent (phentolamine, methyldopa), and (4) an anticholinesterase (isofluorophate) plus a cholinergic blocking drug (atropine).

Certain antagonisms are utilized for minimizing side effects and for their antidotal action. Thus picrotoxin has been used in overdosage with barbiturates; tranquilizers, used with amphetamines, permit appetite depression while minimizing side effects due to CNS overstimulation; caffeine is used to overcome the cerebral depressant action of phenacetin (acetophenetidin); and the miotic (cholinomimetic) pilocarpine is dropped in the eyes to neutralize the mydriatic (antimuscarinic) action of homatropine.

Biological (metabolic) antagonism occurs when a substance, known as an antimetabolite, competes in an enzyme system with a drug that acts through that system. Thus, according to the Woods-Fildes theory, sulfonamides function as anti-infectives by acting as antimetabolites (enzyme antagonists) in the enzyme systems of infecting organisms. By competing with *p*-aminobenzoic acid (PABA), they prevent its incorporation into folic acid which is required by some microorganisms as a nutrient that must be synthesized by them as part of their metabolic processes and not assimilated as a preformed agent. By this means their growth is inhibited. [142,461,462] But on the other hand the antimetabolic activity of the sulfonamides can be destroyed by adding adequate amounts of PABA and certain related agents. Thus, *in vivo,* anesthetics containing the PABA radical antagonize sulfonamides. And *in vitro* in the laboratory, sulfonamides in blood, discharges, and other specimens are inhibited with PABA so that viable microorganisms may be detected.

3. Potentiation of Effects. This term refers to the enhancement of the effect of a drug by another substance, and like inhibition is very broad in its meaning. In some instances the term is used as a synonym for synergism (see below) or supra-addition (see above), or enhancement of the effects of a heterergic drug. Thus, imipramine potentiates *dl*-amphetamine and supersensitizes patients to catecholamines. It may also refer to enhancement of activity by concomitant administration of an adjuvant (see page 64). A potentiating adjuvant may increase rates of absorption (glucosamine) or distribution (hyaluronidase), intensify binding at receptors, or prolong blood levels and duration of action by decreasing the rates of excretion and metabolism. Such adjuvants may or may not possess any physiological activity themselves. [720] Thus probenecid (Benemid), a uricosuric used in treating hyperuricemia associated with gout, is also used as a renal tubular blocking adjuvant to potentiate penicillins and other drugs by elevating and prolonging their blood levels.

An interesting illustration of potentiation is the use of Antabuse (Abstinyl, Averson, disulfiram, Refusal, tetraethylthiuram disulfide) in chronic alcoholism. By competing for the enzyme aldehyde dehydrogenase, it inhibits oxidation of acetaldehyde, an intermediate metabolite of alcohol. Disagreeable symptoms of vasolidation and respiratory difficulties (blurred vision, chest pain, confusion, flushed, hot, scarlet face followed by pallor with shock in severe cases, hypotension, nausea, orthostatic syncope, pulsating headache, vertigo, vomiting, and weakness) lasting from one-half to several hours are produced by potentiating the acetaldehyde effects in the body. These disagreeable effects lessen the desire to drink alcoholic beverages.

Synergism, a type of potentiation, occurs when the combined given effect of two or more drugs acting simultaneously is greater than the algebraic sum of the individual effect that is produced when each drug is administered alone. Some authors reserve the term synergism for heterergic drugs. It is useful, however, to regard it simply as exceptional enhancement of effect when the same effect is produced jointly and concurrently by more than one drug.

The above types of drug interactions may have either beneficial or adverse effects.

Adverse Drug Interactions

An adverse drug interaction occurs when the action of a prescribed drug is modified in the patient by an interactant so that an unfavorable response to the drug is elicited. The drug interactant may be a prescribed or an over-the-counter medication taken previously (perhaps with prolonged action and still lingering in the body), or one taken concurrently or subsequently. By definition, it is always an *administered drug* or an environmental chemical or food ingredient contacting the body and not a naturally occurring chemical endogenously produced, even though the two may be identical. The effects resulting from normal drug action should be differentiated from the abnormal effects of drug interactions. Undesirable effects of drug interactions may sometimes be eliminated or reduced to an acceptable intensity by altering the dosage, but if serious effects can occur it is usually safer to avoid the interacting combination entirely.

It is not always easy to avoid unsafe combinations of drugs. A drug may so sensitize the patient that long after it is withdrawn, an interacting drug may elicit a strong reaction. Nalorphine induces a strong reaction three months after morphine withdrawal,[163] and small doses of iodide induce myxedema as long as six years after radioiodide has been administered.[54] Recall, after 15 years, of a quiescent radiation reaction by administration of adriamycin was reported in the March 6, 1978 issue of *JAMA*. Death resulted. See footnote, page 388.

Anesthetists must be particularly alert to what drugs the patient is taking or has taken, for how long, and when the last doses were taken, especially with reference to antihypertensive therapy. If opiates, meperidine (Demerol), and related drugs are present in the patient when anesthetics are administered, severe hypotension may occur. Nonhypertensive as well as hypertensive patients are at risk when these drugs are used with anesthetics. If tetracyclines are present when methoxyflurane (Penthrane)[471] is administered, renal failure may ensue. If diuretic thiazides have been used they may influence the course of anesthesia by causing hypokalemia. Under normal conditions of excretion, methyldopa, guanethidine, and certain other drugs may persist for more than a week in quantities sufficient to create some risk during anesthesia. If excretion is inhibited in some manner, these drugs may persist in the body much longer. Short-acting agents should be substituted for a period before surgery and withdrawn the day before anesthesia.[8,30]

Some drugs adversely interact with a large number of other agents. Included among such drugs are adrenergic blocking agents, alcohol, anesthetics, antibiotics, anticholinergics, anticoagulants, antidepressants, antidiabetics, antihistamines, antihypertensives, barbiturates, corticosteroids, digitalis glycosides, MAO inhibitors, muscle relaxants, phenothiazines, and sympathomimetics. Extra caution must be exercised when any of these drugs are prescribed.

An adverse interaction may occur when the action of a drug is altered by *substances other than medications*. These interactants, which are absorbed from the environment by the patient, may be constituents of beverages, cosmetics, devices, foods, household chemicals, pesticides, pollutants of air, food, and water, synthetic clothing, etc. Chemical interactants that are inhaled or otherwise received by the body in fumes, solvents, vapors, and forms other than medications may modify drug receptors, enzymes, and tissues so that administered medications produce undesirable effects.

Patients generally lack information about the hazards they face. In one study 2 out of 3 of all patients interviewed were not adequately aware of the nature and probability of hemorrhagic complications that could occur with their anticoagulant therapy. And 1 out of 3 of the patients, many with degenerative and rheumatic heart disease, were taking on an average three other medications that could interact with the anticoagulants they were taking. These included prescribed drugs such as barbiturates and clofibrate and self-selected drugs such as aspirin, known to cause potentially hazardous interactions with anticoagulants. About 17% of the patients had sustained hemorrhagic episodes.[1832]

All types of adverse drug interactions may have serious effects, economic as well as professional, for they often increase the duration of hospitalization, incidences of morbidity and mortality, and patient and physician inconvenience. They often create a potential for legal action against hospitals and physicians, and the requirement for additional medical care. They can therefore greatly increase medical expenses. Iatrogenic disease that is drug-induced via interaction mechanisms unnecessarily overburdens already overtaxed medical facilities.

Adverse Drug Interactions vs. Adverse Drug Reactions

The high probability that many reported *adverse drug reactions* were actually effects induced by *drug interactions* casts doubt on many reports that various adverse reactions were directly produced by the drugs involved. In some instances, medications may have been incorrectly condemned for their toxic effects. This now appears likely with MAO inhibitors where food constituents (tyramine, etc.) interacted and also with other drugs where a variety of subtle nutritive and environmental interactants have been implicated. In the light of this possibility, anyone reporting adverse drug reactions should make certain that all interacting substances were either absent or taken into consideration. This includes not only other drugs, but also the vast array of other natural and synthetic chemicals found in the environment.

The prescribing physician is primarily concerned with avoiding the adverse effects induced by interacting *drugs,* including not only the therapeutic but also preventive and diagnostic agents. This is a very difficult task in itself. Therefore, this chapter provides primarily a presentation of *drug-drug* interactions. Nevertheless, the prescriber of medications must be aware of all types of potential chemical and physical as well as therapeutic incompatibilities that may affect medications.

Chemical and Physical Incompatibilities

The physical and chemical incompatibilities encountered by the formulator of drug products and the compounder of prescriptions are not to be confused with drug interactions. Physicochemical incompatibilities usually occur only as *in vitro* problems in the pharmacy or the laboratory of the pharmaceutical manufacturer. However, similar reactions may occur in the body after a medication has been taken, due to the presence of another drug or other exogenous chemical, and then such reactions are by definition drug interactions.

Chemical incompatibilities *in vitro,* if not avoided, have results like the following during the compounding of medications: (1) cementation into a hard mass through hydration, polymerization, or crystallization, (2) color alteration through a shift in pH or a chemical reaction, (3) explosion through an oxidation reaction, (4) gas evolution through decomposition or reaction of a carbonate with an acid, (5) gelatinization through bonding or polymerization, (6) oxidation through the effects of atmospheric oxygen, heat, incorrect pH, and light especially in the presence of certain catalysts, (7) precipitation through formation of an insoluble substance or the action of microorganisms, (8) racemization through conversion of an optically active drug to a less active racemate, (9) reduction through the effects of light and reducing substances, and (10) separation into immiscible liquids through chemical action.

Some chemical incompatibilities cannot be readily observed or recognized in manufactured drug products. In tablets containing aspirin and phenylephrine or codeine or acetaminophen, for example, the aspirin may acetylate the phenylephrine to form mono-, di, and triacetylated products. Under hot, moist conditions, it may also acetylate the codeine and react with the acetaminophen, to form diacetyl-*p*-aminophenol. These reactions, which may not alter the appearance of the medication, are accelerated in the presence of magnesium sterate, used as a lubricant during tablet manufacture.[262]

Physical incompatibilities *in vitro,* if not avoided, have results like the following during the compounding of medications: (1) incomplete solution because of a low solubility of a solid in the given vehicle, (2) incomplete mixing because liquids prescribed are immiscible, (3) liquefaction because of the formation of a eutectic mixture, and (4) precipitation because the solubility of an ingredient is lowered by adding another vehicle.

Significant incompatibility problems encountered with intravenous medications are outlined in Chapter 8. Additives, in particular, require special handling. [26, 68, 89, 122, 129, 351, 2007]

Many chemical and physical incompatibilities can be potentially hazardous for the patient if they cause the packaged medication to explode, deteriorate rapidly, produce toxic products, or become nonhomogeneous so that toxic doses are given. Such reactions resulting from physicochemical incompatibilities may occur immediately in the vessel used for compounding, or later in the prescription container. They do not require intervention of the human body for their initiation and therefore are not drug interactions.

Therapeutic Incompatibilities

Therapeutic incompatibilities, on the other hand, do require intervention of the human body for their initiation. They are simply *drug-drug interactions* that counteract or *adversely* alter the therapeutic effects of the prescribed medications. Such conflicting chemotherapy may occur because of an error in prescribing, dispensing, or administration whereby combinations of drugs with potentiating, inhibiting, or opposing physiological effects are introduced into the body at the same time. Although it is not logical to do so, some authors also include overdosage, underdosage, various prescribing and compounding errors, and other problems not directly concerned with drug action in the body in their definition of therapeutic incompatibility. The term is more meaningful when applied in its true and more restricted meaning. It then means the opposite of *beneficial* drug-drug interaction.

The frequency with which therapeutic and other types of incompatibilities are allowed to occur can be drastically reduced if multiple drug therapy is always prescribed rationally and then only when essential. The hazards resulting from the large number of drugs received over relatively short periods of time by many patients have been well documented. [304] Even though patients may be under close professional scrutiny, they still may receive dozens of drugs during a few weeks of hospitalization. All members of the health care team, therefore, should always be on the alert to prevent therapeutically incompatible medications from reaching the patient.

It is not unusual for three diuretics to be prescribed simultaneously for resistant edema. Two or three drugs may be required to achieve a satisfactory and sustained reduction in blood pressure in the hypertensive patient. As many as 10 concurrent prescriptions are sometimes written in hospital practice for the patient in which both hypertension and edema coexist. [304, 439] This practice requires careful monitoring, and is to be avoided whenever possible because the number of possible drug interactions may increase exponentially as the number of medications received by a patient in a given period increases (see Table 10-1).

Although some combinations, such as epinephrine and isoproterenol when used together in asthma, are known to be very hazardous and sometimes lethal, [313] and a proprietary cough remedy containing a small dose of a sympathomimetic like phenylpropanolamine may cause a rapid and potentially dangerous rise in blood pressure in a patient receiving a MAO inhibitor like tranylcypromine (Parnate), and numerous other dangerous combinations have been identified, patients nevertheless continue recklessly or through ignorance to overmedicate themselves with both over-the-counter [99] and prescribed medications (see Table 10-7).

Several practitioners may at times treat the same patient concurrently (polymedicine), often without the knowledge of the other physicians involved. Also, several medications may be given to the same patient concurrently (polypharmacy), sometimes including medications to counteract serious side effects of drug products to which they have

Table 10-1 Drug Reaction Frequency vs. Number of Drugs Administered

No. of Drugs Administered	Reaction Rate % Patients
5	4.2
6 - 10	7.4
11 - 15	24.2
16 - 20	40.0
21 or more	45

already reacted adversely. The common but irrational practices of polymedicine and polypharmacy have become untenable in the light of drug interaction information that has been accumulated since about 1960. Rational drug selection and the need for combination drug therapy should always be established on both clinical and pharmacological evidence.[330] The following case history illustrates the problem of polypharmacy.[195]

An 81-year-old patient was prepared for emergency surgery to repair prolapse of the iris through an incision, two weeks after removal of a cataract. His preanesthetic medication consisted of 100 mg. of Nembutal, 50 mg. of Demerol, and 0.4 mg. of scopolamine 1 hr. and 35 min. prior to the induction of anesthesia. Upon arrival in the operating room he was given 30 mg. of Demerol mixed with Lorfan (100:1). Fifteen minutes later he was given 150 mg. of Pentothal followed by 15 mg. of *d*-tubocurarine, but because he began to move as his eye was being prepared for surgery, he was given another 9 mg. of the muscle relaxant. During the course of the operation he received 100 mg. of Pentothal and 30 mg. of the Demerol-Lorfan mixture for a total (within 1 hr. and 15 min. of anesthesia) of 250 mg. of Pentothal, 24 mg. of *d*-tubocurarine and 60 mg. of Demerol in Lorfan. When the patient became *apneic* at the end of the operation the anesthetist gave 2.5 mg. neostigmine IV over a 4½ min. period as a curare antagonist with 0.6 mg. of atropine IV to overcome the muscarinic effects of the antagonist. Respiration still required active assistance. After an additional injection of 1 mg. of Lorfan, the blood pressure rose to 220/110.

One hour and 20 min. after the operation the diaphragm and the lower intercostal muscles began to function and the patient was extubated. When Cheynes-Stokes respiration intervened 500 mg. of caffeine sodium benzoate was injected. Fortunately, the patient finally recovered.

Medical authorities, manufacturers, and government agencies try to keep physicians and therapeutic consultants completely and promptly informed on all possible interactions. But this is difficult to do because new ones are constantly being reported in the literature, often long after they were originally observed and identified. Of course, the longer a drug is in use the lower becomes the probability that any new adverse effect will be reported. Accordingly, conservative practitioners generally use only drugs which have been widely used so that they can abide by all published warnings, thereby circumventing adverse responses and achieving beneficial ones only.

Beneficial Drug Interactions

Some drug interactions may be desirable and intended, as when a combination of medications produces improved therapy, perhaps a greater margin of safety, more appropriate onset or duration of action, lowered toxicity, or enhanced potency with diminished side effects. Extrapyramidal effects of a phenothiazine can be controlled with an antiparkinsonism drug. Excessive hypoprothrombinemia produced by an anticoagulant can be corrected within a few hours by appropriate doses of vitamin K analogs. Tranquilizers counteract CNS effects of central nervous system stimulants functioning as anorexigenics. Probenecid is used to prolong the blood levels of penicillin and certain other drugs by inhibiting renal tubular excretion of the antibiotic. Folate supplements decrease the incidence of hematologic complications in antimalarial therapy. Mestranol is used in oral contraceptives to antagonize the androgenic effects of concomitant medication, and to enhance the anovulatory effects of oral progestational agents such as norethindrone and norethynodrel by suppressing pituitary gonadotropin output. Simultaneous therapy with mercaptopurine, methotrexate, prednisone, and vincristine may provide improved management of acute leukemia. In very resistant diseases which require highly toxic drugs, combinations may provide enhanced therapy with lower toxicity than any one of the drugs given alone.[469]

To achieve beneficial effects from combination therapy, mechanisms of drug interactions must be understood. But adequate information about these mechanisms, the probability of occurence of interactions, severity of adverse effects to be anticipated, and prognoses have not yet been adequately compiled. Investigations to obtain the needed data have been initiated. Evaluation of acute and chronic cellular toxicity through electron microscopy and other advanced instrumentation appears to offer considerable promise as well as investigations in molecular biology. Many drug interaction problems have been identified and are being solved, but better communication tools are urgently needed.

Proper use of terminology is exceedingly important in clarifying a new and rapidly developing discipline. Unfortunately the authors of some publications on drug interactions confuse *action, effect,* and *mechanism,* do not categorize data in mutually exclusive categories, and do not clearly differentiate between adverse drug reactions, adverse drug interactions, clinical laboratory interferences, and physicochemical incompatibilities.

Standardized drug interaction terminology and a universally accepted classification for drug interactions would be helpful in clarifying concepts and improving transmission of pertinent information.

Timing of Observations Important

Timing of observations may be very important in evaluating drug interactions. A beneficial effect may be temporarily masked by an initial brief acute effect that is soon superseded by the desired chronic effect. Thus IV administration of levodopa produces an acute hypertension which is followed by the desired hypotensive effect as therapy is continued. The drug also has an acute mydriatic effect which is replaced with a chronic miotic effect in a short period of time. The acute effects are produced by initial catecholamine release during the adrenergic neuron depletion phase. Once the catecholamines have been largely depleted then chronic hypotensive and miotic effects prevail. In the interaction between phenylephrine and levodopa, mydriasis is initially intense but the miosis produced by levodopa eventually diminishes the mydriasis produced by phenylephrine. Thus different conclusions may be drawn by making observations at different time periods after administration of the interacting drugs. [2027]

Sources of Drug Interaction Information

Most of the publications listed under Sources of Medication Information on pages 111 to 112, as well as a number of textbooks, have carried some information on drug interactions. But the following primary and reference publications have provided most of the important continuing contributions to the literature on the subject:

American Journal of Hospital Pharmacy
Annals of Internal Medicine
British Medical Journal
Clin-Alert
Clinical Pharmacology and Therapeutics
Drug and Therapeutic Bulletin
Drug Intelligence and Clinical Pharmacy
Hospital Formulary
International Pharmaceutical Abstracts
JAMA
Lancet
New England Journal of Medicine
Official Labeling (Drug Package Inserts)
Pharmaceutical Journal
Proceedings of the Royal Society of Medicine
Side Effects of Drugs (Excerpta Medica Foundation)
The Medical Letter
The Pharmacological Basis of Therapeutics

The physician who consistently follows a few publications like the *British Medical Journal, Clin-Alert, Drug Intelligence, Lancet,* and *The New England Journal of Medicine* will usually be able to anticipate the most serious adverse drug interactions.

Anticipating Drug Interactions

The prescriber who is well grounded, not only in pharmacology, physiology, and therapeutics but also in biopharmaceutic and pharmacodynamic properties of the drug he uses, can often predict that certain undesirable drug interactions may occur. He can therefore avoid them. But drug product pharmacology is becoming so sophisticated that even the therapeutic specialist cannot detect every potential hazard. And certainly the average practitioner does not have time to study all the adverse drug data reported in the literature. Furthermore he does not have access to much of the research data which are reported confidentially only to FDA in New Drug Applications.

For these reasons, in the large hospitals, major clinics and other centers where adequate support is available, drug information consultants are becoming established in drug information centers as key sources of precautionary information. They maintain reference libraries, with comprehensive files of readily accessible data on drug reactions and interactions. The carefully classified data are of-

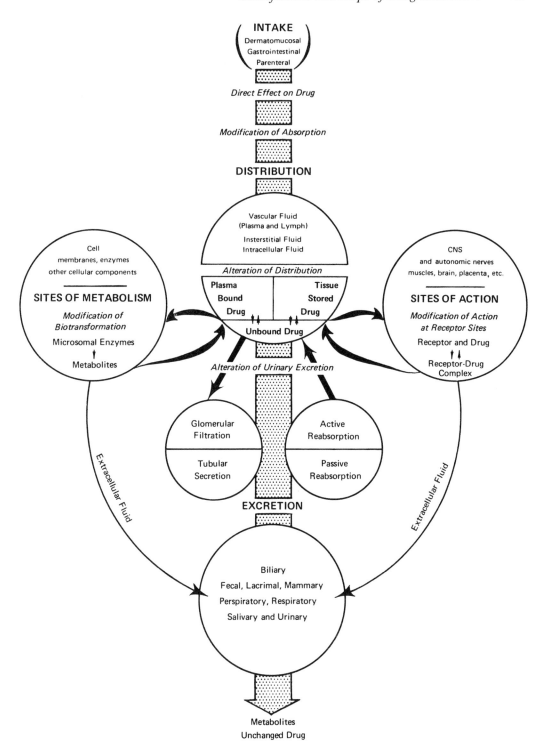

Fig. 10-1. Sites of drug interactions.

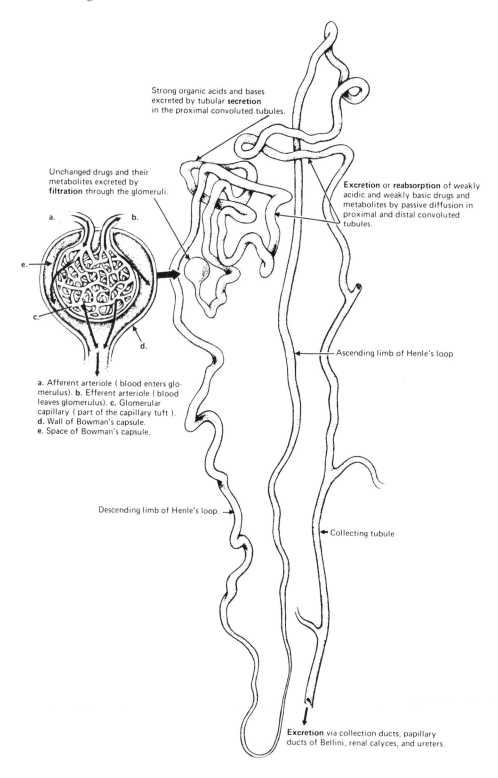

Strong organic acids and bases excreted by tubular **secretion** in the proximal convoluted tubules.

Unchanged drugs and their metabolites excreted by **filtration** through the glomeruli.

Excretion or **reabsorption** of weakly acidic and weakly basic drugs and metabolites by passive diffusion in proximal and distal convoluted tubules.

a.

b.

e.

c.

d.

a. Afferent arteriole (blood enters glomerulus). **b.** Efferent arteriole (blood leaves glomerulus). **c.** Glomerular capillary (part of the capillary tuft). **d.** Wall of Bowman's capsule. **e.** Space of Bowman's capsule.

Ascending limb of Henle's loop

Descending limb of Henle's loop.

Collecting tubule

Excretion via collection ducts, papillary ducts of Bellini, renal calyces, and ureters.

Fig. 10-2. Sites of urinary drug interactions in the nephron. Graphic design of Fig. 10-1 and 10-2 by David S. Quackenbush.

ten semi-automated or fully computerized for practically instantaneous retrieval. This practical approach to the drug information problem is enabling information specialists to assemble useful data on mechanisms of drug interactions. [77, 121, 124, 256, 443]

MECHANISMS OF DRUG INTERACTIONS

An interactant modifies the action of an administered drug by altering either the drug itself or its dynamics. Adequate understanding of these interaction mechanisms enables the physician to make sound judgments when selecting and prescribing combinations of drugs, because he can often predict and avoid adverse drug interactions or engender beneficial ones, and he can also take the most effective countermeasures when unexpected and undesirable interactions do occur.

Although therapeutic incompatibilities have been reported for a century, most information on adverse drug interactions and their mechanisms have appeared in the literature only since about 1960. Since then, many physicians have reported instances when a drug or other chemical that contacted the body has modified the action of a drug given previously, concomitantly, or subsequently.

Sites of Drug Interactions

Theoretically, a drug interaction can occur at any site where any biological, chemical, or physical drug mechanism functions, from the moment of contact or entry of the drug via one of the three main intake routes to the moment of exit by one or more of the eight excretion routes (see Fig. 10-1 and Fig. 10-2). A drug interaction may therefore occur during any of the five stages of drug passage through the body—intake, distribution, action, metabolism, and excretion. An interaction often occurs at the first stage (intake) of medication through alteration of absorption or modification of topical effects. But only the dermatomucosal or gastrointestinal routes are involved. Since an injection or infusion places the medication directly into the body, modification of parenteral intake with an interactant does not occur. See Chapter 8,

however, for *Compatibilities and Incompatibilities of IV Additives.*

After the drug is taken into the body and while it is being distributed via the cardiovascular and lymphatic systems to the various tissues, it acts at receptor sites, or is bound, metabolized, stored or excreted. The drug may directly contact receptors at sites of action or it may first have to cross the blood-brain, placental, or other barriers. Depending on its affinity for proteins and to some extent other constitutents in the plasma, lymph, and tissues, a certain percentage of the drug may be bound either in circulating fluid or in fixed tissues. The circulating unbound (physiologically active) drug is in equilibrium with (1) the bound (inactive) drug in the extracellular fluid (blood plasma and interstitial fluid including the lymph), and (2) the bound (stored) drug in the tissues including the intracellular elements and fluid. As the active drug is metabolized or excreted, circulating bound drug is released to maintain equilibrium, and as this bound drug becomes depleted, stored drug that is not permanently bound may also be released. The equilibria between bound and unbound drug tend to prolong and stabilize the intensity of drug action.

Both unchanged drug and its metabolites are excreted mainly via the urinary system. See page 375 for drug interactions affecting the eight routes of excretion.

Potentiating vs. Inhibiting Mechanisms

Some drug interactions tend to potentiate and some tend to diminish the activity of a drug. When one or more of the following occur, a drug is potentiated: (1) increased rate of absorption, (2) increased rate of distribution to receptor sites, (3) increased affinity, concentration, and rate of action at receptor sites, (4) decreased rate of metabolism, when the metabolites are inactive or less active than the drug, (5) increased rate of metabolism, when the metabolites are more active than the drug, (6) decreased binding of the drug, and (7) decreased rate of excretion. When the opposites occur, the physiological activity of the drug is decreased. If combinations of potentiating and deactivating interactions occur simultaneously, the final effect on the patient may be difficult to foresee. A patient may receive one drug for a given condition, a second drug that stimulates or inhibits the metabolism of the first, and a third that stimulates or inhibits the metabolism of the first or second. When such complex combinations of interactions occur, the net result is not readily predictable. Who can know, for example, the net effect if a diabetic patient receiving tolbutamide to control hyperglycemia and a combination of diphenylhydantoin and phenobarbital to control grand mal seizures is given bishydroxycoumarin postoperatively as a prophylactic against intravascular clotting, especially if the patient often takes a cocktail or two before dinner? Who can possibly know all the indirect and direct effects on each drug, and on any given patient?

Nevertheless, in all types of drug interactions, one or more of the following mechanisms are involved: (1) direct effect on the drug, (2) modification of gastrointestinal absorption, (3) modification of dermatomucosal absorption, (4) alteration of distribution, (5) modification of action at receptor sites, (6) modification of biotransformation, (7) alteration of excretion, and (8) disturbance of water and electrolyte balance. These mechanisms involve an enormous number of combinations of biological, chemical, and physical factors relating to disease, medication, and patient.[298]

Direct Effect on the Drug

Drugs may interact directly with each other, either chemically or physically, after they have been administered. Thus, kanamycin (Kantrex) and methicillin (Staphcillin) inactivate each other directly if they are injected at about the same time. Protein hydrolysates bind barbiturates, digitoxin, digoxin, tetracyclines, and many other drugs. Amino acids like cysteine, and tetracyclines and other potent chelators, can interact with calcium-containing medications, and if intravenously infused rapidly, may cause hypocalcemic tetany. The direct interaction between protamine (strongly basic) and heparin (acidic) is used to counteract excessive dosage of the anticoagulant.[28] However, protamine itself is weakly anticoagulant and overneutralization in patients also receiving oral anticoagulants can result in hemorrhage.[120,180,619,640]

Drug Interaction Mechanisms

1. Direct effect on drug

2. Modification of gastrointestinal absorption
   a. Alteration of tract functions
      (1) Alteration of Motility
      (2) Alteration of Bacterial Flora
   b. Alteration of contents
      (1) Alteration of pH
      (2) Complexation
      (3) Dissolution
      (4) Diffusion
      (5) Osmotic pressure change
      (6) Salt formation
      (7) Sequestration
   c. Alteration of the mucosa
   d. Alteration of transport mechanisms

3. Modification of dermatomucosal absorption

4. Alteration of distribution
   a. Alteration of drug transport
      (1) Fluid flow
      (2) Physical and biochemical factors
      (3) Transmembranal transport
   b. Alteration of drug binding

5. Modification of action at receptor sites
   a. Alteration of drug concentration at its receptors
   b. Alteration of drug reactivity at its receptors
   c. Alteration of concentration of endogenous agent
      (1) Synthesis
      (2) Release
      (3) Uptake

6 Modification of biotransformation
   a. Enzyme induction
   b. Enzyme inhibition

7. Alteration of excretion

8. Disturbance of water and electrolyte balance

Components of a medication other than the primary drug may also interact directly with a drug in another medication. Thus, bisulfite and sulfur dioxide, used as preservatives for sympathomimetic amines such as epinephrine and phenylephrine, inactivate penicillin G if injected at the same time as the antibiotic.

A drug may also be affected by drug interactions when it is applied topically strictly for its local dermal, mucosal, or gastrointestinal effects. It may be adversely affected if some substance prevents it from making proper contact with the surface or prevents it from exerting its effects or destroys or inhibits its activity through some chemical or physical reaction. Thus soap may inhibit the antifungal activity of acrisorcin on the skin. [120]

Modification of Gastrointestinal Absorption

The absorption of drugs from the gastrointestinal tract is modified whenever any drug interaction alters (1) the functions of the tract, (2) the physicochemical characteristics of the contents of the tract which effect oral dosage forms, (3) the condition of the mucosa, and (4) the active and passive transport mechanisms that move drugs from the tract through its lining into the body fluids.

Alteration of Tract Functions. The two major functions of the gastrointestinal tract that affect absorption are the rate of transportation of its contents from stomach to rectum, and the metabolism taking place within its bacterial flora. Accordingly, any drug interaction that markedly influences motility or bacterial balance and growth can have important impacts on some rates of absorption and quantities of some drugs absorbed.

Motility. The emptying time of the stomach varies with the intensity of the gastric motility and therefore the length of time a drug remains in the intestinal tract before it is excreted varies with the intensity of the intestinal peristalsis. Many drugs are readily absorbed directly into the blood from the stomach but many are absorbed much more readily from the intestinal tract. If a drug is absorbed more readily from the stomach then increasing gastric retention by slowing the emptying time tends to increase rate of absorption. On the other hand, if the drug is absorbed more readily from the intestines then decreasing gastric retention by accelerating passage from the stomach into the intestines tends to facilitate absorption. However, since the total absorbing area of the small intestine is roughly equal to that of a football field, even though a drug may be more readily absorbed through the stomach lining, more drug is often absorbed by the intestines with their vastly greater absorbing surface. [475,476]

The total amount of incompletely absorbed drugs like digoxin and tetracyclines that cross the gastrointestinal epithelium varies markedly with gastrointestinal motility. The faster a drug passes through the stomach and intestines, the smaller is the amount of drug absorbed. Thus, cathartics tend to reduce the absorption of any given medication. And incidentally, if cathartics are abused, they may also precipitate or aggravate the toxic effects of some drugs, e.g., digitalis, by inducing excessive potassium loss. [28]

Drugs may also alter gastric motility and emptying time by modifying the contractility of the smooth muscle. Codeine, morphine, and other opiate analgesics that decrease motility, tend to depress absorption of drugs that are absorbed more readily from the intestines and increase absorption of those that are absorbed more readily from the stomach. Ganglionic blocking agents also relax the stomach and inhibit emptying. Chloroquine and iproniazid also delay emptying, but the exact mechanism is still unknown. Anticholinergics inhibit absorption by decreasing gastrointestinal motility. On the other hand, cholinergic stimulants accelerate gastric emptying time, and therefore depress absorption of drugs that are absorbed more readily from the stomach and enhance absorption of those that are absorbed more readily from the intestines. The gastric emptying time is also modified by exercise, temperature, volume and nature of solid and fluid contents, emotional problems, and other factors.

Bacterial Flora. Modifying or eliminating the intestinal flora with antimicrobials may alter the susceptibility of patients to a drug. Because antimicrobial action may diminish bacterial synthesis or metabolism of some drugs in the tract, gastrointestinal absorption and systemic toxicity may be either decreased or increased. Oral anticoagulants may cause bleeding if they are administered after the vitamin K synthesizing flora have been destroyed. [28] And a drug that is metabolized in the intestine and that recirculates enterohepatically, e.g., methotrexate, is markedly more toxic if the flora that normally metabolize it to a nontoxic form are decreased by antimicrobials such as neomycin or sulfathiazole. However, neomycin also appears to decrease the intestinal absorption of methotrexate; urinary excretion is decreased by about 50 percent and fecal excretion is increased by almost 40 percent. This particular antibiotic therefore has one action that tends to increase and one that tends to decrease the systemic toxicity of methotrexate.[468]

Alteration of Contents. A drug interaction may modify gastrointestinal absorption if it alters the physicochemical characteristics of the drug or the contents of the tract, i.e., if it (1) alters the *pH,* (2) forms a nonabsorbable *complex* as certain ions (Al, Ba, Ca, Mg, Sr) do with tetracyclines, (3) modifies rates of *deaggregation* or *dissolution* of the drug in the ambient fluid, (4) modifies rate of *diffusion* of the drug by altering miscibility, viscosity, and other factors given on page 249, (5) exerts an *osmotic force,* as the cathartic magnesium sulfate does when it retains water in the intestinal tract with its slightly absorbable ions, (6) forms a *salt* that is either more or less soluble, stable or absorbable than the original drug, as soluble iron salts do when they form insoluble carbonates on contact with antacids and other drugs containing the CO_3 radical, or (7) sequesters the drug in a *lipoid,* as mineral oil when given as a cathartic dose with oil soluble vitamins A, D, and K, and thus prevents them from having adequate contact with the intestinal epithelium.[35] Of all of these physicochemical mechanisms influencing gastrointestinal absorption, perhaps the most significant ones therapeutically are alteration of pH and complexation.

pH. Alteration of pH in the stomach or intestines by means of an interactant is one of the most important physicochemical changes that can occur. It may modify drug ionization, solubility, and stability, and thereby markedly affect both rate and extent of absorption.

Most drugs are weak electrolytes (weak bases or weak acids) which are most readily absorbed through the lipid-containing membranes of the body when in the most lipid-soluble form, i.e., when nonionized.* There-

---

* Organic acids and bases which are weak electrolytes are characterized by their pK_a values. The pK_a is the negative logarithm of the acidic dissociation constant which is defined by the Henderson-Hasselback equations:

$$pK_a \text{ (for acids)} = pH + \log \frac{\text{nonionized acid}}{\text{ionized acid}}$$

$$pK_a \text{ (for bases)} = pH + \log \frac{\text{ionized base}}{\text{nonionized base}}$$

A low pK_a indicates either a very strong acid or a very weak base, whereas a high pK_a indicates a very weak acid or a very strong base.

---

fore, lowering the pH increases the rate of absorption of weakly acidic drugs and raising the pH increases the rate of absorption of weakly basic drugs, and vice versa. Accordingly, an interaction with an alkaline drug like sodium bicarbonate or an acidic drug like glutamic acid hydrochloride can have important therapeutic implications.[336] The effect of pH on the absorption of weak bases, however, is appreciable only when the pH of the surrounding fluid is lower than the pK of the base, since only then is the base highly ionized. Elevation of the pH above the pK markedly increases absorption because of conversion to the nonionized state. The reverse situation holds true for weak acids.[44] Thus, pK values for weak acids and weak bases govern their degrees of ionization in the strongly acid stomach (pH about 2 ± 1) and in the intestinal tract where the pH of the absorbing surface of the epithelium is about 5.3.

Alkaline antacids in the stomach inhibit absorption of nalidixic acid, nitrofurantoin, oral anticoagulants, phenylbutazone, probenecid, salicylates, secobarbital, some sulfonamides, and other weak acids that are highly nonionized and lipid soluble at the gastric pH. Also, if antacids are given with some orally administered barbiturates, their rate of absorption is lowered sufficiently to nullify their hypnotic effect. Adequate blood levels are not attained even though all the drug may eventually be absorbed over a period of time.[28] Agents that elevate pH usually decrease the absorption of acidic compounds by making them more highly ionized. And the reverse is usually true. But, there are exceptions to these rules. Barbital, although only slightly ionized in the stomach, is not absorbed because it is practically insoluble in lipids. Acidic compounds like bishydroxycoumarin are so insoluble in the gastric acid that they are not absorbed by the mucosa. And drugs like acetanilid, antipyrine and caffeine are so weakly basic that they are partially nonionized even in dilute hydrochloric acid, and are well absorbed from the stomach.[336]

Agents that lower pH tend to decrease the absorption of basic compounds by making them more highly ionized. Thus, the basic drugs aminopyrine, ephedrine, and quinine are not absorbed at the acid pH of the stomach, whereas the acidic drugs antipyrine and secobarbital are absorbed in appreciable amounts, and aspirin, salicylic acid, and thiopental are absorbed even more readily than ethyl alcohol. [325,336,870]

Weak bases are generally more readily absorbed from the intestinal tract than weak acids because at the pH of the tract they are more highly nonionized. However, weak acids are absorbed because of the large surface area. [215]

Administering acidic or alkaline agents to provide an appropriate pH may considerably improve the stability of drugs that are labile at a given pH range as well as the rate of absorption. Thus, penicillin G which is acidlabile may be preserved to some extent from gastric acid by giving an antacid concomitantly. And iron is more readily absorbed at low pH.

Complexation. The gastrointestinal absorption of some drugs may be markedly decreased by chelation with aluminum, barium, calcium, magnesium, strontium and possibly other cations. Thus, tetracyclines may not be absorbed in the presence of antacids (Aluminum hydroxide and aluminum phosphate gels, calcium carbonate, milk of magnesia, etc. and in the presence of dairy products (cottage cheese, milk, yogurt, etc.). In the aluminum phosphate gel, both the aluminum and the phosphate form tetracycline complexes. The aluminum decreases tetracycline absorption whereas phosphates, phoscolic acid, glucosamine, and other agents may increase absorption. [120,508,2011,2012] The fact that sodium bicarbonate decreases tetracycline absorption by 50%, even though it contains no chelating metals, is of interest. [472]

Other types of complexes also diminish or destroy drug activity. Iron may not be absorbed because of complexation with phytic acid which is present in many cereals. Thyroxine and liothyronine are bound by cholestyramine (Cuemid, Questran), a basic anion exchange resin. The resin also impairs the absorption of acidic drugs like aspirin, digitoxin, phenylbutazone, and secobarbital. However, basic drugs like chlorpheniramine, dextromethorphan, dihydrocodeinone, and quinidine, as well as neutral drugs like digoxin, are only slightly bound or not bound at all. [120]

Finally, complexation is purposely used to form sustained release or prolonged action medications. Complexes of sympathomimetic amines and tannic acid, antihistamines and tannic acid, quinidine and polygalacturonic acid, dihydrocodeinone and pectinic acid, and phenyltoloxamine and a cation exchange resin are typical complexes that extend the duration of action of the active ingredient. [303]

On the other hand, formation of a highly lipid-soluble, readily absorbed, and rapidly transported complex tends to increase drug activity and shorten duration and onset of action by enhancing absorption and transport.

Dissolution. The deaggregation and dissolution rates of some drugs may be considerably inhibited or accelerated by interactants, thus causing loss of efficacy on the one hand or increased potency and toxicity on the other. An enteric coated drug like bisacodyl may be extremely irritating to the stomach if its coating is rapidly removed by simultaneous administration of a gastric antacid. The potency and toxicity of a timed release medication such as Ornade may be greatly increased if martinis taken with the medication rapidly dissolve the coating and release the active agents prematurely. Alcohol is a good solvent as well as a good tranquilizer.

Diffusion. Dispersion of a drug in the ambient fluids to its sites of gastrointestinal absorption may be inhibited if an interactant alters any one of a large number of physical properties such as miscibility and viscosity. Thus, drugs may be inhibited by adjuvants such as gelatin or carboxymethylcellulose.

Osmotic Pressure. Increasing the osmotic pressure within the tract tends to offset the osmotic gradient across the absorbing membrane, which tends to force the dissolved drug into the body. This increase in osmotic pressure inhibits absorption. Magnesium sulfate with its slightly absorbable ions tends, by this mechanism, to retain water within the trract as well as hasten its passage through the tract, and thereby prevent absorption of dissolved medication.

Salt Formation. A drug in contact with another chemical may form a salt that is either more or less soluble, stable or absorbable than the original drug. Iron salts, for example, form poorly absorbed insoluble carbonates with antacids and other drugs that contain the carbonate radical.

Sequestration. The absorption of some drugs is prevented when they are sequestered in a lipoid substance. Thus the oil-soluble vitamins A, D and K are prevented by mineral oil from having adequate contact with the intestinal epithelium. This considerably decreases their rates of absorption.

Alteration of the Mucosa. The condition of the gastrointestinal mucosa may affect the absorption from the tract. The rate of transport of drugs into the body is usually highest where surface areas are large and vascularization is profuse as in the peritoneal membrane, pulmonary endothelium, and the intestinal villi. If the intestinal mucosa are destroyed by toxic doses of an agent like tannic acid, the absorption of a drug may be as rapid as when it is given intramuscularly or subcutaneously.

Alteration of Transport Mechanisms. Alteration of active and passive transport from the gastrointestinal tract through its lining into the body fluids may strongly influence drug absorption by this route. Theoretically drug interactions can intervene wherever any of the factors discussed in Chapter 8 (page 249 and 254) pertain. Thus, pore size of the absorbing membrane, lipoid solubility, electrochemical, hydrostatic, osmotic, and pH gradients, and many other factors modify active or passive mechanisms involved in gastrointestinal absorption.

Drug interactions may interfere with an active mechanism by competing in the transport cycle. Thus, amino acids like methyldopa (Aldomet) will only be absorbed slowly from the intestinal tract in the presence of certain natural amino acids ingested in the food because primary phenolic amino acids compete for the same transport sites.[330] The presence of food itself markedly affects rate of absorption. The toxicity of a drug may be closely related to the weight of the intestinal contents.[52]

In general, a drug is poorly absorbed from the gastrointestinal tract, or none may be absorbed if it is (1) rapidly transported through the tract, (2) highly ionized at the ambient pH, and its ions are poorly absorbable, or nonabsorbable, (3) rendered insoluble or poorly diffusible in the gastrointestinal fluid at the site of absorption, (4) converted into an insoluble salt, chelate, or other insoluble complex, (5) rendered unstable by the ambient pH, (6) converted into its nonionized form which is lipid-insoluble, or (7) sequestered from the absorbing tissues by a nonabsorbable lipoid. The opposite situations cause the drug to be well absorbed. These and other mechanisms either enhance intake or interfere with gastrointestinal absorption of drugs and otherwise negate chemotherapy, or exert antidotal and possibly other beneficial effects. See Table 10-2 for a list of some drugs that alter the absorption of other drugs by one or more of the above mechanisms.

Modification of Dermatomucosal Absorption

The full significance of the fact that a drug or other active chemical may be absorbed percutaneously or transmucosally, as well as gastrointestinally, is often overlooked in connection with drug interactions. Obviously, any drug interaction that inhibits or enhances absorption by any of these routes may appreciably affect therapeutic efficacy and toxicity.

The likelihood that a drug interaction may be overlooked, when a topical medication is absorbed in sufficient quantities to interfere with a systemic medication, becomes greater if one specialist, e.g., an ophthalmologist, prescribes a topical medication for the eye while another, e.g., an anesthetist, unaware of the ophthalmic prescription, administers a systemic medication. A dangerous drug reaction may occur when a potent, long acting, irreversible anticholinesterase like echothiophate (Phospholine) iodide is applied topically to the eye for glaucoma and, while the drug is actively inhibiting cholinesterase in the body, a muscle relaxant like succinylcholine is administered prior to general anesthesia. Cholinesterase inhibitors, in general, potentiate the muscle relaxant effects of succinylcholine.[120, 427, 519]

The prescriber should never forget that a topically applied drug that is absorbed through the skin or membranes of the ear, eye, mouth, nose, rectum, urethra, or vagina may interact with drugs administered perorally or parenterally. Therefore, drug interactions that influence rates and sites of dermatomucosal as well as gastrointestinal absorption and function must be anticipated

Table 10-2   Some Drugs that Alter the Absorption of Other Drugs

Acetazolamide (Diamox) [172,179,726]	Cyclamates [619,880]
Acidifying agents [165,325,359,870]	Dietary fats and oils [4]
Alkalinizing agents [165,325,359,870]	EDTA (edetates) [360]
Aluminum salts [178,509,665]	Foods [147,880]
Antacids [28,75,325,870]	Iron salts [359]
Antidiarrheal medications [120]	Magnesium salts [48,421,665]
Bile and bile salts [176,421]	Milk [120,201,665]
Bismuth salts	Mineral oil [35,193,421]
Calcium salts [107,178,509,665]	Neomycin
Cathartics [193,890]	Polysorbate [359]
Cholestyramine (Cuemid, Questran) [120,330,769]	Purgatives [193,890]
Chymotrypsin (oral) [306,508]	Sodium bicarbonate [325,870]
Citric acid [107,270,696]	Sorbitol [359]
Complexing agents [48,178,509,619,665]	Strontium salts [421]

and either avoided or taken into consideration.

Alteration of Distribution

Any of the distribution factors or mechanisms discussed in Chapter 8, may theoretically be modified by a drug interaction and thereby either enhance or seriously reduce the safety and efficacy of a drug. The most important aspects of distribution that can be modified by drug interactions are transport, binding, and redistribution.

Alteration of Drug Transport. The rates and routes of the distribution of a drug from its site of intake to its sites of action, biotransformation, storage, and excretion may be profoundly influenced by another drug or other chemical. Onset, intensity, and duration of action of the drug may be affected by changes in fluid flow, physical factors, and transport across membranes.

Fluid Flow. Any physiologically active chemical that alters the flow rate and volume of fluid in the cardiovascular or lymphatic system may also alter the rate at which a drug is moved from one area of the body to another. Therefore cardiac stimulants, diuretics, hypertensive (pressor) and antihypertensive (hypotensive) agents and other cardiovascular drugs may influence the distribution of other drugs.

Physical and Biochemical Factors. The rate at which an injected or absorbed drug moves from its site of intake to other areas of the body varies appreciably with miscibility, solubility, surface tension, viscosity, and other physical and biochemical characteristics of the ambient fluids. Therefore, modification of

any of these characteristics by means of a drug interaction may cause the drug to remain at its site of entry for a prolonged period or diffuse more rapidly than normal. Thus, estrogens, hyaluronidase, and other drugs act as physical interactants by means of the biochemical activities discussed in Chapter 8.

Transmembranal Transport. Since the transmembranal transport of a drug takes place by means of active transport mechanisms, convective absorption, facilitated or passive diffusion, phagocytosis, and pinocytosis, a drug interaction that modifies any of these also modifies drug distribution in the body. And the rate of transport varies also with the status of the membrane and the forces that drive the drug across the membrane.

The permeability of some membranes, notably the walls of the lymph capillaries, may be increased by histamine and some other chemicals, as well as by massage, sunlight, and warmth to such a degree that the walls present no real barrier between the lymph inside and the interstitial fluid outside the vessels. Transport of a drug across a membrane may theoretically be altered by any drug interaction that alters (1) the cross sectional or surface area of the membrane accessible to the drug, (2) the molecular size and shape, solubility, and other physical characteristics of the drug, (3) the concentration of the drug at the membrane surfaces, (4) the compartment volumes on opposite sides of the membrane, (5) the strength of the electrical charge on the drug ions and the membrane, (6) the size of the pores of the membrane, and (7) the driving forces across the membrane such as electrochemical gradients, hydrodynamic and osmotic pressure gradients, lipoid-water partition coefficients, pH gradients, and active transport mechanisms.

A special type of interference with transmembranal transport involves the norepinephrine pump at the adrenergic neuronal terminals. Certain antidepressants (tricyclic), some antihistamines and various phenothiazines block that active transport mechanism for a number of drugs including guanethidine and its congeners bethanidine (Esbatal) and debrisoquine. Slow reversal of the hypotensive effect induced by these 3 adrenergic neuron blockers occurs when a tricyclic antidepressant or one of the other blockers of the uptake mechanism is added to the antihypertensive therapy. Hypertension occurs and the blocking effect may remain for up to a week after withdrawal of the interactant.[823]

Alteration of Drug Binding. When drugs are bound to proteins and other constituents of the body, three effects may occur. In rare instances, they function as haptens and combine with specific proteins to initiate hypersensitivity reactions. Usually, active drugs attach to specific receptor sites and initiate drug action. This is discussed later under *Modification of Action at Receptor Sites.* Finally, drugs may become inactivated in direct proportion to the percentage of drug bound to inactive receptor sites such as those on serum proteins.

Displacement of a drug from its binding sites in the plasma and the tissues may enhance its activity because it is then free to contact receptor sites, initiate its action, and produce physiological effects. The more tenaciously bound drugs can displace less firmly bound ones from binding sites and thus cause shifts in plasma concentrations and possibly major redistribution of the released drugs in the body compartments. The extent of drug binding and drug displacement is affected by various factors such as pH, inherent affinities, and temperature.

The intensity of effects in the patient caused by displacement varies with the ratio between bound drug and released drug. Only a slight displacement of a highly bound drug like bishydroxycoumarin with agents such as clofibrate (Atromid-S), oxyphenbutazone (Tandearil), and phenylbutazone (Butazolidin) greatly potentiates the anticoagulant ef-

fect and may cause bleeding. Since only 1% of the oral anticoagulant is unbound, if only 2% more of the drug is displaced the activity is increased 200% or 3-fold.[57] See Table 10-3 for a list of some of the more commonly used drugs that displace other drugs from secondary binding sites.

Displacement of a substance from its secondary binding sites may (1) activate or potentiate its physiological activity, (2) increase its toxicity, (3) possibly cause its redistribution into different compartments of the body, or produce a beneficial effect. Thus, clofibrate (Atromid-S) potentiates the oral anticoagulants by displacing them from their protein binding sites and may thereby cause severe hemorrhage. Ethacrynic acid (Edecrin), by displacing oral antidiabetics, may cause hypoglycemic shock. And salicylates, sulfonamides and certain other drugs by displacing bilirubin from protein binding sites may precipitate or exacerbate kernicterus in infants. Such interactions can be very hazardous, even lethal if dosages are sufficiently high in susceptible patients.

On the other hand, the beneficial effects of the nonsteroidal anti-inflammatory agents such as indomethacin (Indocin), phenylbutazone (Butazolidin), oxyphenbutazone (Tandearil) and the salicylates appear to result from their displacement of corticosteroids from secondary binding sites.[137,223,359,393,394,421,1047]

Table 10-3   Drugs That Displace Other Drugs from Plasma Protein-Binding Sites*

Acetaminophen	Indomethacin
p-Aminobenzoic acid	Mefenamic acid
Antidiabetics, oral	Nalidixic acid
Antipyrine	Oxyphenbutazone
Aspirin	Phenylbutazone
Barbiturates	Salicylates (aspirin, etc.)
Chloral hydrate	Sulfinpyrazone
Clofibrate	Sulfonamides
Cyclophosphamide	Tolbutamide
Diazoxide (Hyperstat)	Tranquilizers
Diphenylhydantoin	Triiodothyronine
Ethacrynic acid	

* References to the literature are provided in the Table of Drug Interactions (pages 395 to 618). Some drugs may yield metabolites which actually do the drug displacing. In this table chloral hydrate, which is an enzyme inducer that inhibits some drugs, also forms trichloroacetic acid which displaces some drugs from their secondary binding sites and thereby potentiates them.

The effectiveness of a given drug as a displacer of another drug may be enhanced by several factors. (1) Increasing the dose of the drug tends to make it more effective as a displacing agent, and may even convert it from an ineffective to an effective agent. (2) A drug that is ineffective in displacing a strongly bound drug may be effective in displacing a weakly bound drug. (3) Concomitant therapy with another drug may enhance the effectiveness of a given drug as a displacer. Thus, probenecid (Benemid), sodium salicylate, and tolbutamide (Orinase), when administered alone were ineffective as displacers of sulfadimethoxine (Madribon) but when they were administered together were definitely effective in potentiating the sulfonamide.[1046]

Displacement of a drug from its bound state also makes it available for urinary excretion by means of glomerular filtration and therefore increases its rate of excretion from the body. On the one hand, therefore, the displacement immediately tends to increase drug activity, and on the other hand, tends to remove the drug from the body more rapidly and decrease its duration of action.

Modification of Action at Receptor Sites

Interferences with the mechanisms of drug action at receptor sites may cause hazardous augmentation or reduction of drug effects through activation or inhibition of mechanisms involving enzymes, neurohumors, and other components. A drug interaction that modifies the action of a drug at a receptor site may act: (1) *locally* or *generally* on cells, tissues, or organs, (2) at the *cell surface, extracellularly,* or *intracellularly,* (3) *directly* on effector cells of muscles and other tissues, or *indirectly* by autonomic or vasomotor action, or by antagonizing or stimulating the action of another active chemical, and (4) *biochemically* or *physicochemically.*

An interactant may potentiate the intensity of the action of a drug at its receptors by three general mechanisms: (a) increasing its concentration at its receptors, (b) increasing its reactivity at its receptors, and (c) altering the concentration of an endogenous agent at its receptors.

Alteration of Drug Concentration at its Receptors. There are at least three ways of doing this. Displacement of the drug from its inactive binding sites such as those on serum protein and redistribution of the active drug to its receptors is a common means of potentiation and examples were explained earlier. Preventing the drug from binding to inactive receptors and blocking the action of an enzyme that destroys the drug also produce the same effect. Thus, cholinesterase inhibitors such as edrophonium, neostigmine, and organophosphorus nerve gases and insecticides potentiate the miotic and other cholinergic actions of acetylcholine. Monoamine oxidase (MAO) inhibitors potentiate the hypertensive action of norepinephrine and its releasers such as dextroamphetamine and tyramine. These enzyme inhibitors, by preserving the active agent at its receptors, maintain its concentration and prolong its action.

Alteration of Drug Reactivity at its Receptors. A drug interaction may theoretically enhance drug activity at a receptor site if it: (1) displaces protein-bound endogenous, physiologically active chemicals (cortisol, estradiol, thyroxine, etc.), (2) increases synthesis of active endogenous chemicals, (3) increases release of endogenous stored chemicals (norepinephrine, etc.), (4) prevents binding to secondary receptors, (5) preserves the active agent at its receptor sites, (6) sensitizes effectors to drugs, and (7) enhances the affinity between receptors and drugs.

Apparently, thyroid replacement therapy such as dextrothyroxine and certain anabolic agents like methandrostenolone and norethandrolone potentiate anticoagulants like warfarin by increasing the affinity of the drug for its receptors. A drug interaction may theoretically decrease or destroy drug activity at a receptor site if it: (1) promotes drug binding to protein and drug storage, (2) decreases synthesis of active endogenous chemicals, (3) prevents the release of endogenous stored chemicals (catecholamines, etc.), (4) prevents drug binding at receptor sites, (5) desensitizes effectors to drugs, (6) decreases the amount of drug at receptor sites and its affinity for these sites, and (7) depletes the stores of neurotransmitters and other active chemicals produced in the body.

Drugs and other physiologically active chemicals have their own degree of affinity for receptor sites. When two or more chemicals are competing for the same receptors, the extent to which each is bound depends on the quantity of each present and on their relative binding affinities. The classic example of this is the competition of atropine and acetylcholine for the same population of receptors.

The cholinergic blocking agent atropine has no inherent autonomic activity, but is therapeutically active by virtue of having a higher affinity than the cholinergic transmitter, acetylcholine, for their mutually sought receptors. Thus, atropine antagonizes muscarinic cholinergic stimuli by blocking the neurotransmitter from its receptors. However, a secondary interaction can reverse the blocking action of atropine. A cholinesterase inhibitor like edrophonium or neostigmine can elevate acetylcholine levels by inhibiting cholinesterase, the enzyme that destroys the neurotransmitter.[28]

Alteration of Concentration of Endogenous Agent at its Receptors. Interactants may modify the synthesis, release, or uptake (transport) of a number of active endogenous agents and thereby affect the action of drugs at their receptors.

Synthesis. Apparently, thyroid replacement therapy may inhibit the synthesis and thereby reduce the blood levels of prothrombin and the clotting factors VII, IX and X, and tends to potentiate the anticoagulant action of drugs like warfarin. The synthesis of a false nerve transmitter may create problems for the patient. Thus formation of alpha-methylnorepinephrine from alpha-methyldopa blocks tyrosine hydroxylase and leads to a depletion of norepinephrine (NE), and this increases the risk of vascular collapse during surgery under a general anesthetic.

Release. The release of excessive quantities of NE from the terminals of adrenergic neurons is a hazardous event that may be brought about by interactions. Administration of two NE releasers simultaneously can induce a hypertensive crisis. Yet recognition of this possibility is not always easy. A patient receiving the NE releaser amphetamine for narcolepsy may consume large quantities of a ripe cheese containing tyramine which is also a releaser of NE. The resulting hypertension can be lethal. One physician may prescribe amphetamine as an appetite suppressant for an obese patient and another physician, unaware of the other therapy, may prescribe a MAO inhibitor like pargyline as an antihy-

pertensive for the same patient. Excessive quantities of released NE are then not removed by the usual enzyme activity and once again the resulting hypertension can be lethal.

Uptake. Interactants may potentiate drugs at receptor sites by blocking certain transport mechanisms. Norepinephrine (NE), the transmitter of adrenergic impulses, is synthesized in the terminals of adrenergic neurons and stored there in minute vesicles. While it is stored in these terminal vesicles, it is protected from enzymatic inactivation. When it is released by a stimulus to the adrenergic neurons, it is then usually either inactivated by circulating catechol-O-methyl transferase or bound to receptors until it is taken up again by the vesicles and returned to storage by a so-called "pump" mechanism.

Release of NE and binding to active receptors elevates blood pressure. If a releaser of NE, such as tyramine which is found in many foods, as well as endogenously, is given at the same time as another releaser of NE, e.g., *d*-amphetamine (Dexedrine), severe potentiation of the pressor agent may occur. Normally, the enzyme monoamine oxidase (MAO) found in the liver, deactivates naturally occurring amines such as dopamine, epinephrine, 5-hydroxytryptamine, norepinephrine, tryptamine, and tyramine by oxidative deamination. Also some exogenous substances such as reserpine deplete stored NE. If, however, no reserpine is present, and a MAO inhibitor such as isocarboxazid, nialamide, phenelzine, or tranylcypromine is given, no deactivation occurs and a hypertensive crisis may arise. Neither the releaser of NE nor the intraneuronal NE is inactivated. This is the reason that death has resulted when beer, certain cheeses, Chianti wine, pickled herring, and other foods with high tyramine content or nonprescription cold remedies containing sympathomimetics have been consumed after administration of a MAO inhibitor. See Tyramine-rich foods in the *Table of Drug Interactions.*

The amino uptake mechanism of the terminal neuronal vesicles enters into many drug interactions. Guanethidine (Ismelin) exerts its antihypertensive action when it is taken up by the adrenergic vesicles wherein it contacts sites at which it inhibits release of the neurotransmitter norepinephrine (NE).

But interacting amphetamine and ephedrine are also taken up and antagonize the antihypertensive effects of guanethidine by blocking its vesicular uptake. The same uptake mechanism is also blocked by tricyclic antidepressants, chlorpromazine, cocaine, ouabain, etc. These thereby tend to potentiate responses to adrenergic impulses and to injected pressor agents like epinephrine and levarterenol. They also decrease response to amphetamine, ephedrine, and related indirectly acting sympathomimetic amines.

Blockage of receptors is an interaction mechanism that is frequently applied therapeutically. The action of norepinephrine, the mediator of adrenergic impulses to the blood vessels, eye, heart, glands, smooth muscles and viscera, and of other catecholamines at adrenergic receptor sites may be inhibited by blocking with a drug like phenoxybenzamine (Dibenzyline). Blockage increases peripheral blood flow and lowers both erect and supine blood pressure, and therefore the drug is used in peripheral vascular disorders like diabetic gangrene, frostbite sequelae, and Raynaud's syndrome. Phentolamine (Regitine) is used likewise to control hypertension in pheochromocytoma and in hypertensive crisis due to MAO inhibition, and to prevent norepinephrine sloughs after IV administration.

The first β-adrenergic blocking agent approved for use in clinical practice in the US, propranolol (Inderal), competes with endogenous epinephrine and norepinephrine at myocardial β-receptor sites and thereby prevents these catecholamines from stimulating the heart. Because of the resulting reduction in heart rate (chronotropic effect) and in force of contraction (inotropic effect) produced by the drug, it is useful in cardiac arrhythmias, including the tachyarrhythmias of digitalis intoxication and those associated with anesthesia.[120]

Although drug interactions with adrenergic blocking agents are useful, care must be exercised when administrating them to diabetics. Antagonism of the metabolic effects of catecholamines may potentiate insulin hypoglycemia.

Some drug interactions may occur by increasing the receptor affinity or sensitivity. Although thyroxine has no effect on the clotting factors dependent on vitamin K, on the plasma protein binding of coumarin anticoagulants, or on their half-life, nevertheless it potentiates these anticoagulants and prolongs the prothrombin time, possibly by increasing their affinity for receptors.[394,411]

Modification of Biotransformation

Protective metabolic and excretory forces are marshalled by the body to destroy and eliminate drugs whenever they are administered because it perceives them as foreign substances that pose a threat. This normal response to challenge with a drug includes the biotransformations discussed in Chapter 8. In the absence of inherited abnormalities and interactants these biotransformations effectively handle normal doses of medications. But interactants may interfere with the protective processes and create hazards for the patient by means of enzyme induction or enzyme inhibition.

Enzyme Induction. Stimulation of microsomal drug metabolizing enzymes (enzyme induction) by drugs and other chemicals, which was briefly mentioned in Chapter 8, is one of the most critical drug interaction problems. It has been postulated that it may possibly take place either through increased synthesis of microsomal protein for hepatic enzymes or decreased degradation of this protein. The process increases the size of the liver and markedly influences the rate of biotransformation of drugs and therefore the intensity of their effects. Because metabolites are generally less active than their parent compounds, enzyme induction usually decreases the intensity and duration of drug effects. However, if the metabolites of a given drug happen to be equally or more potent than the drug itself, then enzyme induction either has no effect on patient response or it increases the overall response.

Induction of metabolizing enzymes may be prevented by inhibitors of protein and RNA synthesis, e.g., by ethionine and actinomycin D respectively.[83,1057,1058]

Hundreds of drugs and other chemicals, including certain analgesics, anesthetics, anticonvulsants, antihistamines, anti-inflammatory agents, hormones, hypoglycemics, hypnotics, insecticides, sedatives, and tranquilizers stimulate either the metabolism of themselves or of certain other drugs, or both. In most instances they decrease drug activity in the body. Phenobarbital alone has been shown to stimulate the metabolism of more than 60 chemicals, including widely prescribed drugs like digitoxin, diphenylhydantoin, griseofulvin, glucocorticoids, and oral anticoagulants.[83] In one series of patients the blood levels of diphenylhydantoin dropped 72% when 120 mg. of phenobarbital per day was given. In this instance an enzyme inducer affected a drug which itself is an enzyme inducer. Whether a given drug is an enzyme inducer in man cannot always be predetermined in laboratory animals, however. Thus, tolbutamide is a potent inducer of oxidative drug metabolizing enzymes in rats and dogs, but it has little or no such effect in man.[28,83,297,1057,1058]

For a list of some representative microsomal enzyme inducers see Table 10-4.

Sometimes enzyme induction can be beneficial. Phenobarbital, by stimulating the metabolism of bilirubin, is useful in neonatal hyperbilirubinemia, because it hastens formation of bilirubin metabolites that are readily excreted in the urine.[174,264,1076] Diphenylhydantoin, o,p-DDD,* and certain other inducing drugs, by stimulating the conversion of cortisol to the less potent metabolite, 6β-hydroxycortisol, permit nonsurgical treatment of hyperadrenocorticism and amelioration of the symptoms of Cushing's syndrome.[175] Prescott was tempted to consider giving an occasional dose of DDT to patients who repeatedly attempt suicide with barbiturates.[359,688]

Paradoxically, insecticide residues in man may be reduced by giving enzyme inducing anticonvulsants such as barbiturates and diphenylhydantoin.[1044]

On the other hand, enzyme induction is the basis of many undesirable drug interactions. Griseofulvin, by induction of α-amino levulinic acid synthetase, exacerbates acute intermittent porphyria. Alcohol accelerates the

---

* o,p-DDD (Lysodren) was approved by the FDA, July 8, 1970 for use in adrenal cortical carcinoma (approved on the basis of enzyme induction).[120,271,965]

Table 10-4   Some Drug Metabolizing Enzyme Inducers*

Alcohol (ethanol)	Cotinine	Nitrous oxide
Aldrin	o,p'-DDD	Norethynodrel
Aminopyrine†	DDT†	Orphenadrine (Disipal)†
Amobarbital (Amytal)†	Dieldrin	Oxidized sterols (cholesterol,
Androstenedione	9,10-Dimethyl-1,2-	dihydrocholesterol, or
Anticonvulsants	benzanthracene†	ergosterol)
Antihistamines	Diphenhydramine (Benadryl)	Paramethadione (Paradione)
Barbiturates†	Diphenylhydantoin (Dilantin)†	Pentobarbital (Nembutal)†
Bemegride (Megimide)	Ethchlorvynol (Placidyl)	Pesticides
Benzene†	Fructose	Phenacetin
3,4-Benzpyrene (charcoal broiled	Glutethimide (Doriden)†	Phenaglycodol (Ultran)
meats, cigarette smoke, etc.)†	Griseofulvin (Fulvicin, Grifulvin,	Phenobarbital†
Butabarbital (Butisol)	Grisactin, etc.)	Phenylbutazone (Butazolidin)†
Carbromal (Adalin)	Haloperidol (Haldol)	Prednisolone
Carbutamide	Heptabarbital (Medomin)	Prednisone (Deltasone, Deltra)†
Carcinogens (polycyclic aromatic	Heptachlorepoxide	Probenecid (Benemid)†
hydrocarbons)	Hexachlorocyclohexane	Promazine (Sparine)
Chloral betaine (Beta-chlor)	Hexobarbital (Sombucaps)†	Pyridione (Persedon)
Chloral hydrate	Imipramine (Tofranil)†	Secobarbital (Seconal)†
Chlorcyclizine (Perazil)†	Insecticides, halogenated	Sedatives and hypnotics
Chlorobutanol (Chloretone)	Lindane	Smoking (cigarettes, etc.)
Chlordane	Meprobamate (Equanil, Miltown)†	Steroids
Chlordiazepoxide (Librium)†	Methoxyflurane (Penthrane)†	Stibestrol†
Chlorinated hydrocarbons	Methylphenylethylhydantoin	Testosterone and its derivatives
Chlorinated insecticides	(Mesantoin)	Tolbutamide (Orinase)†
Chlorpromazine (Thorazine)†	Methyprylon (Noludar)	Trifluperidol (Psychoperidol)
Citrus red no. 2†	Nicotine	Triflupromazine (Vesprin)
Cortisone	Nikethamide (Coramine)	Urethane

* References to the literature are provided in the Table of Drug Interactions (page 395).
†These drugs stimulate their own metabolism either in a test animal or in man during long-term administration. Many other microsomal enzyme inducers probably will eventually be shown to have this same property. Some agents are enzyme inducers for some drugs and enzyme inhibitors for others.

metabolism and thereby diminishes the activity of barbiturates, isoniazid, tolbutamide and other widely used drugs. Medication of chronic alcoholics therefore presents special problems. The administration of drugs to heavy users of CNS depressants like the barbiturates also requires special attention. [23,28, 254,674,740]

The metabolism of steroids like cortisol may be stimulated by enzyme inducing agents such as diphenylhydantoin, phenobarbital and phenylbutazone. Halogenated insecticides (chlordane, DDT, etc.) and phenobarbital induce not only the metabolism of cortisol, but also that of androgens, estrogens, and progesterone. These inducers decrease the uterotropic effects of both exogenous and endogenous estrogens. Concern is being created by the possible ineffectiveness of oral contraceptives in women receiving barbiturates, sedatives, tranquilizers, and other drugs that cause enzyme induction.

A classic example of an adverse drug interaction resulting from enzyme induction occurs when a patient who has been receiving an oral anticoagulant and a barbiturate is discharged from the hospital and the sedative is discontinued at the same time. Severe bleeding episodes are often reported within a few weeks if the dosage of anticoagulant is not adjusted accordingly. While the patient is receiving the barbiturate which enhances the hepatic microsomal metabolism of the anticoagulant, the latter is given at a sufficiently high dosage to compensate for the enzyme induction. But if no adjustment is made after withdrawal of the barbiturate the microsomal metabolism returns to its slower rate. The levels of oral anticoagulant then become elevated in the plasma, the prothrombin time becomes prolonged and hemorrhage may ensue. [222] The same situation has occurred with other common inducers such as meprobamate (Equanil, Miltown) and glutethimide (Doriden). [9,69,223,296,297,434]

Some drugs stimulate their own metabolism. Aminopyrine, barbital, chlorcyclizine, glutethimide, meprobamate, orphenadrine, phenobarbital, phenylbutazone and many other drugs are progressively metabolized more rapidly during prolonged administration. These drugs (Table 10-3) also deactivate other drugs through the enzyme induction mechanism. Thus chlorcyclizine shortens the duration of action of hexobarbitol to $\frac{1}{12}$ and phenobarbital shortens the duration of action of zoxazolamine to $\frac{1}{7}$ normal. [336] Tolerance to drugs may therefore be developed through this mechanism. The creation of tolerance in this manner as well as the reduction of true potency through enzyme induction are subjects of vital importance to investigators engaged in testing new drugs. They may arrive at incorrect dosages for individual inducing drugs and for combinations of medications that contain inducing drugs. Morphine, meperidine, and other narcotics do not induce tolerance in this manner, however, but actually inhibit N-dealkylation of the narcotic administered. [28]

When two inducers, e.g., diphenhydramine (Benadryl) and phenobarbital, both of which produce a sedative effect, are administered together it is difficult to predict what their combined effect will be at a given duration of therapy. At first the sedative effect is potentiated, but if the dosage is continued over a prolonged period both the antihistaminic and sedative effects are progressively diminished by mutual and self-induction of the metabolizing enzymes. The net effect of potentiation versus induction at any given time of duration of therapy cannot be predicted accurately.

Accordingly, hepatic microsomal enzyme induction (1) generally decreases patient response to medication, but on occasion may do the opposite, (2) may hasten the removal of undesirable endogenous and exogenous chemicals, (3) may create hazardous situations if undesirable metabolites are produced in excessive quantities too rapidly, (4) may cause the development of tolerance, or (5) may lead to incorrect interpretations of clinical investigations.

Enzyme Inhibition. Inhibition of microsomal drug metabolizing enzymes by drugs and other chemicals is another very critical as well as common drug interaction problem. This type of interaction produces situations exactly the opposite of those described above for enzyme induction.

The list of known microsomal enzyme inhibitors has grown rapidly. Representative examples are listed in Table 10-5, page 374. Most of the inhibiting drugs and other chemicals act directly but some yield metabolites that are the inhibitors. Thus furazol-

Table 10–5   Some Drug Metabolizing Enzyme Inhibitors*

Acetohexamide (Dymelor)	Chlordiazepoxide (Librium)	Norethandrolone (Nilevar)
Allopurinol (Zyloprim)	Chlorpromazine (Thorazine)	Oral anticoagulants (Coumadin,
p-Aminosalicylic acid (PAS)	Chlorpropamide (Diabinese)	Dicumarol, Panwarfin, Sintrom,
Anabolic agents (Dianabol,	Clofibrate (Atromid-S)	etc.)
Durabolin, Maxibolin,	Disulfiram (Antabuse, etc.)	Oral contraceptives
Metandren, Neo-Hombreol,	Estrogens	Pargyline (Eutonyl)
Nilevar, Oreton-M, etc.)	Furazolidone (Furoxone)	Phenelzine (Nardil)
Androgens	Insecticides (fluorophosphates)	Phenyramidol (Analexin)
Anticholinesterases (Floropryl,	Iproniazid (Marsilid)	Prednisolone (Hydeltra,
Humorsol, Mytelase,	Isocarboxazid (Marplan)	Meticortelone, Sterane, etc.)
Phospholine, Prostigmin, etc.)	Isoniazid (Niconyl, Nydrazin)	Procarbazine (Matulane)
Anticoagulants (coumarins)	MAO inhibitors (Eutonyl,	Prochlorperazine (Compazine)
Antidiabetics, oral (Diabinese,	Furoxone, Marplan, Matulane,	Quinacrine (Atabrine)
Dymelor, Orinase, Tolinase,	Nardil, Niamid, Parnate, etc.)	SKF-525A (Proadifen)
etc.)	Methandrostenolone (Dianabol)	Steroids (anabolics, estrogens,
Bishydroxycoumarin (Dicumarol)	Methylphenidate (Ritalin)	etc.)
Calcium carbimide (cyanamide)	Metronidazole (Flagyl)	Sulfonylureas (oral antidiabetics)
citrated (Dipsan, Temposil)	Mushrooms (Coprinus	Sulfaphenazole (Orisul)
Carbon disulfide	atramentarius)	d-Thyroxine
Chloramphenicol	Nialamide (Niamid)	Tolbutamide (Orinase)
(Chloromycetin)	Nitrofurans	Tranylcypromine (Parnate)

* References to the literature are provided in the Table of Drug Interactions (page 395).

idone inhibits monoamine oxidase by virtue of its metabolite that is a MAO inhibitor. Some drugs like aminoazo dyes, meperidine, and morphine are self inhibiting.[28]

Enzyme inhibition may be useful. The potency of methotrexate as an enzyme inhibitor in neoplastic disease is startling. Essentially irreversible competitive inhibition of the entire mass of folic acid reductase in the body is achieved with only about 5 mg. of the antineoplastic. The drug has a 100,000 times greater affinity for the enzyme than folic acid.

Another useful effect of inhibition concerns use of levodopa in parkinsonism.[964] By using an inhibitor of the enzyme L-dopa decarboxylase, investigators have prevented the drug from being degraded in the kidneys and liver of test animals before it reached the brain, and serious side effects were diminished. The inhibitor (compound RO4-4602), developed in Switzerland, greatly potentiates levodopa because it permits more of it to reach its receptors in the brain. Eventually, therefore dosage of the antiparkinsonism drug may be reduced and serious side effects diminished.

Enzyme inhibition, however, is the basis for a large and rapidly increasing number of adverse drug interactions. Inhibition of tolbutamide (Orinase) metabolism by bishydroxycoumarin, phenylbutazone, sulfaphenazole and other drugs, induces hypoglycemia.

Since the two latter drugs are pyrazole derivatives, drugs with this nucleus should be suspect until proven not to interact in this manner.[28]

The oral anticoagulants have been among the most thoroughly investigated drug interactants because they have characteristics that facilitate research. Plasma levels are readily determined and correlate well with physiological activity and their therapeutic index is high. They are converted by the hepatic microsomal enzymes into inactive metabolites and this conversion may be stimulated or inhibited. Their metabolism is stimulated and therefore their activity is decreased by barbiturates such as butabarbital (Butisol), heptabarbital (Medomin), and phenobarbital, also by some antihistamines, ethchlorvynol (Placidyl), glutethimide (Doriden), griseofulvin (Fulvicin), haloperidol (Haldol), and other widely used drugs. The metabolism of the oral anticoagulants is inhibited and therefore their activity is potentiated by aminosalicylic acid (PAS), anabolic steroids like methandrostenolone (Dianabol), methylphenidate (Ritalin), monoamine oxidase inhibitors, phenyramidol (Analexin), and many others. Some potentiate only coumarin anticoagulants whereas some like the MAO inhibitors potentiate also indandiones like phenindione (Danilone).

The oral anticoagulants are not only affected by other drugs; they also affect the metabolism of other drugs. Thus they prolong the hypoglycemic effects of tolbutamide and increase the toxicity of diphenylhydantoin by inhibiting their metabolism.

Diphenylhydantoin is another example of a drug that not only affects the metabolism of other drugs but also is affected itself by other drugs. Many investigators of this anticonvulsant have studied its potentiation by microsomal enzyme inhibitors. Aminosalicylic acid (PAS), bishydroxycoumarin (Dicumarol), disulfiram (Antabuse), isoniazid (Nydrazid, methylphenidate (Ritalin), phenylbutazone (Butazolidin), phenyramidol, sulfaphenazole (Orisul), and some other sulfonamides may produce potentially toxic blood levels of dephenylhydantoin and induce distressing reactions like ataxia, blood dyscrasias, diplopia fatal toxic hepatitis, and nystagmus.[28,222] When oral anticoagulants must be given to patients receiving diphenylhydantoin, one of the indandione anticoagulants may be the drug of choice because they do not inhibit the microsomal enzymes.

If two or more drugs that utilize the same enzyme are given at about the same time, severe potentiation with serious adverse consequences may occur. Thus allopurinol (Zyloprim) which is used in gout because it prevents the biotransformation of hypoxanthine to uric acid by inhibiting xanthine oxidase, may cause severe depression of medullary hematopoiesis if given with azathioprine or 6-mercaptopurine because the same enzyme inactivities these antileukemic agents by oxidizing them to their corresponding thiouric acids.

An interactant may be biphasic in its effects. When N-methyl-3-piperidyl diphenylcarbamate (MPDC) is given up to 12 hours before hexobarbital is administered, the sleeping time is prolonged because of enzyme inhibition. When MPDC is given 24 to 48 hours before hexobarbital is administered, the sleeping time is shortened because of enzyme induction. Thus MPDC can exert either an enzyme inducing or an enzyme inhibiting effect on the barbiturate, depending on the timing.[478] Microsomal enzyme inhibitors, as well as stimulators, urgently require further clinical investigation to generate precise data on their effects on drug action, metabolism, and excretion.

It is essential to learn as soon as possible to what extent (1) long-term exposure to environmental carcinogens induces enzymes that detoxify these and other agents that are harmful to the human body, (2) constituents of cigarette smoke enhance the metabolism of nicotine and produces tolerance to this toxic agent in man, (3) certain drugs induce enzymes responsible for the metabolism of normal body constituents such as bilirubin, fatty acids, and steroid hormones, and (4) common items of the diet such as alcohol and fructose stimulate the metabolism of normal body constituents as well as therapeutic agents.

Alteration of Excretion

Drug interactions may theoretically alter the rate of excretion of drugs via any of the eight excretion routes discussed in Chapter 8. Cathartics may expedite and increase the percentage of *fecal* drug excretion and thereby decrease intake also. Drugs that increase the flow of *perspiration, saliva,* or *tears* may increase the excretion of drugs in these fluids, but these routes are usually of very minor importance as a means of drug elimination. Saliva and tears are largely swallowed and reabsorbed from the intestine. Thus, enterosalivary and enterolacrimal cycling may cause most of the drug in these fluids to be reabsorbed, metabolized, and excreted by the urinary route. Choleretics may significantly increase the excretion of drugs that are removed from the body into the intestinal tract via the *bile.* But enterohepatic cycling may result in metabolism of the drug before it can be fecally excreted. Certain hormones, e.g., lactogenic (prolactin), growth and thyroid hormones, may increase the excretion of drugs via the *mother's milk.* Drugs that alter the partial pressure of a gaseous or volatile drug in the inspired air in the alveoli, or the solubility of the drug in the pulmonary capillary blood, or the rate of the blood flow may alter the rate of excretion of these drugs via the *respiratory route.* Drugs that alter the *exfoliating dermis and the nails and hair* that are removed by trimming could conceivably modify the minor quantities of drug removed in these tissues. But practically no definitive investigations have been conducted to establish accurately the effects and importance of drug interactions associated with these routes. See Fig. 10-1.

The only excretory drug interactions that have received any significant attention by investigators are those involving urinary excretion. Drug interactions may theoretically occur at all stages of urinary excretion by altering any of the factors that control glomerular filtration and tubular secretion on the one hand and active or passive tubular reabsorption on the other. Thus, a drug or other chemical may influence the urinary excretion rate of another drug by altering the dynamics of drug and metabolite transport across the glomerular and tubular membranes. Electrochemical gradients may be altered by varying ionic and membranal charges; hydrostatic gradients by varying blood flow and pressure; osmotic gradients by varying blood constituents; and pH gradients by alkalinizing or acidifying the urine. Solubility, lipid: water partition coefficients, and other factors that influence both active and passive transport of a given drug and its metabolites may also be altered by drugs given concomitantly.

Accordingly, urinary drug interactions may result from the administration of acidifiers, alkalinizers, cardiovascular agents, chelating agents, diuretics, and any other category of drugs that affects the above gradients and physical factors, or the functioning of the glomeruli and tubules. Any drug that causes pathologic changes that destroy the filtration or secretory capacity of a significant percentage of the nephrons of the kidney may significantly decrease urinary drug excretion, thereby elevating blood levels and increasing toxicity. This also holds true for drugs that alter flow, osmolality, pressure, or volume of the cardiovascular and lymphatic fluids. Under such influences, prescribed drugs may repeatedly move in and out of cells, tissues, vessels, and fluid compartments and become temporarily bound and later displaced from binding sites. Major shifts in the factors mentioned above may materially influence drug distribution and redistribution and thus affect its distribution to the urinary apparatus and therefore its excretion rate.

Increasing the glomerular filtration rate or the active transport (secretion) rate of the drug into the proximal convoluted tubules tends to lower blood levels and inhibit drug action. These rates are increased by displacement of drug from plasma binding sites which releases more unbound drug for entry into the glomeruli and filtration into the Bowman's capsules. At the same time, however, such displacement provides more drug for metabolism. Thus, the plasma levels and the overall effects of the drug may be enhanced only temporarily because enhanced excretion and metabolism usually remove the released drug rapidly. The *duration* of the drug in the body is generally decreased significantly when urinary filtration is enhanced.

The opposite effects are achieved and a drug is potentiated when excretion by glomerular filtration and tubular secretion is inhibited. Drugs that alter rates of active transport and thus rates of tubular secretion are especially likely to alter the excretion of other drugs most effectively and to make major changes in safety and efficacy. Thus, probenecid markedly prolongs the half-life of penicillin and various other drugs in the plasma by this mechanism. This drug also increases the uricosuric activity of sulfinpyrazone (Anturane) and the hypoglycemic activity of tolbutamide (Orinase) and other sulfonylureas. Phenylbutazone induces hypoglycemia with acetohexamide, at least in part by decreasing clearance of its active metabolite, hydroxyhexamide.[141] Phenylbutazone also potentiates bishydroxycoumarin by antagonizing its renal excretion.[28] PAS potentiates isoniazid by competing for mechanisms of urinary excretion.[28] These and numerous other examples are listed in the Table beginning on page 395. See also Table 10-6 which lists some drugs that alter the urinary excretion of various other drugs.

Modification of either the active or passive drug reabsorption processes of the urinary tubules also influences the activity and toxicity of medications. Blood levels are elevated and drug toxicity tends to increase most markedly when several or all of the mechanisms that influence drug retention act in unison—inhibition of glomerular filtration and tubular secretion and enhancement of active or passive reabsorption.

The exact mechanisms that pertain to a given drug are often unknown. A great deal of investigation is needed to determine the nature of many drug interactions that affect urinary excretion. Thus, salicylates, used alone, antagonize reabsorption of uric acid and thereby increase its excretion. They nev-

Table 10–6   Some Drugs that Alter Urinary Excretion of Other Drugs

Acetazolamide (Diamox) [172,179,726]	Fatty acids [421]
Acidifying agents [165,325,359,870]	Fruit juices (cranberry, orange, etc.) [120,619]
Alcohol [166]	Phenylbutazone (Butazolidin) [121,141,330]
Alkalinizing agents [165,325,359,870]	Potassium citrate [325,870]
p-Aminohippuric acid (PAHA) [433]	Probenecid (Benemid) [43,160,269,359,650,930,931]
p-Aminosalicylic acid (PAS) [28,179]	Sodium acetate [44,165,325,870]
Ammonium chloride [44,165,325,870]	Sodium acid phosphate [619,689]
Ammonium nitrate [44,165,325,870]	Sodium bicarbonate [44,165,325,870]
Ascorbic acid [325,870,962]	Sodium citrate [44,165,325,870]
Calcium chloride [165,173]	Sodium lactate [44,165,325,870]
Diuretics (Diamox, Diuril, etc.) [120,194]	Thiazides [28,330,870]

ertheless interfere with the uricosuric effect of several drugs including phenylbutazone (Butazolidin), and probenecid (Benemid) via the same mechanisms. [28,40,44,165,330]

Reabsorption is perhaps strongly influenced by changing the pH of the urine. Any drugs that elevate urinary pH (acetazolamide, potassium citrate, sodium acetate, bicarbonate, citrate or lactate, thiazides, etc.) or lower it (ammonium chloride, ammonium nitrate,* calcium chloride, etc.) may have a profound influence on the excretion rates of concurrently administered medications. The results may be adverse or beneficial according to the circumstances. By lowering the pH, ammonium chloride and other acidifiers are useful in eliminating overdosages of amphetamine. And by elevating pH, sodium bicarbonate and other alkalinizers are useful in eliminating overdoses of aspirin, barbiturates, sulfonamides, and other weak acids. [28,330]

The solubility of a drug is another important factor in urinary excretion. Through a chemical reaction or complexation, a prescribed drug may be converted into a much less soluble compound through interaction with another drug or other chemical. Thus, methenamine should not be given with some sulfonamides because the formaldehyde that is liberated from the methenamine may combine with them to form insoluble complexes. [28,280,433,662]

Disturbed Water and Electrolyte Balance

The interactants may affect the action of another drug by producing imbalance of water and electrolytes (Ca^{++}, Cl^-, K^+, Na^+ HCO_3^-, and certain organic ions) in the body. Drugs that produce such imbalance may induce edema or water depletion with hemoconcentration, hyperkalemia or hypokalemia, hypernatremia or hyponatremia, metabolic acidosis, and related conditions. Such drug-induced imbalances, caused by faulty absorption, distribution, excretion, or ventilation, can sometimes create hazardous situations. A few typical examples follow.

A drug that causes excessive diuresis, catharsis, perspiration or vomiting may significantly lower the blood pressure because of fluid and sodium loss. Accordingly, problems may arise with hypotensives and other cardiovascular medications. A drug that produces nephrotoxic effects may not only cause loss of water and sodium but also the retention of certain drugs, and this may produce toxic levels in the blood and tissues. In the presence of drug-induced oliguria resulting from water depletion or kidney damage, any drug may become very toxic. Sodium depletion alone may increase the toxicity of some drugs. Thus, diuretics are contraindicated with lithium carbonate because both types of medication may inhibit tubular reabsorption of sodium and cause its depletion.

Adrenocorticotropic hormone (ACTH), cathartics, corticosteroids, diuretics (carbonic anhydrase inhibitors, ethacrynic acid, furosemide, mercurials, thiazides), outdated tetracyclines (epianhydrotetracycline), and nephrotoxic drugs that cause acute tubular necrosis or renal tubular acidosis may induce a potassium deficiency. Combined use of certain diuretics and corticosteroids is particularly likely to cause a severe loss of potassium. Such loss may cause arrhythmias in cardiac patients receiving digitalis because lowered potassium levels sensitize the heart to the action of the drug. Sometimes more than a third of patients taking diuretics with digitalis experience adverse reactions. This

---

*This explosive chemical is seldom used in medicine except for veterinary therapy.

type of interaction apparently caused the death of a number of patients who were given irrational combinations of drugs to control weight. Several antiobesity medications, which were widely used until condemned, contained various combinations of amphetamine, barbiturates, digitalis, diuretics and thyroid. In the adversely affected patients, severe hypokalemia may have been caused not only by reduced intake of potassium due to the anorexigenic action of amphetamine, but also loss of potassium due to the cathartic and diuretic actions of the other ingredients. This considerably increased the toxicity of the digitalis.

Severe, hazardous hyperkalemia may be produced by the combined use of several potassium-conserving diuretics such as amiloride, spironolactone, and triamterene. Excessive potassium levels, in addition to toxic actions, also tend to diminish the effectiveness of digitalis in cardiac patients, and can be serious in a patient with congestive heart failure, renal failure, or uncontrolled diabetes mellitus.

Elevation of calcium levels above normal also increases the toxicity of digitalis. Injections of calcium salts intravenously into patients receiving the cardiotonic drug have caused several deaths.

MULTIPLICITY OF MECHANISMS

Some drugs are affected by a wide variety of mechanisms. Oral anticoagulants, for example, may have their hypoprothrombinemic action potentiated by (1) decreasing the absorption of vitamin K from the intestine, (2) displacing the anticoagulants from secondary binding sites, (3) inhibiting the hepatic microsomal metabolizing enzymes, (4) increasing the affinity of the anticoagulants for their receptors, or (5) inhibiting the synthesis of vitamin K-sensitive clotting factors.[710] The first mechanism is illustrated by mineral oil,[28,35,120] the second by the acidic pyrazolone derivatives,[3,150,448] the third by phenyramidol,[705,706] and methylphenidate,[156] the fourth by clofibrate, norethandrolone and *d*-thyroxine,[394] and the fifth by aspirin,[712] quinine, and quinidine.[158,260,707,713]

Polymechanistic Drugs

The prediction of patient response to some drug combinations is often exceedingly diffi-

cult because of the multiplicity of pharmacological actions underlying the potential drug interactions. Misinterpretations of responses are frequently made, particularly with new drugs whose mechanisms of action have not been fully elucidated. Consequently, some of the drug interactions reported in the literature appear to be conflicting.* Upon careful analysis, however, a satisfactory explanation can usually be found. Contradictory reports may both be correct under certain circumstances. Sometimes, a patient response may actually be the net effect of several concurrent interactions and since one may predominate at one time and not at another the outcome may not be consistent. Besides, the order in which the doses of one drug are given relative to those of another, as well as dosage level, delay in onset of action, prolonged duration of action following withdrawal, brand of drug product, and other considerations, may be critical in determining the final outcome of combination drug therapy.[117, 120,166,168,170,181,327,550,593,619,823]

Safe administration of medications to the patient often demands considerable knowledge, in depth, of the pharmacology of *all* drugs involved. Excellent examples of the necessity for such understanding are afforded by the adrenergic neuron blocking agents, the monoamine oxidase (MAO) inhibitors, and the tricyclic antidepressants. Although highly useful, these and other drugs with complex mechanisms of action can be extremely hazardous to the patient when improperly used. See Table 10-7 for some potentially lethal drug combinations.

Adrenergic Neuron Blocking Agents. Basically, these agents (guanethidine, methyldopa, reserpine, etc.) function as antihypertensives by inhibiting peripheral adrenergic transmission which constricts blood vessels and tends to elevate the blood pressure. But these drugs do not accomplish this in exactly the same manner.

Reserpine acts (1) by slowly depleting the neurohumoral transmitter, norepinephrine (NE),

---

* Also, the literature may be faulty because some authors perpetuate errors by citing secondary sources without checking back to the original investigations. Thus, metaraminol has repeatedly been described as an indirectly acting pressor sympathomimetic. Like norepinephrine, it mainly acts directly on *alpha*-receptors and depends only partially on norepinephrine release for its pressor action.[168] Because it has only a 3-OH on the ring it has a particularly high ratio of direct to indirect action.

from its total pools (reserve pools and cytoplasmic and granular mobile pools) in the terminals of all postganglionic adrenergic neurons and (2) by blocking the active transport mechanism that is essential for its uptake from extracellular fluid into the cytoplasmic mobile pool of the terminals and thence across the membranes of the osmophilic granules to the intragranular pools where it is stored as the ATP salt. Reserpine also blocks uptake of other catecholamines such as dopamine and serotonin (5-hydroxytryptamine or 5-HT, the tryptaminergic neurohumoral transmitter of the brain) by various tissues, including the adrenal medulla, blood vessels, brain, and heart.

Depletion and blockage of amines, however, are only two of its many actions. Some of its cardiovascular, CNS, endocrinological, gastro-intestinal, and renal effects are due to other mechanisms. These effects may be briefly summarized as follows:

Cardiovascular and Hematic Effects. Reserpine therapy, through depletion of biogenic amines, may reduce cardiac output and myocardial competence may be considerably reduced in the presence of depressants such as anesthetics (in emergency surgery, vagal blocking agents may be used). Its brady-cardiac action may aggravate cardiac failure, but its use in tense patients with tachycardia may be useful.

An angina-like syndrome and ectopic cardiac arrhythmias may occur with reserpine therapy. The arrhythmias are more likely to be encountered when reserpine is administered concurrently with digitalis, quinidine, and similar drugs.

Long latency of onset following initation of therapy and prolonged duration of action following its withdrawal are prominent characteristics of reserpine. The drug acts slowly to reduce hypertension. In the initial stages, particularly after large IV doses, a transient vasopressor effect may result from the released catecholamines. Then with continued depletion and metabolic destruction of the released amines, and also with increased vagal effects, the blood pressure gradually falls. Depletion to negligible catecholamine levels may occur in about 24 hours but full effects of the drug may not be realized for several days to two weeks.

Restoration of the pressor amines is a slow process, and because of the cumulative effect reserpine dosage must be titrated very carefully and supervised very closely. For this reason, too, when the drug is withdrawn, its gradually diminishing effects may still be present for up to a month.

Certain other actions and effects must also be considered. Reserpine inhibits the reflex responses of the veins and decreases peripheral resistance. Peripheral vasodilation with increased cutaneous blood flow, flushing, nasal congestion and postural hypotension may result. Allergic rhinitis and other allergic disorders may be aggravated. Also purpura and lowered platelet counts have been observed as allergic manifestations.

The drug induces a supersensitivity to catecholamines and responses to some sympathomimetics may be exaggerated. This is particularly hazardous in bronchial asthmatics. Finally, because of the catecholamine depletion, patients are rendered more susceptible to infections such as colds, their seizure threshold is lowered, and they are sensitized to shock, stresses, and traumatic conditions such as electroshock therapy and surgery. Deaths have occurred in reserpinized patients in such situations.

CNS Effects. Reserpine induces sedative and tranquilizing effects. It was first used to alleviate psychoneuroses associated with tension and psychoses involving anxiety, compulsive aggression, or hyperkinetic activity. But dosage must be carefully adjusted or paradoxical effects may be produced. The most serious adverse effect caused by reserpine is mental depression, sometimes so severe that patients have committed suicide. Large doses may induce extrapyramidal symptoms, respiratory depression, motor impairment with convulsive episodes, hypothermia, and death. CNS sensitization may be manifested by deafness, dull sensorium, glaucoma, optic atrophy, and uveitis. Epilepsy may be exacerbated.

Endocrinological Effects. Apparently reserpine, by blocking the release of pituitary gonadotropins, inhibits the ovarian cycle (including menstruation) and decreased fertility. Feminization, impotence, and decreased libido have been reported in the male.

Some of the manifestations of hypothyroidism resemble the effects of catecholamines and may be the result of increased sensitivity to sympathomimetics. Reserpine has therefore been used successfully in some patients to suppress the signs and symptoms of this condition (reduction of anxiety, palpitation, and tension as well as tachycardia, tremor and characteristic stare).

Gastrointestinal Effects. Reserpine increases the appetite and gain in weight may become a problem. The drug, due to central cholinergic stimulation, increases salivation and gastrointestinal secretion as well as the tone and motility of the gastrointestinal tract. Thus, it may precipitate ulcers, hemorrhage, cramps and diarrhea, as well as biliary colic in patients with gallstones. The drug is therefore contraindicated in patients with peptic ulcers, ulcerative colitis, or other gastrointestinal disorders, or a history of such conditions, although the Hindus once used the drug in dysentery.

Renal Effects. Reserpine tends to induce sodium and water retention. Dysuria has been reported. If these effects are not checked edematous weight gain and congestive heart failure can result.

Guanethidine, an adrenergic neuron blocker like reserpine, possesses many of the same properties. After administration for 10 days or longer, it sensitizes effector cells to exogenous catecholamines such as epinephrine and levarterenol. Its effect, however, is much more pronounced than that produced by reserpine; it actually intensifies the action of the latter if given subsequently. Like reserpine, too, it decreases response to indirectly acting sympathomimetics like amphetamine, ephedrine and tyramine which depend on release of NE for their effects.

The actions of guanethidine, however, are slightly different; it only partially depletes NE stores and then blocks release of the remainder and prevents further uptake by occupying the NE storage sites. In addition, the lag in its onset of action (a few hours to 3 days for full effect) and its prolonged duration of action (4 to 7 days after withdrawal) are much shorter than those encountered with reserpine. Since it releases the endogenous NE more promptly and releases less of the NE in a deaminated form, the resulting initial hypertension is likely to be more marked, especially if transfer from a ganglionic blocking antihypertensive is not made gradually.

The drug has some properties not possessed by reserpine. It apparently exerts some direct and indirect sympathomimetic actions (hypertension, myocardial stimulation, etc.) which are blocked by prior administration of reserpine or by adrenergic blocking agents. It markedly lowers intraocular pressure in glaucomatous eyes and increases gastrointestinal motility probably through depletion of serotonin in the intestines.

Methyldopa (*levo* isomer), also an adrenergic neuron blocker that depletes biogenic amine stores, apparently functions by a mechanism fundamentally different from that of guanethidine and reserpine. It decreases the concentration of dopamine, norepinephrine and serotonin in the central nervous system and peripheral tissues by theoretically inhibiting amino acid decarboxylase, the enzyme responsible for decarboxylation of dopa and 5-hydroxytryptophan (see Fig. 10-3). The decreases in dopamine and serotonin are transient, however, because the enzyme activity returns to normal, but NE depletion is prolonged because methyldopa is converted by the enzyme it inhibits (decarboxylase) into α-methyldopamine (Fig. 10-3) and by dopamine-beta-oxidase into α-methylnorepinephrine, both of which displace NE and prevent its uptake by tissues. The former metabolite is a vasoconstrictor and the latter is a pressor agent. The pressor agent, often referred to as a weak "false transmitter," actually is almost as active as NE and is released by indirectly acting sympathomimetics.

The major practical differences between methyldopa and the two other drugs just discussed are (1) a much shorter duration of action (48 hours), (2) a marked sedative effect in many patients during the first few days of therapy and after increases in dosage, (3) limited adrenergic neuron blockage, (4) inhibition of response to indirectly acting sympathomimetics without inhibiting response to nerve stimulation, and (5) release of prolactin that stimulates lactation.

MAO Inhibitors. These drugs are so named because one of their major actions is to inactivate irreversibly the *intracellular* metabolizing enzyme (monoamine oxidase or MAO) responsible for the oxidative deamination of certain monoamines (dopamine, epinephrine, norepinephrine, serotonin, tryptamine, tyramine, etc.) that occur in nature but not ephedrine and certain other exogenous amines. MAO inhibitors also inhibit many other drug metabolizing enzymes and thereby cause a wide variety of both endogenous and exogenous drugs and other chemicals to accumulate in the body. Thus the effects of these are potentiated when they are released from storage sites for contact with receptors. See *MAO Inhibitors* in the Table of Drug Interactions.

One result of MAO inhibition is elevation of catecholamine (dopamine, epinephrine and norepinephrine) and serotonin (5-HT) levels in the blood, brain, heart, and intestines. Elevation of these levels appears to be associated with elevation of mood, and as a result the MAO inhibitors became known as psychic energizers. They are mainly used as antidepressants in severe mental depression.

A lag period occurs between initiation of MAO inhibitor therapy and onset of effects; complete inhibition of MAO requires several days. Also, the drug action continues long after its withdrawal; several weeks are required to generate a new enzyme. Because of the prolonged action and potentiation of antidotes, overdosage presents a serious problem.

Cardiovascular Effects. Orthostatic hypotension (dizziness, fainting, palpitation, weakness) is frequently encountered during therapy with all MAO inhibitors. The exact mechanism remains to be determined but many have been postulated. These drugs may decrease peripheral resistance or diminish cardiac output. They may decrease norepinephrine synthesis, slow its turnover, or cause the catecholamine to accumulate perhaps to the point where it blocks ganglionic transmission. They may also cause the false transmitters, dopamine and octopamine, to accumulate. Whatever the mechanism may be, MAO inhibitors in general have a hypotensive action which slowly develops over a period of 3 to 4 weeks.

Some MAO inhibitors induce sympathomimetic effects either by acting directly on receptors or indirectly by catecholamine release. Those with

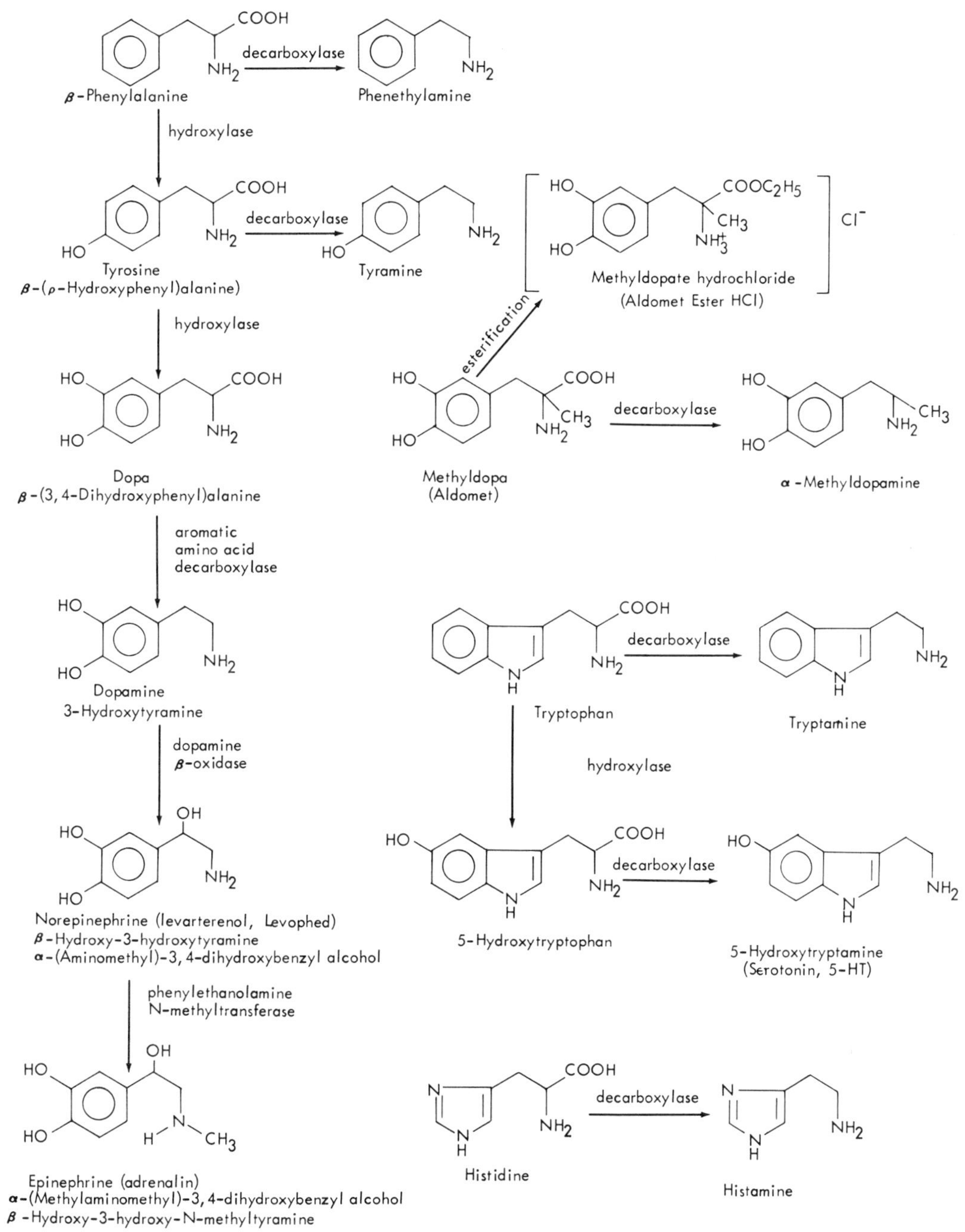

Fig. 10-3. Chemical relationships among the biogenic amines and related drugs and amino acids.

these properties may induce hypertension and cardiac arrhythmias initially, possibly by enhancing the sensitivity of peripheral vessels to vasoconstrictors. In some patients, certain MAO inhibitors induce hypoglycemia. In patients with reduced cardiac reserve, some of these drugs have been associated with congestive heart failure.

The actions of a wide variety of cardiovascular and hematic agents (anticoagulants, antidiabetics, antihypertensives, coronary vasodilators, diuretics, ganglionic blocking agents, sympathomimetics, etc.) are potentiated by MAO inhibitors through inhibition of metabolizing enzymes other than MAO. See pages 522 to 527.

CNS Effects. MAO inhibitors stimulate the central nervous system. with overdosage or some drug interactions, they may induce agitation, tremors, hyperhidrosis, insomnia, nightmares, hallucinations, confusion, hypomanic behavior, psychotic reactions, and sometimes convulsions. They may also cause hyperexcitability, muscular twitching, and other extrapyramidal symptoms. Sweating and headache have also been reported. Many CNS depressants and CNS stimulants are potentiated by MAO inhibitors.

Endocrinological Effects Delayed ejaculation and impotence have been reported.

Gastrointestinal Effects. Increased appetite may create a weight problem. Constipation, nausea and vomiting have been reported.

Other Effects. MAO inhibitors are some of the most toxic and most hazardous drugs in use. Hepatotoxicity, although of low incidence, can be severe because of the potential for hepatocellular degeneration. Blood dyscrasias, dry mouth, weakness, fatigue, and skin rashes have all been reported. These agents should generally be reserved for severely depressed patients. [29,37,74,86-88,134,136,162, 166,293,433,702,745-747,874,877,885]

Tricyclic Antidepressants. These three-ringed drugs are closely related structurally to the phenothiazines and have some of the same properties. Although they are administered for their CNS (psychological) effects they have many actions in the body and enter into a wide variety of drug interactions. The members of this category are listed on page 432 in the Table of Drug Interactions. The proto-type is imipramine (Tofranil, a dibenzazepine derivative). Closely related is amitriptyline (Elavil, a dibenzocycloheptene derivative) with a double-bonded carbon in place of the azepine nitrogen.

As far as drug interactions are concerned the cardiovascular, CNS, and autonomic effects of these drugs are most important.

Cardiovascular Effects. The tricyclic antidepressants lower blood pressure. They frequently induce orthostatic hypotension and, through vagal blockade, tachycardia. Cardiac arrhythmias, congestive heart failure, and myocardial infarction have also been attributed to them. These tricyclics potentiate the action of exogenous epinephrine and levarterenol at peripheral adrenergic receptors. They antagonize the hypotensive action of guanethidine, perhaps by interfering with its neuronal uptake.* They also have a cocaine-like effect (block uptake of NE and super-sensitize to catecholamines).

---

* The tricyclics apparently do not antagonize methyldopa because its mechanism of action is different, and the tricyclic doxepin (Sinequan) with a somewhat different structure from the imipramine-like and amitriptyline-like drugs does not block guanethidine at the usual therapeutic dosages.

CNS Effects. In some patients under some conditions these drugs may lift the patient from his depression to a state where the CNS is unduly stimulated (excitement, delusions, hallucinations, convulsions, etc.). The drugs may also prolong and intensify the sedative, hypnotic or narcotic effects of CNS depressants, impair affectivity, cognition and learning ability, inhibit spontaneous motor activity, sometimes cause weakness, headache, fatigue, and tremors, and apparently sensitize the patient to central adrenergic effects. Thus, they potentiate the augmentation in rate produced by amphetamine in operant conditioning situations and the stimulation of operant behavior by methylphenidate. Overdosage or a potentiating interaction may result in hypertension, hyperpyrexia, convulsions, and coma. In general, the result resembles atropine intoxication.

Autonomic Effects. The anticholinergic (cholinergic blocking) action of these drugs may produce prominent atropine-like symptoms (blurred vision, constipation, dizziness, dry mouth, palpitation, tachycardia, urinary retention, etc.). Such action is hazardous in glaucoma.

From the above discussion on adrenergic neuron blocking agents, MAO inhibitors, and tricyclic antidepressants a number of important conclusions may be deduced.

1. Timing of medication may be of primary importance in determining the outcome of a drug interaction. Because some drugs induce or inhibit enzymes or deplete catecholamines or complete certain other actions slowly their onset of effects is delayed until after a characteristic lag period, and because reversal of such actions is a slow process their duration of effect is prolonged. The outcome of the interaction therefore varies with the points at which the combined drug therapy begins and ceases to overlap.

Interactions with reserpine and with MAO inhibitors are complicated by this situation. The initial action of reserpine is the release of stored catecholamines (norepinephrine, etc.) and serotonin (5-hydroxytryptamine). This release may cause an initial elevation of blood pressure, especially if the drug is given IV. Reserpine then has a prolonged action, i.e., the slow depletion of norepinephrine stored in the postganglionic adrenergic neurons. Full hypotensive effects are achieved only after a depletion period lasting up to 2 weeks. Finally, full recovery from the hypotensive action (regeneration of norepinephrine) is not achieved for as long as a month after the withdrawal of the drug. Accordingly, the exact response to an interaction between reserpine and another drug such as a MAO inhibitor or a vasopressor depends on the timing with respect to reserpine and dosages of the other drug.

If a patient has been on a MAO inhibitor long enough to have his monoamine oxidase sufficiently inhibited, one of the main pathways of metabolism of endogenous pressor amine is inhibited, and NE accumulates in adrenergic nerve endings. If reserpine or another NE releasing adrenergic neuron blocking agent is then added to the regimen, the increased stores of pressor amine (NE) are released and they continue to accumulate. A hypertensive crisis may result. If, however, a MAO inhibitor is given so that its action begins after the norepinephrine is depleted, hypertension cannot be produced by inhibition of metabolism of released endogenous catecholamine. In fact, the hypotensive action of the MAO inhibitor may be additive to the antihypertensive action of reserpine and the resulting potentiation of hypotension may be hazardous.

2. Differences in the mechanism of action of the interactants may alter the outcome of an interaction, even though the primary effects of the interactants are the same. Thus drugs that mainly act directly on receptors often enter into drug interactions that differ from those produced by drugs that mainly act indirectly. Response to an indirectly acting sympathomimetic (amphetamine, cyclopentamine, ephedrine, mephentermine, etc.)* that largely act by releasing norepinephrine (and also α-methylnorepinephrine, the pressor metabolite of methyldopa) is potentiated, during the initial stage of adrenergic neuron blocking therapy, by the catecholamines released. But later when NE stores are depleted, these same sympathomimetics are in-

---

*Sympathomimetics with a prominent direct action on adrenergic receptors possess two hydroxyl groups, either two on the ring at the 3 and 4 position or one hydroxyl at one of these positions and one at the β-position of the ethylamine side chain. Variations in the arrangement of the hydoxyl groups and of the substituents on the side chain modify the intensity of cardiac, central stimulant, metabolic, vasodilator, vasopressor, and other actions.

hibited. However, in some instances an indirectly acting pressor agent such as amphetamine may be antidotal for excessive hypotension with a drug like guanethidine because it, like the tricyclics, prevents neuronal uptake of the drug and it may induce a release of guanethidine. It may exert a direct action also.

If a directly acting vasopressor (epinephrine, isoproterenol, isoxsuprine, levarterenol, levonordefrin, metaraminol, phenylephrine, etc.) is given in the early stages of adrenergic neuron blocking therapy with guanethidine or reserpine it may potentiate the initial hypertension caused by catecholamine release, especially if a MAO inhibitor has increased the stores of catecholamines. If given after depletion occurs it simply antagonizes the hypotensive action of guanethidine or reserpine, but if it is a catecholamine vasopressor a much greater response than that expected may be produced because of the sensitization of the effectors produced by the adrenergic blocking drugs. Also, if the drug levarterenol (Levophed, norepinephrine) is administered, its uptake into sites where it is inactive is prevented, and its action is potentiated several fold.

3. Adverse effects are almost certain to occur when two or more polymechanistic drugs from different pharmacological categories are given concomitantly. It is extremely hazardous to give a MAO inhibitor with a tricyclic antidepressant, for example, although in certain depressed patients the combination has been used successfully.[1049] Even combined therapy with two drugs in the same category demands extreme caution. Such combinations are almost always contraindicated because of the severe hypotension or hypertension that may result, depending on the drugs and the situation. Also shifts from one polymechanistic drug to another requires special precautions. At least a week must elapse before an antidepressant tricyclic like imipramine is substituted for an antidepressant MAO inhibitor, or an adrenergic neuron blocker like guanethidine is substituted for a MAO inhibitor hypotensive.

4. Detrimental properties in one situation may be beneficial in another. The bradycardiac action of reserpine is sometimes utilized to counteract the stimulant action of hydralazine on the heart while the combination promotes mutual hypotensive action. Ched-

dar cheese, containing the NE releasing pressor agent tyramine, and a MAO inhibitor, which prevented metabolism of the tryamine, were successfully used concomitantly to treat severe orthostatic hypotension that was resistant to other therapies because the patient was unable to release stored NE. [1050]

ENVIRONMENTAL FACTORS

The physician must usually consider the environment of his patient carefully, as well as his diet, habits, and occupation before prescribing medications. Essentially, all inhabitants of the world are exposed to numerous potential drug interactants in the air, the fauna and flora used as foods, and in the water, any one of which may lead to altered drug absorption, distribution, metabolism, and excretion, as well as altered activity. On an average, an estimated 3.5 pounds of hundreds of colors, flavors, preservatives, softeners, and other additives are consumed annually per capita.

In the air we breathe are carbon monoxide,* halogenated hydrocarbons, nitrogen oxides, organic phosphates, polycyclic hydrocarbons, sulfur oxides, and many other noxious chemicals. In and on the plants and animals we eat, we may find alkaloids (caffeine, theobromine, theophylline, etc.), antimicrobials (neomycin, phenols, phenotiazines, sulfonamides, tetracyclines, thiazoles, etc.), hormones† (cortisone analogs, etc.), insecticides (chlordane, DDT and other halogenated hydrocarbons; Diazinon, Malathion, parathion, TEPP, and other organic phosphates; naphthalene, etc.), sympathomimetics (Tyramine, etc.), and many other active chemicals.

And although elaborate purification processes are routinely used to provide potable water for most individuals in inhabited areas, errors do occur. Sewage has entered drinking water supplies. Accidental dumping of toxic effluents into sources of drinking water occurs occasionally. In some bodies of water, mercury, microorganisms, plastic intermediates, cancerogenic chloroform from chlorine phosorganic wastes, and other industrial contaminants have reached dangerous levels and created serious health hazards.

No one can predict with any degree of accuracy, how and to what extent most toxic environmental chemicals and other pollutants sensitize patients to drugs or modify the action of drugs in some patients. A major effort is needed to identify, categorize, and explain those types of environmental drug interactions that affect therapeutic efficacy and safety of medications.

Diet Components as Interactants

Essential components of the normal diet—carbohydrates, proteins, lipoids, minerals, oxygen, vitamins, and water may affect drug efficacy and safety when an excess or a deficiency exists. [52] Some common dietary components like caffeine may have additive or synergistic central nervous system effects with medication taken concomitantly. A large dietary intake of sucrose tends to decrease sexual activity and this effect may be accentuated if drugs like aspirin, paracetamol, and phenacetin are also taken. Ingestion of large amounts of sucrose with phenacetin, aspirin, and caffeine compound (PAS) may inhibit growth. Foods containing tyramine or other pressor principles (e.g., beer, Chianti wine, Bovril, strong cheeses like Cheddar and Stilton, pickled herring, or broad bean pods) may be lethal when taken with monoamine oxidase inhibitors like the antihypertensive pargyline hydrochloride (Eutonyl) and antidepressants like isocarboxazid (Marplan), nialamide (Niamid), phenelzine sulfate (Nardil), and tranylcypromine sulfate (Parnate). [25,47,213,265,338,687]

A curious syndrome (pseudoaldosteronism) is caused by excessive ingestion of licorice (glycyrrhiza). Characterized by aldosterone supression, edema, headache, hypertension, muscle weakness, myoglobinuria, paresis and tetany, it may climax in fulminant congestive heart failure. The active principle of licorice is glycyrrhizic acid (glycyrrhetinic acid glycoside), structually and chemically similar to aldosterone and desoxycorticosterone. Apparently, consumption of licorice may unsuspectingly complicate

---

* Poisonings with organic phosphates, carbon monoxide, and other frequently encountered chemicals are constantly being reported. [473,474] Of all poisonings under age 20 reported to the New York City Poison Control Center in one 7 year period 1/3 were due to aspirin (6,190), bleach (2,210), lead (1,367), barbiturates (984), and lye (740). [303]

† Diethylstilbestrol (DES) in animal feeds may lead to vaginal adenocarcinoma in the offspring if contaminated meat is ingested during pregnancy.

treatment in some patients, especially those with pre-existing cardiac compromise. Antihypertensives, thiazide diuretics, and other cardiovascular drugs may require careful monitoring in patients consuming large quantities of licorice. [186,326,667,1088,1089,1090,1993]

Carbohydrates. If animal data are extrapolated to man, either glucose or sucrose administered rapidly on an empty stomach has an oral LD_{50} equivalent to about half a pound of candy in a 10 kg. child. The additive effect of this subtoxicity with that of a drug may produce a fulminating lethal reaction. In rats fed a diet containing 69% sucrose, the time of death with an LD_{50} of benzylpenicillin was shortened from 100 to 3 days. Apparently, diets with a high sugar content lower the body resistance to toxic doses of drugs. [52]

Lipoids. The oral LD_{50} of fresh corn and cottonseed oils in test animals is 250 to 300 ml./kg. when given over a period of 4 to 5 days. Large amounts of oils and fats cause congestion and hemorrhaging of venous capillaries, dehydration, hemolysis, and degenerated changes in some organs. They also interfere with gastrointestinal digestion and alter absorption and distribution patterns of lipoid soluble drugs in the body. When oils and fats turn rancid, their toxic effects may be enhanced in diets deficient in vitamins. A biotin-deficient diet containing 17% of rancid cottonseed and cod liver oils (equivalent to 2 to 5 ounces of rancid oil in a 10 kg. child) was lethal in test animals. Apparently the toxicity was due to the combination of rancid oil and egg-white powder which was used to inactivate the biotin content of the diet. [52]

Proteins. Exceedingly high concentrations of various proteins in the diet can be tolerated by mature individuals, but even milk protein (casein) fed to weanling rats at a diet concentration of 81% was very toxic and increased susceptibility to the toxic effects of DDT and phenacetin. This is of concern to pediatricians and their neonatal patients, particularly when animal experiments indicate that "predigested casein" used in special infant diets, has a much lower oral LD_{50} (25 Gm./kg.). Other animal experiments indicate that soy protein also augments susceptibility to phenacetin toxicity.

Deficiency of dietary proteins may also enhance susceptibility to the toxic effects of drugs, as well as herbicides and pesticides. Thus, phenacetin is more toxic when intake of protein is low, and the pesticide captan is 3,000 times more toxic in animals when dietary protein is eliminated. In addition, growth of the very young is increasingly impaired by such deficiency and diseases such as kwashiorkor are induced. Also the rates of biotransformation of drugs may be lowered because of decreased availability of source material for metabolic enzymes. Because of this lowered capacity to detoxify and eliminate active chemicals from the body, toxicity may be enhanced. The significance of these findings to alcoholics, drug addicts, faddists, and psychopaths is obvious. [52]

Minerals. The oral LD_{50} of potassium and sodium chlorides in laboratory animals is about 3 Gm./kg., equal to only about an ounce for a 10 kg. child. Death is primarily the result of dehydration. The effects of electrolytes, their imbalance, and their ionic effects are discussed in Chapter 8. Probably more people have been killed with sodium chloride than from any disease or drug. Excessive use as an emetic in a child has caused death.

Vitamins. A deficiency of certain vitamins may markedly increase the toxicity of some drugs because of interference with metabolic processes, but definitive studies are lacking in some areas and some studies have been found to be faulty. One series of experiments appeared to indicate that vitamin B deficiency enhanced penicillin toxicity, but then it was discovered that the diets used contained a sugar that caused the problem.

Nevertheless, many of the vitamins influence drug therapy. Vitamin B_{12} prevents the optic neuritis induced by chloramphenicol, [491] and accentuates the hematologic deficiency produced by pyrimethamine. [619] Vitamin B complex increases the prothrombin time and may cause hemorrhage with anticoagulants. [147] Large doses of vitamin C increase the excretion of weak bases like antipyrine, atropine and quinidine, thereby inhibiting them, and decrease the excretion of weak acids like barbiturates, salicylates and sulfonamides, thereby potentiating them. [325,870,962] It also inhibits the oral anticoagulants but the mechanism is obscure. [963] Vitamin K produces the same effect by enhancing the formation of prothrombin and blood-clotting factors. [120,182,330] Pyridoxine decreases the toxic effects of isoniazid. [178,619]

On the other hand, some drugs influence the utilization of some vitamins by the body. Alcohol, colchicine, neomycin and PAS cause malabsorption of vitamin B_{12}. [120,876,880] Antibiotics, when given in large doses or for prolonged periods of time, inhibit the production of vitamin K by the gastrointestinal flora and thereby tend to potentiate anticoagulants by diminishing synthesis of prothrombin and blood-clotting factors VII, IX and X. [182,234,259,433,434,673,898,909,972] Tetracyclines, with their own anticoagulant effect, enhance the action of anticoagulants. Mineral oil and cholestyramine inhibit absorption of the oil-soluble vitamins (A, D, E, K, etc.) and mineral oil may also inhibit the absorption of vitamin C. [28,35,176,486] Cycloserine increases the urinary excretion of vitamin B and PAS inhibits the excretion of vitamin B_{12}. [880]

Water. If extrapolations from laboratory animals are valid, the lethal dose for a 10 kg. child is about 5 liters given intragastrically over a period of 2½ hours. Water intoxication is enhanced by the posteriorpituitary water-retaining hormone and other antidiuretic medications.

The amount of water taken with medication is a significant factor in achieving an optimum degree of efficacy and safety. Too much water dilutes the medciation to such an extent that it interferes with absorption pharmacokinetics. Too little water may interfere with drug distribution and excretion and may cause problems such as crystalluria. An appreciable quantity of water must be administered with certain diuretics, sulfonamides, and other drugs with a low solubility.

Pharmacodynamic Effects. Diet may influence absorption, distribution, biotransformation, and excretion of drugs. [52]

The absorption of drugs across epithelial membranes may be affected by (1) altering the osmotic gradient across the membrane with a high salt or sugar content, (2) inflaming the membrane with spices, oils, and other irritants which increase permeability, (3) sequestering lipid-soluble drugs in dietary oils and fats, and (4) interfering physically with access to the epithelium. Because of these effects on the gastrointestinal lining, timing of drug dosage with respect to food intake may have a very important bearing on drug efficacy.

The distribution of drugs in the body may be altered by a vary large intake of food. This may produce capillary congestion in the brain, heart, kidneys, and lungs as well as local sinusoidal congestion in the liver. These conditions may interfere with both transport mechanisms and access of the drug to metabolizing enzymes in the liver.

The biotransformation of drugs may also be influenced by the diet. Since glucose, predigested casein, and sodium chloride produce varying degrees of hepatic dengeneration when ingested by test animals in lethal doses, these same dietary components when ingested in large amounts by man, may affect the detoxification of drugs. More clinical studies are needed to determine to what extent the extrapolation of animals to man may be valid.

The excretion of drugs from the body via the urinary route may be inhibited if dietary components produce degenerative changes in the kidneys since the rate of urinary excretion varies with the number of functioning glomeruli and tubules.

In general, the toxicity of drugs may be increased by diets that contain (1) high concentrations of certain carbohydates, (2) rancid fats and oils, (3) very high concentrations or inadequate amounts of protein, (4) high concentrations of salt, (5) unsuitable amounts of water, and (6) inadequate amounts of certain vitamins. In addition, excessive quantities of stimulants like tea or coffee and pressor agents like tyramine may be extremely hazardous when taken with some potent medications because of additive, potentiating, or synergistic effects.

Multiplicity of Interactions

Some classes of drugs have such a multiplicity of actions that they enter into a seemingly endless spectrum of interactions with other medications, and environmental components. The phenothiazines, comprised of a large number of related molecular structures, are outstanding in this regard. They possess antihistaminic, antihypertensive, antinauseant, antiparkinsonism, antipruritic, antipsychotic, antipyretic, antishock, antispasmodic, antitussive, local anesthetic, sedative, and tranquilizing properties. In fact, the variations among the phenothiazines are so wide that one of them may be administered to treat Parkinson's disease whereas another one actually induces symptoms of the disease. Because a given phenothiazine may induce combinations of adrenolytic, anticholinergic, ganglionic blocking, CNS depressant and extrapyramidal effects it may potentiate all drugs that induce any one of these effects, and antagonize all that have any one of the opposite effects.

This complex situation clearly illustrates the following: (1) large alterations in therapeutic utility can be achieved by minor molecular manipulations, (2) chemical designations such as "phenothiazines" may not be therapeutically significant or pharmacologically consistent in meaning, (3) each specific drug must be evaluated individually with regard to its own drug actions, reactions, and interactions.

Conclusion

The alarmingly high incidence of iatrogenic problems associated with modern powerful medications provides ample warning that ignorance or apathy cannot be tolerated in chemotherapeutics. The findings of hospital investigating committees and the court dockets underscore this fact. A study of iatrogenic problems in the State of California, completed in 1977 for the California Medical Association, provides a comprehensive analysis of the current situation in that state.

Iatrogenic problems will probably never be completely eradicated. Neither will patient response ever be 100% predictable. Yet, there is no excuse for the present plethora of drug insults to millions of individuals. Concern for the patient is not enough. The physician must also have the necessary education, facilities and information to enable him to avoid adverse drug reactions and interactions. No one should ever prepare or prescribe medications, or administer them without adequate knowledge of their pharmacology.

Hopefully, this volume will not only serve to alert physicians, hospitals, drug manufacturers, pharmacists and all other concerned persons to risks inherent in the preparation, distribution, prescribing and administration of drugs, but will also serve to provide guidance.

Most drugs in some pharmacologic or therapeutic categories (see Table 10-8) have caused the same type of drug interaction. These categories, therefore, appear as Primary Agents and Interactants in the *Table of Drug Interactions,* even though the characteristic drug interaction has not been reported for every member of each category. The entry does, however, alert the physician to the existence of a potential interaction. All drugs in some of the categories are known to cause a given interaction. Thus, all tricyclic antidepressants antagonize the antihypertensive effect of guanethidine (Ismelin).[12] Some of the categories of interactants have been involved in large numbers of extremely hazardous and even fatal drug interactions. Particularly notorious are the coumarin anticoagulants, monoamine oxidase inhibitors, and tricyclic antidepressants. See Table 10-7.

Gaps in information exist but the *Table* does provide the busy prescriber with data that alert him to many pitfalls. Whenever he writes a prescription he can quickly refer to the name of each drug he is prescribing and perhaps locate information he needs to protect his patient from adverse drug reactions. As more information becomes available the table will be revised and updated by automated procedures.

Although the literature has been carefully reviewed and every drug interaction noted has been listed in the *Table of Drug Interactions* given below, obviously no guarantee can be made that every known interaction has been included. On the other hand, the fact that a given drug interaction is not listed under a specific drug does not indicate that it has not occurred or will not occur in the future. The table will be constantly improved as the following deficiencies in our knowledge are removed: (1) Most of the interactions included have not been scientifically verified in both man and laboratory models. Some have been observed and verified only in tissue culture or in animals, and not directly in man. (2) It is unlikely that all the interactions listed will always occur in every patient who receives the agents, but frequencies and probabilities have not been reported. (3) Interactions reported for a given class of drugs have not necessarily been experienced with every member of that class, but with a sufficient number to indicate a hazardous situation. The degree of hazard and clinical significance of each interaction require further evaluation, and all verified interactions should be rated according to the seriousness of the potential hazard. (4) The usual doses of interacting drugs given together may be hazardous, but some adversely interacting drugs may be used concomitantly if their dosages are properly adjusted. The degree of hazard, however, at either the usual or adjusted dosage levels has seldom been accurately determined. (5) Contradictions, misinterpretations, misleading statements, and obvious errors appear frequently in the drug interaction literature. These will only be clarified and questionable data eliminated as more experiences are incorporated into the new and rapidly evolving discipline of hazards of medication.

Table 10-7   Some Potentially Lethal Drug Combinations*

Primary Drug	Interactant
ACTH	Vaccines Antidepressants, tricyclic
Adriamycin[a]	Radiation
Alcohol	Barbiturates Carbamazepine (Tegretol) Carbitral Chloral hydrate CNS depressants (Hypnotics, etc.) Disulfiram and other acetaldehyde dehydrogenase inhibitors Insulin and oral antidiabetics MAO inhibitors plus alcoholic beverages Meprobamate Methotrexate Morphine and narcotic analgesics Muscle relaxants Nitrates and nitrites (nitroglycerin, PETN, etc.)** Quinine, quinidine Sedatives and hypnotics
Aminopyrine	Acetaminophen (long term)
Amitriptyline (Elavil)	Chlordiazepoxide (Librium)
Amphetamines	Cocaine MAO inhibitors Propoxyphene (Darvon) Tyramine-rich foods
Amphotericin B	Other nephrotoxic antibiotics
Analgesics	CNS depressants MAO inhibitors
Anesthetics	Adrenergic neuron blockers Antibiotics (neuromuscular blockers such as aminoglycosides) Antihypertensives Barbiturates Catecholamines CNS depressants Corticosteroids Guanethidine (Ismelin) Kanamycin (Kantrex) MAO inhibitors Mebutamate (Capla) Narcotic analgesics

* Lethal with high dosage or in susceptible patients.
** An outstanding authority has criticized inclusion of these interactions in this table. We repeat, once again, that the purpose throughout *Hazards of Medication* is not to evaluate reports of adverse drug effects critically, but to *alert* physicians and other health professionals to publish serious adverse effects of drugs and to provide prescribers with documentation that will help them to make their own judgments concerning anticipated benefits versus potential risks.[48,120,198,219,398,421,634]

[a] Burdon J., Bell R., Sullivan J., et al.: Adriamycin-induced recall phenomenon 15 years after radiotherapy. *JAMA* 239:931 (Mar. 6) 1978.

Table 10-7 Some Potentially Lethal Drug Combinations *(Continued)*

Primary Drug	Interactant
	Neomycin Oxytocics with vasoconstrictor Propranolol (Inderal) Rauwolfia alkaloids Sedatives and hypnotics Streptomycin
Anorexiants	MAO inhibitors
Antibiotics (neuromuscular blockers) (Bacitracin, clinda- mycin, colistin, gentamicin, gramiciden, kanamycin, inco- mycin, neomycin, polymyxin B, streptomycin, viomycin, etc.)	Anesthetics Antibiotics (neuromuscular blockers) Muscle relaxants Procainamide (Pronestyl) Promethazine (Phenergan) Quinidine
Anticholinesterases	Fluorophosphate insecticides Muscle relaxants (depolarizing)
Anticoagulants (Coumadin, Dicumarol, Panwarfin, Sintrom, etc.)	Analgesics (aspirin, pyrazolones, etc.) Antidiabetics, oral Antineoplastics Carbon tetrachloride Clofibrate (Atromid-S) Dextrothyroxine (Choloxin) Indomethacin (Indocin) Mefenamic acid (Ponstel) Oxyphenbutazone (Tandearil) Phenylbutazone (Butazolidin) Salicylates Thyroid preparations
Anticonvulsants	Methylphenidate (Ritalin) Narcotics
Antidepressants, tricylic (Aventyl, Elavil, Norpramine, Pertofrane, Sinequan, Tofranil, Vivactil)	Alcohol Benzodiazepines Guanethidine (Ismelin) MAO inhibitors Phenytoin (Dilantin) Reserpine Salicylates
Antidiabetics, oral (Diabinese, Dymelor, Orinase, Tolinase)	Anticoagulants (oral) MAO inhibitors Phenylbutazone Salicylates Sulfonamides
Antihistamines	CNS depressants (barbiturates, etc.)
Antihypertensives	Anesthetics MAO inhibitors
Antineoplastics	Attenuated live virus vaccines Radiation (with alkylating agents)
Antipyretics	Narcotic analgesics
Appetite depressants	MAO inhibitors
Barbiturates	CNS depressants
Caffeine (excessive amounts)	MAO inhibitors Propoxyphene (Darvon)
Calcium salts	Digitalis

Table 10-7   Some Potentially Lethal Drug Combinations *(Continued)*

Primary Drug	Interactant
Carbamazepine (Tegretol)	Alcohol MAO inhibitors
Carbon tetrachloride	Barbiturates
Carbital	Alcohol
Catecholamines	Anesthetics Guanethidine (Ismelin)
Cheese (strong, ripe)	MAO inhibitors
Chicken livers	MAO inhibitors
Chloral hydrate	Alcohol
Chloramphenicol (Chloromycetin)	Anticoagulants, oral Antidiabetics, oral
Clofibrate (Atromid-S)	Anticoagulants, oral
CNS depressants	Many hazardous combinations
Cocaine	Sympathomimetics (amphetamines, etc.)
Cold remedies	MAO inhibitors (re sympathomimetics, etc.)
Colistimethate (Coly-Mycin)	Antibiotics (neuromuscular blocking) Muscle relaxants, peripherally acting
Corticosteroids	Anesthetics Sympathomimetics (in asthmatics) Vaccines (live, attenuated)
Curariform drugs	Antibiotics (neuromuscular blocking) Furosemide (Lasix) Quinidine
Cyclopropane	Epinephrine Levarterenol (Levophed)
Dextromethorphan	MAO inhibitors (phenelzine, etc.)
Dextrothyroxine (Choloxin)	Anticoagulants (oral) Epinephrine (coronary insufficiency)
Diazoxide (Hyperstat)	Anticoagulants (oral)
Digitalis	Calcium salts (IV) Diuretics (hypokalemia) Propranolol
Disulfiram (Antabuse)	Alcohol
Diuretics (potent)	Aminoglycosides Muscle relaxants
Dopa	MAO inhibitors
Echothiophate (Phospholine)	Anticholinesterases Succinylcholine
Ephedrine	Ergonovine MAO inhibitors
Epinephrine	Cyclopropane Dextrothyroxine (Choloxin) Fluroxene (Fluoromar) Halothane (Fluothane) Isoproterenol (Isuprel) Levothyroxine Methoxyflurane (Penthrane)

Table 10-7   Some Potentially Lethal Drug Combinations *(Continued)*

Primary Drug	Interactant
	Phenylephrine (Neo-Synephrine)
	Sympathomimetics (status asthmaticus)
	Thyroid preparations
Ethacrynic acid (Edecrin)	Anticoagulants (oral)
	Digitalis
Ether	Neomycin
	Propranolol (Inderal)
Ethyl chloride	Epinephrine
Furosemide (Lasix)	Digitalis
	Muscle relaxants
Guanethidine (Ismelin)	Anesthetics
	Antidepressants, tricyclic
	Catecholamines
	Cough and cold remedies
	MAO inhibitors
Haloperidol	Lithium carbonate
Indomethacin (Indocin)	Anticoagulants (oral)
	Salicylates
Insulin	Alcohol
	Diphamylhydantoin
Isoproterenol (Isuprel)	Epinephrine
	MAO inhibitors
Kanamycin (Kantrex)	Anesthetics
	Antibiotics (neuromuscular blocking)
	Muscle relaxants
	Procainamide
	Quinidine
Levarterenol (Levophed)	Anesthetics (halogenated, cyclopropane, etc.)
	Antidepressants, tricyclic
	Guanethidine (Ismelin)
	MAO inhibitors
	Reserpine (in bronchial asthma)
	Thyroid preparations
Lithium carbonate	Holoperidol
Levodopa	MAO inhibitors
MAO inhibitors (Eutonyl, Furoxone, Marplan, Matulane, Nardil, Niamid, Parnate, etc.)	Amphetamines
	Anesthetics
	Anorexiants
	Antidepressants
	Antidiabetics (oral)
	Caffeine (excessive amounts)
	Carbamazepine (Tegretol)
	Cheese (strong, ripe)
	CNS depressants
	Dextromethorphan
	Dopa
	Dopamine
	Ephedrine
	Guanethidine (Ismelin)
	Insulin
	Isoproterenol (Isuprel)
	Levodopa (Dopar, Larodopa, etc.)
	Livers (beef and chicken)
	MAO inhibitors (combined)

Table 10-7   Some Potentially Lethal Drug Combinations *(Continued)*

Primary Drug	Interactant
	Meperidine (Demerol)
	Metaraminol
	Methotrimeprazine
	Methyldopa (Aldomet)
	Methylphenidate (Ritalin)
	Morphine (narcotics)
	Phenylephrine
	Propranolol (Inderal)
	Reserpine
	Sympathomimetics
	Tyramine-rich foods
Mebutamate	CNS depressants
Mecamylamine	Anesthetics
Meperidine (Demerol)	Anesthetics MAO inhibitors
Metaraminol	MAO inhibitors
Methotrexate	Salicylates Sulfonamides
Methyldopa (Aldomet)	MAO inhibitors
Methylphenidate	Adrenergics MAO inhibitors Phenytoin
Morphine	CNS depressants MAO inhibitors Propranolol (Inderal)
Muscle relaxants, centrally acting	CNS depressants
Muscle relaxants, depolarizing	Anesthetics (fluorine) Antibiotics (neuromuscular blocking) Anticholinesterases Furosemide Quinidine
Narcotic analgesics	CNS depressants
Nitrates and nitrites**	Alcohol
Oxytocics	Vasoconstrictors
Phenytoin (Dilantin)	Analeptics (in overdosage) Disulfiram (Antabuse) Folic acid antagonists (methotrexate, etc.) Methylphenidate Sulfonamides
Quinidine	Antibiotics (neuromuscular blocking) Muscle relaxants
Radiation[a]	Adriamycin

** See footnote on page 388.

Table 10-7   Some Potentially Lethal Drug Combinations *(Continued)*

Primary Drug	Interactant
Reserpine	Anesthetics Antidepressants, tricyclic Digitalis Electroconvulsive therapy MAO inhibitors Stress
Salicylates	Anticoagulants, oral Antidepressants, tricyclic Indomethacin (Indocin) 6-Mercaptopurine (Purinethol) Methotrexate
Sedatives and hypnotics	Alcohol, other CNS depressants Antidepressants
Sulfonamides, long acting	Antidiabetics, oral Folic acid antagonists Methotrexate Phenytoin (Dilantin)
Sympathomimetics	Catecholamines Cocaine Corticosteroids Ergot alkaloids MAO inhibitors Oxytocics
Tetracyclines	Methoxyflurane (Penthrane)
Thyroid preparations	Anticoagulants
Tyramine (foods)	MAO inhibitors
Vaccines	Immunosuppressants (ACTH, antineoplastics, corticosteroids, etc.) X-radiation

Table 10-8   Some Important Categories of Interactants

Acidifying Agents	Antineoplastics	Hyposensitization Therapy
Adrenergic (α, β and Neuronal) Blocking Agents	Antiparkinsonism Drugs Antipyretics	MAO inhibitors Miotic Eyedrops
Adrenocorticosteroids	Antituberculosis Drugs	Muscle Relaxants
Alkalinizing Agents	Antitussives	Narcotic Analgesics
Anabolic Agents	Appetite Depressants	Neuromuscular Blocking Agents
Analgesics	Barbiturates	Oral Contraceptives
Anesthetics, General	Cholinergics	Ototoxic Drugs
Antacids	CNS Depressants	Oxytocics
Antibiotics	CNS Stimulants	Parasympathomimetics
Anticholinergics	Cough and Cold Remedies	Phenothiazines
Anticoagulants	Diuretics	Psychotropic Drugs
Anticonvulsants	Folic Acid Antagonists	Sulfonamides
Antidepressants	Ganglionic Blocking Agents	Sympathomimetics
Antidiabetics	Human Growth Hormones	Tranquilizers
Antihistamines	Hypnotics and Sedatives	Uricosuric Agents
Antihypertensives	Hypoglycemics, Oral	Vaccines
Anti-inflammatory Drugs	Hypotensives	Vasopressors

Table of Drug Interactions

Note—The physician must always give very careful consideration to the advisability of administering two or more medications simultaneously. The following Table of Drug Interactions, arranged in dictionary style, will be helpful as a guide in making his decision. However, in referring to this table, the physician must use his own experience and judgment since this table is compiled from the published literature which does not always agree nor is it always perfectly accurate. Some of the reported interactions occur very rarely. Some may not occur in a particular patient or may be reversed under certain circumstances because of phenotypic and other patient characteristics, the dosage level, order of administration, timing of dosage, and various pharmacokinetic, pharmacodynamic and biopharmaceutic factors. Several interactions may occur simultaneously, some inhibiting, some potentiating. The net effect may be unpredictable. While more definitive information is rapidly becoming available, this table serves mainly as an alerting device. **Interactions that can cause death, teratogenesis, irreversible brain damage, or some other effect with major clinical significance or that can produce a hazardous impact on the therapeutic regimen, are presented in bold face type.**

TABULATION OF DRUG INTERACTIONS

The table beginning on page 397 covers drug interactions puolished since 1955 in the world medical literature for more than 1000 of the most widely prescribed drugs, including the 200 drugs most frequently prescribed in the United States. Interactions have been reported for practically all of the 500 most frequently prescribed drug products which account for well over 80% of all new American prescriptions. Also, it is pertinent that the top 200 drugs which account for 2 out of 3 of these prescriptions, in general appear to exert fewer serious adverse effects than other comparable medications. Physicians apparently tend to prescribe the safest and most efficacious drug products.

The *Table of Drug Interactions* is concisely arranged in three columns under the headings *Primary Agent, Interactant,* and *Possible Interaction.* Under the first heading (Primary Agent) are listed the names of substances for which interactions have been reported. These include both generic and trademarked names of drugs and drug products, the names of foods, food ingredients, natural products, and other chemicals. Under the second heading (Interactant) are listed the drugs or other substances that interact with the primary agents. All interactants are also cross-indexed and listed under Primary Agent. Therefore every interactant may also be a primary agent, depending on the point of view. For every given combination of Primary Agent and Interactant listed, at least one is a drug. Under the third heading (Possible Interaction) are listed the drug interactions which may occur when the specified Primary Agents and Interactants are brought into contact with the human body simultaneously.

Table of Drug Interactions

ACD SOLUTION
See *Sodium Citrate, Neuromuscular Blocking Antibiotics* under *Antibiotics*, and *Glucose.*

ACENOCOUMARIN (Sintrom)
See *Anticoagulants, Oral.*

ACENOCOUMAROL (Sintrom)
See *Anticoagulants, Oral.*

ACETAMINOPHEN
(Datril, Nebs, Paracetamol, Tempra, Tylenol, etc.)
See also *CNS Depressants, Analgesics*, and *Antipyretics.*
Acetaminophen itself is sold under more than 50 brand names and in combinations with other drugs under nearly 200 brand names. Avoid use of acetaminophen with hepatotoxic agents since the drug itself can cause fatal hepatic necrosis. Wide use of the drug as a household analgesic is not without hazard. Prolonged use at high dosage can also induce the microsomal enzymes and thus may antagonize concomitant drugs. [166]

Anticoagulants, oral [147,180,571,572,1161]
(Coumadin, Dicumarol, Panwarfin, Sintrom, etc.)
Anticoagulant response (prothrombinopenic effect) may be slightly enhanced by acetaminophen due to displacement of the anticoagulants from protein binding sites and inhibition of clotting factor synthesis. Acetaminophen, an inducer, may cause hemorrhaging with anticoagulants when it is withdrawn. [1161] Acetaminophen is preferable to aspirin for patients on anticoagulants.

Antihypertensives [166]
Acetaminophen potentiates some antihypertensives (additive CNS depressant effects). See *CNS Depressants.*

Aminopyrine [166]
Serious chronic poisoning and death may occur in individuals who consume medications containing acetaminophen and aminopyrine (or related drugs) over prolonged periods. See *Acetaminophen* under *Aminopyrine.*

N-Acetylcysteine [1987]
N-acetyl-L-cysteine protects against acetaminophen-induced hepatic damage (even when given as long as 4 hours after an overdosage in mice of acetaminophen). But unlike electrophilic scavengers such as cysteamine that interfere with covalent protein binding and thus prevent hepatic cell death due to binding with electrophilic acetaminophen metabolites, acetylcysteine does not act by this mechanism, at least in mice.

Barbiturates
See *Phenobarbital* below.

Cysteamine (mercaptamine)
Cysteamine protects against hepatocellular necrosis after acetaminophen overdosage if given promptly (less than 10 hours after overdosage). Cysteamine affords greater protection than dimercaprol but methionine appears to be a promising substitute.

Dimercaprol
See *Cysteamine* above.

Methionine [1330,1935]
Methionine orally (2.5 Gm. every 4 hr. for 4 doses) effectively counteracts the toxic actions of acetaminophen overdosage, particularly liver damage.

Metoclopramide [1663-4] (Maxolon)
Metoclopramide, by hastening gastric emptying, may facilitate the intestinal absorption of acetaminophen sooner and speed up initiation of analgesia.

Polysorbate 80 [359]
Polysorbate 80 potentiates acetaminophen because its absorption is accelerated in the presence of the polysorbate (surface active agent).

Phenobarbital [166,1985]
Phenobarbital initially may potentiate CNS depressant effects (see *CNS Depressants*). Then, by enzyme induction, may increase the rate of metabolism of acetaminophen into methemoglobin-forming metabolites. The induction decreases the effectiveness of the analgesic, and pretreatment with phenobarbital and other barbiturates greatly potentiates the toxicity of acetaminophen (hepatotoxic metabolites).

Propantheline [1663-4] (Pro-Banthine)
Propantheline, by slowing gastric emptying, may delay the intestinal absorption of acetaminophen and thereby delay its analgesic action.

Sorbitol [359]
Potentiation. Same as for *Polysorbate 80* above.

Vasopressin [172,421] (ADH, Pitressin)
Acetaminophen potentiates vasopressin (in diabetes insipidus).

Warfarin
See *Anticoagulants, Oral* above.

ACETANILID
Chloramphenicol [938] (Chloromycetin)
Chloramphenicol potentiates acetanilid by enzyme inhibition.

ACETAZOLAMIDE (Diamox)
See *Carbonic Anhydrase Inhibitors* and *Diuretics.*
This particular carbonic anhydrase inhibitor may produce some of the same interactions as the sulfonamides since it has a sulfonamide moiety. Acetazolamide and other carbonic anhydrases are potent teratogens. [690]

ACETAZOLAMIDE (Diamox) *(continued)*

Amiloride [690] (Colectril)

The combination of acetazolamide (or other potent carbonic anhydrase inhibitor such as benzolamide, dichlorphenamide [Daranide], ethoxzolamide [Cardrase, Ethamide], or methazolamide [Neptazane]) and very high doses of amiloride (triamterene, etc.) which causes potassium retention, is highly teratogenic (in rats, mice, hamsters). The most sensitive period in hamsters is 204 to 212 hours after mating. Paradoxically, the teratogenic effect of acetazolamide is greatly diminished or abolished when given with triamterene unless the latter is given in amounts that produce hyperkalemia. Do not give acetazolamide in early pregnancy.

Amphetamines [172,719]

Carbonic anhydrase inhibitors like acetazolamide may potentiate weak bases like the amphetamines. See *Alkalinizing Agents* under *Amphetamines*.

Antidepressants, tricyclic [5,78,172,325,330,952]

See *Alkalinizing Agents* under *Antidepressants, Tricyclic*.

Antidiabetics, oral

See *Acetazolamide* under *Antidiabetics, Oral*.

Aspirin [477]

See *Salicylates* below.

Benzolamide [690]

See *Amiloride* above.

Catecholamines [172,325,870]

Acetazolamide potentiates catecholamines and other sympathomimetics (weak bases). For the mechanism see *Alkalinizing Agents* under *Amphetamines*. Some catecholamines may potentiate the anticonvulsant action of acetazolamide. [951]

Dichloroisoproterenol [172] (Dichloroisoprenaline)

Acetazolamide potentiates the β-adrenergic blocker (weak base). For the mechanism see *Alkalinizing Agents* under *Amphetamines*.

Dichlorphenamide [690] (Daranide)

See *Amiloride* above.

Ethoxzolamide [690] (Cardrase, Ethamide)

See *Amiloride* above.

Gallamine [330]

Acetazolamide potentiates gallamine (anticonvulsant plus muscle relaxant). For the mechanism see *Alkalinizing Agents* under *Amphetamines*.

Ganglionic blocking agents [172]

Ganglionic blocking agents and other weak bases are potentiated. See *Alkalinizing Agents* under *Amphetamines* for the mechanism.

Lithium carbonate [120,1851] (Eskalith, Lithane, Lithonate)

Acetazolamide, by decreasing proximal tubular reabsorption of Li^+ and thus increasing lithium excretion, inhibits its action. Adjust dosage as necessary.

MAO inhibitors [950,951]

MAO inhibitors may potentiate the anticonvulsant activity of acetazolamide, by inhibition of metabolism. See *MAO Inhibitors*.

Mecamylamine [137,726] (Inversine)

Acetazolamide potentiates mecamylamine. See *Alkalinizing Agents* under *Amphetamines* for the mechanism.

Methazolamide [690] (Neptazane)

See *Amiloride* above.

Methenamine

See *Acetazolamide* under *Methenamine*.

Procainamide [583,1153,1154,1332]

Acetazolamide, by alkalinizing the urine, tends to decrease procainamide excretion and thus may potentiate its action.

Quinidine

See *Acetazolamide* under *Quinidine*.

Salicylates [172,477]

Carbonic anhydrase inhibitors like acetazolamide may inhibit weak acids like salicylic acid by elevating the urinary pH and thus increasing urinary excretion. The drug should not be used in *late* salicylic poisoning, however, since the carbonic anhydrase inhibitor, which may produce metabolic acidosis, can be detrimental during the late acidosis of salicylate intoxication. The drug in combination with sodium bicarbonate has been recommended for use in the *early* stages of salicylate intoxication (with caution). Acetazolamide also lowers the pH of the ileum and therefore may increase the intestinal absorption of weak acids such as aspirin and salicylates.

Tranylcypromine (Parnate)

See *MAO Inhibitors*.

Triamterene [690,950] (Dyrenium)

Triamterene is a potassium retainer. Same effects as *Amiloride* above.

ACETOHEXAMIDE (Dymelor)

See also *Antidiabetics, Oral*.

Alcohol [120,254,634,674,675,711,740,741]

Alcohol, an enzyme inducer, inhibits acetohexamide. See *Alcohol* under *Antidiabetics, Oral* for other effects.

Allopurinol [421] (Zyloprim)

Acetohexamide increases uricosuria with allopurinol.

Antimicrobial sulfonamides [120,458]

See *Sulfonamides* under *Antidiabetics, Oral*.

MAO inhibitors [86,330,421]

MAO inhibitors potentiate oral antidiabetics like acetohexamide by enzyme inhibition. See *Sulfonylurea Hypoglycemics* under *MAO inhibitors*.

Phenylbutazone [120,121,141,330] (Butazolidin)

Phenylbutazone potentiates acetohexamide. See *Acetohexamide* under *Phenylbutazone*.

Potassium salts [1439]

Potassium enhances acetohexamide efficacy as an antidiabetic, perhaps by facilitating glucose utilization or by increasing insulin secretion.

Probenecid [120] (Benemid)

Probenecid potentiates the hypoglycemic action of acetohexamide by inhibiting urinary excretion of the active metabolite, hydroxyhexamide. Hypoglycemia may result.

Salicylates [141]

Same as given for *Salicylates* under *Antidiabetics, Oral*.

Sulfonamides [120,458]

See *Sulfonamides* under *Antidiabetics, Oral*.

Thiazide diuretics [120] (Anhydron, Diuril, Enduron, Naturetin, Renese, Saluron, etc.)

Thiazide-type diuretics may alter the dosage of acetohexamide required. See *Antidiabetics* under *Thiazide Diuretics*.

ACETOPHENETIDIN

See *Phenacetin*.

ACETYLCHOLINE

Antihistamines [169]

Most antihistamines possess anticholinergic activity and competitively antagonize the action of acetylcholine.

Atropine [57,168]

The antimuscarinic atropine is a highly specific blocking agent (competitive antagonist) for acetylcholine (displacement from parasympathetic receptors).

Decamethonium (Syncurine)
See *Muscle Relaxants* below.

Muscle relaxants [168]
Acetylcholine potentiates depolarizing muscle relaxants like decamethonium. Potentiation may lead to respiratory paralysis.

Nitrites and nitrates [170]
Nitrites, including glyceryl trinitrate (nitroglycerin) and related vasodilator nitro compounds, can act as physiological antagonists to acetylcholine; response may vary from maximal contraction to maximal relaxation of smooth muscle with variations in the relative concentrations of the members of the combination.

Pentaerythritol tetranitrate [170]
(PETN, Peritrate, etc.)
PETN acts as a physiological antagonist to acetylcholine.

Procainamide [120,204] **(Pronestyl)**
Procainamide may antagonize the depolarizing effects of acetylcholine and should be used with caution in patients with muscular weakness.

Quinidine [120]
Same as *Procainamide* above.

Tetraethylammonium chloride [168] **(Etamon)**
Tetraethylammonium displaces acetylcholine from receptors on autonomic ganglion cells (ganglionic blockade).

ACETYLDIGITOXIN (Acylanid)
See also *Digitalis* and *Digitalis Glycosides*.

Digitalis [120]
Acetyldigitoxin should be administered cautiously to patients recently or currently receiving digitalis.

ACETYLSALICYLIC ACID
See *Aspirin*.

ACHLORHYDRIA AGENTS
(Acidulin, Betazole, Hydrion, etc.)

Anticholinergics [168]
Agents used to treat achlorhydria antagonize the inhibitory action of the anticholinergics on gastric HCl secretion.

ACHROMYCIN
See *Tetracycline*.

ACHROSTATIN
See *Nystatin* and *Tetracycline*.

ACIDIC DRUGS

Cholestyramine [120,170] **(Cuemid, Questran, etc.)**
Cholestyramine inhibits intestinal absorption of acidic drugs. See *Acidic Drugs* under *Cholestyramine* for a list of drugs that are sequestered.

ACIDIFYING AGENTS
(Ammonium chloride, ammonium nitrate, ascorbic acid, cranberry juice, lysine HCl, methenamine hippurate, methenamine mandelate, methionine, orange juice, sodium acid phosphate, etc.)
Drugs such as guanethidine, reserpine and others that stimulate the secretion of gastric acid tend to act as acidifying agents in the stomach.
Although acidifying agents tend to inhibit weak bases and potentiate weak acids, only the specific instances appearing in the literature are given below. Compare the list of interactions given below with those given under *Alkalinizing Agents* (opposite effect).
Acidifying agents, by lowering the pH, tend to decrease gas-trointestinal absorption and to increase the urinary excretion of weak bases like meperidine, etc., and thereby *inhibit* their activity. On the other hand, the acidifying agents tend to increase gastrointestinal absorption and to decrease the urinary excretion of weak acids like salicylates and sulfonamides, and thereby *potentiate* their activity. [18,325,870]

Aminoquinolines [325,619,870] **(Antimalarials)**
Acidifiers inhibit aminoquinolines.

Amitriptyline [325,870] **(Elavil)**
Acidifiers inhibit amitriptyline.

Amphetamines [36,312,359,486,870]
Acidifiers inhibit amphetamines.

Anticholinergics [325,870]
Acidifiers inhibit anticholinergics.

Anticoagulants, coumarin [78,325,870,963]
(Coumadin, Dicumarol, Panwarfin, Sintrom, etc.)
Acidifiers in general potentiate coumarin anticoagulants, but ascorbic acid by some other mechanism inhibits agents like warfarin (shortens the prothrombin time).

Antidepressants, tricyclic [28,531,579,870]
Tricyclic antidepressants like imipramine are highly ionized at all physiological pH values and therefore their absorption and excretion are not likely to be altered by changes in pH.

Antidiabetics, oral [421]
Acidifying agents potentiate weak acids like the sulfonylureas by decreasing the rate of their urinary excretion.

Antihistamines [325,870]
Acidifiers inhibit antihistamines.

Antimalarials [325,870]
Acidifiers inhibit antimalarials.

Antimicrobials [578]
(Mandelamine, Furadantin, tetracyclines, etc.)
Methenamine mandelate, nitrofurantoin, tetracyclines and perhaps certain other antimicrobials are more effective in urinary tract infections when the urinary pH is 5.5 or less.

Antipyrine [325,870]
Acidifiers inhibit antipyrine.

Atropine [531]
Acidifiers inhibit atropine.

Barbiturates [325,870]
Acidifiers potentiate barbiturates (weak acids).

Benzodiazepines [325,870] **(Librium, Serax, Valium)**
Acidifiers inhibit benzodiazepines.

Carbamazepine (Tegretol)
See *Antidepressants, Tricyclic* above.

Carbonic anhydrase inhibitors [325,870]
Acidifying agents antagonize carbonic anhydrase inhibitors.

Chlordiazepoxide [325,870] **(Librium)**
Acidifiers inhibit chlordiazepoxide.

Chloroquine [325,870]
Acidifiers inhibit chloroquine.

Clofibrate [325,870] **(Atromid-S)**
Acidifiers potentiate clofibrate.

Clomipramine (Anafranil)
See *Antidepressants, Tricyclic* above.

Colchicine [325,870]
Acidifiers inhibit colchicine.

Desipramine [194,325,870] **(Norpramin, Pertofrane)**
See *Antidepressants, Tricyclic* above.

ACIDIFYING AGENTS *(continued)*

Dibenzazepines [325,870]
See *Antidepressants, Tricyclic* above.

Doxepin (Adapin, Sinequan)
See *Antidepressants, Tricyclic* above.

Ethacrynic Acid [325,870] **(Edecrin)**
Acidifiers potentiate ethacrynic acid.

Imipramine [194,325,870] **(Tofranil)**
Same as for *Antidepressants, Tricyclic* above.

Levarterenol [325,870] **(Levophed)**
Acidifiers inhibit levarterenol.

Levorphanol [325,870] **(Levo-Dromoran)**
Acidifiers inhibit levorphanol.

Mecamylamine [325,870] **(Inversine)**
Acidifiers inhibit mecamylamine.

Mefenamic acid [325,870] **(Ponstel)**
Acidifiers potentiate mefenamic acid.

Mepacrine [325,870]
Acidifiers inhibit mepacrine.

Meperidine [14,28,579] **(Demerol, etc.)**
Acidifiers inhibit meperidine.

Mercurial diuretics [325,870]
Acidifiers potentiate mercurial diuretics.

Methenamine [120]
Acid urinary pH (pH 5.5 or lower) potentiates the antibacterial action of methenamine by increasing the rate of liberation of formaldehyde. Acidic interactants may prematurely decompose the drug.

Methyldopa [325,870]
Acidifiers inhibit methyldopa.

Nalidixic acid [325,870] **(NegGram)**
Acidifiers potentiate systemic effects (toxicity) of nalidixic acid.

Narcotic analgesics [325,870]
Acidifiers inhibit narcotic analgesics.

Nicotine [325,870]
Acidifiers decrease the toxicity of nicotine.

Nitrofurans [325,870]
Acidifiers potentiate nitrofurans.

Norepinephrine [325,870]
Acidifiers inhibit norepinephrine.

Nortriptyline [325,870] **(Aventyl)**
See *Antidepressants, Tricyclic* above.

Pempidine [325,870]
Acidifiers inhibit pempidine.

Pethidine [325,870]
Acidifiers inhibit pethidine (meperidine).

Phenobarbital [579]
Acidifiers potentiate phenobarbital.

Phenylbutazone [28,325,870] **(Butazolidin)**
Acidifiers potentiate phenylbutazone.

Procainamide [583] **(Pronestyl)**
Acidifying agents should theoretically decrease the toxic effects of this weak base. However, alkalinizing agents reverse the toxic effects of procainamide by other mechanisms.

Procaine [325,870] **(Novocain)**
Acidifiers inhibit procaine.

Protriptyline (Vivactil)
See *Antidepressants, Tricyclic* above.

Pyrazolone derivatives [325,870]
Acidifiers potentiate pyrazolone derivatives.

Quinacrine [325,870] **(Atabrine, mepacrine)**
Acidifiers inhibit quinacrine.

Quinine, quinidine [325,581,870]
Acidifiers inhibit quinine (also quinidine).

Salicylic acid [325,870] **(salicylates)**
Acidifiers potentiate salicylic acid.

Sulfonamides [173,325,433]
Acidifying agents decrease urinary excretion of weakly acidic sulfonamides and tend to potentiate them, but decreased solubility as pH of urine is lowered may cause crystalluria and complications in the renal tubules and ureters. Adequate water intake and alkali are essential with the less soluble sulfonamides.

Sulfonylureas [325,870]
Acidifiers potentiate sulfonylureas.

Sympathomimetics [325,870]
Acidifiers inhibit sympathomimetics.

Tetracyclines [578]
Tetracyclines are most active against urinary tract infections at a urinary pH of 5.5 or less.

Theophylline [870]
Acidifiers inhibit theophylline.

Thiazide diuretics [325,421,870]
Acidifiers potentiate thiazide diuretics.

Thyroxine and analogs [421]
Acidifiers potentiate thyroxine and analogs.

Tolazoline (Priscoline) [531]
Acidifiers inhibit tolazoline.

Xanthines [870]
Acidifiers inhibit Xanthines.

ACIDS, FATTY

Pyrazolone derivatives [421]
(Aminopyrine, Anturane, Butazolidin, Tandearil, etc.)
Acidifiers potentiate pyrazolone derivatives by decreasing urinary excretion and increasing gastrointestinal absorption.

ACRISORCIN (Akrinol Cream)

Soap [120]
Soap can considerably reduce the antifungal activity of acrisorcin against *Malassezia furfur* in tinea versicolor.

ACTH
(Adrenocorticotropic hormone, corticotropin, Acthar, Cortigel, Cortrophin, etc.)

Amphotericin B
See *Corticotropin* under *Amphotericin B*.

Anticoagulants, oral [120,147,673,727,903]
ACTH may antagonize oral anticoagulants, possibly by mobilizing or stimulating synthesis of clotting factors, *e.g.*, Factor VII. However, severe hemorrhage has been reported with the combination.

Antidiabetics [120]
ACTH may aggravate diabetes mellitus; higher dosage of antidiabetics may be necessary.

Chlorthalidone [120] **(Hygroton, Regroton)**
ACTH with chlorthalidone and thiazide diuretics causes hypokalemia.

Digitalis [120]
The hypokalemia that may be induced by ACTH may increase the toxicity of digitalis.

Hydrochlorothiazide [120] **(Hydrodiuril)**
Hypokalemia may develop with this combination.

Pyrazinamide
See *ACTH* under *Pyrazinamide.*

Vaccines [120,312,486,619]
ACTH potentiates vaccines. Serious and possibly fatal illness
may develop. See *Immunosupressants* under *Vaccines.*

ACTIDIL
See *Antihistamines* (triprolidine HCl).

ACTIFED— (with or without codeine)
See *Antihistamines* (triprolidine HCl) and *Sympathomimetics*
(pseudoephedrine HCl).

ACTINOMYCIN D (Dactinomycin, Cosmegen)

Antineoplastics [5,120]
The risk of inducing toxic reactions is increased if the antitumor agent actinomycin D is combined with other antineoplastics. Reduce the dosage.

Penicillins
Antinomycin D inhibits penicillin. See *Antibiotics* under *Penicillins.*

Phenobarbital [70,301,709]
Actinomycin D abolishes the induction of microsomal drug
metabolizing enzymes by phenobarbital.

Roentgen radiation [5,101,120]
Enhanced response of the Ridgway osteogenic sarcoma occurs with this combination. Dactinomycin potentiates the effects of X-ray therapy. Severe reactions from this combination
may occur in susceptible patients or when high doses are
used.

ACUTUSS
See *Antihistamines* (chlorpheniramine), *Codeine, Glyceryl
Guaiacolate, Phenylephrine, Phenylpropanolamine.*

ACYLANID
See *Digitalis* and *Digitalis Glycosides* (acetyldigitoxin).

ADIPEX-P
See *Phentermine.*

ADIPHENINE (Trasentine)

Hexobarbital [697] **(Sombucaps, Sombulex)**
Adiphenine potentiates the hypnotic action of hexobarbital.
Lower dosage of hexobarbital is necessary.

ADRENALIN (Adrenaline)
See *Epinephrine* and *Sympathomimetics*

**Antidepressants
(MAO inhibitors and imipramine-like drugs)** [404,423,424]
See *MAO Inhibitors* and *Antidepressants, Tricyclic.*

α-ADRENERGIC BLOCKING AGENTS
See *Phenoxybenzamine, Phentolamine, Tolazoline,* etc.
Some of these agents are useful in hypertension induced by
MAO inhibitors. See also under *Insulin.*

**β-ADRENERGIC BLOCKING AGENTS
(Oxprenolol, propranolol, sotalol, tolamol,
etc.)**
See *Propranolol,* the first β-blocker available in the U.S.
Other β-blockers such as pronetholol and practolol were introduced in Europe but later withdrawn because of tumori-
genicity or other severe adverse effects.

**ADRENERGIC NEURON BLOCKING
AGENTS**
See *Guanethidine, Methyldopa,* and *Reserpine.*
Related drugs are bethanidine and bretylium.

ADRENERGICS
See *Sympathomimetics.*

ADRENOCORTICOSTEROIDS
See *Corticosteroids* and *Hydrocortisone.*

ADRENOCORTICOTROPIC HORMONE
See *ACTH.*

ADRENOSEM SALICYLATE
See *Carbazochrome Salicylate.*

ADRIAMYCIN (Doxorubicin)

Radiation [1967,1980]
Synergistic cardiotoxicity developed in patients who received
the potent radiosensitizer adriamycin (400–475 mg/m² body
surface) plus radiation (400 rads to thoracic spine or 2250
rads whole lung radiation)—severe irreversible congestive
cardiac failure, large pleural effusions, pulmonary edema,
cardiomegaly, splenomegaly, jaundice, etc. A lethal combination.

AEROLONE
See *Sympathomimetics* (cyclopentamine [clopane], isoproterenol HCl).

AEROSPORIN (Polymixin B)
See *Polymyxin B.*

AJMALINE (Rauwolfia alkaloid)

Lidocaine (Xylocaine) [1149]
These drugs have an additive cardiac depressant effect. See
Ajmaline under *Lidocaine.*

AKINETON
See *Antiparkinsonism Drugs* (biperiden HCl).

AKRINOL CREAM
See *Acrisorcin.*

ALADRINE
See *Ephedrine* (ephedrine sulfate) and *Barbiturates* (secobarbital sodium).

ALBAMYCIN
See *Antibiotics* (novobiocin).

ALCOHOL (Ethanol)
See also *CNS Depressants.*
Interactions with alcohol vary from one patient to another,
and with the quantity, timing and duration of consumption.
Acute ingestion inhibits hepatic microsomal drug metabolizing enzymes and decreases the activity of cytochrome P450
reductase. Thus, short term ingestion reduces clearance of
drugs from the blood and total body and enhances the toxicity of drugs, particularly CNS depressants like barbiturates
and meprobamate. This explains the lethal effect. On the other hand, chronic ingestion of alcohol tends to induce the
drug metabolizing enzymes and inhibit drug effects. This explains the tolerance that can develop. Alcohol has enhanced
the rate of clearance from the blood of some drugs (aminopyrine, pentobarbital, meprobamate, tolbutamide, etc.). The in-
ebriated individual reacts differently than the casual drinker
and is more susceptible to the additive or synergistic CNS
effects. In alcoholics the metabolism and toxicity of carbon
tetrachloride is greatly increased. [1966] Two comprehensive
compilations of alcohol interactions have been published. [148,]

ALCOHOL (Ethanol) *(continued)*

[2004] as well as a review,[2032] and a list of 538 oral drug products containing up to 68% alcohol.[2058]

Acetohexamide [254,674,675,711,740,741] **(Dymelor)**
Alcohol, an enzyme inducer, inhibits acetohexamide. The "disulfiram reaction," may follow ingestion of this combination. See *Alcohol* under *Antidiabetics, Oral.*

Adrenergics [537]
See *Alcohol* under *Sympathomimetics.*

Aminopyrine [399]
Aminopyrine increases the toxic effects of alcohol.

Amitriptyline [290,629,729] **(Elavil)**
See *Antidepressants, Tricyclic* below.

Amphetamines
See *CNS Stimulants* below.

Analgesic agents [16,166,619]
Alcohol potentiates narcotic analgesics such as codeine, morphine, propoxyphene, etc., as well as many other types of analgesics. See *CNS Depressants.*

Anesthetics, general [121,166,311,619,634]
In patients with enhanced alcohol tolerance, larger amounts of anesthetic are required but alcohol and anesthetics have additive CNS depressant effects. See *CNS Depressants.*

Antabuse
See *Disulfiram* below.

Anticoagulants, oral [7,120,147,711,1360]
(Coumadin, Dicumarol, Panwarfin, Sintrom)
Alcohol adversely affects the liver and patients with liver disease are sensitive to anticoagulants. Therefore, restrict intake of alcohol. Enzyme induction in alcoholics may decrease prothrombin time by inhibiting the anticoagulant but the response is unpredictable and variable. Avoid this combination.

Antidepressants, tricyclic [71,290,629,729,1566,1638,1639]
(Aventyl, Elavil, Norpramin, Pertofrane, Sinequan, Tofranil, etc.)
A potentially lethal combination. Tricyclic antidepressants potentiate sedation with alcohol, increase gastrointestinal side effects of the tricyclics, and interfere with motor skills. CNS depression and hypothermic coma may occur. The combination, except possibly alcohol with doxepin (Sinequan), adversely affects driving skills during the first few days of therapy. Avoid alcohol with the tricyclic antidepressants.

Antidiabetics, oral [120,121,254,421,633,634,674,675,711,740,741,1360] **(Diabinese, Dymelor, Orinase, etc.)**
Alcohol induces metabolism of oral antidiabetics, thus shortening half-life as much as 50% and inducing hyperglycemia. Antidiabetics (sulfonylureas) block alcohol metabolism and produce a disulfiramlike reaction. Angina pectoris from alcohol intolerance may be produced. See also *Insulin* below. An antihistamine given an hour before a sulfonylurea alleviates the disulfiramlike symptoms[1079]. Excessive amounts of alcohol may produce hypoglycemic convulsions in children.[430]

Antihistamines [121,311,421,634]
Antihistamines potentiate sedation with alcohol; alcohol potentiates the CNS depression caused by antihistamines. See *CNS Depressants.*

Antimalarials [28,121]
See *Quinacrine* and *Quinine* below.

Aspirin [711]
See *Salicylates* below.

Atabrine
See *Quinacrine* below.

Ataractic agents [121]
Alcohol potentiates CNS depressant effects in decreasing order: reserpine, chlorpromazine, propoxyphene, morphine, meprobamate, phenagylcodol, codeine, hydroxyzine.

Atarax
See *Hydroxyzine* below.

Aventyl
See *Antidepressants, Tricyclic* above.

Bactrim
See *Sulfonamides* (sulfamethoxazole) and *Trimethoprim.*

Barbiturates [166,241,244,311,634,730,737,738,1141-3,1566,1580,1633, 1642,1655,1762,1875]
Barbiturates, especially rapidly acting ones, potentiate the sedative effects of alcohol; alcohol potentiates the CNS depression produced by barbiturates. A potentially lethal combination. See *CNS Depressants.* The synergistic CNS depressant action of a rapidly acting barbiturate like secobarbital (Seconal) and alcohol has resulted in many deaths. At least, reaction time is decreased and judgment is impaired while confidence in the judgments made is increased. Apparently in some patients for some unknown reason phenobarbital hastens removal of alcohol from the blood (probably due in part to enzyme induction). Also apparently in acute alcohol intoxication, alcohol inhibits metabolism of barbiturates (at least with pentobarbital) whereas apparently in chronic users of alcohol the reverse is true. This would account for the tolerance to barbiturates that develops in alcoholics. In any event avoid combined use of alcohol and barbiturates.[992]

Benzodiazepines [167,283,330,421,1142,1584,1614]
(Dalmane, Librium, Serax, Valium, etc.)
Benzodiazepines potentiate the sedative, hypotensive and other CNS depressant effects of alcohol and decrease tolerance to alcohol and vice versa. See *CNS Depressants* and *Alcohol* under *Benzodiazepines.*

n-Butyraldoxime
See *Carbon Disulfide* below.

Caffeine
See *CNS Stimulants* below.

Calcium carbimide citrated [121]
Calcium carbimide (cyanamide) has an antialcoholic effect similar to disulfiram in alcoholics. See *Disulfiram* below.

Carbamazepine [48,166,290,629,729] **(Tegretol)**
Carbamazepine, used in the treatment of trigeminal neuralgia and chemically related to the tricyclic antidepressants, may potentiate the sedative effects of the alcohol. The combination with alcohol may be lethal.

Carbon disulfide [354,699]
Workers exposed to carbon disulfide, thiuram derivatives, etc. in the rubber industry and to *n*-butyraldoxime in the printing industry experience disulfiramlike reactions.

Carbon tetrachloride [902,1966]
Alcohol enhances toxicity of carbon tetrachloride; mutual enhancement of CNS depressant, hepatotoxic, and nephrotoxic effects, especially in alcoholics.

Carbrital [120] **(Carbromal)**
Alcohol potentiates Carbrital. May be a lethal combination.

Carbutamide [354] **(Invenol, Nadisan)**
A disulfiramlike reaction occurs when this hypoglycemic inhibits alcohol metabolism past acetaldehyde.

Carisoprodol [120] **(Rela, Soma)**
This combination may cause decreased judgment, alertness, motor coordination, and manual skills. See *CNS Depressants.*

Cartrax [120]
Alcohol may enhance individual sensitivity to the hypotensive effect of PETN in Cartrax with severe responses (nausea, vomiting, collapse, etc.).

Charcoal [1087]
Ingestion of animal charcoal produces a disulfiramlike reaction with alcohol.

Chloral hydrate [28,121,1126,1286,1430,1527,1784]
(Noctec, Somnos)
Chloral hydrate and its derivatives and alcohol all compete for the same enzyme systems and thus mutually inhibit their metabolism; they enter into complex interactions with alcohol. The derivatives, chloral betaine (Beta-Chlor) and triclofos sodium (Triclos), are hydrolyzed in the body to form chloral hydrate and trichloroethanol respectively. Chloral hydrate, taken as such is also reduced to the common product trichloroethanol which has hypnotic properties like those of the parent substance. Some chloral hydrate is also oxidized to another metabolite trichloroacetic acid which potentiates some drugs by displacement from plasma protein binding sites. Alcohol oxidation to acetaldehyde by acetaldehyde dehydrogenase yields a cofactor which accelerates chloral hydrate reduction to trichloroethanol. Alcohol also inhibits trichloroethanol metabolism and excretion as a glucuronide (potentiation of sedative and hypnotic properties). Meanwhile, trichloroethanol inhibits the metabolism of alcohol (competitive inhibition of alcohol dehydrogenase) and thus elevates and prolongs blood alcohol levels. Patients on chloral hydrate who receive alcohol sometimes sustain a disulfiramlike reaction (flushing, nausea, throbbing headache, tachycardia, etc.), although elevated acetaldehyde does not appear to be the cause. The blood levels of both alcohol and trichloroethanol are elevated. Concomitant administration of chloral hydrate and alcohol, both of which are CNS depressants, may synergistically potentiate the sedative effects (impaired motor function). Respiratory arrest and death have occurred with large doses as in the so-called knockout drops (Mickey Finn). Avoid.

Chloramphenicol [28] **(Chloromycetin)**
Chloramphenicol, by enzyme inhibition, produces a disulfiramlike reaction with alcohol.

Chlordiazepoxide [28,167,1142] **(Librium)**
Alcohol potentiates the CNS depressant effects of chlordiazepoxide. See *Alcohol* under *Benzodiazepines.*

Chlormethiazole (Heminevrin)
See *Alcohol* under *Chlormethiazole.*

Chlorpromazine [78,121,311,633,634,731,1139,1140]
Alcohol potentiates the CNS depressant effects of chlorpromazine and vice versa. The combination interferes with coordination and judgment. Chlorpromazine inhibits alcohol metabolism.

Chlorpropamide [120,354,634,675] **(Diabinese)**
See *Antidiabetics, Oral* above.

Chlorprothixene [120,121,731] **(Taractan)**
Alcohol may potentiate the CNS depressant effects of chlorprothixene, an analog of chlorpromazine, and vice versa. See *Chlorpromazine* above and *Phenothiazines* as well as *CNS Depressants.*

CNS depressants [631]
Alcohol combined with a psychotropic drug such as chlorpromazine, diazepam, phenobarbital, thioridazine, trifluoperazine or a tricyclic antidepressant increases the risk of death by impairing psychomotor skills.

CNS stimulants [711,2004,2036]
CNS stimulants like the amphetamines and caffeine antagonize the CNS depressant effects of alcohol, except that they do not improve the decreased motor function induced by alcohol. See *Alcohol* under *Caffeine.* Amphetamines increase the capacity for drinking huge quantities of alcohol without "passing out."

Codeine [121]
Alcohol potentiates codeine. See *CNS Depressants* and *Narcotic Analgesics.*

Compazine
See *Phenothiazines* below.

Coumarin anticoagulants
See *Anticoagulants, Oral* above.

Cyanocobalamin
See *Vitamin B₁₂* below.

Darvon
See *Propoxyphene below.*

Desipramine (Norpramin, Pertofrane)
See *Antidepressants, Tricyclic above.*

Dextropropoxyphene
See *Propoxyphene below.*

Diabinese (Chlorpropamide)
See *Antidiabetics, Oral above*

Diazepam (Valium) [283,1584,1614]
Diazepam may produce supra-additive hypotensive and other CNS depressant effects with alcohol. See *Benzodiazepines above.*

Diazepine derivatives
See *Benzodiazepines above.*

Dibenzazepines [290,629,729] **(Elavil, Tofranil, etc.)**
Dibenzazepines potentiate sedative effects of alcohol. See *Antidepressants, Tricyclic above.*

Dimethindene Maleate (Forhistal Maleate)
See *Antihistamines above.*

Diphenhydramine (Benadryl)
See *Phenothiazines below.*

Disulfiram [120,121,1127,1133] **(Antabuse)**
The disulfiram interaction is potentially lethal. See *Alcohol* under *Disulfiram.* Avoid alcohol.

Diuretics [120]
(Thiazides, Chlorthalidone, Ethacrynic acid, Furosemide, Quinethazone, etc.)
Orthostatic hypotension may occur with these diuretics and it may be potentiated by alcohol. .

Doxepine (Sinequan)
See *Antidepressants, Tricyclic above.*

Dymelor (Acetohexamide)
See *Antidiabetics, Oral above.*

Elavil (Amitriptyline)
See *Antidepressants, Tricyclic above.*

Epinephrine [166]
Alcohol causes increased urinary excretion of epinephrine, norepinephrine, and their metabolites.

Ethacrynic acid [120] **(Edecrin)**
Ethacrynic acid may elevate blood levels of alcohol and potentiate its effects.

Ethchlorvynol [120] **(Placidyl)**
Potentiation of CNS depressant effects. See *CNS Depressants.*

Ethionamide [202] **(Trecator)**
Ethionamide may potentiate the psychotoxic effects of alcohol.

Eutonyl (Pargyline)
See *MAO Inhibitors.*

Fentanyl (Sublimaze)
See under *Morphine below.*

ALCOHOL (Ethanol) *(continued)*

Flagyl
See *Metronidazole* below.

Folic acid
See *Alcohol* under *Folic Acid*.

Folic acid antagonists
See *Methotrexate* below.

Food [166]
Foods (beer, milk, etc.) retard gastric but not intestinal absorption of alcohol.

Fructose [628,873]
Fructose is a very effective compound for increasing the metabolism of ethyl alcohol and lowering blood concentrations.

Furacin (Nitrofurazone)
See *Nitrofurans* below.

Furadantin (Nitrofurantoin)
See *Nitrofurans* below.

Furaltadone (Altafur) [354]
Furaltadone, like furazolidone below, produces a disulfiram-like reaction (neurologic symptoms).

Furazolidone [48,120,202,354,633] **(Furoxone)**
Furazolidone, a MAO inhibitor, produces a disulfiramlike reaction (neurologic symptoms) and hypertension. Avoid alcohol during therapy and for 4 days after.

Ganglionic blocking agents [121]
Alcohol potentiates the antihypertensive effect. Hypotension. See *CNS Depressants.*

Glutethimide [120,1103,1655] **(Doriden)**
This combination may enhance the central nervous system depressant effects. See *CNS Depressants.* Proper supportive care (not dialysis) has prevented death in patients taking as much as 40 Gm of glutethimide with a fifth of whiskey. Apparently glutethimide increases blood alcohol levels even though it is an enzyme inducer (another mechanism must be active). Alcohol, an enzyme inducer, decreases glutethimide blood levels. Preferable not to combine these drugs.

Griseofulvin [1146]
Flushing and tachycardia occurs rarely.

Guanethidine [120,226,421,1622] **(Ismelin)**
Alcohol may aggravate the orthostatic hypotension that is frequently seen with guanethidine therapy. See *CNS Depressants* and also *Alcohol* under *Guanethidine.*

Haloperidol [120] **(Haldol)**
Haloperidol, a butyrophenone major tranquilizer, is potentiated by alcohol and is contraindicated in patients severely depressed by alcohol.

Hexylresorcinol [421]
Alcohol reduces the anthelmintic effect.

Hydralazine [711] **(Apresoline)**
Alcohol potentiates the postural hypotension produced by hydralazine.

Hydrochlorothiazide [120] **(Hydrodiuril)**
See *Diuretics* above.

Hydroxyzine [121,711] **(Atarax, Vistaril)**
The CNS depression with hydroxyzine is potentiated by alcohol. See *CNS Depressants.*

Hypnotics [120]
Toxic interaction; depressed cardiac activity, respiratory failure. See *CNS Depressants.*

Imipramine (Tofranil) [167]
Imipramine prolongs alcohol narcosis. See *Antidepressants, Tricyclic* above.

Insulin [23,121,291,460,1131]
Alcohol decreases glucose tolerance due to impairment of serum glucose disposition (decreased hepatic uptake or decreased peripheral utilization). Insulin response is augmented but the peak serum insulin level is delayed (more likely in prediabetics). Alcohol sometimes tends to produce diabetes (hyperglycemia) but if given to fasting subjects may produce hypoglycemia due to depleted glycogen stores. Alcohol, with its hypoglycemic effect, potentiates antidiabetics (insulin and oral agents). It may induce severe hypoglycemia in diabetics receiving these drugs and may induce irreversible neurological damage, coma and death. It inhibits glyconeogenesis and induces hypoglycemia when this mechanism is required to maintain normal glucose levels. It also inhibits the usual rebound of glucose after hypoglycemia. Small amounts of alcohol have been used in the diet to decrease insulin requirements on the theory that alcohol provides energy without requiring insulin for its metabolism. [291,460]

Iproniazid (Marsilid) [421,874]
See *MAO Inhibitors* below.

Isocarboxazid (Marplan) [874]
See *MAO Inhibitors* below.

Isoniazid [28,121,399] **(Niconyl, Nydrazid, etc.)**
Alcohol inhibits isoniazid; decreases its half-life by increasing its rate of metabolism. See also *MAO Inhibitors* below.

Levarterenol [166] **(Levophed, norepinephrine)**
Alcohol increases the urinary excretion of levarterenol and its metabolites and thus inhibits the drug.

MAO inhibitors [41,120,121,136,404,421,433,874,1593] **(Eutonyl, Marplan, Nardil, Niamid, Niconyl, Nydrazid, Parnate, etc.)**
CNS depressant alcohol may antagonize the antidepressant effect of MAO inhibitors and severe depression may occur with alcohol itself. MAO inhibitors potentiate the hypertensive effect of alcoholic beverages that contain pressor principles (beer, some wines, etc.). See *Tyramine-rich Foods.* Potentially lethal due to hypertensive crisis. MAO inhibitors potentiate the CNS depressant effects of alcohol by inhibiting its metabolism and may cause a disulfiramlike reaction.

Mebutamate [166] **(Capla)**
Mebutamate may enhance the CNS depressant effects of alcohol. See *CNS Depressants.*

Mecamylamine [166] **(Inversine)**
The antihypertensive effect of mecamylamine may be potentiated by alcohol. See *CNS Depressants.*

Meprobamate [121,311,634,732,733,1642,1762,1875] **(Equanil, Miltown)**
Mutual potentiation of CNS depressant effects when meprobamate is combined with alcohol; enhanced impairment of motor activity, coordination and judgment. Can cause drowsiness, lethargy, stupor, ataxia, coma, shock, vasomotor and respiratory collapse and in some instances death with excessive intake. Apparently acute intoxication with alcohol potentiates meprobamate by inhibiting its metabolism whereas chronic use of alcohol, through enzyme induction, inhibits meprobamate by increasing its metabolism. This may explain why alcoholics are able to tolerate higher doses of CNS depressants than nonalcoholics. Avoid use of alcohol with CNS depressants.

Methaqualone [166] **(Quaalude)**
Methaqualone potentiates the effects of alcohol, analgesics, sedatives, and psychotherapeutic drugs. See *CNS Depressants.*

Methotrexate [120,734,1445]
Concomitant use of potentially hepatotoxic drugs like alcohol should be avoided. Respiratory failure and coma have occurred with one cocktail.

Methyldopa[711] **(Aldomet)**
Alcohol potentiates hypotensive effects. Hypotension may be severe. Also increased CNS depression. Better control of hypertension may be achieved in patients who do not drink tyramine-containing beverages like beer and Chianti wine.[368]

Metronidazole (Flagyl)
Metronidazole may produce a disulfiramlike intolerance to alcohol. See *Alcohol* under *Metronidazole*.

Morphine analgesics[121,311,421,634]
Morphine analgesics potentiate sedation with alcohol and they are potentiated by alcohol. Death may occur. However, 60 mg. of morphine in 1 liter of 10% ethanol has been used parenterally as a simple, safe, nonexplosive anesthetic. Fentanyl (0.5-1 mg.) has been substituted for morphine.

Mushrooms[372]
Mushrooms *(Coprinus atramentarius)* cause a disulfiramlike reaction with alcohol.

Muscle relaxants[711]
Additive effects occur with all centrally acting muscle relaxants; may cause increased CNS depression, respiratory arrest and death.

Nalidixic acid[486] **(NegGram)**
This combination may diminish alertness, judgment, motor coordination, and manual skills.

Nalorphine[166] **(Nalline)**
Nalorphine may add to the depressant effects of alcohol.

Narcotic analgesics[121,311,421,634]
Narcotic analgesics prolong the CNS depressive effects of alcohol.

Narcotics[121,311,634]
Narcotics potentiate the CNS effects of alcohol; respiratory arrest may occur.

Nifuroxime (Micofur)[121]
Nifuroxime prevents the oxidation of acetaldehyde, a metabolite of alcohol, thereby producing a disulfiramlike reaction if sufficient of the topical agent is absorbed. See *MAO Inhibitors* above.

Nitrates and nitrites[48,398,634]
Vasodilating effect of nitrates and nitrites is potentiated by alcohol; may result in severe hypotension and cardiovascular collapse.

Nitrazepam (Mogadon)[166]
Nitrazepam potentiates the CNS depressant effects of alcohol. See *CNS Depressants*.

Nitrofurans[28,121]
(Furazolidone, Nitrofurantoin, Nitrofurazone)
Alcohol is potentiated by some nitrofurans (enzyme inhibitors). Contraindicated. See *Furazolidone,* a MAO inhibitor. It prevents the oxidation of acetaldehyde, a metabolite of alcohol, producing a disulfiram (Antabuse)-like reaction.

Nitroglycerin[48,198,398,634,1200]
Severe hypotension when taken with alcohol, due to additive vasodilator effect; may cause cardiovascular collapse. May mistakenly be attributed to coronary insufficiency or occlusion. Avoid alcohol or if an alcoholic preparation is used, monitor closely.

Norepinephrine
See *Levarterenol* above.

Norpramin (Desipramine)
See *Antidepressants, Tricyclic* above.

Opiates
See *Morphine* and *Narcotic Analgesics* above.

Orinase (Tolbutamide)
See *Antidiabetics, Oral* above.

Oxazepam (Serax)[120,166]
See *Benzodiazepines* above and *CNS Depressants*.

Paraldehyde[166]
This combination produces additive CNS depressant effects. See *CNS Depressants* above.

Pargyline (Eutonyl)[711]
Alcohol may induce hypotension (additive effects). Alcoholic beverages containing pressor agents are contraindicated. See *Tyramine-rich Foods* and *MAO Inhibitors*.

Pentaerythritol tetranitrate
See *Alcohol* under *Pentaerythritol Tetranitrate*.

Pentobarbital[737,738]
Dual potentiation of CNS depressant effects occurs with alcohol and barbiturates. See *Barbiturates* above and *CNS Depressants*.

Pentylenetetrazol[166] **(Metrazol, etc.)**
Alcohol suppresses convulsions induced by pentylenetetrazol, but only in amounts that cause general depression of the CNS. This combination is contraindicated.

Phenaglycodol (Ultran)[121,166]
See *CNS Depressants* above.

Phenelzine[41,121,421,874] **(Nardil)**
See *MAO Inhibitors* above.

Phenformin[711,739] **(DBI)**
Alcohol markedly increases the tendency of phenformin to produce lactic acidosis with nausea, vomiting, etc. See *Phenformin*.

Phenobarbital[241,633]
See *Barbiturates* above.

Phenothiazines[78,121,311,633,634,731,1640]
(Chlorpromazine, etc.)
Phenothiazines potentiate the CNS depressant effects of alcohol and vice versa. Impaired psychomotor function (impaired driving and motor skills). Alcohol blocks parkinsonism effects of phenothiazines. See *CNS Depressants*. Some phenothiazines may inhibit the metabolism of alcohol. See *Chlorpromazine* above. Warn patients about the hazards of this combination when driving or operating machinery.

Phenytoin[120,674,1360] **(Dilantin)**
Alcohol inhibits the anticonvulsant action of phenytoin in alcoholics by enhancing its metabolism through enzyme induction.

Procarbazine[120,619] **(Matulane)**
See *MAO Inhibitors* above.

Prochlorperazine[166] **(Compazine)**
See *Phenothiazines* above.

Promazine[166] **(Sparine)**
See *Phenothiazines* above.

Propoxyphene[121,166] **(Darvon)**
See *CNS Depressants*.

Psychotropic drugs[166]
Some psychotropic drugs may inhibit the metabolism of alcohol and thus potentiate its effects. See *CNS Depressants*. The CNS effects may be additive.

Quinacrine[28,121] **(Atabrine, mepacrine)**
Quinacrine, by inhibiting the oxidation of acetaldehyde, a metabolite of alcohol, produces a disulfiramlike reaction.

Quinine[1362]
Quinine and quinidine may produce a synergistic reaction with alcohol. Death has occurred due to a synergism between quinine and alcohol intensified by hyperthermia when a 17-year old girl attempted abortion in a sauna with wine and quinine.

ALCOHOL (Ethanol) *(continued)*

Reserpine and derivatives [121,421]
Reserpine and derivatives potentiate the sedative effects of alcohol; reserpine is potentiated by alcohol. See *CNS Depressants.*

Salicylates [645,711,1222,1257,1327,1570,1656,1912]
(Aspirin, etc.)
Salicylates (aspirin, etc.) given with alcohol increase the probability of gastric hemorrhage. Salicylate buffering reduces the probability of the occurrence of this interaction. Although alcoholic beverages are taken by some patients with little or no ill effects (some bleeding occurs with use of aspirin in most patients), all should be warned of the potential hazard, especially in pre-existing gastrointestinal and other predisposing situations.

Sedatives and hypnotics [166,311,634,711]
(Barbiturates, bromides, chloral hydrate, paraldehyde, etc.)
Serious impairment of coordination may occur. Addiction as well as tolerance may develop. Cross-tolerance develops to sedative effects but not to the respiratory depressant effects. Thus dangerous overdosage can easily occur. Possibly fatal. See *CNS Depressants.*

Sparine
See *Phenothiazines.*

Stelazine
See *Phenothiazines.*

Sulfonamides [121,202]
Sulfonamides may potentiate the psychotoxic effects of alcohol by inhibiting oxidation of acetaldehyde (disulfiramlike reaction).

Sulfonylurea hypoglycemics
See *Antidiabetics, Oral* above.

Temposil
See *Calcium Carbimide Citrated* above.

TETD (Tetraethylthiuram disulfide, Antabuse, disulfiram)
See *Disulfiram* above.

Tetrachloroethylene [711,1387,1752]
(Perchlorethylene)
Tetrachloroethylene can cause symptoms of inebriation (CNS depression). Alcohol may enhance these effects and should not be ingested 24 hours before or after use of tetrachloroethylene.

Tetracyclines [951]
Alcohol may potentiate tetracyclines.

Thiazide diuretics [120]
Alcohol may potentiate the orthostatic hypotension caused by thiazide diuretics.

Thioridazine (Mellaril) [120]
See *CNS Depressants* above.

Thioxanthenes [120]
Administration of thioxanthenes during alcohol withdrawal may lower the convulsive theshold. Caution is necessary.

Thiuram derivatives
See under *Carbon Disulfide* above.

Thorazine (Chlorpromazine)
See *Phenothiazines* above.

Tofranil (Imipramine)
See *Antidepressants, Tricyclic* above.

Tolazamide (Tolinase)
See *Antidiabetics, Oral* above.

Tolazoline (Priscoline) [28,121]
Tolazoline, by preventing the oxidation of acetaldehyde, a metabolite of alcohol, produces a disulfiramlike effect. Avoid this combination if possible.

Tolbutamide (Orinase) [354,634]
See *Alcohol* under *Antidiabetics, Oral.*

Tranquilizers, minor [78,120,619]
Severe hypotension may occur, also deep sedation. See *CNS Depressants.*

Tranylcypromine [421,874] **(Parnate)**
See *MAO Inhibitors* above.

Tricyclic antidepressants
See *Antidepressants, Tricyclic,* above.

Urea derivatives (Bromisovalum, carbromal)
See *Barbiturates* and *CNS Depressants.*

Uricosurics
See *Hyperuricemics* under *Uricosuric Agents.*

Vitamin B$_{12}$ [876]
Alcohol causes malabsorption of vitamin B$_{12}$.

ALCOPHOBIN
See *Disulfiram.*

ALCURONIUM CHLORIDE

Streptomycin [432]
Streptomycin potentiates the muscle relaxant, alcuronium chloride.

ALDACTAZIDE
See *Spironolactone* and *Thiazide Diuretics.*

ALDACTONE
See *Spironolactone.*

ALDOCLOR (Chlorothiazide, Methyldopa)
See *Methyldopa* and *Thiazide Diuretics.*

ALDOMET
See *Antihypertensives* and *Methyldopa.*

ALGIC
See *Antihistamines* and *Ephedrine.*

ALKALINIZING AGENTS
(Sodium bicarbonate, potassium citrate, magnesium hydroxide, calcium carbonate, aluminum and magnesium hydroxide, etc.)
Although alkalinizing agents tend to inhibit weak acids and potentiate weak bases, only the specific instances appearing in the literature are given below. Compare the list of interactions given below with those given under *Acidifying Agents* (opposite effect).
Alkalinizing agents, by raising the pH, tend to decrease gastrointestinal absorption and to increase the urinary excretion of weak acids (carboxylic acids, amides, ureides, etc.) like barbiturates, salicylates and sulfonamides, and thereby *inhibit* their activity. On the other hand, the alkalinizing agents tend to increase gastrointestinal absorption and to decrease the urinary excretion of weak bases (amines, etc.) like antihistamines and narcotic analgesics, and thereby *potentiate* their activity. [325,870]

Allopurinol [120]
Alkalinizing agents should be administered during allopurinol therapy to maintain a neutral or slightly alkaline urine. This avoids urate precipitation and formation of xanthine calculi.

Aminoquinolines [325,619,870] **(Antimalarials)**
Alkalinizers potentiate aminoquinolines.

Amitriptyline (Elavil)
See *Antidepressants, Tricyclic* below.

Amphetamines [36,312,359,486,870]
Alkalinizers potentiate amphetamines.

Antibiotics [619]
See *Antimicrobials* below.

Anticholinergics [325,870]
Alkalinizers potentiate anticholinergics.

Anticoagulants, coumarin [78,325,870]
(Coumadin, Dicumarol, Panwarfin, Sintrom, etc.)
Alkalinizers inhibit these anticoagulants.

Antidepressants, tricyclic [28,531,579]
The antidepressants like imipramine are highly ionized at all physiological pH values and therefore their rates of absorption and urinary excretion are not likely to be significantly altered by change in pH.

Antihistamines [165,325,870]
Alkalinizers potentiate antihistamines.

Antimalarials [325,619,870]
Alkalinizing agents potentiate antimalarials by decreasing urinary excretion.

Antimicrobials [578]
(Chloromycetin, Kantrex, neomycin, streptomycin, etc.)
Alkaline urinary pH enhances the antibacterial activity of chloromycetin, gentamicin, kanamycin, neomycin, streptomycin and perhaps certain other antibiotics when used in urinary tract infections.

Antipyrine [78,870]
Alkalinizers potentiate antipyrines.

Atropine [325,870]
Alkalinizers potentiate atropine.

Barbiturates [325,870,1092]
Alkalinizers inhibit barbiturates, but only a barbiturate with a relatively low pK_a (7.2 for phenobarbital) may be effectively eliminated with alkalinizing agent in barbiturate poisoning.

Chloramphenicol [325,578,870]
Alkalinizers potentiate chloramphenicol.

Chloroquine [78,870]
Alkalinizers potentiate chloroquine.

Colchicine [120,325,870]
Alkalinizers potentiate colchicine.

Erythromycin
The antibacterial activity of erythromycin is enhanced as the urinary pH is elevated. See *Alkalinizers, Urinary* under *Erythromycin*.

Ganglion-blocking agents [325,870]
Alkalinizers potentiate ganglionic blocking agents.

Imipramine (Tofranil) [325,870]
See *Antidepressants, Tricyclic* above.

Kanamycin [120,578] (Kantrex)
Alkalinizers potentiate the urinary antimicrobial activity of kanamycin but neomycin tubular reabsorption is not affected because the antibiotic is not reabsorbed to any appreciable extent.

Levarterenol [325,870]
Alkalinizers potentiate levarterenol.

Levorphanol [325,870]
Alkalinizers potentiate levorphanol.

Lithium carbonate [120]
(Eskalith, Lithane, Lithonate)
Sodium bicarbonate inhibits lithium carbonate action by increasing excretion of lithium.

Mecamylamine (Inversine) [78,870]
Same as for *Antidepressants, Tricyclic* above.

Mepacrine [120,325,870] (Quinacrine)
Alkalinizers potentiate mepacrine.

Meperidine (Demerol, pethidine) [28,78,579,870]
Alkalinizers potentiate meperidine.

Mercurial diuretics [421,870]
Alkalinizing agents antagonize mercurial diuretics.

Methenamine [421]
Alkalinizing agents antagonize the bactericidal action of methenamine. See under *Acidifying Agents*.

Methyldopa [325,870]
Alkalinizers potentiate methyldopa.

Nalidixic acid (NegGram) [78,870]
Increased urinary excretion of weak acids like nalidixic acid with alkalinizers may potentiate urinary antiseptic activity.

Narcotic analgesics [325,870]
Alkalinizers potentiate narcotic analgesics.

Neomycin [578]
Alkalinizers potentiate the urinary antimicrobial activity of neomycin.

Nicotine [325,870]
Alkalinizers decrease urinary excretion of nicotine; potentiate toxicity.

Nitrofurans [78,870]
Alkalinizers inhibit nitrofurans systemically.

Nitrofurantoin [78,325,619,870] (Furadantin)
Alkaline urinary pH inhibits urinary antiseptic activity of nitrofurantoin; more active as an antimicrobial as the pH is lowered.

Pempidine [325,870]
Alkalinizers potentiate pempidine.

Pethidine [325,870]
See *Meperidine* above.

Phenobarbital (phenobarbitone) [325,870]
Alkalinizers inhibit phenobarbital.

Phenylbutazone [28,78,325,870] (Butazolidin)
Alkalinizers inhibit phenylbutazone.

Probenecid (Benemid) [325,870]
Urates tend to crystallize out of an acid urine; alkalinization decreases the possibility of formation of uric acid stones with probenecid.

Procainamide [583]
Alkalinizers reverse toxic effects of procainamide.

Procaine [78,870]
Alkalinizers potentiate procaine.

Pyrazolones [120,325,870]
Akalinizers inhibit pyrazolon derivatives such as oxyphenbutazone, phenylbutazone, and sulfinpyrazone (weak acids) by inhibiting their gastrointestinal absorption and increasing their urinary excretion rates.

Quinacrine [120,325,870] (Atrabrine, mepacrine)
Alkalinizers potentiate quinacrine. Thus sodium bicarbonate, given concomitantly to offset nausea, in large enough doses potentiates the drug.

Quinidine [78,325,581,870,1189-90]
Alkalinizers potentiate quinidine. Toxicity increased. See *Alkalinizing agents* under *Quinidine*.

Quinine [78,325,870,1189-90]
Alkalinizers potentiate quinine. Toxicity increased.

Salicylic acid [78,275,870]
Alkalinizers inhibit salicyclic acid.

ALKALINIZING AGENTS *(continued)*

Streptomycin [120,578]
Alkalinizers potentiate the urinary antibacterial activity of streptomycin. Alkalinization may be necessary only when streptomycin is used to treat urinary tract infections.

Sulfinpyrazone [120,325,870] (Anturane)
Urinary alkalinizers, given concomitantly with sulfinpyrazone to prevent urolithiasis and renal colic, actually decrease the activity of this weak acid.

Sulfonamides [28,78,870]
Alkalinizing agents increase urinary excretion of sulfonamides; may decrease systemic effects, increase urinary antiseptic effects. Also increase solubility and tend to prevent crystalluria.

Sympathomimetics [325,870]
Alkalinizers potentiate all sympathomimetic drugs by enhancing gastrointestinal absorption and decreasing urinary excretion rates.

Tetracyclines [78,198,633]
Antacids inhibit tetracycline absorption. See *Complexing Agents* under *Tetracyclines*. Sodium bicarbonate decreases absorption by 50%.

Theophylline [78,870]
Alkalinizers potentiate theophylline.

Tolazoline (Priscoline) [531]
Same as for *Antidepressants, Tricyclic* above.

Xanthines [870]
Alkalinizers potentiate xanthines.

ALKALOIDS
See *Atropine, Caffeine, Cocaine, Codeine, Ephedrine, Ergotamine, Homatropine, Hyoscine (Scopolamine), Papaverine, Pilocarpine, Physostigmine, Quinine, Quinidine, Reserpine, Theophylline, Tubocurarine, etc.* for specific drug interactions.

ALKA-SELTZER
See *Alkalinizing Agents, Antacids,* and *Salicylates, Buffered.*

ALKERAN
See *Alkylating Agents* (melphalan) and *Antineoplastics.*

ALKYLATING AGENTS
(Alkyl sulfonates such as busulfan [Myleran], ethylenimines such as TEM and thiotepa, nitrogen mustards such as chlorambucil [Leukeran], cyclophosphamide [Cytoxan, Endoxan], mechlorethamine [Mustargen] HCl, melphalan [Alkeran], uracil mustard, etc.)

Other antineoplastics [120,619]
Contraindicated in combination because of the risk of irreversible damage to the bone marrow.

Radiation therapy [120,619]
Radiation therapy with alkylating agents is contraindicated because of the risk of irreversible damage to the bone marrow.

ALLEREST
See *Antihistamines* and *Phenylpropanolamine.*

ALLOPURINOL (Zyloprim)
Allopurinol is an enzyme (xanthine oxidase) inhibitor and thus may potentiate a number of drugs given at or about the same time.

Acetohexamide (Dymelor) [421]
Acetohexamide increases uricosuria with allopurinol.

Alkalinizing agents [120]
Alkalinizing agents should be administered during allopurinol therapy to maintain a neutral or slightly alkaline urine. This avoids urate precipitation and formation of xanthine calculi.

Aminophylline [1931]
Although the xanthine, theophylline is a component of aminophylline and allopurinol is a xanthine oxidase inhibitor, no drug interaction between these drugs has been reported.

Anticoagulants, Oral
See *Allopurinol* under *Anticoagulants, Oral.*

Antidiabetics, Oral
See *Allopurinol* under *Antidiabetics, Oral.*

Antineoplastics
See *Azathioprine* and *6-Mercaptopurine* below.

Antipyrine [82,1879]
Allopurinol inhibits the metabolism of antipyrine and thus prolongs its plasma half-life and increases its toxicity.

Azathioprine [28,421,619,1238] (Imuran)
Allopurinol potentiates the toxicity of azathioprine by inhibiting xanthine oxidase required in the metabolism of 6-mercaptopurine (formed from allopurinol in first metabolic step). Reduce dose of azathioprine to ¼ to ⅓ of the usual dose. Azathioprine enhances allopurinol excretion of uric acid.

Bishydroxycoumarin
See *Allopurinol* under *Anticoagulants, Oral.*

Colchicine [120]
Colchicine or another anti-inflammatory agent may be required in the early stages of allopurinol therapy to counteract gout.

Cyclophosphamide (Cytoxan, Endoxan)
See *Allopurinol* under *Cyclophosphamide.*

Ethacrynic acid [120,421] (Edecrin)
Ethacrynic acid inhibits the uricosuric action of allopurinol.

Iron [120,421,1455]
Allopurinol may increase iron absorption and hepatic iron levels. Iron salts should not be given simultaneously. Allopurinol is not hepatotoxic in presence of adequate hepatic stores of iron. [1455]

6-Mercaptopurine [120,182,421,633,1238] (Purinethol)
Allopurinol inhibits the oxidation of 6-mercaptopurine with xanthine oxidase and thereby potentiates the antineoplastic and toxic effects of 6-mercaptopurine. Thus, reduction to ⅓ or ¼ of the usual dose is necessary.

Penicillins
See *Allopurinol* under *Penicillins.*

Probenecid [421,1391,1855]
Probenecid (Benemid) increases renal excretion of alloxanthine, the active metabolite of allopurinol and this may decrease the effectiveness of the latter antigout drug. Allopurinol inhibits the metabolism of the uricosuric probenecid and thus may enhance the toxicity of the latter drug by increasing plasma levels. This does not appear to be a useful interaction.

Salicylates [120]
Salicylates interfere with tubular clearance and thus decrease urinary excretion of oxypurines (xanthine, uric acid). Uricosuric agents (salicylates, sulfinpyrazone, etc.) may also lower the degree of inhibition of xanthine oxidase by allopurinol and thus enhance oxypurinol (hypoxanthine) excretion.

Sulfinpyrazone [120] (Anturane)
Sulfinpyrazone interferes with tubular clearance and thus decreases urinary excretion of *oxypurines* (xanthine, uric acid, etc.). Renal precipitation of oxypurines may occur with the combined therapy. Uricosuric agents (salicylates, sulfinpyrazone, etc.) may also lower the degree of inhibition of xanthine oxidase by allopurinol and thus enhance *oxypurinol* (hypoxanthine) excretion.

Thiopurines[1238]

See *Azathioprine* and *Mercaptopurine* above.

Thiazide diuretics

See *Allopurinol* under *Thiazide Diuretics.*

Uricosuric agents[120,421]

May result in decrease in urinary excretion of oxypurines (uric acid, etc.). However, the combination may be best for many patients.

Xanthines[421]

Xanthines antagonize antihyperuricemic action of allopurinol.

ALPHA CHYMAR

See *Chymotrypsin.*

ALPHADROL

See *Corticosteroids* (fluprednisolone)

ALPHA-METHYL DOPA

See *Methyldopa.*

Levodopa[724]

α-Methyldopa may defeat the therapeutic purpose of L-dopa in Parkinson's syndrome.

ALPHAPRODINE (Nisentil)

See *Analgesics.*

Anticholinergics[421]

Alphaprodine potentiates side effects of anticholinergics. Hazardous combination in glaucoma.

Chlorpromazine[669] **(Thorazine)**

Chlorpromazine potentiates the narcotic analgesic, alphaprodine. See *CNS Depressants.*

ALSEROXYLON

See *Rauwolfia Alkaloids.*

ALUDROX

See *Antacids.*

ALUDROX SA

See *Antacids, Anticholinergics,* and *Barbiturates.*

ALUMINUM COMPOUNDS (Aluminum hydroxide, etc.)

Quinidine

See *Aluminum Hydroxide* under *Quinidine.*

Tetracyclines[48,198,665] **(Achromycin, Vibramycin, etc.)**

Aluminum hydroxide gels inhibit absorption of tetracyclines. See *Complexing Agents* under *Tetracyclines.*

ALURATE

See *Hypnotics* and *Barbiturates.*

AMANTADINE (Symmetrel)

Anticholinergics[1694,1773]

Amantadine potentiates the side effects of anticholinergics. Confusion and hallucinations may occur. Reduce dosage if necessary.

CNS stimulants and psychopharmacologic agents[120]

Since amantadine may exhibit CNS and psychic side effects, these agents should be used cautiously in combination.

Levodopa[486,1605,1694,1773]

Amantadine enhances the therapeutic effects of levodopa in parkinsonism.

AMBENONIUM (Mytelase)

Atropine[120,619]

Atropine and other parasympatholytics are contraindicated with ambenonium as they may mask the signs of overdosage with the cholinergic (anticholinesterase) agent.

Cholinergics[120]

Other cholinergics should not be given concurrently with ambenonium (additive toxic effects).

Mecamylamine (Inversine)[120,619]

Ambenonium is contraindicated in patients receiving mecamylamine; extreme muscle weakness and sudden inability to swallow may ensue.

AMBENYL EXPECTORANT

See *Acidifying Agents* (ammonium chloride), *Alcohol, Antihistamines* (bromodiphenhydramine and diphenhydramine), and *Guaiacolsulfonates.*

AMBODRYL

See *Antihistamines* (bromodiphenhydramine).

AMCILL

See *Ampicillin.*

AMCILL-S

See *Ampicillin.*

AMESEC

See *Aminophylline, Barbiturates,* and *Ephedrine.*

AMIDOPYRINE

See *Aminopyrine.*

AMIKACIN (Amikin)

See *Aminoglycoside Antibiotics.*

Avoid concurrent or sequential use of topical or systemically neurotoxic (ototoxic) or nephrotoxic antibiotics such as the aminoglycosides, cephaloridine, colistin, polymyxin B, vancomycin, and viomycin. Do not give amikacin concurrently with potent diuretics such as ethacrynic acid, furosemide, mannitol, meralluride sodium, sodium mercaptomerin, etc.

AMILORIDE (Colectril)

Acetazolamide[690] **(Diamox)**

See *Amiloride* under *Acetazolamide.*

AMINO ACIDS

Vinblastine[120,165]

Several amino acids (glutamic acid, tryptophan) reverse antileukemic effects of vinblastine.

p-AMINOBENZOIC ACID (PABA)

_p_-Aminosalicylic acid[178,202] **(PAS)**

PABA decreases PAS activity; goiter and hypothyroidism may ensue because of inhibited iodine accumulation in thyroid.

Aspirin[644]

PABA potentiates aspirin.

Colistin plus sulfafurazole[951]

PABA inhibits bactericidal synergism of colistin plus sulfafurazole.

Folic acid antagonists

See *Methotrexate* below.

Gold therapy[120]

Dermatitis and/or fever associated with gold therapy of arthritis may be aggravated by the PABA.

Methotrexate[120,512]

PABA potentiates methotrexate through displacement from

p-AMINOBENZOIC ACID (PABA) *(continued)*

Methotrexate [120,512]
secondary binding sites. Should be used with caution when given concurrently with methotrexate.

Penicillins [268,269]
PABA potentiates penicillin through displacement from secondary binding sites.

Probenecid [120] (Benemid)
Probenecid elevates the plasma levels of PABA by inhibiting its urinary excretion.

Pyrimethamine [202] (Daraprim)
PABA interferes with the antiplasmodial and antitoxoplasmic effects of the drug which depends on causing a folic acid deficiency for the microorganisms involved.

Salicylates [433,644]
PABA potentiates salicylates. It increases blood levels of salicylates by decreasing urinary excretion through competition for the glycine conjugating enzyme.

Sulfonamides [177,421]
Since sulfonamides are effective antibacterials because they compete with PABA, an increased concentration of the latter will decrease their activity. This holds true also for local anesthetics with a PABA nucleus.

AMINOCAPROIC ACID (Amicar, EACA)

Anticoagulants, oral [901]
Aminocaproic acid antagonizes the anticoagulants because its antifibrinolytic activity decreases prothrombin time. However, large doses IV may induce incoagulability.

Oral Contraceptives
See *Aminocaproic Acid* under *Oral Contraceptives.*

AMINOGLYCOSIDE ANTIBIOTICS
Included in this group of related structures are *Amikacin, Gentamicin, Kanamycin, Neomycin, Paromomycin, Streptomycins,* and *Tobramycin.*
The most serious adverse effects of interactions with these antibiotics include curariformlike neuromuscular blockade, ototoxicity, nephrotoxicity and various hypersensitivity reactions. See under the individual antibiotics such as *Amikacin, Gentamicin,* etc., and see *Aminoglycoside Antibiotics* under *Antibiotics.* Monitor closely renal and 8th nerve function as well as any evidence of neuromuscular blockade in patients receiving these antibiotics.

Calcium salts
See *Kanamycin* under *Calcium Salts.*

Carbenicillin
See *Gentamicin* under *Carbenicillin.*

Cephalosporins
Potentially lethal. See *Gentamicin* under *Cephalosporins.*

Digitalis glycosides
See *Neomycin* under *Digitalis.*

Dimenhydrinate (Dramamine)
See *Aminoglycoside Antibiotics* under *Dimenhydrinate.*

Ethacrynic acid (Edecrin)
See *Aminoglycoside Antibiotics* under *Ethacrynic Acid.*

Methoxyflurane (Penthrane)
See *Aminoglycoside Antibiotics* under *Methoxyflurane.*

Muscle Relaxants
See *Aminoglycoside Antibiotics* under *Muscle Relaxants, Peripherally Acting.*

Penicillin V (Compocillin-V, Ledercillin VK, etc.)
See *Penicillin, Oral* under *Neomycin.*

Vitamin B$_{12}$
See *Neomycin* under *Vitamin B$_{12}$.*

p-AMINOHIPPURIC ACID (PAH)

Ampicillin (Alpen, Omnipen, Penbritin, etc.)
See *Penicillins* below.

Cloxacillin sodium (Tegopen)
See *Penicillins* below.

Dicloxacillin (Dynapen, etc.)
See *Penicillins* below.

Methicillin sodium (Dimocillin-RT, Staphcillin)
See *Penicillins* below.

Nafcillin (Unipen)
See *Penicillins* below.

Oxacillin sodium (Prostaphlin)
See *Penicillins* below.

Penicillins [433] (Ampicillin, Cloxacillin, etc.)
PAH increases penicillin concentration in cerebrospinal fluid and blood (reduces concentration in brain) by inhibiting urinary excretion. Increased potency and toxicity.

Probenecid [43]
Probenecid inhibits excretion of PAH.

6-AMINONICOTINAMIDE
See under *Sulfonamides.*

AMINOPHYLLINE

Lithium carbonate [120,619,1851] (Eskalith, Lithane, Lithonate)
Aminophylline may inhibit the action of lithium carbonate by increasing the urinary excretion of lithium.

Pralidoxime [120,619] (Protopan)
Aminophylline is contraindicated when pralidoxime is used in poisoning with anticholinesterases.

Propranolol (Inderal)
See *Aminophylline* under *Propranolol.*

AMINOPYRINE (Pyramidon)

Acetaminophen [166]
Serious chronic poisoning (fatal agranulocytosis) may occur in individuals who consume medications containing acetaminophen and aminopyrine (or related drugs such as dipyrone) over prolonged periods. Over-the-counter sale of this combination is prohibited.

Alcohol
See *Aminopyrine* under *Alcohol.*

Aminopyrine [555]
Aminopyrine, an enzyme inducer, increases its own metabolic rate. Tolerance thus develops.

p-Aminosalicylic acid [951] (PAS)
PAS (enzyme inhibitor) potentiates aminopyrine.

Androstenedione [555] (Androtex)
Rate of metabolism of the steroid increased by aminopyrine (enzyme induction).

Anticoagulants, oral [673]
Aminopyrine potentiates coumarin anticoagulants (prolongs prothrombin time).

Barbiturates [555,694,695]
Barbiturates increase the rate of metabolism of aminopyrine. Rate of metabolism of barbiturates also increased by aminopyrine. Both drugs are enzyme inducers. Mutual inhibition.

Chloramphenicol [676,938] (Chloromycetin)
Chloramphenicol (enzyme inhibitor) potentiates aminopyrine.

Chlordane [1053]
Chlordane inhibits aminopyrine (enzyme induction).

Chlortetracycline [939] (Aureomycin)
Chlortetracycline potentiates aminopyrine (in rats).

DDT [688]
DDT, an enzyme inducer, inhibits aminopyrine.

Eucalyptol [951]
Eucalyptol given by general route or by aerosol decreases aminopyrine plasma levels in man.

Glutethimide [63,184,694,695] **(Doriden)**
Glutethimide increases the rate of metabolism of aminopyrine, thereby inhibiting its effects.

Fatty acids [421]
Fatty acids potentiate pyrazolones like aminopyrine by decreasing their urinary excretion.

Hexobarbital [555] **(Sombucaps, Sombulex)**
Hexobarbital increases the rate at which aminopyrine is metabolized, and vice versa.

Oxylidine [951] **(3-Quinuclidinol)**
Aminopyrine potentiates oxylidine.

Pentobarbital [555] **(Nembutal)**
Pentobarbital increases the rate at which aminopyrine is metabolized, and vice versa.

Phenobarbital [121,555]
Phenobarbital inhibits aminopyrine by increasing the rate of metabolism of aminopyrine, thus increasing dosage requirements, and vice versa.

Phenylbutazone [16,63,96,133,555,694,701,704] **(Butazolidin)**
Phenylbutazone (enzyme inducer) decreases the effect of aminopyrine. Aminopyrine, also an enzyme inducer, inhibits phenylbutazone.

Propranolol [586] **(Inderal)**
β-adrenergic blocking agents like propranolol inhibit or even abolish the anti-inflammatory action of agents like aminopyrine.

Pyrazolone derivatives [63,555,694]
Pyrazolone derivatives antagonize the effect of aminopyrine and vice versa. See *Phenylbutazone* above.

Testosterone [555]
Aminopyrine increases rate of metabolism of testosterone, thus decreasing the effects of the steroid.

Zoxazolamine [555] **(Flexin)**
Aminopyrine (enzyme inducer) inhibits zoxazolamine. No longer marketed in U.S.

8-AMINOQUINOLINES
See *Primaquine.*

p-AMINOSALICYLIC ACID (PAS)

Acidifying agents
See *Ammonium Chloride* and *Ascorbic Acid* below.

p-Aminobenzoic acid [178,202,1625] **(PABA)**
PABA decreases PAS antimicrobial activity. With prolonged use of compensating high doses, goiter and hypothyroidism may ensue because iodine accumulation in thyroid is inhibited. Avoid concomitant use.

Ammonium chloride [178,1625]
Ammonium chloride, given in doses large enough to acidify the urine, increases the probability of crystalluria with PAS. Use of the sodium salt decreases the probability, and is preferred when NH_4Cl is given.

Aminopyrine [951]
PAS potentiates aminopyrine.

Anticholinergics
Similar interaction as that with *Diphenhydramine* below.

Anticoagulants, oral [193,673,890]
PAS (microsomal enzyme inhibitor) potentiates oral anticoagulants by suppressing prothrombin formation in the liver.

Anticonvulsants, general [951]
PAS decreases the metabolism of anticonvulsants, thereby potentiating them.

Antihistamines
See *Diphenhydramine* below.

Antipyretics [198]
Antipyretics potentiate PAS.

Ascorbic acid [178,1625] **(Vitamin C)**
Same interaction as that given for *Ammonium Chloride* above.

Aspirin [78,202,421]
Aspirin enhances PAS toxicity.

Barbiturates [633]
Same as for *Hexobarbital* below.

Diphenhydramine [1567] **(Benadryl)**
Diphenhydramine, by affecting the motility of the gastrointestinal tract (impairs absorption), or possibly by enzyme induction, inhibits PAS (lowers blood levels). Other drugs with anticholinergic activity should be monitored also.

Hexobarbital [330] **(Sombucaps, Sombulex)**
PAS potentiates hexobarbital, possibly by enzyme inhibition.

Isoniazid [178,202] **(Niconyl, Nydrazid, etc.)**
Combined use of PAS and isoniazid may give rise to an untoward drug interaction causing acute, hemolytic anemia unless the dosage is properly adjusted. PAS action against the tubercle bacillus is potentiated by isoniazid. PAS increases and prolongs the blood levels of isoniazid through competitive acetylation or by competing for the same excretion pathway.

Phenytoin sodium [192,202,294,916,919] **(Dilantin, etc.)**
PAS (microsomal enzyme inhibitor) potentiates phenytoin by inhibiting its parahydroxylation. Toxic reactions may occur. See also under *Antituberculosis Drugs.*

Probenecid [120,1248,1277] **(Benemid)**
Probenecid potentiates PAS by decreasing urinary excretion and increasing plasma levels. Normal doses may be toxic and should be reduced with probenecid.

Pyrazinamide [1311,1787] **(Aldinamide, Zinamide)**
PAS may inhibit the hyperuricemia produced by pyrazinamide, but not markedly.

Rifampin [1249,1306,1350] **(Rifadin, Rimactane)**
PAS powder significantly reduces gastrointestinal absorption of rifampin, perhaps because of the bentonite present in the PAS dosage form (granules). Use other PAS dosage forms or give as far apart timewise as possible (8-12 hours).

Salicylates [78,166,178,202,421,633]
See *p-Aminosalicylic Acid* under *Salicylates.*

Streptomycin [178]
PAS action against the tubercle bacillus is potentiated.

Sulfonamides [421]
PAS may antagonize antibacterial action of sulfonamides.

Vitamin B$_{12}$ [202,880,1469,1481,1572,1692] **(Cyanocobalamin)**
PAS inhibits intestinal absorption of vitamin B_{12} and thus may inhibit B_{12} action when given orally. It also inhibits the urinary excretion of the vitamin and thus potentiates any that is absorbed or injected.

AMISOMETRADINE (Rolicton)

Penicillin [121]
Penicillin diminishes the diuretic effect of amisometradine by interfering with the carrier transport mechanism which facilitates its passage into cells.

AMISOMETRADINE (Rolicton) *(continued)*

Probenecid [950]
Probenecid diminishes amisometradine diuretic activity; mechanism is interference with the carrier transport mechanism which facilitates passage of amisometradine into cells.

AMITRIPTYLINE (Elavil)
See *Antidepressants, Tricyclic.*

AMMONIUM CHLORIDE
See *Acidifying Agents.*

Aminosalicylic Acid
See *Ammonium Chloride* under *p-Aminosalicylic Acid.*

Salicylates
See *Acidifiers, Urinary* under *Salicylates.*

Spironolactone (Aldactone)
See *Ammonium Chloride* under *Spironolactone.*

Sulfonamides [173,174,433]
Crystalluria and the complications thereof may result from a lowering of urinary pH. See under *Acidifying Agents.*

Thiazide diuretics [120]
(Anhydron, Diuril, Enduron, Naturetin, Renese, Saluron, etc.)
Ammonium chloride should not be used to correct hypochloremic alkalosis (caused by the diuretic) in patients with hepatic insufficiency.

AMMONIUM NITRATE
See *Acidifying Agents.*

Sulfonamides [173,174,433]
Crystalluria and the complications thereof, resulting from a lowering of urinary pH. The nitrate is a urinary acidifier; sulfonamides show a decreased solubility as the urinary pH drops. Ammonium nitrate is usually used in veterinary practice.

AMNESTROGEN
See *Estrogens* (conjugated estrogens).

AMOBARBITAL (Amytal)
See *Barbiturates.*

AMPHAPLEX
See *Amphetamines.*

AMPHETAMINE, RACEMIC
See *Amphetamines.*

AMPHETAMINES
(*d*-Amphetamine, *dl*-Amphetamine, racemic amphetamine, [Benzedrine, Biphetamine, Delcobese, Dexedrine, Obetrol, Obotan], benzphetamine [Didrex], methamphetamine [Desoxyn, Fetamin])

Acetazolamide [325,1215,1758]
See *Alkalinizing Agents* below.

Acidifying agents [36,78,312,325,359,486,870]
Gastrointestinal acidifying agents (guanethidine, reserpine, glutamic acid HCL, ascorbic acid, fruit juices, etc.) decrease intestinal absorption of amphetamines, and urinary acidifying agents (ammonium chloride, sodium acid phosphate, etc.) by lowering the pH and shifting the amphetamines towards the ionized form, decrease absorption through the villi and tubular reabsorption, increase urinary excretion, lower the blood levels and thus tend to decrease the effectiveness of the amphetamines.

Adrenergic blockers [168]
Amphetamine inhibits adrenergic blockers.

Alcohol [711]
CNS stimulants like amphetamines antagonize the CNS depressant effects of alcohol, except that they do not improve the decreased motor function induced by alcohol. See *CNS Stimulants* under *Alcohol.*

Alkalinizing agents [325,870,1215,1758]
Gastrointestinal alkalinizing agents (sodium bicarbonate, etc.) increase intestinal absorption of amphetamines, and urinary alkalinizers (such as acetazolamide and some thiazides) decrease the urinary excretion of amphetamines by raising the pH and shifting them toward the nonionized form which is reabsorbed by the tubules. Blood levels are elevated, and metabolism and elimination are shifted more to the liver. The alkalinizers thereby potentiate the amphetamines.

Ammonium chloride.
See *Acidifying Agents* above.

Antidepressants, tricyclic [404,423,424,1027,1724,1923]
Enhanced activity of the tricyclic or sympathomimetic agent may result. The combination of *d*-amphetamine and desipramine or protriptyline and possibly other tricyclics causes striking and sustained increase in the concentration of *d*-amphetamine in the brain; potentiation of the augmentation in rate produced by amphetamines in operant conditioning situations. Cardiovascular effects can be potentiated if *d*-amphetamine, which is apparently an enzyme inhibitor in some patients, is combined with desipramine imipramine, or protriptyline and possibly other tricyclics.

Antihistamines [169]
Amphetamines may be combined with antihistamines to counteract the sedative effects.

Antihypertensives [550,591-596]
Amphetamines and related anorexiants antagonize antihypertensives. However, see discussion of *Amphetamines* under *Antihypertensives.*

Barbiturates
See *Phenobarbital* below.

Cocaine [421]
Cocaine potentiates both CNS and sympathetic stimulation by amphetamines. Vasomotor collapse and respiratory arrest. Lethal.

Bethanidine [117] **(Esbatal)**
Amphetamines antagonize the hypotensive action of bethanidine. The latter, a catecholamine depleter, reduces pressor response to indirectly acting pressor amines like methamphetamine.

Chlorpromazine [1097] **(Thorazine)**
Chlorpromazine is an effective antagonist in poisoning due to amphetamine.

Desipramine [404,423,424] **(Pertofrane)**
Desipramine inhibits the metabolism (hydroxylation) of amphetamine thereby increasing the level of circulating amphetamine and eventually of brain amphetamine.

Ethosuximide [359] **(Zarontin)**
Amphetamines may delay intestinal absorption of ethosuximide.

Furazolidone [633] **(Furoxone)**
Furazolidone potentiates amphetamines. See *MAO Inhibitors* below.

Glucose [1586]
Amphetamines produce no significant change in human blood glucose but they do in laboratory animals. A good example of nonextrapolation of laboratory findings in animals to man.

Guanethidine sulfate [198,327,421,550] **(Ismelin)**
Amphetamine inhibits the hypotensive effects of guanethidine. Hypertension may occur. For full explanation see *Sympathomimetics* under *Reserpine* and *Polymechanistic Drugs* (pages 378-379).

Haloperidol [166,922,1359] (Haldol)
Haloperidol, by inhibiting adrenergic neuronal uptake of amphetamines, inhibits their stimulatory effects.

Hydralazine [421] (Apresoline)
Amphetamines antagonize the antihypertensive action of hydralazine.

Imipramine (Tofranil)
See *Antidepressant, Tricyclic* above.

Lithium carbonate [1426]
(Eskalith, Lithane, Lithonate, etc.)
Lithium carbonate may inhibit the antiobesity and stimulatory effects of amphetamines. The mechanism is not clear.

MAO inhibitors [60,289,355,356,633,745-747,1932]
(Marplan, Niamid, Nardil, etc.)
MAOI antidepressants, as well as a metabolite of the antimicrobial furazolidone (Furoxone), potentiate amphetamines by slowing rate of metabolism, thus increasing their effect on release of norepinephrine from adrenergic nerve endings, and thereby cause headache, subarachnoid hemorrhage, and other signs of a hypertensive crisis. A variety of neurological toxic effects and malignant hyperpyrexia occur. Death may result. See *Amphetamines* under *MAO Inhibitors*.

Marijuana
See *Dextroamphetamine* under *Marijuana*.

Mebanazine [745]
See *MAO Inhibitors* above.

Mecamylamine [169,619,633] (Inversine)
Drugs like methamphetamine, a β-receptor stimulant, tend to antagonize the hypotensive effect of ganglionic blocking agents like mecamylamine. However, the prominent central effects of mecamylamine and the amphetamine (tremors, mental confusion, seizures, mania, and depression) may be additive.

Meperidine (Demerol) [951]
Amphetamine potentiates the analgesic effect of meperidine.

Methenamine therapy [36,120,312,325,329,870]
The urinary excretion of amphetamines is increased by acidifying agents used in methenamine therapy. Amphetamine is thus inhibited.

Methyldopa [421] (Aldomet)
Amphetamines inhibit the hypotensive effect of methyldopa.

Morphine [1441]
See *Dextroamphetamine* under *Morphine*.

Norepinephrine [633]
Enhanced adrenergic effect.

Pargyline HCl (Eutonyl) [633]
See *MAO Inhibitors* above.

Pentolinium [421] (Ansolysen)
Amphetamines inhibit the hypotensive action of pentolinium.

Phenelzine (Nardil) [289]
See *MAO Inhibitors* above.

Phenobarbital [38,359] (Phenobarbitone)
Amphetamines delay intestinal absorption of phenobarbital, followed by synergistic anticonvulsant action. In drug abusers on amphetamines taken in large intravenous doses, barbiturates may increase aggressiveness and violent behavior.

Phenothiazines [1097]
Phenothiazines like chlorpromazine antagonize the CNS stimulant action of amphetamines.

Phenytoin [359] (Dilantin, etc.)
Amphetamines delay intestinal absorption of phenytoin, followed by synergistic anticonvulsant action.

Propoxyphene [120,421] (Darvon)
In propoxyphene overdosage, amphetamine CNS stimulation is potentiated; fatal convulsions may be produced.

Reserpine [600,601,633]
Pressor response to reserpine is antagonized after treatment with amphetamine. The sedative and hypotensive effects of reserpine are inhibited.

Sodium bicarbonate [1215]
See *Alkalinizing Agents* above.

Tyramine [529,533,534]
Hypertensive crisis. See *Tyramine-rich Foods*.

Tranylcypromine [60,120,745] (Parnate)
See *MAO Inhibitors* above. Lethal.

Urinary acidifiers
See *Acidifying Agents* above.

Urinary alkalinizers [325,870]
The magnitude and duration of the effect of amphetamine is significantly greater when the urine is alkaline.

Veratrum alkaloids [421]
Amphetamines inhibit the hypotensive action of veratrum alkaloids.

AMPHICOL
See *Chloramphenicol*.

AMPHOJEL
See *Antacids* and *Aluminum Compounds*.

AMPHOTERICIN B (Fungizone)
See also *Antibiotics*.

Antibiotics, nephrotoxic; Antineoplastics; Corticosteroids; Corticotropin; Mechlorethamine (Mustargen) [120,1290,1453]
Deep fungal infections sometimes emerge in patients being treated with these agents; they should not be given concurrently with amphotericin B unless absolutely necessary to control reactions to the antifungal antibiotic or to treat underlying disease. Such combinations given concurrently can cause blood dyscrasias.

Digitalis and related cardiac glycosides [28,619,1314,1637]
Amphotericin B often causes severe hypokalemia, thus resulting in digitalis toxicity; the cause of the hypokalemia seems to be a reversible potassium-losing nephritis. Monitor patients closely for subnormal potassium levels.

Muscle relaxants [28,120,1314,1448,1637]
Amphotericin often causes a decrease in serum potassium. The hypokalemia has been reported to cause muscular weakness, and, potentially, may increase both the potency and toxicity of skeletal muscle relaxants.

AMPICILLIN
(Alpen, Amcill, Omnipen, Penbritin, Polycillin, Principen, Totacillin, etc.)

Aminohippuric acid [433] (PAH)
PAH elevates serum levels of ampicillin and increases toxicity of the antibiotic.

Carbenicillin [421] (Geopen)
Carbenicillin is inhibited by ampicillin.

Cephalosporins [120,233,1129]
Synergistic antibacterial effect usually, yet cephaloridine, cloxacillin and 6-aminopenicillanic acid antagonize the antimicrobial action of ampicillin against strains of *Escherichia*, *Proteus* and *Pseudomonas*, possibly through receptor site blockage.

AMPICILLIN *(continued)*

Chloramphenicol[748] (Chloromycetin)
Chloramphenicol antagonizes the bactericidal action of this penicillin.

Cloxacillin sodium[382,1129] (Tegopen)
Synergistic antibacterial effect in bacteriuria, yet see under *Cephalosporins* above.

Erythromycin[31,70,301] (Erythrocin, Ilotycin)
Erythromycin antagonizes the bactericidal action of this penicillin against most organisms. Resistant *Staph. aureus* is an exception.

Methicillin[382] (Dimocillin-RT, Staphcillin)
Synergistic antibacterial effect.

Nafcillin (Unipen)[382]
Synergistic antibacterial effect.

Oxacillin sodium[382] (Prostaphlin)
Synergistic antibacterial effect.

Streptomycin[210,492]
Streptomycin potentiates bactericidal activity of ampicillin against enterococci and the combination is therefore useful in diseases such as bacteremia, brain abscess, endocarditis, meningitis and urinary tract infection caused by enterococcus.

Sulfaethylthiadiazole[267-269]
Sulfaethidole lowers the serum concentration of total penicillin but may increase the concentration of unbound, antimicrobially active drug in the serum and body fluids. Relatively large doses of the sulfonamide can reduce the protein binding of this penicillin and thus potentiate it. Sulfonamides in general, may inhibit the antibacterial effect of penicillins.

Sulfamethoxypyridazine (Midicel)
See *Sulfaethylthiadiazole* above. Same interaction for this long-acting sulfonamide.

Tetracyclines[285,301,633,666]
Tetracyclines antagonize the bactericidal actions of this penicillin. See *Antibiotics* under *Penicillins*.

AMYTAL
See *Barbiturates*.

ANABOLIC AGENTS
(Dromostanolone [Drolban], ethylestrenol [Maxibolin], methandriol [Stenediol, etc.], methandrostenolone [Dianabol], nandrolone esters [Deca-Durabolin, Durabolin], norethandrolone [Nilevar], oxandrolone [Anavar], oxymethalone [Adroyd, Anadrol], stanolone [Anabolex, Androlone, Neodrol], stanozolol [Winstrol], testolactone [Teslac], etc.)
See also *Androgens*.
Androgens may be potent anabolic agents (e.g., testosterone) and steroids with these properties vary in their relative potency as anabolic and androgenic agents.

Anticoagulants, oral[9,119,120,198,234,393,394,673,861,907,908,1320,1389,1588,1658,1675,1747]
Anabolic agents like the anabolic steroids methandrostenolone (Dianabol) and norethandrolone (Nilevar), and oxymetholone (Anadrol) potentiate oral coumarin and indandione anticoagulants by inhibiting their metabolism or perhaps by increasing the degradation of clotting factors or decreasing formation of these factors, or increasing the affinity between receptor sites and the anticoagulants. Risk of hemorrhage. Reduce dosage as necessary; monitor closely.

Antidiabetics, oral[120,191,383,1550,1565,1822]
Anabolic steroids may enhance hypoglycemic effect (additive effect). Methandrostenolone (Dianabol) increases plasma insulin response to tolbutamide 3-fold (fall in fasting sugar) but not nandrolone (Durabolin) and methenolone (Primobolan). Reduce the dosage of oral antidiabetics as necessary. Monitor closely.

Clofibrate[383] (Atromid-S)
In some patients with some types of hyperlipidemia some anabolic steroids may tend to increase cholesterol levels and thus antagonize clofibrate and other hypocholesterolemics.

Insulin[120,191,383]
Anabolic steroids enhance hypoglycemic effect (additive effect). Reduce the dosage of insulin.

Oxyphenbutazone[257,448,1029,1502] (Tandearil)
Methandrostenolone (Dianabol) potentiates oxyphenbutazone, the active metabolite of phenylbutazone (Butazolidin), but apparently not the parent compound, by inhibiting glucuronyl transferase and considerably elevates blood levels of the anti-inflammatory agent. Exercise caution and monitor for possible toxic effects.

Phenobarbital
See *Phenobarbital* under *Androgens*.

ANALEPTICS
(Amphetamine, Caffeine and Sodium Benzoate)

Antihistamines[169]
Analeptics are not recommended in antihistamine intoxication as they tend to initiate or potentiate convulsions.

Propoxyphene[120,968] (Darvon)
Analeptics like caffeine and amphetamines should not be used to treat propoxyphene overdosage since fatal convulsions may be produced.

Narcotics[120,968]
Same as for *Propoxyphene* above.

ANALGESICS
(Acetaminophen, aspirin, codeine, morphine, meperidine, etc.)
See also *CNS Depressants* and *Narcotic Analgesics*.

Alcohol[16,166,619]
Analgesics may be potentiated by alcohol. See *CNS Depressants* and *Alcohol* under *Analgesic and Ataractic Agents*.

Analgesics (Narcotics, Salicylates)[166]
Additive effects. See *CNS Depressants*.

Anesthetics[120,619]
General anesthetics potentiate analgesics and vice versa. See *CNS Depressants*.

Anticoagulants, oral[147,150,393,448,571,572,861,896]
Some analgesics (acetaminophen, aspirin, indomethacin, oxyphenbutazone, phenylbutazone) potentiate oral anticoagulants by displacing them from protein binding sites. Prolonged use of narcotic analgesics may enhance the anticoagulant effect. Phenyramidol, by enzyme inhibition, may potentiate the anticoagulants.

Barbiturates[78,147]
Barbiturates, by enzyme induction, may inhibit the action of analgesics but reduced dosage may be necessary in the initial stages of therapy because of additive CNS depressant effects, including respiratory depression, particularly with narcotic analgesics. See *CNS Depressants*.

p-Chlorophenylalanine[421]
p-Chlorophenylalanine reverses analgesic activity.

Chloroquine[120]
Analgesics such as phenylbutazone may cause drug sensitization and should not be given with drugs like chloroquine which cause hypersensitivity reactions.

Chlorprothixene HCl [166] **(Taractan)**
Chlorprothixene potentiates the CNS depressant effects of analgesics.

CNS depressants [120,166,619]
Additive effects are produced with a wide range of CNS depressants, including antihistamines, barbiturates, meprobamate, etc. See *CNS Depressants.*

Cyproheptadine HCl [421] **(Periactin)**
Analgesic activity is reversed by cyproheptadine.

Haloperidol [120] **(Haldol)**
Haloperidol may potentiate the CNS depressant effects of analgesics. See *CNS Depressants.*

MAO inhibitors [633,874,877,878]
Hypotension, ataxia, paresthesia, ocular palsy. Death may occur. See *Meperidine, Narcotic Analgesics,* etc.

Mercurial diuretics [5]
Potent analgesics, by impairing renal function and decreasing urinary output, may interfere with the diuretic action of the mercurials.

Methotrexate [198]
Analgesics containing salicylates potentiate methotrexate. Enhance toxicity.

Methotrimeprazine [120] **(Levoprome)**
Potentiation. Dose of one or both agents may have to be reduced because of additive effect.

Penicillins [198]
Analgesics (salicylates, etc.) potentiate penicillins, displacement from secondary binding site.

Phenobarbital [633]
Phenobarbital may inhibit analgesics (enzyme induction). See also *CNS Depressants.*

Phenothiazines [166]
Phenothiazines potentiate CNS depression by analgesics. See *CNS Depressants.*

Probenecid [198] **(Benemid)**
Analgesics (salicylates, etc.) antagonize probenecid; elevate serum uric acid.

Propranolol [29] **(Inderal)**
This β-adrenergic blocking agent potentiates the depressant effects of the narcotic analgesic, morphine.

Respiratory depressant drugs (Narcotics, etc.) [166]
Enhanced respiratory depression may result; dosage of the narcotic should be reduced. See *CNS Depressants.*

Sedatives and hypnotics [120,198,421,633]
See *CNS Depressants.* The initial effect of such combinations may be potentiation of CNS depressant effects. However, some sedatives and hypnotics (barbiturates, chloral hydrate, glutethimide, etc.) inhibit analgesics by enzyme induction after continued use.

Sulfonamides [198]
Analgesics may potentiate some sulfonamides; displacement from binding site.

Tranquilizers [120,619,878]
Tranquilizers tend to induce additive CNS depressant effects with analgesics. See *CNS Depressants.*

ANALGESIC AND ATARACTIC AGENTS

Alcohol [121]
Alcohol potentiates in decreasing order, reserpine, chlorpromazine, dextropropoxyphene, morphine, meprobamate, phenaglycodol, codeine, hydroxyzine.

ANANASE
See *Bromelains.*

ANAVAR
See *Anabolic Agents* **(oxandrolone).**

ANDROGENS
(Fluoxymesterone [Halotestin, Ora-Testryl, Ultandren], mesterolone [Androviron, Proviron], methyltestosterone [Metandren, Neo-Hombreol-M, Oreton-M, etc.], testosterone [Neo-Hombreol F, Oreton], testosterone esters [Delatestryl, Depo-Testosterone, Neo-Hombreol, Oreton, etc.])
See also *Anabolic Agents.*

Anticoagulants [119,198,330,366]
Norethandrolone and methandrostenolone and certain other androgenic agents (enzyme inhibitors and enhancers of affinity for receptors) potentiate oral anticoagulants.

Barbiturates [198,330,470]
Barbiturates induce the metabolizing enzymes for androsterone, testosterone and similar anabolic and androgenic drugs and thus inhibit their activity.

Calcitonin [181]
Androgens and calcitonin antagonize each other; have opposite effects on calcium retention.

Chlorcyclizine [65,479,485] **(Perazil)**
Chlorcyclizine increases rate of metabolism of (inhibits) testosterone.

Estrogens [181]
Estrogens antagonize anticancer effect of androgens.

Insecticides, halogenated [78]
Halogenated insecticides induce the metabolism of cortisol, estrogens, androgens, and progesterone. They decrease the uterotropic effects of both exogenous and endogenous estrogens.

Oxyphenbutazone [257,448] **(Tandearil)**
Methandrostenolone increases plasma levels of (potentiates) oxyphenbutazone (enzyme inhibition).

Parathormone [181]
Androgens antagonize parathormone. Parathyroid hormone promotes the mobilization of calcium from bone whereas androgens foster retention of calcium in bone.

Pesticides [78]
Pesticides (halogenated) stimulate the metabolism of androgens. See *Insecticides, Halogenated* above.

Phenobarbital
See *Barbiturates* above.

Phenylbutazone [448,470,1029,1502] **(Butazolidin)**
Phenylbutazone increases the rate of metabolism of (inhibits) testosterone; phenylbutazone may be potentiated by methandrostenolone, an enzyme inhibitor. See *Androgens* under *Phenylbutazone.*

ANDROSTENEDIONE (Androtex)
See also *Anabolic Agents* and *Androgens.*

Aminopyrine [555]
Aminopyrine increases the rate of metabolism of androstenedione (enzyme induction inhibits the steroid).

Antihistamines [330]
Antihistamines inhibit androstenedione.

Chlorcyclizine [65,479,485] **(Perazil)**
Chlorcyclizine inhibits androstenedione by increasing the rate at which it is metabolized.

Phenobarbital [330]
Phenobarbital inhibits androstenedione.

ANDROSTENEDIONE (Androtex) *(continued)*

Phenylbutazone [330] **(Butazolidin)**

Phenylbutazone inhibits androstenedione by increasing its rate of metabolism.

ANDROSTERONE

See also *Androgens* and *Anabolic Agents.*

ANECTINE

See *Muscle Relaxants* and *Succinylcholine Chloride.*

ANESTACON

See *Anesthetics, Local.*

ANESTHETICS, FLUORINE

Muscle relaxants, [421] depolarizing type **(Decamethonium, etc.)**

Fluorine anesthetics prolong muscle relaxation with depolarizing type muscle relaxants.

ANESTHETICS, GENERAL

(Chloroform, cyclopropane, divinyl ether, ethyl ether, ethylene, fluroxene [Fluoromar], halopropane, halothane [Fluothane], methoxyflurane [Penthrane], nitrous oxide, etc.)

See also *Ephedrine, Epinephrine, Ganglionic Blocking Agents, Muscle Relaxants,* and specific anesthetics.

β-Adrenergic blocking agents [120,421,619]

β-adrenergic blockers increase the activity of general anesthetics; arrhythmias. Propranolol, a β-adrenergic blocking agent, has been shown to have a synergistic CNS depressant action with various general anesthetics; this synergistic action may occur with other β-adrenergic blocking agents.

Alcohol [120,121,166,311,619,634]

As tolerance to alcohol develops, more anesthetic is required for anesthesia even if the patient is free of alcohol at the time. But, alcohol and anesthetics have additive CNS depressant effects. See *CNS Depressants.*

Analgesics

See *Narcotic Analgesics* below and *CNS Depressants.*

Antibiotics [30,37,55,120,146,311,322,395,499,500,504,505,507,882]

See *Neuromuscular Blocking Antibiotics* under *Antibiotics.* Respiratory depression, apnea, and muscle weakness may occur with certain antibiotics (bacitracin, colistimethate, dihydrostreptomycin, gentamycin, gramicidin, kanamycin, neomycin, paromomycin, polymyxin B, streptomycin and viomycin) which sensitize motor endplates to anesthetics. Topical, oral, and parenteral uses have all been implicated.

Anticholinesterases [692]

Lowered pseudocholinesterase levels create a potential hazard when anesthesia is accompanied by succinylcholine. See also *Anticholinergics* under *Neostigmine.*

Anticoagulants, oral [120,134,147,180]
(Coumadin, Dicumarol, Sintrom, etc.)

Some anesthetics may enhance the anticoagulant effect by inhibiting formation of coagulation factors and increasing the prothrombin time.

Antihistamines [120,619]

Antihistamines potentiate the CNS depressant effects. See *CNS Depressants.*

Antihypertensives [8,30,78,91,120,198,312,619,633]

Antihypertensives are potentiated by anesthetics; severe hypotension or shock and profound cardiovascular collapse may occur during surgery. Halothane and thiopental must be used with caution. Ether and chloroform are contraindicated. The hypotensive effects of some drugs are prolonged and must be discontinued long before surgery (reserpine, 1–3 weeks; guanethidine and methyldopa, 7–10 days; ganglionic

blocking agents, 24 hours) in mild cases. In moderate to severe cases of hypertension, care must be taken to avoid rebound hypertension.

Atropine

See *Anticholinergics* under *Neostigmine.*

Barbiturates [120,312,619]

The combination of barbiturates and some general anesthetics can be hazardous. Recovery from CNS depressant effects may be prolonged and collapse is possible. See *CNS Depressants.*

Catecholamines [772-7,801]
(Epinephrine, dopamine, isoproterenol, nordefrin, norepinephrine or levarterenol, etc.)

Catecholamines with general anesthetics produce the interaction described under *Epinephrine* below.

Chlorpromazine [120] **(Thorazine)**

Chlorpromazine potentiates the CNS depressant effects of general anesthetics.

CNS depressants [120,166]

Anesthetics potentiate CNS depressants. See *CNS Depressants.*

Colistimethate [120,547] **(Coly-Mycin)**

Combination may produce apnea.

Corticosteroids

See *Anesthetics* under *Corticosteroids.*

Cyclophosphamide

See *Anesthetics* under *Cyclophosphamide.*

Doxapram [120] **(Dopram)**

Doxapram, a respiratory stimulant, may cause an increase in epinephrine release to which the heart is more sensitive in the presence of anesthetics like halothane and cyclopropane.

Epinephrine [684,772-7,796,801]

Cardiac arrhythmia; chloroform, cyclopropane, ethyl chloride, trichloroethylene, and halothane sensitize the myocardium to the action of epinephrine and related catecholamines; increases likelihood of ventricular tachycardia or fibrillation when used in combination. Potentially very hazardous. Contraindicated. However, epinephrine used as a vasoconstrictor in small amounts in dental anesthetics is not contraindicated in most cardiac patients. [1087]

Furazolidone [633] **(Furoxone)**

Furazolidone, a MAO inhibitor, potentiates CNS depression produced by general anesthetics. Hazardous.

Guanethidine [120,633] **(Ismelin)**

Guanethidine should not be given during the two weeks prior to surgery to avoid the possibility of collapse (vascular) during anesthesia.

Haloperidol [120] **(Haldol)**

See *CNS Depressants.*

Hydralazine [421] **(Apresoline)**

See *CNS Depressants.*

Isoniazid [330]

Isoniazid potentiates anesthetics.

Isoproterenol

See *Epinephrine* above for the interaction with this catecholamine.

Kanamycin [749]

This antibiotic may cause neuromuscular paralysis with respiratory depression (apnea) when given to patients who have received anesthetics. See *Antibiotics* above.

Levarterenol [773,776,778,796,801]
(Levophed, norepinephrine)
See *Epinephrine* above for the interaction with this catecholamine.

MAO inhibitors [198,330,421,633,878,970]
MAO inhibitors potentiate the CNS depression produced by anesthetics. Patients taking a MAO inhibitor should not undergo surgery requiring general anesthesia. Should spinal anesthesia be essential, consider the possible combined hypotensive effects of the MAO inhibitor and the blocking agent. Also, do not give cocaine or local anesthetic solutions containing sympathomimetic vasoconstrictors. Discontinue the MAO inhibitor at least 10 days to 3 weeks before elective surgery.

Mebutamate [120] **(Capla)**
Mebutamate, a derivative of dimethyl carbamate, may enhance the CNS depressant effects of anesthetics, and in large enough doses or in susceptible patients, cause death.

Mecamylamine [421] **(Inversine)**
Anesthetics enhance the hypotensive action of mecamylamine. See *CNS Depressants.*

Meperidine [399,615] **(Demerol)**
The concurrent or sequential administration of anesthetics with meperidine has produced extreme hypotensive responses. See *CNS Depressants.*

Methotrimeprazine [120] **(Levoprome)**
Additive effects (CNS depression, orthostatic hypotension, etc.) Reduce and critically adjust dosage of each when used concomitantly or when sequence of use results in overlapping drug effects.

Methyldopa [198,421,633] **(Aldomet)**
The hypotensive effects induced by methyldopa are potentiated by anesthetics. See under *Antihypertensives.*

Mio-Pressin [633]
See *Rauwolfia Alkaloids* below. Hypotension may occur up to 2 weeks after withdrawing Mio-Pressin.

Muscle relaxants [120,878]
Cyclopropane, ether, fluroxene, halothane, and methoxyflurane potentiate nondepolarizing muscle relaxants such as *d*-tubocurarine (act synergistically). Reduce the dosage. See *Muscle Relaxants.*

Narcotic analgesics [120,619]
Anesthetics potentiate the hypotension and respiratory depression produced by narcotic analgesics. See *CNS Depressants.*

Neomycin [504,750]
This antibiotic may cause neuromuscular paralysis with respiratory depression (apnea) when given to patients who have received anesthetics. See *Antibiotics* above.

Neostigmine
See *Anticholinergics* under *Neostigmine.*

Nitrous oxide [879]
Combined use of two anesthetics, nitrous oxide with fluroxene increases cardiac output and central venous pressure.

Nordefrin
See *Epinephrine* above for the interaction with this catecholamine.

Norepinephrine [120,773,776,778,796,801]
See *Levarterenol* above.

Pargyline [198,421,878] **(Eutonyl)**
See *MAO Inhibitors* above.

Pentolinium [421] **(Ansolysen)**
Anesthetics potentiate the hypotensive action of the ganglionic blocking agent, pentolinium.

Phenothiazines [120,611]
Effects of the anesthetic and of the phenothiazines are en-

hanced See *CNS Depressants.* Severe hypotension and even circulatory collapse may occur.

Phentolamine [529] **(Regitine)**
Phentolamine antagonizes adrenergic sensitization of the myocardium to anesthetics.

Piminodine [619] **(Alvodine)**
See *Narcotic Analgesics* above.

Procarbazine [330] **(Matulane)**
See *MAO Inhibitors* above.

Propranolol [120,619,633,698] **(Inderal)**
Synergistic CNS depression; the anesthetics sensitize to propranolol. Propranolol should not be used to treat arrhythmias associated with the use of anesthetics that produce myocardial depression.

Quinethazone [120] **(Hydromox)**
Quinethazone decreases arterial responsiveness to norepinephrine and thus potentiates the hypotensive effects of anesthetics and preanesthetic agents. Their dosage should be reduced in emergency surgery when the diuretic cannot be withdrawn well before surgery.

Rauwolfia alkaloids
See *Anesthetics* under *Reserpine.*

Reserpine
See *Anesthetics* under *Reserpine.*

Sedatives and hypnotics [120,312,619]
The combination of sedatives and hypnotics with some general anesthetics can be hazardous. Recovery from anesthesia may be prolonged and collapse is possible. See *CNS Depressants.*

Streptomycin [561]
This antibiotic may cause neuromuscular paralysis with respiratory depression (apnea) when given to patients who have received anesthetics. See *Antibiotics* above.

Sympathomimetics [421,664,684]
Sympathomimetics increase cardiac arrhythmia effect of anesthetics. See *Epinephrine* and *Levarterenol* above.

Thioxanthenes [120]
See *CNS Depressants.*

Tranylcypromine (Parnate)
See *MAO Inhibitors* above.

Tubocurarine
See *Muscle Relaxants* above.

Veratrum alkaloids [120,421]
Anesthetics potentiate the hypotensive action of veratrum alkaloids.

Vasoconstrictors [120] **(Vasopressors)**
If hypotension from anesthetics occurs during obstetrical procedures, use of an oxytocic with a vasoconstrictor may result in severe persistent hypertension. Very hazardous.

Vasopressin [173] **(ADH, Pitressin)**
Anesthetics potentiate vasopressin due to depression of efficiency of baroreceptor reflexes (smaller amounts of the hormone elicit pressor responses).

ANESTHETICS, LOCAL
(Benoxinate [Dorsacaine], butacaine [Butyn], chloroprocaine [Mesacaine], cocaine, cyclomethycaine [Surfacaine], dibucaine [Nupercaine], dimethisoquine [Quotane], dyclonine [Dyclone], ethyl aminobenzoate [Anesthesin, Benzocaine], hexylcaine [Cyclaine], lidocaine [Xylocaine], mepivacaine [Carbocaine], piperocaine [Metycaine], pramoxine [Tronothane], procaine [Novocain], proparacaine [Ophthaine, Ophthetic], tetracaine [Pontocaine], etc.)
Anesthetics, local [950,951]
Enhanced toxicity may occur with combination of local anesthetics. Additive side effects.

ANESTHETICS, LOCAL *(continued)*

Cardiovascular depressants [120]
Effects of these depressant drugs may be enhanced when used simultaneously with local anesthetics. See *CNS Depressants*.

CNS depressants [120]
Effects of these depressant drugs may be enhanced when used simultaneously with local anesthetics. See *CNS Depressants*.

Decamethonium
Same as for *Succinylcholine Chloride* below.

Epinephrine [1087]
Epinephrine may be used safely, even in most cardiac patients, as an additive to local dental anesthetics to strengthen and prolong the anesthetic effect, and to delay systemic absorption. It is, however, contraindicated for such synergistic use in hyperthyroid patients, in cardiac patients in amounts above 0.2 mg. and in those receiving adrenergic neuron blocking agents like guanethidine and reserpine.

Oxytocics [120]
See *Vasoconstrictors* below.

Succinylcholine chloride [435,579,878]
Local anesthetics prolong apnea from succinylcholine chloride; intravenous lidocaine or procaine injections may potentiate the effect of succinylcholine and other depolarizing muscle relaxants, by displacing them from plasma protein binding sites. However, in convulsions (reaction from procaine) succinylcholine and artificial respiration are recommended.

Sulfonamides [167,178,202,433]
Local anesthetics with a PABA moiety (dibucaine, lidocaine, procaine, etc.) inhibit sulfonamides.

Vasoconstrictors [120]
If hypotension occurs during an obstetrical procedure, the use of oxytocics with a vasoconstrictor may result in severe persistent hypertension. A vasoconstrictor (IM or IV) is often used with a local anesthetic like procaine (especially when injected centrally) to combat vasodepressor effects.

Veratrum alkaloids [170]
Local anesthetics inhibit the action of veratrum alkaloids on excitable cells.

ANGIOTENSIN AMIDE (Hypertensin)
See *Vasopressors*.

Levarterenol [117]
In prolonged, severe hypotension caused by an adrenolytic agent, angiotensin is the logical pressor drug since the patient is rendered unresponsive to levarterenol.

Methylphenidate [120] (Ritalin)
Methylphenidate potentiates blood pressure elevating effect with angiotensin amide.

ANHYDRON
See *Thiazide Diuretics* **(cyclothiazide)**

ANORECTICS
(Anorexiants, anorexics, anorexigenics, etc.)
See *Sympathomimetics*.

Antihypertensives [198]
Antihypertensives antagonize anorexigenics and vice versa.

MAO inhibitors [198]
MAO inhibitors potentiate anorexigenics such as amphetamines through monoamine oxidase enzyme inhibition. Contraindicated. Lethal. See *Sympathomimetics* under *MAO Inhibitors*.

ANSOLYSEN
See *Antihypertensives* **(pentolinium).**

ANTABUSE
See *Disulfiram*.

ANTACIDS, ORAL
(Aluminum hydroxide, calcium carbonate, magnesium carbonate, magnesium hydroxide, magnesium trisilicate, sodium bicarbonate, etc.)
See also *Alkalinizing Agents*.
Antacids containing aluminum (hydroxide, aluminates, kaolin, attapulgite, etc.) inhibit intestinal absorption of a variety of drugs, including atropine, homatropine, and sodium pentobarbital either through adsorption or delay in gastric emptying. Simultaneous administration of any drug with alumina gel and related products should probably be avoided. [1959]

Alkaloids [1959]
See introduction to *Antacids, Oral* above. Aluminum hydroxide adsorbs atropine, homatropine and other belladonna alkaloids.

Antibiotics [78]
Antacids markedly decrease the absorption of antibiotics such as penicillin G and tetracycline from the gut.

Anticoagulants, coumarin [147,198,633]
Large doses of antacids inhibit absorption of coumarin anticoagulants, and may decrease their effect.

Barbiturates [28]
Antacids may decrease the rate of absorption of barbiturates, *e.g.* pentobarbital, so markedly that the hypnotic effect is abolished.

Chlorpromazine
See *Antacids* under *Chlorpromazine*.

Digitalis [486,951]
The effects of digitalis and its glycosides are decreased through delayed or decreased gastrointestinal absorption caused by antacids and antidiarrheal agents. See *Antacids* under *Digitalis*.

Indomethacin
See *Antacids* under *Indomethacin*.

Iron [28,928]
Antacids containing carbonates and magnesium trisilicate inhibit the absorption of iron by forming insoluble iron compounds and thus inhibit the effectiveness of iron compounds in iron deficiency anemia. Give these antacids and the iron therapy several hours apart.

Isoniazid
See *Antacids, Oral* under *Isoniazid*.

Levodopa [1335,1419,1742-4]
Oral antacids may increase the effectiveness of levodopa in parkinsonism by hastening gastric emptying time and thus decreasing contact of levodopa with the stomach where it is metabolized. Thus in some patients, oral antacids may facilitate intestinal absorption of levodopa.

Mecamylamine [325,870] (Inversine)
Mecamylamine is potentiated by antacids; increased absorption in alkaline pH.

Meperidine [325,870] (Demerol)
Meperidine is potentiated by antacids; increased absorption in alkaline pH.

Milk [880]
Excessive use of milk and certain antacids may produce hypercalcemia.

Nalidixic acid [78,198,202,633] **(NegGram)**
Antacids inhibit nalidixic acid (decreased absorption).

Nitrofurantoin [198,421,202,633] **(Furadantin)**
Antacids inhibit nitrofurantoin (decreased absorption as pH is lowered).

Penicillins [198,633]
Antacids inhibit penicillins (decreased absorption).

Phenothiazines
See *Antacids* under *Phenothiazines.*

Phenylbutazone [78,198,633]
Antacids inhibit phenylbutazone by decreasing its gastrointestinal absorption.

Quinidine
See *Aluminum Hydroxide* under *Quinidine.*

Salicylates [78]
Antacids inhibit salicylates by decreasing their gastrointestinal absorption.

Sodium polystyrene sulfonate [1421,1771] **(Kayexalate)**
The ion exchange resin binds the magnesium and calcium cations of oral antacids such as Maalox, Aludrox, Alka-2, Tums, etc. With large doses of the antacids, bicarbonate is not adequately bound, plasma CO_2 is elevated, and the patient undergoes systemic alkalosis. This interaction has been used beneficially in systemic acidosis. The elevated pH of the blood and urine, however, may affect absorption and excretion patterns of weakly acidic and weakly basic drugs. See *Alkalinizing Agents* and *Acidifying Agents* for mechanisms.

Sulfonamides [198,202]
Antacids inhibit sulfonamides (weak acids) by decreasing absorption.

Tetracyclines [75,198,359,619,633]
Antacids containing sodium bicarbonate, aluminum, calcium, or magnesium inhibit tetracycline absorption. See *Complexing Agents* under *Tetracyclines.*

ANTAZOLINE (Antistine)
See *Antihistamines.*

Epinephrine [199]
Antazoline may produce an enhanced cardiovascular effect with epinephrine. See under *Antihistamines.*

MAO inhibitors [48,199,311,312]
MAO inhibitors potentiate the antihistamine by decreasing its rate of metabolism; potentiate effect of endogenous norepinephrine. Antihistamine inhibits uptake of NE by tissues causing increased concentration of unbound drug.

Norepinephrine [199] **(Levarterenol, Levophed)**
Antazoline may produce an enhanced cardiovascular effect with norepinephrine. The antihistamine inhibits uptake of norepinephrine by tissues causing increased concentration of unbound drug to be available for interaction with receptors.

ANTHELMINTICS
See *Hexylresorcinol, Piperazine, Primaquine, Quinacrine,* and *Tetrachloroethylene.*

Mineral oil [421]
Mineral oil, by sequestering an antihelmintic, may reduce its effectiveness.

ANTIANGINAL AGENTS
See *Nitrates and Nitrites.*

ANTIARRHYTHMICS
See *Ajmaline, Lidocaine, Procainamide, Propranolol, Quinidine.*

Other antiarrhythmic drugs [120,790,1149]
Delirium may be induced by a combination of certain antiarrhythmic drugs (lidocaine plus procainamide). Certain combinations such as ajmaline and lidocaine exert an enhanced cardiac depressant effect.

ANTIBIOTICS
See also specific drugs such as *Chloramphenicol, Erythromycin, Griseofulvin, Penicillin, Streptomycin, Tetracyclines,* etc.

Alkalinizing agents [619]
Some antibiotics, *e.g.,* gentamicin, have enhanced antimicrobial activity in urine with pH elevated by alkalinizing agents.

Aminoglycoside Antibiotics [120,813]
(Gentamycin, kanamycin, neomycin, paromomycin, streptomycin, tobramycin)
Concomitant use of two or more or sequential use dangerously potentiates inherent nephrotoxicity and ototoxicity. See *Neuromuscular Blocking Antibiotics* below and *Antibiotics, Ototoxic and Neuromuscular Blocking* under *Neomycin.*

Amphotericin B [120,1942]
Amphotericin B should not be given concomitantly with other nephrotoxic antibiotics except with extreme caution and close monitoring. Permanent renal damage that is fatal can result.

Anesthetics
See under *Neuromuscular Blocking Antibiotics* below.

Antacids [78]
Antacids markedly decrease the absorption of antibiotics such as penicillin G and tetracycline from the gut.

Antibiotics [31,70,157,208,233,238,285,301,419,433,444-5,492,633,666, 811,864,1129,1321,1437,1520,1627,1934]
Some combinations of antibiotics act synergistically; others cause inhibitory interactions. See also *Neuromuscular Blocking Antibiotics* below and specific antibiotics. Certain bacteriostatic antibiotics (actinomycin D, *e.g.,* dactinomycin; chloramphenicol; fusidic acid; aminoglycoside antibiotics like the erythromycins, gentamicin, kanamycin, neomycin, and streptomycin; the tetracyclines; etc.) which inhibit protein synthesis, antagonize the bactericidal antibiotics (cephalosporins, penicillins, etc.), certain bacteriostatic antibiotics (cycloserine, vancomycin, etc.), and certain synthetic antimicrobials (nalidixic acid, etc.) because bacteriostatic drugs prevent multiplication of bacteria whereas bactericidal drugs kill only multiplying bacteria. Also they interfere with a mechanism of bactericidal action, the formation of cell wall deficient (CWD) forms. Thus with certain strains of *Escherichia, Proteus,* and *Pseudomonas,* carbenicillin may be antagonized by cephaloridine and 6-aminopenicillanic acid and certain other penicillins may antagonize one another. [1129] And tetracyclines inhibit penicillin in pneumococcal meningitis and in pharyngitis caused by Group A hemolytic streptococcus. However, not all bacteriostatic drugs antagonize bactericidal drugs, *e.g.,* the polymyxins can kill bacteria that are not multiplying. Penicillin G and streptomycin is the therapy of first choice in subacute bacterial endocarditis caused by enterococci *Streptococcus faecalis* and by the viridans group of *Streptococcus.* Synergism may occur when these drugs are given concomitantly in meningitis caused by *Listeria monocytogenes.* Some practitioners use a penicillin with a tetracycline by giving the drugs as far apart as possible. Gentamicin and ticarcillin are synergistically effective in *Pseudomonas aeruginosa* infection. *In vitro,* antagonism has been demonstrated between erythromycin and lincomycin and between nalidixic acid and nitrofurantoin. The degree of inhibition resulting from these interactions depends on dosage conditions, type of patho-

ANTIBIOTICS *(continued)*

genic organism, the relative concentrations of the antibiotics present, the order of therapy, and other factors. Thus neomycin blocks the intestinal absorption of penicillins.

Anticholinesterases

See under *Neuromuscular Blocking Antibiotics* below.

Anticoagulants, oral [120, 182, 193, 234, 259, 433, 434, 673, 898, 909, 972]

Antibiotics (chloramphenicol, kanamycin, neomycin, penicillin, streptomycin, tetracyclines, etc.) given in large doses or for prolonged periods, or malabsorbed, may increase anticoagulant activity by reducing production of vitamin K through supression of normal bacterial flora which produce the vitamin in the intestine. Tetracyclines, with some anticoagulant activity themselves, have an additive effect.

Antidiarrheal medications [120]

Antidiarrheals may be contraindicated with high molecular weight antibiotics because of physical adsorption and poor absorption.

Antineoplastics

See under *Neuromuscular Blocking Antibiotics* below.

Barbiturates

See under *Neuromuscular Blocking Antibiotics* below.

Calcium salts [881]

Respiratory paralysis induced by certain antibiotics, *e.g.*, polymyxin B, may be reversed by calcium chloride IV.

Colistimethate [120, 619]

See *Neuromuscular Blocking Antibiotics* below.

Curare and curariform drugs [421]

See *Neuromuscular Blocking Antibiotics* below.

Cyclamates [619, 880]

Cyclamates inhibit lincomycin by decreasing its absorption.

Dimenhydrinate [120] (Dramamine)

Dimenhydrinate may mask the ototoxic effects of antibiotics such as dihydrostreptomycin, kanamycin, neomycin, ristocetin, streptomycin and vancomycin, and of potent diuretics such as furosemide and ethacrynic acid, until an irreversible condition is reached.

Edrophonium

See *Neostigmine*.

EDTA [360]

EDTA increases the gastrointestinal absorption rate of certain antibiotics and thus potentiates the neuromuscular blockade produced by kanamycin, neomycin, streptomycins, etc. This may produce apnea and muscular weakness.

Ether

See under *Neuromuscular Blocking Antibiotics* below.

Indomethacin [120] (Indocin)

Indomethacin should be used with extra caution in the presence of existing controlled infections because it may mask the signs and symptoms of infection.

Mecamylamine

See under *Neuromuscular Blocking Antibiotics* below.

Milk [120, 665]

Milk and milk products inhibit gastrointestinal absorption of tetracycline antibiotics (calcium complex).

Muscle relaxants

See *Neuromuscular Blocking Antibiotics* below.

Neomycin [421]

Neomycin blocks the intestinal absorption of penicillins. See also under *Antibiotics* above.

Neostigmine [312, 506, 619, 656, 880] (Prostigmin)

The nondepolarizing muscle relaxant properties of certain antibiotics. *e.g.*, kanamycin, neomycin and streptomycin,

produced by competitive blockade, may be reversed by neostigmine. The noncompetitive neuromuscular blockade produced by certain other antibiotics, *e.g.*, colistimethate and polymyxin B is not antagonized by neostigmine and may even be potentiated.

Nephrotoxic antibiotics [120, 1942]

(Aminoglycosides such as gentamicin, kanamycin, *et al.*, amphotericin, cephalosporins, colistimethate, polymyxin, tetracyclines, etc.)

See contraindication under *Aminoglycoside Antibiotics* and *Amphotericin B* above and see *Antibiotics, Ototoxic* and *Neuromuscular Blocking* under *Neomycin*.

Neuromuscular blocking antibiotics [30, 37, 55, 120, 146, 322, 395, 432, 497-508, 813, 882]

Bacitracin, clindamycin, colistimethate, gentamicin, gramicidin, kanamycin, lincomycin, neomycin, paromomycin, polymyxin B, streptomycin, tobramycin, and viomycin may have additive neuromuscular blocking effects among themselves and with other neuromuscular blocking agents. Neuromuscular paralysis is a hazard which leads to respiratory depression, apnea and muscle weakness. These symptoms may be particularly pronounced with curariform and polarizing muscle relaxants, anesthetics, barbiturates, ether, mecamylamine, procainamide, promethazine, quinidine, and sodium citrate, as well as anticholinesterases (echothiophate, organophosphorus insecticides, etc.), antineoplastics (nitrogen mustard, AB-132), etc. Some of these combinations may be potentially lethal.

Ototoxic antibiotics

See *Antibiotics, Ototoxic* under *Neomycin*.

Penicillins [70, 157, 208, 285, 301, 419, 433, 444, 492, 666, 811, 864]

Certain other antibiotics inhibit the bactericidal activity of the penicillins by interfering with their mechanisms of action, *i.e.*, formation of deficient bacterial cell walls or CWD forms (actinomycin D, chloramphenicol, dactinomycin, erythromycin, kanamycin, oleandomycin, paromomycin, tetracyclines) or by blocking absorption of the oral penicillins (neomycin). See *Antibiotics* above.

Physostigmine [950, 951]

Physostigmine antagonizes the curarelike effect of aminoglycoside antibiotics.

Probenecid [120] (Benemid)

Probenecid does not influence the plasma levels of chloramphenicol, chlortetracycline, neomycin, oxytetracycline, or streptomycin. It inhibits tubular reabsorption of erythromycin, and therefore decreases plasma levels and inhibits its action by increasing urinary excretion. On the other hand, probenecid strongly potentiates penicillins by inhibiting their urinary excretion (blocks renal tubular secretion) and promoting higher and more persistent plasma concentrations.

Procainamide [559, 564, 619] (Pronestyl)

Enhanced neuromuscular blocking effect with certain antibiotics. See under *Neuromuscular Blocking Antibiotics* above.

Promethazine (Phenergan)

See *Streptomycin* under *Promethazine* and *Neuromuscular Blocking Antibiotics* above.

Quinidine [447, 559, 564]

See *Neuromuscular Blocking Antibiotics* above.

Sodium citrate

See *Neuromuscular Blocking Antibiotics* above.

Streptokinase-streptodornase [120] (Varidase)

The intramuscular use of streptokinase should be accompanied by the administration of a broad-spectrum antibiotic.

Streptomycin [233]

Streptomycin and benzylpenicillin act synergistically in sub-acute bacterial endocarditis. See *Neuromuscular Blocking Antibiotics* above and *Antibiotics, Ototoxic* under *Neomycin*.

Sulfonamides [883] (Gantanol, Thiosulfil)

Sulfonamides, *e.g.*, sulfamethoxazole and sulfamethizole, potentiate the antimicrobial activity of colistin against *Pseudomonas aeruginosa*.

Vitamin B$_{12}$ [880,1405,1505]

Neomycin inhibits absorption of vitamin B$_{12}$. See *Neomycin* under *Vitamin B$_{12}$*.

Vitamin K [182]

Antibiotics, by their antibacterial action, inhibit production of vitamin K by the intestinal flora. This tends to potentiate anticoagulants and decreases the hepatic synthesis of prothrombin and blood clotting factors VII, IX and X. Severe deficiency of vitamin K, by causing hypoprothrombinemia, may lead to bleeding (gastrointestinal, nasal, intracranial, etc).

ANTICHOLINERGICS
(Cholinergic blocking agents, atropine, scopolamine, trihexyphenidyl, etc.)

The atropinelike (antimuscarinic) anticholinergics inhibit the actions of acetylcholine on autonomic effectors innervated by postganglionic cholinergic nerves and on smooth muscles as well as at the subcortical and cortical levels of the brain. The quaternary ammonium analogs of atropine antagonize the nicotinic actions of acetylcholine in the spinal cord, but since they do not cross the blood brain barrier will have very little central effect. [168]

Anticholinergics tend to delay gastric emptying time and thus depress intestinal absorption of other drugs

Anticholinergics produce a large number of adverse effects including dryness of the mouth, blurred vision, increased ocular tension, urinary retention, tachycardia, dilatation of the pupils, constipation, drowsiness, etc. A wide range of drugs may have additive or potentiating effects, *e.g.*, antihistamines, antiparkinsonism agents, butyrophenones (Haldol, etc.), carbamazepine (Tegretol), glutethimide (Doriden), meperidine (Demerol), phenothiazines, piperazines, etc.

Achlorhydria agents and gastric secretion testing agents [168,421]
(Acidol, Acidulin, Histalog, Hydrionic, etc.)

Agents used to treat achlorhydria antagonize the inhibiting effects of anticholinergics on gastric HCl secretion.

Acidifying agents [165,325,870]

Acidifying agents increase the urinary excretion of weak bases like the anticholinergics, and thus inhibit them.

Adrenergics

See *Sympathomimetics* below.

Alkalinizing agents [165,325,870]

Alkalinizing agents potentiate anticholinergics. Alkalinizing agents have an effect opposite to that of *Acidifying Agents* above.

Alphaprodine [421] (Nisentil)

Alphaprodine potentiates the side effects of anticholinergics. Hazardous combination in glaucoma.

Amantadine (Symmetrel)

See *Anticholinergics* under *Amantadine*.

Anticholinesterases [28,168]

Anticholinergics antagonize the antiglaucoma (miotic) and other actions of cholinesterase inhibitors. See *Anticholinergics* under *Neostigmine*.

Antidepressants, tricyclic [120,194,619]

In susceptible patients receiving anticholinergic drugs (including antiparkinsonism agents), tricyclic antidepressants may potentiate the atropinelike effects (*e.g.*, paralytic ileus). Hazardous in glaucoma.

Antihistamines [198,487,488,633]

Antihistamines potentiate the side effects of anticholinergics. Hazardous in glaucoma.

Benactyzine [120] (Suavitil)

Benactyzine potentiates the side effects of anticholinergics.

Betahistine [421] (Serc)

See *Achlorhydria Agents* above. No longer marketed in U.S.

Betaine HCl [421] (Acidol)

See *Achlorhydria Agents* above.

Betazole [421] (Histalog)

See *Achlorhydria Agents* above.

Buclizine [166] (Softran)

Buclizine may potentiate the atropinelike side effects of anticholinergics. Hazardous in glaucoma.

Cholinergics [168]

Anticholinergics antagonize the cholinesterase inhibitor type of cholinergics.

Corticosteroids [421]

Increased ocular pressure with long-term therapy. Hazardous combination in glaucoma.

Desipramine [120] (Pertofrane)

See *Antidepressants, Tricyclic* above.

Diphenhydramine [120] (Benadryl)

Diphenhydramine may potentiate anticholinergics to produce increased atropinelike complications, *e.g.*, dental caries and loss of teeth from prolonged drug-induced xerostoma (additive anticholinergic effect).

Glutamic acid HCl [421] (Acidulin, etc.)

See *Achlorhydria Agents* above.

Guanethidine [421] (Esimil)

Guanethidine antagonizes the secretion inhibitory effects of anticholinergics.

Haloperidol [120] (Haldol)

Anticholinergics administered with haloperidol, may increase intraocular pressure. Hazardous in glaucoma. The parkinsonism (extrapyramidal) symptoms frequently caused by haloperidol, may be controlled with anticholinergics like benztropine mesylate and trihexyphenidyl HCl.

Histamine [421]

Histamine antagonizes the inhibitory effects of anticholinergics on gastric HCl secretion.

Imipramine [120] (Tofranil)

See *Antidepressants, Tricyclic* above.

Levodopa [715,1419] (Dopar, Larodopa)

Anticholinergics such as trihexyphenidyl often form useful adjuvant therapy in treating all forms of parkinsonism for they potentiate the actions of levodopa in treating the disease. Anticholinergics, however, delay gastric emptying and thus tend to prolong contact of levodopa with the stomach where it is metabolized. Intestinal absorption is decreased and the drug is inhibited. Also the antispasmodic effect of the parasympatholytic homatropine may cause failure of levodopa in parkinsonism. Adjust the dosage as necessary of the effective combinations.

MAO inhibitors [198,950]

MAO inhibitors may intensify the action of anticholinergic drugs (particularly those used in the treatment of parkinsonism) through interference with the mechanisms responsible for their detoxification.

Meperidine [421] (Demerol)

Meperidine and close derivatives potentiate the side effects of anticholinergics. Hazardous combination in glaucoma.

ANTICHOLINERGICS *(continued)*

Methotrimeprazine [120] (Levoprome)
An anticholinergic such as atropine or scopolamine given concomitantly with methotrimeprazine when premedicating a patient may produce tachycardia, lowered blood pressure, and CNS effects such as delirium, and extrapyramidal symptoms may be aggravated.

Methylphenidate [421] (Ritalin)
Methylphenidate enhances anticholinergic effects. Hazardous in glaucoma.

Neostigmine (Prostigmin)
See *Anticholinergics* under *Neostigmine.*

Nitrates and nitrites [421]
Organic nitrates and nitrites potentiate the side effects of anticholinergics. Hazardous combination in glaucoma.

Organophosphate cholinesterase inhibitors [168]
Anticholinergics antagonize the miotic (antiglaucoma) effect of acetylcholinesterase inhibitors.

Orphenadrine [120] (Disipal)
Orphenadrine may potentiate anticholinergics (additive effect).

Phenothiazines
See *Anticholinergics* under *Phenothiazines.*

Pilocarpine
See *Anticholinergics* under *Pilocarpine.*

Primidone [120] (Mysoline)
Primidone may potentiate the central depressant actions of anticholinergics (additive effect).

Procainamide (Pronestyl)
See *Anticholinergics* under *Procainamide.*

Psychotherapeutic agents [166]
See *Benzodiazepines; Butyrophenones; CNS Depressants; Dibenzazepines; Lithium Salts; MAO Inhibitors; Meprobamate; Phenothiazines; Reserpine;* and *Tranquilizers.*

Pyridoxine [1188]
Pyridoxine can counteract the anticholinergic side effects of some drugs. Also See *Pyridoxine* under *Antidepressants, Tricyclic.*

Quinidine [170,619]
Quinidine (vagal blocker) enhances the anticholinergic effects (additive effects).

Reserpine [421]
Reserpine antagonizes the secretion inhibitory effect of anticholinergics.

Sympathomimetics [168,421]
Sympathomimetics enhance the mydriatic and bronchial relaxation effects of anticholinergics. Hazardous combination in narrow angle glaucoma.

Thioxanthenes [120,421,619]
(Navane, Sordinol, Taractan, etc.)
Effects of anticholinergics may be enhanced. See *CNS Depressants.*

Tranquilizers [120,619,633]
(Benzodiazepines, phenothiazines, etc.)
Potentiated sedative effects and additive anticholinergic effects.

Tricyclic antidepressants
See *Antidepressants, Tricyclic* above.

Urinary alkalinizers [325,870]
Enhanced anticholinergic effect because of decreased urinary excretion.

ANTICHOLINESTERASES
(Ambenonium [Mytelase] chloride, demecarium bromide [Humorsol], chloral hydrate intraarterially, isoflurophate [Floropryl], neostigmine [Prostigmin], pyridostigmine, physostigmine, organophosphorus insecticides, echothiophate [Phospholine] iodide, and other cholinesterase inhibitors)

Adrenocorticoids [120,421]
In long term therapy, adrenocorticoids antagonize the antiglaucoma effects of anticholinesterases (increased ocular pressure).

Anesthetics [692]
Lowered pseudocholinesterase levels create a potential hazard in anesthesia accompanied by succinylcholine. See *Succinylcholine* below.

Anticholinergics [28,168]
(Atropine, Benztropine, Caramiphen, Cycrimine, etc.)
Anticholinergics antagonize the miotic (antiglaucoma) and other muscarinic effects of anticholinesterases on the autonomic and central nervous systems.

Antidepressants, tricyclic [120,166,168,619]
(Elavil, Pertofrane, Sinequan, Tofranil, etc.)
Tricyclic antidepressants (anticholinergic effects) antagonize the antiglaucoma (miotic) effects of anticholinesterases in glaucoma.

Antihistamines [120,169,488,619,913,914]
Antihistamines with anticholinergic effects antagonize the miotic (antiglaucoma) and CNS effects of anticholinesterases. Anticholinesterases potentiate tranquilizing and behavioral changes induced by antihistamines.

Atropine [168]
The actions of anticholinesterase agents on autonomic effector cells, and to some extent those on the CNS, are antagonized by atropine, an antidote of choice.

Barbiturates [4,5,966]
Barbiturates are potentiated by anticholinesterases. Although barbiturates may be used cautiously in treating convulsions, extreme care is essential in handling poisonings due to anticholinesterases, particularly organophosphorus pesticides.

Cholinesterase inhibitors [120]
Echothiophate, a cholinesterase inhibitor used as a miotic, potentiates other such inhibitors (malathion, parathion, Sevin, TEPP, etc.) used for other purposes (additive effects) or possibly synergistic. Those exposed to organophosphate insecticides must take strict precautions.

Clofibrate [421] (Atromid-S)
Clofibrate may potentiate the neuromuscular effects of anticholinesterases used in glaucoma.

Colistimethate [120,421] (Coly-Mycin)
Anticholinesterases may potentiate the neuromuscular blocking action of colistimethate.

Contraindicated drugs [966]
Patients poisoned by anticholinesterases should not be given aminophylline, morphine, phenothiazine tranquilizers, reserpine, succinylcholine, theophylline, or large quantities of fluids.

Corticosteroids [120,421]
See *Adrenocorticosteroids* above.

Curare [168]
Anticholinesterases may antagonize the neuromuscular effects of curare and other competitive neuromuscular blocking agents.

Decamethonium [198,421]
Anticholinesterases potentiate the effects of decamethonium, a depolarizing muscle relaxant.

Dexpanthenol [421] **(oral or IV)**
Dexpanthenol potentiates the effects of anticholinesterases.

Fluorophosphate insecticides [2,421,692]
Fluorophosphate insecticides potentiate the effects of other anticholinesterases. Very hazardous. See *Organophosphorus Insecticides* below.

Kanamycin [178]
Anticholinesterases antagonize the curarelike effects of kanamycin.

Morphine (and close derivatives) [166]
Morphine and its close derivatives like meperidine lower intraocular tension and thus enhance the beneficial effects of anticholinesterases in certain categories of glaucoma.

Muscle relaxants, [168,198,421] **competitive and depolarizing**
Anticholinesterases (edrophonium, neostigmine, etc.) *antagonize* the curarelike effects of competitive blocking muscle relaxants (curare, gallamine, kanamycin, neomycin, streptomycin, tubocurarine, etc.), but they *potentiate* the depolarizing type (colistimethate, decamethonium, gramicidin, polymyxin, and succinylcholine). Potentiation may lead to respiratory paralysis.

Neomycin
See *Muscle Relaxants* above.

Organophosphorus insecticides [2,692,966]
Additive anticholinesterase effects. Hazardous. Patients on anticholinesterases (even topical, such as eye drops) should avoid areas where organophosphorus insecticides (cholinesterase inhibitors) have recently been used. See also *Contraindicated Drugs* above.

Parasympathomimetic agents [168]
The cholinergic effects may be enhanced (additive effects) as in certain types of glaucoma.

Phenothiazines [488]
Anticholinesterases extend the tranquilizing action of phenothiazines and this effect is reversed by anticholinergics.

Polymyxin [178]
Anticholinesterases like neostigmine do not antagonize and may potentiate the skeletal muscle blocking effects of polymyxin, a depolarizing muscle relaxant.

Pralidoxime [120,619] **(Protopam)**
Pralidoxime antagonizes fluorophosphates and related anticholinesterases (antidotal).

Procainamide [120,421] **(Pronestyl)**
Procainamide, which possesses anticholinergic activity, is contraindicated in patients with myasthenia gravis. It may potentiate anticholinergic drugs and since it antagonizes the depolarizing effects of acetylcholine, it is antagonistic to anticholinesterases used in myasthenia gravis and may produce a return of the condition.

Procaine [1926]
Procaine, injected into a patient with atypical plasma cholinesterase, may produce peripheral cardiovascular collapse (anaphylactic shock).

Streptomycin
See *Muscle Relaxants* above.

Succinylcholine [2,421,692]
Anticholinesterases, even echothiophate eye drops, potentiate the curarelike effects of succinylcholine. A potential hazard is created during anesthesia.

Sympathomimetics [168]
Anticholinesterases (miotics) antagonize the mydriatic effects of sympathomimetics, and vice versa.

Tricyclic antidepressants [166]
See *Antidepressants, Tricyclic* above.

***d*-Tubocurarine and related blocking agents** [168,198]
d-Tubocurarine, and related competitive blocking agents antagonize the neuromuscular actions and to a lesser extent other actions of anticholinesterases on autonomic ganglia.

ANTICOAGULANTS ORAL
(Coumarin derivatives such as Coumadin, Dicumarol, Liquamar, Panwarfin, Sintrom, and Tromexan; indandione derivatives such as Danilone, Eridione, and Hedulin)
Most of the drug interactions listed below involve the coumarin anticoagulants. The importance of careful monitoring of prothrombin time whenever *any* drug is added to or withdrawn from the regimen of a patient on any anticoagulant cannot be over-emphasized. This class of drugs, with complex pharmacologic and pharmacokinetic properties, has a narrow margin of safety. Outpatients must be warned about taking other medications some of which, like aspirin, are commonly used without prescription.
Extreme caution must be observed if either an inhibitor or a potentiator of an anticoagulant is withdrawn from concomitant use with the anticoagulant. Hemorrhage from withdrawl of the inhibitor (hypoprothrombinemia) or clotting problems from withdrawal of the potentiator (hyperprothrombinemia) may occur. Use of succedanea may be desirable. Thus benzodiazepines (flurazepam, diazepam, etc.) which seem to have little effect on oral anticoagulants may be preferred to barbiturates and other enzyme inducing sedatives and hypnotics. Phenobarbital > glutethimide > methaqualone as inducers of oral anticoagulant metabolizing enzymes.

Acetaminophen [147,571,572,1135,1161,1192]
(Tempra, Tylenol)
See *Anticoagulants, Oral* under *Acetaminophen* which increases response to the anticoagulant. Also see *Distalgesic* below.

Acidifying agents [325,870]
Acidifying agents decrease the urinary excretion of weak acids like coumarin anticoagulants, and thereby potentiate them, but see the different effect of *Vitamin C* (ascorbic acid).

ACTH [120,147,673,727,903]
(Acthar, Cortigel, Cortrophin, etc.)
ACTH theoretically antagonizes oral anticoagulants by mobilizing or replacing coagulant Factor VII. Patients may need larger dosage of the anticoagulant. However, severe hemorrhage has been reported with the combination.

Adrenocorticosteroids [120,147,180,673,903]
Adrenocorticosteroids, possibly by stimulating synthesis of clotting factors, decrease prothrombin time and tend to antagonize oral anticoagulants. See *Corticosteroids* also below.

Alcohol [7,120,147,180,329,345,674,711,991,997,1055,1192,1351,1360]
Alcohol can cause an unpredictable response to coumarin anticoagulants. Alcohol, on the one hand, is a metabolizing enzyme inducer which may inhibit the anticoagulants. On the other hand, it may also adversely affect the liver. Patients with liver disease (alcoholics) are sensitive to anticoagulants. Therefore restrict intake of alcohol. Since alcohol also increases the rate of clearance of warfarin and it may depress the activity of factors VII and X, monitor the net effect closely.

Alkalinizing agents [325,870]
Alkalinizing agents have an effect opposite to that of the *Acidifying Agents* above.

Allopurinol [1879,1929] **(Zyloprim)**
Allopurinol (xanthine oxidase inhibitor), through enzyme inhibition, may triple the half-life of dicumarol and warfarin, and thus potentiate these anticoagulants, and possibly cause bleeding.

ANTICOAGULANTS ORAL *(continued)*

Aminocaproic acid[901] (Amicar, EACA)

Epsilon-aminocaproic acid, with its antifibrinolytic activity, may shorten clotting time and therefore is antagonistic to anticoagulants. However, large doses IV induce incoagulability in some patients.

Aminopyrine[673,1116] (Pyramidon)

Aminopryine prolongs prothombin time as determined by the Quick one-stage test (potentiates anticoagulants), but in the guinea pig decreases the response to the anticoagulants.

p-Aminosalicylic acid[193,673,890,1336,1779,1895]

Aminosalicylic acid (enzyme inhibitor) potentiates oral anticoagulants by supressing prothrombin formation in the liver.

Amobarbital[9,223,296] (Amytal)

Barbiturates, through enzyme induction, inhibit anticoagulants. Increased anticoagulant dosage may be required for therapeutic effect.

Anabolic agents[9,119,147,180,234,393,394,907,908,1135,1320,1389,1588,1658,1675,1682,1747]

(Anadrol, Dianabol, Durabolin, Maxibolin, Metandren, Neo-Hombreol, Nilevar, Oreton-M Steronyl, etc.)

Anabolic steroids such as ethylestrenol, methandrostenolone, norethandrolone and oxymetholone (17-alpha-alkylated) potentiate oral coumarin and indandione anticoagulants by one or several proposed but unconfirmed mechanisms (by inhibiting their metabolism, or by increasing their affinity for receptors or by increasing clotting factor catabolism, or by reducing the concentration of vitamin K-dependent clotting factors through inhibition of their synthesis). The latter is additive or synergistic since the anticoagulants also inhibit synthesis of clotting factors. Risk of hemorrhage. Avoid combination or reduce dosage.

Analgesics[150,393,448,571,572,861,896]

Some analgesics (aspirin, acetaminophen, oxyphenbutazone phenylbutazone, and indomethacin) potentiate oral anticoagulants by displacing them from protein binding sites. Prolonged use of narcotic analgesics may enhance the anticoagulant effect. Phenyramidol may enhance the effects of oral anticoagulants by inhibiting their metabolism.

Androgens[198,330]

Norethandrolone and methandrostenolone and certain other androgenic agents potentiate anticoagulants. See also *Anabolic Agents* above.

Anesthetics[120,134,180,640,997]

Some anesthetics may enhance the anticoagulant effect.

Antacids[147,633,1202,1749]

Large doses of antacids may decrease the effect of coumarin anticoagulants by inhibiting absorption.

Antibiotics[234,259,433,434,898,909,972,1135,1216,1415,1424,1470,1539,1601,1681]

Antibiotics (chloramphenicol, kanamycin, neomycin, penicillins, streptomycin, tetracyclines, etc.) especially when given orally to patients whose vitamin K intake is low, may increase anticoagulant activity by reducing production of vitamin K through suppression of normal bacterial flora which produces the vitamin in the intestine. Tetracyclines themselves possess anticoagulant activity (depress plasma prothrombin activity). Risk of hemorrhage. Decrease dosage of anticoagulants.

Anticonvulsants[189,569,884]

Oral anticoagulants decrease the metabolism of anticoagulants and may thus potentiate them.

Antidepressants, Tricyclic[180,1545,1879]

The tricyclic antidepressants, nortriptyline and amitriptyline, by inhibiting the hepatic microsomal enzymes, may inhibit the metabolism of anticoagulants such as dicumarol and warfarin and potentiate them as much as 4-fold. Be alert to a change in *anticoagulant effect* when the antidepressants are started *(increases)* or withdrawn *(decreases)*. This interaction may occur with other tricyclics in this therapeutic category.

Antidiabetics, oral[120,147,266,330,359,412,449,677,768,976,1285,1412,1545,1702,1713] (Diabinese, Orinase)

The coumarin anticoagulants apparently have no inherent hypoglycemic effect, but they potentiate sulfonylurea hypoglycemics by inhibiting their metabolic degradation and possibly by decreasing urinary excretion. Watch for hypoglycemic reactions. The half-life of chlorpropamide was increased from 40 to 90 hours with bishydroxycoumarin. Oral antidiabetics (sulfonylureas) may potentiate coumarin anticoagulants by displacing them from protein binding sites. The order of administration affects the interaction. See also *Tolbutamide* below. If either type of drug is withdrawn from a patient on both types, monitor carefully.

Antifibrinolytic agents[120,619,901] (Amicar, etc.)

Antifibrinolytic drugs such as aminocaproic acid, by suppressing fibrinolytic activity, antagonize anticoagulants. See *Aminocrapoic Acid* above.

Antihistamines[64,120,223,479,481,555,673]

Antihistamines may decrease the anticoagulant effect of coumarin anticoagulants (enzyme induction) but this has not been well confirmed in the laboratory. However, some antihistamines prolong the prothrombin time as determined by the Quick one-stage test. Their action increases the anticoagulant effect.

Antihypertensives[1832]

Antilipemics[134,619]

(Aluminum nicotinate, Atromid-S, Choloxin, Cytellin, unsaturated fatty acids)

Antilipemics may increase the anticoagulant effect of coumarin anticoagulants, and increase the bleeding tendency.

Anti-inflammatory[3,10,28,78,120,133,147,214,314,330,391,393,434,448,646,673,677,784,814,869,896,903,907,1545,1881,1927]

Anti-inflammatory agents must be given very carefully, if at all, to patients on anticoagulant therapy because of the possibility of enhancing the anticoagulant response. Indomethacin > aspirin or sulfinpyrazone (a uricosuric) > mefenamic acid > flufenamic acid > phenylbutazone in inhibiting serotonin release by connective tissue particles (in blocking platelet function, decreasing aggregation of platelets). See *Indomethacin, Mefenamic Acid,* and *Phenylbutazone* below.

Antimalarials[930]

See *Quinine* below.

Antineoplastics[120,134,619,861,890,2067]

Antineoplastics, by affecting vitamin K, by depressing platelet counts, and by bone marrow depression, tend to potentiate anticoagulants because of the hemorrhagic potential. Hepatotoxic antineoplastics that impair liver function potentiate the hypoprothrombinemic action of coumarin anticoagulants. Potent hepatotoxins include azathioprine, daunorubicin plus cytarabine, doxorubicin, mercaptopurine, and methotrexate. Antineoplastics rarely associated with hepatotoxicity include chlorambucil, cyclophosphamide, and melphalen.

Antipyretics

See *Salicylates* below.

Antipyrine[753,1261,1690,1902]

Antipyrine, a hepatic microsomal enzyme inducer, decreases the activity of oral anticoagulants. Monitor carefully if antipyrine is added to or withdrawn from the regimen. It is not as strong an inducer for the anticoagulants as phenobarbital, however.

Ascorbic acid

See *Vitamin C* below.

Decamethonium [198,421]
Anticholinesterases potentiate the effects of decamethonium, a depolarizing muscle relaxant.

Dexpanthenol [421] **(oral or IV)**
Dexpanthenol potentiates the effects of anticholinesterases.

Fluorophosphate insecticides [2,421,692]
Fluorophosphate insecticides potentiate the effects of other anticholinesterases. Very hazardous. See *Organophosphorus Insecticides* below.

Kanamycin [178]
Anticholinesterases antagonize the curarelike effects of kanamycin.

Morphine (and close derivatives) [166]
Morphine and its close derivatives like meperidine lower intraocular tension and thus enhance the beneficial effects of anticholinesterases in certain categories of glaucoma.

Muscle relaxants, [168,198,421] **competitive and depolarizing**
Anticholinesterases (edrophonium, neostigmine, etc.) *antagonize* the curarelike effects of competitive blocking muscle relaxants (curare, gallamine, kanamycin, neomycin, streptomycin, tubocurarine, etc.), but they *potentiate* the depolarizing type (colistimethate, decamethonium, gramicidin, polymyxin, and succinylcholine). Potentiation may lead to respiratory paralysis.

Neomycin
See *Muscle Relaxants* above.

Organophosphorus insecticides [2,692,966]
Additive anticholinesterase effects. Hazardous. Patients on anticholinesterases (even topical, such as eye drops) should avoid areas where organophosphorus insecticides (cholinesterase inhibitors) have recently been used. See also *Contraindicated Drugs* above.

Parasympathomimetic agents [168]
The cholinergic effects may be enhanced (additive effects) as in certain types of glaucoma.

Phenothiazines [488]
Anticholinesterases extend the tranquilizing action of phenothiazines and this effect is reversed by anticholinergics.

Polymyxin [178]
Anticholinesterases like neostigmine do not antagonize and may potentiate the skeletal muscle blocking effects of polymyxin, a depolarizing muscle relaxant.

Pralidoxime [120,619] **(Protopam)**
Pralidoxime antagonizes fluorophosphates and related anticholinesterases (antidotal).

Procainamide [120,421] **(Pronestyl)**
Procainamide, which possesses anticholinergic activity, is contraindicated in patients with myasthenia gravis. It may potentiate anticholinergic drugs and since it antagonizes the depolarizing effects of acetylcholine, it is antagonistic to anticholinesterases used in myasthenia gravis and may produce a return of the condition.

Procaine [1926]
Procaine, injected into a patient with atypical plasma cholinesterase, may produce peripheral cardiovascular collapse (anaphylactic shock).

Streptomycin
See *Muscle Relaxants* above.

Succinylcholine [2,421,692]
Anticholinesterases, even echothiophate eye drops, potentiate the curarelike effects of succinylcholine. A potential hazard is created during anesthesia.

Sympathomimetics [168]
Anticholinesterases (miotics) antagonize the mydriatic effects of sympathomimetics, and vice versa.

Tricyclic antidepressants [166]
See *Antidepressants, Tricyclic* above.

_d_-Tubocurarine and related blocking agents [168,198]
d-Tubocurarine, and related competitive blocking agents antagonize the neuromuscular actions and to a lesser extent other actions of anticholinesterases on autonomic ganglia.

ANTICOAGULANTS ORAL
(Coumarin derivatives such as Coumadin, Dicumarol, Liquamar, Panwarfin, Sintrom, and Tromexan; indandione derivatives such as Danilone, Eridione, and Hedulin)
Most of the drug interactions listed below involve the coumarin anticoagulants. The importance of careful monitoring of prothrombin time whenever *any* drug is added to or withdrawn from the regimen of a patient on any anticoagulant cannot be over-emphasized. This class of drugs, with complex pharmacologic and pharmacokinetic properties, has a narrow margin of safety. Outpatients must be warned about taking other medications some of which, like aspirin, are commonly used without prescription.

Extreme caution must be observed if either an inhibitor or a potentiator of an anticoagulant is withdrawn from concomitant use with the anticoagulant. Hemorrhage from withdrawl of the inhibitor (hypoprothrombinemia) or clotting problems from withdrawal of the potentiator (hyperprothrombinemia) may occur. Use of succedanea may be desirable. Thus benzodiazepines (flurazepam, diazepam, etc.) which seem to have little effect on oral anticoagulants may be preferred to barbiturates and other enzyme inducing sedatives and hypnotics. Phenobarbital > glutethimide > methaqualone as inducers of oral anticoagulant metabolizing enzymes.

Acetaminophen [147,571,572,1135,1161,1192] **(Tempra, Tylenol)**
See *Anticoagulants, Oral* under *Acetaminophen* which increases response to the anticoagulant. Also see *Distalgesic* below.

Acidifying agents [325,870]
Acidifying agents decrease the urinary excretion of weak acids like coumarin anticoagulants, and thereby potentiate them, but see the different effect of *Vitamin C* (ascorbic acid).

ACTH [120,147,673,727,903] **(Acthar, Cortigel, Cortrophin, etc.)**
ACTH theoretically antagonizes oral anticoagulants by mobilizing or replacing coagulant Factor VII. Patients may need larger dosage of the anticoagulant. However, severe hemorrhage has been reported with the combination.

Adrenocorticosteroids [120,147,180,673,903]
Adrenocorticosteroids, possibly by stimulating synthesis of clotting factors, decrease prothrombin time and tend to antagonize oral anticoagulants. See *Corticosteroids* also below.

Alcohol [7,120,147,180,329,345,674,711,991,997,1055,1192,1351,1360]
Alcohol can cause an unpredictable response to coumarin anticoagulants. Alcohol, on the one hand, is a metabolizing enzyme inducer which may inhibit the anticoagulants. On the other hand, it may also adversely affect the liver. Patients with liver disease (alcoholics) are sensitive to anticoagulants. Therefore restrict intake of alcohol. Since alcohol also increases the rate of clearance of warfarin and it may depress the activity of factors VII and X, monitor the net effect closely.

Alkalinizing agents [325,870]
Alkalinizing agents have an effect opposite to that of the *Acidifying Agents* above.

Allopurinol [1879,1929] **(Zyloprim)**
Allopurinol (xanthine oxidase inhibitor), through enzyme inhibition, may triple the half-life of dicumarol and warfarin, and thus potentiate these anticoagulants, and possibly cause bleeding.

ANTICOAGULANTS ORAL *(continued)*

Aminocaproic acid [901] (Amicar, EACA)

Epsilon-aminocaproic acid, with its antifibrinolytic activity, may shorten clotting time and therefore is antagonistic to anticoagulants. However, large doses IV induce incoagulability in some patients.

Aminopyrine [673,1116] (Pyramidon)

Aminopryine prolongs prothombin time as determined by the Quick one-stage test (potentiates anticoagulants), but in the guinea pig decreases the response to the anticoagulants.

p-Aminosalicylic acid [193,673,890,1336,1779,1895]

Aminosalicylic acid (enzyme inhibitor) potentiates oral anticoagulants by supressing prothrombin formation in the liver.

Amobarbital [9,223,296] (Amytal)

Barbiturates, through enzyme induction, inhibit anticoagulants. Increased anticoagulant dosage may be required for therapeutic effect.

Anabolic agents [9,119,147,180,234,393,394,907,908,1135,1320,1389, 1588,1658,1675,1682,1747]

(Anadrol, Dianabol, Durabolin, Maxibolin, Metandren, Neo-Hombreol, Nilevar, Oreton-M Steronyl, etc.)

Anabolic steroids such as ethylestrenol, methandrostenolone, norethandrolone and oxymetholone (17-alpha-alkylated) potentiate oral coumarin and indandione anticoagulants by one or several proposed but unconfirmed mechanisms (by inhibiting their metabolism, or by increasing their affinity for receptors or by increasing clotting factor catabolism, or by reducing the concentration of vitamin K-dependent clotting factors through inhibition of their synthesis). The latter is additive or synergistic since the anticoagulants also inhibit synthesis of clotting factors. Risk of hemorrhage. Avoid combination or reduce dosage.

Analgesics [150,393,448,571,572,861,896]

Some analgesics (aspirin, acetaminophen, oxyphenbutazone phenylbutazone, and indomethacin) potentiate oral anticoagulants by displacing them from protein binding sites. Prolonged use of narcotic analgesics may enhance the anticoagulant effect. Phenyramidol may enhance the effects of oral anticoagulants by inhibiting their metabolism.

Androgens [198,330]

Norethandrolone and methandrostenolone and certain other androgenic agents potentiate anticoagulants. See also *Anabolic Agents* above.

Anesthetics [120,134,180,640,997]

Some anesthetics may enhance the anticoagulant effect.

Antacids [147,633,1202,1749]

Large doses of antacids may decrease the effect of coumarin anticoagulants by inhibiting absorption.

Antibiotics [234,259,433,434,898,909,972,1135,1216,1415,1424,1470,1539, 1601,1681]

Antibiotics (chloramphenicol, kanamycin, neomycin, penicillins, streptomycin, tetracyclines, etc.) especially when given orally to patients whose vitamin K intake is low, may increase anticoagulant activity by reducing production of vitamin K through suppression of normal bacterial flora which produces the vitamin in the intestine. Tetracyclines themselves possess anticoagulant activity (depress plasma prothrombin activity). Risk of hemorrhage. Decrease dosage of anticoagulants.

Anticonvulsants [189,569,884]

Oral anticoagulants decrease the metabolism of anticoagulants and may thus potentiate them.

Antidepressants, Tricyclic [180,1545,1879]

The tricyclic antidepressants, nortriptyline and amitriptyline, by inhibiting the hepatic microsomal enzymes, may inhibit the metabolism of anticoagulants such as dicumarol and warfarin and potentiate them as much as 4-fold. Be alert to a change in *anticoagulant effect* when the antidepressants are started *(increases)* or withdrawn *(decreases)*. This interaction may occur with other tricyclics in this therapeutic category.

Antidiabetics, oral [120,147,266,330,359,412,449,677,768,976,1285, 1412,1545,1702,1713] (Diabinese, Orinase)

The coumarin anticoagulants apparently have no inherent hypoglycemic effect, but they potentiate sulfonylurea hypoglycemics by inhibiting their metabolic degradation and possibly by decreasing urinary excretion. Watch for hypoglycemic reactions. The half-life of chlorpropamide was increased from 40 to 90 hours with bishydroxycoumarin. Oral antidiabetics (sulfonylureas) may potentiate coumarin anticoagulants by displacing them from protein binding sites. The order of administration affects the interaction. See also *Tolbutamide* below. If either type of drug is withdrawn from a patient on both types, monitor carefully.

Antifibrinolytic agents [120,619,901] (Amicar, etc.)

Antifibrinolytic drugs such as aminocaproic acid, by suppressing fibrinolytic activity, antagonize anticoagulants. See *Aminocrapoic Acid* above.

Antihistamines [64,120,223,479,481,555,673]

Antihistamines may decrease the anticoagulant effect of coumarin anticoagulants (enzyme induction?) but this has not been well confirmed in the laboratory. However, some antihistamines prolong the prothrombin time as determined by the Quick one-stage test. Their action increases the anticoagulant effect.

Antihypertensives [1832]

Antilipemics [134,619]

(Aluminum nicotinate, Atromid-S, Choloxin, Cytellin, unsaturated fatty acids)

Antilipemics may increase the anticoagulant effect of coumarin anticoagulants, and increase the bleeding tendency.

Anti-inflammatory [3,10,28,78,120,133,147,214,314,330,391,393,434, 448,646,673,677,784,814,869,896,903,907,1545,1881,1927]

Anti-inflammatory agents must be given very carefully, if at all, to patients on anticoagulant therapy because of the possibility of enhancing the anticoagulant response. Indomethacin > aspirin or sulfinpyrazone (a uricosuric) > mefenamic acid > flufenamic acid > phenylbutazone in inhibiting serotonin release by connective tissue particles (in blocking platelet function, decreasing aggregation of platelets). See *Indomethacin, Mefenamic Acid,* and *Phenylbutazone* below.

Antimalarials [930]

See *Quinine* below.

Antineoplastics [120,134,619,861,890,2067]

Antineoplastics, by affecting vitamin K, by depressing platelet counts, and by bone marrow depression, tend to potentiate anticoagulants because of the hemorrhagic potential. Hepatotoxic antineoplastics that impair liver function potentiate the hypoprothrombinemic action of coumarin anticoagulants. Potent hepatotoxins include azathioprine, daunorubicin plus cytarabine, doxorubicin, mercaptopurine, and methotrexate. Antineoplastics rarely associated with hepatotoxicity include chlorambucil, cyclophosphamide, and melphalen.

Antipyretics

See *Salicylates* below.

Antipyrine [753,1261,1690,1902]

Antipyrine, a hepatic microsomal enzyme inducer, decreases the activity of oral anticoagulants. Monitor carefully if antipyrine is added to or withdrawn from the regimen. It is not as strong an inducer for the anticoagulants as phenobarbital, however.

Ascorbic acid

See *Vitamin C* below.

Aspirin [330,633,999]

Aspirin potentiates the anticoagulant effect of oral anticoagulants and may cause severe hemorrhage. See *Salicylates* below.

Azapropazone

See *Warfarin* under *Azapropazone*.

Barbiturates [20,63,96,106,183,223,296,297,375,449,685,744,826,1055,1239,1261,1382,1576,1579,1722,1832,1902,1922]

(Butisol, Medomin, etc.)

Barbiturates, by stimulating metabolic degradation of coumarin anticoagulants, through stimulation of microsomal enzyme activity, and by interfering with gastrointestinal absorption inhibit the hypoprothrombinemic effect of the anticoagulants. If barbiturates are withdrawn reduce the dose of the anticoagulant; inhibition may persist for weeks after withdrawal, but the result can be fatal hemorrhage as the inhibiting effect disappears.

Benziodarone [673,930,1114]

(Algocor, Cardivix, Dilafurane, etc.)

Benziodarone prolongs the prothrombin time, as determined by the Quick one-stage test, and potentiates the anticoagulants. A similar effect is not produced by the analog amiodarone (cordarone).

Benzodiazepines [120,330,744,814,894,1135,1561,1748,1817,1902]

(Dalmane Librium, Serax, Valium)

Benzodiazepines (chlordiazepoxide, diazepam, furazepam, etc.) alter the effects of oral anticoagulants according to some authors but some reported studies showed a lack of interaction. The effects reported are variable and in disagreement, but enzyme induction may be involved, and possibly timing of either dosage or observations may alter conclusions. Apparently not a serious problem with Librium or Valium.

Benzpyrene [633]

The carcinogen, benzpyrene, present in charcoal broiled meats and cigarette smoke, is an enzyme inducer that may inhibit oral anticoagulants. See *Smoking* (page 590).

Bile salts [421,1055]

Lack of bile potentiates anticoagulants (decreased vitamin K absorption). This is one mechanism whereby *Cholestyramine* below potentiates the anticoagulants, and the reason why conditions such as obstructive jaundice, external biliary fistula, and associated pancreatitis sensitize patients to the anticoagulants.

Bioflavanoids [134]

Bioflavanoids decrease the response to oral anticoagulants.

Bishydroxycoumarin [1055,1110] **(Dicumarol)**

The rate of metabolism of bishydroxycoumarin is dose-dependent. The drug inhibits its own metabolism with increasing doses.

Blood cholesterol lowering agents [421]

Blood cholesterol lowering agents potentiate oral anticoagulants by drug displacement. See *Clofibrate* and *Dextrothyroxine* below.

Bretylium [180]

Bretylium potentiates the anticoagulants.

Bromelains [5,198,421,619] **(Ananase)**

Bromelains may increase the anticoagulant effect of coumarin derivatives slightly. Concurrent use is not recommended.

Butabarbital sodium [20] **(Butisol)**

Butabarbital sodium inhibits oral anticoagulant therapy presumably through coumarin metabolizing enzyme stimulation. This effect is shown as early as 2 weeks after initiation of butabarbital sodium therapy and persists for 6 weeks after cessation of butabarbital therapy. See *Barbiturates* above.

Carbamazepine [1474] **(Tegretol)**

The anticonvulsant, carbamazepine, induces hepatic microsomal enzymes and thus decreases the action of anticoagulants. See warning under *Barbiturates*.

Carbon tetrachloride [295,898]

Carbon tetrachloride potentiates anticoagulants through hepatic insufficiency. Exposure to carbon tetrachloride can cause hypoprothrombinemia and therefore hemorrhage with coumarin anticoagulants.

Cathartics [193,890,1425,1450,1483]

Drastic cathartics may potentiate anticoagulant therapy by reducing absorption of vitamin K from the gut. This is more likely to occur with anticoagulants like dicumarol which is poorly and unpredictably absorbed.

Cephaloridine [1015,1415,1470,1539] **(Loridine)**

Cephaloridine may prolong prothrombin time. Monitor patients carefully if this antibiotic is given to patients on anticoagulants. Hemorrhase may occur.

Charcoal [1055,1111] **(Activated carbon)**

Large quantities of activated charcoal can cause a deficiency of vitamin K by inhibiting its absorption and thus increases the response to oral anticoagulants.

Chloral betaine [297]

Same as for *Chloral Hydrate* below.

Chloral hydrate [97,297,744,760,1040,1192,1233,1252,1346,1461,1737,1781,1783,1869,1894]

Chloral hydrate, which is reported to increase prothrombin time as determined by the Quick one-stage test, was once believed to stimulate metabolic degradation of coumarin anticoagulants and decrease their effect. It was later found to potentiate them initally through its metabolite, trichloroacetic acid, which displaces them from their plasma protein binding sites. Continued use of the combination seems to produce less interference from the chloral hydrate and more normal action of the anticoagulant. Reduce the dosage of the anticoagulants with choral hydrate to avoid hemorrhage from hypoprothrombinemia if necessary. The relative amounts of the various metabolites, duration of dosage of chloral hydrate, and other factors may alter the outcome, however. Monitor closely.

Chloramphenicol [234,259,676,1135,1415,1424,1470,1539,1681] **(Chloromycetin)**

Chloramphenicol may triple the prothrombin time by inhibiting the hepatic microsomal enzymes, interfering with vitamin K production by gut bacteria, and by damaging hepatic cells. Liver damage may decrease prothrombin production. Alternative antibiotics are often preferably substituted. See also *Antibiotics* above.

Chlorcyclizine [223,555,673] **(Histantine, Perazyl)**

Chlorcyclizine may produce decreased effectiveness of oral anticoagulants by enzyme induction.

Chlordane [83]

Chlordane inhibits oral anticoagulants (enzyme induction).

Chlordiazepoxide [330,744,814,894,1561,1902] **(Librium)**

Chlordiazepoxide may decrease the anticoagulant effect of coumarin derivatives, but variable response has been reported (several conclude there is no interaction). Timing of the two therapies is probably very important to the outcome. See *Benzodiazepines* above.

Chlorinated Insecticides

See *Warfarin* under *Chlorinated Insecticides*.

Chlorobutanol [198]

Chlorobutanol inhibits oral anticoagulants (enzyme induction).

Chloroform [1055]

See *Liver Function Depressors* below.

Chlorpromazine [330,332,453,930,951] **(Thorazine)**

Chlorpromazine diminishes the anticoagulant effect possibly

ANTICOAGULANTS ORAL *(continued)*

Chlorpromazine [330,332,453,930,951] (Thorazine)

Chlorpromazine diminishes the anticoagulant effect possibly by enhancing metabolism of the oral anticoagulants, but solid evidence is lacking. One report states that chlorpromazine enhances the anticoagulant action.[930] See also *Phenothiazines* below.

Chlorpropamide (Diabinese)

See *Antidiabetics, Oral* above.

Chlorthalidone (Hygroton)

See *Diuretics* below.

Cholestyramine [330,769,770,1281,1282,1379,1462,1590,1749] (Cuemid, Questran)

Cholestyramine may decrease the effect of oral anticoagulants by inhibiting or delaying their absorption and thus lowering their blood levels. However, vitamin K absorption may also be decreased and this tends to increase the anticoagulant effect. The resin usually prolongs the prothrombin time as determined by the Quick one-stage test. The anticoagulant should be administered at least 1 hour before or 4 to 6 hours after cholestyramine and the net effect on the specific patient monitored. See *Bile Salts* above.

Choloxin

See *Dextrothyroxine* below.

Chymotrypsin-trypsin [147,421]

Caution should be observed when using concomitantly. Potentiation of the anticoagulants may occur.

Cinchona alkaloids

See *Quinine, Quinidine,* and *Cincophen* below.

Cincophen [1113]

Intensified hypoprothrombinemia caused by cincophen in patients on anticoaguant therapy may be lethal.

Citrates [147,619] (ACD solution, etc.)

Citrates may cause an increase in prothrombin time and thus potentiate anticoagulants.

Clofibrate [137,147,180,223,344,393,394,868,911,999,1192,1338,1718,1820,1832] (Atromid-S)

Clofibrate may potentiate coumarin anticoagulants by displacing them from protein binding sites and by inhibition of hepatic microsomal enzymes. It may also potentiate anticoagulants by lowering lipoprotein and chloesterol levels and thus interfering with vitamin K transport to the liver, and also possibly by enhancing their affinity for their receptors and greatly depressing production of prothrombin and clotting factors VII, IX and X. The actual mechanism(s) have not been proven to cause the potentiation. Caution should be exercised when anticoagulants are given in conjunction with clofibrate. The dosage of the anticoagulant should be reduced by one-third to one-half (depending on the individual case) to maintain the prothrombin time at the desired level and prevent bleeding complications. Frequent prothrombin determinations are advisable until it has been definitely determined that the levels have been stabilized. The hemorrhagic complications have been fatal.

Congo red [147,619]

Congo red inhibits oral anticoagulants if given too rapidly or in excessive dosage (thromboplastic action).

Contraceptives, oral

See *Oral Contraceptives* below.

Contrast media [1834]

(Iodopyracet [Diodone, Diodrast], meglumine diatrizoate [Renografin], meglumine iothalamate [Conray], sodium diatrizoate [Hypaque], sodium methiodal [Skiodan])

Iodine containing drugs used for intravenous angiography and pyelography, during X-ray examinations may bind with coagulation factors in the blood in a transient manner and prolong prothrombin time and partial thromboplastin time,

expecially in the young. Possible additive hypoprothrombinemia.

Corticosteroids and corticotropin [180,646,727,903,905,907,982,1267,1876,1886]

Corticosteroids (adrenocorticosteroids) theoretically decrease the activity of oral coumarin anticoagulants because of their tendency to induce thrombotic episodes to antogonize the hypoprothrombininic effects of the anticoagulants by stimulating synthesis of clothing factors, and to cause adverse vascular effects. However, severe hemorrhage has occurred with the combination, possibly due to gastric erosion and ulcerogenic effects. Monitor patients on this combination carefully.

Dalmane

See *Flurazepam* below.

Dextran [147,912]

High doses of dextran may potentiate oral anticoagulants by decreasing fibrinogen levels.

Dextrothyroxine [147,346,393,394,411,898,1305,1370,1380] (Choloxin)

Dextrothyroxine enhances the anticoagulant effect. It decreases the concentration of clotting factors and platelet activity, and perhaps increases affinity for receptor sites. Reduce the dosage of anticoagulant by $\frac{1}{3}$ when dextrothyroxine therapy is begun, with subsequent adjustment and close monitoring of prothrombin time and other clotting factors. Withdraw the drug prior to surgery if use of anticoagulants is contemplated. See also *Thyroid Preparation* below.

Diazepam (Valium)

See *Benzodiazepines* above.

Diazoxide [180,784,1782] (Hyperstat)

Excessive hypoprothrombinemia and hemorrhage may result because diazoxide potentiates oral anticoagulants like warfarin by displacement from binding sites on human albumin.

Dietary deficiencies [120]

Deficiencies of ascorbic acid, choline, cystine, and protein increase prothrombin time response to oral anticoagulants.

Dietary fats and oils [4]

Dietary fats and oils increase anticoagulant response by decreasing vitamin K absorption.

Digitalis [673,930]

Digitalis should be given with caution to patients receiving oral anticoagulants since it may counteract their effects.

Diphenhydramine [83,120,223,1216] (Benadryl)

Diphenhydramine may decrease the effectiveness of oral anticoagulants through enzyme induction but this has not been confirmed in the laboratory or by controlled clinical studies.

Distalgesic [1161]

This drug, which contains paracetamol (acetaminophen) with Darvon, produced hematuria with warfarin. See *Anticoagulants, Oral* under *Acetaminophen.*

Disulfiram [570,1679,1684,1880] (Antabuse)

Disulfiram may enhance the anticoagulant effect of oral anticoagulants by inhibition of the metabolizing enzymes. Warfarin and disulfiram, for example, require and compete for the limited supply of nadide (nicotinamide adenine dinucleotide) phosphate on which the microsomal enzymes depend in order to metabolize both drugs. Thus the half-life of both drugs is prolonged and they are potentiated. Dosages must be reduced.

Diuretics [619,673,744,861,1135,1683]

Diuretics decrease the prothrombin time as determined by the Quick one-stage test. Drugs like furosemide and ethacrynic acid that cause a rapid diuresis, tend to antagonize anticoagulants because they tend to induce the formation of emboli and vascular thrombosis, decrease plasma water thereby concentrating clothing factors, and increase the excretion rate of the anticoagulant. They increase the activity of the intrinsic clotting system. By reducing hepatic congestion, thiazides improve liver function and thus enhance the synthesis of clotting factors which tend to antagonize oral anticoagulants, especially in patients on long term anticoagulant therapy.

Drugs affecting blood elements[951]
Any drug that interferes with the synthesis, elimination or functioning of clotting factors or other elements involved in the clotting process is likely to influence anticoagulant dosage.

Estrogens[28,134,170,411,619,861,905,906]
See *Oral Contraceptives* below. Estrogens, have a cholesterol lowering effect and tend to potentiate anticoagulants, but on the other hand, their coagulant action (thromboembolic effect) tends to antagonize the anticoagulants. Monitor the net effect carefully, because estrogens may increase vitamin K-dependent clotting factors as the major effect.

Ethacrynic Acid[784,1545,1808] (Edecrin)
See *Diuretics* above. On the other hand, however, ethacrynic acid tends also to potentiate anticoagulants like warfarin by displacement from albumin binding sites and may thus cause excessive hypoprothrombinemia and hemorrhage. Ethacrynic acid may also induce gastrointestinal bleeding. Monitor carefully.

Ethchlorvynol[9,98,120,147,180,1513] (Placidyl)
Ethchlorvynol may decrease anticoagulant response by shortening prothrombin time, possibly through enzyme induction which increases metabolism of coumarin derivatives. If it is withdrawn decrease the anticoagulant dose.

Fatty acids[421]
Fatty acids increase the anticoagulant effect by drug displacement from protein binding sites.

Fibrinolysin[4,5,619]
Fibrinolysin may potentiate anticoagulants.

Flufenamic acid
See *Anti-inflammatory Agents* above.

Flurazepam[1748] (Dalmane)
Flurazepam appears to cause no clinically significant interaction with oral anticoagulants. See *Benzodiazepines* above.

Foods[147,880]
Green leafy vegetables that contain vitamin K antagonize oral anticoagulants. See also *Onions* below.

Furosemide[147,619,673] (Lasix)
Furosemide inhibits oral anticoagulants. See *Diuretics* above.

Glucagon[10,710,1893]
Glucagon may strongly potentiate the anticoagulant effect of warfarin, possibly by increasing the affinity of warfarin for its receptors or by inhibiting synthesis of clotting factors. Use cautiously. Hemorrhaging has been reported.

Glutethimide[9,96,180,223,297,434,867,967,1877,1922] (Doriden)
Gluthethimide, through enzyme induction, increases metabolic degradation of coumarin derivatives and decreases their effect (shortens half-life by 50%). If this drug is withdrawn decrease the anticoagulant dose. Consider use of flurazepam or other benzodiazepine.

Griseofulvin[9,69,96,98,180,330,434,1192] (Fulvicin, Grifulvin, Grisactin)
Griseofulvin, formerly believed to induce the metabolizing enzymes for the oral anticoagulants and thus reduces their anticoagulant effect apparently may antagonize the anticoagulants by inhibiting or interfering with their gastrointestinal absorption. If this drug is withdrawn adjust the anticoagulant dose.

Guanethidine[180]
Guanethidine potentiates the anticoagulants.

Halofenate
See *Anticoagulants, Oral* under *Halofenate*.

Haloperidol[28,96,193,340] (Haldol)
Haloperidol may increase metabolism of coumarin derivatives. It has also been reported to antagonize the anticoagulant effect of phenindione (Danilone, Hedulin). Use with caution even though interference with the effects of phenindione has been reported in very few patients.

Heparin[120,134,673,891,892]
Heparin increases the anticoagulant effect of oral anticoagulants. Note that clinical laboratory results are influenced by heparin. When sodium heparin is given with bishydroxycoumarin, a period of from 4 to 5 hours after the last intravenous dose and 12 to 24 hours after the last subcutaneous (intrafat) dose of sodium heparin should elapse before blood is drawn, if a valid prothrombin time is to be obtained.

Hepatotoxic drugs[120]
Hepatotoxic drugs may increase the anticogulant effect of oral anticoagulants.

Heptabarbital[19,106,826,908,1055] (Medomin)
See *Barbiturates* above. Heptabarbital decreases the response to the anticoagulants largely by interfering with their absorption.

Hydrocortisone
See *Corticosteroids* above.

Hydroxyzine[120,673] (Atarax, Vistaril)
Hydroxyzine increases the prothrombin time as indicated by the Quick one-stage test but the company literature indicates that the drug does not alter patient response to the anticoagulants.

Ibuprofen[1247] (Motrin)
One preliminary study with ibuprofen and phenprocoumon (Liquamar) indicated no significant interaction between these drugs in 24 patients stabilized on long term anticoagulant.

Indomethacin[10,28,120,214,314,393,646,896,907,1545,1881,1927] (Indocin)
Indomethacin competitively displaces highly bound coumarin derivatives from protein binding sites, thus increasing the concentration of free coumarin anticoagulants in the plasma. Displacement of only a relatively small proportion may greatly increase concentration of unbound coumarin derivatives, prolong the prothrombin time, and cause severe bleeding. This has not been well demonstrated. Ulcerogenic medications like indomethacin which also depresses platelet function are hazardous in patients on anticoagulant therapy.

Insecticides[180] (Chlordane, DDT, etc.)
See these enzyme inducers under their specific name. They inhibit anticoagulants.

Insulin[120]
Oral anticoagulants enhance the hypoglycemic effects of insulin.

Iodine[907]
Iodine may potentiate anticoagulants (hypoprothrombinemic effect).

Iothiouracil[120,619] (Itrumil)
Iothiouracil has rarely caused hypoprothrombinemia, and under such circumstances could potentiate anticoagulants.

Isoniazid[421,1336,2066]
Isoniazid may increase the coumarin anticoagulants effect (enzyme inhibition). Studies in dogs show that the antitubercular drug elevates levels and the hypoprothrombinemic action of dicumarol. This interaction was partially confirmed clinically with warfarin in 1977.[2066]

428   *Table of Drug Interactions*

ANTICOAGULANTS ORAL *(continued)*
Kanamycin (Kantrex)
See *Antibiotics* above.

Laxatives
See *Cathartics* above.

Leafy green vegetables [147,880]
Large amounts of leafy green vegetables decrease the anticoagulant effect of oral anticoagulants.

Levothyroxine [330] **(Cytomel, etc.)**
See *Detrothyroxine* above and *Thyroid Preparations* below.

Librium
See *Benzodiazepines* above.

Liotrix [120] **(Levothyronine and Levothyroxine)**
Thyroid replacement therapy may potentiate anticoagulant effects with agents such as warfarin or bishydroxycoumarin. Reduce dosage of the anticoagulant by about ⅓. See *Thyroid Preparation* below.

Liver function depressors [890]
(Amethopterin, amodiaquin [Camoquin], anabolic steroids, cincophens, chlorpropamide [Diabinese], cyclophosphamide [Cytoxan], erythromycin, gold salts, isoniazid, methsuximide [Celontin], methyldopa [Aldomet], oleandomycins [Matromycin, TAO] organic arsenicals, oxyphenbutazone [Tandearil], phenacemide [Phenurone], phenothiazine tranquilizers, phenylbutazone [Butazolidin], pyrazinamide [Aldinamide], probenecid [Benemid], sulfonamides, testosterone and its derivatives and substitutes, tetracyclines, thiouracils, and urethane)
Agents that depress liver function may potentiate (cause hemorrhage with) anticoagulants. A partial list of implicated agents is given in the column to the left. This list is merely indicative and is far from complete. A longer list of hepatotoxic drugs is presented in Chapter 9. Agents such as chloroform and carbon tetrachloride which can induce hepatic necrosis, and diseases such as acute viral hepatitis, hepatic congestion associated with congestive heart failure, and nutritional deficiencies that impair liver function, increase the response to oral anticoagulants and therefore the risk of hemorrhage. [1055]

MAO inhibitors [134,193,223,359,861,885]
MAO inhibitors, particularly nialamide and tranylcypromine, potentiate oral anticoagulants, including acenocoumarol, ethylbiscoumacetate, warfarin, and phenindione, by inhibiting metabolism. Essentially all definitive studies reported have been conducted *in vitro* or in animals. Human studies are needed.

Mefenamic acid [147,673,784,1388,1489,1783] **(Ponstel)**
Mefenamic acid may potentiate oral anticoagulants. The acid itself prolongs prothrombin time and it may displace the anticoagulants from protein binding sites. It may also contribute to gastrointestinal hemorrhage. Severe or fatal hemorrhage may be induced.

Meprobamate [9,96,223,330,1293,1454,1870] **(Equanil, Miltown)**
Meprobamate has been shown to stimulate metabolic degradation of coumarin derivatives and thus decrease their effect although this has not been definitely shown in patients. If the psychochemical is withdrawn monitor the anticoagulant dose carefully.

Mercaptopurine (Purinethol) [180]
Mercaptopurine, probably by inhibiting synthesis of clotting factors as well as inhibiting activity of hepatic microsomal

enzymes, potentiates coumarin anticoagulants. Monitor closely and lower the dosage.

Metandienone [673]
Metandienone prolongs prothrombin time as determined by the Quick one-stage test.

Methandrostenolone [119,120,366] **(Dianabol)**
Methandrostenolone may enhance anticoagulant effect of oral anticoagulants by interfering with their metabolism and by the mechanisms given under *Clofibrate*. Hemorrhagic episodes may occur. See *Anabolic Steroids* above.

Methaqualone [120,619,1902,1922] **(Quaalude)**
Overdosage with the sedative may potentiate oral anticoagulants (enzyme induction) but normal doses appear to have only minor influence on metabolism of the anticoagulants. However, if methaqualone is instituted or withdrawn observe the patient carefully.

Methimazole [120,619] **(Tapazole)**
Methimazole has rarely caused hypoprothrombinemia and under such circumstances could potentiate anticoagulants.

Methotrexate [1294]
Additive hypoprothrombinemic effects may possibly occur. By adversely affecting the liver, methotrexate may induce a hypoprothrombinemia that is not treatable with vitamin K. Monitor both prothromlin time and hepatic function carefully.

Methyldopa [4,5,180,193] **(Aldomet)**
Methyldopa potentiates coumarin anticoagulants like bishydroxycoumarin (Dicumarol), possibly by a hepatic effect.

Methylphenidate [28,156,1466] **(Ritalin)**
Methylphenidate may potentiate the anticoagulant effect of oral anticoagulants by inhibiting the hydroxylating hepatic microsomal enzymes and thus decreasing their metabolism and prolonging their half-life. This CNS stimulant has prolonged the half-life of ethylbiscoumacetate administered in high dose to a patient also receiving phytonadione, but one report states that methylphenidate does not affect the half-life of the biscoumacetate.

Methylthiouracil
See *Thiouracils* below.

Mineral oil [35,120,193,421,1111,1649,1681]
Mineral oil tends to increase the anticoagulant effect by decreasing vitamin K absorption, but variable alterations of anticoagulant effect may occur due to mineral oil effect on anticoagulant absorption. See also *Cathartics* above.

Morphine [193,453,1055]
Morphine potentiates the anticoagulants. See *Narcotic Analgesics* below.

Nalidixic acid [784,1487] **(NegGram)**
Nalidixic acid displaces oral anticoagulants like warfarin from albumin binding sites and may thus cause excessive hypoprothrombinemia and hemorrhage.

Narcotic analgesics [120,134,147,453,861,1115,1216]
Prolonged use of narcotic analgesics may enhance the anticoagulant effect possibly by inhibiting one or more coagulation factors or by inhibiting microsomal enzymes.

Neomycin [234,1192,1415,1424,1470,1539,1601]
Neomycin may potentiate the hypoprothrombinemic action of oral coumarin anticoagulants in some patients. May prolong prothrombin time by impairing vitamin K absorption by inducing steatorrhea, or by acting on the mucosa, or by interfering with vitamin K production by gut bacteria. See also *Antibiotics* above.

Nicotinic acid [170,619,895]
Nicotinic acid may influence anticoagulant therapy. In large doses it may have a transient fibrinolytic activity and it affects the liver and lipoproteins.

Nitrazepam [1239,1351,1902] **(Mogadon)**
Like other benzodiazepines, nitrazepam appears to have little or no effect on oral anticoagulant therapy at usual dosages.

Norethandrolone [120,198,421,633] **(Nilevar)**
See *Anabolic Agents* above.

Nortriptyline [180]
See *Antidepressants, Tricyclic* above.

Onions [895]
Two ounces or more of boiled or fried onions increase fibrinolytic activity and may thus potentiate anticoagulant therapy.

Oral contraceptives [134,147,392,906,1102,1413]
(Estrogen-progestogens)
Oral contraceptives may decrease the anticoagulant effect of oral anticoagulants probably by increasing production of clotting factors. Dosage of the anticoagulants may require an increase. If they are withdrawn under these conditions, reduce the anticoagulant dose to avoid hemorrhage. In some patients, however, some contraceptives have had the opposite effect. Probably desirable for patients on anticoagulants to use another method of contraception.

Organic solvents [295,902]
(Carbon tetrachloride, etc.)
These solvents may cause hypoprothrombinemia through liver damage and thus potentiate coumarin anticoagulants.

Oxazepam (Serax)
See *Benzodiazepines* above.

Oxymetholone
See *Anabolic Agents* above.

Oxyphenbutazone [3,137,150,214,393,421,448,1915]
(Tandearil)
Oxyphenbutazone, a major physiologically active metabolite of phenylbutazone, has the same drug interactions. See *Phenylbutazone* below. However, the metabolite inhibits the clearance of anticoagulants from the plasma.

Papain [5,198,421,619] **(Papase)**
Papain (proteolytic enzymes) may increase anticoagulant effect of coumarin anticoagulants slightly. Concurrent use is not recommended.

Papase
See *Papain*.

Paracetamol [147,571,572]
See *Acetaminophen* above.

Paraldehyde [889]
Paraldehyde inhibits the anticoagulants, probably by its hepatotoxic action.

Penicillins [120,193,1216]
See *Antibiotics* above for oral pencillins. Apparently injected pencillin produces little or no interaction.

Phenformin [1471] **(DBI, Meltrol)**
Phenformin may increase fibrinolytic activity and produce a tendency for the patient to bleed even when prothrombin times are within the normal range. Observe patients on both drugs carefully. This drug was withdrawn from the US market in 1977 because of hundreds of fatal cases of lactic acidosis reported to FDA.

Phenobarbital [9,65,96,106,183,296,297,375,569,709,971]
(Phenobarbitone)
Phenobarbital inhibits the action of oral coumarin anticoagulants by stimulating the hepatic microsomal enzymes responsible for their metabolism. It decreases the biological plasma half-life of the coumarins by 50%. See *Barbiturates*. Serious and fatal hemorrhage has been reported after the withdrawal of phenobarbital in patients on oral anticoagulants. Oral anticoagulants, *e.g.*, dicumarol, inhibit the metabolism (*p*-hy-

droxylation) of phenobarbital and potentiate the sedative effect. Phenindone does not interfere.

Phenothiazines [330,332,453,1055]
Some phenothiazine (enzyme inducers) may inhibit oral anticoagulants, but strong evidence to date is lacking. See also *Antihistamines* above. In one study, in the absence of cholestatic hypersensitivity to the drug, the phenothiazine tranquilizers used did not alter clinical response by the patient to the anticoagulants. One paper indicated that chlorpromazine may potentiate the hypoprothrombinemic effect of acenoncoumarol. This interaction is probably not clinically significant.

Phenylbutazone [3,137,150,166,214,393,448,677,785,898,967,1192, 1267,1410,1680,1690,1914,1927]
Phenylbutazone may displace highly bound coumarin derivatives from protein binding sites (Warfarin is 99.5% bound). Displacement of a relatively small proportion of a coumarin derivative that is highly bound, particularly when given in high dosage, may greatly increase the concentration of unbound drug and acutely increase the anticoagulant effect with severe bleeding. Phenylbutazone also apparently potentiates warfarin in another manner. It inhibits oxidation of S-warfarin, the more potent of the two isomers of warfarin and stimulates elimination of the less potent R-isomer which is an enzyme inducer. Prolonged therapy with phenylbutazone, an enzyme inducer, inhibits drugs like bishydroxycoumarin, and larger doses may be necessary. But if the phenylbutazone is withdrawn, one or two weeks later hemorrhage may occur as the inhibitor (enzyme inducer) no longer is present. Monitor the net effect carefully. Concurrent administration of these two drugs is also very hazardous because of increased risk of gastrointestinal bleeding. The anti-inflammatory agent may induce peptic ulcers and impair platelet function as well as potentiate the prothrombinopenic effect of drugs like warfarin. See also *Oxyphenbutazone* above. The combination is *contraindicated*.

Phenylpropanolamine [466,951] **(Propadrine)**
This decongestant was reported to antagonize the oral anticoagulants.

Phenyramidol [78,120,330,705,706] **(Analexin)**
Phenyramidol may increase the anticoagulant effect by slowing the rate of metabolism in the liver (enzyme inhibition). No longer available in US.

Phenytoin [28,78,189,330,359,379,569,676,884,1213,1473,1816]
(Dilantin)
Phenytoin tends to increase the anticoagulant effect by displacing coumarin derivatives from plasma binding sites and prolonging the prothrombin time in some patients. On the other hand the hydantoin tends to inhibit the anticoagulants through enzyme induction. The net effect must be carefully monitored. Coumarin anticoagulants potentiate Dilantin for a prolonged period by inhibiting its enzymatic para-hydroxylation in the liver and may cause drug intoxication due to the increased serum concentration of the hydantoin. (Phenindione does not interact in this manner.) Because of the complexity of the interaction between phenytoin and dicumarol, usually try to avoid the combination.

Phytonadione [48,120,180,330]
(Vitamin K₁, AquaMephyton, Konakion, Mephyton)
Phytonadione restores prothrombin in the blood and thus tends to antagonize coumarin anticoagulants.

Primidone [120,147,165,619] **(Mysoline)**
Primidone, which is metabolized to a barbiturate (phenobarbital) and phenylethylmalonamide usually inhibits oral anticoagulants by enzyme induction. If it produces blood dyscrasias as side effects it will tend to potentiate the anticoagulants. Close monitoring is necessary with this combination.

ANTICOAGULANTS ORAL *(continued)*

Probenecid [147,930] (Benemid)
Probenecid may potentiate oral anticoagulants by decreasing their rate of excretion.

Propylthiouracil [9,120,134,147,193,330,421,861,893]
See *Thiouracils* below.

Protamine sulfate
See *Protamine Sulfate* under *Heparin.*

Proteolytic enzymes [5,147,198,421,619]

(Bromelains, Chymotrypsin, Papain, Trypsin, Streptodornase, Streptokinase, etc.)
See *Papain.*

Psyllium [1749]
Psyllium (Metamucil) does not affect the gastrointestinal absorption of warfarin.

Pyrazolone derivatives [3,10,150,214,393,1914]

(Antipyrine, Aminopyrine, Phenazone, Oxyphenbutazone, Phenylbutazone, Sulfinpyrazone, etc.)
Pyrazolone derivatives may increase the anticoagulant effect of highly protein bound coumarin anticoagulants by displacing them from the secondary binding sites. Some of these derivatives are also ulcerogenic in the gut. See *Phenylbutazone* above and *Sulfinpyrazone* below.

Quinine, quinidine, and cincophen [158,234,260,582,707,890,898,1055]

Cincophen, quinine and quinidine directly depress prothrombin formation in the liver and inhibit synthesis of clotting factors and thus tend to potentiate the anticoagulant effects of coumarin derivatives (synergistic effect). Hemorrhage has occurred, but the validity of some of the reports has been questioned.

Radioactive compounds [9,134,180,421,861]
Radioactive compounds and X-radiation may prolong prothrombin time and thus tend to cause hemorrhage with anticoagulants. (Potentiation by hepatic damage.)

Reserpine [180,193,453,1680]
Reserpine which may exaggerate prothrombin response has been reported to potentiate coumarin anticoagulants with long-term therapy but antagonizes them with short-term therapy. Monitor patients on oral anticoagulants closely when starting or withdrawing reserpine.

Rifamycin and derivatives [120,725,1306,1355,1685,1874,1969] (Rifampin, Rimactane, Rifadin, etc.)
Rifampin, possibly by enzyme induction, increases the metabolism and elimination of warfarin (doubles dosage requirement) and acenocoumarol (probably other coumarin anticoagulants) and inhibits their anticoagulant activity. Monitor patients on anticoagulants closely when starting or withdrawing rifampin. See also *Antibiotics* above.

Salicylates [9,907,1192,1227,1288,1299,1344,1345,1372,1409,1569,1619,1674,1683,1723,1832,1854]

Contraindicated. Salicylates (aspirin, etc. but not salicylamide) in large doses (>1 Gm. daily) depress prothrombin formation in the liver and also displace oral anticoagulants from protein binding sites. They have an antivitamin K effect (synergistic effect), are ulcerogenic, depress platelet function, and can cause gastrointestinal bleeding. These actions may lead to severe hemorrhage in the presence of anticoagulants. This interaction, although highly variable from one patient to another, may be lethal when a patient on anticoagulants leaves a hospital, for example, and begins to consume OTC drugs containing aspirin. Warn patients carefully.

Secobarbital [9,223,296] (Seconal)
Inhibits the effects of oral coumarin anticoagulants by stimulating the hepatic microsomal enzymes responsible for their

metabolism. It decreases the biologic plasma half-life of the coumarins markedly.

Sedatives and hypnotics [198,421,1055]
Oral anticoagulants are inhibited by sedatives such as barbiturates and glutethimide through enzyme induction. Chloral hydrate may potentiate anticoagulants.

Serax
See *Benzodiazepines.*

Simethicone [1843] (Mylicon)
Simethicone (dimethyl polysiloxanes with silica aerogel) appears to inhibit the action of anticoagulants (warfarin, phenindione) by decreasing gastrointestinal absorption.

Sitosterols [330,619,910]
Sitosterol and other drugs that lower lipoprotein and cholesterol levels may potentiate anticoagulants by interfering with vitamin K transport to the liver.

Skeletal muscle relaxants [890]
Skeletal muscle relaxants may potentiate (cause hemorrhage with) anticoagulants.

SKF 525-A [391,950] (Proadifen)
SKF 525-A, a microsomal enzyme inhibitor, may potentiate coumarin anticoagulants.

Smoking [633]
See *Benzpyrene* above.

Stanozolol (Stromba, Winstrol) [2054]
Stanozolol, an anabolic steroid, potentiates anticoagulants. Apparently this C-17 alkylated steroid impairs synthesis of vitamin-K-dependent clotting factors by diminishing stores of this vitamin which competes metabolically with oral anticoagulants. See *Anabolic Agents* above.

Steroids, anabolic
See *Anabolic Steroids* above.

Streptokinase-streptodornase [120]
See the action of proteolytic enzymes under *Papain* above. Streptokinase parenterally enhances fibrinolytic activity, and thus may potentiate anticoagulants.

Streptomycins [330,1415,1424,1470,1539,1601,1681]
Streptomycin has been associated with production of an inhibitor of blood factor V and thus may potentiate anticoagulants. See also *Antibiotics* above (potentiation).

Sulfamethoxypyridazine [21,433] (Midicel)
Enhanced antibacterial activity and increased toxicity. The acidic drugs displace the long acting sulfonamide from its plasma binding sites. The slowly metabolized and excreted "sulfa" diffuses into skeletal muscle, cerebral spinal fluid and the brain.

Sulfasuxidine
See *Sulfonamides* below.

Sulfinpyrazone [147,180,278,395,930,1521,1690] (Anturane)
Sulfinpyrazone, a uricosuric, may potentiate oral anticoagulants by elevating their blood levels through displacement from protein binding. Sulfinpyrazone also may have value as an adjunct in preventing thromboembolic disorders since it blocks platelet aggregation due to antigen-antibody complexes and collagen (not to ADP or thrombin). See *Pyrazolone Derivatives* above.

Sulfisoxazole [234] (Gantrisin)
See *Sulfonamides* below.

Sulfonamides [21,120,647,869,1415,1424,1470,1539,1601,1681,1974]
Sulfonamides, especially the long-acting, potentiate some anticoagulants by displacing them from secondary binding sites. They may also prolong prothrombin time by interfering with vitamin K synthesis by bacteria in the gut. Reduced dosage of the anticoagulant may be needed. For example, a patient on warfarin for several months was given sulfisoxa-

zole (500 mg. every 6 hours for 14 days). His prothrombin time changed from 20 seconds to 60 seconds during 2 weeks and on admission to the hospital had hematuria, gingival bleeding, and hemoptysis.[1974] Potentiation of anticoagulants by sulfonamides may be delayed for 2 weeks or more. A few highly bound agents such as ethyl biscoumacetate, however, are able to displace the long-lasting, albumin-bound sulfonamides (Gantrisin, Midicel, Sulfabid, Sulla) from plasma protein. These sulfas are not rapidly metabolized or excreted. Thus, displaced sulfonamide molecules diffuse from plasma into tissues with increased antibacterial activity and possibly severe toxicity.

Sulfonylureas [568,677] (Tolbutamide, etc.)
See *Antidiabetics, Oral* above.

Testosterone [930]
Testosterone enhances anticoagulant action.

Tetracyclines [120,234,909,1415,1424,1470,1539,1601,1681,1777]
Tetracyclines may potentiate the effects of oral coumarin anticoagulants. Tetracyclines given IV may reduce prothrombin activity (impaired utilization of prothrombin in the coagulation process). See *Antibiotics* above for the effect on vitamin K synthesis.

Theophylline [6,166,890]
Theophylline and other xanthines may increase formation of prothrombin and clotting factor V and thus tend to antagonize the anticoagulants but significant impact on coagulation has not been demonstrated.

Thiazides [744,1135,1683]
See *Diuretics* above.

Thiouracils [9,120,134,147,180,193,330,421,861,890,893,1112]
(Antibason, Itrumil, Methiocil, Propacil, etc.)
Thiouracils may potentiate anticoagulant response by decreasing vitamin K absorption and possibly by inhibiting prothrombin production. At least one hyperthyroid patient with bleeding, however, was found to have received an overdosage of Dicumarol because of a mix-up with the physically similar antithyroid tablets containing propylthiouracil.

Thioureas [897]
These drugs have a synergistic action with the anticoagulants similar to that of quinidine, quinine and salicylates.

Thrombin [120,619]
Thrombin, a hemostatic blood fraction, antagonizes anticoagulants.

Thyroid preparations [9,330,393,394,408,411,1475,1587,1610,1734,1871,1889]
(Levothyroxine, liothyronine, thyroglobulin, thyroid extract, triiodothyronine, etc.)
Hypothyroid patients tend to be resistant to anticoagulants and require larger doses. Thyroid replacement therapy may potentiate the anticoagulant effects of agents such as warfarin or bishydroxycoumarin by enhancing their affinity for their receptors and greatly reducing the levels of prothrombin and vitamin K-dependent clotting factors VII, IX and X through enhanced catabolism of these factors and reducing availability of vitamin K. Hemorrhage may occur. On the other hand patients already stabilized on a thyroid preparation may be started on carefully titrated anticoagulants with normal precautions. Reduce by one-third the anticoagulant dosage upon initiation of thyroid replacement therapy.

d-Thyroxine [9,408,411] (Choloxin)
See *Dextrothyroxine* and *Thyroid Preparations* above.

Tolbutamide [28,359,568,677,886] (Orinase)
Coumarin compounds may strongly potentiate the hypoglycemic effect of tolbutamide by inhibiting its degradation by drug metabolizing enzymes in the liver. Its half-life is appreciably prolonged. (260% in one study). Tolbutamide potentiates oral anticoagulants by displacement from protein binding sites, but the degree of effect is influenced by order and timing of drug administration. Tolbutamide tends to produce an initial increase in prothrombin time in patients stabilized on an anticoagulant. Monitor carefully. Tolbutamide is an enzyme inducer in some patients and with prolonged therapy may conceivably inhibit the anticoagulant and necessitate higher dosage. If for some reason the patient is switched to insulin, hemorrhage might occur a week or two later.

Triclofos [1233,1781] (Triclos)
A metabolite (trichloroacetic acid) of triclofos (trichloroethyl dihydrogen phosphate) displaces the oral anticoagulant warfarin from plasma protein binding sites and thus potentiates the anticoagulant action initially. The effect diminishes after about a week and practically disappears in two weeks. See also *Chloral Hydrate* above.

Trifluperidol [147] (Psychoperidol)
This antipsychotic agent, by enzyme induction, inhibits oral anticoagulants. Not marketed in the U.S.

Triiodothyronine [421,673] (Cytomel)
See *Thyroid Preparations* above.

Tromthamine [147,619] (Tham-E)
Tromethamine may increase prothrombin time and thus potentiate anticoagulants.

Trypsin [27,180,421]
Proteolytic enzymes like trypsin may potentiate the anticoagulant action of these agents.

Urea [619]
Urea, with its fibrinolytic activity, may potentiate anticoagulants.

Urokinase [901,904]
Urokinase, by its thrombolytic action, may potentiate anticoagulants and cause hemorrhage.

Valium
See *Benzodiazepines* above.

Vitamin B complex [48]
Vitamin B complex increases prothrombin time and may cause hemorrhage with anticoagulants.

Vitamin C [963,1117,1144,1319,1495,1810,1896]
Vitamin C, in large doses, shortens the prothrombin time in patients receiving coumarin anticoagulants. A dose of 1 Gm. daily of the vitamin did not appear to interact in one series of patients.[1144] Some anticoagulants induce the excretion of vitamin C. Monitor patients for change in anticoagulant effect if vitamin C is begun or withdrawn. Some patients consume large quantities of the vitamin in attempts to ward off colds and do not realize they are taking a drug which can interact with other drugs and alter the metabolic situation.

Vitamin E
See *Warfarin* under *Vitamin E.*

Vitamin K [48,120,180,330,1055]
(Fish, green leafy vegetables, polyvitamin preparations)
Vitamin K (in foods and drugs) decreases prothrombin time by stimulating synthesis of clotting factors and thus tends to antagonize coumarin anticoagulants. Phytonadione is highly effective in opposing the action of the coumarin anticoagulants but menadione and its water-soluble salts are relatively ineffective in reversing hypoprothrombinemia induced by anticoagulants. A number of intestinal diseases (chronic diarrhea, intestinal fistula or obstruction, sprue, ulcerative colitis, ulcerative jejunoileitis) prevent vitamin K absorption and thus increase response to the oral anticoagulants. However, these diseases may also decrease absorption of the anticoagulants. The precise net effect must be closely monitored.

X-ray
See *Radioactive Compounds* above.

ANTICOAGULANTS ORAL *(continued)*

Xanthines [120,1740]
(Caffeine, theobromine, theophylline, etc.)
Large doses of xanthines may antagonize the anticoagulant effect. They shorten the prothrombin time (as determined by the Quick one-stage test) by increasing factor V and plasma prothrombin. Response to oral but not IV bishydroxycoumarin (Dicumarol) was decreased by methylxanthines (in rabbits).

ANTICONVULSANTS
(Barbiturates, benzodiazepines [Librium, Valium, etc.], carbamazepine [Tegretol], phenytoin [Dilantin], primidone [Mysoline], etc.)
See *Barbiturates, Phenytoin, Ethosuximide, Glutethimide, Phenacemide,* etc.
Many of the anticonvulsants are enzyme inducers and through this mechanism inhibit many drugs. But acetylureas [Benuride] [166] and benzodiazepines may inhibit excretion (metabolism?) and thus increase plasma levels of some drugs. See *Barbiturates* and *Phenytoin* under *Benzodiazepines.*

Aminosalicylic acid (PAS) [294,884,919]
Aminosalicylic acid decreases the metabolism of anticonvulsants and may thus potentiate them.

Anticoagulants, oral [189,569,884]
(Dicumarol, Panwarfin, Sintrom, etc.)
Oral anticoagulants decrease the metabolism of anticonvulsants and may thus potentiate them. See *Barbiturates* and *Phenytoin* under *Anticoagulants, Oral.*

Antidepressants, tricyclic
(Elavil, Pertofrane, Tofranil, etc.)
High doses of a tricyclic antidepressant may precipitate seizures; dosage of the anticonvulsant may have to be decreased. See *Barbiturates* and *Phenytoin* under *Antidepressants, Tricyclic.*

Barbiturates [78]
Barbiturates inhibit themselves (tolerance) and other anticonvulsants by enzyme induction.

Cycloserine [120] (Seromycin)
Anticonvulsant drugs or sedatives may be effective in controlling symptoms of CNS toxicity, such as convulsions, anxiety, and tremor caused by cycloserine.

Diazepam [120] (Valium)
When diazepam is used as an adjunct in treating convulsive disorders, alteration of the dose of the drugs may be necessary. Barbiturates, narcotics, phenothiazines and some other anticonvulsant agents potentiate diazepam.

Ethamivan [120] (Emivan)
Ethamivan is an antidote for the severe respiratory depression caused by overdosage of CNS depressants like barbiturates. However, this antidote must be continued until the depressant drug is removed by detoxification or dialysis.

Ethosuximide [120] (Zarontin)
Ethosuximide combined with other anticonvulsants may produce an increase in libido.

Folic acid [1229]
Folic acid replacement therapy should only be used with anticonvulsants whose blood levels can be carefully followed. Correction of folic acid deficiency, commonly produced by anticonvulsants, may cause loss of seizure control on the one hand or drug toxicity on the other.

Haloperidol [120] (Haldol)
Haloperidol potentiates the CNS depressant action of barbiturates but not the anticonvulsant action nor that of other anticonvulsants. The dose of the anticonvulsant should not be altered when haloperidol therapy is initiated; however, subsequent adjustment may be necessary.

Hydrocortisone [78,84,330,450]
Some anticonvulsants inhibit hydrocortisone by enzyme induction.

Isoniazid [202,294,333,789]
Isoniazid decreases the metabolism of anticonvulsants and thus may potentiate them.

MAO inhibitors [198,421]
The influence of MAO inhibitors on the convulsive threshold is variable; the dosage of anticonvulsants may have to be lowered because of potentiation.

Methylphenidate [156] (Ritalin)
Methylphenidate potentiates some anticonvulsants and may induce severe toxic reactions (enzyme inhibition).

Narcotic analgesics [120,166,421]
Narcotic analgesics potentiate CNS depressants including anticonvulsants. In susceptible patients or overdosage, severe respiratory depression, coma, and even death may occur. See *CNS Depressants.*

Phenacemide [120] (Phenurone)
Special caution is advised since paranoid symptoms have been induced with ethotoin and phenacemide.

Phenobarbital [63,64,78,83,96,940,647]
Phenobarbital increases the metabolism of some other anticonvulsants and thereby inhibits them. See *Hydantoins* under *Phenobarbital.*

Phenothiazines [120]
Phenothiazines can lower the convulsive threshold in susceptible individuals; an increase in the dosage of the anticonvulsant may be necessary.

Phenytoin [619] (Dilantin)
Phenytoin may potentiate other anticonvulsants which are central nervous system depressants.

Primidone [120] (Mysoline)
Primidone has a synergistic effect with other anticonvulsants such as diphenylhydantoin, mephenytoin, and mephobarbital. As the dosage of other anticonvulsants is maintained or gradually decreased, the dosage of the anticonvulsant primidone should be gradually increased. The transition from other anticonvulsants to primidone should not be completed in less than two weeks.

Rauwolfia alkaloids [120] (Reserpine, etc.)
These agents can lower the convulsive threshold in susceptible individuals; an increase in the dosage of the anticonvulsant may be necessary.

Reserpine
See *Rauwolfia Alkaloids* above.

Thioxanthenes [120]
(Chlorprothixene [Taractan], etc.)
Thioxanthenes, like the phenothiazines, can lower the convulsive threshold in susceptible individuals; an increase in the dosage of the anticonvulsant may be necessary.

Vitamin D [1147,1148]
Anticonvulsant drugs, such as phenobarbital, phenytoin and primidone, through enzyme induction increase the metabolism of vitamin D and increase the requirement for it. Thus osteomalacia tends to develop in treated epileptics. Hypercalcemia and renal calcification due to vitamin D intoxication can be reduced by barbiturates, etc.

ANTIDEPRESSANTS, TRICYCLIC (Dibenzazepine and dibenzocycloheptadiene compounds; amitriptyline [Elavil], clomipramine [Anafranil]; desipramine [Norpramin, Pertofrane], doxepin [Adapin, Sinequan], imipramine [Imavate, Janimine, Presamine, SK-Pramine, Tofranil], nortriptyline [Aventyl], protriptyline [Vivactil]).
These drugs have anticholinergic properties and block the

uptake of some drugs by adrenergic neurons. Also, as weak bases, their gastrointestinal absorption and urinary excretion are influenced by pH. Other properties that are the basis for interactions are the orthostatic hypotension, the vagal blockade, the cocainelike effect (blockade of uptake of administered norepinephrine [Levophed]) which supersensitizes the patient to catecholamines, the psychotogenic action in susceptible individuals, and the parkinsonismlike symptoms that occur in older persons. These tricyclics may also produce ataxia, hypothermia and sedation.

Acetazolamide [325,952,1458,1806] (Diamox)

Acetazolamide, a urinary alkalinizer, tends to shift tricyclic antidepressants to the nonionized state, thereby increasing tubular reabsorption, enhancing blood levels, and increasing the action. Probably only significant with high dosage. See *Alkalinizing Agents* below.

Acidifying agents [172,194,325,870,952,1458,1806]
(Ammonium chloride, ascorbic acid, methionine, sodium acid phosphate, etc.)

Acidifying agents decrease gastrointestinal absorption and increase the urinary excretion of weak bases like the tricyclic antidepressants and thereby tend to inhibit their effects.

Adrenalin
See *Norepinephrine* below.

Adrenergic blockers [433,598]
(Inderal, Priscoline, Regitine, etc.)

β-Adrenergic neuron blockers like guanethidine, bethanidine, etc. are antagonized by tricyclic antidepressants. See *Antidepressants, Tricyclic* under *Guanethidine.* α-Adrenergic blocking agents like phenoxybenzamine, phentolamine, tolazoline, some phenothiazines (chlorpromazine) and butyrophenones (haloperidol), etc., as well as the β-blocker propranol inhibit the hyperthermia induced by a tricyclic antidepressant in fully reserpinized subjects (rats).

Adrenergics
See *Norepinephrine* below.

Alcohol [48,71,290,629,729]

A potentially lethal combination. Contraindicated. Tricyclic antidepressants potentiate the sedative effects of alcohol; CNS depression and severe hypothermic coma may be produced. Motor skills (driving and handling machinery) are impaired.

Alkalinizing agents [194,325,579,870,952,1458,1806,1986]
(Diamox, potassium citrate, sodium bicarbonate, etc.)

Alkalinizing agents tend to increase gastrointestinal absorption (sodium bicarbonate, antacids, etc.) and decrease urinary excretion (acetazolamide, thiazide diuretics, etc.) of weak bases like these tricyclics and thereby potentiate them. Sodium bicarbonate, however, is useful in correcting the acidosis of tricyclic antidepressant overdosage. [1986]

Ammonium chloride
See *Acidifying Agents* above.

Amphetamines [404,423,424,1027,1724,1923]

Enhanced activity of either the tricyclic or sympathomimetic agent may result. Imipramine, like atropine, potentiates the increase in operating rate produced by amphetamine in conditioning situations. The cardiovascular effects of catecholamines can also be potentiated through release of norepinephrine. Amphetamine levels may be enhanced by enzyme inhibition (inhibition of hydroxylation). Exercise caution.

Anticholinergics [5,78,194,619,623,814,1221,1639]
(Antihistamines, antiparkinsonism drugs, Demerol, Doriden, phenothiazines, etc.)

Tricyclic antidepressants potentiate the atropinelike effects of anticholinergics and drugs with anticholinergic side effects (see introduction to *Anticholinergics*). Hazardous in glaucoma. The weak anticholinergic activity of some tricyclics is additive, and may cause paralytic ileus, blurred vision, constipation, urinary retention, tachycardia, drowsiness, pupil dilation, dry mouth, etc. in combination with anticholinergics. Monitor closely when a tricyclic antidepressant such as imipramine is combined with a phenothiazine (Etrafon, Triavil, etc.). Pyridoxine may be useful. See *Pyridoxine* below.

Anticholinesterases [120,166,168,619]

The useful miotic effect of anticholinesterases in glaucoma is antagonized by tricyclic antidepressants with their anticholinergic effect. Physostigmine, an anticholinesterase that crosses the blood-brain barrier, effectively reverses the anticholinergic effects (athetosis, choreoathetosis, coma, delirium, and myoclonus) of tricyclic-antidepressant overdosage.

Anticoagulants, oral
See *Antidepressants, Tricyclic* under *Anticoagulants, Oral.*

Anticonvulsants [120,359]

Tricyclic antidepressants potentiate the effects of anticonvulsants; high doses of a tricyclic may precipitate seizures; dosage of the anticonvulsant may have to be changed. See *Phenytoin* below.

Antidepressants [120]

Combined use of tricyclic antidepressants and other antidepressants may cause hazardous potentiation. Cross sensitization between the tricyclics may occur. MAO inhibitor antidepressants are particularly hazardous and are contraindicated.

Antihistamines [194]

The atropinelike effects of both types of drugs are enhanced (additive effect). Hazardous in glaucoma. One combination drug of imipramine 10 mg. and the antihistamine chloropyramine 10 mg. taken during the first trimester of pregnancy apparently played an etiologic role in congenital malformation.

Antihypertensives [78,120,626]

Tricyclic antidepressants antagonize antihypertensives. Reduced dosage of the antihypertensive is frequently necessary if the tricyclic is withdrawn, in order to prevent profound hypotension. See also *Guanethidine* below and *Doxepin* under *Bethanidine.*

Antiparkinsonism agents [5,78,194,623,814]

Since the tricyclics possess weak anticholinergic activity this effect may be enhanced with antiparkinsonism agents having anticholinergic activity such as trihexyphenidyl and cycrimine. Hazardous in glaucoma.

Antipyrine [82,1879]

Tricyclic antidepressants like nortriptyline inhibit the metabolism of antipyrine and thus prolong its plasma half-life and increase its toxicity.

Aspirin [219]
See *Salicylates* below.

Atropine derivatives [120]

The anticholinergic action of atropine and tricyclics may be enhanced (additive effect). See *Anticholinergics* above.

Barbiturates [71,94,116,194,756,959-961,1198,1273,1365,1472,1665,1759,1799,1805]

The tricyclics may potentiate the hypnonarcotic and sedative effects of barbiturates. Preoperative administration of imipramine (probably other tricyclic antidepressants) potentiates thiopental anesthesia. Severe hypothermia may occur. Barbiturates, taken in excess, may potentiate adverse CNS depressant effects of the tricyclic antidepressants (respiratory depression) but on continued use microsomal enzyme induction by barbiturates eventually tends to inhibit the tricyclic

ANTIDEPRESSANTS, TRICYCLIC *(continued)*

depressants. Use of barbiturates in tricyclic antidepressant overdosage is contraindicated. The convulsions and other toxic effects may be more safely treated with diazepam (Valium) or paraldehyde.

Benzodiazepines [78,120,166,953,954,1358,1468,1544,1799] (Librium, Serax, Valium)

The sedative and atropinelike effects of the benzodiazepines and the tricyclic antidepressants may be potentiated. The depressive syndrome may be potentiated until a clinical picture which simulates brain damage may develop. Although these additive effects are recognized some psychiatrists use chlordiazepoxide with the tricyclics safely with properly adjusted dosage. Monitor patients on these drugs carefully for weakness, drowsiness, and possible increased depression in some patients. High doses may be potentially lethal. Warn patients about impaired motor function in driving and handling machinery.

Bethanidine [327,433,598,823] (Esbatal)

A combination of the adrenergic blocker bethanidine with desipramine or protriptyline and possibly other tricyclics may result in antagonism through blockage of bethanidine uptake into site of action, and may cause complete reversal of the action of the antihypertensive agent. Antagonism may persist for a week after withdrawal of the tricyclic.

Bishydroxycoumarin [1879]

See *Antidepressants, Tricyclic* under *Anticoagulants, Oral.*

Carbamazepine [120] (Tegretol)

Carbamazepine is structurally related to tricyclic antidepressants; therefore, it should not be used with them or for at least one week after discontinuing therapy with one of them.

Carbrital [120]

The tricyclics potentiate carbrital (carbromal plus pentobarbital).

Carisoprodol [599]

The tricyclics potentiate the actions of carisoprodol.

Catecholamines [194,433]

See *Epinephrine, Isoproterenol,* and *Levartenenol (Norepinephrine)* below.

Chlordiazepoxide (Librium)

See *Benzodiazepines* above.

Chlorprothixene (Taractan)

See *Thioxanthenes* below.

Chlorpromazine

See *Antidepressants, Tricyclic* under *Phenothiazines.*

Cholinergics [166,168] (Neostigmine, physostigmine, etc.)

The activity of cholinesterase inhibitor type cholinergics is inhibited by tricyclic antidepressants (anticholinergic activity).

CNS depressants [120,166,421] (Alcohol, phenothiazines, thioxanthenes, etc.)

These drugs may potentiate the sedative and hypotensive effects of the tricyclic antidepressants (additive effects). May be potentially lethal. See *CNS Depressants.*

Corticosteroids [120]

Corticosteroids increase ocular pressure during long-term use with tricyclic antidepressants. Hydrocortisone notably inhibited the metabolism of nortriptyline in a patient who had taken an overdose of this drug.

Debrisoquin [194,598,823]

Same as for *Bethanidine* above.

Dextroamphetamine

See *Antidepressants, Tricyclic* under *Amphetamines.*

Diazepam (Valium)

See *Benzodiazepines* above.

Diazepine derivatives [94] (chlordiazepoxide, diazepam)

The convulsions produced by overdosage of drugs like desipramine can be best controlled with an anticonvulsant like diazepam. See also *Benzodiazepines* above for potential hazard.

Disulfiram [1272,1446,1592,1720] (Antabuse)

The disulfiram reaction with alcohol is potentiated by amitriphyline and probably other tricyclic antidepressants. Exercise caution since this interaction could be lethal.

Diuretics [120,194] (Diamox, Diuril, etc.)

Carbonic anhydrase inhibitors such as acetazolamide, and thiazides and other alkalinizers of the urine may potentiate antidepressants by increasing their tubular reabsorption.

Epinephrine and norepinephrine [404,424,1105,1245-6]

Tricyclic antidepressants enhance adrenergic effects with these catecholamines. The interaction may differ with the antidepressant. Thus, imipramine in low doses potentiates the pressor response to exogenous epinephrine and norepinephrine by enhancing the excitability of the effector cell, but in high doses it has a sympatholytic effect on adrenergic transmission and an adrenolytic effect on the receptor cell. On the other hand, amitriptyline reverses the pressor response to exogenous epinephrine and potentiates the pressor response to exogenous norepinephrine. See also *Norepinephrine* below.

Ethchlorvynol [120,226] (Placidyl)

Transient delirium has been reported with the combination of amitriptyline and ethchlorvynol.

Furazolidine [1098] (Furoxone)

Furazolidone potentiates antidepressants; acute psychosis possible. MAO and microsomal enzyme inhibition. See *MAO Inhibitors* below.

l-Glutavite [120,619]

l-Glutavite potentiates the psychotropic effects (alkalosis and hypokalemia).

Guanethidine (Ismelin)

See *Antidepressants, Tricyclic* under *Guanethidine.*

Haloperidol [166,1456-7] (Haldol)

Tricyclic antidepressants increase the sedative effects of haloperidol. See *CNS Depressants.* Haloperidol may inhibit metabolism and decrease urinary excretion of the tricyclics and thus potentiate their effects.

Hexobarbital [71,116,194] (Sombucaps, Sombulex, etc.)

See *Barbiturates* above.

Hypotensive agents [120] (Thiazide diuretics, phenothiazines, vasodilators)

Since the tricyclics may cause orthostatic hypotension caution should be observed when other agents that lower the blood pressure are given concomitantly.

Isoproterenol [94,1245] (Isuprel)

The severe hypotension produced by overdosage of tricyclic antidepressants may be reversed with isoproterenol. See *Norepinephrine* below.

Levarterenol (Levophed)

See *Norepinephrine* below.

Levodopa [486,715] (Dopar, Larodopa)

Tricyclic antidepressants potentiate the action of levodopa in parkinsonism.

Mandrax [623]

This combination causes disorders of the nasal and oral areas (dry mouth, swollen tongue, cracking at angles of mouth), disorientation, dizziness, etc.

MAO inhibitors
(Eutonyl, Furoxone, Marplan, Matulane, Nardil, Niamid, Parnate, etc.)

See *Antidepressants, Tricyclic* under *MAO Inhibitors*.
The tricyclics supersensitize adrenergic receptors to catecholamines which accumulate because of MAO inhibition and blockage of their uptake by the tricyclics.

MAO inhibitor antidepressants [12,29,53,120,633,874]

See *MAO Inhibitors*. A MAO inhibitor like Eutonyl given for hypertension plus an antidepressant MAO inhibitor can cause agitation, delirium, fever, tremor, opisthotonus, and coma. Two MAO inhibitors such as Eutonyl and Parnate given together can cause a hypertensive crisis, possibly death. However, some physicians recommend the use of such potentially lethal combinations in severely depressed patients. [1049]

Meperidine and analogs [166,194,421]
(Demerol, etc.)

Tricyclic antidepressants potentiate the atropinelike anticholinergic and respiratory depressant effects with meperidine and its analogs. Hazardous in glaucoma. See also *CNS Depressants* above.

Mephentermine [823] (Wyamine)

The potency of indirectly acting pressor agents like mephentermine is diminished by tricyclic antidepressants.

Methyldopa [194,452,823] (Aldomet)

Tricyclics do not alter the hypotensive action of methyldopa since it does not enter the adrenergic neurons by the NE pump.

Methylphenidate [156,194,957,1366,1900,1923] (Ritalin)

Methylphenidate, the psychomotor stimulant, may inhibit the metabolism of imipramine, desipramine and other tricyclics. It should be used cautiously with such antidepressants as it tends to potentiate them, not only their beneficial but also their toxic effects. The tricyclics also potentiate the stimulation of operant behavior by methylphenidate, perhaps by central sensitization to adrenergic action.

Muscle relaxants, centrally acting [166]

Centrally acting muscle relaxants increase the sedative effects of all CNS depressants. The tricyclics have a sedative action.

Narcotic analgesics [120,421]

Tricyclic antidepressants potentiate the CNS depression with narcotic analgesics; narcotic analgesics potentiate the sedation produced by tricyclic antidepressants. See *CNS Depressants* above.

Nitrates and nitrites [421]

Organic nitrates and nitrites potentiate the hypotensive effect of tricyclic antidepressants.

Noradrenaline

See *Norepinephrine* below.

Norepinephrine [166,194,417,433,619,823,941,946,1245-6]
(Levarterenol)

Tricyclic antidepressants increase the pressor effects of norepinephrine (levarterenol), epinephrine (catecholamines), amphetamines and other sympathomimetics many fold, but not isoproterenol (isoprenaline). They block uptake of these amines and supersensitize to catecholamines. The tricyclics intensify the hyperthermia produced by levarterenol. The activity of either the tricyclic or sympathomimetic agents may be enhanced. Desipramine-induced hyperthermia requires the presence of norepinephrine. The tricyclic increases its concentration at receptors.

Oral contraceptives

See *Antidepressants, Tricyclic* under *Oral Contraceptives*.

Organophosphate cholinesterase inhibitors [166]

The tricyclic antidepressants with their anticholinergic properties antagonize the miotic effect of acetylcholinesterase inhibitors.

Oxazepam (Serax)

See *Benzodiazepines* above.

Oxyphenbutazone [85,863,1301] (Tandearil)

The tricyclic antidepressants, like imipramine and desipramine, may inhibit the gastrointestinal absorption of oxyphenbutazone.

Pargyline [120] (Eutonyl)

See *MAO Inhibitors* above.

Parstelin [1077] (Parnate plus Stelazine)

This drug product combined with imipramine has resulted in several fatalities.

Perphenezine [1457] (Trilafon)

See *Antidepressants, Tricyclic* under *Phenothiazines* which have a metabolizing enzyme inhibitory effect on the tricyclics.

Phenothiazines

See *Antidepressants, Tricyclic* under *Phenothiazines*.

Phenylbutazone [85,863,1301] (Butazolidin)

Imipramine or desipramine may delay the intestinal absorption of phenylbutazone, and thus inhibit the drug, because of the anticholinergic action on the gut. Since phenylbutazone is restricted to short term use this interaction can be significant.

Phenylephrine [1245-6] (Neo-Synephrine)

Tricyclic antidepressants increase the pressor response to phenylephrine by infusion 2- or 3-fold. See *Epinephrine* and *Norepinephrine* above.

Phenytoin [120,1056] (Dilantin)

High doses of tricyclics may precipitate seizures. They lower the seizure threshold and dosage of the anticonvulsant may have to be modified accordingly. Tricyclics are displaced from protein binding sites by the anticonvulsant and may thus be potentiated. The highly lipophilic basic antidepressants are extensively bound (91-99%).

Physostigmine

See *Anticholinesterases* above.

Pilocarpine

An antidote for dry mouth. See *Chlorpromazine* under *Pilocarpine*.

Procarbazine [330,619] (Matulane)

Avoid this combination. See *MAO Inhibitors* above.

Propranolol (Inderal)

See *β-Adrenergic Blockers* above.

Pyridoxine [1188]

Pyridoxine (25 mg. 2 to 4 times a day) combats dry mouth, dysuria, urinary retention and other anticholinergic side effects of imipramine and the other tricyclics.

Rauwolfia alkaloids

See *Reserpine* below.

Reserpine

See *Antidepressants, Tricyclic* under *Reserpine*.

Salicylates [219]

A potentially lethal combination. The outcome was fatal for a patient who ingested an overdose of aspirin while receiving imipramine, in spite of every effort to revive her.

Sedatives [166,421]

The sedative effects are potentiated (additive effect). Contraindicated. See *CNS Depressants* above.

ANTIDEPRESSANTS, TRICYCLIC *(continued)*

Sympathomimetics [194,417,433,619,946]
Mutual potentiation; enhanced activity of either agent may result. See *Norepinephrine* above.

Tetrabenazine [399]
Tricyclic antidepressants inhibit the depression induced by tetrabenazine.

Thiazide diuretics [120,166,194]
Since the tricyclics may cause orthostatic hypotension caution should be observed when other agents that lower the blood pressure, such as thiazide diuretics, are given concurrently.

Thioxanthenes [166,1457] (Taractan)
See *CNS Depressants* above. Thioxanthenes such as chlorprothixene (Taractan) may inhibit metabolism (ring hydroxylation) of antidepressants such as nortriptyline and thus potentiate their effects.

Thyroid medications [5,456,529,670,934]
See *Antidepressants, Tricyclic* under *Thyroid Preparations.*

Tranquilizers, minor [194,198,619]
Additive CNS depression and sedation. See *Benzodiazepines* and *CNS Depressants* above. The tricyclics potentiate the anticholinergic and sedative effects of certain tranquilizers. May lower the convulsive threshold and potentiate seizures.

Urinary acidifiers
See *Acidifying Agents* above.

Vasodilators [5]
The hypotension produced by vasodilators may be additive to the orthostatic hypotension produced by the tricyclic antidepressants. Appropriate dosage adjustment may be necessary.

Veratrum alkaloids [421]
The tricyclics diminish the hypotensive action of these alkaloids.

Yohimbine [951]
Tricyclic antidepressants may enhance the toxicity of yohimbine.

ANTIDIABETICS, ORAL

(Acetohexamide [Dymelor], chlorpropamide [Diabinese], tolazamide [Tolinase], tolbutamide [Orinase], etc.).
See also *Acetohexamide, Chlorpropamide, Tolbutamide,* and *Insulin* for specific interactions reported for these drugs.
All oral antidiabetics (oral hypoglycemics) now marketed are sulfonylureas. Tolbutamide is carboxylated in the liver to form a nonhypoglycemic metabolite. Tolazamide and 3 of its 6 metabolites are hypoglycemic. Acetohexamide and its single metabolite are hypoglycemic. [1533]

Acetazolamide [1556]
Acetazolamide may markedly elevate blood glucose in diabetics receiving oral antidiabetics with a prolonged disturbance. Monitor dose carefully.

Acidifying agents [421]
Acidifying agents potentiate weak acids like the sulfonylureas by decreasing the rate of their urinary excretion.

β-Adrenergic blockers [1,42] (Inderal, etc.)
β-Adrenergic blockers increase the activity of oral antidiabetics; mask hypoglycemic symptoms and dampen rebound of plasma glucose levels. See *Antidiabetics* under *Propranolol.*

Adrenocorticosteroids [421]
See *Corticosteroids* below.

Alcohol [144,254,334,381,634,674,675,740,741,1266,1280,1318,1340,1360, 1515,1552,1560,1653,1721,1751,1786,1795,1803,1937-9,2029]
Alcohol, if ingestion is chronic and heavy, induces metabolism of oral antidiabetics, thus shortening their half-lives as much as 50% and inducing hyperglycemia. Acetohexamide may not be affected as much as other oral antidiabetics because its metabolite, produced in large quantities, is also hypoglycemic. Alcohol itself has some potential hypoglycemic action which may be additive. Monitor patients closely. Can be lethal. Alcohol, by inhibiting release of ADH, diminishes the antidiuretic action of chlorpropamide and causes polyuria and polydipsia in patients being treated for ADH-sensitive diabetes insipidus. [1937-9] Sulfonylurea antidiabetics block alcohol metabolism and thereby potentiate the acetaldehyde effects. Angina pectoris and a disulfiramlike reaction may result from the alcohol intolerance produced. This reaction, however, is apparently not due to elevated acetaldehyde levels with chlorpropamide, even though its metabolite (*p*-chlorobenzenesufonamide) is a sulfonamide and this class of chemicals usually causes such a reaction through inhibition of acetaldehyde dehydrogenase. See also *Insulin* under *Alcohol.*

Allopurinol [1702] (Zyloprim)
Allopurinol may potentiate chlorpropamide (possibly other sulfonylureas) perhaps by competing in the renal tubular secretion process.

Anabolic steroids [120,383,1550,1565,1822]
The anabolics in general enhance the hypoglycemic effect of oral antidiabetics through an additive effect and possibly inhibition of the metabolizing enzymes. Exceptions are methenolone (Primobolan) and nandrolone (Durabolin) which do not have a potentiating effect. Reduce the dosage of the oral antidiabetic.

Anticoagulants, oral [28,78,147,266,359,412,633,768,886] (Anticoagulants, coumarin)
Oral anticoagulants enhance the hypoglycemic effect of sulfonylureas by inhibiting drug metabolizing enzymes, and possibly decreasing urinary excretion. Bishydroxycoumarin increases the plasma half-life of chlorpropamide from 40 to 90 hours. The order of administration affects the interaction. See also *Tolbutamide* and *Antidiabetics, Oral* under *Anticoagulants, Oral.* Oral antidiabetics (sulfonylureas but not phenindione) may potentiate coumarin anticoagulants at first by displacing them from protein binding sites, then after a few days induce the hepatic microsomal enzymes to increase their metabolism and decrease their hypoprothrombinemic effect.

Antipyrine
See *Antidiabetics, Oral* under *Antipyrine.*

Aspirin
See *Salicylates* below.

Barbiturates [74,421,433,619,695]
The antidiabetics may prolong the hypnotic and sedative effects of barbiturates. However, tolbutamide reduces the sleeping time with hexobarbital by activation of microsomal enzymes.

Bishydroxycoumarin (Dicumarol)
See *Anticoagulants, Oral* above.

Blood cholesterol lowering agents [421,619] (Clofibrate, etc.)
Blood cholesterol lowering agents potentiate oral antidiabetics by drug displacement.

Chloramphenicol [676,767,1702] (Chloromycetin)
Chloramphenicol may strongly potentiate the hypoglycemic effects of both insulin and the oral hypoglycemic agents by enzyme inhibition. This interaction has prolonged the half-life of tolbutamide several fold to as high as 146 hours and has caused severe hypoglycemia.

Chlorpromazine [243,429] (Thorazine)
See *Phenothiazines* below.

Chlorthalidone [164,386] **(Hygroton)**

Chlorthalidone, by direct toxic effect on the pancreas, may produce hyperglycemia with both insulin and oral antidiabetics by diminishing insulin secretion and reserve. See also *Diuretics* and *Thiazides* below.

Clofibrate [421,619,1378,1383,1702] **(Atromid-S)**

Clofibrate, an antihyperlipidemic, potentiates oral antidiabetics, especially in patients with lowered plasma albumin levels, possibly through drug displacement or because of competition in the renal tubular secretion process, and reduced insulin resistance. Clofibrate decreases fasting plasma glucose and improves glucose tolerance (hypoglycemic effect).

Coffee [1384,1386]

Coffee consumption by a mature-onset diabetic may elevate blood glucose levels by increased stress on the pancreatic β-cells (tend to antagonize oral antidiabetics). The opposite is true (decreased blood glucose) when coffee is drunk by healthy nondiabetics.

Contraceptives, oral

See *Oral Contraceptives* below.

Corticosteroids [4a,120,191,1442,1853]

Corticosteroids, because they cause elevation of blood glucose levels (increase hepatic glycogenesis and gluconeogenesis, decrease peripheral glucose utilization, alter enzyme levels in carbohydrate metabolism, and impair insulin secretion by suppression of β-cell function), may antagonize the hypoglycemic effect of both insulin and the oral antidiabetic agents. See *Diabetogenic Drugs* below. The hyperglycemic action of corticosteroids may be augmented by immunosuppressants. See under *Vaccines*.

Coumarin anticoagulants [78]

See *Anticoagulants, Oral* above.

Cyclophosphamide [203,513] **(Cytoxan)**

Cyclophosphamide potentiates the hypoglycemic effect of insulin possibly by inhibiting formation of antibody to which insulin is bound and freeing insulin from its binding sites.

Dextrothyroxine [120,408,421,1305] **(Choloxin)**

Dextrothyroxine antagonizes the hypoglycemic effect of both insulin and oral hypoglycemics.

Diabetogenic drugs [312]

Corticosteroids, thiazides and other diabetogenic drugs may be contraindicated with oral antidiabetics near the age when maturity-onset diabetes occurs because of the additive insult.

Diazoxide [1514] **(Hyperstat)**

Tolbutamide decreases the hypotensive and oliguric effects of diazoxide.

Disulfiram [1364]

Disulfiram does not affect the metabolism of tolbutamide, according to one report.

Diuretics [152,164,229,386,415,619]

See also *Thiazides* below. Many diuretics (chlorthalidone, ethacrynic acid, furosemide, triamterene, etc.) in addition to thiazides increase blood glucose, perhaps by depressing insulin secretion, and thereby antagonize all antidiabetics. But the acidic drugs like ethacrynic acid potentiate oral antidiabetics by displacing them from secondary binding sites. Monitor the net effect.

Epinephrine [168]

Epinephrine, by its hyperglycemic action (promotes glycogenolysis and inhibits uptake of glucose by peripheral tissues) may inhibit the effects of oral hypoglycemic agents.

Estrogens [181,886]

Estrogens antagonize oral antidiabetics. Blood glucose levels may be increased; higher dosage of the hypoglycemic agent may be necessary.

Ethacrynic acid [421] **(Edecrin)**

See *Diuretics* above.

Fenfluramine [1867]

Fenfluramine, by increasing skeletal muscle uptake of glucose, exerts a hypoglycemic action which can be additive in patients on oral antidiabetics.

Furosemide (Lasix)

See *Diuretics* above.

Glucagon [1264,1670]

Glucagon, a potent hyperglycemic agent in severe hypoglycemia, antagonizes oral antidiabetics. If used in diabetics for its positive inotropic effect in heart failure, monitor patients carefully for possible loss of diabetic control.

Guanethidine [187,1463,1464] **(Ismelin)**

Guanethidine possesses hypoglycemic activity and an increase in antidiabetic dosage may be necessary when guanethidine is withdrawn from diabetics on oral anticoagulants or a decreased dosage when guanethidine is started in such patients. See *Antidiabetics* under *Guanethidine*.

Halofenate [1943] **(Livipas)**

Halofenate, an antihyperlipidemic like clofibrate above, potentiates sulfonylurea antidiabetics.

Insulin [421]

Insulin, in combination with oral antidiabetics, increases the hypoglycemic effect.

Isoniazid [178,191]

Isoniazid in large doses induces hyperglycemia and thus antagonizes the hypoglycemic effect of oral hypoglycemics and insulin.

Levothyroxine [120,421] **(Letter, Synthroid, etc.)**

Levothyroxine antagonizes the hypoglycemic action. Patients taking oral antidiabetics may require increased amounts. See *Thyroid Preparations* below.

MAO inhibitors [86,87,1024,1226,1262]

MAO inhibitors potentiate sulfonylurea hypoglycemics and insulin. Enhanced and possibly dangerous hypoglycemic effects. See *MAO Inhibitors*.

Marijuana [1586,1709,1944]

Marijuana may decrease glucose tolerance and increase the oral antidiabetic requirements of diabetics. Marihuana ingestion has resulted in diabetic ketoacidosis.

Methyldopa [120] **(Aldomet)**

Methyldopa potentiates blood dyscrasias with oral antidiabetics.

Nicotinic acid [182,888]

Large doses of nicotinic acid are diabetogenic and can cause an increase in blood glucose levels and thus antagonize antidiabetics. Larger doses of the antidiabetic drugs are needed.

Oral contraceptives [120,886,1371,1727,1827]

Oral contraceptives, taken with antidiabetics, may increase blood sugar levels and decrease glucose tolerance. The hypoglycemic action of both insulin and oral antidiabetics may be antagonized. Other forms of contraception may be preferable for diabetics.

Oxyphenbutazone [191,359] **(Tandearil)**

Same as for *Phenylbutazone* below.

Oxytetracycline [1484,1636] **(Terramycin)**

Oxytetracycline appears to have some hypoglycemic action and thus potentiates oral antidiabetics. Adjust dosage downward if necessary. See also *Antibiotics* above and *Tetracyclines* below.

Phenformin [120,1373] **(DBI, Meltrol)**

Phenformin, the only biguanide oral antidiabetic made available, potentiates sulfonylurea antidiabetics (additive hypogly-

ANTIDIABETICS, ORAL *(continued)*

cemic effect). However, after phenformin caused several hundred deaths from lactic acidosis over a period of years it was removed from the market by FDA in 1977.

Phenothiazines [120,191,243,421,1218,1380,1381,1852,1928,2013-23]

Some phenothiazines may induce glycosuria and hyperglycemia and thus are antagonistic to antidiabetics, possibly by activating adrenergic mechanisms. Diabetics may go out of control if chlorpromazine or some other phenothiazines are given to some patients. On the other hand hypoglycemia may be produced in some patients. Each patient on both drugs must be closely monitored until mechanisms are better established. In one study chlorpromazine reduced the hypoglycemic effect of tolbutamide in 6 patients. [2013] However, chlorpromazine delayed restoration of normal glucose levels in guinea pigs treated with tolbutamide, phenformin, or buformin. [2014] In some animal studies chlorpromazine had no effect on insulin activity. [2015-7] In other studies it decreased insulin activity. [2018-21] In acute experiments in dogs chlorpromazine antagonized the effect of insulin on glucose utilization whereas in chronic experiments it enhanced the effect of insulin. [2022] In acute experiments in rabbits, chlorpromazine had no effect on insulin whereas in chronic experiments it increased sensitivity to insulin. [2023]

Phentolamine

See *Antidiabetics* under *Phentolamine*.

Phenylbutazone [28,76,141,359,680,768,1315,1382,1479,1689,1807,1845,1864,1954] (Butazolidin)

Phenylbutazone potentiates sulfonylurea hypoglycemics; enhanced hypoglycemic effect by displacing the hypoglycemics from protein binding sites, inhibiting metabolism (e.g., carboxylation of tolbutamide), or inhibiting renal clearance of the drug (chlorpropamide), or inhibiting urinary excretion of metabolites (acetohexamide). Hypoglycemic coma has been reported a number of times. [1382,1479,1845] In one case phenylbutazone appeared to antagonize the hypoglycemic action of tolbutamide. [1689] Monitor dosage closely as death may occur. See *Antidiabetics, Oral* under *Phenylbutazone*.

Phenylpropanolamine [168]

Phenylpropanolamine which tends to elevate blood glucose levels may oppose the action of oral hypoglycemic agents.

Phenytoin [1574,1757,1936,1955,1957]

Phenytoin antagonizes antidiabetics through its hyperglycemic effect caused by inhibition of insulin secretion mediated through the hypothalamus and adrenergic system or a lowering of the beta cell membrane potential. The sulfonylureas increase phenytoin toxicity.

Potassium [1300,1439,1828]

Potassium chloride given by prolonged infusion potentiates the hypoglycemic effect of acetohexamide. Potassium aids glucose utilization and induces insulin secretion.

Probenecid [28,59,418,421,1377,1702] (Benemid)

Probenecid potentiates some oral antidiabetics by inhibiting their urinary excretion (inhibiting renal tubular secretion) but does not interfere with the renal excretion of tolbutamide, and thus does not potentiate this drug unless the glomerular filtration is impaired considerably.

Procarbazine (Matulane)

See *MAO Inhibitors* above.

Propranolol (Inderal)

See *Antidiabetics* under *Propranolol* and *β-Adrenergic Blockers* above.

Pyrazinamide [619] (Aldinamide)

Diabetes mellitus may be more difficult to control during therapy with pyrazinamide. Expect altered dosage of oral antidiabetics in patients on this tuberculostatic drug.

Pyrazolone derivatives [421] (Antipyrine, Butazolidin, etc.)

Pyrazolone derivatives potentiate oral antidiabetics. See *Phenylbutazone* above.

Rifampin [1945-7]

Rifampin, through induction of hepatic microsomal enzymes, increases the rate of metabolism of tolbutamide and probably the other sulfonylurea antidiabetics, thus decreasing their half-lives and necessitating higher doses.

Salicylates [73,350,359,418,458,649,1237,1382,1533,1702]

Salicylates (aspirin, etc.) potentiate sulfonylurea hypoglycemics by drug displacement from protein binding sites [458] and by an additive hypoglycemic action; enhanced hypoglycemic effect. Inhibition of sulfonylurea excretion has also been suggested. Chlorpropamide may increase salicylate blood levels and add to this source of hypoglycemic activity. Aspirin has been reported as a contributor to hypoglycemic coma. [73,350]

Sedatives and hypnotics [78]

Sulfonylureas potentiate sedatives.

Sodium bicarbonate

See *Alkalinizing Agents* above.

Steroids [950,951]

Steroids may increase blood glucose levels.

Sulfaphenazole (Orisul)

See *Sulfonamides* below.

Sulfinpyrazone [120,165,1521,1953] (Anturane)

Sulfinpyrazone may enhance the hypoglycemic effect of antidiabetics by the same mechanisms as *Phenylbutazone* above since they are structurally similar. One case of insulin potentiation with sulfinpyrazone has been reported. See *Pyrazolone Derivatives* and *Phenylbutazone* above.

Sulfisoxazole [76,191,359] (Gantrisin)

See *Sulfonamides* below.

Sulfonamides [76,359,409,680,1237,1316,1797,1865] (Gantrisin, Orisul, etc.)

Some sulfonamides potentiate oral antidiabetics by drug displacement from protein binding and by inhibiting metabolism (carboxylation); enhanced hypoglycemic effect. The interaction between tolbutamide and sulfaphenizole (Sulfabid) is well documented. Hypoglycemic coma may occur. Sulfaphenazole increased the half-life of tolbutamide from 5 to 21½ hours. Some oral antidiabetics may improve the antibacterial action of some sulfonamides.

Tetracyclines [1949-52]

Tetracyclines enhance the hypoglycemic effect of antidiabetic agents (tolbutamide, etc., and insulin), possibly by interfering with carbohydrate metabolism (Krebs cycle, etc.) and by binding insulin within the pancreas. Hypoglycemia may occur. Adjust the dosage.

Thiazides [120,164,386,619] (Diuril, Naturetin, etc.)

See also *Diuretics* above. Thiazides, which may be diabetogenic, may antagonize both insulin and oral antidiabetics; may aggravate glucose intolerance. May cause hyperglycemia. Sulfonylurea and insulin requirements in diabetic patients may be increased, unchanged, or decreased by thiazides depending on various factors. Insulin shock may occur. Chlorpropamide causes hyponatremia with thiazides and may cause resistance to the diuretic action. Monitor closely.

Thyroid preparations [4a,120,421]

In patients with diabetes mellitus, thyroid hormone therapy may necessitate an increase in the required dosage of oral hypoglycemic agents. Decreasing the dose of thyroid hormone may possibly cause hypoglycemic reactions if the dose of oral agents is not adjusted. Oral antidiabetics may increase the effect of thyroid preparations. Careful monitoring is essential.

d-Thyroxine
See *Dextrothyroxine* above.

Tolbutamide [181,257] (Orinase)
Patients may develop a tolerance to a given sulfonylurea by enzyme induction, and a gradual increase in the dosage may be necessary. Use of another sulfonylurea may resolve the problem.

Triamterene [421] (Dyrenium)
See *Diuretics* above.

Vasopressin [421]
Oral antidiabetics potentiate vasopressin.

ANTIDIARRHEAL MEDICATION
(Attapulgite, kaolin, pectin, etc.)

Antibiotics [120,330]
Oral antibiotics of high molecular weight may be contraindicated with some antidiarrheal agents because of physical adsorption and poor absorption.

Lincomycin [330,1042] (Lincocin)
When an attapulgite-pectin suspension (Kaopectate) is given with capsules of lincomycin, only ⅛ of the control level of the antibiotic may be absorbed gastrointestinally due to physical adsorption.

Promazine [1043] (Sparine)
Attapulgite and citrus pectin inhibit the absorption of promazine from the gut. See also *Phenothiazines.*

ANTIEMETICS
(Cyclizine [Marezine], dimenhydrinate [Dramamine], diphenidol [Vontrol], etc.)

Levodopa [724]
Antiemetics are capable of defeating the therapeutic purpose of levodopa in Parkinson's syndrome.

Mepivacaine [120,619] (Carbocaine)
Excessive premedication with antiemetics prior to local anesthesia must be avoided in infants, young children, and the elderly. CNS depression and extrapyramidal effects may cause problems with some medications.

Toxic drugs [5,120]
The toxic effects of some drugs, such as digitalis, may be masked by the antiemetics. Caution is necessary.

ANTIFIBRINOLYTIC AGENTS (Amicar, etc.)

Anticoagulants, oral [120,619,901]
Antifibrinolytic drugs such as aminocaproic acid, by suppressing fibrinolytic activity, antagonize anticoagulants. See *Aminocaproic Acid* under *Anticoagulants, Oral.*

ANTIFUNGALS
See *Amphotericin B, Griseofulvin,* etc.

ANTIGOUT DRUGS
(Allopurinol [Zyloprim]; colchicine; oxyphenbutazone [Tandearil]; phenylbutazone [Azolid, Butazolidin]; probenecid [Benemid]; sulfinpyrazone [Anturane], etc.)
See under specific drugs. Antigout drugs include the anti-inflammatory agent *Colchicine,* used specifically for acute attacks of gout; the inhibitor of uric acid biosynthesis, *Allopurinol;* and the uricosuric drugs which inhibit renal tubular reabsorption of uric acid and thus increase its excretion, *Probenecid, Sulfinpyrazone, Oxyphenbutazone,* and *Phenylbutazone.* The latter two drugs, because of their high toxicity, are used for short-term anti-inflammatory therapy in acute attacks of gout and not for long-term uricosuric action.

Alcohol
See *Hyperuricemics* below.

Allopurinol [120] (Zyloprim)
Concurrent administration may result in a marked decrease in urinary excretion of oxypurines, compared with their excretion with allopurinol alone. However, combination therapy may provide the best control for many patients.

Antineoplastics, cytotoxic
See *Hyperuricemics* below.

Aspirin
See *Salicylates* below.

Chlorothiazide
See *Hyperuricemics* below.

Diuretics [120,421]
(Edecrin, Thiazides, and Xanthines)
Some diuretics antagonize uricosuric agents by decreasing the renal excretion of uric acid. See *Hyperuricemics* below.

Ethacrynic acid [120,421] (Edecrin)
Ethacrynic acid antagonizes the uricosuric action of Benemid, etc. See *Diuretics* above.

Ethambutol
See *Hyperuricemics* below.

Hyperuricemics [172]
Many drugs (alcohol, cytotoxic antineoplastics such as thiotepa, certain diuretics such as chlorothiazide, ethambutol, levodopa, xanthines, etc.) tend to elevate plasma uric acid levels and are therefore antagonistic to uricosuric agents. Avoid these drugs or give higher doses of the uricosurics as necessary.

Levodopa
See *Hyperuricemics* above.

Salicylates [28,120,467,651]
Salicylates (aspirin, etc.) can inhibit the action of uricosuric agents; decreased prophylaxis of gout.

Thiazides
See *Diuretics* and *Hyperuricemics* above.

Thiotepa
See *Hyperuricemics* above and *Uricosurics* under *Thiotepa.*

Xanthines (caffeine, theobromine, etc.)
See *Diuretics* and *Hyperuricemics* above.

ANTIHISTAMINES
(Brompheniramine maleate [Dimetane], carbinoxamine (Clistin) maleate, chlorcyclizine [Perazil] HCl, chlorpheniramine [Chlor-Trimeton], clemizole [Allercur, Reactrol], cyproheptadiene [Periactin] HCl, dextrobrompheniramine maleate [Disomer], dexchlorpheniramine maleate [Polaramine], dimethindene [Forhistal] maleate, diphenhydramine HCl [Benadryl], diphenylpyraline HCl [Diafen, Hispril], methapyrilene [Histadyl, Thenylene, etc.], methdilazine [Tacaryl] HCl, pheniramine maleate [Trimeton], promethazine [Phenergan] HCl, pyrrobutamine [Pyronil] phosphate, trimeprazine tartrate [Temaril], tripelennamine [Pyribenzamine] HCl or citrate, triprolidine HCl [Actidil], etc.). Properties of these drugs that are the basis of interactions with other drugs include the anticholinergic, antihistaminic, adrenergic blocking, CNS depressant, enzyme inducing, ganglionic blocking, and quinidinelike cardiac actions. Antihistamines may or may not possess all of these and they possess them in varying degrees. Some antihistamines have CNS stimulant action.

ANTIHISTAMINES *(continued)*

Acenocoumarol (Sintrom)
See *Anticoagulants, Oral* below.

Acetylcholine
See *Antihistamines* under *Acetylcholine.*

Acidifying agents [325,870]
Acidifying agents increase the urinary excretion of weak bases like the antihistamines and tend to inhibit them.

Adrenergics [169,232,242,483] ·
Some antihistamines may increase the pressor effect of adrenergics. Some antihistamines (chlorpheniramine, tripelennamine, etc.) have a cocainelike effect on adrenergic transmission. They prolong the response to nervous stimulation, potentiate the response to norepinephrine, and inhibit the response to tyramine.

Alcohol [121,311,421,619,634]
Antihistamines potentiate the sedative effects of alcohol. Alcohol potentiates the CNS depression produced by the antihistamines. See *CNS Depressants.*

Alkalinizing agents [165,325,870]
Alkalinizing agents decrease the urinary excretion of weak bases like antihistamines and tend to potentiate them.

Amphetamines [169]
Amphetamines may be combined with antihistamines to counteract the sedative effect.

Androstenedione [330] (Androtex)
Antihistamines inhibit androstenedione.

Analeptics [169]
Analeptics are not recommended in antihistamine intoxication as they tend to initiate or potentiate the convulsive phase.

Analgesics [619]
Potentiation. See *CNS Depressants.*

Anesthetics, general [619]
Potentiation. See *CNS Depressants.*

Anticholinergics [78,198,487,488,633]
Antihistamines (phenothiazine derivatives) potentiate the CNS depressant and atropinelike effects of anticholinergics (atropine, etc.). A hazardous combination in glaucoma. Also, when an antihistamine like diphenhydramine is given with an anticholinergic like trihexyphenidyl or imipramine, the drug-induced xerostoma may cause dental caries, loss of teeth, etc.

Anticholinesterases [169,488,913,914]
(Floropryl, Humorsol, Phospholine, etc.)
Antihistamines with anticholinergic properties antagonize the antiglaucoma (miotic) and CNS effects of anticholinesterases. Anticholinesterases potentiate the tranquilizing and behavioral changes induced by antihistamines.

Anticoagulants, oral [64,223,479,481,555,673]
(Coumadin, Dicumarol, Panwarfin, Sintrom, etc.)
Antihistamines may decrease the anticoagulant effect by enzyme induction.

Antidepressants, tricyclic [194]
See *Antihistamines* under *Antidepressants, Tricyclic.*

Antihypertensives [626]
Tripelennamine and pyrilamine partly reverse the adrenergic blocking action of guanethidine but promethazine has no effect.

Barbiturates [64,116,421,479,481,619,633]
Antihistamines may increase the depth and duration of barbiturate narcosis; preoperative administration of an antihista-mine potentiates thiopental anesthesia. But there may eventually be mutual inhibition with continued use. Chlorcyclizine, diphenhydramine and probably other antihistamines, through enzyme induction, may then decrease the activity of the barbiturate and vice versa. May result in barbiturate tolerance and habituation.

Beta-adrenergic blockers [421] (Inderal, etc.)
Beta-adrenergic blockers antagonize antihistamines.

Betahistine HCl [120,421]
Betahistine antagonizes antihistamines and vice versa; concurrent use not recommended.

Betazole [421] (Histalog)
Betazole antagonizes antihistamines and vice versa.

Caffeine [169]
Caffeine may be prescribed with antihistamines to counteract the sedative effect.

Carbazochrome salicylate [120] (Adrenosem)
Antihistamines antagonize carbazochrome salicylate.

Carbrital [120]
Antihistamines potentiate Carbrital.

Cholinergics [169]
Antihistamines diminish the activity of cholinesterase inhibitor type of cholinergics.

CNS depressants [276,421,621-625]
Antihistamines potentiate the sedative effect of all CNS depressants. Many somnifacient, analgesic and cold remedies sold over-the-counter contain such combinations, *e.g.,* antihistamines plus bromides, scopolamine, salicylates, etc. See also *CNS Depressants.*

Corticosteroids [78,198,421,485]
Antihistamines decrease the effects of the steroids due to enzyme induction. Corticosteroids increase ocular pressure in long term therapy. Dangerous in glaucoma.

Desoxycorticosterone [65,479,485] (Doca, Percorten)
Some antihistamines may inhibit this steroid by enzyme induction (increased hydroxylation).

Diphenhydramine HCl [64,480,555] (Benadryl)
Tolerance develops through induction of its own metabolizing enzyme; results in decreased activity.

Epinephrine [232,242,483,484]
Enhanced adrenergic cardiovascular effects. Same as for *Norepinephrine* below.

Estradiol [65,479,485]
Antihistamines may inhibit estradiol by enzyme induction (increased hydroxylation).

Furazolidone [120] (Furoxone)
Antihistamines should be used in reduced doses and with caution when the MAO inhibitor, furazolidone, is given concomitantly.

Glutethimide [120] (Doriden)
This combination may cause increased CNS depressant effects. With continued use glutethimide may antagonize antihistamines by enzyme induction, and vice versa. See also *CNS Depressants.*

Griseofulvin [64] (Grifulvin, etc.)
Antihistamines (chlorcyclizine, diphenhydramine, etc.) inhibit griseofulvin by enzyme induction.

Guanethidine [626] (Ismelin)
Certain antihistamines, *e.g.,* tripelennamine but not pyrilamine or promethazine, antagonize the adrenergic blocking action of guanethidine. See *Adrenergics* above.

Heparin [181,764]
Antihistamines may antagonize the anticoagulant activity of heparin.

Histamine [169,421]
Antihistamines are competitive antagonists of histamine.

Hydrocortisone [421,485]
Antihistamines inhibit hydrocortisone by enzyme induction.

Hyoscine [168] **(Scopolamine)**
The enhanced sedative effect with this combination is used in many over-the-counter sleeping remedies.

Hyposensitization therapy [78]
Antihistamines interfere with evaluation of therapy and if they are withdrawn during therapy may cause a generalized systemic reaction.

Insecticides, halogenated [485]
(Aldrin, chlordane, DDT, endrin, heptachlor, lindane, etc.)
These insecticides, by enzyme induction, inhibit the action of antihistamines.

Levarterenol [198,421,483] **(Levophed)**
Antihistamines enhance the cardiovascular toxicity of levarterenol. See *Antihistamines* under *Levarterenol*.

Lucanthone [120] **(Miracil D)**
The severity of side effects of lucanthone is reduced by administration of an antihistamine.

MAO inhibitors [48,169,232,242,311,312,433,483,484]
Contraindicated. MAO inhibitors slow the rate of metabolism and potentiate the cardiovascular effects of norepinephrine released by antihistamines and the anticholinergic and other effects of the antihistamines. Free norepinephrine is increased because its uptake at storage sites is blocked by phenothiazine antihistamines.

Methotrimeprazine [120] **(Levoprome)**
Methotrimeprazine and antihistamines have additive CNS depressant effects. See *CNS Depressants*.

Narcotic analgesics [120]
Narcotic analgesics potentiate the CNS depressant effects. See *CNS Depressants*.

Nitrates and nitrites [170,421]
Organic nitrates and nitrites potentiate the physiological antagonism of antihistamines to histamine.

Norepinephrine [169,232,242,400,483,484]
Antihistamines (antazoline, chlorpheniramine, diphenhydramine, tripelennamine) potentiate the cardiovascular effects of norepinephrine by inhibition of norepinephrine uptake by the tissues. Unbound drug for receptors is thus increased. Apparently pyrilamine is an exception; it does not enhance NE toxicity.

Nylidrin HCl [489] **(Arlidin)**
The vasodilator, nylidrin, potentiates the antipsychotic action of phenothiazine therapy by its central vasodilator action and by displacement of the phenothiazine from secondary binding sites.

Organophosphate cholinesterase inhibitors [169,488,913,914]
Antihistamines antagonize the miotic effect of anticholinesterases (cholinesterase inhibitors). See also *Anticholinesterases* above.

Pargyline [48,232,311] **(Eutonyl)**
Antihistamines are potentiated by the MAO inhibitor; severe hypotension; shock. See *MAO Inhibitors* above.

Phenobarbital [633]
Initially enhanced sedation; then inhibition through mutual enzyme induction. See *Barbiturates* above.

Phenothiazines [78,198,421]
Additive CNS depression; potentiated sedation. Urinary retention or glaucoma may be caused when both agents have anticholinergic (atropinelike) effects.

Phenylbutazone [64,485] **(Butazolidin)**
Antihistamines (chlorcyclizine, diphenhydramine, etc.) decrease the effectiveness of phenylbutazone by enzyme induction and protect against its ulcerogenic effects.

Phenytoin [64] **(Dilantin)**
Some antihistamines may decrease the effectiveness of phenytoin by enzyme induction.

Procarbazine [120] **(Matulane)**
Antihistamines should be used with caution. Procarbazine is an enzyme inhibitor (MAO inhibitor).

Progesterone [65,330,479,485,620]
Antihistamines may inhibit progesterone by enzyme induction (increased hydroxylation). Progesterone potentiates phenothiazines, possibly by enzyme inhibition or by blocking them from hepatic cells.

Radiopaque media [486,632]
This combination is incompatible when added to the same IV solution. Not an *in vivo* interaction. Antihistamines, *e.g.,* chlorpheniramine maleate, are commonly injected to reduce side effects of radiopaque media.

Reserpine
Enhanced CNS depression. See *CNS Depressants*.

Scopolamine [168]
Enhanced sedative effect. See *Hyoscine* above.

Sedatives and hypnotics [198,619]
Reinforcement of sedation occurs initially, and then enzyme induction may occur. See *Barbiturates* above, *CNS Depressants*, and specific drugs.

Steroids [65,479,485]
Antihistamines antagonize steroids; decreased activity through increased steroid metabolism (enzyme induction). See *Desoxycorticosterone*, *Estradiol*, and *Progesterone* above and *Testosterone* below.

Sympathomimetics [169,235]
See *Adrenergics* and *Norepinephrine* above.

Testosterone [65,330,479,485]
Antihistamines may inhibit testosterone by enzyme induction (increased hydroxylation).

Thiopental [116]
Potentiation of thiopental anesthesia has occurred from preoperative administration of antihistamines.

Tranquilizers [120,619]
Reinforcement of sedation occurs initially, possibly followed later by reduced effects due to enzyme induction. See *Barbiturates*, *CNS Depressants*, and specific drugs.

Tranylcypromine [120] **(Parnate)**
See *MAO Inhibitors* above.

Trihexyphenidyl HCl [78,487,488] **(Artane)**
Atropinelike effects; additive anticholinergic effect. See *Anticholinergics* above.

ANTIHISTAMINES, SPECIFIC
See *Antazoline, Chlorcyclizine, Chlorpheniramine, Dimenhydrinate, Diphenhydramine, Tripelennamine, etc.*

ANTIHYPERTENSIVES

(*α-Adrenergic blocking agents* such as phentolamine [Regitine] HCl and tolazoline [Priscoline] HCl; *diuretics* such as chlorothiazide [Diuril], diazoxide [Hyperstat], ethacrynic acid [Edecrin], furosemide [Lasix], mercurials [Mercuhydrin, Thiomerin], and quinethazone [Hydromox]; *ganglionic blocking agents* such as chlorisondamine [Ecolid] chloride, hexamethonium chloride, mecamylamine [Inversine], pentolinium [Ansolysen] tartrate, tetraethylammonium chloride, trimethaphan [Arfonad] camsylate, and trimethidinium [Ostensin]; *MAO inhibitors* such as pargyline [Eutonyl], *norepinephrine depleters* and agents that prevent its uptake into inactive sites, *e.g.,* guanethidine and methyldopa, *Rauwolfia alkaloids, vasodilators, e.g.,* agents affecting CNS vasomotor centers such as hydralazine [Apresoline] HCl and mebutamate [Capla], and *Veratrum alkaloids*)

See also specific interactions under *Bethanidine, Debrisoquin, Guanethidine, Hydralazine, Mebutamate, Mecamylamine, Methyldopa, Pargyline, Rauwolfia alkaloids, Reserpine, Veratrum alkaloids,* etc. The major interactants with antihypertensives are CNS depressants such as anesthetics, antidepressants such as the tricyclics and MAO inhibitors, diuretics, phenothiazines, and sympathomimetics.

Drug interactions with these agents hinge on a wide variety of mechanisms because of the multiplicity of pharmacological subcategories of antihypertensives. Careful analysis of the specific pharmacological properties of every drug given concomitantly with antihypertensives is essential.

Acetaminophen (Tempra, Tylenol)
See *Antihypertensives* under *Acetaminophen;* also see *CNS Depressants.*

Alcohol [120]
Alcohol potentiates the hypotensive action of ganglionic blocking agents like pentolinium.

Amphetamines and anorexiants [78,550,591-596,626]
Amphetamines and anorexiants antagonize antihypertensives and vice versa as a general rule. But amphetamines may cause loss of control of blood pressure in the patient on guanethidine because they block guanethidine from its receptor sites and displace the antihypertensive from these sites. They also potentiate the pressor effects of epinephrine and norepinephrine. Amphetamines potentiate ganglionic blockers such as mecamylamine. Hypertensive crisis may occur with antihypertensive MAO inhibitors such as pargyline.

Anesthetics [8,30,78,91,120,198,312,619,633]
Anesthetics potentiate the hypotensive effect of antihypertensives; severe hypotension or shock and profound cardiovascular collapse may occur during surgery, and especially with the use of intermittent positive pressure breathing (IPPB) apparatus. See also under *Anesthetics, General* and *CNS Depressants.*

Antidepressants, tricyclic [120,327,626,823,1414,1672]
Tricyclic antidepressants antagonize antihypertensives, in some instances by inhibiting uptake of antihypertensives (such as the adrenergic neuron blocking agents—bethanidine, debrisoquin, guanethidine) to the site of action in the adrenergic neuron. This has been demonstrated for both desipramine and bethanidine.[327,823] Imipramine reverses the adrenergic blocking action of guanethidine. Reduced dosage of the hypotensive agent is frequently necessary if the tricy-

clic is withdrawn, in order to prevent profound hypotension. Monitor closely or avoid these potentially hazardous combinations.

Antihistamines [626]
Tripelennamine and pyrilamine partly reverse the adrenergic blocking action of guanethidine but promethazine has no effect.

Antihypertensives, other [8]
Antihypertensives combined with other antihypertensives may cause an enhanced hypotensive effect. Reduced dosage of the hypotensive agents is frequently necessary.

Bethanidine (Esbatal)
See *Antidepressants, tricyclic* above and *Doxepin, Ephedrine* and *Phenylpropanolamine* below. Also see main entry *Bethanidine.*

Chlorothiazide [120]
Chlorothiazide potentiates antihypertensives. With ganglionic blocking agents it may cause excessive fall in blood pressure.

Chlorthalidone (Hygroton)
See *Diuretics* below.

Cocaine [626]
Cocaine reverses the adrenergic blocking action of guanethidine but does not antagonize the potentiation of response to sympathomimetics induced by guanethidine.

Debrisoquin
See *Debrisoquin* as main entry, also *Antidepressants, tricyclic* above and *Phenylephrine* below.

Diazepam [619] (Valium)
Diazepam may potentiate the antihypertensive effect of diuretics and antihypertensives. See *CNS Depressants.*

Diazoxide [1782,1785,1910] (Hyperstat, Proglycem)
See *Diazoxide* main entry and *Thiazides* below.

Diethylpropion [550,593] (Tenuate, Tepanil)
Same as for *Methylphenidate* below.

Diuretics [120]
Enhanced hypotensive effect possible. Reduced dosage of the hypotensive agents is frequently necessary. See *Hydrochlorothiazide* below.

Doxepin (Sinequan)
See *Antidepressants, tricyclic* above. Doxepin is not as strong an inhibitor of the antihypertensive action of bethanidine as the other tricyclic antidepressants.

Ephedrine [78,823,1382,1832]
Ephedrine with bethanidine produces symptoms of hypertensive crisis similar to *Amphetamines* above. Avoid or monitor very closely.

Ethacrynic acid [421] (Edecrin)
Ethacrynic acid potentiates antihypertensives (orthostatic hypotension). May require adjustment of dosage.

Ethionamide [178] (Trecator)
Since ethionamide has ganglionic blocking action, it may potentiate the postural hypotension produced by other drugs such as antihypertensives, narcotics like meperidine, etc.

Furosemide [120] (Lasix)
Furosemide potentiates the hypotensive effect of antihypertensives. Reduce the dosage as necessary.

Glycyrrhiza [151,326,667,1088-9,1993]
Daily use of licorice may counteract the antihypertensive effect. Licorice causes a rise in blood pressure. See *Antihypertensives* under *Glycyrrhiza.*

Guanethidine (Ismelin)
See *Guanethidine* as a main alphabetic entry.

Haloperidol [120] (Haldol)
Contraindicated. Potentiation of the hypotensive effect is possible. See *CNS Depressants.*

Hydrochlorothiazide [120,619] (Hydrodiuril)

See *Diuretics* above. Hydrochlorothiazide potentiates the action of other antihypertensive drugs; dosage of these agents, especially of the ganglionic blockers, should reduced by at least 50% as soon as hydrochlorothiazide is added to the regimen.

Imipramine [78,120] (Tofranil)

Imipramine and antihypertensives antagonize each other. See *Antidepressants, tricyclic* above.

Isoniazid [330]

Isoniazid potentiates antihypertensives, probably by enzyme inhibition.

Levarterenol [117,619,633] (Levophed, norepinephrine)

Antihypertensives like guanethidine and methyldopa potentiate levarterenol (exogenous norepinephrine) by preventing its uptake by inactive binding sites in adrenergic neurons. Levarterenol is the drug of choice if a pressor agent is needed in a hypotensive episode with one of these agents since none of these antagonize its action.

MAO inhibitors [120,170,330,421,633]

Some MAO inhibitors and some antihypertensives can mutually lower the blood pressure and there may be an enhanced hypotensive effect. Reduced dosage of the hypotensive agents is then frequently necessary. However guanethidine, methyldopa, and reserpine, which initially release catecholamines suddenly may cause a hypertensive crisis and excitability (severe CNS stimulation) if given during MAO inhibitor antihypertensive or antidepressant therapy. Continued use, with enzyme inhibition, may cause inhibition of metabolism of the antihypertensives and potentiation of hypotensive action, after norepinephrine depletion has occurred.

Methamphetamine [78] (Desoxyn, Methedrine)

Methamphetamine may inhibit antihypertensives like methyldopa and reserpine, but it potentiates ganglionic blockers like mecamylamine. MAO inhibitor type of antihypertensives may cause a hypertensive crisis with the amphetamine. See under *Sympathomimetics*.

Methotrimeprazine [120] (Levoprome)

Concurrent use of methotrimeprazine with antihypertensives is contraindicated; increases orthostatic hypotension.

Methylphenidate [417,550,593,626] (Ritalin)

Methylphenidate antagonizes the hypotensive action of guanethidine by displacing it from its receptors. It does not reverse the adrenergic blocking action of guanethidine but if given first prevents it.

Nasal decongestants [553,626,915,950]

Nasal decongestants antagonize antihypertensives. See under *Sympathomimetics*.

Oral contraceptives [1137]

See *Antihypertensives* under *Oral Contraceptives*.

Ornade

See *Phenylpropanolamine* (one of its ingredients) below. Also contains isopropamide and chlorpheniramine.

Paracetamol [166] (Acetaminophen)

Paracetamol potentiates some antihypertensives. See under *Acetaminophen*. Additive CNS depression.

Phenothiazines [166]

Phenothiazines that are adrenolytic, vasodilating, and cardiac depressant potentiate the hypotensive effect of antihypertensives. Reduced dosage of the hypotensive agent is frequently necessary. See *CNS Depressants*.

Phenylephrine [1212,1703]

Debrisoquin, an adrenergic neuron blocking agent used as an antihypertensive, has MAO inhibitory action which produces a hypertensive crisis with sympathomimetics like phenylephrine.

Phenylpropanolamine [1082] (Propadrine)

Phenylpropanolamine may induce a hypertensive crisis with an antihypertensive like bethanidine (Esbatal) or guanethidine (Ismelin). Avoid this combination or monitor very closely as it is antagonistic to these antihypertensives and may be very hazardous. See *Methyldopa* under *Phenylpropanolamine*.

Procainamide (Pronestyl)

See *Antihypertensive* under *Procainamide*.

Procarbazine [120,330,619] (Matulane)

Concomitant administration of an antihypertensive may potentiate CNS depression caused by MAO inhibition due to procarbazine as well as its hypotensive action.

Propranolol [120,1175] (Inderal)

Propranolol potentiates many antihypertensive agents (guanethidine, thiazides, etc.). See *Antihypertensives* under *Propranolol* for more detail.

Quaternary ammonium compounds [1101]

Orally administered quaternary ammonium antihypertensives may be potentiated by prior administration of biologically inert quaternary ammonium compounds which occupy secondary binding sites in the gastrointestinal tract and thus prevent binding of the antihypertensives at inactive sites and thereby improve their absorption.

Quinethazone [120] (Hydromox)

Same as for *Hydrochlorothiazide* above.

Quinidine [170,619,1176]

Quinidine may potentiate the hypotensive effect of thiazides, related diuretics, and other antihypertensive agents, particularly if it is given parenterally. Dosages should be adjusted accordingly.

Reserpine [120,619]

Reserpine and other antihypertensives when given concomitantly may produce an enhanced hypotensive effect. Reserpine may displace guanethidine from adrenergic nerve endings. Reduced dosage of the hypotensive agent is frequently necessary.

Spironolactone [120] (Aldactone)

Potentiation of the hypotensive effect of other antihypertensive agents may occur with spironolactone. Reduce the dose of these agents, particularly the ganglionic blocking agents, at least 50%.

Sympathomimetics [78,553,626,823,915,1382,1832]

Sympathomimetics and antihypertensives in general antagonize each other. However, bethanidine, methyldopa, guanethidine, and similar antihypertensives may potentiate the pressor response to sympathomimetics like ephedrine, epinephrine and levarterenol, and also the mydriasis with agents like phenylephrine.

Thiazides [78,421,1782,1785,1910]

Thiazide diuretics potentiate antihypertensives. Reduce the dosage of the antihypertensive up to 50% or more. See *Thiazides* under *Diazoxide* and *Thiazide Diuretics* as main entry.

Thioxanthenes [120,166] (Taractan)

Thioxanthenes may potentiate the hypotensive effect. See *CNS Depressants*.

Tranquilizers [78]
(Stelazine, Thorazine, Trilafon, etc.)

An antihypertensive such as pargyline (MAO inhibitor) plus a phenothiazine tranquilizer which is potentiated may cause hypotension and extrapyramidal symptoms.

Triamterene [421] (Dyrenium)

Triamterene potentiates antihypertensive agents. See *Diuretics* above.

Vasodilators [120]

Vasodilators, by lowering the blood pressure, may enhance the hypotensive effect. Reduced dosage of the hypotensive agent is frequently necessary.

ANTIHYPERTENSIVES *(continued)*

Vasopressors[78]

This combination increases the likelihood of occurrence of cardiac arrhythmias. Direct acting vasopressors (levarterenol) given to counteract hypotension in patients on guanethidine, methyldopa or reserpine (antihypertensives that prevent uptake of levarterenol by inactive binding sites) may be strongly potentiated. Indirect acting vasopressors (mephentermine) given to same patients may be inhibited strongly or be completely ineffective because the antihypertensives (guanethidine, methyldopa, reserpine) have depleted the norepinephrine upon release of which these vasopressors depend for their effect. Guanethidine does not inhibit mephentermine or metaraminol, but methyldopa may have a mild potentiating action.

ANTI-INFECTIVES

See *Antibiotics, Sulfonamides,* and specific drugs (chloroquine, furazolidone, nalidixic acid, quinine, etc.)

Probenecid[120,160,269,619]

Probenecid prolongs duration of action of some anti-infectives by inhibiting their tubular reabsorption. It also increases levels of anti-infectives in the aqueous humor and cerebrospinal fluid. See under *Probenecid.*

ANTI-INFLAMMATORY AGENTS
(Enzyme products like Ananase, Buclamase, Chymar, Varidase, etc., also aminopyrine, hydrocortisone, pyrazolones, salicylates, etc.)

Anticoagulants

Anti-inflammatory agents must be given very carefully, if at all, to patients on anticoagulant therapy. See *Anti-inflammatory Agents* under *Anticoagulants, Oral.*

Phenobarbital and some other sedatives and hypnotics[78,421]

Phenobarbital and certain other sedatives and hypnotics (chloral hydrate, glutethimide, meprobamate, etc.) may inhibit many anti-inflammatory drugs by enzyme induction. See *Barbiturates.*

Propanolol[586] (Inderal)

β-Adrenergic blocking agents like propranolol inhibit or even abolish the anti-inflammatory effect of typical anti-inflammatory agents like aminopyrine, hydrocortisone, phenylbutazone, and salicylates.

ANTILIPEMICS
(Aluminum nicotinate, Atromid-S, Choloxin, Cytellin, unsaturated fatty acids, etc.)

Anticoagulants, oral[134,619]

Antilipemics may increase the anticoagulant effect of coumarin anticoagulants. See *Clofibrate* under *Anticoagulants, Oral.*

ANTIMALARIALS

See drug interactions with acidifying agents, alcohol, alkalinizing agents, MAO inhibitors, etc. under *Chloroquine, Primaquine, Pyrimethamine, Quinacrine, Quinidine,* etc.

Quinacrine[177] (Atabrine, mepacrine)

Quinacrine is contraindicated with 8-aminoquinoline antimalarials like primaquine and quinocide. It increases their plasma levels 5- to 10-fold and prolongs their stay in the body. This may occur even when primaquine is given as long as three months after the last dose of quinacrine. Toxic reactions may be induced.

ANTIMETABOLITES
(Folic acid analogs [Methotrexate, etc.], purine analogs [Imuran azathioprine, 6-mercaptopurine, etc.], and pyrimidine analogs [5-fluorouracil, etc.])

Amphotericin B[120] (Fungizone)

Antimetabolites and amphotericin B should not be given concurrently unless absolutely necessary to control reactions to amphotericin B or to treat underlying disease.

ANTIMICROBIALS

See *Antifungals* under specific names, *Antibiotics, Sulfonamides, Antiviral Eye Preparations* and other antimicrobials under specific names such as *Amantadine, Penicillins,* etc.

ANTINAUSEANTS

See *Antiemetics.*

ANTINEOPLASTICS

See *Alkylating Agents, Azathioprine, Cyclophosphamide, Dactinomycin, Folic Acid Antagonists, 6-Mercaptopurine, Methotrexate, Nitrogen Mustards, Thiotepa,* etc.

Amphotericin B

Antineoplastics with this antifungal are generally contraindicated. See under *Amphotericin B.*

Anticoagulants, oral[120,134,861,890]

Antineoplastics, by affecting vitamin K, depressing platelet counts, and by bone marrow depression, tend to potentiate anticoagulants (hemorrhagic potential). See *Antineoplastics* under *Anticoagulants, Oral.*

Bone marrow depressants[120]

Excessive bone marrow depression may result if other bone marrow depressants are given concomitantly. Some antineoplastics are used in combination but concurrent use with some agents may be contraindicated.

Chloroquine[120]

Chloroquine is contraindicated in patients receiving bone marrow depressants.

Insulin[120]

Some antineoplastics like cyclophosphamide, may enhance hypoglycemia through additive effect.

Marijuana[1197]

Δ-9-Tetrahydrocannabinol is reported to relieve the nausea and vomiting in some cancer patients on chemotherapy but the data appear to be equivocal. In some leukemia patients and in some who have undergone mastectomy and have evidence of metastatic bone disease, smoking marijuana intensifies the pain.

Other antineoplastics[120]

Mutual potentiation by additive cytotoxic effect. Often contraindicated.

Succinylcholine

See *Antineoplastics* under *Muscle Relaxants, Peripherally Acting, Depolarizing.*

Uricosuric agents

See *Hyperuricemics* under *Uricosuric Agents.*

Vaccines[120,312,377,486,619]

Vaccinia may develop following smallpox vaccination because of the immunosuppressive effect of the antineoplastics. Vaccines should not be administered to patients receiving immunosuppressant drugs which depress resistance to disease and reduce the effectiveness of the vaccination. Serious and possibly fatal illness may develop.

X-radiation[120,198]

Mutual potentiation (additive cytotoxic effects). Hazardous with alkylating antineoplastics.

ANTIPARKINSONISM DRUGS
(Trihexyphenidyl, Benztropine, Chlorphenoxamine, Ethopropazine, Orphenadrine, Procyclidine [Kemadrin])

Antidepressants, tricyclic [194]
Since the tricyclics also possess weak anticholinergic activity the atropinelike effects may be enhanced. Paralytic ileus, damage to glaucomatous eyes, xerostoma, etc. may occur.

Furazolidone [202,633] (Furoxone)
Furazolidone (used more than 4 days) potentiates antiparkinsonism drugs. See *MAO Inhibitors* below.

Haloperidol [120] (Haldol)
Antiparkinsonism drugs may be used concurrently with haloperidol to control extrapyramidal symptoms.

Imipramine (Tofranil)
See *Antidepressants, Tricyclic* above.

Isoniazid [330]
Isoniazid potentiates antiparkinsonism drugs, possibly by enzyme inhibition.

MAO inhibitors [202,421,633]
MAO inhibitors potentiate antiparkinsonism drugs. Tremor, profuse sweating and neurological symptoms are intensified.

Nortriptyline (Aventyl)
See *Antidepressants, Tricyclic* above.

Pargyline (Eutonyl)
See *MAO Inhibitors* above.

Phenothiazines [120]
Antiparkinsonism drugs are frequently used concurrently with phenothiazines and various other psychotherapeutic agents to control extrapyramidal symptoms. Anticholinergic effects may be additive.

Phenothiazine antihistamines [120]
Constipation and dryness of mouth may occur because of additive anticholinergic effects.

Procarbazine [330]
See *MAO inhibitors* above.

Thioxanthenes [120] (Taractan, etc.)
Antiparkinsonism agents are frequently used concurrently with thioxanthenes to control extrapyramidal symptoms sometimes caused by the thioxanthenes.

ANTIPSORIATICS

Chloroquine [120,421] (Aralen)
Chloroquine may antagonize the action of antipsoriatics, and may actually precipitate a severe attack of psoriasis in patients with the disease. Avoid its use in such patients.

ANTIPYRETICS
(Acetaminophen, Salicylates, etc.)

p-Aminosalicylic acid [198] (PAS)
Antipyretics potentiate PAS.

Anticoagulants, oral [198]
Antipyretics potentiate oral anticoagulants.

Methotrexate [198]
Some antipyretics potentiate methotrexate. See under *Salicylates.*

Narcotic analgesics
Narcotic analgesics potentiate all CNS depressants, including the antipyretic analgesics. If the additive effect is strong enough, severe respiratory depression, hypopyrexia, coma, and possibly death may occur. See *CNS Depressants.*

Penicillins [198]
Antipyretics potentiate penicillins.

Phenobarbital [198]
Some antipyretics inhibit phenobarbital and vice versa.

Probenecid [198] (Benemid)
Antipyretics inhibit probenecid. See *Salicylates* under *Probenecid.*

Sulfonamides [198]
Antipyretics potentiate sulfonamides. See *Salicylates* under *Sulfonamides.*

Sulfonylureas [198]
Antipyretics potentiate oral antidiabetics. See Salicylates under *Antidiabetics, Oral* and *Antidiabetics, Oral* under *Antipyrine.*

ANTIPYRINE
(Analgesine, anodynine, parodyne, phenazone, phenylone, pyrazoline, sedatine)
Antipyrine and dipyrone (methanesulfonate methylamine derivative of antipyrine) have similar properties and adverse effects with interactants.

Acidifying agents [325,870]
Acidifying agents increase urinary excretion of weak bases like antipyrine and thus tend to inhibit them.

Alkalinizing agents [325,870]
Alkalinizing agents decrease urinary excretion of weak bases like antipyrine and thus tend to potentiate them.

Allopurinol [82,1879]
Allopurinol inhibits the metabolism of antipyrine and thus prolongs its plasma half-life and increases its toxicity.

Anticoagulants, oral (Coumadin, etc.)
See *Antipyrine* under *Anticoagulants, Oral.*

Antidepressants, tricyclic [82,1879]
Antidepressants like nortriptyline inhibit the metabolism of antipyrine and thus increase its toxicity.

Antidiabetics, oral [166]
Some pyrazolon derivatives (dipyrone, and possibly others) may aggravate a prothrombin deficiency and increase a bleeding tendency. The combination with an antidiabetic may cause hemorrhage.

Barbiturates [65,96,184,222,694,695,1261,1837]
Barbiturates stimulate the metabolism of antipyrine (enzyme induction) and thus inhibit it. See *Barbiturates.* Antipyrine, also an enzyme inducer, diminishes sleeping time with pentobarbital and probably other barbiturates.

Estrogens
See *Antipyrine* under *Oral Contraceptives.*

Fatty acids [951]
Fatty acids potentiate antipyrine by decreasing its urinary excretion.

Glutethimide [184,222,694,695] (Doriden)
Glutethimide stimulates the metabolism of antipyrine (enzyme induction) and thus inhibits it and other pyrazolon derivatives. See under *Dipyrone.*

Oral contraceptives
See *Antipyrine* under *Oral Contraceptives.*

Phenobarbital [65,96]
Phenobarbital inhibits antipyrine (enzyme induction).

Phenothiazines
See *Chlorpromazine* under *Dipyrone* for a possible hypothermic reaction with pyrazolon derivatives.

Phenylbutazone [222,694,695] (Butazolidin)
Phenylbutazone stimulates the metabolism of antipyrine (enzyme induction) and thus inhibits it.

Spironolactone
See *Antipyrine* under *Spironolactone.*

ANTIPYRINE *(continued)*

Vitamin C [274,616,870]

Antipyrine can cause an increased excretion of vitamin C and thus inhibit it and vice versa.

ANTIRHEUMATIC DRUGS (Anti-inflammatory Agents)

Cortisol [57,198,421] (Hydrocortisone)

All the antirheumatic drugs so far examined have displaced cortisol and presumably driven it into tissues (presumed to be the mechanism of action.)

ANTISTINE (Antazoline phosphate)

See *Antihistamines.*

ANTITHYROID DRUGS

See the specific drugs as listed in Chapter 8 (Table 8-3).

ANTITUBERCULOSIS DRUGS (Cycloserine [Seromycin], isoniazid, PAS, etc.)

Combination therapy [120]

Several antituberculosis agents should be used in combination to improve effectiveness of therapy and to reduce the possibility of bacterial resistance developing.

Corticosteroids [120,421]

Corticosteroids are usually contraindicated in patients with tuberculosis; however, the concurrent administration with antitubercular agents may be life saving in certain cases.

Phenytoin [916] (Dilantin)

The antituberculosis drug, isoniazid, a very strong inhibitor of phenytoin metabolism causes accumulation of unmetabolized anticonvulsant and potentiates the toxic effects. Other antituberculosis drugs that enter into the same interaction include cycloserine and *p*-aminosalicylic acid. See under *Phenytoin.*

ANTITUSSIVES (Benzonatate [Tessalon], carbetapentane citrate [Toclase], chlophedianol HCl [Ulo], codeine phosphate or sulfate, dextromethorphan [Methorate, Romilar] HBr, dihydrocodeinone bitartrate [Dicodid, Hycodan, Mercodinone], dimethoxanate [Cotheral], diphenhydramine HCl [Benadryl], levopropoxphene [Novrad] napsylate, methadone [Adanon, Amidone, Dolophine] HCl, meperidine [Demerol], morphine, noscapine [Nectadon], pipazethate [Theratuss] HCl, Tripelennamine [Pyribenzamine] citrate, etc.)

The antitussives may possess the same drug interaction potentials as anticholinergics, antihistamines, local anesthetics, or narcotics since they individually possess one or more of these characteristics. [120,166,619,689]

The precise interactions for a given antitussive can be determined by examining its specific pharmacological properties. Note whether it is a centrally acting narcotic or nonnarcotic agent, a peripherally acting agent (demulcent, local anesthetic), or an expectorant (iodide, ipecac, ammonium chloride, terpin hydrate, glyceryl guaiacolate, etc.).

ANTIVIRAL EYE PREPARATIONS (Stoxil, etc.)

Corticosteroids [120,421]

Corticosteroids are usually contraindicated in viral infections of the eye (e.g., herpes simplex keratitis) because they can accelerate spread of the infections.

ANTRENYL

See *Anticholinergics* (oxyphenonium bromide).

ANTROCOL

See *Atropine Sulfate* and *Phenobarbital.*

ANTURANE

See *Sulfinpyrazone* and *Uricosuric Agents.*

APAMIDE

See *Acetaminophen.*

APOMORPHINE

Levodopa [838]

Apomorphine, a catecholamine analog of dopamine, eliminates the tremor and decreases the akinesia and choreoathetosis caused by levodopa.

APPETITE DEPRESSANTS (Amphetamines, chlorphentermine HCl [Pre-Sate], dethylpropion HCl [Tenuate, Tepanil], phendimetrazine tartrate [Plegine], phenmetrazine HCl [Preludin HCl], phentermine, etc.)

See *Sympathomimetics.*

MAO inhibitors [198]

A potentially hazardous, possibly lethal combination. See *Sympathomimetics* under *MAO Inhibitors.*

APRESOLINE

See *Antihypertensives* and *Hydralazine.*

APRESOLINE—ESIDRIX

See *Hydralazine, Hydrochlorothiazide,* and *Thiazide Diuretics.*

AQUACHLORAL

See *Chloral Hydrate.*

AQUACORT

See *Corticosteroids* (hydrocortisone acetate) and *Tyrothrycin.* Also contains phenylmercuric acetate, 9-aminoacridine HCl, urea, etc.

AQUALIN

See *Theophylline.*

AQUATAG (Benzthiazide)

See *Thiazide Diuretics.*

ARALEN

See *Chloroquine.*

ARAMINE

See *Metaraminol* and *Sympathomimetics.*

ARGININE GLUTAMATE (Modumate) or Hydrochloride (R-gene)

Malic acid [619]

Combination of arginine and malic acid is more effective than arginine alone in lowering blood ammonia levels. Many drugs, including barbiturates, narcotics and diuretics may produce ammonia or interfere with its excretion.

ARISTOCORT

See *Glucocorticoids* and *Triamcinolone.*

ARISTOSPAN

See *Glucocorticioids* and *Triamcinolone.*

ARTANE

See *Antiparkinsonism Drugs* and *Trihexyphenidyl.*

ARTARAU
See *Rauwolfia Alkaloids* (whole root).

ARTHRALGEN
See *Acetaminophen* and *Salicylamide.*

ARTIFICIAL SWEETENERS
See *Cyclamates* and *Saccharin.*

ASBRON
See *Glyceryl Guaiacolate, Phenylpropanolamine* and *Theophylline.*

ASCODEEN (Codeine phosphate, aspirin)
See *Aspirin* and *Codeine.*

ASCORBIC ACID
See *Vitamin C.*

ASCRIPTIN
See *Aluminum Compounds, Antacids, Aspirin, Codeine,* and *Magnesium Salts.*

ASMINYL
See *Ephedrine, Phenobarbital,* and *Theophylline.*

ASMOLIN
See *Epinephrine.*

ASPARTIC ACID

Vinblastine [120]
Aspartic acid protects test animals from lethal doses of vinblastine, but does not reverse the antitumor action.

ASPIRIN (Acetylsalicylic acid)
See *Salicylates.*

Aspirin [108]
Death occurred when a patient previously hypersensitized to the drug ingested 2 tablets.

ASTHMA METER
See *Epinephrine.*

ASTHMA PREPARATIONS

Chloroquine [421]
Chloroquine potentiates some asthma preparations.

ASTRAFER
See *Iron Salts* (dextriferron).

ATARACTIC AGENTS
See *CNS Depressants* and *Tranquilizers.*

Alcohol [121]
Alcohol potentiates the CNS depressant effects in decreasing order: reserpine, chlorpromazine, propoxyphene, morphine, meprobamate, phenaglycodol, codeine, hydroxyzine.

ATARAX
See *Hydroxyzine* and *Tranquilizers.*

ATARAXOID
See *Hydroxyzine* and *Prednisolone.*

ATENOLOL (Tenormin)
See *Propranolol* under *Insulin.*

ATHROMBIN
See *Anticoagulants, Oral.*

ATROMID-S
See *Clofibrate.*

ATROPINE
See *Anticholinergics.*

Acetylcholine
See *Atropine* under *Acetylcholine.*

Ambenonium [120,619] (Mytelase)
Atropine or other parasympatholytic drugs are contraindicated with ambenonium because they may mask signs of cholinergic overdosage.

Antacids, oral
See *Alkaloids* under *Antacids, Oral.*

Anticholinesterases [168]
The actions of anticholinesterases on autonomic effector cells, and to some extent those on the CNS, are antagonized by atropine.

Antidepressants, tricyclic [120] (Aventyl, Elavil, Pertofrane, Tofranil, etc.)
In susceptible patients receiving anticholinergic drugs (atropine, etc.) tricyclic antidepressants may potentiate the atropine-like effects (*e.g.* paralytic ileus).

Bethanechol [168,619] (Urecholine)
Atropine readily blocks the cholinergic effects of the parasympathomimetic agent bethanechol.

Chlorpromazine [120,166] (Thorazine)
Because chlorpromazine also has anticholinergic activity it must be used with caution in persons receiving atropine (additive effects).

Cholinergics [168,619] (Pilocarpine, etc.)
The miotic action of a cholinergic is used to counteract the mydriatic action of atropine.

Cocaine
See *Atropine* under *Cocaine.*

Echothiophate iodide [120,619] (Phospholine Iodide)
Atropine IV or SC is an effective antidote for echothiophate overdosage.

Isoniazid [202]
Isoniazid has been reported to have an additive anticholinergic effect when given with atropine. A hazardous combination in glaucoma.

Lucanthone [177] (Miracil D)
Severity of side effects of lucanthone is reduced by administration of atropine.

MAO inhibitors [128]
MAO inhibitors may potentiate atropine; do not use together nor within 2 or 3 weeks following treatment with MAO inhibitors.

Meperidine [633]
Atropine and meperidine have additive effects (*e.g.,* dryness of mucous membranes, flushing, depressed respiration, etc.).

Methacholine chloride [168] (Mecholyl Chloride)
Atropine is a competitive antagonist of methacholine. See *Acetylcholine* above.

Methotrimeprazine [120] (Levoprome)
Should be used concomitantly with caution in that tachycardia and fall in blood pressure may occur and undesirable CNS effects such as stimulation, delirium and extrapyramidal symptoms may be aggravated.

Morphine [166,168]
Atropine antagonizes the respiratory depression and increases the gastrointestinal responses to morphine.

Neostigmine (Prostigmin)
See *Anticholinergics* under *Neostigmine.*

ATROPINE *(continued)*

Oral medications[1791]
Atropine tends to delay gastric emptying time and thus depresses drug absorption.

Phenothiazines[78,120,198,421]
Atropine potentiates some phenothiazines in psychiatric treatment and counteracts the extrapyramidal symptoms produced by them. Urinary retention or glaucoma may be induced when the phenothiazine also has anticholinergic (atropinelike) effects.

Pilocarpine[168]
Atropine effectively blocks pilocarpine from receptors at parasympathetic nerve endings and thus acts as a competitive antagonist.

Propanidid[527] (Bayer 1420, Epontol)
Two cases of marked peripheral vasodilation and severe hypotension were ascribed to a combination of intravenous atropine followed by the systemic anesthetic propanidid.

Propranol
See *Atropine* under *Propranolol.*

Pyridostigmine[120] (Mestinon)
In the event of cholinergic crisis induced by excessive dosage of pyridostigmine, atropine should be given immediately as an antidote. But atropine used to control gastrointestinal muscarinic side effects of pyridostigmine can lead to inadvertent induction of cholinergic crisis by masking signs of overdosage.

Reserpine[120]
Vagal blocking agents like atropine are used to prevent and treat vagal circulatory responses in patients receiving reserpine when emergency surgery must be performed. Reserpine and its derivatives antagonize the antisecretory effects of anticholinergics. Anticholinergics given concomitantly counteract the abdominal cramps and diarrhea resulting from the increased gastrointestinal motility and tone produced by reserpine.

Veratrum alkaloids[120,170]
Atropine abolishes the bradycrotic effect of cryptenamine and diminishes its hypotensive effect.

Vitamin C[274,616,870]
Atropine may cause increased excretion of vitamin C; inhibition of the vitamin and vice versa.

ATROPINE DERIVATIVES

Antidepressants, tricyclic[120]
Mutual anticholinergic action should indicate cautious use. Potentiation of atropinelike effects may induce urinary retention, paralytic ileus, etc.

ATROPINE EYEDROPS
See *Atropine, Miotic Eyedrops,* and *Mydriatic Eyedrops.*

ATTAPULGITE

Phenothiazines
See *Attapulgite* under *Phenothiazines*

ATTENUVAX
See *Neomycin* and *Vaccines* (measles).

AUREOMYCIN
See *Antibiotics, Chlortetracycline,* and *Tetracyclines.*

AVAZYME
See *Chymotrypsin.*

AVENTYL
See *Antidepressants, Tricyclic,* also *Dibenzazepine Derivatives* and *Nortriptyline.*

AYR
See *Barbiturates, Ephedrine,* and *Theophylline.*

AZAPETINE (Ilidar)

Epinephrine and norepinephrine[529]
Azapetine, an adrenergic blocking agent, reverses the pressor effect of epinephrine and reduces the vasoconstrictor effect of norepinephrine.

AZAPROPAZONE (Rheumox)
This nonsteroidal anti-inflammatory agent is a chemical congener of phenylbutazone and may eventually be found to enter into the same drug interactions. See *Phenylbutazone.*

Warfarin[1991,2051]
Azapropazone potentiates oral anticoagulants, probably by the same mechanism as phenylbutazone (increased clearance of the R isomer of warfarin which is 5 times less potent an anticoagulant than the S isomer, the metabolism of which is inhibited). This combination of azapropazone and warfarin caused hematemesis in a gastric ulcer patient on oral anticoagulants. The prothrombin time may continue to increase for several weeks after azapropazone is withdrawn. The drug is contraindicated in patients already on warfarin.

AZASERINE

6-Chloropurine[951]
Synergistic antineoplastic activity.

AZATHIOPRINE (Imuran)

Allopurinol[28,619,1348,1662] (Zyloprim, Zyloric)
Azathioprine potentiates allopurinol toxicity and excretion of uric acid by inhibiting its metabolism. The uricosuric is an enzyme inhibitor (inhibits xanthine oxidase) and thereby inhibits conversion of 6-mercaptopurine, the active metabolite of azathioprine, into inactive products. High blood levels of the metabolite can be lethal by exerting highly toxic effects on the bone marrow, etc. The dose of azathioprine should be reduced to $\frac{1}{3}$ to $\frac{1}{4}$ of the usual dose.

Corticosteroids[619,755] (Prednisone)
This combination in prolonged therapy may cause negative nitrogen balance and muscle wasting, also possible development of reticular cell sarcoma.

6-AZAURIDINE

Chloramphenicol[951]
Chloramphenicol potentiates the immunosuppressive activity of 6-azauridine (enzyme inhibition).

AZO GANTANOL
See *Sulfonamides* (sulfamethoxazole) and *Phenazopyridine.*

AZO GANTRISIN
See *Sulfonamides* (sulfisoxazole) and *Phenazopyridine.*

AZO-MANDELAMINE
See *Methenamine* and *Phenazopyridine.*

AZOTREX (Capsules)
See *Phenazopyridine, Sulfonamides* (sulfamethizole), and *Tetracyclines.*

BACITRACIN

Muscle relaxants, depolarizing or polarizing[421]
Bacitracin prolongs the muscle relaxant effect of drugs such as decamethonium and succinylcholine. See *Neuromuscular Blocking Antibiotics* under *Antibiotics.*

Neomycin [120,322,499]
This combination, used as an irrigating solution during surgery, may cause respiratory depression. See *Neuromuscular Blocking Antibiotics* under *Antibiotics*.

Procainamide [619]
Procainamide may potentiate the neuromuscular blocking action of bacitracin. The resulting respiratory depression may be hazardous.

BACTRIM
See *Sulfonamides* and *Trimethoprim*.

BANANAS
See *Tyramine-rich Foods*.

BANCAPS (with or without codeine)
See *Acetaminophen, Barbiturates, Codeine,* and *Mephenesin*.

BARBIDONNA
See *Atropine, Barbiturates, Hyoscyamine, Phenobarbital,* and *Scopolamine*.

BARBITAL
See *Barbiturates*.

BARBITURATES
See *Barbital, CNS Depressants, Hexobarbital, Phenobarbital*. Additional pertinent interactions are given under *Anticonvulsants*.

Acenocoumarol (Sintrom)
See *Anticoagulants, Oral* below.

Acetaminophen (Datril, Nebs, Tylenol, etc.)
See *Phenobarbital* under *Acetaminophen* for potentiation of acetaminophen toxicity, etc.

Acidifying agents [28,165,325,870]
Acidifying agents potentiate weak acids like the barbiturates because they tend to increase gastrointestinal absorption and tubular reabsorption in the urinary tubules.

Alcohol [166,241,244,311,631,634,730,737,738]
Alcohol potentiates barbiturates and the combination is potentially lethal. Dual potentiation of CNS depressant effects. See *Barbiturates* under *Alcohol*.

Alkalinizing agents [165,325,870]
Opposite effect to that of *Acidifying Agents* above. Antacids, by decreasing the absorption rate severely, may nullify the hypnotic effect.

Amphetamine [359]
Amphetamine delays the intestinal absorption of phenobarbital, then synergistically enhances anticonvulsant effects.

Aminopyrine [555]
Barbiturates increase the rate at which aminopyrine is metabolized. Also, the rate of metabolism of barbiturates is increased by aminopyrine. Mutual inhibition.

Analgesics [78,147]
Barbiturates may decrease effects of some analgesics (enzyme induction) but they potentiate the CNS depressant effects of narcotic analgesics. See *CNS Depressants*.

Androgens [198,330]
Barbiturates induce the metabolism of drugs like androsterone and testosterone and thus inhibit androgenic activity.

Anesthetics [120,312,619]
Barbiturates potentiate the CNS depressant effects of anesthetics (delayed recovery, possible collapse). See *CNS Depressants*.

Antibiotics [360]
Barbiturates (amobarbital, etc.) may produce apnea, muscle weakness and enhanced neuromuscular blockage with aminoglycoside antibiotics such as neomycin, kanamycin and streptomycin.

Anticholinesterases [4,5,155,966]
Barbiturates, which are potentiated by anticholinesterases, must be used very cautiously in treating convulsions caused by poisoning with these agents (insecticides, etc.). Anticholinesterases may increase the rate of entry of long-acting barbiturates into the brain.

Anticoagulants, oral [9,20,63,78,106,223,434,677,685,744,826,1055,1513,1682] (Coumadin, Dicumarol, Sintrom, etc.)
Barbiturates inhibit anticoagulants through enzyme induction. Inhibition may last for 6 weeks after withdrawal of barbiturate. They may also inhibit absorption of the anticoagulants when given orally but not IV (e.g., heptabarbital plus bishydroxycoumarin). They may also affect coagulation factors IX and X. Monitor dosage of anticoagulant carefully when barbiturates are added to or withdrawn from the regimen to avoid hemorrhagic episodes.

Anticonvulsants [78]
Barbiturates inhibit other anticonvulsants through enzyme induction. See *Phenytoin*.

Antidepressants, tricyclic [71,116,194,756]
See *Barbiturates* under *Antidepressants, Tricyclic*.

Antidiabetics, oral [421,433]
See *Barbiturates* under *Antidiabetics, Oral*.

Antihistamines [64,78,116,479,481,619,633]
Some antihistamines and barbiturates inhibit each other through enzyme induction, possibly after initial potentiation of CNS depressant effects. See *CNS Depressants*. Preoperative administration of antihistamines potentiates thiopental anesthesia. Tolerance may be induced by enzyme induction (both drugs).

Anti-inflammatory agents [78]
Barbiturates inhibit anti-inflammatory agents.

Antipyrine [65,96,222,1837]
Barbiturates stimulate the metabolism of antipyrine and antipyrine stimulates the metabolism of barbiturates. See *Barbiturates* under *Antipyrine*.

Barbiturates [28,63]
Tolerance to barbiturates is developed by continued administration because of lessening response due to enzyme induction.

Benzodiazepines [330,421] (Librium, Valium)
Benzodiazepines may potentiate the sedative and respiratory depressant effects of barbiturates and vice versa. See *CNS Depressants*.

Bishydroxycoumarin [78] (Dicumarol)
See *Anticoagulants, Oral* above.

Black widow spider venom [120]
The neurotoxic venom can cause respiratory paralysis. Use barbiturates with caution.

Carbamazepine (Tegretol)
See *Barbiturates* under *Carbamazepine*.

Carbon tetrachloride [902]
Barbiturates sensitize to the toxic effects of carbon tetrachloride 100-fold.

Carisoprodol [120] (Rela, Soma)
Possible potentiation of CNS depressant effects initially, followed by inhibition due to enzyme induction. See *CNS Depressants*.

Chloramphenicol [83,330] (Chloromycetin)
Chloramphenicol potentiates barbiturates.

Chlorcyclizine [640]
Chlorcyclizine and barbiturates mutually potentiate the CNS depressant effects and then with continued dosage mutually inhibit each other through enzyme induction.

BARBITURATES *(continued)*

Chlordiazepoxide [78,120] **(Librium)**
See *Benzodiazepines* above.

Chlorinated insecticides [198]
Chlorinated insecticides inhibit barbiturates by enzyme induction.

Chlorphenoxamine [120,619] **(Phenoxene)**
Chlorphenoxamine, an antiparkinsonism drug, potentiates CNS depressant effects of barbiturates. See *Antihistamines* above.

Chlorpromazine [120,668,669] **(Thorazine)**
See *CNS Depressants*, and *Barbiturates* under *Phenothiazines*.

Chlorpropamide [120] **(Diabinese)**
Chlorpropamide may prolong the hypnotic and sedative effect of barbiturates.

Chlorthalidone [120] **(Hygroton)**
Barbiturates potentiate the orthostatic hypotension caused by chlorthalidone. See *Thiazide Diuretics*.

CNS depressants [38,120,166]
Alcohol, benzodiazepines, and other depressants of the central nervous system are contraindicated in patients receiving barbiturates (enhanced CNS depressant effects). See *CNS Depressants*.

Codeine
See *Barbiturates* under *Codeine*.

Corticosteroids [78,198,421]
Barbiturates increase the rate of metabolism and thereby inhibit the steroids. These steroids may potentiate the sedative effect of barbiturates.

Coumarin anticoagulants [106,371,421,434,640,673]
Barbiturates inhibit these anticoagulants through enzyme induction. Coumarin anticoagulants potentiate the effects of barbiturates. See *Barbiturates under Anticoagulants, Oral*.

Cyclophosphamide [359] **(Cytoxan)**
Barbiturates, by enzyme induction, *potentiate* cyclophosphamide by markedly increasing its rate of conversion *in vivo* into an active alkylating agent. Cautious monitoring is essential if a barbiturate is added to or withdrawn from the regimen.

Cyclopropane [120]
Thiopental reduces the cardiac arrhythmias produced by cyclopropane.

Desoxycorticosterone [421]
This steroid, by increased rate of metabolism, is inhibited by barbiturates.

Dextrothyroxine [330]
Increased barbiturate dosage is required when thyroid hormonal therapy is initiated (increased metabolism).

Diazepam (Valium) [78,120]
Additive or super-additive CNS depressant effects may occur with diazepam plus barbiturates. See *CNS Depressants* above.

Diazepine derivatives (Chlordiazepoxide, Diazepam)
See *CNS Depressants* above.

Digitalis glycosides
See *Barbiturates* under *Digitalis and Digitalis Glycosides*.

Diphenhydramine [695] **(Benadryl)**
Barbiturates and diphenhydramine inhibit each other through enzyme induction.

Diphenoxylate [120] **(in Lomotil)**
The sedative action of barbiturates may be potentiated by diphenoxylate.

Dipyrone [184,694,695]
Barbiturates inhibit dipyrone through enzyme induction.

Disulfiram [1210] **(Antabuse)**
Disulfiram, through enzyme inhibition and decreased metabolism of barbiturates, may potentiate them.

Doxapram [120] **(Dopram)**
Barbiturates may be used to manage excessive CNS stimulation caused by doxapram overdosage.

Estrogen-progestogens [78] **(Oral Contraceptives)**
Barbiturates, through enzyme induction, increase the rate of metabolism of the steroids and thus inhibit them.

Ethamivan [120] **(Emivan)**
Ethamivan is an antidote for the severe respiratory depression caused by overdosage of CNS depressants like barbiturates.

Ethchlorvynol [120]
See *CNS Depressants* above. Patients who respond unpredictably to barbiturates (excitement, release of inhibitions, etc.) may react the same way to ethchlorvynol.

Ethyl biscoumacetate [685] **(Tromexan)**
See *Anticoagulants, Oral* above.

Flurorthyl [935] **(Indoklon)**
An unfruitful seizure (ICT) may be caused by the use of amobarbital or thiopental which greatly elevate the convulsive threshold during Indoklon convulsive treatment.

Folic acid antagonists
See *Methotrexate* below.

Furazolidone [202,633]
Furazolidone potentiates barbiturates (enzyme inhibition). See *MAO Inhibitors* below.

Griseofulvin [66,78,640] **(Fulvicin, Grifulvin, Grisactin)**
Barbiturates inhibit this antifungal agent through enzyme induction.

Halogenated insecticides [83,485]
Insecticidal sprays containing chlordane, DDT, etc. stimulate the metabolism of hexobarbital, etc.

Haloperidol [120,421] **(Haldol)**
Haloperidol potentiates the sedative effects of barbiturates and vice versa. See *CNS Depressants* above.

Hexobarbital [63,695] **(Cyclonal, Evipan, etc.)**
The metabolizing enzymes for hexobarbital are induced so strongly by phenobarbital that the sedative and hypnotic effect is eliminated.

Hydrochlorothiazide [120] **(Hydrodivil)**
The orthostatic hypotension produced by hydrochlorothiazide may be potentiated by barbiturates.

Hydrocortisone [633]
Barbiturates inhibit hydrocortisone through enzyme induction.

Hydroxyzine [120,166] **(Atarax)**
Hydroxyzine potentiates barbiturates. See *CNS Depressants* above.

Hypnotics [78,120]
Barbiturates may inhibit hypnotics through induction after an initial potentiation of the mutual CNS depressant effects. Respiratory depression may be severe. See *CNS Depressants* above.

Imipramine [756] **(Tofranil)**
See *Antidepressants, Tricyclic* above.

Iproniazid [743]
Iproniazid potentiates barbiturates. See *MAO Inhibitors* below.

Levodopa
See *Hexobarbital* under *Levodopa.*

Lidocaine
See *Barbiturates* under *Lidocaine.*

MAO inhibitors [633,743,874]
These enzyme inhibiting antidepressants potentiate barbiturates; barbiturate intoxication results.

Mephenesin [120,166] **(Tolserol)**
The combination of barbiturates and mephenesin may cause marked sedation and respiratory depression.

Mephenytoin [120] **(Mesantoin)**
Barbiturates, by enzyme induction, inhibit the anticonvulsant action of mephenytoin. See *Hydantoins* under *Phenobarbital.*

Meprobamate [640] **(Equanil, Miltown)**
See *CNS Depressants* above and *Barbiturates* under *Meprobamate.*

Methotrexate [166,950,951]
Enhanced toxicity. Some barbiturates, such as thiopental which is highly bound to plasma albumin, may displace methotrexate from its protein (plasma albumin) binding sites and thus increase the blood levels of active unbound folic acid antagonist.

Methotrimeprazine [120,166] **(Levoprome)**
Additive CNS depressant effects. Reduce the dosage of both drugs when used concurrently.

Methyldopa (Aldomet)
See *Barbiturates* under *Methyldopa.*

Nalorphine [166]
Nalorphine may add to the depressant effects of barbiturates. See *CNS Depressants* above.

Oral contraceptives [78,222]
(Estrogens-Progestogens)
Concern is being created by the possible ineffectiveness of oral contraceptives in women receiving barbiturates and other drugs that cause enzyme induction.

Pantothenyl alcohol [120] **(Ilopan)**
According to the manufacturer, concomitant use of barbiturates with pantothenyl alcohol causes allergic reactions. No substantiating reports exist in the literature as of 1977.

Pargyline [633] **(Eutonyl)**
Pargyline, an enzyme inhibitor, potentiates barbiturates.

Pentylenetetrazol [120] **(Metrazol, etc.)**
Pentylenetetrazol, a CNS stimulant, is used as an antidote to counteract the respiratory depression or failure caused by poisoning with barbiturates.

Phenothiazines [78,116,421,633,668,669]
Phenothiazines potentiate barbiturates but not their anticonvulsant action. Barbiturates decrease the effects of phenothiazines by increasing their metabolism after initial mutual potentiation of CNS depressant effects. Barbiturates antagonize parkinsonism effects of phenothiazines. Preoperative administration of phenothiazines potentiates thiopental anesthesia.

Phenylbutazone [330,555] **(Butazolidin)**
Barbiturates inhibit phenylbutazone through enzyme induction, and vice versa.

Phenytoin [63,78,96,640] **(Dilantin)**
See *Hydantoins* under *Phenobarbital.*

Piminodine [120,619] **(Alvodine)**
Barbiturates potentiate piminodine. See *CNS Depressants* and *Narcotic Analgesics.*

Pipazethate [950] **(Theratuss)**
Pipazethate, chemically related to the phenothiazines, may enhance CNS depressant effects of barbiturates.

Primidone [120,166] **(Mysoline)**
Since primidone is a barbiturate analog and is partially metabolized to phenobarbital, patients receiving the drug should be monitored for possible barbiturate interactions.

Proadifen [165]
See under *SKF-525A.* Proadifen is a drug potentiator which strongly inhibits the metabolism of other drugs.

Procaine [120] **(Novocain)**
Barbiturates (ultra-short acting, IV, slow infusion) may be used to control convulsions in severe reactions caused by procaine.

Procarbazine HCL [120] **(Matulane)**
Barbiturates should be used with caution in patients receiving this antineoplastic, to minimize CNS depression and possible synergism. See *MAO Inhibitors* above.

Progesterone [78]
Barbiturates inhibit progesterone (enzyme induction).

Propiomazine HCL [120] **(Largon)**
Propiomazine, a sedative, enhances the effects of central nervous system depressants. Therefore, the dose of barbiturates should be eliminated or reduced by at least ½ in the presence of propiomazine.

Pyrimethamine [120] **(Daraprim)**
Parenteral barbiturate followed by folinic acid is used to control CNS stimulation (convulsions) caused by an overdosage of pyrimethamine.

Reserpine [137]
Reserpine may potentiate CNS depression of barbiturates (hypotension and bradycardia) and decrease their anticonvulsant activity. The clinical importance of these effects has not been established.

Sodium bicarbonate
See *Alkalinizing Agents* above.

Steroids [78,421]
Barbiturates inhibit steroids through enzyme induction.

Steroids, ovarian [257,617]
Because of the resulting acceleration of the metabolism of ovarian steroids, administration of barbiturates to some patients may be contraindicated.

Sulfonamides
See *Barbiturates* under *Sulfonamides.*

Sulfonylurea hypoglycemics [78,633]
Sulfonylurea hypoglycemics potentiate barbiturates.

Tetracyclines
See *Barbiturates* under *Tetracyclines.*

Thiazide diuretics [120]
Orthostatic hypotension may be potentiated when the thiazides are given with barbiturates.

Thyroid drugs [330]
Increased barbiturate dosage is required when thyroid replacement therapy is initiated (increased metabolism).

Tranquilizers, minor [116,619]
Additive CNS effects; respiratory depression and sedation. Preoperative administration of minor tranquilizers potentiates thiopental anesthesia. See *CNS Depressants* above.

Vitamin C [274,325,616,962]
Vitamin C (ascorbic acid) by lowering the pH of the urine and decreasing urinary excretion, potentiates the sedative. Barbiturates increase the excretion of vitamin C.

Vitamin D
See *Barbiturates* under *Vitamin D.*

Warfarin sodium [120,223,434] **(Coumadin, Panwarfin)**
See *Anticoagulants, Oral* above.

BARBITURATES *(continued)*

X-Ray, cephalic [951]
X-Ray accelerates onset and prolongs duration of hypnosis by barbiturates.

BAR-TROPIN TABLETS
See *Atropine* and *Barbiturates.*

BECOTIN
See *Ascorbic Acid* and *Vitamin B Complex.*

BEEF LIVER

MAO inhibitors [757]
A meal of beef liver with MAO inhibitor therapy may cause a hypertensive crisis.

BEER
See *Tyramine-rich Foods* and MAO Inhibitors.
A patient who takes MAO inhibitors and drinks beer may have severe headaches and possibly suffer a hypertensive crisis.

BELBARB
See *Atropine, Hyoscyamine, Phenobarbital,* and *Scopolamine.*

BELLADENAL
See *Alcohol, Belladonna,* and *Phenobarbital.*

BELLERGAL
See *Belladonna, Ergotamine,* and *Phenobarbital.*

BEMINAL
See *Ascorbic Acid* and *Vitamin B Complex.*

BENACTYZINE (Suavitil)

Anticholinergics [120]
Benactyzine, an anticholinergic used as a sedative, potentiates the side effects of other anticholinergics. The additive effects are hazardous in glaucoma.

Meprobamate [125]
A small but significant inhibition of microsomal metabolism of meprobamate is caused by benactyzine.

Psychotherapeutic drugs [618]
Avoid concomitant administration of other psychotherapeutic drugs, particularly phenothiazines and MAO inhibitors. See *CNS Depressants* and *MAO Inhibitors.*

BENADRYL
See *Antihistamines* and *Diphenhydramine.*

BENDECTIN
See *Antihistamines, Doxylamine (Decapryn),* and *Pyridoxine.*

BENDROFLUMETHIAZIDE (Benuron, Naturetin)
See *Thiazide Diuretics.*

Diazoxide [117,120] **(Hyperstat)**
The antihypertensive effect of diazoxide may be augmented by thiazide diuretics. A combination of diazoxide with another benzothiadiazine (bendroflumethiazide) has proved useful in treating hypoglycemia produced by insulin-secreting tumors.

BENEMID
See *Probenecid* and *Uricosuric Agents.*

BENORYLATE [1984]

D-Penicillamine
See *Benorylate* under *Penicillamine.*

BENTYL HCl
See *Alcohol, Acidifying Agents,* and *Phenobarbital.*

BENYLIN
See *Alcohol, Acidifying Agents,* and *Antihistamines.*

BENZEDRINE
See *Amphetamine* and *Sympathomimetics.*

BENZODIAZEPINES (Chlordiazepoxide [Librium], clonazepam [Clonopin], clorazepate [Tranxene], diazepam [Valium], flurazepam [Dalmane], oxazepam [Serax], etc.
See also *Chlordiazepoxide* (Librium), *Diazepam* (Valium), and *Oxazepam* (Serax).

Alcohol [120,167,283,330,421,1142,1584,1614]
Warn patients about the hazards of this combination. Alcohol may potentiate the sedative and other CNS depressant effects of benzodiazepines, especially chlordiazepoxide, and vice versa. The effects may be supra-additive, particularly respiratory depression and impairment of motor skills.

Anticoagulants, oral [330,814,894]
Benzodiazepines may have variable effects on oral anticoagulants. See *Benzodiazepines* under *Anticoagulants.*

Antidepressants, tricyclic [78,120,166,330,421,953,954]
Antidepressants may potentiate the sedative and anticholinergic effects of benzodiazepines and vice versa. A syndrome resembling brain damage may appear.

Barbiturates [120,166,421]
Barbiturates may potentiate the sedative effects of benzodiazepines and vice versa. Benzodiazepines, by inhibiting metabolism, may increase the plasma levels of barbiturates. See *CNS Depressants.*

Haloperidol [120,421] **(Haldol)**
This combination produces potentiated CNS depressant effects. See *CNS Depressants.*

Levodopa [1498,1909]
Diazepam and possibly other benzodiazepines antagonize the therapeutic effectiveness of levodopa in parkinsonism. Monitor patients on this combination closely.

Lidocaine
See *Diazepam* under *Lidocaine.*

Lithium carbonate
See *Benzodiazepines* under *Lithium Carbonate.*

Mandrax [783] **(Diphenhydramine plus methaqualone)**
Diazepam (Valium) given to a patient with high dosage of Mandrax may develop apnea, respiratory depression and paralysis.

MAO inhibitors [120,330,421,1988,2008]
MAO inhibitors may potentiate the sedative effects of benzodiazepines. Phenelzine and diazepam were reported to cause severe edema [1988] but the interaction has been questioned. [2008] See *Benzodiazepines* under *MAO Inhibitors.*

Muscle relaxants [781,1331,1891]
Diazepam (Valium) may influence the duration of action of muscle relaxants (increase that of gallamine, decrease that of succinylcholine) or may have no effect depending on dosage, route of administration, etc.

Narcotics [421]
See *CNS Depressants.*

Phenothiazines [120,330,421]
Phenothiazines may potentiate the sedative effects of benzodiazepines and vice versa. See *CNS Depressants.* Severe atropinelike reactions may occur.

Phenytoin [884]
Benzodiazepines, by inhibiting metabolism of the hydantoin, potentiate the anticonvulsant and increase its toxicity.

Sedatives and hypnotics [421]
See *CNS Depressants.*

BENZOLAMIDE
See *Amiloride* under *Acetazolamide.*

BENZOTHIADIAZIDES
See *Thiazide Diuretics.*

3,4-BENZPYRENE

Anticoagulants, oral [633]
Benzpyrene inhibits oral anticoagulants probably through enzyme induction.

BENZQUINAMIDE (Quantril)
See *Reserpine.*
This benzoquinolizine derivative is similar to reserpine except it does not deplete stores of norepinephrine and serotonin in the brain. Benzquinamide probably has many interactions similar to those given for reserpine.

BENZTROPINE MESYLATE (Cogentin)
See *Anticholinergics, Antiparkinsonism Drugs,* and *Phenothiazines.*
Since this drug is related structurally to atropine (anticholinergic) and diphenhydramine (antihistamine) it possesses both types of drug interaction potentials.

Alcohol [120]
See *Alcohol* under *Anticholinergics* and *Phenothiazines.*

Haloperidol [120,619]
Haloperidol and benztropine may cause gynecomastia. Benztropine antagonizes the extrapyramidal effects of haloperidol.

Phenothiazines [120]
Benztropine relieves the parkinsonism that may be induced by phenothiazine therapy.

Reserpine [120]
Same as for *Phenothiazines* above.

BENZYL PENICILLIN

Cephalosporin antibiotics [120]
(Keflin, Loridine, etc.)
Cross-allergenicity (possibly death) may occur. Patients who are allergic to penicillin may also be allergic to cephalothin, cephaloridine, and related antibiotics.

Sodium cloxacillin [382] **(Tegopen)**
Synergistic antibacterial effect.

Sodium Methicillin [382] **(Dimocillin-RT, Staphcillin)**
Synergistic antibacterial effect.

Sodium nafcillin [382] **(Unipen)**
Synergistic antibacterial effect.

Sodium oxacillin [382] **(Prostaphlin)**
Synergistic antibacterial effect.

BEROCCA-C
See *Ascorbic Acid* and *Vitamin B Complex.*

BESTA
See *Ascorbic Acid* and *Vitamin B Complex.*

BETA-ADRENERGIC BLOCKERS
See *β-Adrenergic Blocking Agents.*

BETA-CHLOR
See *Chloral Betaine* and *Chloral Hydrate.*

BETACREST
See *Ascorbic Acid* and *Vitamin B Complex.*

BETAHISTINE HCl (Serc)

Anticholinergics [421]
The inhibitory action of the anticholinergics on hydrochloric acid secretion is antagonized by betahistine.

Antihistamines [120,421]
Betahistine antagonizes antihistamines and vice versa. Do not use concurrently.

BETAINE (Acidol)

Anticholinergics [421]
The inhibitory action of the anticholinergics on hydrochloric acid secretion is antagonized by betaine.

BETALIN COMPLEX
See *Vitamin B Complex.*

BETAMETHASONE (Celestone)
See *Corticosteroids.*

BETAZOLE (Histalog)

Anticholinergics [421]
The inhibitory action of the anticholinergics on the hydrochloric acid secretion is antagonized by betazole.

Antihistamines [421]
Betazole, an analog of histamine, antagonizes antihistamines and vice versa.

BETHANECHOL (Urecholine)
See *Parasympathomimetics.*

Atropine [168,619]
Atropine readily blocks the effects of the muscarinic agent bethanechol.

BETHANIDINE (Esbatal)
See *Antihypertensives* and *Guanethidine.*
Since bethanidine is an adrenergic neuron blocking agent like guanethidine, many of their interactions are identical.

Amphetamines [550,626,797]
Amphetamines antagonize the hypotensive action of bethanidine.

Antidepressants, tricyclic [327,598,823,1414,1672]
Tricyclic antidepressants inhibit bethanidine, an adrenergic blocking agent, and may completely reverse its antihypertensive action. See *Antidepressants, Tricyclic* under *Antihypertensives.*

Doxepin [1672] **(Sinequan)**
See *Antidepressants Tricyclic* under *Antihypertensives.* Doxepin inhibits uptake of bethanidine by adrenergic neurons to the site of its action, but not as strongly as other tricyclic antidepressants. It therefore antagonizes bethanidine's antihypertensive actions and caution must be exercised.

Ephedrine [823,1382,1832]
Ephedrine, given to patients on bethanidine, may produce symptoms of hypertensive crisis (severe headache, visual disturbances, etc.). Avoid or monitor very closely.

Levarterenol [117] **(Levophed)**
Bethanidine increases the pressor response to levarterenol 2- or 3-fold.

Methamphetamine [117]
(Desoxyn, Drinalfa, Methedrine, etc.)
Bethanidine, by causing depletion of catecholamines, reduces the pressor response to indirectly acting pressor amines like methamphetamine which act by releasing norepinephrine from its storage sites.

BETHANIDINE (Esbatal) *(continued)*

Methyldopa [951] **(Aldomet)**
Synergistic antihypertensive activity; effective in patients resistant to methyldopa.

Phenylpropanolamine [1082] **(Propadrine)**
This sympathomimetic (constituent of Ornade, etc.) antagonizes bethanidine. Severe hypertension may occur in a hypertensive patient under control. On one hypertensive patient both Ornade and bethanidine had to be stopped and methyldopa used. Avoid the combination or monitor very closely.

BICARBONATE OF SODA
See *Alkalinizing Agents*

Tetracyclines [75,633]
Absorption of tetracycline is reduced by 50% when a patient takes bicarbonate of soda. See *Antacids* and *Tetracyclines*.

BICILLIN
See *Penicillin*.

BIGUANIDES
See *Phenformin DBI*.

Insulin [421]
Biguanides increase the hypoglycemic effect of insulin.

BILAMIDE
See *Dehydrocholic Acid, Homatropine*, and *Phenobarbital*.

BILE SALTS

Anticoagulants, oral [421]
Lack of bile potentiates anticoagulants (decreased absorption of vitamin K).

Vitamins [176]
Bile salts enhance the absorption of vitamins A and K and other fat soluble vitamins.

BILIRUBIN

Corticosteroids [198]
Bilirubin potentiates corticosteroids by displacing them from secondary binding sites.

DDT [264,1076]
DDT has been used to accelerate the conjugation of bilirubin in neonatal hyperbilirubinemia, sometimes caused by displacement from protein binding sites with drugs like sulfonamides.

BIOLOGICALS
See *Vaccines*.

BIOMYDRIN (Antibiotic Nasal Spray, Drops)
See *Phenylephrine*.

BISACODYL (Dulcolax)

Dioctyl sodium sulfosuccinate [433,951]
The combination may induce abdominal cramps.

BISHYDROXYCOUMARIN (Dicumarol)
See *Anticoagulants, Oral*.

BISMUTH SALTS
See *Complexing Agents* under *Tetracyclines*.

BLACK WIDOW SPIDER VENOM

Barbiturates [120]
The neurotoxic venom can cause respiratory paralysis. Use morphine and barbiturates with caution.

Morphine [120]
See *Barbiturates* above.

Calcium gluconate [689]
Calcium gluconate relieves the pain and muscle spasm caused by the venom.

BLOOD CHOLESTEROL LOWERING AGENTS
See *Cholestyramine, Clofibrate, Dextrothyroxine, Triiodothyronine*, etc.

BONE MARROW DEPRESSANTS
See *Antineoplastics* and *Chloroquine*.

BONINE
See *Antihistamines* (meclizine HCl).

BONTRIL
See *Phendimetrazine*.

BOVRIL
See *Tyramine-rich Foods* [758]

BRETYLIUM (Bretylan, Darenthin, Ornid, etc.)
See *Antihypertensives* and *Guanethidine*.
Since bretylium is an adrenergic neuron blocking agent like guanethidine, many of their interactions are identical. [550]

BRINALDIX
See *Clopamide*.

BRISTURON
See *Thiazide Diuretics*.

BROAD BEAN PODS
See *Tyramine-rich Foods* [213,633,759] and under *MAO Inhibitors*.

BROMELAINS (Ananase)

Anticoagulants, oral [120,421]
Oral anticoagulants are potentiated by bromelains. The latter should be used cautiously in patients with abnormal clotting mechanisms, but are usually not recommended in this combination.

BROMISOVALUM (Bromural)
See *CNS Depressants*.

BROMPHENIRAMINE (Dimetane)
See *Antihistamines*.

BROMSULPHALEIN (BSP) SOLUTION
See *Sulfobromophthalein*.

BROMURAL (Bromisovalum)
See *Hypnotics* and *Sedatives*.

BRONCHOBID
See *Ephedrine* and *Theophylline*.

BRONDECON
See *Glyceryl Guaiacolate* and *Xanthines*.

BRONKOLIXIR
See *Ephedrine, Glyceryl Guaiacolate, Phenobarbital*, and *Theophylline*.

BRONKOSOL
See *Isoetharine* and *Phenylephrine*.

BRONKOTABS
See *Ephedrine, Glyceryl Guaiacolate, Barbiturates*, and *Theophylline*.

B-SCORBIC
See *Ascorbic Acid* and *Vitamin B Complex*.

BUCLADIN-S
See *Buclizine*.

BUCLIZINE (Bucladin-S, Softran)

Anticholinergics[166]
Buclizine potentiates the side effects of anticholinergics such as dryness of the mouth. Hazardous in glaucoma.

BUFF-A-COMP
See *Aspirin, Barbiturates, Caffeine* and *Phenacetin*.

BUFFERIN
See *Salicylates, Buffered*.

BULBOCAPNINE
Bulbocapnine, which blocks central dopamine receptors and which has been used for 4 centuries to control tremor, is a cataleptic agent whose action is prevented by pretreatment with amantadine, imipramine, trihexyphenidyl, or diphenhydramine. Both apomorphine and levodopa antagonize bulbocapnine-induced catalepsy.[166]

BUSULFAN (Myleran)

Other antineoplastics[120]
Busulfan should not be administered if other similar antineoplastics have recently been administered. Possible additive cytotoxic or myelosuppressive effects.

BUTABARBITAL (Butisol)
See *Barbiturates*.

BUTACAINE (Butyn)
See *p-Aminobenzoic Acid* and *Anesthetics, local*.

BUTALBITAL (Lotusate, Sandoptal)
See *Barbiturates*.

BUTAZOLIDIN
See *Phenylbutazone*.

BUTAZOLIDIN ALKA
See *Aluminum, Magnesium*, and *Phenylbutazone*.

BUTIBEL
See *Barbiturates* and *Belladonna*.

BUTIBEL-ZYME
See *Barbiturates, Belladonna*, and *Enzymes*.

BUTICAPS
See *Barbiturates*.

BUTISERPAZIDE
See *Barbiturates, Hydrochlorothiazide, Reserpine*, and *Thiazide Diuretics*.

BUTISOL SODIUM
See *Barbiturates*.

BUTIZIDE
See *Barbiturates, Hydrochlorothiazide*, and *Thiazide Diuretics*.

BUTYN
See *p-Aminobenzoic Acid (analog)* and *Anesthetics, local*.

BUTYROPHENONES
See *Haloperidol* (Haldol), the first in this series of tranquilizers.

CAFERGOT P-B
See *Belladonna, Caffeine, Ergot Alkaloids*, and *Pentobarbital*.

CAFFEINE
See also *CNS Stimulants*.

Alcohol[166,711,2004,2024]
CNS stimulants like caffeine antagonize the CNS depressant effects of alcohol, except that they do not improve the decreased motor function induced by alcohol. One study did not support caffeine antagonism of alcohol, but showed that the alkaloid increased impairment of performance. Severe alcoholic intoxication must be treated like other acute central depressions (IV mannitol, spinal fluid drainage, ventilatory assistance, hemodialysis, etc.). Certain phenothiazines may be indicated for hyperactive, violent alcoholics.

Diazepam[120] **(Valium)**
Caffeine and sodium benzoate combats CNS depressant effects caused by overdosage of diazepam.

MAO inhibitors[120]
Dosage of caffeine-containing medications should be reduced. Excessive use of caffeine can cause hypertensive reaction.

Pargyline (Eutonyl)
See *MAO Inhibitors* above.

Propoxyphene[120,421] **(Darvon)**
Caffeine increases CNS stimulation in overdosage of propoxyphene. Fatal convulsions may be produced.

CALCIDRINE
See *Calcium Salts, Codeine* and *Ephedrine*.

CALCITONIN

Androgens[181]
Calcitonin and androgens potentiate each other; have similar effects on calcium retention. Calcitonin directly inhibits bone resorption.

Parathormone[181]
The hypocalcemic effect of calcitonin antagonizes the hypercalcemic effect of parathormone.

CALCIUM CARBIMIDE CITRATE (Dipsan, Temposil)

Alcohol[121]
Calcium carbimide citrate prevents oxidation of acetaldehyde, a metabolite of ethyl alcohol, thus producing a disulfiramlike reaction after ingestion of alcohol.

CALCIUM SALTS (Calcium chloride, calcium gluconate, calcium lactate, milk, etc.)

Black widow spider venom[689]
Calcium gluconate relieves the pain and muscle spasm caused by the venom.

Cephalothin[120] **(Keflin)**
Cephalothin is incompatible with calcium, magnesium, strontium, and other alkaline earth elements.

Digitalis[120,633,634]
Elevated serum calcium increases digitalis toxicity. Death has resulted after calcium IV. See *Calcium Salts* under *Digitalis*.

Kanamycin[178,421,494-498]
Calcium may reduce the neuromuscular blockade (neuromuscular paralysis and respiratory depression) produced by the aminoglycoside antibiotics kanamycin, neomycin, polymyxin, and streptomycin.

Milk[61]
This combination in excess may cause the milk-alkali syndrome described for *Milk* under *Sodium Bicarbonate*.

CALCIUM SALTS *(continued)*

Narcotic analgesics [166]
The intracisternal injection of calcium ions antagonizes the analgesic action of narcotic analgesics (opioids).

Neomycin
See *Kanamycin* above.

Streptomycin
See *Kanamycin* above.

Tetracyclines [48, 421]
Calcium inhibits tetracycline absorption and thus its antimicrobial action.

Vitamin D [182]
Vitamin D enhances the Intestinal absorption of dietary calcium.

CALPHOSAN
See *Calcium Salts.*

Digitalis [120]
Calphosan is contraindicated with digitalis; both have similar action on the contractility and excitability of the heart muscle.

CALSCORBATE
See *Calcium Salts.*

CANCER THERAPY
See *Antineoplastics,* individual chemotherapeutic agents, *X-radiation,* etc.

CANTIL (with or without phenobarbital)
See *Anticholinergics, Bromides, Mepenzolate Bromide,* and *Phenobarbital.*

CARBAMAZEPINE (Tegretol)
See also *Antidepressants, Tricyclic.*
This drug, used in treating trigeminal neuralgia, is structurally related to the imipramine type of drugs, and its interactions are similar.

Alcohol [48, 139, 166, 290, 629, 729]
Carbamazepine may potentiate the sedative effect of alcohol. The combination of alcohol and a tricyclic antidepressant has been fatal.

Anticoagulants, oral
See *Carbamazepine* under *Anticoagulants, Oral.*

Antidepressants, tricyclic [120]
Carbamazepine should not be used with or for at least one week after discontinuing therapy with amitriptyline, desipramine, imipramine, etc. A latent psychosis and confusion or agitation in elderly patients may be activated.

Barbiturates [120, 1289]
Barbiturates may be used parenterally to treat hyperirritability caused by overdosage of the drug, but use caution because barbiturates may induce respiratory depression, especially in children. Contraindicated if MAO inhibitors have been given recently. In combined therapy of carbamazepine and barbiturate, the latter as an enzyme inducer enhances the metabolism of the former and lowers its plasma levels and potency. Adjust dosage as necessary.

Digitalis glycosides
See *Carbamazepine* under *Digitalis and Digitalis Glycosides.*

MAO inhibitors [120]
Concurrent use with MAO inhibitors is contraindicated because of its structural relationship to tricyclic antidepressants. Discontinue the MAO inhibitors at least 7 days before giving carbamazepine.

Phenytoin
See *Carbamazepine* under *Phenytoin.*

Propoxyphene
See *Carbamazepine* under *Propoxyphene.*

Tetracyclines
See *Carbamazepine* under *Tetracyclines.*

CARBAZOCHROME SALICYLATE (Adrenosem Salicylate)

Antihistamines [120, 421]
Antihistamines inhibit the antihemorrhagic effects of carbazochrome salicylate and should be discontinued 2 days before the drug is administered.

CARBENICILLIN (Geopen)

Ampicillin [421, 1129] **(Alpen, Polycillin, etc.)**
Ampicillin inhibits the antibiotic carbenicillin.

Gentamicin [1402, 1506, 1540, 1549, 1575, 1611, 1612, 1738, 1739, 1767, 1908] **(Garamycin)**
Carbenicillin in high concentrations inhibits the antibacterial activity of gentamicin *in vitro* if allowed to remain in contact over a period of time and this could be a problem in some patients when carbenicillin levels become high (as in renal impairment). However, the combination of carbenicillin and gentamicin is a drug of choice in severe infections due to *Pseudomonas aeruginosa.* Do not mix the antibiotics ahead of time and allow them to stand for a prolonged period before administration.

CARBENOXOLONE (Biogastrone, Bioral, Duogastrone)

Spironolactone **(Aldactone)**
See *Carbenoxolone* under *Spironolactone.*

CARBOCAINE
See *Anesthetics, Local* and *Mepivacaine.*

CARBON DIOXIDE

Mecamylamine [349] **(Inversine)**
Administration of CO_2 potentiates mecamylamine.

d-**Tubocurarine** [1075]
Excess CO_2 potentiates *d*-tubocurarine.

CARBONIC ANHYDRASE INHIBITORS (Acetazolamide [Diamox], dichlorphenamide [Daranide, Oratrol], ethoxzolamide [Cardrase, Ethamide], methazolamide [Neptazane])
For drug interactions typical of this category see *Acetazolamide.*

Acidifying agents [325, 870]
Acidifying agents antagonize the alkalinizing carbonic anhydrase inhibitors.

CARBON TETRACHLORIDE

Alcohol [902]
Alcohol and carbon tetrachloride may mutually enhance hepatotoxic, nephrotoxic and CNS depressant effects.

Anticoagulants [48, 295, 433]
Because of its hepatotoxic effects, carbon tetrachloride may cause hypoprothrombinemia (hemorrhage) with coumarin anticoagulants.

Barbiturates [902]
Barbiturates sensitize to the toxic effects of carbon tetrachloride 100-fold.

CARBRITAL
See *Barbiturates (Pentobarbital)* and *Carbromal*

Alcohol [120]
Alcohol potentiates the CNS depressant effects of Carbrital. Death possible.

BUCLADIN-S
See *Buclizine.*

BUCLIZINE (Bucladin-S, Softran)

Anticholinergics [166]
Buclizine potentiates the side effects of anticholinergics such as dryness of the mouth. Hazardous in glaucoma.

BUFF-A-COMP
See *Aspirin, Barbiturates, Caffeine* and *Phenacetin.*

BUFFERIN
See *Salicylates, Buffered.*

BULBOCAPNINE
Bulbocapnine, which blocks central dopamine receptors and which has been used for 4 centuries to control tremor, is a cataleptic agent whose action is prevented by pretreatment with amantadine, imipramine, trihexyphenidyl, or diphenhydramine. Both apomorphine and levodopa antagonize bulbocapnine-induced catalepsy. [166]

BUSULFAN (Myleran)

Other antineoplastics [120]
Busulfan should not be administered if other similar antineoplastics have recently been administered. Possible additive cytotoxic or myelosuppressive effects.

BUTABARBITAL (Butisol)
See *Barbiturates.*

BUTACAINE (Butyn)
See *p-Aminobenzoic Acid* and *Anesthetics, local.*

BUTALBITAL (Lotusate, Sandoptal)
See *Barbiturates.*

BUTAZOLIDIN
See *Phenylbutazone.*

BUTAZOLIDIN ALKA
See *Aluminum, Magnesium,* and *Phenylbutazone.*

BUTIBEL
See *Barbiturates* and *Belladonna.*

BUTIBEL-ZYME
See *Barbiturates, Belladonna,* and *Enzymes.*

BUTICAPS
See *Barbiturates.*

BUTISERPAZIDE
See *Barbiturates, Hydrochlorothiazide, Reserpine,* and *Thiazide Diuretics.*

BUTISOL SODIUM
See *Barbiturates.*

BUTIZIDE
See *Barbiturates, Hydrochlorothiazide,* and *Thiazide Diuretics.*

BUTYN
See *p-Aminobenzoic Acid (analog)* and *Anesthetics, local.*

BUTYROPHENONES
See *Haloperidol* (Haldol), the first in this series of tranquilizers.

CAFERGOT P-B
See *Belladonna, Caffeine, Ergot Alkaloids,* and *Pentobarbital.*

CAFFEINE
See also *CNS Stimulants.*

Alcohol [166, 711, 2004, 2024]
CNS stimulants like caffeine antagonize the CNS depressant effects of alcohol, except that they do not improve the decreased motor function induced by alcohol. One study did not support caffeine antagonism of alcohol, but showed that the alkaloid increased impairment of performance. Severe alcoholic intoxication must be treated like other acute central depressions (IV mannitol, spinal fluid drainage, ventilatory assistance, hemodialysis, etc.). Certain phenothiazines may be indicated for hyperactive, violent alcoholics.

Diazepam [120] **(Valium)**
Caffeine and sodium benzoate combats CNS depressant effects caused by overdosage of diazepam.

MAO inhibitors [120]
Dosage of caffeine-containing medications should be reduced. Excessive use of caffeine can cause hypertensive reaction.

Pargyline (Eutonyl)
See *MAO Inhibitors* above.

Propoxyphene [120, 421] **(Darvon)**
Caffeine increases CNS stimulation in overdosage of propoxyphene. Fatal convulsions may be produced.

CALCIDRINE
See *Calcium Salts, Codeine* and *Ephedrine.*

CALCITONIN

Androgens [181]
Calcitonin and androgens potentiate each other; have similar effects on calcium retention. Calcitonin directly inhibits bone resorption.

Parathormone [181]
The hypocalcemic effect of calcitonin antagonizes the hypercalcemic effect of parathormone.

CALCIUM CARBIMIDE CITRATE (Dipsan, Temposil)

Alcohol [121]
Calcium carbimide citrate prevents oxidation of acetaldehyde, a metabolite of ethyl alcohol, thus producing a disulfiramlike reaction after ingestion of alcohol.

CALCIUM SALTS (Calcium chloride, calcium gluconate, calcium lactate, milk, etc.)

Black widow spider venom [689]
Calcium gluconate relieves the pain and muscle spasm caused by the venom.

Cephalothin [120] **(Keflin)**
Cephalothin is incompatible with calcium, magnesium, strontium, and other alkaline earth elements.

Digitalis [120, 633, 634]
Elevated serum calcium increases digitalis toxicity. Death has resulted after calcium IV. See *Calcium Salts* under *Digitalis.*

Kanamycin [178, 421, 494-498]
Calcium may reduce the neuromuscular blockade (neuromuscular paralysis and respiratory depression) produced by the aminoglycoside antibiotics kanamycin, neomycin, polymyxin, and streptomycin.

Milk [61]
This combination in excess may cause the milk-alkali syndrome described for *Milk* under *Sodium Bicarbonate.*

CALCIUM SALTS *(continued)*

Narcotic analgesics [166]
The intracisternal injection of calcium ions antagonizes the analgesic action of narcotic analgesics (opioids).

Neomycin
See *Kanamycin* above.

Streptomycin
See *Kanamycin* above.

Tetracyclines [48,421]
Calcium inhibits tetracycline absorption and thus its antimicrobial action.

Vitamin D [182]
Vitamin D enhances the intestinal absorption of dietary calcium.

CALPHOSAN
See *Calcium Salts*.

Digitalis [120]
Calphosan is contraindicated with digitalis; both have similar action on the contractility and excitability of the heart muscle.

CALSCORBATE
See *Calcium Salts*.

CANCER THERAPY
See *Antineoplastics*, individual chemotherapeutic agents, *X-radiation*, etc.

CANTIL (with or without phenobarbital)
See *Anticholinergics, Bromides, Mepenzolate Bromide,* and *Phenobarbital*.

CARBAMAZEPINE (Tegretol)
See also *Antidepressants, Tricyclic*.
This drug, used in treating trigeminal neuralgia, is structurally related to the imipramine type of drugs, and its interactions are similar.

Alcohol [48,139,166,290,629,729]
Carbamazepine may potentiate the sedative effect of alcohol. The combination of alcohol and a tricyclic antidepressant has been fatal.

Anticoagulants, oral
See *Carbamazepine* under *Anticoagulants, Oral*.

Antidepressants, tricyclic [120]
Carbamazepine should not be used with or for at least one week after discontinuing therapy with amitriptyline, desipramine, imipramine, etc. A latent psychosis and confusion or agitation in elderly patients may be activated.

Barbiturates [120,1289]
Barbiturates may be used parenterally to treat hyperirritability caused by overdosage of the drug, but use caution because barbiturates may induce respiratory depression, especially in children. Contraindicated if MAO inhibitors have been given recently. In combined therapy of carbamazepine and barbiturate, the latter as an enzyme inducer enhances the metabolism of the former and lowers its plasma levels and potency. Adjust dosage as necessary.

Digitalis glycosides
See *Carbamazepine* under *Digitalis and Digitalis Glycosides*.

MAO inhibitors [120]
Concurrent use with MAO inhibitors is contraindicated because of its structural relationship to tricyclic antidepressants. Discontinue the MAO inhibitors at least 7 days before giving carbamazepine.

Phenytoin
See *Carbamazepine* under *Phenytoin*.

Propoxyphene
See *Carbamazepine* under *Propoxyphene*.

Tetracyclines
See *Carbamazepine* under *Tetracyclines*.

CARBAZOCHROME SALICYLATE (Adrenosem Salicylate)

Antihistamines [120,421]
Antihistamines inhibit the antihemorrhagic effects of carbazochrome salicylate and should be discontinued 2 days before the drug is administered.

CARBENICILLIN (Geopen)

Ampicillin [421,1129] (Alpen, Polycillin, etc.)
Ampicillin inhibits the antibiotic carbenicillin.

Gentamicin [1402,1506,1540,1549,1575,1611,1612,1738,1739,1767,1908] (Garamycin)
Carbenicillin in high concentrations inhibits the antibacterial activity of gentamicin *in vitro* if allowed to remain in contact over a period of time and this could be a problem in some patients when carbenicillin levels become high (as in renal impairment). However, the combination of carbenicillin and gentamicin is a drug of choice in severe infections due to *Pseudomonas aeruginosa*. Do not mix the antibiotics ahead of time and allow them to stand for a prolonged period before administration.

CARBENOXOLONE (Biogastrone, Bioral, Duogastrone)

Spironolactone (Aldactone)
See *Carbenoxolone* under *Spironolactone*.

CARBOCAINE
See *Anesthetics, Local* and *Mepivacaine*.

CARBON DIOXIDE

Mecamylamine [349] (Inversine)
Administration of CO_2 potentiates mecamylamine.

d-Tubocurarine [1075]
Excess CO_2 potentiates *d*-tubocurarine.

CARBONIC ANHYDRASE INHIBITORS (Acetazolamide [Diamox], dichlorphenamide [Daranide, Oratrol], ethoxzolamide [Cardrase, Ethamide], methazolamide [Neptazane])
For drug interactions typical of this category see *Acetazolamide*.

Acidifying agents [325,870]
Acidifying agents antagonize the alkalinizing carbonic anhydrase inhibitors.

CARBON TETRACHLORIDE

Alcohol [902]
Alcohol and carbon tetrachloride may mutually enhance hepatotoxic, nephrotoxic and CNS depressant effects.

Anticoagulants [48,295,433]
Because of its hepatotoxic effects, carbon tetrachloride may cause hypoprothrombinemia (hemorrhage) with coumarin anticoagulants.

Barbiturates [902]
Barbiturates sensitize to the toxic effects of carbon tetrachloride 100-fold.

CARBRITAL
See *Barbiturates (Pentobarbital)* and *Carbromal*

Alcohol [120]
Alcohol potentiates the CNS depressant effects of Carbrital. Death possible.

Antidepressants, tricyclic [120]
(Amitriptyline, imipramine, etc.)
Tricyclic antidepressants potentiate Carbrital.

Antihistamines [120]
Antihistamines potentiate Carbrital.

Corticosteroids [120]
Corticosteroids potentiate Carbrital.

MAO inhibitors [120]
MAO inhibitors potentiate Carbrital.

Narcotic analgesics [120]
Narcotic analgesics potentiate Carbrital.

Rauwolfia alkaloids [120]
Rauwolfia alkaloids potentiate Carbrital.

Tranquilizers [120]
Tranquilizers potentiate Carbrital.

CARBROMAL
See *CNS Depressants*.
This drug is a monoureide which is a short-acting sedative and hypnotic. It has the additive CNS depressant effects of other drugs in its class.

CARDIAC GLYCOSIDES
See *Digitalis*.

CARDILATE-P
See *Erythrityl Tetranitrate, Nitrates* and *Nitrites*, and *Phenobarbital*.

CARDIOQUIN
See *Quinidine*.

CARDIOVASCULAR DEPRESSANTS

Anesthetics, local [120]
Cardiovascular depressant effects may be enhanced when used simultaneously with local anesthetics.

CARISOPRODOL (Rela, Soma)
See *Muscle Relaxants*.

Alcohol [120]
The CNS depressant effects of alcohol and carisoprodol may be additive and impair the mental and physical abilities required for driving automobiles, operating machinery, and other hazardous tasks.

Antidepressants, tricyclic [599]
Tricyclic antidepressants like imipramine potentiate the actions of carisoprodol.

Barbiturates [120]
Possible potentiation of CNS depressant effects initially, followed by inhibition due to enzyme induction. See *CNS Depressants*.

Carisoprodol [120]
Tolerance to the sedative and hypnotic effects of the drug may develop (enzyme induction).

Chlorcyclizine [565]
Chlorcyclizine inhibits carisoprodol by enzyme induction.

CNS stimulants [120]
Central nervous system stimulants (caffeine, pentylenetetrazol) may be used cautiously to counteract the shock and respiratory depression caused by overdosage of carisoprodol.

Diphenhydramine [950] **(Benadryl)**
Diphenhydramine may decrease the effects of the meprobamate analog by enzyme induction.

MAO inhibitors [599,950]
MAO inhibitors may potentiate the muscle relaxant and CNS depressant effects of carisoprodol.

Meprobamate [120]
Cross hypersensitivity reactions may occur with these drugs which have similar structures, *e.g.*, meprobamate. Also, due to enzyme induction, decreased effectiveness may result.

Phenobarbital [120]
See *Barbiturates* above.

CAROID AND BILE SALTS TABLETS
See *Cathartics, Papain*, and *Phenolphthalein*.

CARPHENAZINE
See *Phenothiazines* (proketazine).

CARTRAX
See *Hydroxyzine, Pentaerythritol Tetranitrate*, and *Tranquilizers*.

Acetylcholine [120]
Cartrax can act as a physiologic antagonist to acetylcholine.

Alcohol [120]
Alcohol may enhance individual sensitivity to the hypotensive effects of the PETN. Severe responses (nausea, vomiting, weakness, restlessness, pallor, and collapse).

CNS depressants [120]
Hydroxyzine potentiates other central nervous system depressants. Caution—reduce dosage of the depressants since Cartrax contains hydroxyzine.

Histamine [120]
Cartrax can act as a physiologic antagonist to histamine.

Nitrates and nitrites [120]
Tolerance to pentaerythritol tetranitrate (PETN) and cross tolerance to other nitrates and nitrites may develop.

Norepinephrine [120]
Cartrax can act as a physiologic antagonist to norepinephrine and many other drugs.

CATECHOLAMINES
(Dopamine [Intropin], epinephrine, isoproterenol [Isuprel], levarterenol [Levophed, norepinephrine], nordefrin [Cobefrin], protokylol, etc.)
See *Epinephrine, Levarterenol*, and *Sympathomimetics*.

Acetazolamide [172,325,870]
Catecholamines potentiate the anticonvulsant activity of acetazolamide. Acetazolamide, by its alkalinizing action potentiates these amines.

Anesthetics
See *Catecholamines* and *Epinephrine* under *Anesthetics, General*.

Furazolidone [198] **(Furoxone)**
MAO and microsomal enzyme inhibition; furazolidone potentiates catecholamines.

Guanethidine [117] **(Ismelin)**
Contraindicated. Guanethidine may augment responses to epinephrine, isoproterenol, levarterenol (norepinephrine), and other catecholamines. Cardiovascular (pressor) effects are intensified, glycogenolysis occurs, blood glucose levels are increased and many other effects of these sympathomimetic agents are enhanced. See *Polymechanistic Drugs* (page 378).

Levothyroxine [120]
Careful observation is required if catecholamines are administered to patients with coronary artery disease receiving thyroid preparations. An episode of coronary insufficiency may be precipitated.

CATECHOLAMINES *(continued)*

Propranolol [42,165,263]
Propranolol (adrenergic blocker) inhibits the glycogenolytic (hyperglycemic) action of epinephrine and related catecholamines.

Reserpine [168]
Reserpine and its derivatives reduce tissue levels of catecholamines.

Theophylline [168]
Theophylline potentiates the contractile response to catecholamines.

CATHARTICS
See also *Mineral Oil.*

Anticoagulants, oral [193,890]
Drastic cathartics may potentiate anticoagulant therapy by reducing absorption of vitamin K from the gut.

Dextrose [359]
Cathartics inhibit intestinal absorption of dextrose.

Digitalis [28,691]
Cathartics, by increasing the rate of passage of digitalis glycosides, inhibit their absorption and thus their cardiac action, but the hypokalemia produced increases the toxicity of the absorbed digitalis, and its potency. Monitor patients closely.

Glucose [359]
Some purgatives inhibit the intestinal absorption of glucose.

Muscle relaxants [28]
Laxative-induced hypokalemia potentiates muscle relaxants.

Oral medications [950,951]
Medications administered by the gastrointestinal route tend to be inhibited by cathartics because of hastened passage through the gut.

Tetracyclines [28]
Cathartics, especially magnesium sulfate, inhibit absorption and thus their antimicrobial action. See also *Complexing Agents.*

CAUSALIN
See *Salicylates.*

CECON
See *Ascorbic Acid.*

CEDILANID
See *Digitalis* and *Lanatoside C.*

CELESTONE
See *Betamethasone* and *Corticosteroids.*

CEPHALOSPORINS
(Cephaloridine [Loridine], sodium cephalothin [Keflin], etc.)

Aminoglycoside antibiotics
See *Gentamicin* below.

Ampicillin [120,233,1129]
Synergistic antibacterial effect. See *Penicillin* below re cross-sensitivity. Extemporaneous mixtures of cephalosporins with other antibiotics are not recommended as a rule, especially with others with a high nephrotoxic potential. See also *Cephalosporins* under *Ampicillin.*

Benzyl penicillin [120]
Synergistic antibacterial effect. See *Ampicillin* above and *Penicillins* below.

Calcium chloride
Cephalosporins are incompatible in parenteral mixtures with alkaline earth metals (calcium, magnesium, strontium, etc.). See Chapter 8.

Colistin [1546] (Coly-Mycin)
Cephalosporins such as cephalothin (Keflin) may potentiate the nephrotoxicity of colistin. A potentially very dangerous interaction. Monitor patients closely for impaired renal function.

Erythromycin
Cephalosporins are incompatible in parenteral mixtures with compounds of high molecular weight. See Chapter. 8.

Ethacrynic acid [1328] (Edecrin)
Ethacrynic acid may increase the nephrotoxicity of cephalosporins such as cephaloridine (Loridine).

Furosemids [1274,1328,1435,1541,1802] (Lasit)
Furosemide increases the nephrotoxicity of cephalosporins such as cephaloridine (Loridine). Potentially very dangerous. Monitor patients closely.

Gentamicin [1223,1251,1271,1274,1540,1541,1542,1668,1669,1678,1971] (Garamycin)
Cephalosporins (cephaloridine, cephalothin, etc.) and gentamicin (probably other aminoglycosides) have additive, possibly synergistic, nephrotoxicity, especially in older patients and those with renal impairment or on high dosage, or receiving probenecid. Monitor patients closely. A lethal interaction.

Erythromycin
Cephalosporins are incompatible in parenteral mixtures with compounds of high molecular weight. See Chapter 8.

Kanamycin [233,252,253]
Synergistic antibacterial effect on *E. coli.* Synergistic activity in treatment of multiple antibiotic-resistant, methicillin-resistant *Staph. aureus.*

Magnesium
See *Calcium* above.

Oxacillin, sodium [120] (Prostaphlin)
Cross-resistance with cephalosporins occur frequently.

Penicillins [120]
(Ampicillin, cloxacillin, methicillin, penicillin G, etc.)
Cross-sensitivity occurs between penicillins and cephalosporins. Death may occur in persons hypersensitive to either group. Cross-resistance also occurs with penicillinase-resistant penicillins.

Probenecid [1353,1620,1862] (Benemid)
Probenecid, by reducing the renal clearance of cephalosporins (especially cephalothin), potentiates the nephrotoxicity of these antibiotics. A very dangerous interaction. Renal damage is possible. Monitor patients closely and reduce dosage as necessary.

Streptomycin [252,253]
Synergistic activity against *Str. viridans* and *Str. faecalis.*

Tetracyclines
Incompatible in parenteral mixtures.

CEREALS
See *Cereals* under *Iron Salts.*

CEREBRO-NICIN
See *Niacinamide, Nicotinic Acid, Pentylenetetrazole,* and *Vitamin B.*

CEREMIA
See *Nicotinic Acid* and *Papaverine.*

CERESPAN
See *Papaverine.*

CHARCOAL
See *Charcoal* under *Anticoagulants, Oral.*

CHARCOAL BROILED MEATS
See *Smoking.*

CHARDONNA
See *Belladonna* and *Phenobarbital.*

CHEESE
See *Tyramine-rich Foods.*

CHELATING AGENTS (Citric acid, glucosamine, phosphates, etc.)

Tetracyclines [421]
Chelating agents that bind bivalent and trivalent ions enhance the absorption of tetracyclines by preventing these ions from forming insoluble complexes with the antibiotics. See *Complexing Agents.*

CHENODEOXYCHOLIC ACID

Vitamin C [1999]
Long-term administration of vitamin C may improve treatment of gallstones with chenodeoxycholic acid by accelerating transformation of cholesterol to bile acids and shortening the half life of plasma and liver cholesterol. Vitamin C may increase secretion of bile unsaturated in cholesterol both by the action of the chenoacid and by synthesis of the acid from cholesterol.

CHEMOVAG SUPPS
See *Sulfisoxazole* and *Sulfonamides.*

CHIANTI WINE
See *Tyramine-rich Foods*

CHICKEN LIVERS
See *Tyramine-rich Foods* and under *MAO Inhibitors* [120,207,421]

CHICKEN POX

Indomethacin
See *Chicken Pox* under *Indomethacin.*

CHLORAL BETAINE (Beta-chlor)

Anticoagulants, oral (Warfarin, etc.)
See *Chloral Hydrate* below. Chloral is both an enzyme inducer and, via its metabolite trichloroacetic acid, a displacer of some drugs from their protein binding sites.

CHLORAL HYDRATE (Noctec, Somnos)

Alcohol ("Mickey Finn")
See *Chloral Hydrate* under *Alcohol.*

Anticoagulants, oral [78,83,96,97,120,166,297,421,633,640,673,753,760,1135]
Chloral betaine or hydrate once believed to induce the hepatic microsomal enzymes and inhibit oral anticoagulants was later found to potentiate them through its metabolite, trichloracetic acid, which displaces them from their plasma protein binding sites.[753,760] This elevates anticoagulant blood levels and also expedites their metabolism (shortens half-life). Reduce the dosage of anticoagulants with chloral hydrate to avoid hemorrhage. See also *Chloral Hydrate* under *Anticoagulants, Oral.*

Bishydroxycoumarin [120]
See *Anticoagulants, Oral* above.

Corticosteroids [198]
Chloral hydrate decreases the activity of corticosteroids by enzyme induction.

Furazolidone [120,633] (Furoxone)
Furazolidone, a MAO inhibitor, may potentiate chloral hydrate. Reduce the dosage of the sedative as necessary if there is enhanced CNS depression.

Furosemide (Frusemide, Lasix)
See *Chloral Hydrate* under *Furosimide.*

Hexamethonium [166]
Chloral hydrate, if injected intraarterially, is a potent anticholinesterase, capable of reversing the effects of hexamethonium.

MAO inhibitors [120,633] and MAO inhibitor antidepressants
MAO inhibitors potentiate chloral hydrate. Reduce the dosage of the sedative.

Pargyline [120] (Eutonyl)
See *MAO Inhibitors* above.

Phenothiazines [120,166,608]
Some phenothiazines (antihistamines, etc.) potentiate the sedative (CNS depressant) effects of hypnotics. See *CNS Depressants.*

Steroids [198]
Steroids are inhibited by chloral hydrate (enzyme induction).

Tubocurarine [166]
Same action as with hexamethonium above.

CHLORAMBUCIL (Leukeran)
See *Alkylating Agents.*

CHLORAMPHENICOL (Chloromycetin)
See *Antibiotics.*

Acenocoumarol (Sintrom)
See *Anticoagulants, Oral.*

Acetanilid [938]
Chloramphenicol potentiates acetanilid by enzyme inhibition.

Alcohol [28]
Chloramphenicol, an enzyme inhibitor, produces a disulfiramlike reaction with alcohol by inhibiting aldehyde dehydrogenase and causing acetaldehyde, formed from alcohol, to accumulate.

Alkalinizing agents [578]
Alkaline urinary pH potentiates the antibacterial action of chloramphenicol.

Aminopyrine [676,938]
Chloramphenicol potentiates aminopyrine by enzyme inhibition.

Ampicillin [157,208,301,748] (Alpen, Polycillin, etc.)
Chloramphenicol inhibits the bactericidal action of penicillins.

Anticoagulants, oral [120,673,676]
Chloramphenicol may prolong the prothrombin time by interfering with vitamin K production by the gut bacteria and by enzyme inhibition; this reduces the dosage of anticoagulant needed. Hypoglycemic coma has occurred. Chloramphenicol inhibits the metabolism of dicumarol.

Antidiabetics, oral [676,767,1802] (Diabinese, Dymelor, Orinase, Tolinase, etc.)
Chloramphenicol potentiates the hypoglycemic effect of oral hypoglycemic agents. The half-lives of the sulfonylurea antidiabetics (chlorpropamide, tolbutamide, etc.) are prolonged when these drugs are administered simultaneously with chloramphenicol (enzyme inhibition). Hypoglycemic collapse may occur. Monitor patients closely and substitute insulin if necessary in those very few instances when chloramphenicol may be a drug of choice.

CHLORAMPHENICOL (Chloromycetin) (continued)

6-Azauridine [951]
Chloramphenicol, a drug metabolizing enzyme inhibitor, potentiates the immunosuppressive activity of 6-azauridine.

Barbiturates [83,330]
Chloramphenicol potentiates barbiturates (enzyme inhibition).

Chlorpropamide [767] (Diabinese)
See *Antidiabetics, Oral* above.

Cloxacillin [301,444,748]
Chloramphenicol inhibits the bactericidal action of this penicillin.

Codeine [676,938]
Chloramphenicol potentiates codeine (enzyme inhibition).

Cyclophosphamide [938,1045] (Cytoxan)
Chloramphenicol pretreatment reduces the lethality of cyclophosphamide; effect is apparently due to an inhibition of microsomal enzymes which are responsible for the *in vivo* activation of cyclophosphamide.

Dicloxacillin [748]
Chloramphenicol inhibits the bactericidal action of penicillins.

Diphtheria toxoid [633]
Chloramphenicol interferes with the immune response to the toxoid.

Erythromycin [951] (Erythrocin, Ilotycin)
This combination is highly effective against most strains of *Staph. aureus.*

Folic acid [633,1512,1626]
Chloramphenicol may inhibit folic acid activity in patients with a folic acid deficiency.

Hexobarbital [938]
Chloramphenicol potentiates hexobarbital (enzyme inhibition).

Iron [633,1626,1764]
Chloramphenicol inhibits the action of iron in iron deficiency anemia. Select an alternate antibiotic.

Methicillin [748]
Chloramphenicol inhibits the bactericidal action of this penicillin. See *Penicillins* below.

Oxacillin [748]
Chloramphenicol inhibits the bactericidal action of this penicillin. See *Penicillins* below.

Penicillins [238,301,421,445,492,633,1321,1437,1627]
Chloramphenicol, a bacteriostatic drug, inhibits the bactericidal activity of penicillin in pneumococcal infections and in subacute bacterial endocarditis. The degree of inhibition depends on dosage, order of administration, and other factors. Ampicillin plus chloramphenicol is a useful combination in typhoid, especially if the penicillin is begun several hours before chloramphenicol.

Phenylalanine [230,920]
Phenylalanine may ameliorate bone marrow depression caused by chloramphenicol.

Phenytoin [676,1225,1716,2053] (Dilantin)
Chloramphenicol, by enzyme inhibition, potentiates the anticonvulsant action and toxic effects of phenytoin. The antibiotic inhibits biotransformation of phenytoin into its metabolite, 5-(*p*-hydroxyphenyl)-5-phenylhydantoin. The neurological status of one patient with brain tumor and seizures obscured the recurrent phenytoin intoxication.

Pyridoxine [120]
Pyridoxine may prevent chloramphenicol-induced optic neuritis.

Riboflavin [491,920] (Vitamin B₂)
Riboflavin may ameliorate chloramphenicol-induced bone marrow depression; reduced incidence of chloramphenicol-induced optic neuritis.

Sulfonamides [178] (Gantrisin, sulfadiazine)
Chloramphenicol plus sulfadiazine or sulfisoxazole is a highly effective combination against *H. Influenzae.*

Tetanus toxoid [633]
Chloramphenicol interferes with the immune response to the toxoid.

Thiotepa [120]
Increased depression of the bone marrow may result. See under *Thiotepa.*

Tolbutamide (Orinase)
See *Chlorpropamide* above.

Vitamin B₁₂ [491,633,1626,1764]
Vitamin B₁₂ may prevent chloramphenicol-induced optic neuritis. Chloramphenicol inhibits the action of vitamin B₁₂ in pernicious anemia. Select another antibiotic.

CHLORCYCLIZINE (Perazil)
See *Antihistamines* also.

Androgens [65,121,479,485,1123]
Chlorcyclizine, an enzyme inducer, increases the rate of metabolism of androgens and thus inhibits these steroids.

Anticoagulants, oral [223,555,673]
Chlorcyclizine, through enzyme induction, may inhibit oral anticoagulants. Monitor patients on anticoagulants closely when chlorcyclizine is added to the regimen or withdrawn.

Barbiturates [565,640]
See *Barbiturates, Antihistamines,* and *CNS Depressants.*

Carisoprodol [65,555,565,576] (Rela, Soma)
Chlorcyclizine inhibits the muscle relaxant due to enhanced metabolism through enzyme induction.

Chlorcyclizine [64,704] (Perazil)
Patients develop tolerance to chlorcyclizine through enzyme induction and enhanced metabolism of itself.

Corticosteroids
See *Cortisone* and *Desoxycortisone* below.

Cortisone (Cortone) [198]
Chlorcyclizine inhibits cortisone through enzyme induction.

Desoxycorticosterone [198,421]
Chlorcyclizine may increase hydroxylation through enzyme induction and decrease the activity of the hormone.

Estradiol [198]
Chlorcyclizine may increase hydroxylation and decrease the activity of estradiol through enzyme induction.

Estrogen-progestogens [198] (Oral contraceptives)
Increased rate of metabolism. See *Estradiol* above. The contraceptive action may be inhibited by chlorcyclizine.

Griseofulvin [199] (Fulvicin, Grifulvin, Grisactin)
Chlorcyclizine may decrease the effectiveness of griseofulvin and vice versa since both are enzyme inducers.

Hexobarbital [481,640] (Sombucaps, Sombulex)
Chlorcyclizine and hexobarbital may inhibit each other through enzyme induction. See *Barbiturates* under *Antihistamines* and also *CNS Depressants.*

Hydrocortisone [198,950,951]
Chlorcyclizine may inhibit hydrocortisone.

Oral contraceptives
See *Estrogen-Progestogens* above.

Pentobarbital [640]
Chlorcyclizine and pentobarbital may inhibit each other through enzyme induction. See *Barbiturates* under *Antihistamines.*

Phenylbutazone (Butazolidin) [64,485]
Chlorcyclizine may decrease the effectiveness of the drug through enzyme induction.

Phenytoin [199] **(Dilantin)**
Chlorcyclizine may decrease the effectiveness of phenytoin through enzyme induction.

Progesterone [330]
Chlorcyclizine, through enzyme induction, may increase hydroxylation and decrease the activity of the hormone.

Testosterone [198,421,1123]
Chlorcyclizine, through enzyme induction, may increase hydroxylation and decrease the activity of the hormone.

CHLORDANE
(Octa-klor, Toxichlor, Velsicol 1068, etc.)
See also *Halogenated Insecticides.*
Chlordane has a prolonged enzyme inducing effect because it is stored in body fat.

Aminopyrine [1053]
Chlordane stimulates the metabolism of aminopyrine (inhibition).

Anticoagulants, oral [83]
(Coumadin, Dicumarol, Panwarfin, Sintrom, etc.)
Chlordane, by enzyme induction, inhibits oral anticoagulants like bishydroxycoumarin.

Bishydroxycoumarin [83] **(Dicumarol)**
See *Anticoagulants, Oral* above.

Chlorpromazine [1053] **(Thorazine)**
Chlordane stimulates the metabolism of chlorpromazine (inhibition of the tranquilizer).

Cyclophosphamide [114,619] **(Cytoxan)**
Increased cyclophosphamide toxicity. Enzyme induction hastens conversion to active metabolites (aldophosphamide, phosphoramide mustard, and acrolein).

Dextrothyroxine [421] **(Choloxin, D-Thyroxine)**
Chlordane decreases rate of metabolism of thyroxine, and potentiates its action.

DL-Ethionine [1053]
The amino acid antagonist, DL-ethionine blocks the microsomal enzyme induction by chlordane.

Hexobarbital [1053]
Same as for *Aminopyrine* above.

Phenylbutazone [83,485,1053] **(Butazolidin)**
Chlordane inhibits phenylbutazone by enzyme induction.

CHLORDIAZEPOXIDE (Librium)

Acidifying agents [325,870]
Acidifying agents increase urinary excretion of weak bases like chlordiazepoxide.

Alcohol [78,167]
See *Alcohol* under *Benzodiazepines.*

Amitriptyline [120,953]
Mutual enhancement of side effects; weakness, drowsiness, increased depression; possibly fatal. See also *Antidepressants, Tricyclic* below. Amitriptyline potentiates chlordiazepoxide.

Anticoagulants, oral [753,894]
Variable effects on blood coagulation have been reported rarely. The timing of both therapies is probably important. See *Benzodiazepines* under *Anticoagulants, Oral.*

Antidepressants, tricyclic [953]
(Elavil, Tofranil, etc.)
Chlordiazepoxide and amitriptyline (and other tricyclic antidepressants) are mutually potentiated. The depressive syndrome may be intensified with a clinical picture which simulates brain damage.

Barbiturates [78,120]
Possibly combined (additive) CNS effects. Deep sedation, lethargy, and other hazardous effects may occur.

CNS depressants [120]
(Barbiturates, Alcohol, Narcotics, etc.)
Mutual potentiation of CNS depression.

Codeine [120,443]
Coma may ensue with narcotic analgesics combined with chlordiazepoxide.

Diazepam [120,951,1124] **(Valium)**
Enuresis may occur when chlordiazepoxide and diazepam are given with drugs such as disulfiram.

Imipramine
See *Antidepressants, Tricyclic* above.

MAO inhibitors [78,120,834,874,1086]
Additive or super-additive effects may occur with chlordiazepoxide. Deep sedation, seizures, or other hazardous effects such as excitement, chorea, stimulation and acute rage may occur, but with careful dosage a dramatic response may be achieved with this combination in certain types of anxiety and in initial stages of depression.

Narcotics [120]
Chlordiazepoxide may tend to lower blood pressure and may potentiate the hypotensive effects of narcotics. See *Codeine* above.

Phenobarbital [120]
See *Barbiturates* above.

Phenothiazines [78,120]
Phenothiazines potentiate the CNS depressant effects of chlordiazepoxide. Sedation, seizures, or severe atropinelike effects may occur.

CHLORETONE
See *Chlorobutanol.*

CHLORIDE ION

Diuretics, mercurial [172]
Chlorides enhance the diuresis produced by mercurial diuretics.

CHLORINATED INSECTICIDES
(Aldrin, Chlordane, DDT, etc.)
See *Halogenated Insecticides.*

CHLORMETHIAZOLE (Heminevrin)

Alcohol [2060]
A lethal combination. Deaths have been reported in alcoholics in whom chlormethiazole edisylate, a sedative, hypnotic and anticonvulsant widely used in the treatment of depression was consumed by alcoholics, sometimes even at therapeutic levels.

CHLOROBUTANOL

Acenocoumarin [198] **(Sintrom)**
Chlorobutanol inhibits acenocoumarin by enzyme induction.

CHLOROFORM
See *Anesthestics, General.*
Chloroform, which is carcinogenic, is being avoided scrupulously in cough remedies, as a solvent residue in manufacturing medications, in drinking water, etc. During 1977 chloroform was banned from all foods and drugs.

CHLOROGUANIDE (Paludrine)

Pyrimethamine[619]
Cross-resistance may occur.

CHLOROMYCETIN

See *Chloramphenicol.*

p-CHLOROPHENYLALANINE

Narcotic analgesics[421]
p-Chlorophenylalanine reverses the analgesic activity of narcotic analgesics.

CHLOROPROCAINE (Nesacaine)

See ***p**-Aminobenzoic Acid Analogues* and *Anesthetics, Local.*

CHLOROQUINE (Aralen)

See *Antimalarials* and *Primaquine.*

Acidifying agents[120,325,870]
(Ammonium chloride, etc.)
Acidifying agents increase urinary excretion of weak bases like chloroquine. Inhibition.

Alkalinizing agents
Opposite effect of *Acidifying Agents* above. With alkaline urine a large proportion of the drug is present in the nonionized and therefore lipid-soluble form which is reabsorbed and only small quantities appear in the urine. Potentiation.

Analgesics[120]
Phenylbutazone and other agents known to cause drug sensitization and dermatitis should not be given concurrently with chloroquine.

Antipsoriatics[120,421]
Chloroquine antagonizes the action of antipsoriatics and may actually precipitate a severe attack of psoriasis in patients with the disease.

Asthma preparations[421]
Chloroquine potentiates some asthma preparations.

Bone marrow depressants[120]
The antimalarial is contraindicated in patients receiving depressants of myeloid elements of the bone marrow.

Folic acid antagonists[421] **(Methotrexate, etc.)**
Chloroquine potentiates folic acid antagonists.

Gold[120]
Concomitant use of drugs containing gold that are known to cause drug sensitization and dermatitis should be avoided.

Hemolytic drugs[4]
The antimalarial is contraindicated in patients receiving other potentially hemolytic drugs, particularly patients with a G6PD deficiency.

Hepatotoxic drugs[120]
Since the antimalarial concentrates in the liver it should be used with caution with known hepatotoxic drugs.

MAO inhibitors[74,433]
Chloroquine is stored in large quantities in the liver even after a short period of use. In view of the known effects of MAO inhibitors on liver enzyme systems, prudence is necessary if concurrent therapy is contemplated. Increased chloroquine toxicity and possible retinal damage may occur.

Oral medications[1791]
Chlorquine tends to delay gastric emptying time and thus depresses drug absorption.

Phenylbutazone[120]
Concomitant use of drugs like phenylbutazone that are known to cause drug sensitization and dermatitis should be avoided.

Quinacrine[4]
See under *Primaquine.*

X-ray, total body[1125]
Chloroquine protects against lethality of X-rays.

CHLOROTHIAZIDES (Diuril, etc.)

See *Hydrochlorothiazide* and *Thiazide Diuretics.*

Antihypertensive drugs[120]
Chlorothiazides potentiate the antihypertensive effect of rauwolfia and veratrum alkaloids, hydralazine, and ganglionic blocking agents. With the latter agents it may cause excessive fall in blood pressure.

Cholestyramine[120] **(Cuemid, Questran, etc.)**
Absorption of chlorothiazides is inhibited by the resin. Administer cholestyramine at least 1 hour before or 4 to 6 hours after the diuretics.

Digitalis[120,580]
Potassium loss potentiates the action of digitalis drugs and may aggravate disturbances in heart rhythm associated with coronary-artery insufficiency. Dosage of these diuretic drugs should be reduced in patients taking digitalis.

Ganglionic blocking agents[120,633]
Potentiated antihypertensive activity.

Guanethidine[120]
Potentiated antihypertensive activity.

Hydralazine[421,633]
Potentiated antihypertensive activity.

Reserpine[117]
Potentiated antihypertensive activity.

Uricosurics
See *Hyperuricemics* under *Uricosuric Agents.*

Veratrum alkaloids[421,619]
Potentiated antihypertensive activity.

CHLORPHENESIN (Maolate)

CNS stimulants[120]
Chlorphenesin antagonizes the convulsive effects of strychnine but not pentylenetetrazol.

Penicillin[951]
Chlorphenesin reduces hypersensitivity to penicillin.

CHLORPHENIRAMINE
(Chlor-Trimeton, Polaramine, etc.)
See *Antihistamines.*

CHLORPHENOXAMINE (Phenoxene)

Barbiturates[120,619]
The parasympatholytic, chlorphenoxamine, with antihistaminic and anticholinergic properties potentiates the CNS depressant effects of barbiturates.

CHLORPHENTERMINE (Pre-Sate)

Chlorpromazine[765]
Chlorpromazine inhibits the anorectic activity of chlorphentermine.

MAO inhibitors[120]
Chlorphentermine, a sympathomimetic drug, is contraindicated in patients who are receiving MAO inhibitors. See *Sympathomimetics* under *MAO Inhibitors.*

Phenothiazines
Same as for *Chlorpromazine* above.

CHLORPROMAZINE (Thorazine)
See *Phenothiazines.*

Alcohol [121,731]
Alcohol potentiates CNS depressant effects of chlorpromazine and vice versa. The combination interferes with coordination and judgment.

Alphaprodine [669] **(Nisentil)**
Chlorpromazine potentiates the synthetic narcotic analgesic alphaprodine. See *CNS Depressants.*

Amobarbital [669]
See *Barbiturates* below.

Amphetamines
See *Amphetamines* under *Phenothiazines.*

Anesthetics [120] **(general)**
Chlorpromazine potentiates CNS depressant effects of anesthetics. See *CNS Depressants* below.

Antacids [1408]
Antacids decrease the intestinal absorption of chlorpromazine and thus reduce its blood levels and potency.

Anticholinergics
See *Anticholinergics* under *Antihistamines.*

Anticoagulants, oral [330,332,453]
Chlorpromazine diminishes the anticoagulant effect by inducing metabolism of the oral anticoagulants.

Antidiabetics [191]
See *Phenothiazines* under *Antidiabetics, Oral.*

Atropine [120,166]
Use chlorpromazine with caution in persons receiving atropine (additive anticholinergic effects).

Barbiturates [120,669]
See *Barbiturates* under *Phenothiazines.*

Chlorphentermine [765] **(Pre-Sate)**
Chlorpromazine inhibits the anorexic activity of chlorphentermine.

CNS depressants [120]
(Alcohol, anesthetics, barbiturates, narcotics, etc.)
The combination of the phenothiazine with other CNS depressants may severely potentiate the CNS effects. Hypotension, coma can occur.

Cocaine
See *Chlorpromazine* under *Cocaine.*

Diazoxide
See *Chlorpromazine* under *Diazoxide*

Dipyrone [166,184] **(Narone, Pyrilgin)**
Dipyrone should not be used with chlorpromazine. The antipyretic effect is potentiated, possibly resulting in severe hypothermia.

Dopa [120]
Dopa antagonizes the cataleptic effect of chlorpromazine.

Epinephrine [120,166,1074]
Epinephrine and other pressor agents, except Levophed and Neo-Synephrine, should never be used to treat a hypotensive reaction from chlorpromazine as a paradoxical further lowering of blood pressure may be produced. Chlorpromazine inhibits many of the peripheral actions of epinephrine but does not affect its hyperglycemic action.

Estradiol [92]
Chlorpromazine may inhibit estrogens by enzyme induction. Estradiol potentiates chlorpromazine by inhibiting its rate of metabolism.

Guanethidine
Chlorpromazine, like the tricyclic antidepressants, antagonizes the antihypertensive action of guanethidine by inhibiting its uptake into the adrenergic neurons. Chlorpromazine has the same effect on the indirectly acting pressor agent tyramine. See under *Guanethidine.*

Hexobarbital [669,697] **(Evipal)**
Chlorpromazine potentiates the hypnotic action of hexobarbital. See *Barbiturates* above.

Insulin [951]
Chlorpromazine antagonizes the hypoglycemic effect.

Levodopa
See *Chlorpromazine* under *Levodopa.*

Levorphanol [669] **(Levo-Dromoran)**
This synthetic narcotic analgesic is potentiated by phenothiazine. See *CNS Depressants.*

Lysergic acid diethylamide [166] **(LSD)**
Chlorpromazine antagonizes the behavioral effects of LSD.

Morphine [166]
Chlorpromazine potentiates the miotic and sedative effects of morphine.

Narcotics [120,669] **(Meperidine, morphine, etc.)**
Chlorpromazine potentiates narcotics. See *CNS Depressants.*

Nialamide [162,198] **(Niamid)**
Nialamide antagonizes cataleptic effect of chlorpromazine.

Orphenadrine [528,619]
When orphenadrine is given concomitantly with chlorpromazine, severe hypoglycemia may develop and coma may be induced.

Pargyline [162] **(Eutonyl)**
Chlorpromazine potentiates the hypotensive effect of pargyline.

Pentobarbital [640,669]
The hypnotic effect of barbiturates is potentiated by chlorpromazine. See *Barbiturates* under *Phenothiazines.*

Phenmetrazine [765] **(Preludin)**
Chlorpromazine inhibits anorexic activity of phenmetrazine.

Phenobarbital [83]
Hypnotic effect is potentiated by chlorpromazine but, by enzyme induction, phenobarbital inhibits chlorpromazine.

Phenytoin [884] **(Dilantin)**
Chlorpromazine, which has some anticonvulsant activity, may potentiate phenytoin.

Phosphorus insecticides [120]
Chlorpromazine potentiates the toxic effects of phosphorus insecticides.

Piperazine [660,766]
Piperazine in patients receiving chlorpromazine may induce convulsions that may be fatal, but this has been questioned. This could not be confirmed by FDA in animal studies. The authors of the sole report in the literature[766] were unable to duplicate their results. A diagnosis of brain tumor was made at one time.

Psilocybin [951]
Chlorpromazine counteracts the mydriasis and visual distortion produced by psilocybin.

Rauwolfia alkaloids [633]
Chlorpromazine potentiates the hypotensive effect of the reserpine group of alkaloids.

Reserpine
See *Rauwolfia Alkaloids* above.

Secobarbital [669]
See *Barbiturates* under *Phenothiazines.*

CHLORPROMAZINE (Thorazine) *(continued)*

Sedatives and hypnotics [120] and analgesics
Chlorpromazine potentiates the CNS depressant action of sedatives, hypnotics, and analgesics. See *CNS Depressants.*

Thiamylal [669] (Surital)
See *Barbiturates* under *Phenothiazines.*

Thiopental [668, 669]
See *Barbiturates* under *Phenothiazines.*

Toxic drugs [120]
Chlorpromazine may obscure the signs of overdosage and toxic effects of other drugs.

CHLORPROPAMIDE (Diabinese)
See *Antidiabetics, Oral* (sulfonylureas). Chlorpropamide differs from other sulfonylureas in degree of protein binding, location of binding, duration of activity, extent of metabolism, and activity of metabolites.

Alcohol [120, 354, 634, 675]
See *Antidiabetics, Oral.* A disulfiram type of reaction may occur.

Allopurinol
See *Allopurinol* under *Antidiabetics, Oral.*

Anticoagulants, oral [120, 768]
Coumarin compounds, by inhibiting drug metabolizing enzymes in the liver, can cause hypoglycemia when used with chlorpropamide. They cause chlorpropamide to accumulate and more than double its half life. See *Antidiabetics, Oral* under *Anticoagulants, Oral.*

Aspirin [120]
Toxic interaction; hypoglycemia. See *Salicylates* below.

Barbiturates [120]
The action of barbiturates may be prolonged by therapy with chlorpropamide.

Bishydroxycoumarin [120, 768] (Dicumarol)
The oral anticoagulant potentiates the oral antidiabetic by inhibiting the microsomal enzymes.

Chloramphenicol [767]
Potentiation of hypoglycemic effect. The half-lives of sulfonylureas like chlorpropamide are prolonged by chloramphenicol.

MAO inhibitors [120]
MAO inhibitors potentiate chlorpropamide.

Oxyphenbutazone and phenylbutazone [120]
The anti-inflammatory agents potentiate chlorpropamide; hypoglycemia.

Probenecid [120]
Probenecid potentiates the hypoglycemic effect of chlorpropamide.

Propranolol [42, 263]
May cause hypoglycemia; potential danger may be increased because propranolol may prevent the premonitory signs and symptoms of acute hypoglycemia.

Salicylates [120, 350, 359, 418, 649]
(Acetylsalicylic acid, sodium salicylate)
Salicylates potentiate the hypoglycemic action of sulfonylureas like chlorpropamide. The highly bound salicylate may displace chlorpropamide from its albumin binding sites. Also the hypoglycemic effect of salicylate may be additive.

Sedatives [120]
Chlorpropamide may prolong hypnotic and sedative effects.

Sulfonamides [120]
Hypoglycemia may result from potentiation of chlorpropamide.

Thiazides
See *Thiazides* under *Antidiabetics, Oral.*

Vasopressin [421, 722, 723] (Pitressin)
Chlorpropamide potentiates the antidiuretic effect of vasopressin (small amounts but not large amounts of vasopressin).

Warfarin
See *Anticoagulants, Oral,* above and under *Antidiabetics, Oral.*

CHLORPROTHIXENE (Taractan)
See *Phenothiazines* and *Tranquilizers.*
Chlorprothixene, a thioxanthene has many interactions like the phenothiazines.

Alcohol
See *CNS Depressants* below.

Analgesics
See *CNS Depressants* below.

Anesthetics, general
See *CNS Depressants* below.

CNS depressants [120, 121, 731]
Chlorprothixene potentiates CNS depressants like alcohol, anesthetics, hypnotics and opiates. Circulatory collapse and coma may ensue.

Epinephrine [120]
Chlorprothixene may reverse the action of epinephrine. Do not use epinephrine as a vasopressor in severe cases of hypotension caused by chlorprothixene.

Hypnotics
See *CNS Depressants* above.

Opiates
See *CNS Depressants* above.

Phenothiazines
See *Phenothiazines* (because of structural similarity) and *CNS Depressants* above.

CHLORTETRACYCLINE (Aureomycin)
See *Antibiotics* and *Tetracyclines.*

Aminopyrine [939]
Chlortetracycline may potentiate aminopyrine by enzyme inhibition. It does so in rats.

Hexobarbital [939]
Same as for *Aminopyrine* above.

Penicillin [285, 666]
Chlortetracycline inhibits the bactericidal activity of penicillin.

CHLORTHALIDONE (Hygroton)

ACTH [120]
See *Adrenocorticosteroids* below.

Adrenocorticosteroids [120, 1853]
Guard against excessive potassium depletion when chlorthalidone is used with adrenocorticosteroids and ACTH.

Alcohol [120]
See *CNS Depressants* below.

Antidiabetics [120, 164, 386]
Hyperglycemia and glycosuria may develop. See *Insulin* below.

Antihypertensives [120]
Reduce the dosage of the potent antihypertensives by half when initiating chlorthalidone therapy because of potentiation of the hypotensive effect.

Barbiturates [120]
See *CNS Depressants* below.

CNS depressants [120]
The orthostatic hypotension induced by chlorthalidone may be potentiated by CNS depressants such as alcohol, barbiturates, and narcotics.

Corticosteroids
See *Adrenocorticosteroids* above.

Curariform drugs [120,330]
(Curare, gallamine, tubocurarine)
Reduce the dosage of the muscle relaxant by half when initiating chlorthalidone therapy because of potentiation of the relaxant effect.

Digitalis [120,1234,1451,1508,1766,1780]
Potassium, and possibly magnesium, depletion caused by chlorthalidone increases the toxic effects of digitalis. The toxicity increases as K^+ decreases. Monitor carefully all patients receiving diuretics and digitalis and provide K^+ supplementation as necessary.

Gallamine [120,330]
See *Curariform Drugs* above.

Ganglionic blocking agents [120]
Chlorthalidone potentiates these antihypertensive agents. Reduce their dosage by one-half when initiating therapy with chlorthalidone.

Insulin [120,164,386]
Hyperglycemia and glycosuria may develop. The dosage requirement of insulin in a controlled diabetic may be increased. Implies a lowered rate of insulin secretion and diminished reserve of insulin. A direct toxic effect has been demonstrated on the pancreas of animals.

Narcotics [120]
See *CNS Depressants* above.

Sulfonylureas [120]
Hyperglycemia. See *Insulin* above.

Tubocurarine [120]
See *Curariform Drugs* above.

CHLOR-TRIMETON
See *Antihistamines* and *Chlorpheniramine*.

CHLOR-TRIMETON EXPECTORANT
See *Ammonium Chloride, Antihistamines, Chlorpheniramine, Glyceryl Guaiacolate,* and *Phenylephrine.*

CHLORZOXAZONE (Paraflex)

Testosterone [951]
Testosterone inhibits the muscle relaxant chlorzoxazone.

CHOCOLATE
See *Tyramine-rich Foods.*

MAO inhibitors [120,265]
Excessive amounts of chocolate with MAO inhibitors can cause hypertensive reactions.

CHOLAN-HMB
See *Dehydrochloric Acid, Homatropine Methylbromide,* and *Phenobarbital.*

CHOLEDYL (Oxtriphylline)
See *Xanthines.*

CHOLESTYRAMINE (Cuemid, Questran, etc.)

Acidic drugs [28,120,170,330,421,672-3,769,770,1361,1848]
Cholestyramine inhibits the absorption of many medications (chlorothiazide, digitalis glycosides, iron preparations, phenobarbital, phenylbutazone, tetracyclines, thiazides, thyroid products such as liothyronine and thyroxine, vitamins that are fat soluble, warfarin, etc.), especially the acidic drugs. Such drugs should be ingested at least one hour before cholestyramine. Patients stabilized on any drug inhibited by cholestyramine may experience toxic effects from these drugs when cholestyramine is withdrawn, particularly drugs like digitalis which must be titrated accurately. Do not give other drugs for at least 4 to 6 hours after cholestyramine. Cholestyramine enhances elimination of phenprocoumon an oral anticoagulant, by interrupting its enterohepatic recycling. The resin is useful in intoxication with this anticoagulant and probably others.

Anticoagulants, oral [120,330,421,673,769,770,1462,2056]
(Warfarin, etc.)
Cholestyramine, an anion exchange resin which has a strong affinity for acid substances, may decrease the effect of oral anticoagulants like warfarin by inhibiting or delaying absorption and thus lowering blood levels. However, vitamin K absorption may also be decreased (cholestyramine sequesters bile acids and thus inhibits absorption of fat-soluble vitamins such as vitamin K) and this tends to increase the anticoagulant effect. Hypoprothrombinemia and hemorrhage may occur. Administer the anticoagulants at least one hour before cholestyramine and monitor the net effect on the specific patient. Do not give other drugs for at least 4 to 6 hours after cholestyramine. Cholestyramine enhances elimination of phenprocoumon an oral anticoagulant, by interrupting its enterohepatic recycling. The resin is useful in intoxication with this anticoagulant and probably others.

Chlorothiazide [120]
See *Acidic Drugs* above. The absorption of chlorothiazide is not inhibited by the resin if it is given at least 60 minutes before the diuretic.

Digitalis glycosides [120]
See *Cholestyramine* under *Digitalis* and see *Acidic Drugs* above.

Iron preparations [1848]
See *Acidic Drugs* above.

Liothyronine [28,672]
See *Acidic Drugs* above.

Phenobarbital [120]
See *Acidic Drugs* above.

Phenprocoumon (Liquamar)
See *Anticoagulants, Oral* above.

Phenylbutazone [120,769]
See *Acidic Drugs* above.

Tetracyclines [120]
See *Acidic Drugs* above.

Thiazides [120]
See *Acidic Drugs* above.

Thyroid products [28,672] **(Thyroxine, etc.)**
See *Acidic Drugs* above.

Vitamins, fat soluble [120,1462]
See under *Anticoagulants, Oral* above. The absorption of fat soluble vitamins may be decreased by the resin. Hypoprothrombinemic hemorrhage may be caused by inhibition of absorption of vitamin K.

Warfarin [120]
See *Anticoagulants, Oral* above.

CHOLINERGICS (Direct type)
See also *Anticholinesterases* (indirect type of cholinergics) and specific agents (acetylcholine, ambenomium [Mytelase], bethanechol, carbachol, demecarium [Humorsol], echothiophate iodide [Phospholine], edrophonium [Tensilon], methacholine, neostigmine [Prostigmin], physostigmine, pilocarpine, pyridostigmine bromide [Mestinon], etc.). Some drugs (e.g., edrophonium) have both direct and indirect cholinergic action.

CHOLINERGICS (Direct type)   *(continued)*

Adrenergics[421]
Adrenergics (mydriatic, etc.) antagonize cholinergics (miotic, etc.).

Antihistamines[169]
Antihistamines diminish the activity of cholinesterase inhibitor type of cholinergics.

Atropine[168,619]
The miotic action of a cholinergic is used to counteract the mydriatic action of atropine. Atropine abolishes the cholinergic actions of cholinergics.

**Cholinergics, indirect type
   (Cholinesterase inhibitors)**[168]
Cholinergic effects are potentiated when cholinesterase inhibitors are given with direct type cholinergics.

Corticosteroids[421]
Corticosteroids may decrease cholinergic effects.

Muscle relaxants, polarizing type[168]
Diminished activity of cholinesterase inhibitor type cholinergics with polarizing type muscle relaxants.

Nitrates, nitrites[170]
Cholinergics antagonize the effects of organic nitrates and nitrites.

Procainamide[120,619]
Procainamide, with its anticholinergic activity, inhibits cholinesterase inhibitor type cholinergic in myasthenia gravis patients.

Quinidine[170]
Quinidine with its anticholinergic properties may antagonize cholinergics.

Sympathomimetics
See *Adrenergics* above.

CHOLINESTERASE INHIBITORS (Anticholinesterases, indirect type cholinergics)
See *Anticholinesterases* and specific agents (ambenonium, demecarium, echothiophate, isoflurophate, physostigmine, etc.). See also *Cholinergics (direct type)*.

CHOLOXIN
See *Dextrothyroxine*.

CHYMOLASE
See *Chymotrypsin* below.

CHYMOTRYPSIN

Anticoagulants, oral[147,421]
Caution should be observed when using concomitantly as chymotrypsin potentiates the anticoagulants.

Penicillins[27]
Elevated blood level of penicillin through enhanced absorption.

Phenethicillin[27]
Chymotrypsin may potentiate phenethicillin. It elevates the blood levels of the antibiotic.

Tetracyclines[27,397]
Chymotrypsin elevates the antibiotic blood levels and may potentiate them by facilitating blood-tissue exchange.

CIGARETTE SMOKE
See *Smoking*.

CIMETIDINE (Tagamet)
See *Cimetidine* under *Pancreatin*.

CINCHONA ALKALOIDS (Quinidine, Quinine)

Muscle relaxants, depolarizing[255,324,390,447]
Respiratory depression leading to apnea (potentiation of depolarizing and nondepolarizing agents). The neuromuscular blocking effect of quinidine seems to be related to a curariform activity at the myoneural junction as well as a depression of muscle action potential.

Quinidine[619]
The other cinchona alkaloids may potentiate quinidine.

CITANEST
See *Anesthetics, Local* (Prilocaine).

CITRA
See *Antihistamines, Caffeine, Phenlephrine, Phenacetin,* and *Salicylamide.*

CITRATES

Oxytocin[421]
Erratic and unpredictable results occur when these agents are given together.

Sulfinpyrazone[120] **(Anturane)**
Citrates antagonize the uricosuric action of sulfinpyrazone and are contraindicated.

CITRIC ACID

Tetracyclines[107,270,696]
Citric acid elevates the antibiotic blood level through enhanced absorption of the antibiotic.

CLINDAMYCIN (Cleocin)

Erythromycin[4b,808,809,1343]
(Erythrocin, Ilosone, Ilotycin, etc.)
Avoid concomitant use of these two antibiotics as they, like lincomycin, are competitors for the same ribosomal protein binding sites. The full significance is not known but they may be antagonistic.

CLINICAL LABORATORY INTERFERENCES
See Chapter 7.

CLOFIBRATE (Atromid-S)

Acidifying agents[325,870]
Acidifying agents decrease the urinary excretion of clofibrate; potentiation.

Anabolic Steroids
See *Clofibrate* under *Anabolic Steroids.*

Anticholinesterases[421]
Clofibrate potentiates the effects of anticholinesterases. Hazardous in glaucoma.

Anticoagulants, oral[78,120,137,223,359,393,394,411]
(Warfarin, other coumarin derivatives, etc.)
Caution: Clofibrate potentiates oral anticoagulants by displacing them from protein binding sites or by inhibiting the metabolizing enzymes, and also possibly by enhancing their affinity for their receptors and markedly depressing production of prothrombin and clotting factors VII, IX and X. Reduce the dosage of the anticoagulant by $\frac{1}{3}$ to $\frac{1}{2}$ to maintain the prothrombin time at the desired level to prevent bleeding complications.

**Antidiabetics, oral
   (Diabinese, Dymelor, Orinase, Tolinase, etc.)**
Clofibrate potentiates oral antidiabetics. See *Clofibrate* under *Antidiabetics, Oral.*

Contraceptives, oral[421]
Oral contraceptives antagonize the antihyperlipidemic effect of clofibrate.

Dextrothyroxine [589]
Potentiation of the hypocholesterolemic effects. See *Thyroxine* below.

Estrogens [170,421]
Estrogens, by inducing hyperlipemia, antagonize the effect of clofibrate.

Furosemide [1263] **(Lasix)**
Concomitant use of clofibrate and furosemide may produce pain and stiffness of the muscles and enhanced diuresis, particularly in patients with hypoalbuminemia. These drugs appear to compete for plasma protein binding sites. Thus increased levels of unbound drugs are produced.

Neomycin [170,421]
Neomycin, which causes a drug-induced malabsorption syndrome, potentiates clofibrate by inhibiting cholesterol absorption.

Oral contraceptives [170]
OCs that contain estrogen elevate plasma lipoproteins and triglyceride values and thus antagonize clofibrate and other hypolipemics. See *Estrogens* above.

Organophosphate cholinesterase inhibitors [421]
Clofibrate potentiates miotic effect of the cholinergics.

Phenformin [421] **(DBI)**
Clofibrate may potentiate phenformin. Coagulation irregularities and hemorrhage may be induced.

Phenindione [951] **(Danilone, Hedulin)**
Blood coagulation irregularities, hemorrhagic episodes.

Puromycin [421]
Puromycin potentiates clofibrate.

Sitosterols [421]
Sitosterols potentiate clofibrate. Additive effect.

Sulfonylureas [421,619]
Caution should be observed in giving clofibrate to diabetic patients since the hypoglycemic effect in a patient taking tolbutamide was enhanced. See *Clofibrate* under *Antidiabetics, Oral*.

Thyroxine [421,589]
Clofibrate potentiates thyroxine by slowing its rate of metabolism or by drug displacement.

Tolbutamide (Orinase)
See *Antidiabetics, Oral* above.

Warfarin (Coumadin)
See *Anticoagulants, Oral* above.

CLOPAMIDE (Aquex)

Spironolactone [950,951] **(Aldactone)**
Clopamide potentiates spironolactone.

CLOXACILLIN, SODIUM (Tegopen)

Acetylsalicylic acid [267-269] **(Aspirin)**
Aspirin potentiates penicillin by displacing it from protein binding sites.

Aminohippuric acid (PAHA) [433]
Elevated serum levels of penicillin and increased toxicity.

Ampicillin [382] **(Policyllin)**
Synergistic antibacterial effect.

Benzyl penicillin [382]
Synergistic antibacterial effect.

Cephalosporins and penicillins [120]
Cross-sensitivity occurs. A patient who is allergic to one cephalosporin or penicillin, including cloxacillin, may be allergic to the others.

Chloramphenicol [301,492,748,864]
Chloramphenicol inhibits the bactericidal action of this penicillin.

Sulfaethylthiadiazole [267-269] **and other sulfonamides**
Relatively large doses of the sulfonamide can reduce the protein binding of this penicillin and increase the level of antimicrobially active drug in serum and body fluids.

Sulfamethoxypyridazine
See *Sulfaethylthiadiazole* above.

Tetracyclines [233,285,301,633,666]
Tetracyclines inhibit the bactericidal action of penicillins.

CNS DEPRESSANTS

The CNS depressants include (1) *general depressants* such as alcohol (ethyl and other aliphatic alcohols), general and regional anesthetics, barbiturates, hypnotics, and sedatives; (2) *specific depressants* such as analgesics, antipyretics, narcotic analgesics, and psychotropic agents such as benzodiazepines, butyrophenones, meprobamate group, phenothiazines, Rauwolfia alkaloids and thioxanthenes; and (3) *miscellaneous agents* in which CNS depression is incidental, *e.g.*, certain anticonvulsants, antidepressants, antihistamines, antihypertensives, antineoplastics (procarbazine, etc.), and centrally acting muscle relaxants.
Many of the combinations possible with these CNS depressants are contraindicated. Considerable caution must be exercised when any combination is used. Hazardous potentiation of CNS depression is always a possibility, with resulting conditions ranging from excessive sedation through hypnosis, hypotension, and general anesthesia to coma and death. Other effects may be enhanced, *e.g.*, seizures or severe atropinelike reactions with the phenothiazines plus the minor tranquilizers (chlordiazepoxide, diazepam and oxazepam). Also potentiators of CNS depressants are often contraindicated for use with these drugs. If such a combination acts synergistically and permits the use of lower dosages the results can be beneficial. If, as with the MAO inhibitors and reserpine or methyldopa, complete reversal of effects occurs with hazardous potential, the combination is contraindicated. Certain sedatives and hypnotics, also antihistamines, are enzyme inducers. Thus tolerance and mutual inhibition may develop. [38,78,166,945] See under specific drugs such as *Acetaminophen, Alcohol, Analgesics, Anesthetics, Anticonvulsants, Antidepressants, Antihistamines, Antihypertensives, Antineoplastics* (Matulane, etc.), *Antipyretics, Aspirin, Barbiturates, Beazodiazepines* (Librium, Valium, etc.), *Butyrophenones* (Haldol, etc.), *Hypnotics, Meprobamates* (Carisoprodol, Equanil, Miltown, etc.), *Muscle Relaxants, Narcotic Analgesics, Phenothiazines* (Compazine, Mellaril, Thorazine, etc.), *Rauwolfia Alkaloids* (Reserpine, etc.), *Sedatives, Thioxanthenes* (Narane, Taractan, etc.), etc.

CNS STIMULANTS
(Doxapram [Dopram], ethamivan [Emivan], fluorothyl [Indoklon], methylphenidate [Ritalin], nikethamide [Coramine, Nikorin], pentylenetrazol [Metrazol, etc.], picrotoxin, xanthines, etc.)

Amantadine [120] **(Symmetrel)**
Since amantadine may exhibit CNS and psychic side effects, these agents should be used cautiously in combination.

Antidiabetics, oral
See *Coffee* under *Antidiabetics, Oral*

Bulbocapnine [166]
CNS stimulants counteract the cataleptic effects of bulbocapnine.

CNS STIMULANTS *(continued)*

Carisoprodol [120]
CNS stimulants may be used cautiously to counteract shock and respiratory depression resulting from carisoprodol overdosage.

Phenothiazines [166]
Phenothiazines like chlorpromazine antagonize the central nervous system stimulant activity of amphetamines but do not protect against the convulsive action of pentylenetetrazol, picrotoxin, or strychnine.

COCAINE

Amphetamines [167,421]
Cocaine, readily absorbed through mucous membranes, potentiates the central nervous system stimulants (additive effects). Vasomotor collapse and respiratory arrest is possible with death.

Atropine [167]
Atropine and cocaine have an additive mydriatic effect.

Chlorpromazine [2068]
Chlorpromazine protects against lethal overdoses of cocaine by preventing cocaine-induced changes in cardiovascular function and antagonizes production of hyperpyrexia and decline in arterial pH.

Epinephrine [167,633]
Cocaine produces sensitization to epinephrine. See *Sympathomimetics* below.

Furazolidone [633] (Furoxone)
Furazolidone potentiates cocaine.

Guanethidine [626]
Cocaine antagonizes the hypotensive effect of guanethidine.

Iproniazid [633]
Iproniazid potentiates the CNS effects of cocaine.

MAO inhibitor antidepressants [633]
These antidepressants potentiate the CNS effects of cocaine.

Norepinephrine [167] (Levarterenol, Levophed)
Cocaine produces sensitization to norepinephrine. See *Sympathomimetics* below.

Pargyline [633]
Pargyline potentiates the CNS effects of cocaine.

Propranolol [1995,2068]
The dopaminergic crisis (hypertension, tachycardia, anxiety, paranoia, disorientation) produced by cocaine overdosage is reversed by the β_1-blocking action of propranolol. Propranolol may serve as an antidote for moderate overdosage of cocaine, but is not as effective as chlorpromazine (see above). [2068]

Sympathomimetics [167,633]
Cocaine with sympathomimetics if received systemically may induce cardiac arrhythmia, convulsions, and vasomotor collapse. By blocking the uptake of catecholamines, such as epinephrine and norepinephrine, at adrenergic nerve endings, cocaine potentiates the responses (excitatory and inhibitory) of organs innervated with sympathetic nerves to these agents and to sympathetic stimuli. Epinephrine is combined with cocaine for topical anesthesia for its vasoconstrictor effect.

Heroin [771]
An additive effect is produced, unpredictable in extent.

CODALAN
See *Acetaminophen, Caffeine, Codeine,* and *Salicylamide*.

CODEINE
See *CNS Depressants* and *Narcotic Analgesics*.
Drugs with interactions similar to those of codeine include hydrocodone (dihydrocodeinone) and dihydrocodeine.

Alcohol [121]
CNS depression due to codeine is potentiated by alcohol.

Aspirin [166]
Better analgesia than with either alone.

Barbiturates [2028]
Codeine may interact synergistically with barbiturates to produce a stimulant effect on onset and duration of sleep.

Chloramphenicol [676,938]
Chloramphenicol potentiates codeine.

Chlordiazepoxide [120,443]
The combination may induce coma.

Nalorphine [39] (Nalline)
Nalorphine is a potent antagonist of the respiratory depressant effects of codeine, morphine, and other narcotic derivatives.

Oral medications [1791]
Codeine tends to delay gastric emptying time and thus depresses drug absorption.

CODIMAL DH
See *Antihistamines, Codeine, Guaiacolsulfonate, Phenylephrine, Potassium,* and *Sodium Citrate*.

COFFEE
See *CNS Stimulants* and *Xanthines*.
Coffee is an enzyme inducer. [1094]

CO-GEL TABLETS
See *Aluminum, Antacids,* and *Magnesium*.

COGENTIN
See *Anticholinergics (Antiparkinsonism Drugs)*.

COLA DRINKS
See *CNS Stimulants* and *Xanthines*.

COLBENEMID
See *Probenecid* and *Uricosuric agents*.

COLCHICINE

Acidifying agents [325,870]
Acidifying agents inhibit colchicine.

Alkalinizing agents [325,870]
Alkalinizing agents potentiate colchicine.

Allopurinol [120] (Zyloprim)
Colchicine or anti-inflammatory agents may be required during early stages of allopurinol therapy to counteract attacks of gout.

Antigout drugs [166]
No interactions of an inhibiting or potentiating nature have been reported between colchicine and other antigout drugs. See *Antigout Drugs*.

CNS depressants [166]
Colchicine may increase sensitivity to the depressants.

Probenecid [120]
Colchicine helps to prevent the acute attacks of gout that may temporarily occur during the early stages of probenecid therapy.

Sympathomimetics [226]
Colchicine may enhance response to sympathomimetic agents.

Vitamin B_{12} [166,1405]
Colchicine may interfere with the absorption of vitamin B_{12} from the gut. There has been no evidence of deficiency as a result of concurrent use, but the interaction is accentuated by prolonged administration of colchicine. See also *Neomycin* under *Vitamin B_{12}*.

COLD AND COUGH REMEDIES

These preparations contain one or more of a vast array of drugs including *analgesics* and *antipyretics* (acetaminophen, aspirin, phenacetin, salicylamide, sodium salicylate, etc.), *anticholinergics* (atropine, homatropine methylbromide, hyoscyamine, methscopolamine, etc.), *antihistamines* (brompheniramine, bromodiphenhydramine, chlorpheniramine, dexchlorpheniramine, diphenhydramine, doxylamine, phenindamine, pheniramine, phenyltoloxamine, pyrilamine, thenyldiamine, etc.), *antipruritics* (camphor, menthol, etc.), *antitussives* (codeine, dextromethorphan, hydrocodone bitartrate, noscapine, etc.), *CNS stimulants* (caffeine, etc.), *decongestants* (ephedrine, naphazoline, phenylephrine, phenylpropanolamine, propylhexedrine, pseudo-ephedrine, xylometazoline, etc.), *expectorants* (ammonium chloride, carbonate or citrate, chloroform, creosote, glyceryl guaiacolate, iodides, ipecac, squill, terpin hydrate, etc.), *mucolytics* (acetylcysteine, etc.), *sedatives* (alcohol up to 50%, barbiturates, opium and other CNS depressants), *vitamins* (ascorbic acid, vitamin B complex, etc.), etc.

More medications are available for the relief of cough than for any other symptom. Hundreds of complex preparations for coughs, colds, hay fever, and other respiratory conditions are available both over-the-counter and on prescription. Many of them are available only on prescription because they are abused by those seeking "kicks" and because they possess the potential for a vast number of drug interactions. Ingredients include enzyme inducers (antihistamines, barbiturates, etc.) neuromuscular agents (anticholinergics, CNS stimulants and depressants), cardiovascular agents (decongestants, etc.), nephrotoxic agents (phenacetin, etc.), and other potent and toxic pharmacologic categories. Medications for respiratory diseases probably cause more iatrogenic problems than any other single class of therapeutic agents. Particular caution should be observed when cold remedies are used with MAO inhibitors, tricyclic antidepressants, and other hazardous interactants.

Guanethidine

See *Cold Remedies* under *Guanethidine Sulfate.*

COLD, HAY FEVER, REDUCING, AND OTHER OTC REMEDIES

MAO inhibitors [78,96,99,311,431]

Contraindicated. Potentially lethal because of the possible interactions wherein MAO inhibitors potentiate antihistamines, sympathomimetics, and other potent drugs.

COLESTIPOL (Colestid)

Thiazides

See *Colestipol* under *Thiazide Diuretics.*

COLISTIMETHATE
(Sodium colistin methanesulfonate and dibucaine HCl [Coly-Mycin M]).

Colistin sulfate [Coly-Mycin S Oral Suspension] is the corresponding sulfate salt.
See also *Anesthetics, Local, Colistin,* and *Neuromuscular Blocking Antibiotics* (under *Antibiotics*)

Anesthetics [120,547]

Apnea may result. See *Antibiotics* and *Muscle Relaxants* below for discussion of mechanism.

Antibiotics [120,619]

Certain antibiotics (dihydrostreptomycin, kanamycin, neomycin, polymyxin, and streptomycin) as well as colistimethate itself interfere with nerve transmission at neuromuscular junctions (competitive blockade plus reduction in acetylcholine release) and should not be given concomitantly except with the greatest caution. Potentiation of this action may result in apnea.

Anticholinesterases [120,421]

Anticholinesterases like edrophonium and neostigmine may potentiate the neuromuscular blocking action of colistimethate.

Cephalothin

Potentiation of nephrotoxicity. See *Colistin* under *Cephalosporins.*

Dihydrostreptomycin

See *Antibiotics* above.

Edrophonium [421] (Tensilon)

See *Anticholinesterases* above.

Kanamycin

See *Antibiotics* above.

Muscle relaxants [120,421,619]

Curariform muscle relaxants and colistimethate both interfere with nerve transmission at neuromuscular junctions. Concomitant use can lead to apnea requiring assisted respiration. Use extreme caution. See *Colistin* under *Muscle Relaxants, Peripherally Acting.*

Neomycin

See *Antibiotics* above.

Neostigmine [421]

See *Anticholinesterases* above.

Organophosphates [120,421] (Cholinesterase inhibitors)

Anticholinesterases potentiate the neuromuscular blocking action. See *Antibiotics* and *Muscle Relaxants* above for discussion.

Polymyxin [120]

See *Antibiotics* above. There is complete cross-resistance between colistin and polymyxin.

Streptomycin

See *Antibiotics* above.

Succinylcholine [421]

Colistimethate potentiates succinylcholine.

Tubocurarine [421]

See *Muscle Relaxants* above.

Sulfonamides [883,1107] (Sulfamethomidine, sulfafurazole, etc.)

This combination of antibiotics has synergistic antibacterial activity against *Proteus* and *Pseudomonas* species.

COLISTIN PLUS SULFAFURAZOLE

See *Sulfonamides* under *Colistimethate* above.

p-Aminobenzoic acid (PABA)

PABA inhibits bactericidal synergism of colistin plus sulfafurazole.

COLISTIN SULFATE (Coly-Mycin S)

See *Colistimethate.*
The antibiotic, colistin (Coly-Mycin) forms a sulfate and a methanesulfonate (colistimethate).

COLREX DECONGESTANT

See *Antihistamines, Phenylephrine,* and *Phenylpropanolamine.*

COLY-MYCIN

See *Colistimethate.*

COMBID (Compazine and Darbid)

See *Phenothiazines* (prochlorperazine) and *Anticholinergics* (isopropamide).

COMPAZINE

See *Phenothiazines* (prochlorperazine).

COMPLEX DIGESTANTS

Some digestant products are complex mixtures of ingredients such as barbiturates, berberis, betaine HCl, bismuth salts, calcium salts, cascara, cellulase, charcoal, diastase, glutamic acid, hydrastis, methionine, methscopolamine nitrate, mycozyme, nux vomica, ox bile, pancreatin, papain, pepsin, strychnine, etc.

Determine the specific ingredients of each medication and make certain that no adverse drug interaction with prescribed or other medication can occur.

COMPLEXING AGENTS

Tetracyclines
See *Complexing Agents* under *Tetracyclines*.

COMPOCILLIN
See *Penicillin* (hydrabamine phenoxymethyl penicillin).

COMPOZ
See *Sleeping Pills* and *Hallucinogenic Medications*.

COMYCIN CAPSULES
See *Tetracyclines* and *Nystatin*.

CONAR
See *Noscapine* and *Phenylephrine*.

CONSOTUSS
See *Antihistamines* (decapryn), *Dextromethorphan*, and *Glyceryl Guaiacolate*.

CONTAINERS

Medicaments[89]
Some drugs interact adversely with various container components. See also *Plastic Containers* and *Rubber Caps*.

CONTRACEPTIVES, ORAL
See *Oral Contraceptives*.

COPE
See *Aluminum, Antihistamines, Magnesium,* and *Salicylates*.

CORICIDIN
See *Antihistamines* (chlorpheniramine), *Aspirin,* and *Caffeine*.

CORIFORTE
See *Antihistamines* (chlorpheniramine), *Caffeine, Phenacetin,* and *Salicylamide*.

CORILIN
See *Antihistamines* and *Salicylates*.

COROVAS TYMCAPS
See *Barbiturates* (secobarbituric acid) and *Pentaerythritol Tetranitrate*.

CORTEF
See *Corticosteroids* (hydrocortisone).

CORTENEMA
See *Hydrocortisone*.

CORTICOSTEROIDS
(Adrenocortical steroids, adrenocorticosteroids, glucocorticoids, betamethasone, cortisone, desoxycorticosterone, dexamethasone, fluocinolone, hydrocortisone, prednisone, prednisolone, triamcinolone, etc.)
See also *Hydrocortisone*.

Adrenergics [120,421,728,940]
Increased ocular pressure in long-term corticosteroid use. Potentiated smooth muscle response.

Amphotericin B [120]
Deep fungal infections sometimes emerge in patients being treated with amphotericin B (and corticosteroids). The latter should not be given concurrently unless absolutely necessary to control reactions to amphotericin B or treat underlying disease.

Anesthetics [16,37,311,1448]
Anesthetics, given to patients on corticosteroids (other than interarticularly), produce profound, refractory, potentially lethal hypotension during and after anesthesia. Any patient who has received corticosteroid therapy within the past 2 years and certainly during the past 6 months (even on a short-term course) prior to surgery should be given hydrocortisone preoperatively, intraoperatively, and in diminishing doses postoperatively because of possible adrenocortical atrophy.

Anticholinergics [421]
Corticosteroids increase ocular pressure with anticholinergics (long term therapy). Hazardous in glaucoma.

Anticholinesterases [120,421]
In long term therapy corticosteroids antagonize effects of anticholinesterases in glaucoma.

Anticoagulants, oral [120,147,673,903]
Corticosteroids and ACTH decrease prothrombin time and inhibit oral coumarin anticoagulants. However, severe hemorrhage has been reported with the combination.

Antidepressants, tricyclic [120]
Corticosteroids with tricyclic antidepressants increase ocular pressure. Hazardous in glaucoma. Hydrocortisone inhibits the metabolism of nortriptyline and thus may potentiate the tricyclic antidepressant.

Antidiabetics, oral [4a,120,191]
Corticosteroids may cause an increase in blood glucose levels, thus antagonizing antidiabetics; increased dosage of the hypoglycemic agents may be necessary.

Antihistamines [78,198,421]
Antihistamines, e.g., chlorcyclizine (Perazil), increase the rate of metabolism of corticosteroids, and thus inhibit their action. Corticosteroids with antihistamines increase ocular pressure in long term therapy. Hazardous in glaucoma.

Antituberculars [120,421]
Tuberculosis is usually an absolute contraindication for corticosteroids which tend to spread infections but may be life saving in certain cases.

Antiviral eye preparations [120,421] (Stoxil, etc.)
Corticosteroids antagonize antiviral eye preparations and increase spread of infection.

Azathioprine [755] (Imuran)
See *Azathioprine* under *Prednisone*.

Barbiturates [83,198,421,633,1265,1404,1824]
Barbiturates decrease activity of corticosteroids by increasing the rate of their metabolism through induction of hepatic microsomal enzymes. Possibly, also, in asthmatics dependent on corticosteroids a vicious cycle is formed wherein barbiturate inhibits corticosteroid, the asthma is exacerbated with increased hypoxemia, and the hypoxemia induces the metabolizing enzymes. Corticosteroids may potentiate sedation of barbiturates. Monitor patients closely.

Bilirubin [198]
Bilirubin potentiates corticosteroids by displacing them from secondary binding sites.

Carbitral [120]
Corticosteroids potentiate Carbitral.

Chloral hydrate[198]
Chloral hydrate decreases the activity of corticosteroids by enzyme induction.

Chlorcyclizine
See *Antihistamines* above.

Chlorthalidone[120,1853]
This combination may cause severe hypokalemia. See under *Diuretics*.

Cholinergics[421]
Corticosteroids antagonize cholinergics (pilocarpine, physostigmine, etc.).

Cholinesterase inhibitors[120]
Corticosteroids antagonize cholinesterase inhibitors (increased ocular pressure on long usage).

Cyclophosphamide[359,1100] **(Cytoxan, Endoxan)**
Cyclophosphamide may be inhibited by prednisolone and some other corticosteroids due to enzyme inhibition (not transformed into active metabolites).

o,p′-DDD[78]
o,p′-DDD inhibits the steroids by stimulating their metabolism.

Digitalis[580,619]
Prolonged corticosteroid therapy may produce hypokalemia and thus enhance digitalis toxicity.

Diphenhydramine[198]
Diphenhydramine may decrease steroid effects of enzyme induction; increases hydroxylation of hydrocortisone and related corticosteroids.

Diuretics[120,1853]
Excessive potassium depletion may occur since both the corticosteroids and diuretics can cause hypokalemia. See *Corticosteroids* and *Diuretics*.

Estrogens[1659,1826]
Estrogens (oral contraceptives, etc.) enhance the glucosuric and anti-inflammatory effects of hydrocortisone (3- to 20-fold for the latter effect). They do not potentiate the glucosuric effect of dexamethasone, methylprednisolone, prednisone, or prednisolone. Possibly the potentiation of hydrocortisone may be due to decreased rate of metabolism because of increased plasma protein binding in the presence of increased levels of a binding globulin produced by estrogens. Monitor patients closely for corticosteroid side and extension effects.

Ethacrynic acid
See *Corticosteroids* under *Diuretics*.

Furosemide (Lasix)
See *Corticosteroids* under *Diuretics*.

Glutethimide[198]
Glutethimide decreases the activity of corticosteroids by enzyme induction.

Gold therapy[1482,1760] **(Solganol, etc.)**
Corticosteroids inhibit the therapeutic efficacy of gold and increase its toxicity.

Halogenated insecticides[83,485]
(Aldrin, chlordane, DDT, dieldrin, heptachlor, methoxychlor, TDE, etc.)
Halogenated insecticides (see chlordane, DDT, etc.) induce the metabolism of cortisol and also other steroids, *e.g.*, estrogens and progesterone. The effects of both exogenous and endogenous steroids may be reduced.

Human growth hormone[181]
Corticosteroids inhibit the anabolic actions of human growth hormone but augment the other actions.

Hydrochlorothiazide[120] **(Hydrodiuril)**
See *Diuretics* above.

Immunizing agents
See under *Vaccines*.

Idoxuridine[120] **(Dendrid, Herplex, Stoxil)**
Corticosteroids can accelerate the spread of a viral infection. They should not be used in combination with idoxuridine unless absolutely necessary.

Indomethacin[1047,1396] **(Indocin)**
Indomethacin potentiates corticosteroids by displacing them from their plasma protein binding sites and this combination may increase the incidence and severity of gastrointestinal ulcers that may be produced. Avoid this combination or monitor patients very closely.

Insulin[120,181,191]
Corticosteroids may antagonize the hypoglycemic effect of insulin.

Levothyroxine[120]
Levothyroxine is contraindicated in the presence of uncorrected adrenal insufficiency because it increases the tissue demands for adrenocortical hormones and may cause an acute adrenal crisis in such patients.

Meperidine[421] **(Demerol)**
Corticosteroids with meperidine increase ocular pressure in long term therapy. Hazardous in glaucoma.

Nicotine (smoking)[951]
Nicotine increases the blood levels of endogenous corticosteroids and may have an additive effect with administered corticosteroids.

Organophosphates[120,421]
(Cholinesterase inhibitors)
Corticosteroids may antagonize the miotic effects of the inhibitors.

Oxyphenbutazone (Tandearil)
See *Phenylbutazone* below.

Parathormone[181]
Corticosteroids antagonize parathormone induced hypercalcemia.

Pentobarbital[78,633]
Pentobarbital (enzyme inducer) inhibits glucocorticoids. See *Barbiturates* above.

Pesticides[83,485] **(Chlorinated)**
These pesticides (enzyme inducers) inhibit glucocorticoids. See *Halogenated Insecticides* above.

Phenobarbital[84] **(Phenobarbitone)**
Phenobarbital (enzyme inducer) increases rate of metabolism of corticosteroids and thus inhibits them. See *Barbiturates* above.

Phenylbutazone[83,421,1047] **(Butazolidin)**
The anti-inflammatory action of phenylbutazone may be due to its ability to displace corticosteroids from plasma protein binding sites, thus allowing much freer dispersal into tissues. The metabolism of steroids like cortisol (urinary excretion of the metabolite 6-beta-hydroxycortisol) may be stimulated by inducing action of phenylbutazone and thus their activity diminished. The net effect of these two mechanisms (immediate effect is potentiation) determines dosage.

Phenytoin[78,83,84,192,450] **(Dilantin)**
Phenytoin, through enzyme induction, inhibits the ability of corticosteroids (dexamethasone) to suppress endogenous hydrocortisone. See also *Corticosteroids* under *Phenytoin*.

Pyrazolone derivatives
(Aminopyrine, Antipyrine, Phenylbutazone, etc.)
See *Phenylbutazone* above. Corticosteroid displacement occurs only with anti-inflammatory pyrazolones.

CORTICOSTEROIDS *(continued)*

Rifampin
See *Corticosteroids* under *Rifampin*.

Salicylates [421,618,1047,1393,1396]
The anti-inflammatory action of salicylates may be due to their ability to displace corticosteroids from plasma protein binding sites, thus allowing greater dispersal of free steroids into the tissues. Salicylates may also potentiate corticosteroids by inhibiting their metabolic conjugation Both corticosteroids and salicylates have an ulcerogenic effect on the gastric mucosa which may be additive. Corticosteroids may increase the urinary clearance rate of salicylates by increasing their glomerular filtration rate and decreasing their tubular reabsorption and their withdrawal may lead to signs of salicylate intoxication. Monitor patients closely for this toxic effect when corticosteroids are withdrawn from patients also receiving salicylates.

Sympathomimetics [120,421,728]
Corticosteroids with sympathomimetics increase ocular pressure in long term therapy. Hazardous in glaucoma. Aerosols of sympathomimetics with corticosteroids may be lethal in asthmatic children.

Sedatives and hypnotics [198,421]
Corticosteroids potentiate sedatives and hypnotics. Some sedatives and hypnotics inhibit corticosteroids by enzyme induction.

Tetracyclines
See *Corticosteroids* under *Tetracyclines*.

Thiazide diuretics
See *Corticosteroids* under *Diuretics*.

D-Thyroxine [120] (Dextrothyroxine, choloxin, etc.)
Thyroid preparations increase tissue demands for adrenocortical hormones and may cause an acute adrenal crisis in patients with adrenocortical insufficiency. Correct adrenal insufficiency with corticosteroids before administering thyroid hormones.

Tuberculin test [486]
Temporary depression of tuberculin response.

Vaccines, live attenuated virus (Measles, smallpox, rabies, yellow fever) [312,486,619]
Serious and possibly fatal illness may develop. Discontinue corticosteroids at least 72 hours prior to vaccination and do not resume for at least 14 days after vaccination. Corticosteroids also depress immunological response to vaccines of all types.

Vitamin A [486,1496,1836]
Topically applied vitamin A overcomes the antihealing effect of corticosteroids and promotes wound healing in patients on corticosteroids by enhancing tissue lysosome production of healing enzymes. Systemically administered vitamin A may inhibit the anti-inflammatory action of corticosteroids. Administer vitamin A with caution to patients on the steroids.

CORTICOTROPIN (ACTH, adrenocorticotropic hormone, Achthar, etc.)
See *ACTH*.

CORTIPHATE
See *Hydrocortisone*.

CORTISOL (Hydrocortisone)
See *Corticosteroids* and *Hydrocortisone*.
Some drugs displace cortisol from plasma protein binding sites and presumably drive it into the tissues. The actions and interactions of a number of drugs can be explained on this basis, *e.g.*, antirheumatics.

CORTISONE ACETATE
See *Hydrocortisone* and *Corticosteroids*.

CORTISPORIN
See *Hydrocortisone, Neomycin,* and *Polymyxin B.*

CORTRIL
See *Hydrocortisone.*

CORYBAN-D SYRUP
See *Acetaminophen, Antihistamines* (chlorpheniramine), *Dextromethorphan, Glyceryl Guaiacolate,* and *Phenylephrine.*

CO-SALT
See *Ammonium Chloride* and *Potassium Salts.*

COSMEGEN
See *Actinomycin D* (dactinomycin) and *Antineoplastics.*

CO-TYLENOL
See *Acetaminophen, Antihistamines* (chlorpheniramine), and *Ephedrine.*

COUGH AND COLD REMEDIES
See *Cold and Cough Remedies.*

MAO inhibitors [99]
Phenylpropanolamine may cause a rapid and potentially dangerous rise of blood pressure with MAO inhibitors.

COUMADIN
See *Anticoagulants* (sodium warfarin).

Vitamin E
See *Warfarin* under *Vitamin E.*

COUMARIN ANTICOAGULANTS
See *Anticoagulants, Oral.*

COVANAMINE
See *Antihistamines* (chlorpheniramine and pyrilamine) *Phenylephrine,* and *Phenylpropanolamine.*

COVANGESIC
See *Antihistamines* (chlorpheniramine), *Aspirin, Phenylephrine,* and *Phenylpropanolamine.*

CO-XAN
See *Antihistamines* (methapyrilene), *Codeine, Ephedrine, Glyceryl Guaiacolate,* and *Theophylline.*

C-RON FA
See *Ascorbic Acid* and *Iron Salts.*

CRYSTICILLIN A.S.
See *Penicillin.*

CRYSTIFOR 400
See *Penicillin.*

CRYSTODIGIN
See *Digitalis* (digitoxin).

CURARE AND CURARIFORM DRUGS (Dimethyl tubocurarine [Mecostrix] chloride, dimethyl tubocurarine [Metubine] iodide, gallamine [Flaxedil] triethiodide, *d*-tubocurarine [Tubadil, Tubarine] chloride, etc.)
See *Muscle Relaxants, Peripherally Acting, Competitive Type.*

Antibiotics [421]
Certain antibiotics (colistin, dihydrostreptomycin, gramicidin, kanamycin, neomycin, polymyxin, and streptomycin) interfere

with nerve transmission at neuromuscular junctions (competitive blockade plus reduction in acetylcholine release) and none of these should be given concomitantly or with curariform muscle relaxants except with extreme caution. Potentiation may result in apnea requiring assisted respiration.

Anticholinesterases [168]
Anticholinesterases (neostigmine, edrophonium, etc.) antagonize the effects of curare.

Colistin
See *Antibiotics* above.

Chlorthalidone [120,330] **(Hygroton)**
Chlorthalidone potentiates curariform drugs. Reduce their dosage by half.

Diazepam [950,951] **(Valium)**
Diazepam potentiates the muscle relaxing effect of curare.

Dihydrostreptomycin
See *Antibiotics* above.

Edrophonium [168]
Edrophonium reverses the neuromuscular blocking action of curare (an antagonist).

Furosemide [120]
Great caution should be exercised in administering curare or its derivatives to patients being treated with furosemide.

Gramicidin
See *Antibiotics* above.

3-Hydroxyphenyltriethylammonium [57]
3-Hydroxyphenyltriethylammonium is said to be a potent anticurare drug.

Kanamycin
See *Antibiotics* above.

Muscle relaxants, depolarizing type [168]
Diminished activity of depolarizing type muscle relaxants with curare.

Narcotic analgesics [421]
Respiratory depression reversed only by methylphenidate or naloxone.

Neomycin
See *Antibiotics* above.

Polymyxin
See *Antibiotics* above.

Procaine [168]
The neuromuscular blocking effects of procaine and curare are additive.

Quinidine [447]
If curare is administered during surgery, quinidine should not be administered during recovery; recurarization may occur.

Streptomycin
See *Antibiotics* above.

CYANOCOBALAMIN
See *Vitamin B₁₂*

CYCLAMATES

Lincomycin [619,880,1385,1887]
Cyclamates inhibit lincomycin by decreasing its intestinal absorption.

MAO inhibitors
See *Cyclamates* under *MAO Inhibitors*.

CYCLAZOCINE

Methylphenidate [166] **(Ritalin)**
Respiratory depression produced by the analgesic, cyclazocine, is reversed by methylphenidate.

Morphine [166]
Cyclazocine, a narcotic antagonist, inhibits morphine.

Naloxone [166,237] **(Narcan)**
Naloxone antagonizes the miosis, psychotomimetic effects and the respiratory depression produced by cyclazocine. See also *Alkylating Agents* and *Antineoplastics*.

CYCLIZINE (Marezine)

Heparin [764]
Large doses of cyclizine antagonize the action of heparin.

CYCLOMYDRIL
See *Anticholinergics* (Cyclopentolate) and *Sympathomimetics* (phenylephrine).

CYCLOPHOSPHAMIDE (Cytoxan, Endoxan)
See also *Alkylating Agents* and *Antineoplastics*.

Allopurinol [1256,1591] **(Zyloprim)**
Addition of allopurinol to regimens of cytotoxic drugs such as cyclophosphamide may be hazardous due to increased depression of the bone marrow. Avoid or monitor patients very closely.

Anesthetics [1979]
Combination of cyclophosphamide and inhalation anesthetics, particularly halothane, and even nitrous oxide, are lethal (mice and rabbits). Discontinue the antineoplastic at least 12 hours before general anesthesia is administered.

Antidiabetics [203]
See *Cyclophosphamide* under *Antidiabetics, Oral*.

Barbiturates [359,1526]
Barbiturates, *e.g.*, phenobarbital, by means of enzyme induction, *potentiate* cyclophosphamide by markedly increasing the metabolic cleavage of the drug by the cytochrome P-450 mixed-function oxidase system in the liver into an active nitrogen mustard alkylating agent. Cautious monitoring of dosage is essential with this combination, especially if the barbiturate is discontinued.

Chloramphenicol [1045] **(Chloromycetin)**
Animal studies indicate that chloramphenicol pretreatment can reduce the lethality of cyclophosphamide; effect is apparently due to an inhibition of microsomal enzymes which are responsible for the *in vivo* activation of cyclophosphamide.

Chlordane [114]
Increased cyclophosphamide toxicity. May induce the metabolism of cyclophosphamide to produce increased cyclophosphamide toxicity due to more rapid formation of the active metabolite.

Corticosteroids [359,1100]
Animal studies suggest that the activation of cyclophosphamide can be inhibited by prednisolone. See below under *Prednisolone*.

Halothane
See *Anesthetics* above.

Insulin [203]
See *Antidiabetics* above.

Nitrous oxide
See *Anesthetics* above.

Other alkylating agents [120]
Combinations with other alkylating agents may cause irreversible bone marrow damage.

Oxytocin [421]
Oxytocin is potentiated by cyclophosphamide.

Prednisolone [359,1100,1526]
Cyclophosphamide, inactive itself, is metabolized in the liver to several active metabolites (aldophosphamide, phosphor-

CYCLOPHOSPHAMIDE (Cytoxan, Endoxan)
(continued)

amide mustard, and acrolein) with potent cytotoxic activity, but the metabolism of cyclophosphamide is inhibited by prednisolone in the rat. If these two drugs are given concomitantly to patients with malignant disease, and if a similar interaction happens in man, the effects of cyclophosphamide will be reduced. Conversely, serious toxicity may develop if prednisolone and other similarly acting steroids are discontinued while the dose of cyclophosphamide remains unchanged.

Radiation[120]
Radiation plus cyclophosphamide therapy may cause irreversible bone marrow damage.

Succinylcholine[1646,1814,1888,1917,1925]
(Anectin, Quelicin)
Cyclophosphamide may decrease plasma levels of the enzyme pseudocholinesterase which metabolizes succinylcholine. The potency of the muscle relaxant may thus be enhanced, with the hazard of apnea occurring. Avoid this combination where levels of the enzyme are depressed.

Vasopressin[421]
Cyclophosphamide inhibits vasopressin by increasing its excretion.

CYCLOPROPANE OR HALOGENATED ANESTHETICS

Adrenergics[120,684,799,806]
Sensitization to arrhythmias.

Barbiturates
See *Thiopental* below.

Epinephrine[683,684,763,772-777]
Epinephrine induces cardiac arrhythmias with cyclopropane. Death has occurred.

Levarterenol[120,683,772,778] **(Norepinephrine)**
Cyclopropane sensitizes the myocardium to the action of norepinephrine; possibility of ventricular tachycardia or fibrillation exists with combined use. Death has occurred.

Thiopental[120]
Thiopental reduces the cardiac arrhythmia produced by cyclopropane.

Tubocurarine[878]
Enhanced effect of tubocurarine; dosage should be reduced.

CYCLOSERINE (Seromycin)

Anticonvulsant drugs[120] **or sedatives**
Anticonvulsant drugs or sedatives may be effective in controlling symptoms of CNS toxicity, such as convulsions, anxiety, and tremor, due to cycloserine, but see *Diphenylhydantoin* below.

Ethionamide[619,1207] **(Trecator)**
Ethionamide potentiates the toxic CNS effects of cycloserine. Monitor patients closely.

Isoniazid[1884]
Cycloserine antagonizes the MAO inhibition produced by isoniazid, the opposite of its effect on pheniprazine and tranylcypromine.

Pheniprazine[1884] **(Catron, Cavodil)**
Cycloserine potentiates MAO inhibition produced by pheniprazine (rat liver and brain). Pheniprazine is no longer marketed.

Phenytoin[919] **(Dilantin)**
The anticonvulsant drug, phenytoin, is potentiated by cycloserine.

Tranylcypromine[1884] **(Parnate)**
Cycloserine potentiates MAO inhibition produced by tranylcypromine (rat liver and brain).

Vitamin B complex[880]
Cycloserine increases excretion of vitamin B.

CYCLOSPASMOL
See *Vasodilators* (cyclandelate).

CYCLOGESTERIN
See *Progesterone.*

CYPROHEPTADINE (Periactin)
See *Antihistamines.*
This drug is not a phenothiazine and does not enter into many of the phenothiazine interactions although its tricyclic configuration resembles that of amitriptyline.

Analgesics[421]
Analgesic activity reversed by cyproheptadine.

CNS depressants[120]
Periactin has the same additive CNS depressant effects as certain antihistamines. Avoid alcohol, etc. See *CNS Depressants.*

MAO inhibitors[120]
Contraindicated. See *Antihistamines* under *MAO Inhibitors.*

Narcotic analgesics[421]
Cyproheptadine reverses analgesic activity of narcotic analgesics.

CYSTEAMINE (mercaptamine)

Acetaminophen
See *Cysteamine* under *Acetaminophen.*

CYTARABINE HCL
(Cytosar, cytosine arabinoside)
See *Antineoplastics* and *Immunosuppressants* (under vaccines).

Deoxycytidine[949]
Deoxycytidine inhibits the immunosuppressive activity of cytarabine (cytosine arabinoside).

Tetanus toxoid[120]
Cytarabine is immunosuppressive and inhibits antibody synthesis with tetanus toxoid.

CYTELLIN
See *Sitosterols.*

CYTOXAN
See *Cyclophosphamide.*

DACTINOMYCIN
See *Actinomycin D.*

DAINITE
See *Aluminum, Aminophylline, Barbiturates, Benzocaine.*

DANILONE
See *Anticoagulants, Oral* and *Phenindione.*

DANTEN
See *Phenytoin.*

DAPSONE (Avlosulfon)

Probenecid[925]
Probenecid, by blocking renal tubular excretion of dapsone, enhances its antileprotic potency and its toxicity.

DARAPRIM
See *Antimalarials* and *Pyrimethamine.*

DARBID
See *Anticholinergics* (isopropamide iodide).

MAO inhibitors [198]
See *Anticholinergics* under *MAO Inhibitors*.

PBI test [120]
Discontinue one week prior to PBI test—may alter PBI test results and will suppress iodine uptake (see Chapter 7).

DARICON PB
See *Anticholinergics* (oxyphencyclimine) and *Phenobarbital*.

DARVON
See *Narcotic Analgesics* and *Propoxyphene*.

DARVON COMPOUND
See *Narcotic Analgesics, Caffeine, Phenacetin, Propoxyphene,* and *Salicylates*.

DARVO-TRAN
See *Narcotic Analgesics, Aspirin, Phenaglycodol* and *Propoxyphene*.

DBI
See *Phenformin*.

o,p′-DDD

Cortisol [271]
o,p′-DDD, an enzyme inducer, accelerates the metabolism of cortisol.

Hexobarbital [271]
Same as for *Cortisol* above.

DDT
See also *Chlorinated Insecticides*.

Anticonvulsants [1044] **(Barbiturates, Dilantin)**
Certain anticonvulsants tend to decrease the storage of DDT in the body (enzyme induction).

Bilirubin [264, 359, 1076]
DDT has been used to accelerate the conjugation of bilirubin in neonatal hyperbilirubinemia, sometimes caused by displacement from protein binding sites with drugs like sulfonamides.

Various drugs [83, 180, 335, 688]
(Aminopyrine, anticoagulants, hexobarbital, pentobarbital, zoxazolamine, etc.)
DDT, an enzyme inducer, inhibits various drugs by stimulating microsomal enzyme metabolism. DDT, inactivated by absorption from the environment and storage in body fat, may be mobilized and activated by fasting. It was shown by this means to accelerate the metabolism of drugs (chlordiazepoxide, meprobamate, and methyprylon in one study).

DEBRISOQUIN (Isocaramidine) SULFATE
See also *Antihypertensives*.

Amphetamines [78]
Amphetamines antagonize the hypotensive action of debrisoquine.

Antidepressants, tricyclic [598, 823]
Tricyclic antidepressants antagonize the hypotensive action of debrisoquine. See *Antidepressants, Tricyclic* under *Antihypertensives* for discussion.

Phenylephrine [1212, 1703] **(Neo-Synephrine)**
Debrisoquin (adrenergic blocking agent used as an antihypertensive) has MAO inhibitory action which can produce a hypertensive crisis with sympathomimetics like phenylephrine. Controllable with phentolamine. This severe reaction should be avoided if possible or monitor extremely closely.

DECADRON
See *Corticosteroids* (dexamethasone).

DECAGESIC
See *Antacids, Aluminum, Aspirin, Dexamethasone,* and *Salicylates*.

DECAMETHONIUM (Syncurine)
See *Muscle Relaxants, Peripherally Acting, Depolarizing*.

DECHOLIN
See *Dehydrocholic Acid*.

DECLOMYCIN
See *Tetracyclines* (demethylchlortetracycline).

DECONAMINE
See *Antihistamines* (chlorpheniramine), and *Ephedrine*.

DECONGESTANTS
See *Nasal Decongestants*.

DEHIST
See *Antihistamines* (chlorpheniramine), *Phenylephrine,* and *Phenylpropanolamine*.

DEHIST INJECTABLE
See *Antihistamines* (chlorpheniramine) *Atropine,* and *Phenylpropanolamine*.

DELADUMONE
See *Estradiol* and *Testosterone*.

DELALUTIN
See *Progestogens* (hydroxyprogesterone)

DELATESTRYL
See *Testosterone*.

DELESTROGEN
See *Estradiol*.

DEMAZIN
See *Antihistamines* (chlorpheniramine) and *Phenylephrine*.

DEMEROL
See *Meperidine*.

DEOXYCYTIDINE

Cytarabine [949] **(Cytosar)**
Deoxycytidine inhibits the immunosuppressive activity of cytarabine (cytosine arabinoside).

DEPO-ESTRADIOL CYPIONATE
See *Estradiol*.

DEPO-HEPARIN
See *Heparin*.

DEPO-MEDROL
See *Corticosteroids* (methylprednisolone).

DEPO-PROVERA
See *Progesterone* (medroxyprogesterone).

DEPO-TESTADIOL
See *Estradiol* and *Testosterone*.

DEPO-TESTOSTERONE
See *Testosterone*.

DEPROL
See *Antidepressants* (benactyzine) and *Meprobamate*.

DERFULE
See *Aspirin, Atropine Sulfate, Ipecac, Phenacetin,* and *Salicylates*.

DESA-HIST PF
See *Antihistamines* (chlorpheniramine) and *Phenylpropanolamine*.

DESIPRAMINE (Pertofrane)
See *Antidepressants, Tricyclic*.

DESOXYCHOLIC ACID

Reserpine [603]
Desoxycholic acid increases the blepharoptotic effect of reserpine by enhancing its absorption.

Vitamins [603]
Desoxycholic acid, through its surface activity or its ability to form inclusion compounds (clathrates), increases the solubility of the fat-soluble vitamins (A, D, E, K).

DESOXYCORTICOSTERONE (Percorten)
See *Corticosteroids*.

DESOXYN
See *Methamphetamine* and *Sympathomimetics*.

DEXAMETHASONE (Decadron)
See *Corticosteroids* (main section) and under *Phenytoin, Barbiturates*, etc.)

Phenytoin [450-1,1232,1477,1518,1733,1897] (Dilantin)
Phenytoin, an enzyme inducer, may inhibit the effect of dexamethasone by accelerating its hepatic conjugation and biliary excretion. See *Corticosteroids* under *Phenytoin*.

Secobarbital
See *Barbiturates* under *Corticosteroids*.

DEXAMYL
See *Amphetamines* (dextroamphetamine) and *Barbiturates* (amobarbital).

DEXBROMPHENIRAMINE (Disomer)
See *Antihistamines*.

DEXEDRINE
See *Amphetamines* (dextroamphetamine).

DEXPANTHENOL
(Dextro-pantothenyl alcohol)

Anticholinesterases [421]
Dexpanthenol potentiates the effect of anticholinesterases.

Muscle relaxants, [421] depolarizing type (Decamethonium, succinylcholine, etc.)
Dexpanthenol enhances the activity of depolarizing type muscle relaxants and should not be given within one hour after administration of agents like succinylcholine.

Organophosphate cholinesterase inhibitors [421]
Dexpanthenol potentiates the miotic effect of cholinergics.

Parasympathomimetics [421]
Dexpanthenol should not be given for 12 hours after use of a parasympathomimetic because of the possibility of hyperperistalsis.

Succinylcholine
See *Muscle Relaxants, Depolarizing* above.

DEXTRAN

Anticoagulants [912]
Dextran (large dose) may potentiate anticoagulants (prolonged prothrombin time and hemorrhage). See *Dextran* under *Heparin*.

Tromethamine [486] (Tham-E)
The action of tromethamine in systemic acidosis is potentiated by dextran.

DEXTROAMPHETAMINE
See *Amphetamines*.

DEXTROMETHORPHAN

Phenelzine [779] (Nardil)
Death may be caused by this combination (muscular rigidity, apnea, hyperpyrexia, laryngospasm). Reversed by succinylcholine in genetically suitable patients. Cough medicines and other dosage forms containing dextromethorphan are contraindicated in patients on MAO inhibitors such as phenelzine.

DEXTROPROPOXYPHENE (Darvon)
See *Propoxyphene*.

DEXTROSE
See *Glucose*.

DEXTROTHYROXINE (Choloxin)
See *Thyroid Preparations* also.

Anticoagulants, oral [9,120,134,330,346,393,394,411,434,780,861,911,1305]
Dextrothyroxine potentiates the anticoagulant response by increasing the affinity of the anticoagulant for its receptor site, by inhibiting protein binding, by decreasing levels of factors VII, VIII and IX, and by depressing platelet activity. Also, the availability of vitamin K is reduced as serum cholesterol and lipoproteins are reduced. Reduce the anticoagulant dosage by one-third when dextrothyroxine therapy is initiated and adjust as necessary to avoid hemorrhage.

Antidiabetics [120,588]
Increase the doses of the hypoglycemic agents if necessary since dextrothyroxine antagonizes the hypoglycemic effect in some patients.

Clofibrate [589]
Summation of hypocholesterolemic effects. Blood cholesterol lowering agents like clofibrate may potentiate thyroxine by displacement from binding sites.

Digitalis [787]
Thyroxine may increase the toxic effects of digitalis.

Epinephrine [120]
Injections of epinephrine in patients with coronary heart disease may precipitate an episode of coronary insufficiency; the likelihood of this occurring may be increased in patients taking dextrothyroxine.

Insulin [120]
Dextrothyroxine antagonizes the hypoglycemic effect.

Norepinephrine [590]
Thyroxine augments rate of oxidation of epinephrine and norepinephrine. This is manifested by an augmentation of epinephrine and norepinephrine response.

Reserpine and sympatholytics [590]
Reserpine abolishes the angina induced by dextrothyroxine in patients with coronary artery disease.

Thyroid preparations [120]
Dosage of other thyroid preparations used concomitantly must be carefully adjusted (additive effects).

DEXTRO-TUSSIN
See *Ammonium Chloride, Antihistamines* (chlorpheniramine) *Dextromethorphan Hydrobromide* and *Phenylephrine*.

D.H.E. 45
See *Adrenergic Blockers* and *Dihydroergotamine*.

DIABETOGENIC DRUGS
See under *Antidiabetics, Oral*.

DIABINESE
See *Antidiabetics, Oral* and *Chlorpropamide*.

DIACETYLCHOLINE CHLORIDE (Anectine Chloride)
See *Succinylcholine Chloride*.

DIAFEN
See *Antihistamines* (diphenylpyraline).

DIALOG
See *Acetaminophen* and *Barbiturates* (allobarbital).

DIAMOX
See *Acetazolamide* and *Diuretics*.

DIANABOL
See *Methandrostenolone*.

DIA-QUEL
See *Anticholinergics* (homatropine) and *Opium*.

DIASAL
See *Potassium Salts*.

DIAZEPAM (Valium)
See also *Benzodiazepines*.

Alcohol [78,120]
Diazepam potentiates the hypotensive effects of alcohol. Deep sedation or seizures may occur, unless tolerance has developed in a social drinker on benzodiazepines. Still risky, however. See *Alcohol* under *Benzodiazepines*.

Anticoagulants [120,330,814,894]
See *Benzodiazepines* under *Anticoagulants, Oral*.

Anticonvulsants [120,283]
When diazepam is used as an adjunct in treating convulsive disorders, an increase in the dose of standard anticonvulsant medication may be necessary because of the possibility of increased severity and/or frequency of grand mal seizures.

Antidepressants, tricyclic [94,120]
Antidepressants may potentiate the sedative action of diazepam. However, the convulsions produced by overdosage of a tricyclic antidepressant may be best controlled with diazepam.

Antihypertensives [619]
Diazepam may potentiate the antihypertensive effects of thiazides, other diuretics, and other antihypertensives.

Barbiturates [78,120,166]
Hazard of synergistic CNS depression. Deep sedation and other hazardous effects may occur.

Caffeine and sodium benzoate [120]
Caffeine and sodium benzoate combats CNS depressant effects caused by overdosage of diazepam.

Chlordiazepoxide [120] (Librium)
Enuresis may occur with the combination in about 1% of patients.

CNS depressants [78,120,166]
Diazepam may potentiate effects of CNS depressants such as alcohol, barbiturates, narcotics, and phenothiazines.

Curare [782]
Diazepam potentiates the muscle relaxing effect of curare. Malignant hyperthermia may be induced.

Gallamine [781,782]
Diazepam potentiates the muscle relaxant effect of gallamine and may induce neuromuscular block.

Imipramine
See *Antidepressants* above.

Levarterenol [120] (Levophed)
Levarterenol combats hypotension caused by overdosage of diazepam.

Levodopa
See *Levodopa* under *Benzodiazepines*.

Lidocaine
See *Diazepam* under *Lidocaine*.

Mandrax-B [783]
This combination may induce apnea, respiratory depression and paralysis.

MAO inhibitors [78,120]
MAO inhibitors may potentiate the action of diazepam. Severe sedation, seizures, excitement, stimulation, acute rage, or other hazardous effects may occur.

Metaraminol [120] (Aramine)
Metaraminol combats hypotension caused by overdosage of diazepam.

Methylphenidate [120] (Ritalin)
Methylphenidate combats CNS depressant effects caused by overdosage of diazepam.

Muscle relaxants [486]
Diazepam IV may briefly potentiate *d*-tubocurarine.

Narcotics [120,166]
Diazepam may potentiate hypotensive effects of narcotics and narcotics may potentiate the CNS depressant effects of diazepam.

Phenothiazines [78,120]
Additive or super-additive effects may occur with diazepam. Deep sedation, seizures or severe atropinelike effects may occur.

Tubocurarine [781]
The same interaction given above for gallamine may be expected.

DIAZEPINE DERIVATIVES
See *Benzodiazepines* (chlordiazepoxide, diazepam, and oxazepam).

DIAZOXIDE (Hyperstat)
See also *Antihypertensives* and *Thiazides*.

Anticoagulants, oral [784]
Diazoxide may potentiate the oral anticoagulants. Severe or fatal hemorrhage is possible.

Antidiabetics [120,191,1941] (Oral drugs and insulin)
Because diazoxide inhibits pancreatic insulin release, it is diabetogenic, tends to increase blood glucose, and is antagonistic to all antidiabetics and potentiates hyperglycemics such as furosemide. Pretreatment with tolbutamide prevents the hyperglycemic effect of diazoxide.

Bendroflumethiazide [117,1940-1] (Naturetin)
A combination of diazoxide with a thiazide diuretic (bendroflumethiazide) has proved useful in treating hypoglycemia produced by insulin-secreting tumors. But see *Thiazides* below for enhanced diabetogenic and other side effects.

Chlorpromazine [1940-1]
Chlorpromazine may strongly potentiate the hyperglycemic effect of diazoxide and other thiazides. A single oral dose of 30 mg. of chlorpromazine in a 20 month old patient on diazoxide and bendroflumethiazide produced blood glucose up to 403 mg./100 ml. and somnolence for 2 days.

Furosemide [1941]
Diazoxide produces severe hyperglycemia with furosemide. See *Antidiabetics* above.

Hydralazine (Apresoline, Dralzine, Hydralyn, Lopress) [2050]
Hydralazine, given after diazoxide, to lower a blood pressure of 240/150 mm. Hg (furosemide and methyldopa also given) produced a deep hypotension (60 mm. Hg) and bradycardia (36 beats /min.). Atropine IV and dopamine drip reversed the situation.

DIAZOXIDE (Hyperstat) (continued)

Lithium carbonate
See Benzodiazepines under Lithium Carbonate.

MAO inhibitors
See Diazoxide under MAO Inhibitors.

Hydrochlorothiazide[117] **(Hydrodiuril)**
See Bendroflumethiazide and Thiazides below.

Thiazides[117,1940-1]
See Bendroflumethiazide above. Diazoxide (a rapidly acting antihypertensive thiazide which acts by directly dilating peripheral arterioles when rapidly injected IV, or which acts as a strong antihypoglycemic orally), when combined with a thiazide diuretic (e.g., to treat diazoxide-induced sodium retention), produces potentiated antihypertensive, hyperglycemic, and hyperuricemic effects. These are caused by displacement of diazoxide from plasma protein binding sites. The enhanced hyperglycemic effect is also caused by inhibition of insulin secretion.

Tolbutamide[1514]
Tolbutamide decreases the hypotensive and oliguric effects of diazoxide.

DIBENZAZEPINES

See Antidepressants, Tricyclic.

Thiopental[116,194]
Potentiation of thiopental anesthesia has occurred from preoperative administration of dibenzazepines such as imipramine.

DIBENZYLINE

See Adrenergic Blockers and Phenoxybenzamine.

DIBUCAINE

Sulfonamides[178,421]
The local anesthetic (PABA analog) antagonizes the antibacterial activity of sulfonamides.

DICARBOSIL

See Antacids, Calcium, and Magnesium.

DICHLORALANTIPYRINE (Sominat)

Anticoagulants, oral[753,785]
Warfarin is inhibited by the hypnotic.

DICHLORPHENAMIDE (Daranide, Oratrol)

See Carbonic Anhydrase Inhibitors.

DICHLOROISOPROTERENOL (Dichloroisoprenaline)

Acetazolamide[172] **(Diamox)**
Dichloroisoproterenol potentiates the anticonvulsant action of the acetazolamide.

DICLOXACILLIN (Dynapen, sodium dicloxacillin monohydrate)

See also Penicillins.

Aminohippuric acid (PAH)[433]
Elevated serum levels of penicillin and increased toxicity.

Chloramphenicol[433,748]
Antagonism to the bactericidal action of this penicillin. See Penicillins.

Erythromycin[811]
Antagonism to the bactericidal action of this penicillin. See Penicillins.

Sulfaethylthiadiazole
See Sulfonamides below.

Sulfamethoxypyridazine
See Sulfonamides below.

Sulfonamides[268,269,433]
Lowered serum concentration of total penicillin but increased concentration of unbound, antimicrobially active drug in serum and body fluids. Relatively large doses of the sulfonamide reduce the protein binding of this penicillin and thus potentiate it.

Tetracycline[301]
Antagonism to the bactericidal action of this penicillin.

DICORVIN

See Ascorbic Acid and Vitamin B_2 and Estrogens.

DICUMAROL

See Anticoagulants, Oral and Bishydroxycoumarin.

DIETARY FATS AND OILS

Anticoagulants, oral[4,182]
Dietary fats and oils increase anticoagulant response by decreasing vitamin K absorption.

DIETARY SUPPLEMENTS

Various antianemic, geriatric and other dietary supplemental medications contain one or more of the following: alcohol, ascorbic acid, calcium, copper, iron, magnesium, manganese, potassium, and zinc salts, choline, cyanocobalamin (B_{12}), dexpanthenol, liver (dessicated or extract), inositol, iodide, folic acid, lysine, niacinamide, pantothenic acid, phosphorus (as phosphate), pyridoxine (B_6), riboflavin (B_2), sodium, thiamine (B_1), and vitamins A, D, and E, etc.
When other drugs are administered with one of these complex mixtures, the specific formula should be studied carefully to determine whether a potential drug interaction may occur. See, for example, the interactions under Calcium Salts, Iron Salts, Magnesium Salts, Dexpanthenol, Folic Acid, Pantothenic Acid, Vitamins A, B, C, D, E, etc.

DIETHYLPROPION (Tenuate)

See also Sympathomimetics.

Guanethidine[550,593]
Diethylpropion inhibits the hypotensive effect of guanethidine.

MAO inhibitors[120]
Contraindicated. MAO inhibitors potentiate the hypertensive and other effects of this sympathomimetic. See Sympathomimetics under MAO Inhibitors.

DIETHYLSTILBESTROL

See Estrogens.

DIGITALINE NATIVELLE

See Digitalis Glycosides (digitoxin).

DIGITALIS AND DIGITALIS GLYCOSIDES (Acetyldigitoxin [Acylanid], deslanoside [Cedilanid-D], digitoxin [Crystodigin, Digitalline Nativelle, Myodigin, Purodigin], digoxin [Davoxin, Lanoxin, Saroxin], gitalin [Gitaligen], lanatoside C [Cedilanid]), etc.

Acetyldigitoxin[120] **(Acylanid)**
Administer acetyldigitoxin cautiously to patients recently or presently receiving digitalis. Additive effects.

Adrenergics[170,619]
Ephedrine, epinephrine, and probably other sympathomimetics may produce cardiac arrhythmias in digitalized patients.

Aminoglycosides
See *Neomycin* below.

Amphotericin B [28,619,1314,1637] (Fungizone)
Often causes severe hypokalemia, thus giving rise to digitalis toxicity. See *Digitalis* under *Amphotericin B*.

Antacids and antidiarrheal agents [486,2034,2041]
Digitalis effects are decreased through delayed or decreased gastrointestinal absorption. Bioavailability of digoxin was considerably decreased by aluminum hydroxide and magnesium hydroxide (Maalox) and by kaolin-pectin (Kaopectate).

Anticholinergics [1597]
(Anisotropine, belladonna alkaloids, dicyclomine, glycopyrrolate, hexocyclium, isopropamide, methantheline, methscopolamine, metoclopramide, oxyphencyclimine, oxyphenonium, pipenzolate, piperidolate, propantheline, tridihexethyl, valethamate, etc.)
Anticholinergics, by inhibiting gastrointestinal motility, tend to slow the passage of digitalis glycoside tablets through the gut and thus tend to increase bioavailability (elevated blood levels of digoxin, digitoxin) although this effect is not as significant as it formerly was before rigid bioavailability standards for these tablets were adopted. See *Metoclopramide* and *Propantheline* below.

Anticoagulants, oral [673]
Give digitalis preparations with caution to patients receiving oral anticoagulants since they may counteract the effects of the anticoagulants.

Barbiturates [1509,1818]
Barbiturates, such as phenobarbital, may decrease the effectiveness of digitoxin by accelerating, through enzyme induction, the conversion of digitoxin to digoxin which has a shorter half-life then digitoxin. With this combination (or digitoxin plus any other enzyme inducer) monitor patients for underdigitalization.

Calcium salts [170,446,619,633,1667,1766,1793]
Deaths have been reported after intravenous calcium in digitalized patients. Elevated serum levels (hypercalcemia) increase some effects of digitalis and its toxicity. Arrhythmias may occur with digitalis therapy plus calcium and large doses of vitamin D or plus calcium supplements with estrogens for osteoporosis. One author de-emphasizes the seriousness of this interaction, but avoid elevated serum calcium levels in patients on digitalis or its glycosides.

Calphosan [120]
Calphosan is contraindicated with digitalis; both drugs have similar action on the contractility and excitability of cardiac muscle.

Carbamazepine [1537] (Tegretol)
Concomitant use of carbamazepine and a digitalis glycoside may produce bradycardia.

Cathartics [28]
Purgatives decrease the effects of digitalis by markedly increasing passage through the gut and thus decreasing absorption. Cathartics tend to potentiate absorbed digitalis by causing hypokalemia.

Chlorothiazide [120,580] (Diuril)
Cardiac arrhythmias. See *Diuretics* below.

Chlorthalidone [120] (Hygroton)
See *Diuretics* below.

Cholestyramine [1230,1276,1850] (Cuemid, Questran)
Cholestyramine, by binding the digitalis glycoside digitoxin in the intestinal tract and thereby cutting off the enterohepatic cycle, tends to shorten the half-life of the glycoside and pro-

duce underdigitalization. In rats digoxin behaves differently from digitoxin. Monitor patients carefully.

Corticosteroids [580,619]
Prolonged corticosteroid therapy may produce hypokalemia and thus enhance digitalis toxicity.

Diuretics [78,410,579,580,1234,1451,1508,1766,1780]
(Thiazides, Furosemide, Ethacrynic acid, etc.)
Diuretics, which induce hypercalcemia, hypomagnesemia and hypokalemia, such as chlorthalidone (Hygroton), ethacrynic acid (Edecrin), furosemide (Lasix), metolazone (Zaroxolyn), and thiazides (Anhydron, Diurils, Naturetin, etc.), enhance digitalis toxicity. With hypokalemia, the most frequent cause of digitalis intoxication, as well as with low serum magnesium levels, the heart becomes more sensitive to effects of digitalis, possibly resulting in toxicity, cardiac arrythmia, etc. Sometimes fatal. The hazard may be reduced by adding a potassium-conserving diuretic such as spironolactone or triamterene. In one study, 4 out of 5 patients experiencing a toxic reaction to digitalis were also receiving diuretics. [410]

EDTA [634]
(Salts of ethylenediaminetetraacetic acid)
Sodium versenate (sodium edetate) given IV is considered to be the best antidote for digitalis intoxication. It chelates the calcium ions upon which digitalis depends in part for its cardiac action.

Epinephrine
See *Sympathomimetics* below.

Ephedrine
See *Sympathomimetics* below.

Ethacrynic acid
See *Diuretics* above.

Furosemide
See *Diuretics* above.

Glucose [1793]
Infusion of large quantities of glucose, which tends to shift potassium into the cells and decrease serum levels, may cause digitalis toxicity from hypokalemia. See *Diuretics* above.

Guanethidine [120] (Ismelin)
Additive effect; both drugs decrease heart rate.

Heparin [1574]
Digitalis' glycosides may inhibit the anticoagulant action of hyparin.

Insulin [619]
Prolonged insulin therapy, by producing hypokalemia, may increase the toxicity of digitalis.

Isoproterenol [16] (Isuprel)
Isoproterenol is contraindicated in tachycardia; digitalis intoxication is induced.

Laxatives [28,691] (prolonged use)
Laxatives may increase digitalis effects and its toxicity.

Magnesium [619]
Hypomagnesemia potentiates digitalis by increasing sensitivity of the myocardium and may result in toxicity.

Mercurial diuretics [120,691]
Mercurial diuretics enhance the activity of digitalis due to hypokalemia.

Metoclopramide [1596-7,1613,1634,1849]
(Maxolon, Primperan)
Metoclopramide, which shortens gastric emptying time and enhances gastrointestinal motility, may decrease intestinal absorption and thus decrease the efficacy of slowly dissolving digoxin products. New bioavailability requirements for all

DIGITALIS AND DIGITALIS GLYCOSIDES
(continued)

digoxin products may diminish the significance of this interaction, since all must meet the same dissolution standard, except when metoclopramide is added to or withdrawn from the regimen.

Neomycin [1582]
Neomycin may antagonize digitalis glycosides by decreasing their gastrointestinal absorption. Monitor blood levels and give the drugs at different times as far apart as possible.

Oxyphenbutazone (Tandearil)
Same as for *Phenylbutazone* below.

Phenylbutazone [1819] (Butazoldin)
Phenylbutazone, an enzyme inducer, may increase digitalis glycoside metabolism and decrease the activity of the cardiac drug. Sodium retention, induced by the anti-inflammatory agent, may also be a factor in view of the relationship of cardiac glycoside activity and the Na,K-ATPase system. Monitor carefully for underdigitalization.

Phenytoin [786] (Dilantin)
Enhanced digitalis effect. Bradycardia may be induced. See also under *Digitoxin* and *Digitalis glycosides* under *Phenytoin*.

Potassium salts [120,580]
Hyperkalemia may result in decreasing the toxicity and action of digitalis. Hypokalemia, as induced by many diuretics, may result in increasing the toxicity and action of digitalis.

Pressor agents [619]
Digitalis glycosides combined with adrenergic drugs such as ephedrine and epinephrine predisposes the patient to cardiac arrhythmias.

Procainamide [583,619] (Pronestyl)
Procainamide may be useful in treating tachyarrhythmias of digitalis intoxication, but extreme caution must be used to avoid ventricular fibrillation or further depression of cardiac function. Effects may be additive. Avoid overdosage.

Propantheline [1596-7,1613,1634,1849] (Pro-Banthine)
The antimuscarinic drug, propantheline, which decreases gastrointestinal motility, tends to increase absorption of digitalis glycosides and thus enhance their effectiveness. Adjust dosages of the glycosides carefully when propantheline is added to or withdrawn from the regimen.

Propranolol [584,1162-4,2057]
Bradycardia. Enhanced digitalis effect (additive). Avoid overdosage. May cause cardiac arrest in patients with pre-existing partial heart block due to digitalis. See also *Digitalis* under *Propranolol* for use of the combination in angina pectoris. The two drugs may be combined to control a difficult tachyarrhythmia. Digitalis may be used for therapy of atrial fibrillation in a patient receiving propranolol for hypertension or to treat heart failure induced by propranolol, according to two authors.[2057] Since digitalis increases myocardial contractility and propranolol has the opposite effect the two should not be used to alter the inotropic state of the myocardium. In some patients propranolol may mask digitalis toxicity.

Quinethazone [120] (Hydromox)
Quinethazone, particularly during concomitant use of ACTH or corticosteroids, may induce hypokalemia which considerably increases the toxicity of digitalis.

Quinidine [619]
Enhanced digitalis effect (additive). Avoid overdosage.

Rauwolfia derivatives
See *Reserpine* below.

Reserpine and derivatives [110,120,619,691]
Reserpine and derivatives increase the likelihood of bradycardia and cardiac arrhythmia; reserpine enhances digitalis toxicity. Both release catecholamines from the myocardium.

Spironolactone [120,396] (Aldactone)
Hyperkalemia induced by spironolactone may result in decreasing the effectiveness and cardiotoxicity of digitalis. See under *Digitoxin* below.

Succinylcholine [120,783,1242,1312] (Anectine, Quelicin)
Succinylcholine may induce cardiac arrhythmias in digitalized patients. The depolarizing neuromuscular blocking agent may potentiate cardiac conduction and enhance ventricular irritability, perhaps by inducing cholinergic receptors to release catecholamines and by producing a sudden shift in potassium from intracellular to extracellular fluid. Avoid this combination if possible.

Sympathomimetics [912,1793]
Sympathomimetics, especially beta-adrenergics like epinephrine and isoproterenol, given concomitantly with digitalis glycosides, may produce cardiac arrhythmias by causing ectopic pacemaker activity. Use caution.

Thiazide diuretics [78]
See *Diuretics* above. Hazardous.

Thyroid preparations [330,619]
Thyroid preparations may potentiate the toxic effects of digitalis. Increased digitalis dosage is required when thyroid hormonal therapy is initiated (increased metabolism).

Triamterene [120,580] (Dyrenium)
Hyperkalemia induced by triamterene may result in decreasing the effectiveness of digitalis.

Veratrum alkaloids [120,170]
Cardiac arrhythmias are more likely to occur with the combination.

Thyroxine [787]
Thyroxine may increase the toxic effects of digitalis.

DIGITORA
See *Digitalis.*

DIGITOXIN
See *Digitalis.*

Phenylbutazone [950,951] (Butazolidin)
Phenylbutazone may markedly decrease plasma level of digitoxin (enzyme induction).

Phenytoin [786,1700,1818-9,1962] (Dilantin)
Phenytoin, an antiarrhythmic agent as well as an enzyme inducing anticonvulsant, may accelerate conversion of digitoxin to digoxin and markedly decrease the plasma concentration of digitoxin (enzyme induction) on prolonged use, but in the initial stages of the combined therapy may enhance digitalis effects (bradycardia). In one report a patient had ataxia, nystagmus, and rigidity suggesting brain damage, and could not walk after receiving this combination but this was reported in only one patient, a mongoloid. On the other hand with suitable parenteral dosage phenytoin has been useful in treating digitalis glycoside induced cardiac arrhythmias.

Spironolactone [120,396] (Aldactone)
Spironolactone counteracts digitalis glycoside toxicity by competitive inhibition of aldosterone. A potent antidote. May interfere with digitalization, although it is often given with the glycosides to cardiac patients.

DIGOLASE
See *Amylase, Pancreatin* and *Papain.*

DIGOXIN
See *Digitoxin* and *Digitalis and Digitalis Glycosides.*

DIHYCON
See *Phenytoin.*

DIHYDROXYPHENYLALANINE
See *dl-Dopa*.

DI-ISOPACIN
See *Aminosalicyclic Acid* (PAS) and *Isoniazid*.

DILANTIN
See *Anticonvulsants* and *Phenytoin*.

DILAUDID
See *CNS Depressants, Hydromorphone and Narcotic Analgesics*.

DILOCOL
See *Dihydromorphinone* and *Narcotic Analgesics*.

DILOR
See *Xanthines*.

Ephedrine and Sympathomimetics [120]
Xanthines with adrenergics can cause excessive CNS stimulation.

DIMENHYDRINATE (Dramamine)
See *Antihistamines*.

Aminoglycoside Antibiotics [120]
(Gentamicin, Kanamycin, Neomycin, Paromomycin, Streptomycin, Tobramycin)
Dimenhydrinate may mask the ototoxicity of aminoglycosides which may occur. Extra alertness is essential to detect the side effect. See also *Ototoxic Antibiotics* below.

Dihydrostreptomycin
See *Ototoxic Antibiotics* below.

Kanamycin (Kantrex)
See *Ototoxic Antibiotics* below.

Neomycin (Mycifradin)
See *Ototoxic Antibiotics* below.

Ototoxic antibiotics [120,421]
Dimenhydrinate may mask the ototoxic symptoms of the ototoxic antibiotics such as kanamycin, neomycin, ristocetin, the streptomycins and vancomycin, and an irreversible state may be reached before it is recognized.

Ristocetin (Spontin)
See *Ototoxic Antibiotics* above.

Streptomycin
See *Ototoxic Antibiotics* above.

Vancomycin (Vancocin)
See *Ototoxic Antibiotics* above.

DIMERCAPROL (BAL, British anti-Lewisite)

Cadmium salts [926]
Dimercaprol increases the toxicity of cadmium salts.

Iron salts [619,926]
Dimercaprol increases the toxicity of ferrous sulfate and other iron salts (toxic iron chelate formed).

Selenium compounds [926]
Dimercaprol increases the toxicity of selenium compounds.

Uranium salts [926]
Dimercaprol increases the toxicity of uranium salts.

Various other metals [120,175]
Dimercaprol is a useful antidote in poisoning by arsenic, gold, lead and mercury.

DIMETANE
See *Antihistamines* (brompheniramine).

DIMETANE EXPECTORANT-DC
See *Antihistamines* (brompheniramine), *Codeine, Glyceryl Guaiacolate, Phenylephrine,* and *Phenylpropanolamine*.

DIMETAPP
See *Antihistamines* (brompheniramine) *Phenylephrine,* and *Phenylpropanolamine*.

DIMETHYL SULFOXIDE

Neomycin [788]
Deafness can be caused by potentiation of the ototoxicity of neomycin applied topically.

DIOCTYL SODIUM SULFOSUCCINATE (Colace, DDS, etc.)

Bisacodyl [443,951] **(Dulcolax)**
The combination of stool softener and contact laxative may produce abdominal cramps.

Danthron [1118] **(Anavac, Dorbane, etc.)**
DSS increases the absorption of Danthron, oxyphenisatin, and other compounds and greatly increases their toxicity (LD_{50} of danthron reduced to only 9 mg./kg. in rats in the presence of DSS).

Mineral oil [120,4d]
Absorption of mineral oil may be increased. Do not give concurrently for long periods.

Oxyphenisatin [1118] **(Prulet, etc.)**
See *Danthron* above.

DIPAXIN (Diphenadione)
See *Anticoagulants, Oral*.

DIPHENYDRAMINE (Benadryl)
See also *Antihistamines*.

Alcohol [78,120]
See *CNS Depressants* below.

Aminosalicylic Acid
See *Diphenhydramine* under *p-Aminosalicylic Acid*.

Anticholinergics [78]
(Atropine, trihexyphenidyl, imipramine, etc.)
Diphenhydramine has atropinelike side effects and with trihexyphenidyl, imipramine, and other anticholinergics may produce increased atropinelike complications, e.g., dental caries and loss of teeth from prolonged drug-induced xerostoma because of additive anticholinergic effect.

Anticoagulants, oral [120,223]
Diphenhydramine, through enzyme induction may decrease the effectiveness of oral anticoagulants.

Barbiturates [695]
Diphenhydramine and barbiturates, both enzyme inducers, may decrease the effectiveness of both drugs.

Carisoprodol [120,166,555,558,576] **(Rela, Soma)**
Decreased effect of relaxant due to enhanced metabolism via enzyme induction.

CNS depressants [78,120]
Diphenhydramine produces potentially hazardous additive effects with alcohol, hypnotics, sedatives, tranquilizers and other CNS depressants.

Corticosteroids [198]
Diphenhydramine, through enzyme induction, increases hydroxylation of corticosteroids and decreases the steroid effects.

Diphenhydramine [64,480,704] **(Benadryl)**
Diphenhydramine may produce a decrease in its own activity (tolerance) because enzyme induction speeds up its own metabolism.

DIPHENYDRAMINE (Benadryl) *(continued)*

Epinephrine[120]
Diphenhydramine may be used to supplement epinephrine. Enhanced cardiovascular effect.

Griseofulvin[199]
Diphenhydramine and griseofulvin may decrease the effectiveness of each other by mutual enzyme induction.

Halogenated hydrocarbon insecticides[485] **(Chlordane, DDT, etc.)**
Diphenhydramine and halogenated hydrocarbon insecticides may decrease the activity of each other by mutual enzyme induction.

Heparin[764]
Large doses of the antihistamine, diphenhydramine, have an antiheparin action.

Hydrocortisone[198]
Diphenhydramine may decrease the steroid effects of hydrocortisone; enzyme induction increases hydroxylation of the steroid.

Hypnotics
See *CNS Depressants* above.

Imipramine (Tofranil)
See *Anticholinergics* above.

MAO inhibitors[48,199,312]
MAO inhibitors potentiate the antihistamine by decreasing its rate of metabolism.

Norepinephrine[235,400] **(Levarterenol, Levophed)**
Diphenhydramine may enhance cardiovascular effects of norepinephrine (NE); the antihistamine inhibits uptake of NE causing increased concentration of unbound drug which interacts with receptors.

Phenobarbital[695]
Diphenhydramine and phenobarbital, both enzyme inducers, may decrease antihistamine activity and decrease barbiturate activity. Enhanced sedation is a primary (additive) effect.

Phenothiazines[120]
Diphenhydramine antagonizes parkinsonismlike extrapyramidal syndrome induced by certain ataractic phenothiazines.

Phenylbutazone[64,485] **(Butazolidin)**
Decreased effectiveness of both drugs (enzyme induction).

Phenytoin[199] **(Dilantin)**
Diphenhydramine and phenytoin through mutual enzyme induction, may decrease the effectiveness of each other.

Reserpine[78]
See *CNS Depressants* above.

Sedatives
See *CNS Depressants* above.

Thioridazine[623] **(Mellaril)**
The side effects of thioridazine (dryness of mouth, furred tongue, cracking of the angles of the mouth, dizziness and disorientation) are potentiated by diphenhydramine. (Additive anticholinergic effects). The symptoms subside upon the withdrawal of diphenhydramine even when the psychotropic drug is continued.

Tranquilizers
See *CNS Depressants* above.

Trihexyphenidyl[526]
See *Anticholinergics* above.

DIPHENIDOL (Vontrol)

Digitalis[120]
See *Drugs, Overdosage* below.

Drugs, overdosage[120]
Diphenidol, through its antinauseant and antiemetic actions may mask overdosage of other drugs such as digitalis.

DIPHENOXYLATE (in Lomotil)

Barbiturates[120]
Lomotil may potentiate the CNS depressant action of barbiturates.

DIPYRIDAMOLE (Persantine)

Heparin
See *Dipyridamole* under *Heparin*.

DIPYRONE (Narone, Pyrilgin)
See also under *Antipyrine* for other *interactions*.

Antidiabetics, Oral
See *Antidiabetics, Oral* under *Antipyrine*.

Barbiturates[65,96,184,222,694,695]
Barbiturates, enzyme inducers, inhibit dipyrone.

Chlorpromazine[120,166,184,421] **(Thorazine)**
Contraindicated. The potentiating effect of chlorpromazine on the antipyretic action of dipyrone can result in severe hypothermia.

Glutethimide[184,222,694,695]
Glutethimide, an enzyme inducer, inhibits diprone and other pyrazolon derivatives. See under *Antipyrine*.

Phenothiazines[120,421]
Dipyrone should not be used with chlorpromazine and related compounds. The hypothermia is potentiated. See *Chlorpromazine* above.

Phenylbutazone[166,222,694,695] **(Butazolidin)**
Phenylbutazone may increase the rate of metabolism of dipyrone and thus inhibit it. Dipyrone may increase any bleeding (gastrointestinal tract, etc.) caused by phenylbutazone.

DISIPAL (Orphenadrine HCl)
See *Anticholinergics* and *Antiparkinsonism Drugs*.

Propoxyphene
See *Propoxyphene* under *Orphenadrine*.

DISOMER (Dexbrompheniramine maleate)
See *Antihistamines*.

DISOPHROL (Dexbrompheniramine maleate plus *d*-Isoephedrine sulfate)
See *Antihistamines*.

Alcohol and other CNS depressants[120]
Possible additive effects.

DISULFIRAM (Antabuse TETD, tetraethythiuram disulfide)

Alcohol[120,121,127,144,1133] **(Even in the form of aftershave lotions, back rubs, cough syrups, fermented foods, sauces, and any other substances that contain alcohol that may be absorbed)**
Disulfiram increases acetaldehyde concentration in the blood by inhibiting acetaldehyde dehydrogenase. The severity of the resulting unpleasant reaction varies with the individual and the amount of alcohol. *Never administer to a patient when he is in a state of alcohol intoxication or without his full knowledge.* The patient should carry an identification card and his physician should be prepared to institute supportive measures to restore blood pressure and to treat shock. Can be lethal.

The so-called "disulfiramlike reaction" may be caused by a large variety of other drugs and other chemicals. A true disulfiram type of reaction with alcohol (acetaldehyde levels elevated) is produced with oral antidiabetics (sulfonylureas except chlorpropamide), cyanamide, impurity in animal charcoal, certain pyrazoline derivatives (irgopyrine), certain imidazoline derivatives (tolazoline), antimalarials (quinacrine), carbon disulfide and thiuram derivatives in the rubber industry, n-butyraldoxine in the printing industry, chloramphenicol, MAO inhibitors including furaltadone [Altafur], furazolidone [Furoxone], nifuroxime [Micofur], procarbazine [Matulane], and tranylcypromine [Parnate], metronidazole [Flagyl], sulfonamides, etc. The reaction with some drugs (carbutamide, chlorpropamide, etc.) does not seem to be a true disulfiram type of reactions since acetalehyde is not elevated.

Anesthetics [120]
Disulfiram increases the risks of anesthesia.

Anticoagulants, oral [10,359,570]
Disulfiram may enhance the anticoagulant effect of oral anticoagulants (enzyme inhibition).

Antidepressants, tricyclic
See *Disulfiram* under *Antidepressants, Tricyclic.*

Antidiabetics, oral
See *Disulfiram* under *Antidiabetics, Oral.*

Ascorbic acid [144]
Ascorbic acid may abolish the toxic effects of disulfiram without lowering blood acetaldehyde levels.

Barbiturates
See *Disulfiram* under *Barbiturates.*

Digitalis [120]
Hypokalemia, induced by the alcohol-disulfiram reaction, may increase digitalis toxicity.

Isoniazid [718,1138]
This combination (disulfiram plus isoniazid) by altering the metabolism of brain catecholamines, causes coordination difficulties and changes in behavior with a variety of neurological symptoms. However, see *Rifampin* under *Isoniazid.*

Mephenytoin [342,343] (Mesantoin)
Same as for *Phenytoin* below.

Metronidazole [791] (Flagyl)
Metronidazole produces a psychotic reaction when administered with disulfiram (visual and auditory hallucinations).

Paraldehyde [120,166,1465]
Disulfiram should not be given to patients who have been recently treated with paraldehyde and vice versa. Since paraldehyde depolymerizes to acetaldehyde and since disulfiram, by inhibiting the enzyme acetaldehyde dehydrogenase, causes acetaldehyde to accumulate, toxic levels of the aldehyde may be produced with paraldehyde plus disulfiram.

Phenytoin [113,294,342,343,359,916] (Dilantin, diphenlhydantoin)
Disulfiram potentiates phenytoin and increases its toxicity. Phenytoin and related compounds given in the presence of disulfiram involves a serious risk of poisoning. It requires about 3 weeks after the withdrawal of disulfiram before the serum concentrations (up to 500% rise) of phenytoin return to normal because of inhibition of enzymatic p-hydroxylation.

Rifampin
See *Rifampin* under *Isoniazid.*

Sedatives and hypnotics [198]
Disulfiram, an enzyme inhibitor, potentiates sedatives and hypnotics.

DIUPRES
See *Antihypertensives, Chlorothiazide, Reserpine,* and *Thiazide Diuretics.*

Cardiac drugs [580] (Digitalis, Quinidine)
Use cautiously; cardiac arrhythmias.

CNS depressants [120] (Alcohol, Barbiturates, Narcotics, etc.)
Orthostatic hypotension may occur and be potentiated by these drugs.

Other antihypertensives [120]
Diupres potentiates the action of other antihypertensive drugs—dosage must be reduced by at least 50%.

DIURETICS
See also *Acetazolamide, Chlorthalidone, Ethacrynic Acid, Furosemide, Mercurial Diuretics, Quinethazone, Spironolactone, Thiazide Diuretics,* and *Triamterene.*

Alcohol [120]
Orthostatic hypotension may be potentiated.

Aminoglycoside antibiotics [120]
Do not give potent diuretics (ethacrynic acid, furosemide, mannitol, meralluride sodium, sodium mercaptomerin, etc.) with amikacin, gentamicin, kanamycin, neomycin, paromomycin, streptomycin, or tobramycin. The toxicity of the antibiotics (neurotoxicity, ototoxicity, nephrotoxicity) is increased. Some of the potent diuretics are ototoxic themselves.

Ammonium chloride
Possible systemic acidosis. See *Ammonium Chloride* under *Spironolactone.*

Anticoagulants, oral [673]
Diuretics may inhibit oral anticoagulants.

Antidepressants, tricyclic [120,194,325,870]
The antihypertensive effect of both the tricyclics and diuretics is additive. The elevated pH of the urine caused by acetazolamide and thiazides, etc. increases tubular reabsorption of the tricyclics and thus potentiates them.

Antidiabetics, oral [74,120,164,191,386,433,619]
Diuretics (chlorthalidone, ethacrynic acid, furosemide, thiazides, triamterene, etc.) antagonize antidiabetics by increasing blood glucose levels and possibly by depressing insulin secretion.

Antihypertensives [120]
Enhanced hypotensive effect possible. Reduced dosage of the hypotensive agent is frequently necessary.

Antipyrine
See *Antipyrine* under *Spironolactone.*

Carbenoxolone
See *Carbenoxolone* under *Spironolactone.*

Chlorides [172]
Chlorides potentiate mercurial diuretics. The acidifying agent, ammonium chloride, is often used to supply chloride ions and combat alkalosis.

Clofibrate (Atromid-S)
See *Clofibrate* under *Furosemide.*

Cholestyramine
See *Cholestyramine* under *Thiazide Diuretics.*

Corticosteroids [120,1853]
Excessive potassium depletion may occur when corticosteroids and a potassium depleting diuretic such as chlorthalidone (Hygroton), ethacrynic acid (Edecrin) or a thiazide diuretic (Aquatag, Amhydron, Diuril, Naturetin, etc.) are given concomitantly. Both the corticosteroids and diuretics can cause hypokalemia, especially in patients with inadequate potassium intake. Correct the hypokalemia and monitor patients closely.

DIURETICS *(continued)*

Digitalis [120,579,580]
Diuretics in general may enhance digitalis toxicity through excessive loss of potassium and cause arrhythmias.

Dopamine
See *Diuretics* under *Dopamine.*

Furosemide [120,152] (Lasix)
Other diuretics with furosemide enhance the hypotensive effects and with some the hypokalemic action.

Insulin [120]
Diuretics may antagonize the hypoglycemic effect of insulin. See *Antidiabetics, Oral* above.

Kanamycin [120,250]
Kanamycin plus potent diuretics such as ethacrynic acid, particular IV, cause rapid and irreversible deafness.

Levarterenol [951] (Levophed, norepinephrine)
Diuretics may decrease arterial responsiveness to levarterenol.

Lithium carbonate [120,619,1499,1701,1851,1970,2061] (Eskalith, Lithane, Lithonate)
Diuretics are usually contraindicated (potentiated toxicity because of decreased electrolytes). Sodium depletion, when produced by diuretics like furosemide or by dietary restriction, depresses lithium excretion and may severely increase its toxicity. Also, thiazide diuretics used over prolonged periods potentiate lithium because of increased reabsorption resulting from increased proximal tubular reabsorption of sodium, a compensatory effect. Increased blood levels of lithium may produce toxic effects (confusion, disorientation, slurred speech). Maintain normal sodium fluid levels, particularly during periods of loss due to sweating, and monitor lithium levels closely. In lithium poisoning, its excretion may be increased by forced osmotic diuresis with IV infusions of mannitol or urea, or by administering large quantities of sodium or potassium. See also *Lithium Carbonate* under *Acetazolanide.* If a diuretic is required to treat hypertension or to control lithium-induced effects (diabetes insipiduslike state) in manic-depressive patients on long-term lithium therapy where there is a strong tendency for elevation of lithium levels as urine volume falls, maintain close laboratory control of these levels as elevation is prompt with diuretic therapy. Lower lithium dose.

MAO inhibitors [74,433,633]
This combination has an additive hypotensive effect. Shock has been produced with furosemide and thiazides when they are given concomitantly with MAO inhibitors.

Methyldopa [117]
Enhanced hypotensive effect; the diuretics also counteract weight gain and edema which may occur with methyldopa therapy.

Muscle relaxants [28,433,1364]
Diuretics such as ethacrynic acid, furosemide and thiazide diuretics which tend to deplete potassium may induce prolonged paralysis of respiratory muscles with muscle relaxants. See *Muscle Relaxants* under *Furosemide.*

Narcotics
Orthostatic hypotension may be potentiated. See *CNS Depressants.*

Norepinephrine
See *Levarterenol* above.

Phenothiazines [166,633]
Thiazide diuretics with phenothiazines have caused shock. See *CNS Depressants.* When attempts have been made to reverse the hypotensive shock with metaraminol, the condition was exacerbated because phenothiazines block part of metaraminol action (peripheral vasoconstriction prevented by α-adrenergic blockade).

Phenytoin
See *Furosemide* under *Phenytoin.*

Potassium chloride
See *Potassium Chloride* under *Spironolactone.*

Reserpine [117]
Enhanced hypotensive effect; reduced dosage of the hypotensive agent is frequently necessary.

Salicylates
See *Salicylates* under *Spironolactone.*

Sodium salts [2039]
Administration of IV and oral sodium rapidly reverses hyponatremia with sodium deficit (lethargy, weakness, slowing of cerebration, anorexia, and nausea, progressing to coma and convulsions) induced in patients by various diuretics (amiloride, bendrofluazide, cyclopenthiazide, furosemide, etc.) but is not to be given in the common dilutional hyponatremia of cardiac failure resulting from depressed free water production.

Spironolactone [120,172] (Aldactone)
Spironolactone is frequently combined with a thiazide or mercurial diurectic to reduce potassium loss caused by the other diuretics and to obtain an additive and more prompt effect. However, hyponatremia may be caused or aggravated by such a combination. Sometimes glucocorticoids are also added as a third component of the regimen to increase the glomerular filtration rate.

Tetracyclines
See *Diuretics* under *Tetracyclines.*

Tranylcypromine [120] (Parnate)
Contraindicated. Enhanced hypotensive effect may be induced by this MAO inhibitor.

Triamterene [120] (Dyrenium)
Triamterene, a potassium-conserving diuretic, is frequently combined with a thiazide diuretic to reduce potassium loss and to enhance the diuretic effect.

Tubocurarine [120,691]
Diuretics may enhance the muscle relaxant effect of tubocurarine.

Uricosuric agents [120]
Some diuretics (Edecrin, xanthines) antagonize uricosurics and decrease the renal excretion of uric acid. Higher doses of uricosuric agents may be required.

Urinary acidifiers [120,325,870]
Urinary acidifiers, *e.g.*, ammonium chloride, increase the diuretic effect of mercurial diuretics.

DIURIL
See *Chlorothiazide* and *Thiazide Diuretics.*

DIUTENSEN-R
See *Antihypertensives, Cryptenamine, Reserpine,* and *Thiazide Diuretics.*

Atropine sulfate
Atropine sulfate reverses the bradycrotic effect of cryptenamine.

DOLONIL
See *Barbiturates, Hyoscyamine,* and *Phenazopyridine.*

DOLOPHINE
See *Methadone HCl.*

DONNAGEL
See *Atropine, Hyoscine, Hyoscyamine.*

DONNATAL
See *Atropine, Hyoscine, Hyoscyamine,* and *Phenobarbital.*

DONNAZYME
See *Atropine, Enzymes* (Proteolytic), *Hyoscine, Hyoscyamine,* and *Phenobarbital.*

DOPA (Dihydroxyphenylalanine)
(Amino acid occurring in beans, pods and seedlings of *Vicia faba* [broad bean] in the L–form)

Chlorpromazine[120] (Thorazine)
Dopa antagonizes the cataleptic effect of chlorpromazine.

Haloperidol[120] (Haldol)
Dopa antagonizes the cataleptic effect of haloperidol.

Isocarboxazid (Marplan)
See *MAO inhibitors* below.

MAO inhibitors[792]
Increased toxicity. Flushing, hyperthermia, tachycardia, hypertensive crisis and associated distress, *e.g.,* headache, myocarditis, cerebral hemorrhage, respiratory arrest, coma. See *Tyramine-rich Foods.*

Nialamide (Niamid)
See *MAO inhibitors* above.

Pargyline (Eutonyl)
See *MAO inhibitors* above.

Phenelzine (Nardil)
See *MAO inhibitors* above.

Tranylcypromine (Parnate)
See *MAO inhibitors* above.

DOPAMINE (Intropin)
See *Sympathomimetics.*

Anesthetics[120]
Cyclopropane and halogenated hydrocarbon anesthetics sensitize the myocardium to catecholamines such as dopamine and enhance the pressor and beta-adrenergic effects, thus producing arrhythmias. Use extreme caution with concomitant usage.

Diuretics[120]
Dopamine exerts an additive or potentiating effect with diuretics. (Dilation of renal vasculature increased glomerular filtration rate, renal blood flow, and sodium excretion).

MAO inhibitors[120,793]
MAO inhibitors potentiate and prolong the stimulatory effects of pressor amines like dopamine and tryamine on blood pressure and on the contractile force of the heart. The potentiation by MAO inhibitors is even more important after oral administration than after intravenous injection. Hypertension.

Morphine[643]
Dopamine antagonizes the analgesic effects of morphine, which depletes catecholamines.

Pargyline
See *MAO inhibitors* above.

DOPRAM
See *Doxapram* HCl.

DORIDEN
See *Glutethimide.*

DOXAPRAM HCL (Dopram)
See also *CNS Stimulants.*

Anesthetics, general[120]
Doxapram may increase the release of epinephrine and thus stimulate respiration and pulse rate in patients with postanesethetic respiratory depression. The anesthetics may make the heart more sensitive to doxapram.

Barbiturates[120]
Barbiturates may be used to manage excessive CNS stimulation caused by doxapram overdosage.

MAO inhibitors[120] or sympathomimetics
MAO inhibitors or sympathomimetics should be administered cautiously since a synergistic pressor effect may occur.

Narcotic analgesics[120]
Doxapram *does not* block respiratory depression of narcotic analgesics (or muscle relaxants).

DOXEPIN (Sinequan)
See *Antidepressants, Tricyclic* and *Doxepin* under *Antihypertensives, Bethanidine,* and *Guanethidine.*

Anticholinesterases[2052]
(Neostigmine, physostigmine, etc.)
Physostigmine (2 mg. IV) is very effective in controlling the symptoms (agitation, disorientation, hallucination, myoclonus, tachycardia) of doxepin overdosage. Neostigmine has also been useful but one patient, with the characteristic recurring symptoms of tricyclic intoxication, well controlled with physostigmine, did not respond when neostigmine was given in error.

Neostigmine
See *Anticholinesterases* under *Antidepressants, Tricyclic.*

Physostigmine
See *Anticholinesterases* under *Antidepressants, Tricyclic.*

DOXYCYCLINE (Vibramycin)
See *Barbiturates, Iron Salts,* and *Complexing Agents* under *Tetracyclines.*

DRAMAMINE
See *Antihistamines* and *Dimenhydrinate.*

Antibiotics[120]
Dramamine may mask signs of ototoxicity caused by some antibiotics; an irreversible state may be reached.

DRINUS
See *Antihistamines, Chlorpheniramine Maleate, Methscopolamine Nitrate* and *Phenylephrine.*

DRIXORAL
See *Antihistamines* (dexbrompheniramine maleate) and *Ephedrine.*

DRIZE M CAPSULES
See *Antihistamines* (chlorpheniramine maleate).

l-DROMORAN (Levo-Dromoran)
See *Levorphanol.*

DROPERIDOL (Inapsine)

MAO inhibitors[352]
MAO inhibitors such as phenelzine potentiate the tranquilizer.

Phenoperidine[951]
Droperidol counteracts the respiratory depression caused by phenoperidine.

DUADACIN
See *Antihistamines* (chlorpheniramine maleate and pyrilamine maleate), *Ascorbic Acid, Caffeine, Acetaminophen, Phenylephrine HCl,* and *Salicylamide.*

DULARIN
See *Acetaminophen.*

DULARIN-TH
See *Acetaminophen* and *Barbiturates* (butabarbital) and *Caffeine.*

DUO-MEDIHALER
See *Isoproterenol HCl* and *Phenylephrine Bitartrate*.

Epinephrine [6,120,370,547]
Epinephrine should not be administered with isoproterenol. Since both drugs are direct cardiac stimulators, their combined effects may produce serious arrhythmias.

DUOSTERONE
See *Estrogens (ethinyl estradiol)* and *Corpus Luteum Hormone (ethisterone)*.

DUOTRATE 45
See *Nitrates* and *Nitrites, Pentaerythritol tetranitrate*.

Acetylcholine, histamine, norepinephrine and many agents [120,170]
Duotrate acts as a physiological antagonist to these smooth muscle stimulants.

DUOVENT
See *Ephedrine, Glyceryl Guaiacolate, Phenobarbital* and *Theophylline*.

DUPHASTON
See *Progestogens (dydrogesterone)*.

DURABOLIN
See *Anabolic Agents (nandrolone phenpropionate)*.

DURACILLIN
See *Penicillin*.

DURAGESIC
See *Magnesium* and *Salicylates (aspirin, salicylsalicylic acid)*.

DYAZIDE
See *Thiazide Diuretics (hydrochlorothiazide)* and *Triamterene*.

DYCLONE
See *Dyclonine HCl*.

DYCLONINE HCL

Pyelographic contrast agents
Dyclonine HCl causes precipitation of iodine in pyelographic contrast agents. See Chapter 8.

DYMELOR
See *Acetohexamide, Antidiabetics,* and *Sulfonylureas*.

DYNAPEN
See *Penicillin (sodium dicloxacillin)*.

DYRENIUM
See *Diuretics* and *Triamterene*.

ECHOTHIOPHATE IODIDE (Phospholine iodide)

Anticholinesterases
See *Cholinesterase Inhibitors* below.

Atropine [120]
Atropine is an effective antidote for echothiophate iodide.

Cholinesterase inhibitors [120]
Echothiophate, a cholinesterase inhibitor, used as a miotic potentiates other such inhibitors (malathion, parathion, Sevin, TEPP and other organophosporus insecticides) as well as anticholinesterases such as edrophonium chloride (Tensilon) and methacholine chloride (Mecholyl) used in myasthenia gravis, and related agents used for other purposes (additive effects or possibly synergistic). Those exposed to organophosphate and carbamate insecticides must take strict precautions.

Pilocarpine [120]
Prior pilocarpine administration may prevent the formation of lens opacities with echothiophate therapy.

Pralidoxime
See *Anticholinesterases* under *Pralidoxime*.

Procaine [1926] (Novocain, etc.)
Procaine injections may cause severe reactions (unconsciousness, cardiovascular collapse, anaphylactic shock) when given to a patient who has been receiving echothiophate, a cholinesterase inhibitor. The latter reduces the activity of pseuducholinesterase which metabolizes procaine and greatly enhances the toxicity of the local anesthetic.

Succinylcholine [120,979,1031,1297,1538,1585,1646] (Anective, Quelicin)
Echothiophate iodide, like other cholinesterase inhibitors, potentiates succinylcholine, which should not be used prior to general anesthesia in patients receiving such inhibitors. Prolonged paralysis of respiratory muscles and a protracted apnea may occur. The anticholinesterase echothiophate can depress the activity of serum cholinesterase to dangerously low levels on prolonged use and thus depress the metabolism of succinylcholine.

ECOTRIN
See *Aspirin* and *Salicylates*.

EDECRIN
See *Ethacrynic Acid*.

EDROPHONIUM (Tensilon Chloride)
See *Anticholinesterases*.

Antibiotics [421]
Edrophonium may antagonize the neuromuscular blocking effect of certain antibiotics (dihydrostreptomycin, kanamycin, neomycin, and stretomycin).

Anticholinesterases [120]
Edrophonium (a cholinergic) must be used with caution in patients receiving other anticholinesterases since cholinergic crisis (overdosage) may mimic underdosage (myasthenic weakness) and administration of the drug may exacerbate their condition.

Curare [120]
Edrophonium reverses the neuromuscular blocking action of curare.

Dihydrostreptomycin
See *Antibiotics* above.

Gallamine triethiodide [120] (Flaxedil)
Edrophonium antagonizes the neuromuscular blocking action of gallamine triethiodide (competitive antagonist).

Colistimethate [421]
Colistimethate potentiates anticholinesterases like edrophonium and neostigmine.

Kanamycin
See *Antibiotics* above.

Neomycin
See *Antibiotics* above.

Streptomycin
See *Antibiotics* above.

Succinylcholine chloride [168] (Anectine)
Edrophonium may prolong the muscle relaxant effect of succinylcholine.

Tubocurarine or dimethyl tubocurarine [168]
Edrophonium antagonizes the neuromuscular blocking action of tubocurarine (competitive antagonist).

EDTA
(Ethylenediaminetetraacetic acid as calcium disodium edathamil, calcium disodium edetate, Calcium Disodium Versenate, etc.)

Antibiotics[360]
EDTA increases the gastrointestinal absorption rate of certain antibiotics and thus potentiates the neuromuscular blockade produced by kanamycin, neomycin, streptomycins, etc. This may produce apnea and muscular weakness.

Decamethonium[161] **(Syncurine)**
EDTA increases the gastrointestinal absorption rate of decamethonium (potentiation).

EDTA[161]
EDTA increases its own gastrointestinal absorption rate. This chelating agent probably enhances the gastrointestinal absorption of some substances by altering the permeability of the intestinal epithelium.

Heparin[161,870]
EDTA increases the gastrointestinal absorption rate of heparin (potentiation).

Inulin[161]
EDTA increases the gastrointestinal absorption rate of inulin.

Kanamycin[360]
See *Antibiotics* above.

Mannitol[161]
EDTA increases the absorption rate of mannitol.

Nalidixic acid[360,421] **(NegGram)**
EDTA increases the grastrointestinal absorption rate and thereby potentiates nalidixic acid against *Ps. aeruginosa*.

Neomycin[360]
See *Antibiotics* above. EDTA potentiates the antibacterial action of neomycin against *Ps. aeruginosa*.

Streptomycin[360]
See *Antibiotics* above.

Sulfonic acids[161,360]
EDTA increases the gastrointestinal absorption rate of sulfonic acids.

EGGS

Iron salts[359]
Egg protein inhibits the absorption of iron.

EKKO
See *Phenytoin*.

ELAVIL
See *Amitriptyline HCl* and *Antidepressants, Tricyclic*.

ELECTROCONVULSIVE THERAPY (ECT)

Reserpine[794,795]
Apnea, respiratory depression, paralysis and death may be caused by combined reserpine-electroshock therapy.

ELIXOPHYLLIN
See *Theophylline*.

ELIXOPHYLLIN-KI
See *Potassium Iodide* and *Theophylline*.

Other theophylline preparations
Do not use Elixophyllin-KI with other theophylline preparations (additive effect).

EMFASEEM
See *Dyphylline* and *Glyceryl Guaiacolate*.

EMPIRIN COMPOUND WITH OR WITHOUT CODEINE
See *Aspirin, Caffeine, Codeine,* and *Phenacetin*.

EMPRAZIL WITH OR WITHOUT CODEINE
See *Aspirin, Caffeine, Codeine, Ephedrine* and *Phenacetin*.

E-MYCIN
See *Antibiotics* (erythromycin).

ENARAX
See *Hydroxyzine, Oxyphencyclamine,* and *Tranquilizers*.

ENDOXAN
See *Cyclophosphamide*.

ENDURON
See *Thiazide Diuretics* (methyclothiazide).

ENDURONYL
See *Deserpidine* and *Methyclothiazide*.

ENOVID
See *Estrogens, Progestogens* (norethynodrel and mestranol).

ENURETROL
See *Atropine* and *Ephedrine*.

ENZYMES, PROTEOLYTIC
See *Papain*.

ENZYME INDUCERS
See *Table 10-4*.
Many enzyme inducers, including barbiturates, phenytoin, glutethimide, meprobamate, phenylbutazone, probenecid, and tolbutamide can accelerate their own metabolism. Thus tolerance may develop.[96,257,311,703]

Oral contraceptives[78]
Concern is being created by the possible ineffectiveness of oral contraceptives in women receiving barbiturates, sedatives, tranquilizers, and other drugs that induce enzymes.

ENZYME INHIBITORS
See Table 10-5.

EPHEDRINE

Bethanidine
See *Ephedrine* under *Bethanidine*.

Digitalis[170,619]
Digitalis glycosides combined with adrenergic drugs such as ephedrine and epinephrine predisposes the patient to cardiac arrhythmias.

Epinephrine[552] **(Adrenalin)**
Enhanced (additive) sympathomimetic effects with the phenylisopropanolamine (ephedrine) and the catecholamine (epinephrine) may occur.

Ergonovine[120,609] **(Ergotrate)**
A vasoconstrictor with ergonovine may induce postpartum hypertension; sometimes extremely hazardous.

Furazolidone[120] **(Furoxone)**
Contraindicated. The pressor effects of the monoamine sympathomimetic are potentiated by the MAO inhibitor furazolidone. Possible hypertensive crisis.

Guanethidine[797]
Ephedrine inhibits the hypotensive effects of guanethidine. Guanethidine suppresses the α and β adrenergic responses to ephedrine.

Halothane[796] **(Fluothane)**
Ephedrine with halothane produces cardiac arrhythmias.

EPHEDRINE *(continued)*

Isocarboxazid (Marplan)
See *MAO Inhibitors* below.

Kaolin [1589]
See *Pseudoephedrine* under *Kaolin.*

MAO inhibitors [136,211]
(See *MAO Inhibitors* for generic and brand names.)
Acute hypertensive crisis with possible intracranial hemorrhage, hyperthermia, convulsions, coma and in some cases death. MAO may be irreversibly inhibited and metabolism of monoamines blocked, thus causing their accumulation. This prolongs and potentiates action of tyramine, dopamine, and related pressor amines which release norepinephrine from peripheral stores. This release and the central additive stimulation cause the hypertensive crisis.

Methyldopa
See *Ephedrine* under *Methyldopa.*

Nialamide [211] (Niamid)
See *MAO Inhibitors* above. Has caused subarachnoid hemorrhage.

Oxytocin [120]
Ephedrine plus oxytocin may cause postpartum hypertension.

Pargyline (Eutonyl)
See *MAO Inhibitors* above.

Phenelzine (Nardil)
See *MAO Inhibitors* above.

Procaine (Novocain)
Ephedrine IM or IV counteracts the vasodilator effects of procaine.

Reserpine [636]
Reserpine inhibits the vasopressor action of ephedrine.

Theophylline [1892]
Ephedrine may increase the side effects of theophylline (gastrointestinal upset, insomnia, irritability and other CNS stimulant effects) without enhancing its efficacy. Probably best to avoid this combination.

Tranylcypromine (Parnate)
See *MAO Inhibitors* above.

Trifluoperazine [120] (Stelazine)
Collapse and death may occur with this combination.

EPHOXAMINE
See *Antihistamines* (phenyltoloxamine) and *Ephedrine.*

E-PILO
See *Epinephrine* and *Pilocarpine.*

EPINEPHRINE

α-Adrenergic blocking agents [120]
Epinephrine should not be used to treat overdosage since a further drop in blood pressure may occur (epinephrine reversal).

Alcohol [166]
Alcohol causes increase in urinary excretion of epinephrine.

Anesthetics, general [684]
Cardiac arrhythmias may occur with epinephrine plus certain halogenated and other anesthetics.

Antazoline
See *Antihistamines* below.

Antidepressants, tricyclic [404,424]
Enhanced adrenergic effect. See *Epinephrine* under *Antidepressants, Tricyclic.*

Antidiabetics [168]
Epinephrine may antagonize the action of oral hypoglycemic agents.

Antihistamines [232,235,483]
Antihistamines with epinephrine may produce an enhanced cardiovascular (pressor) effect. The antihistamine inhibits uptake of norepinephrine and causes increased concentration of unbound drug for interaction with receptors.

Azapetine [619] (Ilidar)
The α-adrenergic blocking agent tends to reverse the pressor effects of epinephrine and prevent cardiac arrhythmias induced by the catecholamine.

Chloroform [684,761-763]
Chloroform sensitizes the myocardium to the action of epinephrine; increased likelihood of ventricular tachycardia or fibrillation when used in combination. Death may occur. Chloroform, a carcinogen, is being avoided. See under *Chloroform.*

Chlorpheniramine (Chlor-Trimeton) and dexchlorpheniramine (Polaramine) maleates
See *Antihistamines* above.

Chlorpromazine [120,166] (Thorazine)
Epinephrine (and other adrenergics except levarterenol and phenylephrine) should never be used to treat reactions from intravenous doses of chlorpromazine as the adrenolytic action of the chlorpromazine may cause epinephrine reversal and further paradoxical lowering of blood pressure.

Chlorprothixene (Taractan)
Same effect as *Chlorpromazine* above.

Cocaine [633]
Cocaine produces sensitization to epinephrine.

Cyclopropane [683,684,763,772-777]
Epinephrine enhances the ventricular irritability and may increase the cardiac arrhythmias produced by cyclopropane. Death may occur. *

Detrothyroxine [120] (Choloxin) sodium
See *Thyroid Preparations* below.

Digitalis [170,619]
Digitalis glycosides, combined with adrenergic drugs such as ephedrine and epinephrine, predispose the patient to cardiac arrhythmias.

Diphenhydramine (Benadryl)
See *Antihistamines* above.

Ephedrine [552]
Enhanced pressor, myocardial stimulant, and other sympathomimetic effects.

Ethyl chloride [684]
Same as for *Cyclopropane* above and *Halothane* below.

Fluroxene [683,806] (Fluoromar)
The halogenated anesthetic (trifluoroethyl vinyl ether) produces cardiac arrhythmias with epinephrine. May be fatal.

Haloperidol [421,619] (Haldol)
Epinephrine should not be used as an intravenous vasopressor to correct hypotension caused by haloperidol since the latter may block its vasoconstrictor effect and an increased fall in blood pressure may occur (epinephrine reversal).

Halothane [120,683,796,799-804] (Fluothane)
Halothane sensitizes the myocardium to the action of epinephrine; the likelihood of ventricular tachycardia or fibrillation increases when used in combination. May be fatal.

Histamine [169]
Epinephrine IM, or in severe poisoning IV, is the antidote of choice in histamine overdosage with bronchoconstriction in asthmatics (aminophylline and isoproterenol are also used).

Hydralazine [421] **(Apresoline)**
Hydralazine may reduce the pressor responses to epinephrine.

Insulin [549,805]
Insulin may antagonize the cardiac and hyperglycemic actions of epinephrine. Epinephrine may inhibit the hypoglycemic effect of insulin.

Iproniazid
See *MAO Inhibitors* below.

Isoprenaline (Isoproterenol)
See *Isoproterenal* below.

Isoproterenol [6,120,185,313,370,547,693] **(Isuprel) HCl**
Epinephrine and isoproterenol should not be used simultaneously since both are direct cardiac stimulants and combined use may produce arrhythmias and death; $\frac{1}{15}$ of the safe dose of isoproterenol for healthy heart-lung preparations has killed the failing heart. These drugs should be administered alternately.

Levothyroxine sodium [539,590] **(Synthroid)**
See *Thyroid Preparations* below.

MAO Inhibitors [136,312]
See *Epinephrine* under *MAO Inhibitors*.

Mephenterime [120,619] **(Wyamine)**
Contraindicated combination. Mephentermine potentiates and prolongs the vasopressor effects of epinephrine.

Methotrimeprazine [120] **(Levoprome)**
Epinephrine should not be used to alleviate severe hypotensive effects that may develop with methotrimeprazine because of a paradoxical reversal of the pressor effects of epinephrine by phenothiazines.

Methoxyflurane [806,807] **(Penthrane)**
This halogenated anesthetic causes cardiac arrhythmias and possibly death with epinephrine.

Miotics [548]
Epinephrine antagonizes the beneficial effects of miotics in glaucoma. Glaucoma (acute closed angle) has been precipitated by epinephrine plus a miotic.

Nitrites [170]
Hypotensive nitrates and nitrites can counteract the marked pressor effects of large doses of epinephrine.

Phenothiazines [120,619]
(Sparine, Taractan, Thorazine, etc.)
Epinephrine should not be used to treat hypotension caused by a phenothiazine or thioxanthene since agents have been found to reverse its action, resulting in a further lowering of blood pressure.

Phenoxybenzamine [120] **(Dibenzyline)**
Epinephrine is contraindicated as a treatment for shock induced by phenoxybenzamine α-adrenergic blockade of the sympathetic nervous sytem and of circulating epinephrine. Because epinephrine stimulates both α and β adrenergic receptors, the net effect is vasodilation and a further drop in blood pressure (epinephrine reversal).

Phentolamine [619] **(Regitine)**
Phentolamine inhibits adrenergic sensitization of the myocardium to anesthetics.

Phenylephrine [120] **(Neo-Synephrine) HCl**
Epinephrine, administered with phenylephrine or other sympathomimetic amines, may produce lethal pressor effects.

Prenylamine [170] **(Segontin)**
This vasodilator augments the response to epinephrine and norepinephrine.

Promazine (Sparine)
See *Phenothiazines* above.

Propiomazine [120]
The pressor response to epinephrine is usually reduced and may even be reversed in the presence of propiomazine.

Propanolol
See *Epinephrine* under *Propranolol*.

Sympathomimetics [6,120,185,313,370,547]
It is dangerous to use excessive amounts of any sympathomimetic amine for asthma and giving epinephrine for status asthmaticus to patients who have been using excessive amounts of such drugs can be lethal.

Thioxanthenes [120,619] **(Taractan)**
Epinephrine should not be used to treat hypotension caused by phenothiazine or thioxanthene since these agents have been found to reverse its action, resulting in a further lowering of blood pressure.

Thyroid preparations [120,590]
(Choloxin, Synthroid, etc.)
Injection of epinephrine in patients with coronary artery disease may precipitate an episode of coronary insufficiency. This may be enhanced in patients receiving thyroid preparations. Careful observation is required if catecholamines are administered to patients in this category.

Trichloroethylene [683,684]
Same as for *Cyclopropane* and *Halothane* above.

Tripelennamine [232,235,242,483] **(Pyribenzamine)**
See *Antihistamines* above.

EPITRATE
See *Epinephrine*.

EPPY
See *Epinephrine*.

EQUAGESIC
See *Analgesics* (ethoheptazine), *Aspirin* and *Meprobamate*.

EQUANIL
See *Meprobamate*.

EQUANITRATE
See *Meprobamate*, *Nitrates and Nitrites*, and *Pentaerythritol Tentranitrate*.

EQUILET
See *Alkalinizing Agents* and *Antacids* (calcium carbonate, magnesium trisillicate).

ERGOMETRINE
See *Oxytocics* (ergonovine).

ERGONOVINE MALEATE (Ergotrate)

Ephedrine [120,609]
Postpartum hypertension. Same as for *Methoxamine* below.

Methoxamine [120,609] **(Vasoxyl)**
Postpartum hypertension and severe headaches are induced by use of a vasoconstrictor with an oxytocic.

Vasopressors [120,609]
Excessively high blood pressure may result. Same as for *Methoxamine* above.

ERGOT ALKALOIDS
(Ergotamine [Cafergot, Gynergen, Medihaler-Ergotamine], ergonovine [Ergotrate], etc.)
See also *Oxytocics*.

ERGOT ALKALOIDS *(continued)*

Propranolol [1166-8]
This combination may cause severe, painful peripheral vasoconstriction and increase the severity and frequency of migraine headaches. See *Ergot alkaloids* under *Propranolol.*

Sympathomimetics [173,609,611]
Sympathomimetics (pressor agents) with ergot alkaloids may cause extreme elevation of blood pressure. This will subside promptly with chlorpromazine IV.

ERGOTAMINE TARTRATE (Cafergot, Gynergen)

Triacetyloleandomycin [359,682] (TAO, troleandomycin)
The antibiotic triacetyloleandomycin may inhibit the metabolism of ergotamine and thus potentiate the antimigraine drug (acute ergotism).

ERGOTRATE
See *Oxytocics* (ergonovine).

ERYTHROCIN
See *Erythromycin.*

ERYTHROMYCIN (Erythrocin, Ilotycin)

Acetazolamide (Diamox)
See *Alkalinizers, Urinary* below.

Acid beverages [421,619] (Fruit juices, etc.)
Since the activity of erythromycin is decreased as the pH is lowered due to hydrolysis, acidifying drinks should not be taken concomitantly.

Alkalinizers, urinary [120,1763,1924]
Antibacterial activity of erythromycin is enhanced as the urinary pH is made more alkaline. Thus both acetazolamide and sodium bicarbonate enhance the urinary antibacterial activity of erythromycin against *Escherichia coli, Proteus mirabilis, Pseudomonas aeruginosa,* etc. In one study, elevation of urinary pH to 8.5 with sodium bicarbonate enabled erythromycin estolate to reduce urinary organisms 99.99% or more in 92% of a series of patients.

Ampicillin (Alpen, Polycillin, etc.)
See *Penicillins* below.

Cephalothin (Keflin) sodium
Erythromycin and cephalothin are incompatible in parenteral mixtures. See Chapter 7.

Chloramphenicol [811] (Chloromycetin)
This combination is effective against some strains of resistant *Staph. aureus.*

Clindamycin
See *Erythromycin* under *Clindamycin,* and *Lincomycin* below.

Cloxacillin (Tegopen)
See *Penicillins* below.

Dicloxacillin (Veracillin)
See *Penicillins* below.

Lincomycin [46,808,809,1343] (Lincocin)
Erythromycin and lincomycin are antagonistic regarding antibacterial activity. Avoid concomitant use.

Methicillin
See *Penicillins* below.

Oxacillin
See *Penicillins* below.

Penicillins [31,70,238,301,419,811,1437,1520,1627] (Ampicillin, cloxacillin, dicloxacillin, methicillin, oxacillin, etc.)
Erythromycin, which is bacteriostatic in normal doses, tends to inhibit the bactericidal activity of penicillins but it potentiates their activity against resistant strains of *Staph aureus.* High bactericidal doses of erythromycin, started a few hours after penicillin has been started, may act synergistically against certain organisms such as streptococci.

Probenecid [120] (Benemid)
Probenecid inhibits tubular reabsorption of erythromycin in animals and thereby potentiates the antibiotic.

Streptomycin [178]
This combination is effective against the enterococcus in bacteremia, brain abscess, endocarditis, meningitis, and urinary tract infections.

Tetracyclines
Erythromycin and tetracyclines are incompatible in parenteral mixtures. See Chapter 7.

ESGIC
See *Acetaminophen, Barbiturates* (butalbital) and *Caffeine.*

ESIDRIX
See *Thiazide Diuretics* (hydrochlorothiazide).

ESIMIL
See *Guanethidine* and *Thiazide Diuretics* (hydrochlorothiazide).

ESKABARB
See *Barbiturates* (phenobarbital).

ESKATROL
See *Amphetamines* (dextroamphetamine) and *Phenothiazines* (prochlorperazine).

Alcohol [120]
See *Amphetamines* and *Phenothiazines,* both under *Alcohol.*

CNS depressants [120]
Possible potentiation of effects of CNS depressants. See *CNS Depressants* and *Phenothiazines* under *Amphetamines.*

Epinephrine [120,619,950]
If hypotension should occur, epinephrine should not be used, since there may be a reversal of its usual hypertensive effect. See *Antihistamines* under *Epinephrine.*

MAO inhibitors [120]
Do not use Eskatrol in patients taking MAO inhibitors because of the content of amphetamine which is potentiated by inhibition of metabolizing enzymes. See *Sympathomimetics.*

Organic phosphate insecticides [120]
Possible potentiation of toxicity of organic phosphate insecticides through metabolizing enzyme inhibition.

ESTINYL
See *Estrogens.*

ESTRADIOL

Chlorcyclizine [198] (Perazil)
Chlorcyclizine, through enzyme induction, increases hydroxylation of the hormone, and thereby inhibits its action.

Chlorpromazine [92,951] (Thorazine)
Chlorpromazine may inhibit estradiol through enzyme induction. Estradiol potentiates chlorpromazine by enzyme inhibition.

Phenobarbital [287,330,812]
Phenobarbital inhibits estradiol through enzyme induction.

Phenylbutazone [950]
Phenylbutazone inhibits estradiol through enzyme induction.

ESTRADURIN
See *Estrogens* (polyestradiol).

ESTRATAB
See *Estrogens, Conjugated.*

ESTRATEST
See *Androgens* and *Estrogens.*

ESTROGEN-PROGESTOGENS
(Oral contraceptives)
See *Oral Contraceptives.*

ESTROGENS

Anticoagulants, Oral
See *Estrogens* under *Anticoagulants, Oral.*

Antidiabetics, oral [421]
Estrogens potentiate oral antidiabetics.

Antipyrine
See *Antipyrine* and reaction due to estrogen under *Oral Contraceptives.*

Blood cholesterol lowering agents [421]
Estrogens inhibit antihypercholesterolemics by inducing hyperlipemia.

Corticosteroids
See *Estrogens* under *Corticosteroids.*

Folic acid antagonists [421]
Estrogens potentiate folic acid antagonists.

Insulin [120]
Estrogen can cause an increase in blood glucose levels (decreased glucose tolerance).

Oxytocin [173] (Pitocin)
In presence of estrogen, oxytocin augments electrical and contractile activity of uterine smooth muscle; when estrogen levels are low, effect of oxytocin is much reduced.

Meprobamate [78]
Meprobamate, by enzyme induction, may inhibit the action of estrogens during menopausal therapy.

Parenteral medications
Estrogenic hormones reduce the rate of spreading of injected drugs and thus are inhibitory (Ref. 113, Chap. 8).

Phenobarbital [78,287]
Phenobarbital induces the metabolism of steroids and thus decreases the uterotropic effects of both exogenous and endogenous estrogens.

Rifampin
See *Corticosteroids* and *Estrogens* under *Rifampin.*

ETHACRYNIC ACID (Edecrin)

Acidifying agents [325,870]
Acidifying agents decrease the urinary excretion of the weak acid, ethacrynic acid, and thereby potentiate it.

Alcohol [120]
Ethacrynic acid may elevate blood levels of alcohol and may possibly augment the effects of alcohol ingestion.

Allopurinol [120,421] (Zyloprim)
Ethacrynic acid may antagonize the uricosuric action of allopurinol.

Aminoglycoside Antibiotics [653,813,1604,1618,1705,1717,1774]

(Gentamicin, Kanamycin, Neomycin, Paromomycin, Streptomycin, Tobramcyin, etc.)
The ototoxic side effects of both ethacrynic acid and these antibiotics are additive and may cause permanent deafness, especially in renal impairment. Potentiated ototoxicity may be prolonged after discontinuation of the antibiotic. Extreme caution is essential.

Anticoagulants, oral [784]
See *Diuretics* under *Anticoagulants, Oral.*

Antidiabetics, oral [421]
Ethacrynic acid potentiates oral antidiabetics by displacing them from protein binding sites.

Antihypertensives [120,421] (Hypotensives)
Ethacrynic acid potentiates other antihypertensives. The combination may cause orthostatic hypotension. Ethacrynic acid and antihypertensives coadministered may require adjustment.

Corticosteroids
See *Corticosteroids* under *Diuretics.*

Digitalis [120,421]
Ethacrynic acid may precipitate cardiac arrhythmias if it induces hypokalemia in digitalized patients.

Furosemide (Lasix)
See *Ethacrynic Acid* under *Furosemide.*

Gallamine [330]
See *Muscle Relaxants* below.

Gentamicin
See *Aminoglycoside Antibiotics* above.

Hydralazine [421] (Apresoline)
See *Antihypertensives* above.

Hypotensive agents
See *Antihypertensives* above.

Kanamycin
See *Aminoglycoside Antibiotics* above.

Mecamylamine [421] (Inversine)
See *Antihypertensives* above.

Mercurial diuretics [120]
This combination enhances diuresis (additive effect).

Muscle relaxants, competitive [330]
Ethacrynic acid potentiates the competitive type of peripherally acting muscle relaxants.

Neomycin
See *Aminoglycoside Antibiotics* above.

Ototoxic drugs [120,653,813]
Ethacrynic acid administered to patients also receiving ototoxic drugs has caused permanent deafness. See *Aminoglycoside Antibiotics* above.

Paromomycin
See *Aminoglycoside Antibiotics* above.

Pentolinium [421] (Ansolysen)
See *Antihypertensives* above.

Probenecid [421] (Benemid)
Probenecid tends to antagonize the diuretic action of ethacrynic acid. Ethacrynic acid inhibits the uricosuric action of probenecid.

Streptomycin [653]
See *Aminoglycoside Antibiotics* above.

Tobramycin
See *Aminoglycoside Antibiotics* above.

Tubocurarine [330]
See *Muscle Relaxants* above.

Uricosuric agents [421]
Ethacrynic acid antagonizes uricosuric agents.

Veratrum alkaloids [421]
See *Antihypertensives* above.

ETHAMBUTOL (Myambutol)

Uricosurics
See *Hyperuricemics* under *Antigout Agents*.

ETHAMIVAN (Emivan)

An analeptic no longer readily available in the U.S.

Anticonvulsants [120]
The metabolism of anticonvulsants and depressant drugs, *e.g.*, barbiturates, is not affected by ethamivan. Therefore, the CNS depressant (barbiturate) must be removed by detoxification or hemodialysis during use of this antidote.

Curariform drugs [120]
Ethamivan has no effect on respiratory paralysis produced by blockade of the myoneural junction in curariform drug overdosage.

MAO inhibitors [120,421]
MAO inhibitors potentiate the respiratory stimulant action of ethamivan (additive stimulant action and possibly enzyme inhibition). Convulsions possible.

ETHANOL

See *Alcohol*.

ETHAVERINE

See *Papaverine*.

ETHCHLORVYNOL (Placidyl)

Alcohol
See *CNS Depressants* below.

Amitriptyline (Elavil)
See *Antidepressants, Tricyclic* below.

Anticoagulants, oral [9,421,814]
Ethchlorvynol has been reported to decrease the anticoagulant response, probably by enzyme induction. If it is withdrawn, decrease the anticoagulant dosage.

Antidepressants, tricyclic [120]
Transient delirium has been reported with the combination of amitriptyline and ethchlorvynol.

Barbiturates [120]
See *CNS Depressants* below. Patients who respond unpredictably to barbiturates (excitement, release of inhibitions, etc.) may react the same way to ethchlorvynol.

CNS depressants [120]
Ethchlorvynol exaggerates the effects (blurred vision, hypnosis, paralysis of accomodation) produced by CNS depressant drugs.

MAO inhibitors [120]
Enhanced sedative effect with ethchlorvynol; dosage of ethchlorvynol should be reduced.

Warfarin
See *Anticoagulants, Oral* above.

ETHER

See *Anesthetics, General*.

Muscle relaxants, peripheral action, depolarizing type [878] **(Decamethonium, succinylcholine)**
Diminished relaxant activity with ether.

Muscle relaxants, competitive type [878] **(Curare, gallamine, *d*-tubocurarine)**
Enhanced (synergistic) relaxant activity with ether. Dose of relaxant must be reduced.

Neomycin [358,815-817]
Neomycin and ether given simultaneously may cause apnea, respiratory depression and possibly arrest, and paralysis (neuromuscular block).

Norepinephrine [543] **(Levarterenol)**
Ether increases the plasma level of norepinephrine and of sympathetic activity.

Propranolol [4c,198,698,818] **(Inderal)**
It is risky to use propranolol to treat arrhythmias associated with the use of anesthetics since most of them produce myocardial depression. Hazardous potentiation of depression may occur.

Tubocurarine [878]
Ether enhances the effect of tubocurarine; dosage should be reduced.

X-ray contrast agents [951] **for bronchography**
Decerebration-type syndromes occur in children when anesthetized with ether in presence of these agents.

ETHIONAMIDE (Trecator, Trescatyl)

Alcohol [202,511]
Ethionamide may potentiate psychotoxic effects of alcohol. Avoid alcohol during therapy with the tuberculostatic drug.

Antihypertensives [178]
Since ethionamide has ganglionic blocking action, it may potentiate the postural hypotension produced by other drugs such as antihypertensives, narcotics like meperidine, etc.

Antituberculosis drugs [120]
Ethionamide may intensify the adverse effects (convulsions, etc.) of other antituberculosis drugs given concomitantly.

Cycloserine [619] **(Seromycin)**
Ethionamide may potentiate the toxic CNS effects of cycloserine.

ETHIONINE

o,p'-DDD [271]
Ethionine inhibits o,p'-DDD stimulation of pentobarbital metabolism.

ETHOSUXIMIDE (Zarontin)

***dl*-Amphetamine** [359]
dl-Amphetamine inhibits intestinal absorption of ethosuximide; decreases the anticonvulsant activity.

Anticonvulsants [120]
Ethosuximide combined with other anticonvulsants produced an overwhelmingly increased libido.

ETHOTOIN (Peganone)

See also *Phenytoin*.

Phenacemide [120] **(Phenurone)**
Caution is advised since paranoid symptoms have been reported during therapy with this combination.

Disulfiram [342] **(Antabuse)**
Disulfiram, by enzyme inhibition, potentiates ethotoin. Effect is prolonged for about 3 weeks after withdrawal of disulfiram.

Ethoxzolamide (Cardrase, Ethamide)
See *Carbonic Anhydrase Inhibitors*.

ETHYL ALCOHOL

See *Alcohol*.

ETHYL BISCOUMACETATE (Tromexan)

Discontinued coumarin anticoagulant
See *Anticoagulants, Oral*.

ETHYL CHLORIDE

Epinephrine [684]
Ethyl chloride may sensitize the myocardium to the action of epinephrine. The combination increases the likelihood of arrhythmias and may be fatal.

ETHYLESTRENOL (Maxibolin)

Anticoagulants, oral [819]
See *Anabolic Steroids* under *Anticoagulants, Oral.*

ETRAFON
See *Antidepressant, Tricyclic* (amitriptyline) and *Phenothiazines* (perphenazine).

Alcohol, antihistamines, barbiturates, narcotics, and other CNS depressants [120]
These drugs enhance CNS depression with Etrafon; therefore, Etrafon is contraindicated with these drugs.

Anticonvulsants [120]
Increased dosage of concomitantly used anticonvulsants may be required.

Epinephrine [120]
If hypotension develops with Etrafon, do not use epinephrine because its action is blocked by the phenothiazine and partly reversed.

Other drugs [120]
The antiemetic effect of Etrafon can obscure signs of toxicity dur to overdosage with other drugs. The phenothiazine also potentiates the effects of phosphorus insecticides.

EUCALYPTOL

Aminopyrine [82,951]
Eucalyptol given by general route or by aerosol decreases aminopyrine plasma levels in man.

EUTHROID
See *Thyroid* (sodium levothyroxine and sodium liothyronine).

EUTONYL
See *Antihypertensives* (pargyline) and *MAO Inhibitors.*

EUTRON
See *Antihypertensives* (pargyline), *MAO Inhibitors,* and *Thiazide Diuretics.*

EVEX
See *Estrogens, Conjugated.*

EVIPAL
See *Hexobarbital.*

EXCEDRIN
See *Acetaminophen, Caffeine, Salicylamide* and *Salicylates* (aspirin).

EXCIPIENTS

Phenytoin
See *Excipients* under *Phenytoin.*

EXNA
See *Thiazide Diuretics* (benzthiazide).

EXNA-R
See *Reserpine* and *Thiazide Diuretics* (benzthiazide).

EXOGENOUS AMINES

Furazolidone [120,356,633] (Furoxone)
Furazolidone has MAO inhibitor effects; it may induce susceptibility to hypertensive attacks caused by exogenous amines such as tyramine in cheese and wine; the problem is more likely to arise when furazolidone is used in prolonged treatment.

EXTENDRYL
See *Antihistamines* (chlorpheniramine), *Methscopolamine,* and *Phenylephrine.*

FATTY ACIDS

Anticoagulants, oral [421]
Fatty acids increase the anticoagulant effect by drug displacement from protein binding sites.

FEDAHIST
See *Antihistamines* (chlorpheniramine) and *Ephedrine.*

FELSOL
See *Antipyrine.*

FELSULES
See *Hypnotics* (chloral hydrate).

FEMOGEN
See *Estrogens, Conjugated.*

FENFLURAMINE (Pondimin)
See *Sympathomimetics* [927]
A MAO inhibitor (phenelzine) has produced a severe hypertensive reaction with this anorexigenic.

Antidiabetics, Oral
See *Fenfluramine* under *Antidiabetics, Oral.*

FENOPROFEN (Nalfon)

Salicylates
See *Fenoprofen* under *Salicylates.*

FENTANYL (Sublimaze)
See *Narcotic Analgesics.*

CNS depressants [120]
Fentanyl may potentiate other CNS depressants such as alcohol, anesthetics, antihistamines, narcotics, sedatives, and tranquilizers. Severe respiratory depression may occur.

Dextromethorphan [120] (Methorate, Romilar)
Muscular rigidity may be increased, and apnea, bronchospasm and laryngospasm induced. This rigidity may be reversed by succinylcholine (Anectine) in patients without inherited sensitivity to the drug.

MAO inhibitors
This combination is contraindicated. See *CNS Depressants* under *MAO Inhibitors.*

Nalorphine (Nalline) [120] and levallorphan (Lorfan)
These drugs antagonize the respiratory depression produced by fentanyl and also its analgesic effect.

FEOSOL
See *Iron Salts* (ferrous sulfate)

Milk [120]
Feosol Elixir should not be mixed with milk since iron forms insoluble complexes with certain constituents of milk.

Fruit juices [120]
Feosol Elixir should not be mixed with fruit juices since the formulation is incompatible with vitamin C.

FEOSTAT
See *Iron Salts* (ferrous fumarate)

FEOSTIM
See *Iron Salts* (ferrous fumarate) and *Vitamin B₁₂.*

FERAMEL
See *Ascorbic Acid* and *Iron Salts* (ferrous carbonate).

FERANCEE
See *Ascorbic Acid* and *Iron Salts* (ferrous fumarate).

FERGON WITH OR WITHOUT VITAMIN C
See *Ascorbic Acid* and *Iron Salts* (ferrous gluconate).

FER-IN-SOL
See *Iron Salts* (ferrous sulfate).

FERMALOX
See *Iron Salts* (ferrous sulfate) and *Magnesium* (magnesium and aluminum hydroxides).

FERNISOLONE
See *Glucocorticoids* (prednisolone).

FERO-FOLIC-500
See *Ascorbic Acid, Folic Acid,* and *Iron Salts* (ferrous sulfate).

FERO-GRAD-500
See *Ascorbic Acid* and *Iron Salts* (ferrous sulfate).

FERO-GRADUMET
See *Iron Salts* (iron sulfate).

FERRITRINSIC
See *Iron Salts* (ferrous sulfate) and *Vitamins.*

FERRO-GENT
See *Ascorbic Acid, Iron Salts* (ferrous fumarate), and *Vitamins B_1 and B_{12}.*

FERROLIP
See *Iron Salts* (ferrocholinate).

FERRONORD
See *Iron Salts* (ferrous iron amino acid complex).

FERRO-SEQUELS
See *Iron Salts* (ferrous fumarate).

FERROSPAN
See *Ascorbic Acid* and *Iron Salts* (ferrous fumarate).

FERROUS IRON
See *Iron Salts.*

FESTALAN
See *Atropine* (atropine methyl nitrate), *Bile Acids and Salts,* and *Enzymes* (amylolytic and proteolytic).

FETAMIN
See *Barbiturates* (pentobarbital),*Calcium, Iron Salts* (ferrous gluconate), *Methamphetamine* and *Vitamins* (B complex).

FIGS
See *Tyramine-rich Foods.*

FILIBON FORTE
See *Calcium, Iron Salts* (ferrous fumarate), *Magnesium,* and *Vitamins* (B complex).

FIORINAL WITH OR WITHOUT CODEINE
See *Barbiturates* (butalbital), *Caffeine, Codeine, Phenacetin,* and *Salicylates* (aspirin).

FISH
See *Vitamin K* and *Anticoagulants, Oral.*

FLAGYL
See *Metronidazole.*

Alcohol [120,354,735,736]
Alcoholic beverages should not be consumed during Flagyl therapy. Enzyme inhibition causes a disulfiramlike reaction.

FLORINEF
See *Corticosteroids* (fludrocortisone acetate or hemisuccinate).

FLUFENAMIC ACID (Arlef)

Aspirin [120]
Aspirin inhibits the anti-inflammatory effect of flufenamic acid.

FLUORINE ANESTHETICS

Muscle relaxants, depolarizing type [120,421] (Decamethonium, succinylcholine, etc.)
Fluorine anesthetics prolong muscle relaxation with the depolarizing type of muscle relaxants. See under *Muscle Relaxants.*

FLUOROPHOSPHATE INSECTICIDES
See *Anticholinesterases.*

Anticholinesterases [421]
Fluorophosphate insecticides potentiate the effects of other anticholinesterases.

Muscle relaxants, depolarizing type [204] (Decamethonium, succinylcholine, etc.)
Fluorophosphate insecticides increase muscle relaxation with depolarizing type of muscle relaxants. See *Muscle Relaxants.*

5-FLUOROURACIL

Methotrexate [951]
Synergistic antineoplastic activity.

Methylmitomycin [951]
Synergistic antineoplastic activity.

Mitomycin [951]
Synergistic antineoplastic activity against ascites cell neoplasms.

FLUOTHANE
See *Halothane.*

FLUPHENAZINE HCl (Prolixin)
See *Phenothiazines.*

FLUROTHYL (Indoklon)

Barbiturates [935] (Amytal, Pentothal)
An unfruitful seizure with Indoklon convulsive treatment (ICT) may be caused by the use of amobarbital or thiopental which greatly elevates the convulsive threshold.

Phenothiazines [935]
Prolonged or multiple seizures may occur with flurothyl if phenothiazine potentiation is present. These drugs lower the seizure threshold.

Rauwolfia alkaloids [935] (Reserpine, etc.)
Same as for *Phenothiazines* above.

FLUROXENE (Fluoromar)
See *Anesthetics, General* and *Halothane* (similar interactions).

Epinephrine [683]
Cardiac arrhythmias are produced when this vasopressor is used to correct the hypotension caused by fluroxene.

Nitrous oxide [879]
Combined use of these two general anesthetics increases cardiac output and central venous pressure.

Phenytoin (Dilantin, etc.)
See *Fluroxene* under *Phenytoin.*

Tubocurarine [120,878]
This type of halogenated inhalation anesthetic enhances the muscle relaxing effect of tubocurarine.

FOLBESYN
See *Ascorbic Acid* and *Vitamins* (B complex and B_{12}).

FOLIC ACID (Vitamin B$_c$, vitamin M)

Alcohol [1136]
Alcohol may produce folic acid deficiency via poor diet, defective liver function (poor storage and excessive loss in the urine), or inhibition of the enzyme (pteroylpolyglutamate hydrolase) that functions in folate utilization.

Anticonvulsants
See *Folic Acid* under *Anticonvulsants*.

Oral contraceptives [924]
Malabsorption of folate has been associated with oral contraceptives.

Phenytoin [198,421,444,633,880] (Dilantin)
Phenytoin depresses folic acid levels in the body and potentiates folic acid antagonists.

Pyrimethamine [619]
Folic acid is contraindicated for use with pyrimethamine, a folic acid antagonist, because it interferes with the mechanism of pyrimethamine action.

FOLIC ACID ANTAGONISTS (Methotrexate, etc.

Alcohol [120]
Concomitant use of alcohol and other potentially hepatotoxic drugs should be avoided because folic acid antagonists may themselves be hepatotoxic.

p-Aminosalicylic acid [120] (PAS)
Same interaction as for *Salicylates* below.

Chloroquine [421]
Chloroquine potentiates folic acid antagonists such as methotrexate.

Estrogens [28,421,924]
Estrogens potentiate folic acid antagonists. This includes oral contraceptives containing estrogen which causes malabsorption of folate.

Oral contraceptives
See *Estrogens* above.

Phenobarbital [421]
Phenobarbital potentiates folic acid antagonists.

Phenytoin [444,880,1087,1229] (Dilantin)
See *Folic Acid* under *Phenytoin*.

Primidone [421] (Mysoline)
Primidone potentiates folic acid antagonists.

Salicylates [120]
Salicylates enhance the activity and toxicity of methotrexate through displacement from protein binding.

Sulfonamides [120]
Synergistic activity in coccidiosis. Sulfonamides potentiate folic acid antagonists in same manner as PAS and salicylates.

FOLVRON
See *Folic Acid* and *Iron Salts* (ferrous sulfate).

FOOD ADDITIVES

Barbiturates and certain other drugs [78]
Some food additives decrease the duration of action of some drugs by enzyme induction.

FOODS
See *Alcohol, Beer, Cereals, Cheese, Eggs, Fish, Fruit Juices, Licorice, Milk, Mushrooms, Onions, Tyramine-rich Foods, Wines, Xanthines* (coffee, cola, tea, etc.), *Yogurt, etc.*

Griseofulvin [619,921]
A high fat diet enhances griseofulvin activity by increasing absorption from the gut.

FOODS CONTAINING PRESSOR AMINES
See *Tyramine-rich Foods.*

FORHISTAL
See *Antihistamines* (dimethindene maleate).

Alcohol [120]
Same as for *Hypnotics* below.

Hypnotics [120]
Administer CNS depressant drugs cautiously to patients receiving dimethindene (additive CNS depressant effects).

Narcotics [120]
Same as for *Hypnotics* above.

Sedatives [120]
Same as for *Hypnotics* above.

FORMATRIX
See *Androgens* (methyltestosterone), *Ascorbic Acid,* and *Estrogens, Conjugated.*

FOSFREE
See *Calcium Salts* (carbonate, gluconate, lactate), *Iron Salts* (ferrous gluconate), and *Vitamins* (B complex, B$_{12}$, A, D).

FRUCTOSE

Alcohol [873]
Fructose is the most effective compound for increasing the metabolism of ethyl alcohol.

FRUIT JUICE
See *Acid Drinks* under *Erythromycin.*

Feosol Elixir [120]
Feosol Elixir should not be mixed with fruit juices since the formulation is incompatible with vitamin C.

FULVICIN-U/F
See *Griseofulvin.*

FUMARAL SPANCAP
See *Ascorbic Acid* and *Iron Salts* (ferrous fumarate).

FUMASORB
See *Iron Salts* (ferrous fumarate).

FURADANTIN
See *Nitrofurantoin.*

FURAZOLIDONE (Furoxone)
See also *MAO Inhibitors.* [335]
Furazolidone yields a metabolite, 2-hydroxyethyl hydrazine (HEH), which acts as a MAO inhibitor if given for 4 or 5 days or longer. [1932]

Alcohol [28,48,120,354,633,1687,1859]
See *CNS Depressants* below. Avoid ingestion of alcohol in any form during oral furazolidone therapy and for 4 days thereafter. A disulfiramlike reaction (flushing, throbbing headache, nausea, vomiting, sweating, with hypotension and neurologic symptoms) may occur due to inhibition of aldehyde dehydrogenase and consequent accumulation of acetaldehyde.

Amitriptyline [1098] (Elavil)
Combined therapy of furazolidone (MAO inhibitor) and a tricyclic antidepressant such as amitriptyline causes blurred vision, profuse perspiration followed by alternating chills and hot flashes, motor hyperactivity, restlessness, persecutory delusions, auditory hallucination, and visual illusions.

Amphetamines [633]
See *Sympathomimetic Amines* below.

Anesthetics, general
See *CNS Depressants* below.

FURAZOLIDONE (Furoxone)   *(continued)*

Antidepressants, tricyclic [1098]
Furazolidone (MAO inhibitor) potentiates these antidepressants. See *Amitriptyline* above.

Antihistamines
See *CNS Depressants* below.

Antiparkinsonism drugs [202,633]
Furazolidone potentiates antiparkinsonism drugs.

Barbiturates [120,202,633]
See *CNS Depressants* below.

Broad beans [633]
See *Tyramine-rich Foods.*

**Catecholamines
(Epinephrine, dopamine, norepinephrine, isoproterenol, etc.)** [198]
See *Sympathomimetic Amines* below.

Cheese [633]
See *Tyramine-rich Foods.*

Chianti wine [633]
See *Tyramine-rich Foods.*

Chloral hydrate [120,198,633]
See *CNS Depressants* below.

Cocaine [633]
Furazolidone potentiates cocaine.

CNS depressants [120,198,633]
Furazolidone potentiates CNS depressants by microsomal enzyme inhibition. Orthostatic hypotension, hazardous CNS depression, and hypoglycemia may occur. Use alcohol, antihistamines, barbiturates, chloral hydrate, narcotics, sedatives, and tranquilizers, if they must be given, in reduced dosages. See also *CNS Depressants.*

Ephedrine [120]
Contraindicated. See *Sympathomimetic Amines* below.

Exogenous amines
See *Sympathomimetic Amines* below.

Guanethidine [120]
Contraindicated. See *Guanethidine* under *MAO Inhibitors.*

Herring [633]
See *Tyramine-rich Foods.*

Insulin [202,633]
Furazolidone potentiates insulin. See *MAO Inhibitors* under Insulin.

Liver [633]
See *Tyramine-rich Foods.*

MAO inhibitors [633]
Additive MAO inhibition (furazolidone may act as a MAO inhibitor if given for more than 4-5 days). (Hypertension with furazolidone plus tranylcypromine and other MAO inhibitors).

Meperidine [202,633] **(Demerol)**
Meperidine inhibits furazolidone; furazolidone potentiates meperidine.

Methyldopa [633] **(Aldomet)**
Excitation and hypertension may occur when this catecholamine is given with furazolidone.

Narcotics [120]
Should be used in reduced dosages and with caution. See *CNS Depressants* above.

Phenothiazines [120,198,633]
Furazolidone potentiates phenothiazines. See *CNS Depressants* above.

Phenylephrine [120,136] **(Neo-Synephrine, etc.)**
Contraindicated. See *Sympathomimetic Amines* below.

Reserpine [633]
Excitation initially. Contraindicated. See *Reserpine* under *MAO Inhibitors.*

Sedatives [120,198]
Should be used in reduced dosages and with caution. See *CNS Depressants* above.

Sympathomimetic amines [120,198,354-356,633]
Contraindicated. Furazolidone potentiates sympathomimetic amines, including catecholamines, through enzyme inhibition. Furazolidone is a MAO inhibitor. A hypertensive crisis may occur if it is given with pressor amines like tyramine and others found in some foods (see *Tyramine-rich Foods*), in nasal decongestants (ephedrine, phenylephrine, etc.), and in anorectics (amphetamines).

Thiazide diuretics [120,633]
This combination may potentiate the orthostatic hypotension which may be caused by both the thiazides and furazolidone. Furazolidone potentiates the diuretics.

Tranquilizers [120]
Should be used in reduced dosages and with caution. See *CNS Depressants* above.

Tyramine-rich foods [633]
Tyramine sensitivitiy is potentiated by the MAO inhibitor, furazolidone; hypertensive crisis possible. See *Tyramine-rich-Foods.*

Vasopressors [120,198,356,633]
Furazolidone potentiates vasopressors; severe hypertension. See *Sympathomimetic Amines* above.

FUROSEMIDE (Frusemide, Lasix)
See *Diuretics.*
Furosemide enters into the interactions of the sulfonamide diuretics.

Allopurinol
See *Uricosurics and Other Antigout Drugs* below.

Anticoagulants, oral [147]
Furosemide inhibits oral anticoagulants.

Antidiabetics [120,152,986,1013]
Furosemide can cause an elevation of blood glucose levels and may precipitate diabetes mellitus in persons with latent diabetes. Increased doses of antidiabetics may be necessary.

Antihypertensives [120,152,1013]
Furosemide potentiates the hypotensive effect of antihypertensives. Reduce their dosage.

Aspirin [120]
High doses of aspirin given concurrently with furosemide may produce salicylate toxicity because of competition for renal excretory sites.

Cephaloridine [120] **(Loridine)**
Diuretics such as furosimide enhance the nephrotoxicity of cephaloridine. See *Furosemide* under *Cephalosporins.*

Chloral hydrate [1972]
Chloral hydrate given simultaneously with or up to 12 hours before furosemide produces hypertension, tachycardia, hot flushes and sever diaphoresis. Contraindicated, especially in patients with acute coronary disease, within same 24-hour period.

Clofibrate (Atromid-S)
See *Furosemide* under *Clofibrate.*

Curare [120,152,1013]
Utmost caution should be exercised in administering curare or its derivatives to patients undergoing therapy with furosemide. These muscle relaxants are potentiated by sulfonamide diuretics.

Corticosteroids [120,1013,1853]
Excessive potassium depletion may occur when corticosteroids are given with furosemide. See *Corticosteroids* under *Diuretics*.

Diazoxide
See *Furosemide* under *Diazoxide*.

Digitalis [120,152,1013]
Digitalis toxicity may be precipitated in patients receiving furosemide because of excessive loss of potassium. Cardiac arrhythmias may be precipitated in patients with myocardial ischemia.

Diuretics, other [120]
Furosemide enhances the hypotensive effects of other diurectics. Dehydration from excessive diuresis may cause reversible elevation of blood urea.

Ethacrynic acid [120,1978] **(Edecrin)**
Hypokalemia plus nodal tachycardia may occur with this combination of diuretics. Other adverse effects that may be additive with these potent diuretics are ototoxicity (tinnitus, deafness), metabolic alkalosis, hypotension, thromboembolic episodes, etc. The ototoxic effects appear to be dose related and reversible (cats).

Gallamine [330]
See *Muscle Relaxants* below.

Insulin [120]
Furosemide may cause hyperglycemia. The dosage requirements of a controlled diabetic may have to be increased.

Lithium carbonate
See *Lithium Carbonate* under *Diuretics* regarding toxicity produced by the combination.

MAO inhibitors [120,184,404]
May cause an augmented hypotensive effect approaching shock levels. Additive effect.

Muscle relaxants [120,152,330,1013,1364]
(Gallamine, tubocurarine, etc.)
Prolonged paralysis of respiratory muscles may occur with ethacrynic acid, furosemide, thiazide diuretics, chlorthalidone, etc with peripherally acting competitive type of muscle relaxants. Persistent curarization. Potassium depletion may be involved. Discontinue oral furosemide for one week and parenteral furosemide for two days prior to surgery. Potentially lethal.

Ototoxic drugs [120]
Transient deafness is more likely to occur in patients receiving drugs also known to be ototoxic. See *Ototoxic Drugs* and *Antibiotics with Ototoxic Effects* under *Neomycin*.

Oxyphenbutazone
See *Uricosurics* below.

Phenylbutazone
See *Uricosurics* below.

Phenytoin (Dilantin)
See *Furosemide* under *Phenytoin*.

Pressor amines [120,1013]
Sulfonamide diuretics like furosemide have been reported to decrease arterial responsiveness to pressor amines. Discontinue oral furosemide for one week and parenteral furosemide for two days prior to surgery.

Probenecid [152,986] **(Benemid)**
Probenecid prolongs the diuretic action of furosemide by inhibiting its excretion, and it tends to correct the hyperuricemia produced by the diuretic. See *Uricosurics* below.

Salicylates [120]
Patients receiving high doses of salicylates in conjunction with furosemide may experience salicylate toxicity at lower doses because of competition for renal excretory sites.

Spironolactone [986,1013] **(Aldactone)**
Spironolactone enhances the diuretic action of furosemide while preventing excessive potassium excretion.

Spironolactone-hydrochlorothiazide [443]
(Aldactazide)
Severe electrolyte imbalance may occur if furosemide is given concurrently with this other diuretic.

Steroids
See *Corticosteroids* above.

Sulfinpyrazone
See *Uricosurics* below.

Sulfonamides [120]
Patients known to be sensitive to sulfonamides may also be sensitive to furosemide, itself a sulfonamide. Take precautions if an anti-infective sulfonamide is used with this diuretic sulfonamide.

Triamterene [986,1013] **(Dyrenium)**
Same as for *Spironolactone* above.

Tubocurarine [152,330,1013]
Furosemide potentiates tubocurarine. See *Curare* and *Muscle Relaxants* above.

Uricosurics and other antigout drugs
Furosemide, since it elevates blood uric acid and tends to produce gout, is antagonistic to uricosurics such as probenecid, oxyphenbutazone, phenylbutazone and sulfinpyrazone as well as allopurinol, the inhibitor of uric acid synthesis.

FUROXONE
See *Furazolidone*.

GALLAMINE TRIETHIODIDE
(Flaxedil Triethiodide)
See *Muscle Relaxants, Peripherally Acting, Competitive Type*.
The drug interactions of gallamine are like those given under *Curare*.

Aminoglycosides
See *Streptomycin* below.

Diazepam
See *Muscle Relaxants* under *Benzodiazepines*

Diuretics
See *Muscle Relaxants* under *Furosemide*.

Gallamine [120]
Cumulative effects occur with gallamine.

Streptomycin [330,654]
Streptomycin, kanamycin, and other aminoglycoside antibiotics potentiate neuromuscular blockade by gallamine; prolonged paralysis of respiratory muscles may occur. See *Neuromuscular Blocking Antibiotics* under *Antibiotics*.

GANGLIONIC BLOCKING AGENTS
(Mecamylamine [Inversine] HCl, pentolinium [Ansolysen] tartrate, tetraethylammonium bromide and chloride, trimethaphan [Arfonad] camsylate, trimethidinium methosulfate [Ostensin], etc.
See also *Antihypertensives*.

Acidifying agents [325,870]
Opposite effect to *Alkalinizers* below.

Alcohol [120]
Alcohol potentiates the antihypertensive effect of ganglionic blocking agents. See *CNS Depressants*.

GANGLIONIC BLOCKING AGENTS *(continued)*

Alkalinizers[325,870]

Elevation of pH potentiates because with alkaline urine a large proportion of a drug like mecamylamine is present in the nonionized and therefore lipid-soluble form which is reabsorbed and only small quantities appear in the urine.

Anticholinesterases[168]

The actions of anticholinesterases on autonomic ganglia are generally readily blocked by ganglionic blocking agents such as hexamethonium and its congers.

Chlorthalidone[120,619] **(Hygroton)**

Although this sulfonamide diuretic is not a thiazide, it has the same interactions as *Thiazide Diuretics* below.

Levarterenol[117,947] **(Levophed)**

The pressor effects of levarterenol (norepinephrine) are augmented by ganglionic blocking agents which sensitize the effector cells to these hypotensive agents and may account for the tolerance that develops to them.

MAO inhibitors[120]

MAO inhibitors may potentiate ganglionic-blocking agents; do not use together or within 2 or 3 weeks following treatment with MAO inhibitors.

Reserpine[117]

Reserpine potentiates the hypotensive action of ganglionic blocking agents.

Thiazide diuretics[120,633]
(Anhydron, Diuril, Naturetin, Renese, Saluron, etc.)

Thiazide diuretics enhance the hypotensive effect of ganglionic blocking drugs. Reduce their dosage by about half when initiating therapy with a thiazide.

Vasopressin[173] **(ADH, Pitressin)**

Ganglionic blocking agents markedly increase snesitivity to the pressor effects of vasopressin.

GANTANOL

See *Sulfonamides* (sulfamethoxazole)

GANTRISIN

See *Sulfonamides* (sulfisoxazole)

GARAMYCIN

See *Antibiotics* (gentamicin)

GAYSAL

See *Acetaminophen, Aluminium* (hydroxide), *Barbiturates,* (phenobarbital, and secobarbital), and *Salicylates* (sodium salicylate)

GELATIN

Methenamine[619]

Methenamine may slowly combine with gelatin capsules, and gradually become insoluble.

GELUSIL

See *Antacids* (aluminum hydroxide plus magnesium trisilicate).

GEMONOL

See *Barbiturates* (metharbital).

GENTAMICIN SULFATE (Garamycin)

See *Aminoglycoside Antibiotics.*

Carbenicillin

See *Gentamycin* under *Carbenicillin.*

Cephalosporins (Loridine, Keflin, etc.)

See *Gentamicin* under *Cephalosporins.*

Dimenhydrinate[120] **(Dramamine)**

Dimenhydrinate may mask the ototoxicity of aminoglycosides that may occur. Extra alertness is essential to detect the side effect.

Ethacrynic Acid (Edecrin)

See under *Ethacrynic Acid.*

Kanamycin, neomycin, and paromomycin[178]

Gentamicin has been shown to possess cross-resistance between itself and other aminoglycoside antibiotics such as kanamycin, neomycin, paromomycin, and streptomycin.

Methoxyflurane (Penthrane)

See under *Methoxyflurane.*

GERAMINE

See *Ethinyl Estradiol, Methyltestosterone, Thyroid, Vitamins.*

GERANDREST

See *Androgens* (methyltestosterone) and *Estrogens, Conjugated.*

GERILETS FILMTABS

See *Iron Salts* (ferrous sulfate) and *Vitamins.*

GERITAG CAPSULETTES

See *Androgens, Estradiol, Estrogens,* and *Testosterone.*

GITALIGIN

See *Digitalis* (gitalin).

GLAUCON

See *Epinephrine* (*l*-epinephrine).

GLUCAGON (Hyperglycemic factor)

Anticoagulants, oral[10,710]

Glucagon potentiates oral anticoagulants such as warfarin.

Antidiabetics, oral

See *Glucagon* under *Antidiabetics, Oral.*

Insulin[184,421]

Glucagon in large doses stimulates insulin secretion but in small doses promotes glycogenolysis and glyconeogenesis. It is therefore used to counteract hypoglycemia induced by insulin.

GLUCARIC ACID
(Saccharic acid, D-tetrahydroxyadipic acid)

In drug interactions involving hepatic microsomal enzyme induction, excretion of glucaric acid is increased. The extent of the increase is an index of microsomal enzyme activity.

GLUCOCORTICOIDS

See *Corticosteroids.*

Digitalis glycosides

See *Glucose* under *Digitalis* and *Digitalis Glycosides.*

GLUCOSE

Diuretics[120]

Many diuretics such as furosemide and the thiazide diuretics decrease glucose tolerance and may aggravate or provoke diabetes mellitus with hyperglycemia and glycosuria. Blood glucose levels must be monitored closely when such diuretics are used with antidiabetic therapy. See *Diuretics* under *Antidiabetics, Oral.*

Purgatives[359]

Purgatives may inhibit the intestinal absorption of glucose.

GLUTAMIC ACID HCL

Anticholinergics[421]

Glutamic acid may antagonize the anti-HCl acid secretory effect of anticholinergics.

Vinblastine[120,179]

Glutamic acid blocks both toxic and antineoplastic activity of vinblastine.

Vincristine [120,179]
Glutamic acid blocks both toxic and antineoplastic activity of vincristine.

L-GLUTAVITE
(Monosodium L-glutamate and vitamins)

Meprobamate [950,951] **(Equanil, Miltown)**
L-Glutavite potentiates the psychotropic activity of meprobamate.

Nortriptyline [120,619] **(Aventyl)**
L-Glutavite potentiates the psychotropic effect of nortriptyline.

Perphenazine [950,951] **(Trilafon)**
L-Glutavite potentiates the psychotropic activity of perphenazine.

GLUTEST
See *Glutamic Acid, Testosterone,* and *Vitamin B₁.*

GLUTETHIMIDE (Doriden)

Alcohol [120]
Possible combined CNS depressant effects. See *CNS Depressants,* and also *Glutethimide* under *Alcohol.*

Aminopyrine [63,184]
Glutethimide inhibits aminopyrine by stimulating its metabolism.

Anticoagulants, oral [78,223,297,434,633,673,814]
Glutethimide inhibits coumarin anticoagulants. It accelerates the metabolism of the coumarins in the same manner as do the barbiturates. The dosage of the anticoagulants must be adjusted during and upon cessation of glutethimide therapy.

Antidepressants, tricyclic [166,194]
This combination produces additive atropinelike effects (mydriasis, inhibition of salivary secretions and intestinal motility). Hazardous in glaucoma.

Antihistamines [198]
Glutethimide inhibits antihistamines by enzyme induction. Also, potentiated CNS depressant action. See *CNS Depressants.*

Antipyrine [222]
Glutethimide stimulates the metabolism of antipyrine and thus inhibits the analgesic.

Coumarin anticoagulants
See *Anticoagulants, Oral* above.

CNS depressants [120]
Possible combined CNS depressant effects. See *CNS Depressants.*

Corticosteroids [198]
Glutethimide decreases the activity of corticosteroids by enzyme induction.

Dipyrone [184,694,695] **(Narone, Pyrilgin, etc.)**
Glutethimide inhibits dipyrone by enzyme induction.

Ethyl biscoumacetate [436] **(Tromexan)**
See *Anticoagulants, Oral* above.

Glutethimide [63]
Patients develop tolerance to glutethimide. Decreases its own effects by enzyme induction.

Griseofulvin [198] **(Fulvicin, Grifulvin, etc.)**
Glutethimide inhibits griseofulvin by enzyme induction.

Hypnotics [78,120]
Glutethimide inhibits hypnotics by enzyme induction. Possible combined CNS depressant effects.

Meprobamate [198,950]
Glutethimide inhibits meprobamate by enzyme induction and the reverse may also be possible.

Phenothiazines [120]
Potentiation of CNS depressant effects may be experienced initially with enzyme induction later.

Phenytoin [198] **(Dilantin)**
Glutethimide inhibits phenytoin by enzyme induction.

Steroids [198]
Glutethimide inhibits steroids by enzyme induction.

Warfarin [223,297,434] **(Coumadin)**
Glutethimide inhibits warfarin. See *Anticoagulants, Oral* above.

Zoxazolamine [198] **(Flexin)**
Glutethimide inhibits zoxazolamine (no longer marketed in the U.S.) by enzyme induction.

GLYCERYL GUAIACOLATE
See *Cold and Cough Remedies.*
This expectorant, an ingredient of many proprietary cold and cough remedies, interferes with clinical laboratory diagnostic tests. See Chapter 7.

Heparin
See *Glyceryl Guaiacolate* under *Heparin.*

GLYCYRRHIZA (Licorice)

Antihypertensives [151,326,667,1088,1089,1993]
Patients who regularly consume 20 Gm. or more of licorice daily experience hypoaldosteronism, depressed renin activity and an elevation in blood pressure. Continued use of moderate amounts of licorice by hypertensive individuals can cause potentially serious metabolic effects, can aggravate their condition, and might counteract the effect of antihypertensive medication. Steroidal constituents of licorice such as glycyrrhetinic acid which is chemically related to corticosteroids tends to induce hypokalemia and sodium retention. This widely used flavoring agent can induce a toxic reaction. See page 384. Cardiac drugs like digitalis may become more toxic. Hypertensive patients should avoid licorice.

MAO inhibitors
See *Licorice* under *MAO Inhibitors.*

Thiazide diuretics [186,667,1088,1089]
(Anhydron, Diuril, Naturetin, Renese, Saluron, etc.)
Severe hypokalemia may occur if a patient consumes licorice in large quantities or for prolonged periods during or while being maintained on thiazide therapy.

GLYTINIC
See *Iron Salts* (ferrous gluconate) and *Vitamins* (niacinamide, panthenol).

GOITROGENIC MEDICATIONS

Thyroid preparations [181]
Avoid the goitrogenic medications listed in Table 8-3 (page) as they may act as physiological antagonists to thyroid preparations.

GOLD THERAPY (Solganal, etc.)

***p*-Aminobenzoic acid** [120] **(PABA)**
Dermatitis and fever associated with chrysotherapy of arthritis may be aggravated by the PABA.

Chloroquine [120]
Concomitant use should be avoided, because of increased toxicity.

Corticosteroids
See *Gold Therapy* under *Corticosteroids.*

Hydroxychloroquine (Plaquenil)
See *Gold Compounds* under *Hydroxychloroquine.*

GOURMASE PB CAPSULES
See *Belladonna, Bile Acids and Salts, Enzymes* (amylase, pancreatin, pepsin) and *Phenobarbital.*

GRAMICIDIN
Systemic interactions have been reported but this antibiotic should only be used topically. It is a potent hemolytic agent.[178]

GRIFULVIN
See *Griseofulvin.*

GRISACTIN
See *Griseofulvin.*

GRISEOFULVIN
(Fulvicin, Grifulvin, Grisactin)

Alcohol[1146]
Flushing and tachycardia occur rarely.

Anticoagulants, oral[69,78,98,223,330,633]
Griseofulvin inhibits oral anticoagulants through enzyme induction. See a discussion of this problem with *Barbiturates* under *Anticoagulants, Oral.*

Barbiturates[64-67,83,490,633,640,821,1842]
Barbiturates inhibit griseofulvin through inhibition of intestinal absorption and enzyme induction. Griseofulvin potentiates the CNS depressant action of barbiturates. See *CNS Depressants.*

Chlorcyclizine[199] **(Perazil)**
Chlorcyclizine may decrease effectiveness of griseofulvin through enzyme induction.

Coumarin anticoagulants
See *Anticoagulants, Oral* above.

Diphenhydramine[199] **(Benadryl)**
Diphenhydramine may decrease the effectiveness of griseofulvin by enzyme induction and possibly vice versa.

Food[619,921]
A diet high in fat enhances griseofulvin action by increasing absorption from the gut.

Glutethimide (Doriden)[198]
Glutethimide inhibits griseofulvin by enzyme induction.

Methotrexate[951]
Griseofulvin inhibits methotrexate.

Orphenadrine[529] **(Disipol)**
Orphenadrine may inhibit griseofulvin via enzyme induction.

Phenobarbital[66,67,821] **(Phenobarbitone)**
Phenobarbital (enzyme inducer) inhibits griseofulvin; inadequate antifungal therapy due to a decrease in griseofulvin blood levels. See also *Barbiturates* above. One study demonstrated that inhibition of griseofulvin was due entirely to decrease in its absorption caused by the barbiturate.

Phenothiazines[822]
Acute porphyria may be induced.

Phenylbutazone[64,65,490]
Phenylbutazone inhibits griseofulvin through enzyme induction.

Phenytoin[619] **(Dilantin)**
Phenytoin may potentiate griseofulvin by displacement of the antifungal from protein binding sites.

Sedatives and hypnotics[198,421]
Some sedatives and hypnotics inhibit griseofulvin by enzyme induction.

Warfarin[69,98,223]
See *Anticoagulants, Oral* above.

GUAIACOLSULFONATES
See Chapter 7 for interferences with clinical laboratory tests.

GUANETHIDINE SULFATE (Ismelin)
See also *Antihypertensives.*
Many of the antagonists of guanethidine listed below possess CNS stimulant and sympathomimetic activity (antidepressants, antianxiety agents, anorexiants, etc.).

Alcohol[120,226,421,1622]
Alcohol (a vasodilator) may aggravate the orthostatic hypotension that is frequently seen with guanethidine therapy. Avoid alcohol or limit intake to circumvent possible syncope.

Amitriptyline (Elavil)
See *Antidepressants, Tricyclic* below.

Amphetamines[550,593,626,797,871,872]
(Dexedrine, Methedrine, Paredrine, etc.)
Amphetamines decrease the hypotensive effect by antagonizing the antiadrenergic effect of guanethidine. Control of blood pressure may be lost since amphetamines block guanethidine uptake, directly affect vasoconstrictor receptors, and also displace guanethidine and norepinephrine at sites of action. See also *Sympathomimetics* below. Avoid use of dextroamphetamine, methamphetamine, and other amphetamines in patients on guanethidine.

Anesthetics[120,619,633]
Guanethidine should not be given during the 2 weeks prior to surgery to avoid the possibility of vascular collapse (potentiated hypotension) during anethesia. Depletion of catecholamines by guanethidine increases the hazard of cardiac arrest during anesthesia. The hypotensive effects of guanethidine may persist for 10 days or longer.

Anticholinergics[421]
Guanethidine antagonizes the hyposecretory effect of anticholinergics.

Antidepressants, tricyclic[12,28,78,281,327,417,421,742, 797,823,946,955,1137,1253,1369,1376,1414,1563,1621,1643,1672,1673,1707,1905]
(Aventyl, Elavil, Norpramin, Pertofrane, Sinequan, Tofranil, Vivactil, etc.)
The hypotensive action of guanethidine may be antagonized (sometimes after a delay) or completely reversed by the action of desipramine, protriptyline, and possibly other tricyclics (inhibition of guanethidine and norepinephrine uptake into the adrenergic neurons). The tricyclics tend to block the hypotensive action of guanethidine and other similar antiadrenergics, and to potentiate exogenous and endogenous norepinephrine because of the blockage of the NE pump. They tend also to antagonize the prolonged depletion of tissue catecholamines produced by guanethidine. Hypotensive shock and unresponsive cardiac standstill may occur up to a week after the tricyclic drug is withdrawn. This combination is contraindicated. Note that addition of a tricyclic to guanethidine therapy may cause hypertension but this does not occur when guanethidine is added to tricyclic antidepressant therapy. Doxepin appears to be an exception; it may not always enter into this interaction at usual dosages.

Antidiabetics[187,1463-4]
Guanethidine, which is related chemically to biguanide, has some antidiabetic action which may produce an additive hypoglyemic effect with antidiabetics. Immediate effect of guanethidine IV is liberation of catecholamine and production of hyperglycemia but continued administration causes a depletion of tissue catecholamines and a fall in blood sugar. Monitor diabetic patients closely if guanethidine is added to or withdrawn from a regimen.

Antihistamines [626,823]
Antihistamines antagonize the adrenergic blocking (hypotensive) action of guanethidine.

Catecholamines [117,120,1504]
Guanethidine given systemically augments responses to epinephrine, isoproterenol, levarterenol (norepinephrine), and other catecholamines. Cardiovascular (pressor) effects are intensified, glycogenolysis occurs, blood glucose levels are increased and many other effects of these sympathomimetic agents are enhanced due to sensitization of receptors to the catecholamines. Hypertensive crisis is a possibility. A hazardous interaction. Guanethidine applied topically in the eye as a pretreatment potentiates the mydriatic effect of phenylephrine and catecholamines (neosynephrine and epinephrine).

Chlorpromazine
See *Phenothiazines* below. Chlorpromazine affects guanethidine like the *Antidepressants, Tricyclic* above.

Chlorthiazide [120] (Diuril)
Guanethidine and chlorothiazide induce synergistic antihypertensive activity.

Cocaine [417,550,593,626,1813]
Cocaine inhibits the hypotensive effect of guanethidine. It potentiates responses to adrenergic impulses.

Cold remedies [168,1082,1270]
Guanethidine sensitizes to some sympathomimetics such as phenylpropanolamine (Propadine) found in "cold remedies" and can thus induce a very hazardous hypertensive crisis. Over 100 widely used remedies contain this sympathomimetic, ranging from Alclear Anti-Allergy Tablets and Allerest Tablets and Capsules to Tussaminic Tablets and Vernate Capsules, Injection, and Tablets.

Contraceptives, oral [80]
See *Oral Contraceptives* below.

Desipramine [327,391,823] (Pertofrane)
Desipramine reverses the antihypertensive effect of guanethidine. See *Antidepressants, Tricyclic* above.

Dexamphetamine [550,593] (dexedrine, etc.)
See *Amphetamines* above.

Diethylpropion [550,593] (Tenuate)
Diethylpropion inhibits the hypotensive effect of guanethidine.

Digitalis glycosides [120]
Guanethidine and digitalis both decrease the heart rate (additive effect). Caution is necessary.

Diuretics [120,1956]
Diuretics potentiate the hypotensive action of guanethidine. The combination of a thiazide diuretic and guanethidine is clinically useful. Reduced dosages are effective and adverse effects such as orthostatic hypotension are minimized.

Dopamine [871,872]
Guanethidine ophthalmic drops antagonize the mydriatic action of dopamine in the eye.

Doxepin [1672] (Sinequan)
See *Antidepressants, Tricyclic* under *Antihypertensives*. Doxepin may inhibit uptake of guanethidine by adrenergic neurons to the site of its action, but not as strongly as other tricyclic antidepressants. It therefore may antagonize guanethidine's antihypertensive action. Exercise caution.

Ephedrine [550,593,797,871,872,1832]
Ephedrine decreases the hypotensive effect of guanethidine (similar to amphetamines). Guanethidine ophthalmic drops antagonize the mydriatic action of ephedrine in the eye.

Ephinephrine [871]
Guanethidine in ophthalmic drops potentiates the mydriatic action of epinephrine in the eye.

Furazolidone [120] (Furoxone)
Contraindicated. See *MAO Inhibitors* below.

Haloperidol [1347] (Haldol)
Haloperidol, like some phenothiazines (see below), antagonizes the antihypertensive action of guanethidine. Monitor patients closely.

Hydralazine [1790] (Apresoline)
Guanethidine and hydralazine used concomitantly produce a greater hypotensive effect than either drug alone, especially when the patient is recumbent.

Hydrochlorothiazide
See *Thiazide Diuretics* below.

Hydroxyamphetamine [550,593,871] (Paredrine)
See *Amphetamines* above.

Imipramine [281,330,341,626] (Tofranil)
Imipramine inhibits guanethidine and vice versa. See *Antidepressants, Tricyclic* above.

Insulin [191]
Guanethidine may potentiate insulin.

Isocarboxazid [74,433] (Marplan)
Contraindicated. See *MAO Inhibitors* below.

Levarterenol [117,421,633,1657] (Levophed, norepinephrine)
Guanethidine by sensitizing the α-receptors for this sympathomimetic, potentiates the catecholamine levarterenol and may greatly enhance the hypertension; bradycardia, cardiac arrhythmia. See *Catecholamines* above.

Levodopa [1497,1648] (Dopar, Larodopa, etc.)
Levodopa may potentiate the antihypertensive action of guanethidine. Monitor patients closely.

MAO inhibitors [162,550,593,797,1399,1831] (Eutonyl, Furoxone, Marplan, Nardil, Niamid, and Parnate)
Concomitant use of a monoamine oxidase inhibitor and guanethidine is contraindicated. Due to sudden release of catecholamines with guanethidine a hypertensive crisis may occur. Metabolism of norepinephrine and serotonin is inhibited. Serotonin levels in the brain are markedly elevated. Guanethidine should not be given for at least a week after a MAO inhibitor has been withdrawn from a patient. Some MAO inhibitors have shown weak antagonistic action against guanethidine. If phenelzine, pheniprazine or tranylcypromine are given before guanethidine the expected hypotensive response may be prevented. If guanethidine or bretylium are given first they are able to restore blood pressure and responses to adrenergic stimulation to normal levels.

Mephentermine [550,593,633] (Wyamine)
Guanethidine inhibits the pressor effect of mephentermine and mephentermine inhibits the hypotensive effect of guanethidine.

Mepyramine [626] (Pyrilamine)
See *Antihistamines* above.

Metaraminol [633,824] (Aramine)
Metaraminol may inhibit the hypotensive effects of guanethidine. Headache and nausea may occur with severe hypertension due to sensitization of adrenergic neurons to the α-adrenergic sympathomimetic by guanethidine.

Methamphetamine [117,550,593,626,797] (Desoxyn, Methedrine, etc.)
See *Amphetamines* above. The pressor response to amines like methamphetamine is abolished by guanethidine that depletes norepinephrine from nerve endings since the pressor

GUANETHIDINE SULFATE (Ismelin)

(continued)

action is mediated by release of norepinephrine from stores. Methamphetamine antagonizes the hypotensive action and the postural hypotensive produced by guanethidine.

Methotrimeprazine [120] (Levoprome)

Methotrimeprazine, with its side effect of orthostatic hypotension, may potentiate the antihypertensive action of guanethidine which also has the same side effect. Avoid this combination, if possible.

Methoxamine [871] (Vasoxyl)

Guanethidine in ophthalmic solution potentiates the mydriatic action of methoxamine in the eye.

Methylphenidate [120,550,593,595,626,797,823] (Ritalin)

Methylphenidate, a CNS stimulant with properties similar to those of amphetamine, inhibits the hypotensive effect of guanethidine by antagonizing its adrenergic neuron blocking action. Cardiac arrhythmias may occur. See the mechanism under *Amphetamines* above.

Neo-Synephrine

See *Phenylephrine below.*

Nialamide [797] (Niamid)

Contraindicated. See *MAO Inhibitors* above.

Norepinephrine [120] (Levophed)

Responsiveness to norepinephrine is increased with guanethidine. See *Levarterenol* above. Guanethidine should not be used in patients with pheochromocytoma.

Nortriptyline (Aventyl)

See *Antidepressants, Tricyclic* above.

Oral contraceptives [80]

Satisfactory control of hypertension with guanethidine is difficult or may be impossible when oral contraceptives are also being taken. In 80% of cases, when oral contraceptives are withdrawn a substantial decrease in the dosage requirements of guanethidine occurs.

Pargyline [74,433] (Eutonyl)

Contraindicated. See *MAO Inhibitors* above.

Phenelzine [74,433] (Nardil)

Contraindicated. See *MAO Inhibitors* above.

Phenmetrazine [871]

Guanethidine in ophthalmic solution antagonizes the mydriatic action of phenmetrazine eye drops.

Phenothiazines [593,633,823,922,1304,1347,1406,1411,1563,1673,1863]

Some phenothiazines, in varying degrees, antagonize the hypotension induced by guanethidine because of their blocking action on the norepinephrine pump, whereas other phenothiazines without this action may have additive hypotensive effects. See also *Antidepressants, Tricyclic* above for mechanisms of action. Chlorpromazine antagonizes guanethidine.

Phenylephrine [553,871,1504] (Neo-Synephrine)

Guanethidine, a sympathomimetic receptor sensitizer, potentiates phenylephrine (a powerful α-receptor stimulant and to some extent a norepinephrine releaser), *e.g.,* prolongs mydriasis with eye drops such as Phenelzin and may greatly potentiate the hypertensive effects. Also phenylephrine inhibits the hypotensive effect of guanethidine and may induce cardiac arrhythmias. See *Sympathomimetics* below.

Phenylpropanolamine [168,1082] (Propadrine)

See *Cold Remedies* above.

Pipradol HCl (Meratran HCl) [417]

Pipradol, which is related to methylphenidate, also inhibits the hypotensive effect of guanethidine.

Protriptyline [327,823] (Vivactil)

Protriptyline inhibits the hypotensive effect of guanethidine.

Rauwolfia alkaloids [120,421,824]

Concomitant use of reserpine and other similar rauwolfia alkaloids with guanethidine may exaggerate orthostatic hypotension, bradycardia, and mental depression.

Reserpine

See *Rauwolfia Alkaloids* above.

Sympathomimetics [30,117,550,633,871,872]

Guanethidine potentiates some sympathomimetic actions; sympathomimetics inhibit guanethidine; hypertension may occur but see full discussion on *Sympathomimetics* under *Reserpine.* Guanethidine, through its sympathomimetic sensitizing action, potentiates the mydriasis produced by α-receptor stimulants such as epinephrine bitartrate, and phenylephrine HCl in ophthalmic drops such as Epitrate and Neo-Synephrine Hydrochloride (ophthalmic). It antagonizes the mydriasis produced by indirectly acting sympathomimetics (release norepinephrine from adrenergic neuronal storage sites) such as amphetamine sulfate, dopamine, ephedrine HCl, hydroxyamphetamine HBr, methamphetamine, methylphenidate, phenmetrazine HCl, and tyramine HCl. Amphetamine prevents or reverses the hypotensive action of guanethidine. Methamphetamine (also dexamphetamine, ephedrine and mephentermine but not epinephrine, norepinephrine and pheylephrine) abolishes the postural hypotension due to guanethidine.

Thiazide diuretics [120,421,1790] (Anhydron, Aquatag, Diuril, Metahydrin, Renese, Saluron, etc.)

Thiazide diuretics synergistically enhance the hypotensive activity of guanethidine, but they also increase symptoms due to postural hypotension. Reduce dosage accordingly.

Thiothixene [1347] (Navane)

Thiothixene, an antipsychotic thioxanthene, interacts with guanethidine similarly to the phenothiazines (see above) and may reverse the antihypertensive action.

Tranylcypromine [74,433] (Parnate)

Contraindicated. See *MAO Inhibitors* above.

Tripelennamine [626] (Pyribenzamine)

Tripelennamine may antagonize the adrenergic blocking action of guanethidine.

Tyramine [117,633]

This pressor amine which is a catecholamine (norepinephrine) releaser antagonizes the hypotensive effect of guanethidine. See *Tyramine-rich Foods.*

Vasopressors [20,117,120]

Guanethidine may enhance the response to vasopressors and increase the likelihood of cardiac arrhythmias occurring.

HALDOL

See *Haloperidol.*

HALDRONE

See *Corticosteroids* (paramethasone acetate).

HALEY'S M-O

See *Antacids* (milk of magnesia) and *Mineral Oil.*

HALLUCINOGENIC AGENTS

Phenothiazines [120,619]

Some phenothiazines reduce mydriasis and the unusual visual experiences. The CNS depressant action of phenothiazine tranquilizers antagonizes the CNS stimulation of hallucinogenic agents.

HALODRIN

See *Androgens* (fluoxymesterone) and *Estrogens* (ethinyl estradiol).

HALOFENATE (Livipas)

Anticoagulants, oral [1943]
Halofenate potentiates the anticoagulant action of warfarin.

Antidiabetics, oral [1943]
The hypolipemic and uricosuric agent, halofenate, elevates the blood levels of (potentiates) sulfonylureas after about a month of combined therapy.

Thyroid hormones [1943]
Halofenate displaces both thyroxine and triiodothyronine from protein binding sites and may potentiate them.

HALOGEN ANESTHETICS
See *Anesthetics, Halothane, Methoxyflurane,* etc.

HALOGENATED INSECTICIDES (Aldrin, chlordane, DDT, dieldrin, heptachlor, methoxychlor, TDE, etc.)

Antipyrine [1059]
The metabolism of antipyrine is stimulated by DDT and lindane.

Barbiturates [83,485,1053]
Insecticide sprays containing DDT and chlordane stimulated the metabolism of hexobarbital.

Cortisol [83,271,485] (Hydrocortisone)
Halogenated insecticides induce the metabolism of cortisol (related compounds are useful in Cushing's syndrome), and also other steroids, *e.g.,* estrogens and progesterone. The effects of both exogenous and endogenous steroids may be reduced.

Diphenhydramine [485,1053] (Benadryl)
These insecticides may decrease the antihistamine activity of diphenhydramine by enzyme induction and vice versa.

Estrogen-progestogens [485,1053] (Oral contraceptives, etc.)
Halogenated insecticides induce the metabolism of estrogens, androgens, and progesterone, and thereby decrease the uterotropic and other effects of these steroids, both exogenous and endogenous.

Phenylbutazone [83,485] (Butazolidin)
Small doses of chlordane (in dogs) stimulate the metabolism of phenylbutazone up to 5 months after withdrawal of the insecticide.

Warfarin [2044]
Chlorinated hydrocarbon insecticides (toxaphene, benzene hexachloride) decreased the hypoprothrombinemic effect of warfarin (enzyme induction).

HALOPERIDOL (Haldol)

Alcohol [120]
This combination should be avoided. The tranquilizer haloperidol, is potentiated by alcohol, and is definitely contraindicated in patients depressed by alcohol. See *CNS Depressants* below.

Amphetamines
See *Haloperidol* under *Amphetamines.*

Analgesics
See *CNS Depressants* below.

Anesthetics [120]
Haloperidol potentiates the depressant effects of anesthetics. See *CNS Depressants* below.

Anticholinergics [120,1804] (Benztropine, trihexyphenidyl, etc.)
Anticholinergics, administered with haloperidol, may increase intraocular pressure and enhance anticholinergic effects. The parkinsonism (extrapyramidal) symptoms frequently caused by haloperidol may be controlled with anticholinergics like benztropine mesylate and trihexyphenidyl HCl. The combination is contraindicated in glaucoma.

Anticoagulants, oral [147,198,421]
Haloperidol may stimulate the hepatic microsomal enzymes which metabolize coumarin anticoagulants. This increases the dosage of anticoagulant needed. Same mechanism as with phenobarbital. Haloperidol also interferes with the anticoagulant activity of phenindione.

Anticonvulsants [120]
The dose of anticonvulsant should not be altered when haloperidol therapy is initiated; however, subsequent adjustment may be necessary as haloperidol may alter the convulsive threshold.

Antidepressants, tricyclic [421]
Tricyclic antidepressants increase the sedative effects of haloperidol.

Antihypertensives [120]
Contraindicated. Potentiation of hypotensive effect possible.

Barbiturates [120,421]
Barbiturates increase the sedative effects of haloperidol and vice versa. See *CNS Depressants* below.

Benzodiazepines [120,421]
Benzodiazepines increase the sedative effects of haloperidol. See *CNS Depressants* below.

Antiparkinsonism drugs [120]
Antiparkinsonism drugs may be used with haloperidol to control the drug-induced extrapyramidal symptoms.

Benztropine mesylate [120,619,1804] (Cogentin Mesylate)
Haloperidol and benztropine may produce gynecomastia and additive anticholinergic effects (blurred vision, urinary retention, diaphoresis, etc.). Benztropine antagonizes the extrapyramidal effects of haloperidol (parkinsonlike symptoms, e.g., akinesia, akathisia, rigidity, tremor, etc.). In one series of patients the combination produced increased social avoidance behavior.

CNS depressants [120]
Haloperidol is contraindicated in patients depressed by CNS depressants. Haloperidol may potentiate (additive effects) CNS depressants such as alcohol, analgesics, anesthetics, barbiturates, narcotics, sedatives and tranquilizers. Observe caution to avoid overdosage. See *CNS Depressants.*

dl-Dopa [120]
dl-Dopa antagonizes the cataleptic effect of haloperidol.

Epinephrine [120,421]
Haloperidol blocks the vasopressor effects of epinephrine, and epinephrine reversal with a fall rather than a rise in blood pressure may occur. Thus epinephrine should not be used as a vasopressor if hypotension occurs with haloperidol.

Guanethidine
See *Haloperidol* under *Guanethidine Sulfate.*

Levarterenol [120,421] (Levophed)
Levarterenol antagonizes the hypotensive effects of haloperidol. Antidotal.

Levodopa [724,922,923,2001]
Haloperidol may defeat the therapeutic action of levodopa in Parkinson's syndrome by interfering with dopamine synthesis or by blocking its receptors.

Lithium carbonate [1145]
Severe encephalopathic syndrome may develop with irreversible brain damage and persistent dyskinesias. See *Haloperidol* under *Lithium Carbonate.*

MAO Inhibitors [120,352]
MAO inhibitors decrease the rate of metabolism of haloperidol and thus may potentiate the tranquilizer.

HALOPERIDOL (Haldol) *(continued)*

Methyldopa[1996]
Haloperidol, added to a methyldopa regimen for hypertensive patients, may produce a dementia syndrome in one week. Withdrawal of haloperidol corrects the condition within about 3 days.

Narcotic analgesics
See *CNS Depressants* above.

Norepinephrine (Levarterenol)
See *Levarterenol*.

Phenindione[340,703,814] **(Danilone, Hedulin, Indon)**
Haloperidol (enzyme inducer) inhibits phenindione (shortens the prothrombin time). See *Anticoagulants, Coumarin* above.

Phenothiazines[420]
Phenothiazines increase sedative effects of haloperidol. See *CNS Depressants* above.

Phenylephrine[120,421] **(Neo-Synephrine)**
Phenylephrine antagonizes the hypotensive effect of haloperidol. Antidotal.

Sedatives
See *CNS Depressants* above.

Tranquilizers
See *CNS Depressants* above.

Trihexyphenidyl[1804] **(Artane)**
See *Anticholinergics* and *Benztropine Mesylate* above.

HALOTESTIN
See *Androgens* and *Anabolic Agents* (fluoxymesterone).

HALOTHANE (Fluothane)

Desoxyephedrine[796]
See *Methamphetamine* below.

Ephedrine[796]
Same as for *Methamphetamine* below.

Epinephrine[683,796,799-804,917]
Halothane seems to sensitize the myocardium to the action of epinephrine. Ventricular tachycardia or fibrillation may occur with combined use. May be fatal (cardiac standstill). An immune mechanism may be involved in halothane hypersensitivity.

MAO inhibitors[1498] **(Phenelzine, etc.)**
MAO inhibitors elevate biogenic amines (5-HT, norepinephrine) and this may increase anesthetic requirements. Also drugs like phenelzine have a hypotensive effect that may be additive to the same effect of the anesthetic. Cease MAOI therapy at least 2 weeks prior to anesthesia if possible. Although no interaction has been reported caution is essential.

Mephentermine[120,820] **(Wyamine)**
Cardiac arrhythmias are produced when this vasopressor is used to correct halothane-induced hypotension.

Methamphetamine[796]
(Desoxyephedrine, Desoxyn, Methedrine, etc.)
Cardiac arrhythmias are induced by this combination.

Methoxamine[120,820]
Same as for *Mephentermine* above.

Nitrous oxide[166]
Anesthesia with 50:50 nitrous oxide and oxygen mixtures together with halothane or methoxyflurane in low concentration causes an increase in the inspired tension of nitrous oxide and may produce appreciable depression of blood pressure, heart rate, and muscle tone.

Nordefrin[803] **(Cobefrin)**
Cardiac arrhythmias may be induced when nordefrin is used with halothane. No longer promoted in the U.S.

Norepinephrine[120,773,776,778,796,801]
(Levarterenol, Levophed)
Halothane sensitizes the myocardium to the action of norepinephrine. Ventricular tachycardia or fibrillation may occur with combined use. May cause death.

Phenytoin (Dilantin, etc.)
See *Halothane* under *Phenytoin*.

Rifampin
See *Halothane* under *Rifampin*.

Succinylcholine[657,658]
Malignant hyperpyrexia may be induced with this combination.

Sympathomimetics[120,796,801]
Some sympathomimetics are contraindicated. See *Epinephrine* and *Norepinephrine* above.

Tubocurarine[878,1930]
Halothane enhances the muscle relaxant effect of tubocurarine; dosage should be reduced. See also *Halothane* under *Muscle Relaxants, Peripherally Acting, Competitive Type*.

HARMONYL
See *Rauwolfia Alkaloids* (deserpidine).

HEDULIN
See *Phenindione*.

HEMATOVALS
(Liver desiccated plus Vitamins B and C plus calcium)
See *Ascorbic Acid, Calcium Salts, Iron Salts* (ferrous sulphate), and *Vitamins* (B complex and B_{12}).

HEMINEVRIN
See *Chlormethiazole*.

HEMO-VITE
See *Iron Salts* (ferrous furmarate) and *Vitamins* B_1 and B_2.

HEPARIN
See *Anticoagulants*.

Anticoagulants, oral[673]
Heparin increases the anticoagulant effect of oral anticoagulants. See *Heparin* under *Anticoagulants, Oral*.

Antihistamines[181,764]
Large doses of antihistamines antagonize the anticoagulant action of heparin.

Ascorbic Acid[2025]
About 2 mg. of ascorbic acid eliminates the anticoagulant effect of 1 unit of heparin. This antagonism may be the reason for heparin-induced depression of aldosterone synthesis and development of osteoporosis.

Aspirin[28]
Avoid aspirin with heparin therapy since the salicylate inhibits platelet adhesiveness, one of the bases for hemostasis.

Chlorpheniramine[764]
(Chlor-Trimeton, Polaramine, etc.)
See *Antihistamines* above.

Cyclizine[764] **(marezine)**
See *Antihistamines* above.

Dextran[1964]
Dextran and heparin may exert synergistic anticoagulant activity. Monitor patients carefully. High doses of dextran prolong prothrombin time.

Digitalis[120]
Digitalis glycosides may inhibit the anticoagulant activity of heparin.

Diphenhydramine [764] **(Benadryl)**
See *Antihistamines* above.

Dipyridamole [28, 1839] **(Persantine)**
Avoid use of dipyridamole in patients receiving heparin. The antianginal agent inhibits the hemostatic platelet function and increases the risk of hemorrhage with the anticoagulant heparin.

EDTA [161, 870]
EDTA (calcium disodium edetate, etc.) increases the absorption rate of heparin.

Glyceryl guaiacolate [1339, 1800] **(Guaifenesin)**
Guaifenesin, the USAN (US Adopted Name) for glyceryl guaiacolate beginning in 1977, inhibits the hemostatic platelet function and increases the risk of hemorrhage with the anticoagulant heparin.

Hexadimethrine bromide [180] **(Polybrene)**
Hexadimethrine bromide is a heparin antagonist.

Hyaluronidase [180]
Hyaluronidase stimulates heparin absorption.

Hydroxyzine [764] **(Atarax, Vistaril)**
Hydroxyzine antagonizes the anticoagulant action of heparin.

Injections
See *Parenteral Drugs* below.

Nicotine [120]
Same as for *Digitalis* above.

Parenteral drugs [1438, 1882]
Parenteral medications given intramuscularly to patients, especially the elderly, who are receiving heparin may produce hematomas and bleeding into tissues at the point of injection.

Penicillin [433]
Penicillin inhibits heparin. Withdrawal of penicillin IV may cause severe hemorrhage.

Perphenazine [764] **(Trilafon)**
See *Phenothiazines* below.

Phenothiazines [764]
Phenothiazine tranquilizers antagonize the anticoagulant action of heparin.

Polymyxin B
Heparin and polymyxin B are incompatible in parenteral mixtures. See Chapter 7.

Promazine [764] **(Sparine)**
See *Phenothiazines* above.

Promethazine [764] **(Phenergan)**
See *Phenothiazines* above.

Protamine sulfate [153, 180, 619, 640, 2006]
Protamine sulfate which is strongly basic, powerfully antagonizes heparin by forming a complex with the strongly acidic heparin. But protamine is weakly anticoagulant and overneutralization in patients can result in hemorrhage, particularly if they are also receiving oral anticoagulants or they are hypoprothrombinemic.

Quinacrine
See *Heparin* under *Quinacrine*.

Quinine [180, 1208]
Theoretically the strongly acidic moieties (sulfuric acid) of the heparin molecule may react with the basic N of quinine and nullify its anticoagulant activity. This remains to be demonstrated.

Salicylates [120, 1322, 1661] **(Aspirin, PAS, etc.)**
Salicylates, by decreasing the prothrombin time (hypoprothrombinemia) potentiate heparin and increase the hemorrhagic tendency. See *Heparin* under *Salicylates*.

Tetracycline
See *Heparin* under *Tetracyclines*.

Thyroxin [120]
Heparin strikingly elevates the levels of free thyroxin and to some extent total thyroxin. Concurrent medication with heparin and thyroxin may be a factor precipitating arrhythmias, especially in a myocardium predisposed because of an infarct.

Vitamin C
See *Ascorbic Acid* above.

HEPATHROM
See *Heparin*.

HEPATOTOXIC AGENTS
See Table 9-20 (page 331) and *Liver Function Depressors* under *Anticoagulants, Oral*.
The agents interfere with many functions of the liver. They may cause hypoprothrombinemia and hemorrhage with anticoagulants, and potentiate many drugs because they depress metabolic processes, etc.

Hydroxychloroquine [120]
Use hydroxychloroquine with caution in patients receiving other drugs known to be hepatotoxic. Additive toxic effects.

Methotrexate [120]
Avoid administration of methotrexate with other drugs known to be hepatotoxic. Additive toxic effects.

HEPTABARBITAL (Medomin)
See *Barbiturates*.

Acenocumarol (Sintrom)
See *Anticoagulants, Oral* below.

Anticoagulants, oral [78, 83, 106, 825, 826, 1055]
Heptabarbital, by enzyme induction, inhibits the anticoagulant action of the oral anticoagulants. It also inhibits the intestinal absorption of bishydroxycoumarin.

Bishydroxycoumarin (Dicumarol)
See *Anticoagulants, Oral* above.

HEPTUNA PLUS CAPSULES
See *Ascorbic Acid, Calcium Salts, Iron Salts* (ferrous sulfate), *Magnesium Salts,* and *Vitamin B Complex*.

HEROIN

Cocaine [771]
An additive effect, unpredictable in consequences, occurs.

Nalorphine [166]
Nalorphine antagonizes the depressant effects of heroin; nalorphine can precipitate an acute abstinence syndrome in postaddicts who have received heroin for brief periods.

Quinine [771]
An additive effect, unpredictable in consequences, occurs.

HERRING, PICKLED
See *Tyramine-rich Foods*.

HEXADIMETHRINE BROMIDE (Polybrene)

Heparin [180]
Hexadimethrine bromide is a heparin antagonist.

HEXADROL
See *Corticosteroids* (dexamethasone).

HEXAFLUORENIUM (Mylaxen)

Muscle relaxants, depolarizing type [421]
Hexafluorenium prolongs muscle relaxation of the depolarizing type of muscle relaxants such as decamethonium and succinylcholine.

HEXALET
See *Methenamine* and *Salicylates* (sulfosalicylate).

HEXALOL
See *Atropine, Gelsemium* (CNS stimulant), *Hyoscyamine, Methylene Blue,* and *Salol.*

HEXOBARBITAL (Sombucaps, Sombulex)
See *Barbiturates* also.

Adiphenine [697] **(Trasentine)**
Hexobarbital is potentiated by adiphenine; a lower dose is required.

Aminopyrine [555]
Aminopyrine increases the rate at which hexobarbital is metabolized, and therefore inhibits the sedative effects, and vice versa.

p-Aminosalicylic acid [330] **(PAS)**
PAS potentiates hexobarbital (enzyme inhibition).

Barbiturates [63,695] **(Barbital, phenobarbital, etc.)**
Other barbiturates may induce the metabolizing enzymes for hexobarbital so strongly that its hypnotic effect is abolished.

Chloramphenicol [330] **(Chloromycetin)**
Chloramphenicol, an enzyme inhibitor, potentiates hexobarbital.

Chlorcyclizine [481,640] **(Perazil)**
Chlorcyclizine increases the rate at which hexobarbital is metabolized, and therefore inhibits the sedative effects, and possibly vice versa. See also *CNS Depressants.*

Chlorpromazine [669,697] **(Thorazine)**
Chlorpromazine potentiates the hypnotic action of hexobarbital. Lower the dosage.

DDT [688]
DDT, an enzyme inducer, inhibits hexobarbital.

Hexobarbital [63,695,1070]
Patients develop tolerance to repeated doses of hexobarbital (enzyme induction).

Imipramine [599] **(Tofranil)**
Imipramine prolongs hexobarbital sleeping time.

Iproniazid [827]
Iproniazid, an enzyme inhibitor, potentiates the sedative and hypnotic effects of hexobarbital.

Levarterenol [544]
(Levophed)
Repeated use of levarterenol may enhance the effect of hexobarbital via microsomal enzyme depression.

Orphenadrine [555] **(Disipal)**
Orphenadrine strongly inhibits hexobarbital by enzyme induction.

Phenobarbital [83,330]
Phenobarbital induces the metabolizing enzymes for hexobarbital so strongly that the pharmacological activity of subsequent doses is almost abolished. May mutually inhibit each by enzyme induction.

Phenylbutazone [330,555]
Phenylbutazone increases the rate at which hexobarbital is metabolized, and thereby inhibits its action. May thus inhibit each other.

Phenytoin
See *Hydantoins* under *Phenobarbital.*

Propranolol [818] **(Inderal)**
Hexobarbital markedly increases the toxicity of propranolol in mice, and the combination may be lethal. Use caution if patients are given both of these drugs.

SKF-525A
See *SKF-525A.*

Testosterone [83,330,421]
Testosterone inhibits hexobarbital and vice versa.

Urethan [695]
Urethan (enzyme inducer) inhibits hexobarbital.

HEXOBARBITAL PLUS AMINOPYRINE

Norepinephrine [544] **(Levophed)**
Enhanced effect of hexobarbital via microsomal enzyme depression by repeated norepinephrine.

HEXOBARBITAL PLUS METHAMPHETAMINE

Antidepressants, tricyclic [71,116,194]
Tricyclic antidepressants potentiate hexobarbital-methamphetamine hypnonarcosis effects.

HEXYLRESORCINOL

Alcohol [421]
Alcohol reduces the anthelmintic effect of hexylresorcinol.

Mineral oil [421]
Mineral oil reduces the anthelmintic effect of hexylresorcinol.

Santonin [421]
Santonin antagonizes hexylresorcinol.

HGH
See *Human Growth Hormone.*

HIPREX
See *Methenamine* (methenamine hippurate).

HISPRIL
See *Antihistamines* (diphenylpyraline HCl).

HISTABID
See *Antihistamines* (chlorpheniramine maleate), *Phenylephrine HCl, Phenylephrine,* and *Phenylpropanolamine HCl.*

HISTA-DERFULE
See *Antihistamines* (methapyrilene), *Atropine, Caffeine, Ipecac, Phenacetin,* and *Salicylamide.*

HISTADYL
See *Antihistamines* (methapyrilene).

HISTAMINE

Anticholinergics [421]
Histamine may antagonize the anti-HCl acid secretory effect of anticholinergics.

Antihistamines [421]
Histamine antagonizes antihistamines.

Bulbocapnine [951]
Bulbocapnine enhances the increase in the capillary permeability produced by histamine.

Epinephrine [169]
Epinephrine HCl IM, or in severe poisoning IV, is the antidote of choice in histamine overdosage with bronchoconstriction in asthmatics (also aminophylline and isoproterenol).

Imipramine [166]
Imipramine blocks the spasmogenic effects of histamine (guinea pig ileum).

Isosorbide dinitrate [120] **(Isordil, Sorbitrate)**
These drugs are physiological antagonists.

Nitrates, nitrites [170]
Nitrates and nitrites are antagonistic physiologically to histamine; the response may vary from maximal contraction to

maximal relaxation with variations in the relative concentrations of the members of any such pair.

Papaverine[951]
Papaverine enhances the increase in capillary permeability produced by histamine.

HOMATROPINE

Antacids[1959]
See *Alkaloids* under *Antacids, Oral.*

Levodopa[1419]
See *Levodopa* under *Anticholinergics.*

HORMONES
See *Anabolic Agents, Androgens, Corticosteroids, Estrogen-Progestins, Desoxycorticosterone, Insulin, Oral Contraceptives, Oxytocin, Thyroid Preparations, Vasopressin,* etc.

HORMONIN
See *Estradiol, Estriol* and *Estrone.*

HUMAN GROWTH HORMONE

Cortisone[181]
Cortisone inhibits most anabolic actions of human growth hormone but augments the other actions.

HYALEX
See *p-Aminobenzoic Acid, Magnesium Salts, Salicylates,* and *Vitamins.*

HYASORB
See *Penicillin.*

HYALURONIDASE

Parenteral medications
Hyaluronidase increases the rate of spreading of injected drugs and thus tends to enhance their effect and offset the decreased absorption caused by the histamine and 5-HT released through trauma caused by nonphysiologic foreign fluids, the needle, injection pressure, and sometimes by the injected drug (Ref. 113, Chap. 8).

HYBEPHEN
(Atropine sulfate plus hyoscine hydrobromide plus hyoscyamine sulfate plus phenobarbital)
See *Atropine, Hyoscine, Hyoscyamine,* and *Phenobarbital.*

HYCODAN
See *Hydrocodone Bitartrate* and *Homatropine Methylbromide.*

HYCOMINE COMPOUND
See *Acetaminophen, Antihistamines,* (chlorpheniramine maleate), *Caffeine, Hydrocodone Bitartrate,* and *Phenylephrine HCl.*

HYDANTOINS
(Dilantin, Mesantoin, Peganone)
See *Phenytoin.*
Similar interactions probably occur with all hydantoins.

HYDELTRA
See *Corticosteroids (prednisolone).*

HYDRALAZINE (Apresoline)
See *Antihypertensives.*

Amphetamines[421]
Amphetamines antagonize the hypotensive action of hydralazine.

Anesthetics[421]
Anesthetics potentiate the hypotensive action of hydralazine.

Antidepressants, tricyclic[421]
These antidepressants may affect the action of hydralazine. Adjust the dosage. May be contraindicated in some patients.

Diazoxide
See *Hydralazine* under *Diazoxide.*

Epinephrine[120,421]
Pressor response to epinephrine may be inhibited.

Ethacrynic acid[421] **(Edecrin)**
Ethacrynic acid potentiates the hypotensive action of hydralazine.

Guanethidine
See *Hydralazine* under *Guanethidine.*

Levarterenol[117]
Hydralazine reduces the pressor response to levarterenol.

MAO inhibitors[421]
MAO inhibitors such as nialamide may potentiate the vasodilator action of hydralazine but this has not been established in man. Monitor patients closely if this combination is used.

Pyridoxine[120]
Hydralazine has an antipyridoxine action and pyridoxine may be added to the regimen to relieve peripheral neuritis (numbness, tingling, etc.) if it develops.

Reserpine[1352]
The combination of reserpine and hydralazine is considerably more effective as an antihypertensive agent than reserpine alone in moderately severe hypertension.

Spironolactone[421]
Spironolactone enhances the hypotensive action of hydralazine.

Sympathomimetics[421]
Sympathomimetics antagonize the hypotensive action of hydralazine. Hydralazine reduces the pressor response to epinephrine.

Thiazide diuretics[421,633]
Thiazide diuretics potentiate the hypotensive action of hydralazine.

Tolbutamide
See *Hydralazine* under *Tolbutamide.*

Triamterene[421] **(Dyrenium)**
This diuretic potentiates the hypotensive action of hydralazine.

HYDREA (Hydroxyurea)

Iron salts[120]
Hydroxyurea delays plasma iron clearance and reduces the rate of iron utilization by erythrocytes.

HYDROCHLOROTHIAZIDE (Hydrodiuril)
See *Thiazide Diuretics.*

ACTH[120]
Hypokalemia may develop with this combination.

Alcohol[120]
Orthostatic hypotension with hydrochlorothiazide may be potentiated by alcohol. See *CNS Depressants.*

Antihypertensives, other[120]
Hydrochlorothiazide potentiates the action of other antihypertensive drugs; dosage of these agents, especially of the ganglionic blockers, should be reduced by at least 50% as soon as hydrochlorothiazide is added to the regimen.

HYDROCHLOROTHIAZIDE (Hydrodiuril)
(continued)

Barbiturates [120]
Orthostatic hypotension with hydrochlorothiazide may be potentiated by barbiturates.

Diazoxide [117,120] (Hyperstat)
Enhanced diabetogenic effect of diazoxide.

Glycyrrhiza [667] (Licorice)
Severe hypokalemia has been reported in a patient who consumed 30-40 Gm of licorice daily while maintained on hydrochlorothiazide. See *Antihypertensives* under *Glycyrrhiza*.

Insulin [120]
Insulin requirements in diabetic patients receiving hydrochlorothiazide may increase, decrease or remain unchanged.

Methyldopa [117,120]
Synergistic antihypertensive activity.

Narcotics [120,166]
Orthostatic hypotension with hydrochlorothiazide may be potentiated by narcotics. See *CNS Depressants*.

Norepinephrine [330,421] (Levarterenol, Levophed)
Hydrochlorothiazide decreases arterial responsiveness to norepinephrine.

Potassium salts [120]
Inflammation and stenosis of small intestine.

Quinethazone [120] (Hydromox)
Cross photosensitivity has occurred between quinethazone and hydrocholorothiazide.

Spironolactone [120] (Aldactone)
Facilitates management of hypertension. The two drugs act independently and additively in their antihypertensive effect, and spironolactone conserves potassium.

Steroids [120]
Hypokalemia may develop with the combination.

Triamterene [120,172] (Dyrenium)
Synergistic activity in diuresis and sodium excretion, with minimal potassium excretion; combination reduces hypokalemia and alkalosis produced by hydrochlorothiazide, and hyperkalemic metabolic acidosis produced by triamterene.

HYDROCORTISONE
(Cortef, Hydrocortone, Lipo-Adrenal Cortex, etc.)
See also *Corticosteroids*.

Anticonvulsants [78,330,450]
Anticonvulsants inhibit hydrocortisone.

Antihistamines [633]
The enzyme inducing antihistamines inhibit hydrocortisone.

Antirheumatic drugs [198,421]
Antirheumatic drugs displace hydrocortisone from protein binding and drive it into the tissues (mechanism of action).

Barbiturates [28,359,633]
Barbiturates (enzyme inducers) inhibit hydrocortisone (stimulation of 6-β-hydroxylation) and inhibit production of hydrocortisone (interference with ACTH production). Monitor patients closely since both exogenous and endogenous hydrocortisone are affected.

Butabarbital (Butisol, etc.)
See *Barbiturates* above.

Chlorcyclizine [198]
Chlorcyclizine (enzyme inducer) inhibits hydrocortisone.

Diphenhydramine [198] (Benadryl)
Diphenhydramine may decrease the steroid effect; enzyme induction increases hydroxylation of hydrocortisone.

Methandrostenolone [181] (Dianabol)
Methandrostenolone potentiates the anti-inflammatory activity of hydrocortisone.

Nortriptyline HCl [120,359] (Aventyl HCl)
Hydrocortisone notably inhibited the metabolism of nortriptyline in a patient who had taken an overdosage of this drug.

Phenobarbital [28,359]
See *Barbiturates* above.

Phenylbutazone [359]
Phenylbutazone inhibits hydrocortisone. It increases the urinary excretion of 6-*beta*-hydroxycortisol, a metabolite of hydrocortisone.

Phenytoin [28,198,359,633]
Phenytoin inhibits hydrocortisone. It increases the urinary excretion of 6-*beta*-hydroxycortisol, a metabolite of hydroxycortisone. A useful interaction in hyperadrenocorticism (Cushing's syndrome).

Propranolol [586]
Propranolol abolishes the anti-exudative effects of hydrocortisone.

HYDROCORTISONE SODIUM SUCCINATE (Solu-Cortef)
See *Hydrocortisone*.

HYDROCORTONE
See *Hydrocortisone*.

HYDRODIURIL
See *Thiazide Diuretics* (hydrochlorothiazide).

HYDROMOX
See *Diuretics* (quinethazone).

HYDROPRES
See *Thiazide Diuretics* (hydrochlorothiazide) and *Resperine*.

HYDROXYAMPHETAMINE (Paredrine)
See *Amphetamines*.

HYDROXYCHLOROQUINE (Plaquenil)

Gold compounds and other drugs known to cause sensitization and dermatitis. [120]
The drugs listed in Tables 9-9 to 9-18 should not be used concomitantly with antimalarial compounds such as hydroxychloroquine sulfate.

Hepatotoxic drugs [120]
Use with caution in patients receiving other drugs known to be hepatotoxic.

Phenylbutazone [120] (Butazolidin)
Phenylbutazone and other agents known to cause drug sensitization and dermatitis should not be given concurrently with hydroxychloroquine. See *Gold Compounds* above.

HYDROXYUREA (Hydrea)

Iron salts [120]
Hydroxyurea may delay the clearance of iron from the plasma and reduce the rate of iron utilization by erythrocytes.

HYDROXYZINE (Atarax, Vistaril)
See *Tranquilizers* and *CNS Depressants*.

Alcohol [121,711]
The CNS depressant effect of hydroxyzine and alcohol are potentiated.

Anticoagulants, oral[673]
Hydroxyzine potentiates the coumarin anticoagulants.

Barbiturates[120]
Hydroxyzine potentiates the CNS depressant effects of barbiturates. Reduce barbiturate dosage.

CNS depressants[120]
Hydroxyzine potentiates CNS depressants.

Heparin[764]
Large doses of hydroxyzine antagonize the anticoagulant effect of heparin.

HYDRYLLIN COMPOUND
See *Antihistamines, Aminophylline, Diphenhydramine,* and *Ephedrine.*

HYGROTON
See *Diuretics.*

HYOSCINE (Scopolamine)
See also *Solanaceous Alkaloids.*

Antihistamines[168]
Antihistamines with scopolamine produce an enhanced sedative effect. See *CNS Depressants.*

Methaqualone[4,5] **(Quaalude)**
The sedative action of methscopolamine may be prolonged by methaqualone.

Methotrimeprazine[120,1014]
Should be used with caution concomitantly in that tachycardia and fall in blood pressure may occur and undesirable CNS effects such as stimulation, delirium and extrapyramidal symptoms may be aggravated.

Morphine[951]
Synergistic hypnotic and narcotic activity.

Phenothiazine[120]
Phenothiazines with anticholinergic action may have additive effects with the anticholinergic solanaceous alkaloid hyoscine (blurred vision, constipation, dry mouth, impotence, urinary retention, etc.).

HYOSCYAMINE
See *Solanaceous Alkaloids.*
dl-Hyoscyamine is *Atropine* (see it also). *l*-Hyoscyamine is twice as active an antimuscarinic as atropine.

HYPERLOID
See *Rauwolfia Alkaloids.*

HYPERTENSIN
See *Vasopressor* (angiotensin amide).

HYPERURICEMICS
See under *Uricosuric Agents.*

HYPNOTICS AND SEDATIVES
See *CNS Depressants* and *Sedatives and Hypnotics.*

HYPOGLYCEMICS
See *Antidiabetics, Oral,* also *Insulin.*

HYPOSENSITIZATION THERAPY

Antihistamines[78]
Antihistamines interfere with evaluation of hyposensitization therapy.

HYPOTENSIVES
See *Antihypertensives.*

HYPTRAN TABLETS
See *Barbiturates* (secobarbital) and *Antihistamines* (phenyltoloxamine).

HYTAKEROL
See *Dihydrotachysterol.*

IBERET
See *Complex Supplements* and *Iron Salts.*

IBUPROFEN (Motrin)

Anticoagulants, oral
See *Ibuprofen* under *Anticoagulants, Oral.*

IDOXURIDINE (Stoxil)

Boric acid[120]
Boric acid should not be administered in the presence of idoxuridine antiviral ophthalmic solution since the combination may cause irritation.

Corticosteroids[120]
Corticosteroids can accelerate the spread of a viral infection such as herpes simplex keratitis; they should not be used in combination with idoxuridine unless absolutely necessary. After they are withdrawn idoxuridine therapy should be continued for a few days.

Other medications[120]
To insure stability do not mix idoxuridine ophthalmic solution with other medications.

ILETIN
See *Insulin.*

ILOPAN (with or without choline)
See *Dexpanthenol*

ILOSONE
See *Erythromycin*

ILOTYCIN
See *Erythromycin*

ILX PREPARATIONS
See *Complex Supplements.*

IMFERON
See *Iron Dextran*

IMIPRAMINE (Tofranil)
See *Antidepressants, Tricyclic*

Acidifying agents[165]
Acidifying agents do not significantly alter the rate of urinary excretion of imipramine.

Alcohol[167]
Imipramine increases alcohol narcosis. A lethal combination.

Alkalinizing agents[165]
Alkalinizing agents do not significantly alter the rate of urinary excretion of imipramine.

***dl*-Amphetamine**[424]
Imipramine potentiates augmentation in rate produced by amphetamines in operant conditioning situations.

Anticholinergic drugs[120] **(Atropine, etc.)**
Anticholinergic (atropinelike) effects of both may become more pronounced (paralytic ileus). Adjust doses carefully.

Antidepressants, tricyclic[120]
Other tricyclic antidepressants may potentiate imipramine (additive) and cross-hypersensitivity may occur.

Antihypertensives[78,120]
Imipramine inhibits hypotensive agents like guanethidine. See *Antidepressants, Tricyclic* under *Guanethidine.*

Antiparkinsonism drugs[120,194]
Anticholinergic (atropinelike) effects may become more pronounced (paralytic ileus). Adjust doses carefully.

IMIPRAMINE (Tofranil) *(continued)*

Aspirin[48]
Possible synergism. May be fatal.

Atropine
See *Anticholinergic* Drugs above.

Barbiturates[599]
Imipramine potentiates CNS depressant effects and prolongs hexobarbital sleeping time.

Carisoprodol[599] **(Rela, Soma)**
Imipramine potentiates the action of carisoprodol.

Chlordiazepoxide[120] **(Librium)**
Additive or superadditive effects may occur with chlordiazepoxide.

Diazepam[94,120] **(Valium)**
Additive or superadditive effects may occur with diazepam.

Dibenzazepines[120] **(Tricyclic antidepressants)**
Cross-hypersensitivity to other dibenzazepine compounds is possible.

Guanethidine[28,327,341,417,594,597,626]
Imipramine inhibits the antihypertensive effect of guanethidine and similar agents. Guanethidine antagonizes the antidepressants.

Hexobarbital[599]
See *Barbiturates* above.

Histamine[166]
Imipramine blocks the spasmogenic effects of histamine on the ileum (guinea pig).

Isocarboxazid (Marplan)
See *MAO Inhibitors* below.

Levarterenol (Levophed)
See *Norepinephrine* below.

MAO inhibitors[53,218,251,756,828-830]
Concurrent use of MAO inhibitors with imipramine may result in central adrenergic signs such as severe anxiety, profuse sweating, hyperexcitation or coma, and serious or fatal hyperpyretic crisis or fatal convulsive seizures. A minimum interval of 14 days should elapse between therapy with a MAO inhibitor and imipramine. Use low doses with the new therapy.

Meperidine[194,421] **(Demerol)**
Imipramine enhances the respiratory depression produced by meperidine, and potentiates the adverse effects (increased ocular pressure and mydriatic effect) of meperidine in glaucoma.

Meprobamate[599]
Imipramine potentiates the actions of meprobamate.

Methylphenidate[194] **(Ritalin)**
Methylphenidate slows the metabolism of imipramine and thus has a potentiating effect.

Morphine[166]
Additive effect with morphine. Depressant action of morphine and related narcotics are exaggerated and prolonged.

Nialamide (Niamid)
See *MAO Inhibitors* above.

Norepinephrine[166,169,232] **(Levarterenol)**
Imipramine blocks uptake of administered norepinephrine which results in supersensitization to the catecholamine.

Oxyphenbutazone[85] **(Tandearil)**
Imipramine apparently inhibits oxyphenbutazone by reducing its gastrointestinal absorption.

Pargyline[829] **(Eutonyl)**
Dangerous potentiation. See *MAO Inhibitors* above.

Pentobarbital[599]
See *Barbiturates* above.

Phenelzine (Nardil)
Phenelzine potentiates imipramine; possibly fatal. See *MAO Inhibitors* above.

Phenylbutazone[85] **(Butazolidin)**
Imipramine apparently reduces the gastrointestinal absorption of phenylbutazone.

Procarbazine[619] **(Matulane)**
See *MAO Inhibitors* above.

Reserpine[633]
Reserpine may cause mental depression and affect activity of imipraminelike drugs. It could be highly toxic, if not fatal, in patients receiving these tricyclic drugs. Such toxicities are seldom observed, probably because of the relatively small doses of reserpine given to man. See *Polymechanistic Drugs* (page 378).

Salicylates[48]
A potentially lethal combination.

Sympathomimetics[194,424,541]
Imipramine potentiates sympathomimetics. Great caution is mandatory, particularly in narrow-angle glaucoma.

Thiopental[116] **(Pentothal)**
See *Barbiturates* above.

Thyroid medications[120,456,670,671,934,1337,1486,1715,1901]
Imipramine must be given with caution to patients who are taking thyroid medication; cardiac arrhythmias may occur. T_3 (L-triiodothyronine) increases receptor sensitivity and enhances imipramine antidepressant acitivity. See also *Antidepressants, Tricyclic* under *Thyroid Preparations*.

Tranquilizers[619] **(Meprobomate type)**
The meprobamate tranquilizers are potentiated by the imipramine group of drugs.

Tranylcypromine (Parnate)
See *MAO Inhibitors* above.

Triiodothyronine[456] **(Cytomel)**
The speed and efficacy of imipramine in the treatment of clinical depression was enhanced by the addition of triiodothyronine to the treatment program. See also *Thyroid Medications* above.

IMMUNOSUPPRESSANTS
See *Antineoplastics, Corticosteroids, Diphenylhydantoin,* and *Immunosuppressants* under *Vaccines*

INAPSINE
See *Droperidol.*

INDERAL
See *Propranolol.*

INDOCIN
See *Analgesics* and *Indomethacin.*

INDOMETHACIN (Indocin)
See also *Analgesics*

Antacids[1397]
Antacids may delay by as much as 50% the peak serum levels of indomethacin.

Antibiotics[120]
Indomethacin should be used with extra caution in the presence of existing controlled infections because it may mask the signs and symptoms of infection.

Anticoagulants, oral
See *Anti-inflammatory Agents* under *Anticoagulants, Oral.*

Aspirin[708]
Aspirin inhibits the anti-inflammatory effect of indomethacin. See also *Salicylates* below.

Chicken pox[1594]
Same reaction with this disease as with smallpox vaccine below.

Corticosteroids[1396]
Indomethacin probably displaces corticosteroids from their plasma-protein binding sites and thereby potentiates them. Ulcerogenic effect is potentiated. Monitor patients closely for ulcer formation.

Cortisone
Indomethacin potentiates cortisone. See *Corticosteroids* above.

Coumarin anticoagulants
See *Anticoagulants, Oral* above.

Phenylbutazone (Butazolidin)
Administration of phenylbutazone and indomethacin concomitantly potentiates their ulcerogenic effect.

Probenecid[421,1048,1397] **(Benemid)**
Probenecid may dangerously potentiate the analgesic effect of indomethacin by inhibiting renal excretion which produces an elevation of blood levels and increases the half life of the anti-inflammatory agent. The latter does not appear to affect the uricosuric activity of probenecid. A combination that may be desirable if dosage is carefully adjusted.

Propranolol
See *Indomethacin* under *Propranolol*.

Pyrazolone derivatives[421]
Pyrazolone derivatives potentiate the analgesic effect of indomethacin by displacing it from protein binding sites.

Salicylates[120,708,1284] **(Aspirin, etc.)**
Both indomethacin and salicylates have an ulcerogenic effect on the gastric mucosa and their combined use may therefore be especially dangerous, even fatal. Aspirin interferes with the gastrointestinal absorption of indomethacin, increases its fecal excretion, and tends to decrease its efficacy. However, aspirin appears to prolong the serum half-life of indomethacin and thus potentiates drug that is absorbed.

Smallpox vaccine[1594]
Indomethacin may increase the severity of reactions to smallpox vaccination, including the production of hemorrhage.

Thyroid medication[120]
Indomethacin with thyroid medication increases the potential for cardiovascular toxicity.

INFLAMASE
See *Prednisolone*.

INNOVAR
See *Droperidol, Fentanyl* and *Narcotics*.

INSECTICIDES, CHLORINATED
See *Halogenated Insecticides*.

INSECTICIDES, ORGANOPHOSPHORUS
See also *Anticholinesterases* and *Halogenated Insecticides*.

Muscle relaxants, polarizing[198]
Anticholinesterase (organophosphorus) insecticides antagonize competitive blocking muscle relaxants. See *Contraindicated Drugs* and *Muscle Relaxants* under *Anticholinesterases*.

Phenothiazines[120]
Phenothiazines may enhance the toxic effects of organophosphorus insecticides.

Thioxanthenes[120] **(Taractan, etc.)**
Thioxanthenes may enhance the toxic effects of organophosphorus insecticides.

INSULIN
See *Antidiabetics, Oral*.
Insulin secretion is inhibited by a number of drugs (diazoxide, epinephrine, thiozide diuretics, etc.) and stimulated by others (glucagon, glucose, sulfonylureas, theophylline, etc.).[1571]

α-Adrenergic blockers[168,1992] **(Phentolamine, etc.)**
Adrenergic blockade restores insulin response to glucose after stress and has a hypoglycemic effect in juvenile diabetes (probably antagonizes adrenergic suppression of insulin release).

β-Adrenergic blockers[421] **(Inderal, etc.)**
β-Adrenergic blockers increase the activity of insulin and mask the symptoms of serious hypoglycemia. See also *Propranolol* below.

Alcohol[23]
See *Insulin* under *Alcohol*.

Aminophylline[1156]
See effect of aminophylline on plasma insulin levels under *Aminophylline* in the section on *Propranolol*.

Anabolic steroids[120,191]
The steroids potentiate the hypoglycemic effect of insulin.

Anticoagulants, oral[120] **(Coumadin, Dicumarol, Panwarfin, Sintrom, etc.)**
The anticoagulants potentiate the hypoglycemic effect of insulin.

Antidiabetics, oral[421] **(Diabinese, Dymelor, Orinase, Tolinase, etc.)**
Insulin potentiates the hypoglycemic effect of oral antidiabetic compounds.

Antineoplastics[120]
Antineoplastics may induce hypoglycemia by liberating insulin from binding sites.

Atenolol (Tenormin)
See *Propranolol* below.

Beta-adrenergic blocking agents
See *β-Adrenergic Blockers* above.

Biguanides[421] **(DBI, etc.)**
Biguanides potentiate the hypoglycemic effect of insulin.

Chlorthalidone[120] **(Hygroton)**
Chlorthalidone antagonizes the hypoglycemic effect of insulin; hyperglycemia.

Corticosteroids[181]
Corticosteroids antagonize the hypoglycemic effect of insulin; hyperglycemia.

Dextrothyroxine[120] **(Choloxin)**
Dextrothyroxine antagonizes the hypoglycemic effect of insulin; hyperglycemia.

Diuretics[120]
Thiazide diuretics, which tend to be diabetogenic, antagonize the hypoglycemic effect of insulin; hyperglycemia may occur also. Insulin requirements in diabetic patients receiving thiazide diuretics may be increased, decreased, or remain unchanged.

Epinephrine[549,805] **(Adrenalin)**
Insulin modifies the cardiac and hyperglycemic effects of epinephrine. Epinephrine may inhibit the hypoglycemic effect of insulin.

INSULIN *(continued)*

Furazolidone (Furoxone)
See *MAO Inhibitors* below.

Furosemide [120] (Lasix)
Furosemide may induce hyperglycemia. The insulin requirements of a controlled diabetic may have to be increased.

Glucagon [181,421] (Hyperglycemic factor)
Glucagon in large doses stimulates insulin secretion, but in small doses promotes glycogenolysis and glyconeogenesis. It is therefore used to counteract hypoglycemia induced by insulin.

Isocarboxazid (Marplan)
See *MAO Inhibitors* below.

Isoniazid [178,330]
Isoniazid potentiates the hypoglycemic effect of insulin. However, large doses of isoniazid antagonize the hypoglycemic action of insulin by elevating blood sugar levels.

Levothyroxine [120] (Letter, Synthroid, etc.)
Diabetic patients may require an increased dosage of insulin with thyroid preparations. See *Thyroid Preparations*.

MAO inhibitors [78,86-89,162,330,421,1134]
A hazardous combination. MAO inhibitors of the hydrazine variety potentiate the hypoglycemic activity of sulfonylureas by interfering with homeostatic adrenergic mechanisms and they may significantly potentiate and prolong insulin-induced hypoglycemia. Tranylcypromine but not the other MAOIs may cause a 20-fold rise in plasma insulin (in mice), depresses liver glycogen, and inhibits conversion of lactate to glucose, and thus causes a profound hypoglycemia. Both phenelzine and pargyline lower insulin blood levels (but not by MAO inhibition) and abolish the rise in insulin levels that usually follows glucose administered to fasting subjects (in rats). Probably pancreatic insulin secretion is inhibited as well as release to the blood by accumulation of biogenic amines (epinephrine, serotonin) in the β-cells by MAO inhibition. Nonhydrazine MAO inhibitors do not potentiate the hypoglycemic effect of insulin, but, like the hydrazines, greatly delay the time of recovery. Thus, when using a MAO inhibitor in a diabetic, the dose of the antidiabetic drug should be carefully regulated.

Mebanazine
See *MAO Inhibitors* above.

Methamphetamine [120] (Desoxyn, Methedrine, etc.)
Methamphetamine plus insulin induces lower blood glucose levels than insulin alone. Amphetamines may increase the metabolic rate and also plasma corticosteroids and immunoreactive growth hormone both of which impair glucose tolerance.

Methotrexate [120]
Antineoplastics may potentiate insulin and cause hypoglycemia by displacement of the bound hormone.

Oral contraceptives [181]
Oral contraceptives may increase blood sugar levels and decrease glucose tolerance.

Oxyphenbutazone [120] (Tnadearil)
Oxyphenbutazone may potentiate the hypoglycemic action of insulin.

Pargyline (Eutonyl)
See *MAO Inhibitors* above.

Penelzine (Nardil)
See *MAO Inhibitors* above.

Phentolamine [1992]
See *Antidiabetics* under *Phentolamine* for effectiveness of α-adrenergic blockade in juvenile diabetics.

Phenylbutazone [120] (Butazolidin)
Phenylbutazone potentiates the hypoglycemic effect of insulin.

Phenylpropanolamine [549] (Propadrine)
Phenylpropanolamine may oppose the action of insulin and thus potentiates it.

Phenyramidol [951] (Analexin)
Phenyramidol slows rate of metabolism of insulin.

Phenytoin [1957]
Phenytoin, by inhibiting insulin secretion, may cause a severe hyperglycemia, possibly progressing to hyperosmolar nonketotic coma.

Procarbazine [330] (Matulan)
See *MAO Inhibitors* above.

Propranolol [263,681] (Inderal)
Propranolol potentiates insulin; a prolonged hypoglycemic reaction can occur because rebound of plasma glucose levels is inhibited (propranolol-induced suppression of blood glucose recovery rate). See also *Antidiabetics* under *Propranolol*. The new selective β_1-blocking drugs like atenolol (Tenormin), specifically produce only β_1-adrenergic antagonism and are free of the prolonging effect on insulin-induced hypoglycemia. Atenolol does not impair blood glucose recovery (hepatic glycogenolysis, gluconeogenesis, decreased peripheral glucose).

Pyrazinamide [619] (Aldinamide)
Diabetes mellitus may be more difficult to control during therapy with pyrazinamide because the dose of insulin in patients on this tuberculostatic drug is altered.

Salicylates [421]
Salicylates potentiate the hypoglycemic effect of insulin.

Sulfinpyrazone [120] (Anturane)
Sulfinpyrazone may potentiate the hypoglycemic effect of insulin.

Sulfonamides [120]
Sulfonamides enhance the hypoglycemic effect of insulin.

Sulfonylureas [421]
Sulfonylureas potentiate the hypoglycemic effect of insulin.

Sympathomimetics [549,805]
See *Epinephrine* above.

Thiazide diuretics [120]
(Anhydron, Aquatag, Diuril, Methahydron, Saluron, Renese, etc.)
These diuretics inhibit the hypoglycemic effect of insulin and its requirements may therefore be increased in some patients, but in others insulin requirements may be decreased or unchanged.

Thyroid preparations [120]
Thryoid hormones may increase the required dosages of insulin and oral hypoglycemic agents. Decreasing the dose of thyroid hormone may possibly cause hypoglycemic reactions if the dosage of insulin or the oral agents is not adjusted.

Tranylcypromine (Parnate)
See *MAO Inhibitors* above.

INTERACTIONS *IN VITRO*
See *Incompatibilities* (page 355), Chapter 7 on Clinical Laboratory Testing Errors, and IV Additive Problems in Chapter 8.

INTERFERON

Puromycin [951]
Interferon inhibits the antiviral activity of puromycin.

INTRAMUSCULAR INJECTIONS

Heparin
See *Parenteral Drugs* under *Heparin*.

INTROPIN
See *Dopamine*.

INULIN

EDTA[951]
EDTA increases the absorption rate of inulin.

INVERSENE
See *Antihypertensives* (mecamylamine).

IN VITRO INTERACTIONS
See *Chapters 7 and 8 and page 355*.

IODIDES

Lithium carbonate
See *Potassium Iodide* under *Lithium Carbonate*.

IODINE

Estrogens
Estrogens increase protein bound iodine. See Chapter 7.

Progesterones
Progesterones increase protein bound iodine. See Chapter 7.

Radioiodine[54]
Patients, euthyroid after radioiodine treatment, become hypothyroid when given small doses of iodine. A defect in organic binding induced by radioiodine may further enhance susceptibility to iodide myxedema.

IODOPYRACET (Diodrast)

Probenecid[120] (Benemid)
Probenecid inhibits the urinary excretion of iodopyracet and thus elevates its blood levels.

IOPHENOXIC ACID (Teridax)
Sulfonamides[21,202,359]
Iophenoxic acid displaces certain weakly bound sulfonamides from their protein binding sites and thereby potentiates them and enhances their toxicity.

IPRONIAZID
See *MAO Inhibitors*.

IRON SALTS
(Ferrous bromide, carbonate, fumarate, gluconate, iodide, lactate, sulfate, etc.)

Allopurinol[120,421]
Allopurinol may increase hepatic iron concentration. Iron salts should not be given simultaneously. Hemosiderosis may be caused when allopurinol blocks the enzyme that metabolizes iron.

Antacids[28]
Antacids containing carbonates inhibit the absorption of iron by forming insoluble iron carbonate.

Asorbic acid
See *Vitamin C* below.

Cereals[28]
Phytic acid in cereals forms a complex with iron which prevents its absorption.

Cholestyramine
See *Iron Salts* under *Cholestyramine*.

Dimercaprol[619,926]
Dimercaprol increases the toxicity of ferrous sulfate and other iron salts (toxic iron chelate formed).

Eggs[359]
Eggs can inhibit the absorption of iron.

Estrogen-progestogens (Oral contraceptives)
Estrogens and progestogens increase protein bound iron. See Chapter 7.

Hydroxyurea[120] (Hydrea)
Hydroxyurea may delay the clearance of iron from the plasma and reduce the rate of iron utilization by erythrocytes.

Magnesium trisilicate[928]
Magnesium trisilicate inhibits the absorption of iron.

Milk[120]
Milk reduces the absorption of iron salts.

Pancreatic extracts[1325]
Pancreatic enzymes, extracts and other preparations may inhibit the intestinal absorption of iron and decrease its effectiveness.

Tetracyclines[48,198,421,665]
Iron salts may interfere with the absorption of tetracyclines. See *Complexing Agents* under *Tetracyclines*.

Vitamin C[180,1963] (Ascorbic acid)
Vitamin C in doses of 1 Gm. or more facilitates absorption of ferrous iron. In anemic patients desired iron blood levels are reached more rapidly.

Vitamin E[1616]
Vitamin E may decrease the therapeutic efficacy of iron preparations in patients with iron deficiency anemia.

ISMELIN
See *Guanethidine*.

ISOCARBOXAZID (Marplan)
See *MAO Inhibitors*.

ISOETHARINE (Bronkometer, Dilabron)
See *Sympathomimetics*.
The β-adrenergic receptor activity of this bronchodilator should alert the prescriber to the interactions and precautions given for drugs like epinephrine and isoproterenol.

ISOFEDROL
See *Ephedrine*.

ISONIAZID (INH, Niconyl, Nydrazid, etc.)
See also *Antituberculosis Drugs*.

Adrenergics[202,619]
Additive CNS stimulation. Aggravated side effects.

Alcohol[28,1631]
Chronic use of alcohol decreases the half-life of isoniazid and, therefore, inhibits its action. Alcoholics metabolize isoniazid more rapidly than those who seldom drink. Also, INH through enzyme inhibition, may tend to produce a disulfiram type of intolerance to alcohol.

p-Aminosalicylic acid[202,619] (PAS)
PAS increases and prolongs the blood levels of isoniazid because of competition for the same pathway of excretion and thus potentiates the antitubercular effect. Combined use may induce hemolytic anemia.

Anesthetics[330]
Isoniazid potentiates anesthetics.

Antacids, oral[1500]
Aluminum hydroxide gel (Amphojel) and magaldrate (Riopan) decrease gastrointestinal absorption of isoniazid, possibly due to delayed gastric emptying time. Give INH at least an hour prior to an antacid. For some unknown reason this interaction may be reversed in an alcoholic.

ISONIAZID (INH, Niconyl, Nydrazid, etc.)
(continued)

Anticoagulants, oral [421]
Isoniazid may potentiate coumarin anticoagulants.

Anticonvulsants [202,333,789]
Isoniazid inhibits the metabolism of anticonvulsants and thereby potentiates them.

Antidiabetics [178,191,330]
Isoniazid in very large doses antagonizes the hypoglycemic effect of oral hypoglycemics but in small doses may potentiate these drugs by enzyme inhibition.

Antihypertensives [330]
Isoniazid potentiates antihypertensives.

Antiparkinsonism drugs [330]
Isoniazid potentiates antiparkinsonism drugs.

Atropine [619,633]
Isoniazid has an additive anticholinergic effect with atropine. Hazardous in glaucoma.

Cycloserine
See *Isoniazid* under *Cycloserine*.

Disulfiram [718,1433,1757,1884]
This combination (disulfiram plus isoniazid), by increasing the metabolism of brain catecholamines such as dopamine through inhibition of the enzymes beta-hydroxylase (by disulfiram) and MAO (by isoniazid) followed by enhanced dopamine metabolism with catecholamine-O-methyltransferase to produce elevated levels of dopamine metabolites such as norepinephrine) can cause coordination difficulties and changes in behavior, with a variety of neurological symptoms. Avoid concomitant use of these drugs.

Insulin [178,330]
Large doses of isoniazid antagonize the hypoglycemic effect of insulin by elevating blood sugar levels. In lower doses isoniazid may potentiate the hypoglycemic effect of insulin.

Meperidine [120,619,1206,1884] (Demerol)
Meperidine and isoniazid combined result in increased side effects. MAO inhibition by isoniazid may be a factor. Hazardous in glaucoma.

Narcotics [330]
Isoniazid potentiates narcotics.

Penicillamine [421]
Penicillamine potentiates isoniazid.

Phenobarbital [178,333]
Excessive sedation is produced by this combination.

Phenytoin [28,178,192,333,359,789,916,919]
Isoniazid potentiates phenytoin by inhibition of metabolizing enzymes (*p*-hydroxylation inhibited). Excessive sedation and toxic effects may be induced. Increased likelihood of thromboembolism, especially in slow acetylators. Death has occurred. See also *Isoniazid* under *Phenytoin*.

Pyridoxine [178,619,880]
Pyridoxine reduces the neurotoxicity (peripheral neuritis) caused by isoniazid but in large doses may antagonize the tuberculostatic activity.

Reserpine [831]
Isoniazid inhibits reserpine.

Rifampin [178,1306,1564]
(Rifadin, Rifomycin, Rimactine, Rimactazid)
Isoniazid, probably through MAO inhibition, tends to potentiate the toxicity of rifampin but shortens its half-life because of increased biliary excretion of acetylated product in the enterohepatic cycle. The combination may be hepototoxic. Monitor patients closely, especially those with liver impairment and those who are slow metabolizers of isoniazid. One report, however, notes that rifampin, although it tends to be hepatotoxic, was given to an alcoholic being treated with disulfiram, and isoniazid also was given. Although both of the latter drugs interfere with hepatic enzymes no untoward hepatic effects were observed.

Sedatives [330]
Isoniazid potentiates sedatives.

Streptomycin [120]
Isoniazid and streptomycin have synergistic activity against tuberculosis.

Sulfonamides [443]
The combination may give rise to an acute, hemolytic anemia.

Sympathomimetics [619,1206,1884]
Isoniazid potentiates sympathomimetics, probably through MAO inhibition and sympathomimetics increase the side effects of isoniazid.

Tricyclic antidepressants [330]
Isoniazid potentiates tricyclic antidepressants.

Vitamin B complex
See *Pyridoxine* above.

ISOPRENALINE (Isuprel)
See *Isoproterenol*.

ISOPROPAMIDE IODIDE
See *Anticholinergics* under *MAO Inhibitors*, and *Darbid*.

ISOPROTERENOL (Isuprel)
See also *Sympathomimetics*.

Adrenergics [313,370]
Isoproterenol potentiates the bronchial relaxation produced by adrenergics. Lethal with epinephrine.

Antidepressants, tricyclic [94]
The severe hypotension produced by overdosage of a tricyclic antidepressant such as imipramine or its active metabolite desipramine may be reversed with isoproterenol.

Digitalis [16]
Isoproterenol is contraindicated in tachycardia caused by digitalis intoxication. Puzzling arrhythmias may arise with this combination.

Epinephrine [6,120,185,313,370,693]
This combination has been lethal in the treatment of asthma or has caused serious arrhythmias. These cardiac stimulants may be administered alternately. See under *Epinephrine*.

Isoproterenol [155] (when used too frequently)
This is a drug interaction between doses of one drug. Isoproterenol is converted to 3-methoxyisoproterenol by catechol 0-methyl transferase of the liver and the lung. The metabolite is a beta-adrenergic blocking agent (antagonist) and produces the reverse effect of isoproterenol which is used in asthma because it is a beta-adrenergic agonist.

MAO inhibitors [136,162,184,211,217,289,431]
This combination may induce an acute hypertensive crisis with possible intracranial hemorrhage, hyperthermia, convulsions, coma and in some cases death. The metabolism of the monoamine is blocked causing its accumulation. This prolongs and potentiates release of norepinephrine from peripheral stores. This release and the central additive stimulation causes the hypertensive crisis.

Prenylamine [170] (Segontin)
Prenylamine antagonizes isoproterenol and may reverse the pressor action of the amine.

Propranolol (Inderal)
See *Isoproterenol* under *Propranolol*.

Sympathomimetics [6,48,185,547]
Isoproterenol, a β-adrenergic agonist, enhances the bronchial dilating effect of other sympathomimetics.

ISOSORBIDE DINITRATE (Isordil)
See *Nitrates and Nitrites.*

β-Adrenergic blockers [421]
β-Adrenergic blocking agents potentiate isosorbide dinitrate (synergistic effects) when treating angina pectoris. See *Propranolol* below.

Acetylcholine [120]
These are physiological antagonists.

Alcohol [120]
Alcohol enhances the sensitivity of the patient to the hypotensive effects (nausea, vomiting, weakness, restlessness, pallor, perspiration, and collapse).

Histamine [120]
These are physiological antagonists.

Isosorbide dinitrate [120] (Isordil)
Tolerance develops with repeated use.

Nitrates and nitrites [120]
Cross tolerance may occur with nitrites and other nitrates.

Norepinephrine [120] (Levophed)
These are physiological antagonists.

Propranolol [120]
Synergistic effects in treating angina pectoris have been reported; however, the potential benefit of using these agents in combination has been disputed.

ISUFRANOL
See *Barbiturates* (phenobarbital), *Sympathomimetics* (benzylephedrine, isoproterenol) and *Xanthines* (theophylline).

ISUPREL
See *Sympathomimetics* (isoproterenol).

KANAMYCIN SULFATE (Kantrex)
See also *Neuromuscular Blocking Antibiotics* under *Antibiotics.*

Alkalinizing agents [578]
Alkaline urinary pH potentiates kanamycin by enhancing antimicrobial activity.

Amobarbital [360]
This combination of antibiotic and barbiturate enhances the neuromuscular blockade and induces apnea and muscle weakness.

Anesthetics [749]
Neuromuscular paralysis with apnea and respiratory depression may occur when kanamycin sulfate is injected concomitantly with anesthetics.

Antibiotics, other [120,250] (Neomycin, streptomycin, polymyxin, viomycin, etc.)
With certain other antibiotics, the ototoxic and neuromuscular blocking effects may be additive. See under *Antibiotics.*

Anticholinesterases [178] (Prostigmin, etc.)
Anticholinesterases antagonize the curarelike effects of kanamycin (reverses neuromuscular block).

Calcium salts [178,494-498]
Calcium salts inhibit the neuromuscular blockade induced by kanamycin.

Cephalothin [252,253] (Keflin)
Synergistic activity in treatment of multiple antibiotic-resistant and methicillin-resistant *Staph. aureus* and of *E. coli* infections.

Cephalosporins [210,252,253]
Synergistic antibacterial effect on *E. coli* and resistant *Staph. aureus.*

Colistimethate (Coly-Mycin)
See *Ototoxic Drugs* below and *Neuromuscular Blocking Antibiotics* under *Antibiotics.*

Curariform muscle relaxants and other neurotoxic drugs [250,832]
Contraindicated for concurrent use. See *Muscle Relaxants* below.

Dimenhydrinate [120] (Dramamine)
Dimenhydrinate may mask ototoxic symptoms of the aminoglycoside antibiotic. Extra alertness is essential to detect the side effect.

Diuretics [120,250]
Kanamycin plus potent diuretics such as ethacrynic acid, particularly IV, cause rapid and irreversible deafness.

Edrophonium chloride [421] (Tensilon)
Edrophonium antagonizes kanamycin; (reverses neuromuscular block).

EDTA [360]
Edetates may enhance absorption and produce apnea and muscle weakness.

Ethacrynic acid (Edecrin)
Concurrent use may cause rapid and sometimes irreversible deafness. See *Aminoglycoside Antibiotics* under *Ethacrynic Acid.*

Gallamine [832]
See *Muscle Relaxants* below.

Gentamicin [178] (Garamycin)
Contraindicated. Same as for *Colistimethate* above.

Kanamycin [120] (Kantrex)
The ototoxic and neuromuscular effects of kanamycin may be additive. See *Ototoxic Drugs* below.

Mannitol [813]
This combination may cause deafness.

Methicillin [210,239]
Mutual inactivation in IV mixtures. See Chapter 7. Antagonism in some infections; potentiation in others.

Methoxyflurane (Penthrane)
See under *Methoxyflurane.*

Muscle relaxants [120,178,250,832] (Decamethonium, ether, gallamine, sodium citrate, succinylcholine, tubocurarine, etc.)
Kanamycin has a curarelike effect and potentiates neuromuscular blockade by muscle relaxants and other neuromuscular blocking drugs. See also *Neuromuscular Blocking Antibiotics* under *Antibiotics.* Neuromuscular paralysis with apnea and respiratory depression may occur when kanamycin is injected concomitantly.

Neomycin
See *Ototoxic Drugs* below.

Neostigmine [178,494-498,656]
Neostigmine reduces neuromuscular blockade by kanamycin.

Organophosphate cholinesterase inhibitors [178]
Cholinesterase inhibitors antagonize neuromuscular blocking effects of kanamycin.

Other neurotoxic or nephrotoxic drugs [120]
Additive effects. See *Ototoxic Drugs* below.

Ototoxic drugs [120,250]
The major toxic effect of parenteral kanamycin is deafness produced by its action on the auditory portion of the 8th nerve. Concurrent use of other ototoxic or nephrotoxic drugs, particularly the antibiotics gentamicin, neomycin, polymyxins B and E (colistin), streptomycin, and viomicin, and the diuret-

KANAMYCIN SULFATE (Kantrex) *(continued)*
ics ethacrynic acid and furosemide may cause bilateral, irreversible (reversible with furosemide) deafness and should be avoided. Prior administration of kanamycin or other ototoxic agents which may have induced subclinical damage to the 8th nerve may contraindicate use of kanamycin.

Penicillins [210,239]
Penicillin bactericidal activity is often inhibited by bacteriostatic antibiotics such as kanamycin but against some organisms kanamycin may potentiate pencillins. See *Antibiotics* under *Penicillin.*

Polymyxins B and E
See *Ototoxic Drugs* above.

Potent diuretics [120] **(Ethacrynic acid)**
Kanamycin plus potent diuretics such as ethacrynic acid, particularly IV, may cause rapid and irreversible deafness.

Procainamide [619]
Procainamide may increase the neuromuscular blocking action of kanamycin and produce apnea and muscle weakness. A potentially hazardous combination.

Promethazine [360] **(Phenergan)**
Promethazine enhances the neuromuscular blockade produced by kanamycin and thus induces apnea and muscle weakness.

Sodium citrate [120]
See *Muscle Relaxants* above.

Quinidine [447,559]
Quinidine may increase the neuromuscular blocking action of kanamycin and produce apnea and muscle weakness. A potentially hazardous combination.

Streptomycin
See *Ototoxic Drugs* above.

Succinylcholine
See *Muscle Relaxants* above.
d-**Tubocurarine**
See *Muscle Relaxants* above.

Viomycin
See *Ototoxic Drugs* above.

KANTREX SULFATE
See *Kanamycin.*

KANUMODIC
See *Complex Digestants,* also *Glutamic Acid, Hyoscine,* and *Barbiturates* (pentobarbital).

KAOCHLOR LIQUID
See *Potassium Salts* (KCl).

KAOLIN

Lincomycin [330,1108] **(Lincocin)**
Kaolin inhibits absorption of lincomycin just as for *Pseudoephedrine* below.

Pseudoephedrine [1589] **(Sudafed)**
Kaolin, through its adsorptive action, inhibits the intestinal absorption of some drugs, such as ephedrine and pseudoephedrine, and may inhibit their therapeutic effectiveness significantly in some patients under some conditions of dosage.

KAON ELIXIR OR TABLETS
See *Potassium Salts* (K gluconate).

KATO
See *Potassium Salts* (KCl).

KAY CIEL
See *Potassium Salts* (KCl).

KAYEXALATE
(Sodium polystyrene sulfonate)

Digitalis [120]
Potassium deficiency may occur and in patients with lowered potassium blood levels, the action of digitalis, particularly its toxicity, is likely to be exaggerated.

K-CILLIN
See *Penicillin.*

KEFLIN
See *Cephalothin.*

KEMADRIN
See *Anticholinergics,* and *Antiparkinsonism Drugs* (procyclidine HCl).

KENACORT
See *Triamcinolone.*

KENALOG
See *Triamcinolone* (acetonide).

KESSO-BAMATE
See *Meprobamate.*

KESSODANTEN
See *Phenytoin.*

KESSODRATE
See *Chloral Hydrate.*

KESSO-PEN
See *Penicillin.*

KESSO-TETRA
See *Tetracycline.*

KETAMINE (Ketajet, Ketalar)

Thyroid
See *Ketamine* under *Thyroid Preparations.*

17-KETOGENIC STEROIDS

Phenothiazines
Drug enters into color-forming reaction and may falsely elevate 17-KS determination. See Chapter 7.

KIE
See *Ephedrine, Iodides* (KI) and *Potassium Salts.*

K-LYTE
See *Potassium Salts.*

KOLANTYL
See *Aluminum Salts* (hydroxide), *Antacids,* and *Magnesium Salts* (hydroxide).

KONAKION
See *Vitamin K* (phytonadione).

K-PEN
See *Penicillin.*

K-PHOS
See *Acidifying Agents* and *Potassium Salts* (KH_2PO_4).

K-10
See *Potassium Salts* (KCl).

KUDROX TABLETS
See *Aluminum Salts* (hydroxide), *Antacids,* and *Magnesium Salts* (carbonate).

LANOXIN
See *Digitalis* (digoxin).

LARGON
See *Propiomazine*.

LASIX
See *Diuretics* and *Furosemide*.

LAUD-IRON TABLETS
See *Iron Salts* (ferrous fumarate).

LAXATIVES

Digitalis[28] and its glycosides
Laxatives may decrease digitalis action (reduced absorption due to rapid passage through the gut). However, laxative-induced hypokalemia increases the toxicity of absorbed digitalis.

Mecamylamine[120] (Inversine)
Laxatives overcome the constipation caused by mecamylamine which could lead to paralytic ileus, but do not use bulk laxatives.

LEAFY GREEN VEGETABLES

Anticoagulants, oral[147,880]
Large amounts of leafy green vegetables decrease the anticoagulant effect of oral anticoagulants.

LEDERCILLIN VK
See *Penicillin*.

LEDPERPLEX
See *Complex Supplements*.

LESTEMP
See *Acetaminophen*.

LETTER
See *Levothyroxine*.

LEUCOVORIN

Methotrexate[120]
Leucovorin antagonizes the effects of methotrexate and can be used as an antidote for overdosage if given within 4 hours, before the cells become too damaged to respond.

LEUKERAN
See *Alkylating Agents* (chlorambucil).

LEVALLORPHAN TARTRATE (Lorfan)

Narcotic analgesics[120,166]
(Alphaprodine [Nisentil], levorphanol [Levo-Dromoran], meperidine [Demerol, etc.], and morphine)
Levallorphan reverses the respiratory depression produced by narcotic analgesics without abolishing analgesia. It will not reverse respiratory depression caused by sedatives, hypnotics, anesthetics, etc. and it may cause respiratory depression if given without a narcotic.

Propoxyphene[120] (Darvon)
Levallorphan is an antidote of choice for overdosage with propoxyphene.

Scorpion venom[120]
Levallorphan enhances the toxicity of scorpion venom.

LEVARTERENOL
(Levophed, noradrenaline, norepinephrine)

α-Adrenergic blockers[120,330,421,542]
α-Adrenergic blocking agents like phentolamine and phenoxybenzamine antagonize the hypertensive effect of levarterenol. However, see the opposite effects with guanethidine, methyldopa, and reserpine, adrenergic neuron blockers, under *Polymechanistic Drugs* (page 378).

Alcohol[166]
Alcohol increases the urinary excretion of levarterenol and thus inhibits the drug.

Amphetamines[633]
Amphetamines potentiate the adrenergic effects of levarterenol. Hazardous.

Anesthetics[120,773,776,778,796,801]
Certain anesthetics such as cyclopropane, halothane, and methoxyflurane sensitize the myocardium to levarterenol (norepinephrine) and thus combined use is contraindicated because of the risk of producing ventricular tachycardia or fibrillation. May be lethal.

Angiotensin[117]
In prolonged, severe hypotension caused by an adrenolytic agent, angiotensin is the logical pressor drug since the patient is rendered unresponsive to levarterenol.

Antazoline[199] (Antistin)
See *Antihistamines* below.

Antidepressants, tricyclic[221,404,424,541,942]
These antidepressants potentiate the hyperthermic and other adrenergic effects produced by levarterenol. The cardiovascular effects of catecholamines can be potentiated 9-fold with combination of levarterenol and desipramine or protriptyline and possibly other tricyclics.

Antihistamines[169,232,235,242,400,483]
Some antihistamines like chlorpheniramine and tripelennamine, potentiate levarterenol and increase its cardiovascular toxicity. They inhibit uptake of norepinephrine by the tissues and at the neuronal membrane thus increasing the concentration of unbound drug available for receptors.

Antihypertensives[117]
Antihypertensives and levarterenol have opposite effects. Levarterenol is the drug of choice if a pressor agent is needed in a hypotensive episode with an antihypertensive since none of these drugs antagonizes its action. In fact the sensitivity of the patient to levarterenol may be increased, and its duration of action prolonged.

Azapetine[619] (Ilidar)
Azapetine, an α-adrenergic blocking agent antagonizes the vasoconstrictor action of levarterenol.

Bethanidine[117]
Same as for *Reserpine* below.

Brompheniramine (Dimetane, Disomer)
See *Antihistamines* above.

Chlorcyclizine (Perazil)
See *Antihistamines* above.

Chlorpheniramine (Chlor-Trimeton, Teldrin)
See *Antihistamines* above.

Clemizole (Allercur, Reactrol)
See *Antihistamines* above.

Cocaine[167]
Cocaine sensitizes the patient to levarterenol.

Cyclopropane
See *Anesthetics* above.

Cyproheptadine (Periactin)
See *Antihistamines* above.

Desipramine (Norpramine, Pertofrane)
See *Antidepressants, Tricyclic* above.

Dexchlorpheniramine (Polaramine)
See *Antihistamines* above.

LEVARTERENOL *(continued)*

Dextrothyroxine [120] **(Choloxin)**
See *Thyroid Preparations* below.

Dimethindene [120] **(Forhistal)**
See *Antihistamines* above.

Diazepam [120] **(Valium)**
Levarterenol combats the hypotension caused by diazepam overdosage.

Diphenhydramine (Benadryl)
See *Antihistamines* above.

Diphenylpyraline (Diafen, Hispril)
See *Antihistamines* above.

Diuretics [950]
Diuretics may decrease arterial responsiveness to levarterenol (hypertensive effect).

Ether [543]
Ether tends to increase plasma levels of norepinephrine.

Guanethidine [117,421,663] **(Ismelin)**
Guanethidine increases responsiveness to exogenously administered norepinephrine (levarterenol) 2- or 3-fold; bradycardia, cardiac arrhythmias and hypertension. See *Polymechanistic Drugs* (page 378).

Haloperidol [120,421] **(Haldol)**
Levarterenol antagonizes the hypotensive effects of haloperidol.

Halothane (Fluothane)
See *Anesthetics* above.

Hexobarbital [544]
Repeated use of levarterenol may enhance the effect of hexobarbital via microsomal enzyme depression.

Hexamethonium [117]
The effect of levarterenol is moderately increased.

Hydralazine [117] **(Apresoline)**
Hydralazine slightly reduces the pressor effects of levarterenol.

Imipramine
See *Antidepressants, Tricyclic* above.

Iproniazid [546]
See *MAO Inhibitors* below.

Isocarboxazid (Marplan)
See *MAO Inhibitors* below.

Levothyroxine [590]
See *Thyroid Preparations* below.

MAO inhibitors [117,166,546,793]

MAO inhibitors given concomitantly with sympathomimetic amines, intensify the sympathomimetic effects. Some of the sequelae are elevated blood pressure, cerebral hemorrhage, headache, tachycardia, nausea, vomiting, neck stiffness, and coma. The resulting hypertensive crisis can be fatal with a directly acting agent or with a norepinephrine releaser. However, since administered catecholamines (levarterenol, epinephrine) are largely destroyed by catechol-O-methyl transferase, MAO inhibitors may only slightly intensify and prolong their action. The reaction can be reversed by administration of an alpha-adrenergic blocking agent such as phentolamine (Regitine). MAO inhibitor activity may remain for 7 to 10 days after withdrawal of the drug.

Mecamylamine [117]
The effect of levarterenol is moderately increased.

Methapyrilene (Histadyl, Semikon, etc.)
See *Antihistamines* above.

Methdilazine (Tacaryl)
See *Antihistamines* above.

Methoxyflurane (Penthrane)
See *Anestethics* above.

Methyldopa [117,421,633] **(Aldomet)**
Methyldopa potentiates the pressor effects of levarterenol. See *Polymechanistic Drugs* (page 378).

Nialamide (Niamid)
See *MAO Inhibitors* above.

Nitrous oxide [166]
Nitrous oxide (80%) in oxygen slightly increases the response of vascular smooth muscle to the sympathetic mediator levarterenol (norepinephrine).

Organic nitrates and nitrites [120]
Nitrates and nitrites which relax smooth muscle can act as physiological antagonists to levarterenol (norepinephrine). The actual response of the muscle may vary with variations in the relative concentrations of the members of the combination.

Pargyline (Eutonyl)
See *MAO Inhibitors* above.

Pempidine [117]
The effect of levarterenol is moderately increased.

Pentolinium [117]
The effect of levarterenol is moderately increased.

Phenelzine (Nardil)
See *MAO Inhibitors* above.

Pheniramine (Trimeton)
See *Antihistamines* above.

Phenothiazines [421]
Levarterenol antagonizes the hypotensive effect of the CNS depressant phenothiazines.

Phenoxybenzamine [117,619] **(Dibenzyline)**
Phenoxybenzamine, an α-adrenergic blocking agent, blocks the α-adrenergic action produced by levarterenol; reduces blood pressure, increases blood flow, etc.

Phentolamine [117,619] **(Regitine)**
Phentolamine, an α-adrenergic blocking agent, has actions similar to phenoxybenzamine above, and therefore is an antagonist of levarterenol.

Prenylamine [170]
Prenylamine augments response to levarterenol.

Promethazine (Phenergan)
See *Antihistamines* above.

Propranolol [120] **(Inderal)**
Propranolol, a β-adrenergic blocking agent, blocks the β-adrenergic action produced by levarterenol (norepinephrine), particularly on the myocardium.

Pyrrobutamine (Pyronil)
See *Antihistamines* above.

Rauwolfia alkaloids [117,330,633]
The antihypertensive rauwolfia alkaloids potentiate arterial responsiveness to levarterenol. See *Polymechanistic Drugs* (page 378).

Reserpine [117,198,330,421,633]
Reserpine may increase arterial responsiveness to norepinephrine 2- or 3- fold. Because reserpine depletes the catecholamine, special care must be exercised when treating patients with a history of bronchial asthma. See *Polymechanistic Drugs* (page 378).

Thyroid preparations [120,539,590]

Injection of catecholamines such as epinephrine and norepinephrine into patients receiving thyroid preparations increases the risk of precipitating an episode of coronary insufficiency, especially in patients with coronary artery disease.

Thiazide diuretics[330,421]
Thiazide diuretics tend to antagonize the hypertensive effect of levarterenol.

Trimeprazine (Temaril)
See *Antihistamines* above.

Tripelennamine (Pyribenzamine)
See *Antihistamines* above.

Triprolidine (Actidil)
See *Antihistamines* above.

LEVODOPA (Dopar, Larodopa, Parda, etc.)

See *Antiparkinsonism Drugs*.
The following drugs can be safely given with levodopa: ampicillin, antacids, benzodiazepines, chlorpropamide, dexamphetamine, digoxin, diuretics, general anesthetics, insulin, paracetamol, phenindione, prednisolone, sulfadimidine, and thyroxine.[1497] The following drugs reduce the efficacy of levodopa: butyrophenones (haloperidol), papaverine, phenothiazines, pyridoxine, reserpine, and thioxanthenes (thiothixene).[2001]

Alpha-methyl dopa
See *Methyldopa* below.

Amantadine[486] **(Symmetrel)**
Amantadine enhances the effect of levodopa in parkinsonism.

Antacids
See *Levodopa* under *Antacids*.

Antiemetics[724]
Antiemetics defeat the therapeutic purpose of levodopa in Parkinson's syndrome.

Anticholinergics[715,1419]
Some anticholinergics may enhance the effect of levodopa in parkinsonism but see also *Levodopa* under *Anticholinergics*.

Antidepressants, tricyclic[715,1497]
These tricyclic drugs potentiate levodopa in parkinsonism. This combination should be given with caution in cardiac disease because of the possibility of cardiac arrhythmias.

Antiparkinsonism drugs[1038]
(Artane, Cogentin, Kemadrin, etc.)
Levodopa may be used in combination with these drugs at reduced dosages.

Apomorphine[838]
Apomorphine, a catecholamine analog of dopamine, eliminates the tremor and decreases the akinesia and choreoathetosis caused by levodopa.

Benzodiazepines
(Dalmane, Librium, Serax, Valium, etc.)
See *Levodopa* under *Benzodiazepines*.

Butyrophenones (Haloperidol, etc.)
See introduction to *Levodopa* above.

Chlorpromazine[724,922,923,1510,1648,1918-9,2001]
(Thorazine)
Phenothiazines may defeat the therapeutic effects of levodopa in Parkinson's syndrome by interfering with dopamine synthesis from levodopa *in vivo* (caudate nucleus and limbic system).

Diazepam
See *Levodopa* under *Benzodiazepines*.

Guanethidine
See *Levodopa* under *Guanethidine Sulfate*.

Haloperidol[922,923]
Same as for *Chlorpromazine* above.

Hexobarbital[2031]
Long-term levodopa therapy may increase the drug metabolizing activity of the liver (rats).

Homatropine[1419]
See *Levodopa* under *Anticholinergics*.

MAO inhibitors and psychoenergizers[724,792,1038]
These are potentially dangerous combinations. See under *MAO Inhibitors*. Hypertensive crisis may be induced, and interaction may occur for a prolonged period after withdrawal of one of the drugs.

Methyldopa[724] **(Aldomet)**
Methyldopa is capable of defeating the therapeutic purpose of levodopa in Parkinson's syndrome.

Multivitamin preparations[686,715]
(containing pyridoxine)
Pyridoxine inhibits the effects of levodopa.

Papaverine[2001]
See introduction to *Levodopa* above.

Phenelzine
See *MAO Inhibitors* above.

Phenothiazines[724,2001]
Phenothiazines may defeat the therapeutic purpose of levodopa in Parkinson's syndrome. See *Levodopa* under *Phenothiazines*.

Phenylbutazone[1909] **(Butazolidin)**
Phenylbutazone may decrease the therapuetic effectiveness of levodopa.

Phenylephrine[717,2027]
Levodopa (or its metabolites), by competitive α-adrenergic receptor blockade, reduces the mydriatic action of phenylephrine after a brief intensified miotic effect.

Propranol[1171-4]
This drug produces several important interactions, some harmful, some beneficial. See *Levodopa* under *Propranolol*.

Pyridoxine[120,686,715,724,1241,1278,1302-3,1403,1568,1600,1693,2001]
Pyridoxine in a single dose has only a slight effect on levodopa but prolonged oral therapy markedly reduces or completely abolishes the clinical benefits of levodopa. Vitamin preparations containing even small amounts of pyridoxine may be contraindicated. The inhibiting action of pyridoxine on levodopa (stimulation of L-amino acid decarboxylase during intestinal absorption, which converts levodopa through decarboxylation to more dopamine in the periphery and less in the CNS where it exerts its therapeutic effect) may be prevented by a peripheral metabolic inhibitor such as *dl-α-*methyl dopahydrazine (MK 485).

Reserpine[724,2001]
Reserpine may defeat the therapeutic purpose of levodopa in Parkinson's syndrome.

Tranquilizers[724]
Tranquilizers may defeat the therapeutic purpose of levodopa in Parkinson's syndrome.

Thioxanthenes[2001]
Thiothixene and probably other thioxanthenes may significantly reduce the therapeutic efficacy of levodopa.

Uricosurics
See *Hyperuricemics* under *Uricosuric Agents*.

Vitamin B complex[686,715]
The interaction is due to *Pyridoxine* (see above).

LEVO-DROMORAN
See *Levorphanol Tartrate*.

LEVOMEPROMAZINE (Levoprome)
See *Phenothiazines* (methotrimeprazine)

LEVOPHED
See *Levarterenol.*

LEVOPROME
See *Phenothiazines* (methotrimeprazine).

LEVORPHANOL TARTRATE (Levo-Dromoran)

Acidifying agents [325,870]
Acidifying agents antagonize levorphanol by increasing the urinary excretion rate.

Alkalinizing agents [325,870]
Alkalinizing agents potentiate levorphanol by decreasing the urinary excretion rate.

Chlorpromazine [669]
Chlorpromazine potentiates levorphanol.

Nalorphine [39]
Nalorphine can precipitate acute abstinence syndromes in patients physically dependent on levorphanol, and related synthetics.

LEVOTHYROXINE (Letter, Synthroid, etc.)
See *Thyroid Preparations.*

LEVSIN
See *Hyoscyamine* and *Phenobarbital.*

LEVULOSE
See *Fructose.*

LIAFON
See *Ascorbic Acid, Folic Acid* and *Iron Salts* (ferrous sulfate).

LIBRAX
See *Anticholinergic* (clidinium bromide) and *Chlordiazepoxide.*

LIBRITABS
See *Chlordiazepoxide.*

LIBRIUM
See *Chlordiazepoxide* and *Benzodiazepines.*

LICORICE
See *Glycyrrhiza.*

LIDOCAINE (Xylocaine, lignocaine, etc.)
See *Anesthetics, Local* and *Antiarrhythmics.*

Ajmaline [1149]
Lidocaine, especially in high doses rapidly administered IV, plus the antiarrhythmic Rauwolfia alkaloid ajmaline exerts an additive cardiac depressant effect.

Anesthetics [120]
Preanesthetic medications potentiate local anesthetics like lidocaine. Other CNS depressants and cardiovascular depressant drugs may be potentiated by lidocaine.

Barbiturates [1150,1326]
Lidocaine effects are decreased by increased metabolism due to enzyme induction by barbiturates (man and dogs).

Diazepam [1151] (Valium)
Prior IV administration of diazepam may enhance the antiarrhythmic effect of lidocaine (in dogs).

Muscle relaxants [421,435,640,790] (Decamethonium, succinylcholine, tubocurarine)
Lidocaine, particularly in high doses, enhances the neuromuscular blocking action of peripherally acting muscle relaxants, both competitive and depolarizing.

Pargyline [120] (Eutonyl)
Some patients receiving pargyline for a prolonged period of time become refractory to the nerve blocking effects of lidocaine.

Phenytoin [1150,1152] (Dilantin)
Phenytoin decreases the action of lidocaine through enzyme induction. These drugs may have serious additive cardiac depressant effects, especially when the hydantoin is administered rapidly.

Procainamide [120,721] (Pronestyl)
These two antiarrhythmic drugs have a synergistic effect on the CNS and may produce restlessness, visual hallucinations, etc. Cross sensitivity may occur.

Quinidine [120]
Cross sensitivity may occur between lidocaine and quinidine.

Sulfonamides [178,421]
Lidocaine inhibits the antibacterial activity of sulfonamides.

LIDOSPORIN
See *Lidocaine* and *Polymyxin B.*

LINCOMYCIN (Lincocin)
See also *Antibiotics.*

Antidiarrheal medication [330,633,1042] (Attapulgite, kaolin, pectin, etc.)
When an attapulgite-pectin suspension (Kaopectate) is given with capsules of lincomycin, only ⅑ of the control level is absorbed due to physical absorption.

Cyclamates [619,880,1385,1887]
Cyclamates inhibit lincomycin given orally by inhibiting intestinal absorption of the anti-infective.

Erythromycin [808,809]
Lincomycin and erythromycin are antagonistic antibacterially.

Kaolin [330,1042,1108]
Kaolin with pectin in such products as Kaopectate strongly inhibits absorption of lincomycin given orally. Give lincomycin at least 2 hours after or 3 to 4 hours before a kaolin-pectin product is taken. Avoid the combination if possible.

LINCOCIN
See *Lincomycin.*

LINDANE
See *Halogenated Insecticides.*

LIOTHYRONINE
See *Liotrix* and *Thyroid Preparations.*

LIOTRIX (Euthroid [sodium levothyroxine plus sodium liothyronine], Thyrolar, etc.)

Anticoagulants, coumarin [120]
Thyroid replacement therapy may potentiate anticoagulant effects of bishydroxycoumarin, warfarin, and other coumarin anticoagulants. Reduce dosage of the anticoagulant by ⅓, monitor closely, and adjust on basis of prothrombin determinations.

Cholestyramine [28,672] (Cuemid, Questran)
Cholestyramine inhibits absorption of liothyronine.

LIPO-HEPIN
See *Heparin.*

LIQUAMAR
See *Anticoagulants, Oral* (phenprocoumon).

Cholestyramine
See *Anticoagulants, Oral* under *Cholestyramine.*

LIRUGEN
See *Vaccines* (live measles).

LISTICA
See *Tranquilizers* (hydroxyphenamate).

LITHIUM CARBONATE
(Eskalith, Lithane, Lithonate)

Acetazolamide[120]
Acetazolamide inhibits the action of lithium carbonate by increasing its urinary excretion.

Alkalinizing agents[120]
Sodium bicarbonate inhibits lithium carbonate by increasing its excretion.

Aminophylline[120,619]
Aminophylline may inhibit the action of lithium carbonate by increasing the urinary excretion of lithium. Useful in toxicity due to overdosage.

Amphetamines
See *Lithium Carbonate* under *Amphetamines*.

Benzodiazepines[2055]
Profound hypothermia has been produced on several occasions with combined lithium carbonate and diazepam therapy.

Flupenthixol[1983] **(Depixol)**
See *Neuroleptics* below.

Haloperidol[1145,1983] **(Haldol)**
Lithium carbonate combined with haloperidol produces severe encephalopathic symptoms (persistent parkinsonism, dementia and dyskinesias) with fever, confusion, lethargy, weakness, tremulousness, hyperglycemia, leukocytosis, and elevated BUN and serum enzymes. Two patients suffered irreversible devastating, widespread, brain damage. See *Neuroleptics* below.

Diazepam
See *Benzodiazepines* above.

Caffeine[619]
Same as for *Aminophylline* above.

Diuretics[619,1970]
Diuretics are usually contraindicated because they enhance the toxicity of lithium (electrolyte depletion). Elevated blood levels of lithium caused by hyponatremia induced by diuretics, *e.g.*, spironolactone plus hydrochlorothiazide (Aldactazide), with low salt diet and excessive water intake produces Li^+ toxicity—confusion, disorientation, and indistinct speech. See also *Lithium Carbonate* under *Diuretics*. In poisoning due to overdosage, lithium excretion may be increased by forced osmotic diuresis with IV infusions of mannitol or urea.

Methyldopa (Aldomet)
See *Lithium Carbonate* under *Methyldopa*.

Neuroleptics[1145,1982-3]
Neuroleptics (flupenthixol, haloperidol, etc.) are powerful blockers of cerebral dopamine receptors and related dopamine sensitive adenylate cyclase, which is probably responsible for extrapyramidal side effects. Lithium synergistically enhances the inhibition of the adenylate cyclase and the combination may produce a severe adverse drug interaction. See *Haloperidol* above.

Phenothiazines
See *Lithium Carbonate* under *Phenothiazines*.

Potassium iodide[1796]
Potassium iodide and lithium carbonate act synergistically to produce hypothyroidism. This combination may be contraindicated in susceptible patients.

Sodium bicarbonate[1851]
Sodium bicarbonate enhances the urinary excretion of lithium. See *Sodium Chloride* below.

Sodium chloride[1243,1356,1499,1708,1970]
The urinary excretion of lithium varies with intake of sodium salts. Salt-free diets decrease excretion and potentiate the toxicity of lithium. Large amounts of sodium (used by some as an antidote for lithium poisoning) increase excretion and depress therapeutic efficacy. Do not give lithium carbonate to patients on a salt-free diet, only to patients with normal sodium levels and monitor lithium and sodium blood levels closely.

Thiazide diuretics
See *Lithium Carbonate* under *Diuretics*, and *Diuretics* above.

Tricyclic antidepressants[619,1921]
Probably contraindicated. Patients on lithium carbonate maintenance therapy may shift from depression to mania when given the tricyclics for moderate depressive relapses. However, one report[1921] indicates that lithium in combination with tricyclics or MAO inhibitors is more effective than lithium alone.

Urea[120,1851]
Urea antagonizes lithium carbonate by increasing its excretion.

Vasopressin
See *Lithium Carbonate* under *Vasopressin*.

LIVER
See *Tyramine-rich Foods*.

LIVER FUNCTION DEPRESSORS
See under *Anticoagulants, Oral*.

LIVITAMIN
See *Complex Supplements*.

LOCAL ANESTHETICS
See *Anesthetics, Local*.

LOMOTIL
See *Atropine* and *Diphenoxylate*.

LORFAN
See *Levallorphan Tartrate*.

LORIDINE
See *Cephaloridine*.

LORYL
See *Chloral Hydrate* and *Tranquilizers* (phenyltoloxamine).

LOTUSATE
See *Barbiturates* (talbutal).

LSD
See *Lysergic Acid Diethylamide*.

LUCANTHONE (Miracil-D)

Antihistamines[120]
Severity of side effects of the antischistosomal, lucanthone, is reduced by administration of an antihistamine.

Atropine[177]
Severity of side effects of lucanthone is reduced by administration of atropine.

LUFYLLIN-EPG
See *Ephedrine, Glyceryl Guaiacolate, Phenobarbital,* and *Theophylline* (diphylline).

LUMINAL
See *Phenobarbital*.

LYSMINS
See *Complex Supplements* (methionine, dietary supplement).

LYSERGIC ACID DIETHYLAMIDE (LSD, lysergide)

Chlorpromazine (Thorazine) [166]
Chlorpromazine antagonizes the undesirable behavioral effects of LSD.

Perphenazine [482] (Trilafon)
This combination (perphenazine plus LSD) induces major chromosome abnormalities (breaks, gaps, and hypodiploid cells).

Propranolol [1130] (Inderal)
Propranolol (10 mg. t.i.d.) quickly banishes the anxiety symptoms (tachycardia, feelings of doom, etc.) and depression with suicidal ideas induced by LSD (up to 2500 mcg. at one dose).

Reserpine
See *LSD* under *Reserpine*.

MAALOX
See *Aluminum Salts, Antacids* and *Magnesium Salts*.

MACRODANTIN
See *Nitrofurantoin*.

MADRIBON
See *Sulfonamides* (sulfadimethoxine).

MAGNESIUM SALTS

Coumarin anticoagulants [814]
Magnesium antacids inhibit absorption of coumarin anticoagulants.

Digitalis [619]
Hypomagnesemia potentiates digitalis by increasing sensitivity of the myocardium and may result in toxicity.

Iron salts [928]
Magnesium trisilicate inhibits the absorption of iron.

Muscle relaxants
See *Magnesium Salts* under *Muscle Relaxants, Peripherally Acting*.

Procainamide [619] (Pronestyl)
Magnesium enhances the neuromuscular blocking effect of procainamide.

Tetracyclines [48,421]
Magnesium inhibits tetracycline absorption. See *Complexing Agents* under *Tetracyclines*.

MAGNATRIL
See *Aluminum Salts, Antacids,* and *Magnesium Salts*.

MALIC ACID

Arginine [619]
The combination of arginine and malic acid is more effective than arginine alone in lowering blood ammonia levels. Many drugs, including barbiturates, narcotics, and diuretics may produce ammonia or interfere with its excretion.

MANDALAY
See *Methenamine* and *Phenazopyridine*.

MANDELAMINE
See *Methenamine*.

MANDRAX
See *Methaqualone* and *Diphenhydramine*.

Amitriptyline (Elavil) [623]
Similar as for *Thioridazine* below.

Diazepam [783] (Valium)
Apnea, respiratory depression and paralysis may be produced by this combination.

Thioridazine [623] (Mellaril)
Side effects (dryness of mouth, swelling of tongue, furred tongue, cracking of the angles of the mouth, dizziness, disorientation) are potentiated by Mandrax. Symptoms subside upon withdrawal of Mandrax even when the psychotropic drug is continued. Diphenhydramine has anticholinergic properties and may be the potentiating component of Mandrax.

MANNITOL

EDTA
(Calcium disodium edetate, edathamil, Versenate)
Ethylenediaminetetraacetate increases the absorption rate of mannitol.

Kanamycin [813] (Kantrex)
This combination may cause deafness.

MAO INHIBITORS
(Isocarboxazid [Marplan], furazolidone [Furoxone], Isoniazid [Niconyl, Nydrazid], mebanazine, nialamide [Niamid], pargyline [Eutonyl], phenelzine [Nardil], procarbazine [Matulane], Tranylcypromine [Parnate], etc.)
Note: The effects of MAO inhibitors may not occur for several weeks after therapy is started and may last to 1 to 3 weeks after they are discontinued. Every patient on MAO inhibitors should be warned against taking any other medication unless his physician approves. Through enzyme inhibition MAOI potentiate a very long list of drugs.

Acetanilid [166]
MAO inhibitors potentiate acentanilid.

Acetazolamide [951] (Diamox)
MAO inhibitors may potentiate acetazolamide.

Acetohexamide (Dymelor)
See *Sulfonylurea Hypoglycemics* below.

α-Adrenergic blockers [136]
See *Phentolamine* below. One of these agents should be administered promptly when a hypertensive crisis occurs in any patient receiving a MAO inhibitor.

β-Adrenergic blockers [74,120]
β-adrenergic blockers potentiate monoamine oxidase inhibitors.

Adrenergics
See *MAO Inhibitors* under *Sympathomimetics*.

Alcohol [44,78,120,121,136,404,433,874,1593]
This is a very hazardous combination. See *MAO Inhibitors* under *Alcohol*.

Aminopyrine [166]
MAO inhibitors potentiate aminopyrine.

Aminoquinolines [74,433]
(Chloroquine, quinacrine [Atabrine], etc.)
MAO inhibitors potentiate the toxic effects (retinal damage, etc.).

Amitriptyline
See *Antidepressants, Tricyclic* below.

Amphetamines [60,78,120,162,289,355-6,633,745-747]
MAO inhibitors potentiate amphetamine, its derivatives, and other sympathomimetic amines. MAO inhibitors increase the amount of norepinephrine stored in adrenergic nerve endings. If an indirectly acting sympathomimetic like amphet-

amine, chlorphentermine, ephedrine, or tyramine is given after a MAO inhibitor has been taken for a period of time the sudden release of stored catecholamines, such as norepinephrine (with levels highly elevated by MAOI) can produce an extremely intense pressor response. In addition some MAO inhibitors exert an additive amphetaminelike action (*e.g.*, phenelzine and tranylcypromine). The combination of amphetamine and a MAOI may cause a hypertensive crisis with tachycardia, and seizures. May be fatal (subarachnoid hemorrhage). Hyperpyrexia (104.9°F) occurred with an amphetamine plus tranylcypromine. Note that many anorexiants, nasal decongestants, and other drug products contain these and related sympathomimetic amines. Contraindicated. See *Sympathomimetics* below. Phentolamine (Regitine), an alpha-adrenergic blocker counteracts the potentiated norepinephrine effect on alpha-receptors and is short-acting.

Analgesics [619,874,877]
MAO inhibitors plus these CNS depressants may induce hypotension, ataxia, paresthesia, ocular palsy, etc., especially severe with narcotic analgesics (see *Meperidine* below).

Anesthetics, general [37,120,198,330,421,970]
Enhanced sedation. MAO inhibitors decrease metabolism of anesthetics and potentiate their CNS depressant effects. Patients taking a MAO inhibitor should not undergo surgery requiring general anesthesia. Should spinal anesthesia be essential, consider the possible combined hypotensive effects of the MAO inhibitor and the blocking agent. Also, do not give cocaine or local anesthetic solutions containing sympathomimetic vasoconstrictors. Discontinue the MAO inhibitor at least 10 days to 3 weeks before elective surgery.

Anorexiants [198]
MAO inhibitors potentiate the cardiac, central, and other sympathomimetic actions of anorexiants by enzyme inhibition. Very hazardous. See MAO *Inhibitors* under *Sympathomimetics*.

Antazoline (Antistine)
See *Antihistamines* below.

Anticholinergics [78,166,312,330,404]
The effects of the anticholinergics (particularly the antiparkinsonism effect) are potentiated by the MAO inhibitors which block detoxification of these drugs by the liver. Tremors and profuse sweating may occur.

Anticoagulants, oral [134,359,861,885,890]
MAO inhibitors enhance the effects of oral anticoagulants.

Anticonvulsants [198,421]
The influence of MAO inhibitors on the convulsive threshold is variable; the dosage of anticonvulsants may have to be altered.

Antidepressants, tricyclic [12,29,53,78,103,162,290,293,352,395,404,634,823,956,1231,1369,1543,1765,1772,1801,1907,1988,2008]

(Amitriptyline [Elavil]; carbamazepine [Tegretol]; clomipramine [Anafranil]; desipramine [Norpramin, Pertofrane]; doxepin [Adapin, Sinequan]; imipramine [Imavate, Janimine, Presamine, SK-Pramine, Tofranil]; nortriptyline [Aventyl]; protriptyline [Vivactil]; other dibenzazepines, cycloheptadienes, etc.
MAO inhibitors decrease the rate of metabolism of tricyclic antidepressants (amitriptyline, desipramine, imipramine, nortriptyline, protriptyline, etc.) and a toxic interaction may occur: agitation, clonic convulsions, delirium, hyperpyrexia, rapid pulse and respiration, tremors, coma, and vascular collapse. These tricyclics should not be given for at least 2 weeks after discontinuing therapy with a MAO inhibitor. Combined use can apparently cause fluid retention (massive edema, ascites) and produce other reactions although this has been questioned.[2008] It has caused death. Some physicians use this hazardous combination in low oral doses and avoid

the more potent MAO inhibitors such as clomipramine, imipramine, and tranylcypromine, but the patients must be very closely monitored and the risks are high, both therapeutically and legally.

Antidiabetics [86-88,191]
MAO inhibitors plus insulin or a sulfonylurea is a dangerous combination. Hypoglycemic collapse has occurred. MAO inhibitors of the hydrazine type and probably the nonhydrazine type (not with insulin) potentiate these hypogylcemics because they exert a hypoglycemic action of their own, and all MAO inhibitors tend to prevent a normal rebound from the hypoglycemic state by interfering with adrenergic homeostatic mechanisms. In some cases the MAO inhibitor can function as the hypoglycemic and the antidiabetic can be withdrawn.

Antihistamines [48,311,421]
MAO inhibitors, by decreasing the rate of metabolism of antihistamines, potentiate their sedative, anticholinergic, and other effects, depending on the agent. Usually contraindicated. Hazardous in glaucoma. See *Antihistamines*.

Antihypertensive [330,421] (Hypotensives)
MAO inhibitors potentiate antihypertensives. Since both types of agents lower the blood pressure, there may be an enhanced hypotensive effect. Reduced dosage of the hypotensive agent is frequently necessary.

Antimalarials [74,433]
MAO inhibitors increase the toxicity (retinal damage) caused by antimalarials like chloroquine and quinacrine.

Antiparkinsonism drugs [78,330,421]
MAO inhibitors potentiate antiparkinsonism drugs by inhibiting their metabolism (tremor, profuse sweating, etc.).

Appetite depressants
See *MAO Inhibitors* under *Sympathomimetics*.

Atropine [128]
MAO inhibitors potentiate atropine. Do not use together nor within 2 or 3 weeks following treatment with MAO inhibitors.

Barbiturates [78,166,404,743]
MAO inhibitors potentiate barbiturates, probably by inhibiting detoxication and elimination. Prolonged sedation and CNS depression occur with a normal dose. Respiratory arrest and coma may occur. See *CNS Depressants* below.

Beer [41]
Severe headaches and hypertensive crisis may be induced. See *Tyramine-rich Foods*.

Bendroflumethiazide [331] (Naturetin)
See *Diuretics* below.

Benzodiazepines [330,421] (Librium, Valium, etc.)
MAO inhibitors may enhance the sedative and other CNS depressant effects of benzodiazepines. Phenelzine and diazepam have been reported to cause severe edema.[1988] This interaction has been questioned,[2008] since phenelzine alone may cause edema in the elderly.

Biogenic amines and their precursors [166]
The precursors of biogenic amines, such as 5-hydroxytryptophan (for serotonin) and dopa (for norepinephrine and epinephrine), if given in the presence of MAO inhibition, increase the catecholamine and serotonin levels in the brain and stimulate the CNS excessively.

Broad beans [759]
See *Tyramine-rich Foods*.

Brompheniramine (Dimetane, Disomer)
See *Antihistamines* above.

MAO INHIBITORS *(continued)*

Caffeine[120]
Dosages of medications containing caffeine should be reduced. Excessive use of caffeine with MAO inhibitors can cause a hypertensive reaction.

Carbamazepine[120] **(Tegretol)**
Concurrent use of this anticonvulsant with MAO inhibitors is not recommended because of its structural relationship to the tricyclic antidepressants. See *Antidepressants, Tricyclic* above.

Carbinoxamine (Clistin)
See *Antihistamines* above.

Carisoprodol (Rela, Soma)[951]
The combination enhances relaxation via enzyme inhibition.

Cheeses[11,25,34,45,46,105,162,220,284,352,428,634,687]
Strong ripened cheeses such as Brie, Cheddar, Camembert, and Stilton contain high levels of tyramine which can cause a hypertensive crisis with MAO inhibitors. Deaths have been reported. See *Tyramine-rich Foods.*

Chianti wine
See *Tyramine-rich Foods.*

Chicken livers
See *Tyramine-rich Foods.*

Chloral hydrate[78,633]
MAO inhibitors potentiate and prolong the CNS depressant effects of chloral hydrate.

Chlorcycline (Perazil)
See *Antihistamines* above.

Chlordiazepoxide[834,874,1086] **(Librium)**
Additive or superadditive effects (coma) may occur when chlordiazepoxide is combined with MAO inhibitors. Chorea occurred with chlordiazepoxide and phenelzine (Nardil). However, with careful dosage, a dramatically beneficial response may be achieved in certain types of anxiety and depression. In some patients MAOI alone produce best results, in others chlordiazepoxide alone, but in some the combination provides optimum therapy.

Chloroquine[74,128,433]
Do not use together or within 2 or 3 weeks following treatment with MAO inhibitors to avoid increased toxicity and possible retinal damage. See *MAO Inhibitors* under *Chloroquine.*

***d*-Chlorpheniramine (Polaramine)**
See *Antihistamines* above.

Chlorphentermine[120] **(Pre-Sate)**
Chlorphentermine, an anorexiant, is contraindicated in patients who are receiving MAO inhibitors. See *Sympathomimetics* below.

Chlorpromazine[162,198,330] **(Thorazine)**
MAO inhibitors (nialamide) antagonize the cataleptic effect of chlorpromazine. Chlorpromazine potentiates the hypotensive effect of pargyline.

Chlorpropamide (Diabinese)
See *Sulfonylurea Hypoglycemics* below.

CNS depressants[30,96,162,311,352,399,634,701,702]
MAO inhibitors potentiate CNS depressants by physicochemical reactions or by enzyme inhibition. MAO inhibitors taken concomitantly with alcohol, anesthetics, barbiturates, codeine, glutethimide, morphine, meperidine, other sedatives and hypnotics, and other depressants (see *CNS Depressants*) can cause severe hypotension, respiratory arrest, coma, shock, and possibly death.

Cocaine[78,166]
MAO inhibitors including MAO inhibitor antidepressants potentiate cocaine.

Coffee
See *Tyramine-rich Foods.*

Cola drinks
See *Tyramine-rich Foods.*

Cold, hay fever, reducing and other OTC remedies[78,99,305,431]
Warn against their use concomitantly with MAO inhibitors. Very hazardous because of their content of antihistamines, sympathomimetics and other drugs that can be potentiated.

Coronary vasodilators[950]
MAO inhibitors decrease metabolism of coronary vasodilators and thus potentiate them.

Cream[41]
Hypertensive crisis with severe headaches may occur.

Cyclamates[1385]
Cyclamates are metabolized to cyclohexylamine, a pressor amine which may be potentiated by MAO inhibitors. This interaction should be kept in mind if pending modifications of the Delaney Amendment are enacted and these sweeteners are allowed back on the market.

Cycloserine[1884]
See *Isoniazid, Tranylcypromine,* etc. under *Cycloserine* for its varying effects on different MAO inhibitors.

Desipramine (Norpramin, Pertofrane)
See *Antidepressants, Tricyclic* above.

Dextromethorphan[120,779]
Death has apparently been caused by this combination (apnea, hyperpyrexia, laryngospasm, muscular rigidity) but proof is unsubstantial. MAO inhibitors may potentiate the CNS depressant effect of high doses. See *CNS Depressants* above.

Diazepam[78,120,1988] **(Valium)**
Additive or superadditive CNS effects may occur with diazepam. See also *Benzodiazepines* above.

Diazoxide[1197] **(Hyperstat)**
MAOI with diazoxide produces confusion, tremors, choreiform movements, and at times death.

Dibenzazepines[12,29,53,103,120,162,293]
Toxic interaction, sweating, salivation, excitement, hyperthermia, coma, possibly fatal. See *Antidepressants, Tricyclic* above.

Diethylpropion[120] **(Tepanil)**
Contraindicated. See *MAO Inhibitors* under *Sympathomimetics.*

Diphenhydramine (Benadryl)
See *Antihistamines* above.

Diuretics[74,162,331,433,633] **(Lasix, thiazides, etc.)**
Hypotensive shock may be induced by this combination. It accentuates both recumbent and postural blood pressure—lowering effects. At times fibrillation and hypertension occur. The result is unpredictable.

Dopa[792] **(Levodopa, *dl*-dopa)**
Increased toxicity, flushing, coma, hyperthermia, hypertension, cerebral hemorrhage.

Dopamine[120,793] **(Intropin)**
See *MAO inhibitors* under *Sympathomimetics.* MAOI potentiate dopamine at least 10-fold.

Doxapram[120,166,1349] **(Dopram)**
MAO inhibitors should be used cautiously with doxapram since a synergistic pressor effect (hypertension, arrhythmias) may occur.

Ephedrine[28,136,162,211,404,1599]
See *MAO Inhibitors* under *Sympathomimetics.* Ephedrine, orally or IV, is strongly potentiated by agents like phenelzine (a hydrazine) or tranylcypromine (a nonhydrazine) because these inhibitors increase the stores of norepinephrine in the

adrenergic neuronal terminals which are released in increased amounts by indirectly acting sympathomimetics like ephedrine. See *Amphetamine* above for mechanism. This interaction has been lethal. Phentolamine (Regitine), an alpha-adrenergic blocking agent, is antidotal.

Epinephrine [162,404,1245-6] (Adrenalin)
Exogenous epinephrine is not appreciably affected by MAO inhibitors at usual dosage levels because administered catecholamines like epinephrine are destroyed by COMT and thus MAO inhibitors will have relatively little effect (except for "denervation sensitivity" produced by MAOI). See also *Sympathomimetics* below.

Ethchlorvynol [120] (Placidyl)
MAO inhibitors enhance the sedative effect of ethchlorvynol. The dosage of ethchlorvynol should be reduced.

Ethamivan [421] (Emivan)
MAO inhibitors potentiate the central respiratory stimulant effect of ethamivan.

Fenfluramine [927]
See *MAO Inhibitors* under *Sympathomimetics*. A MAO inhibitor (phenelzine) has produced a severe hypertensive reaction with this anorexigenic.

Fentanyl [120] (Sublimaze)
This analgesic is contraindicated with MAO inhibitors. See *CNS Depressants* above.

Figs, canned [421]
See *Tyramine-rich Foods*.

Foods
See under *Tyramine-rich Foods*.

Furazolidone [633] (Furoxone)
Additive MAO inhibition; hypertension. Reduce dosage.

Furosemide [120] (Lasix)
This combination may cause an augmented hypotensive effect approaching shock levels. Additive effect.

Ganglionic-blocking agents [74,120,330,421]
MAO inhibitors may potentiate ganglionic blocking agents. Do not use together nor within 2 or 3 weeks following treatment with the MAO inhibitors.

Glutethimide [184] (Doriden)
This combination may cause respiratory arrest, shock, and coma. See *CNS Depressants* above.

Guanethidine [120]
Parenteral guanethidine is contraindicated during or for at least one week after discontinuing therapy with a MAO inhibitor, as the injected drug may cause hypertensive reactions from sudden release of catecholamines. See also *Polymechanistic Drugs* (page 378).

Haloperidol [120,352] (Haldol)
MAO inhibitors decrease rate of metabolism of haloperidol and potentiate its CNS depressant effects; hypotension, sedation, extrapyramidal effects.

Herring, pickled
See *Tyramine-rich Foods*.

Hydralazine (Apresoline)
See *Antihypertensives* above.

Hydroxyamphetamine (Paredrine)
See *Sympathomimetics* below and *Amphetamines* above.

Hypotensives
See *Antihypertensives* above.

Imipramine [53]
Imipramine, taken concomitantly with MAO inhibitors, may cause hyperpyrexia. Death has occurred. See *Antidepressants, Tricyclic* above.

Insulin [78,86-89,162,330,421]
A hazardous combination. See *MAO Inhibitors* under *Insulin*.

Isoproterenol [136,162,404,1245-6] (Isoprenaline)
See *MAO Inhibitors* under *Sympathomimetics*.

Levarterenol (Levophed, norepinephrine)
See *MAO Inhibitors* under *Sympathomimetics*. Like epinephrine (see above), exogenously administered levarterenol (norepinephrine) is not appreciably affected by MAO inhibitors, except in instances when MAO inhibitors have lowered the blood pressure. Then the response to levarterenol is increased somewhat. MAO inhibitors increase the stores of norepinephine (NE) but not the released or exogenously received NE nor do they affect the mechanism for its release, except for the limitations or uptake imposed by increased stores. The duration of action of NE is not determined by enzymatic action at the neuronal terminal. MAO merely inactivates excess NE within the neuronal cytoplasm. The metabolism of extraneuronal NE is due to the activity of (COMT) catechol-O-methyltransferase, another enzyme.

Levodopa [691,724,792,833,922,1302,1433,1449,1551,1789] (Dopar, Larodopa)
Hypertensive crisis may occur with MAO inhibitors and this precursor of the pressor catecholamines. This combination is contraindicated. Levodopa, by means of the enzyme L-amino acid decarboxylase, is converted to the neurotransmitter dopamine, a catecholamine. The latter is converted into norepinephrine by dopamine—β-hydroxylase. On the one hand MAO inhibition of catecholamine metabolism and on the other hand the accumulation of catecholamines produced from levodopa (increased storage and release of both dopamine and norepinephrine) in the presence of MAOI produces severe cardiovascular effects. If inadvertently an indirectly acting sympathomimetic (amphetamine, ephedrine, or tyramine) is also taken the effect is particularly lethal. See *Sympathomimetics* below.

Licorice [667]
MAO inhibitors with large licorice intake may produce hypertension.

Livers (chicken, beef, etc.) [207,757]
See *Tyramine-rich Foods*. Bacterial contamination of liver kept in a refrigerator but not frozen markedly increases the tyramine content. A concentration of 274 mcg. per gram was recorded in contaminated beef liver that caused a hypertensive crisis with phenelzine.

MAO inhibitors [56,120,166,633,1197]
Two MAO inhibitors should not be given simultaneously as they potentiate each other (hypertensive crisis hyperpyrexia, cyanosis, death). Two weeks should elapse between the discontinuation of therapy with one and initiation of therapy with the other.

Marmite
See *Tyramine-rich Foods*.

Mecamylamine (Inversine)
See *Antihypertensives* above.

Mepacrine [74,433] (Quinacrine)
MAO inhibitors may potentiate mepacrine and increase its toxicity. Quinacrine is stored in large quantities for prolonged periods in the liver. Since MAO inhibitors inhibit hepatic enzyme systems, they may potentiate the adverse effects of the drug, including explosive eczematoid skin reactions and other severe dermatitides, aplastic anemia and other severe blood dyscrasias, psychotic episodes, etc.

Meperidine (Demerol)
See *MAO Inhibitors* under *Meperidine*.

Mephentermine [847] (Wyamine)
Tachycardia and hypertension are produced by MAO inhibitor potentiation of the pressor agent (norepinephrine releaser).

MAO INHIBITORS *(continued)*

Meprobamate [198,421]
These agents mutually increase sedation (*e.g.,* pargyline). See *CNS Depressants* above.

Metaraminol [217,404] **(Aramine)**
MAO inhibitors plus this indirectly acting pressor agent may induce an acute hypertensive crisis with possible intracranial hemorrhage, hyperthermia, convulsions, coma and in some cases death. Avoid this combination. See *Amphetamine* above and *Sympathomimetics* below for the mechanism. Levarterenol would be a safer pressor agent to use with MAO inhibitors.

Methamphetamine [137]
Hypertensive crisis. See *Amphetamines* above and *MAO Inhibitors* under *Sympathomimetics*.

Methionine [532]
Hypertension with tranylcypromine.

Methotrimeprazine [120,404,1007] **(Levoprome)**
Concurrent use of MAO inhibitors with methotrimeprazine is contraindicated. Death has been reported as a result of this combination.

Methoxamine (Vasoxyl)
Use of a MAO inhibitor with the vasoconstricting catecholamine, methoxamine, is hazardous. See *Sympathomimetics* below.

Methyldopa (Aldomet)
Contraindicated. MAO inhibitors may reverse the hypotensive action of α-methyldopa and produce a hypertensive crisis and severe CNS stimulation. See *Polymechanistic Drugs* (page 378) and *MAO Inhibitors* under *Methyldopa.*

Methylphenidate [120,404] **(Ritalin)**
MAO inhibitors plus the CNS stimulant may induce acute hypertensive crisis with possible intracranial hemorrhage, hyperthermia, convulsions, coma and in some cases death. Both drugs inhibit drug metabolizing enzymes and methylphenidate acts like *Amphetamine* (see above).

Morphine [128,854]
MAO inhibitors potentiate morphine (analgesia, side effects). See *Narcotics* below.

Muscle relaxants [950,951]
MAO inhibitors enhance the activity of muscle relaxants.

Narcotics [120,198,330,421,633]
(Morphine, meperidine, etc.)
Narcotics may potentiate MAO inhibitor antidepressant effects by increasing norepinephrine release in the CNS. MAO inhibitors potentiate the CNS depressant effects of narcotics by enzyme inhibition; prolonged and intensified CNS depression may occur. Potentially very hazardous.

Nitrates and nitrites [421]
This combination may produce a false sense of cardiac strength and ability.

Norepinephrine
See *Levarterenol* above.

Nortriptyline (Aventyl)
See *Antidepressants, Tricyclic* above.

Pargyline [470] **(Eutonyl)**
See *MAO Inhibitors* above.

Pentolinium (Ansolysen)
See *Antihypertensives* above.

Pethidine [60,128] **(Meperidine)**
See *Meperidine* above.

Phenelzine (Nardil)
See *MAO Inhibitors* above.

Phenmetrazine [120] **(Preludin)**
Contraindicated. Excessive CNS stimulation may occur with this anorexiant.

Phenobarbital [633]
MAO inhibitors potentiate the sedative effects of phenobarbital. The latter antagonizes the antidepressant action of MAO inhibitors.

Phenothiazines [162,198,330,404,1480]
Phenothiazines such as trifluoperazine when given in proper dosage with MAO inhibitors may decrease the side effects of both drugs. And some phenothiazines protect patients against a hypertensive crisis due to tyramine, probably through α-adrenergic blocking action. However, MAO inhibitors tend to potentiate CNS depression and, depending on the drug, the anticholinergic, extrapyramidal, and other effects produced by phenothiazines. Exercise caution and monitor patients closely if such combined therapy is administered.

Phentolamine [120,136,166] **(Regitine)**
Hypertensive crisis with MAO inhibitors may be counteracted by the antiadrenergic phentolamine.

Phenylephrine [136,404,1245-6,1562]
This combination may cause an acute hypertensive crisis. Contraindicated. See *Sympathomimetics* below. Phenylephrine, after *oral* administration, is enormously potentiated either by hydrazines like phenelzine or nonhydrazines like tranylcypromine because of enzyme inhibition. The drug after IV administration is not potentiated nearly as much because of lower doses since exposure to hepatic and intestinal MAO is circumvented.

Phenylpropanolamine [99,115,431,535,1494]
(Propadrine)
See *MAO Inhibitors* under *Sympathomimetics* and *Amphetamines* above. This combination of phenylpropanolamine, an indirectly acting sympathomimetic, and a MAO inhibitor is contraindicated because of the potential for hypertensive crisis.

Phenyramidol (Analexin)
Contraindicated. No longer marketed in the U.S.

Pickled or kippered herring [338,421]
See *Tyramine-rich Foods.* This food with a MAO inhibitor has caused profound palpitation, severe chest pain, intense pain on top of the head and other symptoms of hypertensive crisis.

Pressor agents
See *Catecholamines* (dopamine, isoproterenol, nordefrin, etc.), *Amphetamines, Ephedrine, Phenylephrine, Sympathomimetic Vasopressors, Tyramine-rich Foods,* etc. All produce potentially lethal interactions with MAO inhibitors. *Epinephrine* and *Norepinephrine* do not appreciably interact (see above).

Primidone [633] **(Mysoline)**
MAO inhibitors potentiate the anticonvulsant, primidone.

Procaine [120] **(Novocain)**
Effects of procaine may be enhanced with MAO inhibitors.

Procarbazine [633] **(Matulane)**
See *MAO Inhibitors* above.

Propranolol [74,120,1179-80] **(Inderal)**
Propranolol should not be used concurrently or during the 2 week withdrawal period following MAO inhibitors. See *MAO Inhibitors* under *Propranolol.*

Quinacrine
See *MAO Inhibitors* under *Quinacrine.*

Rauwolfia alkaloids [104,120,604,633,639,640]
See *Reserpine* below.

Reserpine [104,331,604,637]

Parenteral reserpine may initially cause hypertensive reactions from sudden release of catecholamines. Through enzyme inhibition, MAO inhibitors potentiate the pressor effects and reverse the hypotensive action. A hypertensive crisis and severe CNS stimulation may be produced. Reserpine therapy is contraindicated during and for at least one week following treatment with a MAO inhibitor. However, combined use of reserpine and isocarboxazid in one study produced an additive blood pressure lowering effect. See *Polymechanistic Drugs* (page 378).

Romilar capsules

See *Phenelzine* under *Romilar Capsules*.

Sedatives and hypnotics [330,421]

MAO inhibitors potentiate sedatives by decreasing their rate of metabolism.

Sinutabs

See *Phenelzine* under *Sinutabs*.

Succinylcholine [855] **(Anectine, Quelicin)**

Succinylcholine, a neuromuscular blocking agent which is metabolized with pseudocholinesterase, may be potentiated by at least one MAO inhibitor, phenelzine, which has been reported to decrease levels of the metabolizing enzyme in the plasma. Use this combination, if it is necessary to do so, with caution.

Sulfonylurea hypoglycemics [86,330,421]
(Diabinese, Dymelor, Orinase, etc.)

MAO inhibitors potentiate these hypoglycemics by enzyme inhibition. Severe hypoglycemia may occur.

Sympathomimetics [48,78,99,115,117,136,162,211,305,399,1245]
(Amphetamines, metaraminol, methylphenidate, phenmetrazine, phenylephrine, phenylpropanolamine, etc.)

See also *Tyramine-rich Foods*.
See *MAO Inhibitors* under *Sympathomimetics*.

Tea

See under *Tyramine-rich Foods*.

Tetrabenazine [874]

This combination may produce agitation and delirium.

Thiazide diuretics [633]

MAO inhibitors potentiate the hypotensive effect of these diuretics.

Tolbutamide (Orinase)

See *Sulfonylurea Hypoglycemics* above.

Tranquilizers, minor [74,633]

MAO inhibitors including MAO antidepressants potentiate minor tranquilizers (Librium, Valium, etc.) by inhibiting their metabolism.

Tranylcypromine [120] **(Parnate)**

See *MAO Inhibitors* above. Hypertensive crisis with convulsions and possibly death.

Tripelennamine

See *Antihistamines* above.

Thiopental

See *Barbiturates* above.

Tubocurarine [198]

MAO inhibitors potentiate the muscle relaxant action of tubocurarine.

Tranquilizers

See under *Phenothiazines* and *CNS Depressants*.

Tryptophan [1197]

MAOI with tryptophan, a precursor of serotonin (5-HT), elevates the levels of the latter and causes drowsiness and ataxia.

Tyramine-rich foods [16,45-47,49]

MAO inhibitors enhance and prolong the stimulatory effects of tyramine (inhibition of metabolism of stored norepinephrine) on blood pressure and the contractile force of the heart. Severe headache, hypertension, subarachnoid hemorrhage, perhaps death. See *Sympathomimetics* above and *Tyramine-rich Foods*.

Vasopressors [78]

Severe hypertension with indirect acting vasopressors like mephentermine and metaraminol and a MAO inhibitor like pargyline. Cold, hay fever and weight reducing preparations, nasal decongestants, and other products containing pressor agents are contraindicated.

Veratrum alkaloids [421]

See *Antihypertensives*.

Wine

See under *Alcohol* and *Tyramine-rich Foods*.

Yeast extract [47,120,493,687]

See *Tyramine-rich Foods*.

Yogurt [486]

MAO inhibitors with yogurt may produce hypertension.

MAOLATE

See *Chlorphenesin*.

MARAX

See *Ephedrine, Hydroxyzine,* and *Theophylline*.

MARBLEN

See *Aluminum Salts, Calcium Salts,* and *Magnesium Salts*.

MAREZINE

See *Antihistamines* (cyclizine lactate).

MARIJUANA (Marihuana)

See *the review covering many drug interactions with marijuana.* [2046]

Antidiabetics, oral

See *Marijuana* under *Antidiabetics, Oral*.

Antineoplastics

See *Marijuana* under *Antineoplastics*.

Dextroamphetamine [2048]

Marijuana smokers who add other drugs may encounter additional risks. Studies in animals showed that higher doses of tetrahydrocannabinol (THC) increased the toxicity of dextroamphetamine (DAMP) in mice (4/cage) but not in isolated mice and reduced DAMP lethality in small doses. THC enhanced the locomotor activity induced by DAMP. Driving performance and motor skills may be impaired.

MARMITE

See *Tyramine-rich Foods*.

MARPLAN

See *MAO Inhibitors* (isocarboxazid).

MATULANE

See *Procarbazine*.

MAXIPEN

See *Penicillin* (potassium phenethicillin).

MAXOLON

See *Metoclopramide*.

MEASLES VIRUS VACCINE

See *Vaccines, Live Virus, Attenuated*.

Measles virus vaccine (live) [1051]

In patients previously exposed to *inactivated* measles virus vaccine, vaccination with *live* vaccine may cause a delayed dermal hypersensitivity.

MEASLES VIRUS VACCINE *(continued)*
PPD tuberculin skin test [120]
Live measles virus, when added to PPD sensitive lymphocytes, has been shown to reduce significantly the mean response of these cells to PPD. The PPD skin test should not be given concomitantly with live measles virus vaccine. See Chapter 7.

MEBANAZINE
See *MAO Inhibitors.*

MEBARAL
See *Barbiturates* (mephobarbital).

MEBROIN
See *Barbiturates* (mephobarbital) and *Diphenylhydantoin.*

MEBUTAMATE (Capla)
See *Antihypertensives.*

Alcohol
See *CNS Depressants* below.

Anesthetics
See *CNS Depressants* below.

Barbiturates
See *CNS Depressants* below.

CNS depressants [120,166]
Exercise caution if mebutamate is used with other CNS depressants such as alcohol, anesthetics, barbiturates, hypnotics, sedatives, etc. because additive depression may produce stupor, coma, respiratory depression and, with large enough doses, death.

Hypnotics
See *CNS Depressants* above.

Sedatives
See *CNS Depressants* above.

MECAMYLAMINE (Inversine)
See *Antihypertensives* and *Ganglionic Blocking Agents.*

Acetazolamide [137,726] (Diamox)
Acetazolamide inhibits renal carbonic anhydrase, thereby producing an alkaline urine, reducing the excretion rate of mecamylamine, and potentiating the hypotensive effect. See *Alkalinizing Agents* below.

Acidifying agents [325,529,726,870]
Acidifying agents by increasing renal excretion, inhibit mecamylamine.

Alcohol [619]
Alcohol potentiates the antihypertensive effect of mecamylamine.

Alkalinizing agents [325,529,726,870]
(Acetazolamide, sodium bicarbonate, etc.)
Alkalinizing agents, by causing an alkaline urinary pH, slow the rate of renal excretion and potentiate mecamylamine.

Ambenonium [120] (Mytelase)
Ambenonium is contraindicated in patients receiving mecamylamine because extreme muscle weakness and sudden inability to swallow may occur with the combination.

Amphetamines [421,633] (Desoxyn, Methedrine, etc.)
Amphetamines potentiate ganglionic blocking agents like mecamylamine. See *Amphetamines* under *Antihypertensives.*

Anesthetics [8,30,78,91,421]
Anesthetics potentiate the hypotensive action of the antihypertensive; severe hypotension, shock, and cardiovascular collapse may occur during surgery.

Antacids [325,870]
Mecamylamine is potentiated by antacids. See *Alkalinizing Agents* above.

Antidepressants, tricyclic [421]
These antidepressants antagonize the hypotensive action of mecamylamine.

Antihypertensives [5,120]
See *Reserpine* and *Thiazide Diuretics.*

Antimicrobials [120] (Antibiotics, Sulfonamides)
Ganglionic blocking agents are contraindicated in patients with chronic pyelonephritis being treated with these antimicrobials.

Carbon dioxide [349]
Carbon dioxide inhalation potentiates mecamylamine.

Diuretics [529,619]
Diuretics such as the thiazides, through salt depletion (Na, K), loss of fluids, and reduced arteriolar tension, potentiate the hypotensive action of mecamylamine. Reduce the dosages.

Ethacrynic acid [421] (Edecrin)
The diuretic potentiates the hypotensive.

Laxatives [120]
Laxatives overcome the constipation caused by mecamylamine which could lead to paralytic ileus, but do not use bulk laxatives.

Levarterenol [117]
Mecamylamine potentiates the pressor effects of levarterenol.

MAO inhibitors [950]
MAO inhibitors potentiate mecamylamine.

Methamphetamine (Desoxyn, Methedrine)
See *Sympathomimetics* below.

Reserpine [619]
An advantageous combination. Mecamylamine dosage may be reduced because of additive hypotensive effects.

Spironolactone [421] (Aldactone)
This diuretic potentiates mecamylamine.

Sympathomimetics [120,529,619,633]
Sympathomimetics may reverse the hypotensive effect of mecamylamine. Potentiation of sympathomimetic pressor effects. Ganglionic blocking agents like mecamylamine tend to potentiate the action of epinephrine on the vasculature.

Thiazide diuretics [421,633]
(Benuron, Diuril, Exna, Esidrix, etc.)
Thiazides potentiate the hypotensive activity of mecamylamine.

Triamterene [421] (Dyrenium)
This diuretic potentiates the hypotensive action of mecamylamine.

MECHLORETHAMINE (Mustargen)
See *Alkylating Agents.*

Amphotericin B [120]
Antineoplastics agents such as mechlorethamine should not be given concurrently with amphotericin B which also causes many blood dyscrasias.

Sedatives [120]
Chlorpromazine, alone or with barbiturates, given prior to mechlorethamine helps control the nausea and vomiting it causes.

Sodium thiosulfate [619]
Sodium thiosulfate (2% solution) neutralizes the vesicant effect of mechlorethamine on dermatomucosal surface.

MECHOLYL
See *Methacholine*.

MEDIATRIC
See *Androgens* (methyltestosterone), *Estrogens, Conjugated, Iron Salts* (ferrous sulfate), *Methamphetamine*, and *Vitamins* (B complex and B$_{12}$).

MEDIHALER-EPI
See *Epinephrine* (bitartrate).

MEDIHALER-ERGOTAMINE
See *Ergotamine* (tartrate).

MEDIHALER-ISO
See *Isoproterenol* (sulfate).

MEDROL
See *Corticosteroids* (methylprednisolone).

MEFENAMIC ACID (Ponstel)

Acidifying agents [165,529]
Acidifying agents, by decreasing urinary excretion of the weak acid (mefenamic acid), potentiate it.

Anticoagulants, oral
See *Anti-inflammatory Agents* under *Anticoagulants, Oral*.

MELLARIL
See *Phenothiazines* (thioridazine).

MELPHALEN (Alkeran)
See *Alkylating Agents*.

MENADIONE
See *Vitamin K*.

MENEST
See *Estrogens, Conjugated*.

MENRIUM
See *Chlordiazepoxide* and *Estrogens, Conjugated*.

MEPACRINE
See *Quinacrine*.

MEPERGAN
See *Meperidine* and *Promethazine*.

MEPERIDINE
(Demerol, Dolantin, isonipecaine, pethidine, etc.)

Acidifying agents [28,579,633,870]
Acidifying agents, by increasing urinary excretion, inhibit meperidine.

Alkalinizing agents [28,579,633,870]
Alkalinizing agents, by decreasing urinary excretion, potentiate meperidine.

Amphetamine [950]
Amphetamine potentiates the analgesic effect of meperidine.

Anesthetics, general [399,615]
The concurrent or sequential administration of anesthetics with meperidine has produced extreme hypotensive responses.

Antacids [325,870]
Meperidine is potentiated by antacids; increased tubular reabsorption in alkaline pH.

Anticholinergics [421] **(Atropine, etc.)**
Meperidine with its atropinelike action increases the adverse mydriatic effects of anticholinergics in glaucoma.

Anticholinesterases and Parasympathomimetics [120]
Meperidine antagonizes the beneficial miotic effects of anticholinesterases in glaucoma.

Antidepressants, tricyclic [194,421]
Tricyclic antidepressants with their anticholinergic activity potentiate the adverse effects of meperidine in glaucoma (increased ocular pressure and mydriatic effect). They also enhance the respiratory depression caused by meperidine.

Atropine [633]
Atropine and meperidine have additive effects such as mydriasis, blurred vision, dryness of the mouth, etc. Hazardous in glaucoma. See *Anticholinergics*.

Corticosteroids [421]
Corticosteroids increase ocular pressure with meperidine in long term therapy. Hazardous in glaucoma.

Furazolidone [202] **(Furoxone)**
Furazolidone, a MAO inhibitor, potentiates meperidine. Orthostatic hypotension and hypoglycemia may occur.

Imipramine (Tofranil)
See *Antidepressants, Tricyclic* above.

Iproniazid [839-842] **(Marsilid)**
See *MAO Inhibitors* below. This drug is no longer available in the U.S.

Isocarboxazid (Marplan)
See *MAO Inhibitors* below.

Isoniazid [120,202]
Isoniazid, with some MAO inhibitor activity, potentiates meperidine. Enhanced anticholinergic effects. Hazardous in glaucoma. See *MAO Inhibitors* below.

Levallorphan [120] **(Lorfan)**
Specific antidote against respiratory depression caused by overdosage of or hypersensitivity to meperidine.

MAO inhibitors [120,162,404,441,633,634,834-836,839-842,874,875, 1197,1342,1401,1440,1517,1883]
MAO inhibitors decrease the rate of detoxification of some narcotics (especially meperidine), causing a prolongation and intensification of CNS depression and increase in toxicity. The latter is caused by an accumulation of 5-HT (serotonin) in the brain. Serious reactions may occur including coma, severe hypotension, severe respiratory depression, violent convulsions, malignant hyperpyrexia (due to release of serotonin) excitation, peripheral vascular collapse, and even death. A variety of neurologic symptoms and dangerous blood pressure changes (both hypotension and hypertension depending on the conditions) have been reported. Contraindicated. Do not use meperidine within 2 or 3 weeks following treatment with MAO inhibitors. Chlorpromazine reduces the toxicity if given an hour before the meperidine is given. [1440]

Methotrimeprazine [120] **(Levoprome)**
Meperidine and methotrimeprazine have analgesic and sedative effects. Reduce the dosage of both drugs when used concurrently.

Nalorphine [120] **(Nalline)**
Nalorphine is a specific antidote against respiratory depression caused by meperidine overdosage or hypersensitivity to the drug.

Neostigmine [204] **(Prostigmin)**
Neostigmine, a cholinergic stimulant, increases the intensity and duration of analgesia produced by meperidine.

Nialamide (Niamid)
See *MAO Inhibitors* above.

Nitrates, nitrites [633]
Nitrates and nitrites, vasodilators, potentiate the hypotensive effect of meperidine.

MEPERIDINE *(continued)*

Oral contraceptives[92]
Oral contraceptives may potentiate meperidine by decreasing the urinary excretion of the analgesic and its metabolites.

Organophosphate cholinesterast inhibitors
See *Anticholinesterases* above.

Pargyline (Eutonyl)
See *MAO Inhibitors* above.

Phenelzine [60,425,835,843] (Nardil)
See *MAO Inhibitors* above.

Pheniprazine (Catron)
See *MAO Inhibitors* above.

Phenobarbital[83]
Initially, the combined effect may be enhanced CNS depression, but by enzyme induction by phenobarbital tends to inhibit meperidine.

Phenothiazines [78,633,669,844-846]
Enhanced CNS depression; sedation, hypotension. IV and IM administration of promazine (Sparine) and meperidine results in shock, collapse, and death, including fetal death.

Promazine (Sparine)
See *Phenothiazines* above.

Promethazine (Phenergan)
See *Phenothiazines* above.

Propiomazine [120] (Largon)
Propiomazine, a sedative, potentiates the CNS depressant effects of meperidine. The dose of meperidine should be reduced by ¼ to ½ in the presence of propiomazine.

d-Thyroxine [951] (Choloxin)
d-Thyroxine potentiates meperidine.

Tranylcypromine [120,834] (Parnate)
See *MAO Inhibitors* above.

MEPHENESIN (Myanesin, Tolserol)
This drug is no longer marketed in the U.S. but the information on interactions is given below because the actions of mephenesin have been studied more than practically any other muscle relaxant.

Barbiturates [120,166] (Hypnotics, Sedatives)
Concomitant use of this muscle relaxant with a sedative or hypnotic (barbiturates, etc.) may cause marked sedation and respiratory depression. Death may occur with high dosages. See *CNS Depressants*. Although mephenesin is no longer used it is the prototype of the centrally acting muscle relaxants. See *Muscle Relaxants, Centrally Acting*.

MEPHENTERMINE (Wyamine)
See *Sympathomimetics*.
No longer marketed in the U.S. The drug interactions given below are retained, however, to indicate the variability and complexity when a pressor agent like mephentermine has both directly acting (on α-receptors) and indirectly acting by release of endogenous norepinephrine.

Guanethidine [330,421,550,633] (Ismelin)
Guanethidine, an adrenergic blocking hypotensive agent, may inhibit or potentiate mephentermine, an indirect-acting pressor agent depending on the timing. Mephentermine may or may not antagonize the hypotensive effects of guanethidine. See *Polymechanistic Drugs* (page 378).

MAO inhibitors[847]
Tachycardia and hypertension are produced as a result of potentiation of the pressor agent (norepinephrine releaser) by MAO inhibitors.

Methyldopa [168,633] (Aldomet)
Methyldopa may or may not have a potentiating or antagonizing action on the indirectly acting pressor agent, mephentermine, depending on the timing. See *Polymechanistic Drugs* (page 378).

Rauwolfia alkaloids [633,636]
Mephentermine, an indirect-acting pressor agent, inhibits the hypotensive effects of the reserpine group of alkaloids. These catecholamine depleters inhibit mephentermine which depends on release of stored catecholamines for its action. See *Polymechanistic Drugs* (page 378).

MEPHENYTOIN (Mesantoin)
Same as for *Diphenylhydantoin*

MEPIVACAINE HCL (Carbocaine HCl)
See *Anesthetics, Local*.

Tetracaine [120,166] (Pontocaine)
Enhanced toxicity may result from the combination.

MEPROBAMATE (Equanil, Miltown)

Alcohol [121,311,634,732,733]
See *CNS Depressants* below. Impaired ability, coordination and judgment.

Anticoagulants, oral [96,223,330]
Meprobamate can induce metabolizing enzymes; larger doses of the anticoagulant may be required but decrease them if meprobamate is withdrawn.

Antidepressants, tricyclic [120,198,421]
Meprobamate may be useful as a tranquilizer in controlling manic episodes caused as an adverse effect with tricyclics. Tricyclic antidepressants may potentiate the response to CNS depressants such as meprobamate.

Barbiturates [198,421,640,1310,2010]
See *CNS Depressants* below. The net effect of interaction between a barbiturate and meprobamate in a given patient may be unpredictable because the CNS depressant effects of both are additive and yet inhibition occurs because of enzyme induction. Meprobamate inhibits plasma protein binding of thiopental (Pentothal) and thus potentiates the anesthetic effect of the barbiturate.

Benactyzine[951]
Benactyzine inhibits microsomal meprobamate metabolism, conversion to the metabolites hydroxymeprobamate and the N-glucuronide may be slowed, and the effect of meprobamate potentiated.

Carisoprodol [83,565] (Rela, Soma)
Carisoprodol decreases the effect of meprobamate via enzyme induction. Crosshypersensitivity reactions may occur with these drugs which have similar structures.

CNS depressants [166]
The CNS depressant effects of meprobamate and other CNS depressants are additive or synergistic. When alcohol and meprobamate are taken together the half-life of the tranquilizer may be prolonged significantly (competitive inhibition of the meprobamate oxidizing enzymes). However, in chronic consumers of alcohol, the metabolizing enzymes of the tranquilizer are induced and the half-life is decreased (tolerance develops). Thus caution must be exercised when psychotropic drugs, alcohol, etc., are given concomitantly. Potentiation or overdosage can lead to drowsiness, lethargy, stupor, ataxia, coma, shock, vasomotor and respiratory collapse, and in some instances death.

l-Glutavite [950,951]
l-Glutavite potentiates the psychotropic activity of meprobamate.

Glutethimide[951]
Glutethimide inhibits meprobamate by enzyme induction. The reverse action may also be possible.

MAO inhibitors[599]
MAO inhibitors increase the sedation and other CNS depressant effects of meprobamate.

Meprobamate[63,118]
Patients develop tolerance to meprobamate; decreases its own effect by enzyme induction.

Methotrimeprazine
Additive effect. Reduce dosage of both drugs when used concurrently. See *CNS Depressants* above.

Muscle relaxants
See *Carisoprodol* above.

Pentylenetetrazol[120] **(Metrazol, etc.)**
Pentylenetetrazol, a CNS stimulant, is used as an antidote to counteract the respiratory depression or failure caused by poisoning with meprobamate.

Sedatives and hypnotics
See *CNS Depressants* above.

Steroid hormones[78]
(Estrogens, oral contraceptives, etc.)
Meprobamate may inhibit the action of estrogens during the menopause, by enzyme induction, as well as the effectiveness of oral contraceptives.

Thiopental (Pentothal)
See *Barbiturates* above.

Warfarin
See *Anticoagulants, Oral* above.

MEPROSPAN
See *Meprobamate.*

MEPROTABS
See *Meprobamate.*

MEPYRAMINE MALEATE
See *Antihistamines* (pyrilamine maleate).

MERALLURIDE (Mercuhydrin)
See *Mercurial Diuretics.*

MERCAPTOPURINE (Purinethol)

Allopurinol[28,120,181,330,633,1002,1238,1275,1295] **(Zyloprim)**
Allopurinol potentiates both the antineoplastic action and toxic effects of mercaptopurine by inhibiting its metabolic oxidation with xanthine oxidase. Reduce dose of the antineoplastic to ⅓ or ¼ of the usual dose to reduce toxic effects. Large IV doses of mercaptopurine do not appear to be affected as much as oral doses.

Anticoagulants, oral
See *Mercaptopurine* under *Anticoagulants, oral.*

Methotrexate[120,443]
Leukopenia plus thrombocytopenia may occur; both agents depress the hematopoietic system.

Prednisone[443]
Hyperuricemia may occur with this combination.

Salicylates[470]
Salicylates (aspirin) potentiate mercaptopurine and induce pancytopenia.

Sulfonamides[470]
Sulfonamides potentiate mercaptopurine and induce pancytopenia.

MERCUHYDRIN (Meralluride)
See *Mercurial Diuretics* below.

MERCURIAL DIURETICS
(chlormerodin [Neohydrin], meralluride [Mercuhydrin], mercaptomerin [Thiomerin], mercurophylline [Mercupurine], merethoxylline [Dicurin], etc.)

Acidifying agents, urinary[172]
Urinary acidifying agents (ammonium chloride, etc.) increase the diuretic effects of mercuhydrin.

Alkalinizing agents[165,421]
Alkalinizing agents reduce the diuretic effects of mercurial diuretics.

Analgesics[5]
Potent analgesics, by impairing renal function and decreasing urinary output, may interfere with the action of mercurial diuretics.

Chloride ion[172]
Chloride ion enhances diuresis with mercurial diuretics.

Digitalis[120,172]
Mercurial diuretics enhance the activity of digitalis and its toxicity through hypokalemia if it is induced (cardiac arrhythmias).

Ethacrynic acid[120]
The diuretic, ethacrynic acid, enhances the diuretic effects of mercurial diuretics.

MESCALINE

Histamine[169,950,951]
Mescaline enhances the increase in blood pressure produced by histamine in some animals. In man and some other species histamine causes a dramatic fall in systemic blood pressure.

MESANTOIN
See *Anticonvulsants* (mephenytoin).

MESTINON
See *Parasympathomimetics* (pyridostigmine Br).

METAHYDRIN
See *Thiazide Diuretics* (trichlormethiazide).

METALEX
See *Niacin* and *Pentylenetetrazol.*

METAMINE WITH BUTABARBITAL
See *Barbiturates* (butabarbital) and *Nitrates and Nitrites* (aminotrate phosphate).

METANDREN
See *Androgens* (methyltestosterone).

METAPROTERENOL (Alupent, orciprenaline)

Compound lobelia powder[849]
The bronchodilator (β-receptor activator) metaproterenol caused sudden death in an asthmatic patient using compound lobelia powder.

METARAMINOL (Aramine)

Diazepam[120] **(Valium)**
Metaraminol combats the hypotension caused by overdosage of diazepam.

Guanethidine[550,633,824] **(Ismelin)**
Guanethidine does not appreciably inhibit the vasopressor action of metaraminol, a directly acting sympathomimetic. Metaraminol may antagonize the hypotensive effects of guanethidine which functions by partial depletion of norepinephrine stores in adrenergic neurons and blockage of the release of the remainder (adrenergic blocking agent). The combina-

METARAMINOL (Aramine) *(continued)*
tion may cause severe headaches and nausea with severe hypertension due to sensitization of adrenergic neurons to the α-adrenergic sympathomimetic by guanethidine. See *Polymechanistic Drugs* (page 378).

MAO inhibitors[217]
MAO inhibitors combined with vasopressors such as metaraminol can cause an acute hypertensive crisis with possible intracranial hemorrhage, hyperthermia, convulsions, coma and in some cases death. MAO is irreversibly inhibited. Metabolism of monoamines is blocked causing their accumulation. This prolongs and potentiates the action of agents like tyramine which release norepinephrine from peripheral stores. This release and the central additive stimulation causes the hypertensive crisis.

Methyldopa[633] **(Aldomet)**
Metaraminol may cause hypertension during the early catecholamine-releasing stage of methyldopa therapy. After such depletion, the pressor drug antagonizes the antihypertensive. See *Polymechanistic Drugs* (page 378).

Pargyline
See *MAO Inhibitors* above.

Reserpine[633,640]
Reserpine, an adrenergic blocking agent, has interactions similar to those of guanethidine and methyldopa. See *Polymechanistic Drugs* (page 378).

Thioxanthenes[120]
Hypotension induced by thioxanthenes responds to metaraminol.

METATENSIN
See *Antihypertensives* (reserpine) and *Thiazide Diuretics* (trichlormethiazide).

METHACHOLINE (Mecholyl)
See *Cholinergics*.

METHADONE (Dolophine)
See *CNS Depressants* and *Narcotic Analgesics*.

Nalorphine[39] **(Nalline)**
Nalorphine can precipitate acute abstinence syndromes in addicts who have received methadone therapy for brief periods or in patients physically dependent on methadone.

Neostigmine[204]
Neostigmine increases the intensity and duration of analgesia.

Nitrous oxide[166]
Narcotics are often given with nitrous oxide to provide adequate anesthesia since 70% N_2O is the maximum concentration that can be used without producing hypoxia.

Rifampin[1973,2049]
Rifampin, an enzyme inducer, lowers the plasma levels of methadone and may alter its distribution. Thus former heroin addicts on methadone experience narcotic withdrawal symptoms when they are treated for tuberculosis with rifampin. Symptoms range from yawning, irritability, rhinorrhea, and abdominal cramps to anorexia, joint pains, nausea, vomiting, tremulousness, and severe anxiety. However, a short course of rifampin may be the best initial approach for methadone patients with active, advanced tuberculosis.

METHAMPHETAMINE (Desoxyn, Methedrine, etc.)
See *Vasopressors*.

Antihypertensives[78]
Antihypertensives of the MAO inhibitor type potentiate methamphetamine; methamphetamine, a vasopressor and central stimulant, inhibits the antihypertensive effect of other types of hypotensives, except ganglionic blockers which it may potentiate under certain situations. See *Polymechanistic Drugs* (page 378).

Bethanidine[117]
See *Methamphetamine* under *Bethanidine*.

Guanethidine[117,626,633,797]
Loss of control of blood pressure may occur if an amphetamine is given to a patient receiving guanethidine because amphetamine blocks guanethidine from sites of action and also displaces it from those sites. Methamphetamine antagonizes the adrenergic neuron blocking action of guanethidine.

Halothane[796] **(Fluothane)**
Cardiac arrhythmias are induced.

Hydralazine[117]
Hydralazine reduces the pressor response to methamphetamine.

Hexamethonium[117]
Hexamethonium increases the pressor effects of methamphetamine.

Insulin[120]
Methamphetamine plus insulin induces lower blood glucose levels than insulin alone. Amphetamines may increase the metabolic rate and also plasma corticosteroids and immunoreactive growth hormone both of which impair glucose tolerance.

MAO inhibitors[41,60,305,850,851]
See *Sympathomimetics* and *MAO Inhibitors*.

Mecamylamine[117,633] **(Inversine)**
Sympathomimetic drugs reverse the hypotensive effect of mecamylamine. Mecamylamine increases the pressor effects of methamphetamine.

Methyldopa[117,633] **(Aldomet)**
Methamphetamine inhibits the hypotensive effect of methyldopa.

Pempidine[117]
Pempidine increases the pressor effects of methamphetamine.

Pentolinium[117]
Pentolinium increases the pressor effects of methamphetamine.

Reserpine[633,636]
Methamphetamine inhibits the hypotensive effect of reserpine and vice versa.

Tranylcypromine[137] **(Parnate)**
See *MAO Inhibitors*. Hypertensive crisis, and associated distress, *e.g.*, headache, myocarditis, cerebral hemorrhage, respiratory arrest, coma.

METHANDROSTENOLONE (Dianabol)

Anticoagulants, oral[119,366]
Methandrostenolone potentiates the effects of phenindione and coumarin anticoagulants; may cause hemorrhagic episodes in combination.

Hydrocortisone[181]
Methandrostenolone potentiates the anti-inflammatory activity of hydrocortisone.

Oxyphenbutazone[330,421,448,852] **(Tandearil)**
Methandrostenolone increases plasma levels of oxyphenbutazone by enzyme inhibition of glucuronyl transferase.

Warfarin (Coumadin, Panwarfin)
See *Anticoagulants, Oral* above.

METHAQUALONE (Melsedin, Optimil, Parest, Quaalude Somnifac, Sopor)

Alcohol[166]
See *CNS Depressants* below.

Anticoagulants, oral[120,619]
Excessive dosage of the sedative potentiates oral anticoagulants.

CNS Depressants[166]
Care should be used if methaqualone is administered with alcohol, analgesics, anesthetics, hypnotics, sedatives, psychotropic drugs, and other CNS depressants. Potentiation may occur. See *CNS Depressants*.

Methscopolamine[4,5] **(Hyoscine methylbromide)**
The sedative action of methscopolamine may be prolonged by methaqualone.

METHAZOLAMIDE (Neptazane)
See *Carbonic Anhydrase Inhibitors*.

METHDILAZINE (Tacaryl)
See *Phenothiazines*.

METHEDRINE
See *Methamphetamine*.

METHENAMINE

Acetazolamide[120] **(Diamox)**
Acetazolamide, which renders the urine alkaline, is antagonistic to methenamine which requires an acid urine (pH $\leq$ 5.5) in order that formaldehyde, the active urinary anti-infective, may be released.

Acidifiers, urinary[120,578]
Acid urinary pH (pH 5.5 or less) potentiates the antibacterial action of methenamine by increasing the rate of liberation of formaldehyde. Acidic interactants may prematurely decompose the drug.

Alkalies and ammonium salts[619]
Methenamine is discolored by ammonium salts and alkalies. See Chapter 7.

Alkalinizing agents[120,421]
Alkalinizing agents (sodium bicarbonate, etc.) inhibit methenamine by decreasing liberation of formaldehyde in the urine. See *Acetazolamide* above.

Alkaloids[619]
Methenamine is incompatible with most alkaloids.

Amphetamines[325,870]
The acidifying agents used with methenamine inhibit amphetamines by increasing their urinary excretion.

Gelatin[619]
Methenamine may slowly combine with gelatin, even gelatin capsules, and gradually become insoluble.

Metallic salts[619]
Ferric, mercuric, and silver salts are incompatible with methenamine.

Sodium bicarbonate
See *Alkalinizing Agents* above.

Sulfamethizole[280]
See *Sulfonamides* below.

Sulfonamides[28,120,280,433,662,1367,1628]
Formaldehyde, liberated from methenamine, condenses with sulfonamides (sulfamethizole, sulfathiazole, etc.) to form insoluble amorphous precipitates of formaldehyde-sulfonamide combinations in the urine, particularly at lower pH. Drug combinations like methenamine mandelate and sulfonamides are probably reduced in effectiveness as urinary antibacterials and may possibly increase the potential hazard of renal blockage or calculus formation. Sulfonamides such as sulfadiazine, sulfamerizine and sulfapyridine are likely to produce

crystalluria in the presence of the acid urine required with methenamine therapy.

METHERGINE
See *Oxytocics*

METHICILLIN SODIUM (Staphcillin)
See *Penicillin*.

Aminohippuric acid[433] **(PAH)**
Elevated serum levels of penicillin and increased toxicity.

Ampicillin[382]
Synergistic antibacterial effect.

Benzyl penicillin[382] **(Penicillin G)**
Synergistic antibacterial effect.

Cephalosporins[120]
Cross sensitivity occurs.

Chloramphenicol[240,301,444,492,864] **(Chloromycetin)**
Chloramphenicol inhibits the bactericidal action of this penicillin.

Erythromycin[31,70,301,419,811] **(Erythrocin, Ilotycin)**
Erythromycin inhibits the bactericidal action of this penicillin.

Fusidic acid[1122]
For methicillin-sensitive resistant staphylococci a combination of fusidic acid and methicillin is highly effective, whereas for methicillin-resistant strains of these organisms, fusidic acid is used with erythromycin, novobiocin, or rifamycin.

Kanamycin[210,239] **(Kantrex)**
Mutual inactivation in IV mixtures. See Chapter 7. Inhibition in some infections, potentiation in others.

Penicillins[382]
The combination of natural and semisynthetic penicillins have synergistic activity against *Strep. pyogenes* and *Staph. aureus*.

Probenecid[43,160,269] **(Benemid)**
Probenecid elevates and prolongs duration of blood concentration of methicillin by blockade of the renal tubular secretion of penicillins.

Tetracyclines[470]
Incompatible. Do not give together IV. Tetracyclines inhibit the bactericidal action of this penicillin.

METHIONINE
See *Urinary acidifiers*.

Acetaminophen[1330,1935]
See *Methionine* under *Acetaminophen*.

MAO inhibitors[532]
Methionine caused severe hypertension in patients receiving tranylcypromine.

METHISCHOL
See *Dietary Supplements*.

METHOCARBAMOL
See *Muscle Relaxants*.

METHOTREXATE (Amethopterin)
See also *Antineoplastics*.

Alcohol[120,734,1445,1691,1857]
Concomitant use of alcohol with this folic acid antagonist should be avoided because of the additive hepatotoxic potentials. Methotrexate-induced cirrhosis of the liver appears to be increased. Respiratory failure and coma have occurred with one cocktail. Avoid alcohol with methotrexate.

***p*-Aminobenzoic acid**[120,512] **(PABA)**
PABA enhances methotrexate toxicity by displacing it from protein binding sites. These drugs should be used with cau-

METHOTREXATE (Amethopterin) *(continued)*

tion when given concurrently. PABA is present in a large number of medications, both prescription and over-the-counter.

Analgesics [120,198]
Analgesics containing salicylates potentiate methotrexate.

Antipyretics [120,198]
Antipyretics containing salicylates potentiate methotrexate.

Aspirin [120,198,633]
Pancytopenia may occur. The effects of methotrexate are potentiated by aspirin. See *Salicylates* below.

Barbiturates [203]
Barbiturates potentiate methotrexate toxicity via displacement from protein binding sites.

5-Fluorouracil [951]
Synergistic antineoplastic activity results with the combination.

Griseofulvin (Grifulvin, Grisactin) [951]
Griseofulvin inhibits methotrexate via enzyme induction.

Hepatotoxic drugs, other [120]
Concomitant use of other drugs with hepatotoxic potential should be avoided.

Insulin [120]
Antineoplastics, *e.g.,* cyclophosphamide, tend to potentiate insulin and produce hypoglycemia by displacement of bound hormone.

Leucovorin [120]
Calcium leucovorin is the antidote of choice to antagonize the toxic effects of methotrexate overdosage if given within 4 hours before the affected cells become too damaged to respond.

Mercaptopurine [120] (Purinethol)
Leukopenia and thrombocytopenia may occur with this combination.

Other antineoplastics [120]
Combination of antineoplastics produces additive cytotoxic effects.

Phenytoin [203] (Dilantin)
Phenytoin potentiates methotrexate toxicity via displacement from protein binding sites.

Salicylates [78,120,330,359,512,633,1224,1334,1581]
Salicylates increase the plasma levels of methotrexate by displacing it from binding sites on plasma protein and by blocking its renal tubular secretion. This may lead to serious toxic reactions (pancytopenia and hepatotoxicity). A potentially lethal combination to be avoided. Special alertness is essential because salicylates are present in a host of prescription and OTC medications.

Smallpox vaccine
See *Immunosuppressants* under *Vaccines*.

Sulfamethizole (Mesulfin)
See *Sulfonamides* below.

Sulfisoxazole (Gantrisin, etc.)
See *Sulfonamides* below.

Sulfonamides [78,202,330,359,512,633]
Pancytopenia may occur. Same action on methotrexate as *Salicylates* above. A potentially lethal combination.

Tranquilizers [198,512,619]
Tranquilizers enhance methotrexate toxicity via displacement from protein binding sites.

Triamterene (Dyrenium) [120]
Triamterene potentiates methotrexate. Both are folic acid antagonists.

Vaccines (smallpox vaccine, tetanus toxoid, and other immunizing agents) [120,203,377,619,1199]
Methotrexate exerts an immunosuppressive effect which lowers resistance to disease as well as the immunity produced. See *Immunosuppressants* under *Vaccines*. A potentially lethal interaction, to be avoided.

Vincristine [433,443] (Oncovin)
This combination may cause melena and hypotension.

METHOTRIMEPRAZINE (Levoprome)
See *Analgesics* and *Phenothiazines*.

Acetylsalicylic acid
See *Analgesics* below.

Alcohol [120]
Potentiation of alcohol (CNS depression) occurs with phenothiazines.

Alkaloids
Incompatible with most alkaloids. Atropine and scopolamine are exceptions.

Analgesics [120,1014] (Aspirin, etc.)
Analgesics have an additive effect with methotrimeprazine. Reduce the dosage of one or both drugs if used concurrently. See *CNS Depressants* below.

Anesthetics, general [120]
See *CNS Depressants* below.

Anticholinergics
See *Methotrimeprazine* under *Anticholinergics*.

Antihistamines [120]
See *CNS Depressants* below.

Antihypertensives [120]
Concurrent use of antihypertensives, particularly the MAO inhibitor type, is contraindicated because of the hazard of increased orthostatic hypotension.

Atropine [120,1014]
Atropine must be used with caution if it is given concomitantly with phenothiazines which have varying degrees of anticholinergic activity also. Potentiation of atropine may induce tachycardia and fall in blood pressure may occur. Other effects, such as delirium and aggravated extrapyramidal symptoms may occur.

Barbiturates
See *CNS Depressants* below.

CNS Depressants [120,1014]
The phenothiazine, methotrimeprazine, has both sedative and analgesic effects and it occasionally causes orthostatic hypotension, all of which effects are additive with those of other CNS depressants, including morphine, meperidine, aspirin, other salicylates, and other analgesics, general anesthetics, sedatives such as antihistamines and the barbiturates, antihypertensives such as reserpine, and tranquilizers such as meprobamate. When used in combination the dosage of one or both drugs should be decreased and closely monitored. Combinations that produce severe hypotension or other serious effects are contraindicated.

Epinephrine [120,619,1014]
Epinephrine should not be used to alleviate severe hypotensive effects that may develop with methotrimeprazine because of a paradoxical reversal of the pressor effects of epinephrine by phenothiazines.

Guanethidine
See *Methotrimeprazine* under *Guanethidine Sulfate*.

Heavy metals
Incompatible. See Chapter 7.

Hyoscine [120,1014] (Scopolamine)

Hyoscine and methotrimeprazine should be used with caution concomitantly in that tachycardia and fall in blood pressure may occur and undesirable CNS effects such as stimulation, delirium and extrapyramidal symptoms may be aggravated.

MAO inhibitors [120,1014]

Concurrent use of MAO inhibitors with methotrimeprazine is contraindicated; excessive hypotension.

Meperidine
See *CNS Depressants* above.

Meprobamate
See *CNS Depressants* above.

Methyldopa (Aldomet)
See *Methotrimeprazine* under *Methyldopa*.

Morphine
See *CNS Depressants* above.

Muscle relaxants [120,1014]

Peripherally acting muscle relaxants such as succinylcholine and the curare type are potentiated by methotrimeprazine. Toxicity may be increased and the muscle relaxant effect prolonged. Use concomitantly with caution in that tachycardia and fall in blood pressure may occur and undesirable CNS effects (delirium, extrapyramidal symptoms, and stimulation) may be aggravated.

Narcotics and narcotic analgesics
See *CNS Depressants above.*

Oxidizing agents
Incompatible. See Chapter 7.

Organophosphorus insecticides [120]
Same warning given for *Atropine* above.

Reserpine
See *CNS Depressants* above.

Salicylates
See *CNS Depressants* above.

Scopolamine [120]
Same warning as given for *Hyoscine* above.

Sedatives and hypnotics [120]
See *CNS Depressants* above.

Succinylcholine [120,1014]
See *Muscle Relaxants* above.

Trioxsalen [120] (Trisoralen)
No photosensitizing agent like methotrimeprazine should be given with trioxsalen. Serious burning may occur.

METHOXAMINE (Vasoxyl)
See *Sympathomimetics* and *Vasopressors*.

Ergonovine [609] (Ergotrate)
Severe hypertension may occur if methoxamine, a sympathomimetic pressor agent is injected soon after parenteral use of ergot alkaloids such as ergonovine and methylergonovine.

Halothane [820] (Fluothane)
Cardiac arrhythmias are induced by this combination.

MAO inhibitors [793]
Severe hypertension may be produced. See *MAO Inhibitors* under *Sympathomimetics*.

Methylergonovine [609] (Methergine)
See *Ergonovine* above.

Oxytocin [609] and other oxytocics
Postpartum hypertension may occur. Same warning as that given for *Ergonovine* above.

METHOXYFLURANE (Penthrane)
See *Anesthetics, General*

Aminoglycoside Antibiotics [1291,1307,1429] (Gentamycin, Kanamycin, Neomycin, Paromomycin, Streptomycin, Tobramycin, etc.)
Administration of these antibiotics following anesthesia with methoxyflurane may produce additive nephrotoxicity. Exercise extreme caution for permanent renal insufficiency may occur.

CNS depressants [120,166]
Use barbiturates, narcotics and other CNS depressants with this anesthetic cautiously to avoid respiratory depression.

Epinephrine [806,807]
Halogenated anesthetics cause cardiac arrhythmias and possibly death with sympathomimetics like epinephrine.

Gentamicin
See *Aminoglycoside Antibiotics* above.

Kanamycin
See *Aminoglycoside Antibiotics* above.

Levarterenol (Levophed)
See *Epinephrine* above.

Neomycin
See *Aminoglycoside Antibiotics* above.

Nitrous oxide [166]
Anesthesia with 50:50 nitrous oxide and oxygen mixture, together with methoxyflurane in low concentration causes increase in tension of inspired nitrous oxide and may produce appreciable depression of blood pressure, heart rate and muscle tone.

Paromomycin
See *Aminoglycoside Antibiotics* above.

Streptomycin
See *Aminoglycoside Antibiotics* above.

Tetracyclines [471,1191,1307]
Methoxyflurane anesthesia combined with tetracycline parenterally may seriously impair renal function and lead to death. Methoxyflurane potentiates the nephrotoxicity of antibiotics such as the aminoglycosides, amphotericin, cephalosporins, colistin, tetracyclines, etc. if these are prescribed during the preoperative, operative, and postoperative periods. Contraindicated. If they are used the patient must be monitored very closely for renal damage and the risk fully understood.

Tobramycin
See *Aminoglycoside Antibiotics* above.

Tubocurarine and other nondepolarizing muscle relaxants [878]
This anesthetic potentiates the effect of tubocurarine. Reduce the dosage of the muscle relaxant by about half.

METHSCOPOLAMINE
See *Hyoscine*.

METHYLAMPHETAMINE
See *Methamphetamine*.

MAO inhibitors [41,60,305,850,851]
Methylamphetamine administered to patients receiving MAO inhibitors may cause symptoms similar to those evoked in patients having a pheochromocytoma or subarachnoidal bleeding. Side effects (severe occipital headache, sweating, stiff neck, palpitations, paradoxical hypertension) can be severe. Deaths have been reported in patients receiving both tranylcypromine and an amphetaminelike compound.

METHYLDOPA (Aldomet)

See *Antihypertensives.*

Acidifiers, urinary [325,870]
Acidifiers inhibit the hypotensive activity of methyldopa by increasing its renal excretion.

Adrenergics [117,168,421,633]
Adrenergics may antagonize the hypotensive effect of methyldopa. The vasopressor effect may or may not be potentiated, depending on the timing and type of adrenergic agent. See *Polymechanistic Drugs* (page 378).

Alcohol
See *CNS Depressants* below.

Alkalinizing agents [325,870]
Opposite effect to *Acidifying Agents* above.

Amino acids [330]
The absorption of methyldopa may be inhibited by other amino acids ingested in the diet.

Amitriptyline [194,452]
Tricyclic antidepressants may inhibit the hypotensive effect of methyldopa. The combination of amitriptyline and methyldopa may cause agitation, hand tremors, and increased pulse rate and blood pressure.

Amphetamines [117,633]
Amphetamines, sympathomimetics that act indirectly by releasing norepinephrine from adrenergic neuronal storage sites, may antagonize the hypotensive effect of methyldopa. See *Adrenergics* above and exercise caution.

Anesthetics, general [633]
See *CNS Depressants* below.

Anticoagulants, oral [421]
Methyldopa potentiates coumarin anticoagulants like bishydroxycoumarin. Hemorrhage may occur.

Antidepressants [194,452,823,1524]
Methyldopa with antidepressants such as the MAO inhibitors and tricyclics may cause headache, hypertension and related symptoms in some patients. Combined use should be avoided or at least carefully monitored. See *Amitriptyline* above and *Polymechanistic Drugs* (page 378).

Antidiabetics [120]
Methyldopa increases the incidence of blood dyscrasias with oral antidiabetics.

Barbiturates [1523,1533,1553,1554]
Barbiturates may reduce methyldopa blood levels, possibly by enzyme induction, but proof at present is inadequate. Some authorities disagree with this mechanism. [1533]

Bethanidine [951]
Because of the synergistic antihypertensive activity, this combination may be effective in reducing blood pressure in resistant patients.

CNS Depressants [633]
The combined hypotensive effects of methyldopa and a CNS depressant such as a general anesthetic, alcohol, narcotic analgesic, etc., may be hazardous. Catecholamine depletion increases the risk of vascular collapse during surgery. Cardiac arrest may occur.

Diuretics
See *Thiazide Diuretics* below.

Dopa [168]
Methyldopa inhibits pressor and other responses to dopa by inhibiting its decarboxylation by aromatic L-amino acid decarboxylase (forms the pressor catecholamine, dopamine, normally).

Ephedrine [1815]
Ephedrine, an indirectly acting synepathomimetic via norepinephrine release from adrenergic neuronal storage sites, may be antagonized in patients receiving methyldopa which produces a metabolite α-methyl-norepinephrine. The latter (acting as a "false transmitter") in some circumstances, through storage in sympathetic nerve endings, decreases the amount of norepinephrine available for release by ephedrine. Thus the mydriatic effect of ephedrine in the eye is decreased.

Furazolidone [633] **(Furoxone)**
Excitation and hypertension may be produced with this MAO inhibitor plus methyldopa. See *MAO Inhibitors* below.

Haloperidol
See *Methyldopa* under *Haloperidol.*

Hydrochlorothiazide [117,120] **(Hydrodiuril)**
Synergistic antihypertensive activity.

Hypotensives [120]
Methyldopa may have an additive hypotensive effect with other hypotensives. Adjust the dose carefully.

Levarterenol [117] **(Levophed, norepinephrine)**
Methyldopa potentiates levarterenol 2- or 3-fold by preventing its uptake into its inactive storage sites in adrenergic neurons. The metabolite of methyldopa (α-methyl-norepinephrine) acts as a "false transmitter." According to one theory, it is stored in sympathetic nerve endings instead of the naturally occurring catecholamine norepinephrine and thus pressor effects of norepinephrine, infused as a drug, are greatly enhanced as well as its other α-adrenergic effects. Administer with caution.

Levodopa [433,633,724,872,922,1417,1418,1443,1547,1647,1648,1840,1917]
Methyldopa is capable of defeating the therapeutic purpose of levodopa in Parkinson's syndrome, perhaps through replacement of dopamine (normally replenished from levodopa) with a "false transmitter" (α-methyl-norepinephrine, a methyldopa metabolite). See under *Levarterenol* and *Ephedrine* above. The inhibiting effect of methyldopa has been used intentionally to modify the antiparkinsonism action of levodopa. Another concurrent interaction to be considered is the additive hypotensive effects of both drugs. Monitor each patient carefully.

Lithium carbonate [1975]
Methyldopa, used to control hypertension in a patient on lithium carbonate (1800 mg. lithium carbonate and 1 Gm. methyldopa daily) produced elevated lithium blood levels and toxicity (diarrhea, tremors, blurred vision, confusion, slurred speech). The methyldopa had to be discontinued and the lithium carbonate dosage decreased 50%.

MAO inhibitors [120,166,170,348,633,663,1878]
MAO inhibitors may reverse the hypotensive effect of methyldopa and produce a strong and prolonged excitation of the CNS resembling amphetamine overdosage. Headache, hallucinations, hypertension and related symptoms may develop; combined use should be avoided. See *Polymechanistic Drugs*

Mephentermine [168,633] **(Wyamine)**
Same as for *Metaraminol* below.

Metaraminol [633] **(Aramine)**
Metaraminol inhibits the hypotensive effect of methyldopa. Methyldopa may have a mild potentiating effect on the pressor agents mephentermine and metaraminol.

Methamphetamine [117,633] **(Desoxyn, Methedrine)**
Methamphetamine inhibits the antihypertensive effect of methyldopa.

Methotrimeprazine [120] **(Levoprome)**
Methotrimeprazine, with its commonly occurring side effect orthostatic hypotension, should not be given with the hypotensive methyldopa because of the additive effects.

Norepinephrine
See *Levarterenol* above.

Pargyline (Eutonyl)
See *MAO Inhibitors* above.

Phenothiazines [1899]
Phenothiazines may block uptake of the "false transmitter" α-methyl-norepinephrine (methyldopa metabolite) and thereby reverse the action of methyldopa and produce hypertension. Monitor patients closely if phenothiazines such as trifluoperazine (Stelazine) are added to the regimen.

Phenylpropanolamine
See *Methyldopa* under *Phenylpropanolamine*

Propranolol (Inderal)
See *Antihypertensives* under *Propranolol*.

Sympathomimetics [30,117,421,633]
Sympathomimetics inhibit the hypotensive effect of methyldopa; methyldopa potentiates sympathomimetics; hypertension may occur but see full discussion of *Sympathomimetics* under *Reserpine*. See also *Polymechanistic Drugs* (page 378).

Thiazide diuretics [117,120]
Enhanced hypotensive effect. The diuretic also counteracts weight gain and edema which may occur with methyldopa therapy. Decrease methyldopa dosage by as much as 50%.

Tolbutamide [421] (Orinase)
This combination may cause blood dyscrasias. See *Anticoagulants, Oral* above.

Urinary acidifiers [325,870]
Acidifiers inhibit the activity of methyldopa by increasing its renal excretion.

METHYLERGONOVINE (Methergine)
See under *Methoxamine* and *Oxytocics*.

Vasopressin [120] (Pitressin)
Excessively high blood pressure may result from this combination.

METHYLMITOMYCIN

5-Fluorouracil [951]
This combination has synergistic antineoplastic activity against ascites cell neoplasms.

METHYLPHENIDATE (Ritalin)

Adrenergics [156]
Methylphenidate, a sympathomimetic agent and psychomotor stimulant which is also an enzyme inhibitor potentiates many drugs. It should not be given concomitantly with pressor agents such as epinephrine and levarterenol (hazardous in glaucoma and may precipitate a hypertensive crisis).

Angiotensin [120] (Hypertensin)
Methylphenidate potentiates the adverse effect of anticholinergics. Hazardous in glaucoma.

Anticholinergics [421]
Methylphenidate potentiates the adverse effect of anticholinergics. Hazardous in glaucoma.

Anticoagulants, oral [156,359,705] (Coumadin, Dicumarol, Hedulin, etc.)
Methylphenidate may potentiate the anticoagulant effect of oral anticoagulants by inhibiting their metabolism.

Anticonvulsants [156]
Methylphenidate may potentiate anticonvulsants.

Antidepressants, tricyclic
Methylphenidate should be used cautiously with antidepressants; it may inhibit metabolism of drugs like imipramine and desipramine and thereby potentiate them. See *Methylphenidate* under *Antidepressants, Tricyclic*.

Cyclazocine [166,421]
Methylphenidate reverses the respiratory depression produced by cyclazocine.

Diazepam [120] (Valium)
Methylphenidate combats the CNS depressant effects caused by diazepam overdosage.

Epinephrine
See *Adrenergics* above.

Guanethidine [595,626,797] (Ismelin)
Methylphenidate antagonizes the hypotensive effect of guanethidine. Cardiac arrhythmias may occur.

Imipramine [194] (Tofranil)
Methylphenidate inhibits the metabolism of imipramine, thus potentiating this tricyclic antidepressant, and producing a synergistic effect. Use caution.

MAO Inhibitors [74,874]
Acute hypertensive crisis with possible intracranial hemorrhage, hyperthermia, convulsions, coma and in some cases death may occur. MAO is irreversibly inhibited. Metabolism of monoamines is doubly blocked, causing their accumulation. This prolongs and potentiates release of norepinephrine from peripheral stores. This release and the central additive stimulation cause the hypertensive crisis.

Pentazocine [166] (Talwin)
Methylphenidate blocks the respiratory depression produced by pentazocine.

Phenobarbital [156]
Methylphenidate potentiates the anticonvulsant action of phenobarbital by enzyme inhibition.

Phenytoin [155,1641]
Methylphenidate may produce potentially toxic blood levels of phenytoin and induce distressing reactions like ataxia, blood dyscrasias, diplopia, fatal toxic hepatitis, and nystagmus (enzyme inhibition). This interaction was questioned by two investigators. [1641]

Pressor agents [120,619]
Pressor response may be enhanced with methylphenidate. See *Adrenergics* above.

Primidone [156,359] (Mysoline)
Methylphenidate potentiates the anticonvulsant action of primidone (enzyme inhibition).

Serotonin [853]
Methylphenidate potentiates the blood pressure response to serotonin.

Sympathomimetics [421]
Methylphenidate potentiates the adverse effects on glaucoma and the pressor effects of sympathomimetics.

Zoxazolamine [156] (Flexin)
Methylphenidate, by enzyme inhibition, potentiates zoxazolamine (no longer marketed in the U.S.).

METHYLTHIOURACIL

Anticoagulants, coumarin [147,421,673]
Methylthiouracil increases the activity of the anticoagulants; hemorrhage may occur if methylthiouracil is added to a stabilized anticoagulant regimen.

METHYSERGIDE (Sansert)

Narcotic analgesics [421]
Methysergide, an analog of the ergot alkaloids structurally related to LSD, reverses the analgesic activity of narcotic analgesics.

METICORTELONE
See *Prednisolone*.

METOCLOPRAMIDE (Maxolon)

Acetaminophen
See *Metoclopramide* under *Acetaminophen*

Digitalis glycosides
See *Metoclopramide* under *Digitalis*.

METOPROLOL
See *Epinephrine* under *Propranolol*.

METRANIL-AM
See *Barbiturates* (Amobarbital) and *Nitrates and Nitrites* (Pentaerythritol Tetranitrate).

METRONIDAZOLE (Flagyl)

Alcohol [354,427,735,736,1412,1503,1698,1846]
Metronidazole inhibits the enzyme aldehyde dehydrogenase and slows the rate of metabolism of alcohol. Disulfiramlike intolerance to alcohol may ensue. A variety of neurologic symptoms appear. In one long term trial the disulfiramlike reaction was not encountered according to the investigator yet many side effects were reported (headache, nausea, foul taste, etc.) with the combination. Warn patients not to consume alcohol while taking Flagyl for amebiasis or trichomoniasis.

Disulfiram [791,1452]
Combined use has led to the development of acute psychoses and confusional states. Avoid concomitant use.

X-radiation [2002]
See *Metromidazole* under *X-radiation*.

METUBINE
See *Muscle Relaxants* (Dimethyltubocurarine).

METYRAPONE (Metopirone)

Phenytoin
See *Metyrapone* under *Phenytoin*

MI-CEBRIN T
See *Dietary Supplements*.

MIDRIN
See *Acetaminophen, Dichloralphenazone*, and *Isometheptene mucate*.

MILK

Antibiotics [665] **(Tetracyclines)**
Milk and milk products inhibit absorption of tetracycline antibiotics (calcium complex).

Feosol Elixir [120]
Feosol Elixir should not be mixed with milk since iron forms insoluble complexes with certain constituents of milk.

Sodium bicarbonate [61,1085] **(absorbable alkali)**
Prolonged intake of a combination of milk and absorbable alkali (sodium bicarbonate) produces hypercalcemia, renal insufficiency. See a fuller discussion under *Sodium Bicarbonate*.

MAO inhibitors [687]
Canned milk taken by patients on MAO inhibitors has produced headache and hypertension.

MILONTIN
See *Anticonvulsants* (Phensuximide).

MILPATH
See *Anticholinergics* (Tridihexethyl chloride) and *Meprobamate*.

MILTOWN
See *Meprobamate*.

MILTRATE
See *Meprobamate* and *Nitrates and Nitrites* (Pentaerythritol Tetranitrate).

MINERAL OIL

Anthelmintics [421]
Reduced anthelmintic effect because of reduced absorption.

Anticoagulants, oral [128,120,421,673]
Variable alterations of the anticoagulant effect have occurred on rare occasions. Enhanced activity of the anticoagulant may occur through sequestering of vitamin K synthesized in the gut and thus preventing gastrointestinal absorption. On the other hand, the oil may decrease absorption of the anticoagulants under certain conditions. Also, up to 60% of a dose of mineral oil may be absorbed in some individuals, and the oil thus becomes available to affect prothrombin levels. [35]

Dioctyl sodium sulfosuccinate [4d]
Absorption of mineral oil may be increased; should not be given concurrently for long periods.

Hexylresorcinol [421]
Reduced anthelmintic effect through solution in the oil and reduced absorption.

Oral contraceptives
See *Mineral Oil* under *Oral Contraceptives*.

Poloxalkol (Magcyl, Polykol)
This surface active agent may increase the absorption of mineral oil and should not be given with it for prolonged periods.

Sulfonamides [421]
Mineral oil antagonizes the antibacterial action of sulfonamides in GI tract infections only.

Vitamins [28,35,198,616,1296]
Prolonged administration of mineral oil may reduce the absorption of fat-soluble vitamins (A, D, E, K) and possibly others (B, C, etc.). See *Mineral Oil* under *Vitamin A*.

Warfarin [120] **(Coumadin)**
See *Anticoagulants, Oral* above.

MIO-PRESSIN
See *Antihypertensives* (phenoxybenzamine), *Rauwolfia Alkalodis* and *Veratrum Alkaloids*.

Anesthetics [120]
Hypotension from this combination may last up to 2 weeks after withdrawal of Mio-Pressin.

MIOTICS

Epinephrine [548]
Epinephrine antagonizes the beneficial effects of miotics in glaucoma.

MI-PILO
See *Miotics* (Pilocarpine).

MIRADON
See *Anticoagulants* (Anisindione).

MISSION PRENATAL
See *Calcium Salts, Dietary Supplements*, and *Iron Salts* (Ferrous Gluconate).

MITOMYCIN

5-Fluorouracil [951]
Synergistic antineoplastic activity against ascites cell neoplasms.

6-Thioguanine [951]
Synergistic antineoplastic activity against ascites cell neoplasms.

MOL-IRON
See *Dietary Supplements* and *Iron Salts*.

MONACET
See *Caffeine*, *Phenacetin*, and *Salicylates* (Aspirin).

MONOAMINE OXIDASE INHIBITORS
See *MAO Inhibitors*.

MONOMEB
See *Anticholinergics* (Penthienate) and *Barbiturates* (Mephobarbital)

MONOSODIUM GLUTAMATE (MSG)
See *L-Glutavite*.

MORPHINE

β-Adrenergic Blocking Agents[698]
β-Adrenergic blocking agents like propranolol have a synergistic CNS depressant action with morphine.

Alcohol[121,311,634]
Synergistic CNS depression. See *CNS Depressants* below.

Anticoagulants[453]
Morphine potentiates the coumarin anticoagulants.

Atropine[166,168]
Atropine antagonizes the respiratory depression produced by morphine.

Black widow spider venom[120]
The venom is a neurotoxin that can cause respiratory paralysis; use morphine and other CNS depressants such as barbiturates with caution.

Chlorpromazine[166] **(Thorazine)**
Chlorpromazine potentiates the sedative and miotic effects of morphine.

CNS Depressants[78,633]
The use of more than one CNS depressant (alcohol, analgesics, general anesthetics, antihistamines, barbiturates, hypnotics, narcotics, phenothiazines, psychotropic agents, sedatives, etc.) simultaneously may result in additive effects with enhanced CNS depression (coma, respiratory paralysis, and possibly death), particularly in sensitive patients and in large doses. Some antihistamines, however, may inhibit morphine through enzyme induction with continued use.

Cyclazocine[166]
Cyclazocine inhibits morphine. See, however, *CNS Depressants* above.

Dextroamphetamine[1441]
Analgesia is augmented 2-fold when 10 mg. of dextroamphetamine is given IM with morphine for postoperative pain (1 1/2 times) when 5 mg. is given, and undesirable side effects are reduced.

Hyoscine[166] **(Scopolamine)**
Synergistic hypnotic and narcotic activity.

Imipraminelike drugs[166]
These drugs potentiate and prolong the depressant action of morphine and related narcotics.

Isopropylaminonitrophenylethanol (INPEA)[951]
Morphine enhances the toxicity of INPEA.

MAO inhibitors[854]
MAO inhibitors potentiate morphine analgesia and CNS depression. See *Narcotics* under *MAO Inhibitors*.

Methotrimeprazine[120]
Additive effect. Reduce dosage of both drugs when used concurrently.

Nalorphine[39]
Nalorphine is used as a morphine (narcotic) antagonist.

Neostigmine[168,204]
Neostigmine increases the intensity and duration of morphine analgesia.

Oral medications[1791]
Morphine tends to delay gastric emptying time and thus depresses drug absorption.

Papaverine[619]
Morphine antagonizes the relaxant effect of papaverine.

Phenelzine[854] **(Nardil)**
See *MAO Inhibitors* above.

Phenothiazines[633]
See *CNS Depressants* above.

Propiomazine[120] **(Largon)**
Morphine dosage should be reduced by 1/4 to 1/2 in the presence of the sedative propiomazine.

Propranolol[818]
Synergistic CNS depression. May cause death.

Reserpine[643]
Reserpine inhibits the analgesic activity of morphine.

Tyramine-rich foods[643]
Tyramine antagonizes the analgesic effects of morphine which depletes catecholamines.

Veratrum alkaloids[120,619]
The bradycrotic effect of veratrum alkaloids is additive to that produced by morphine and related drugs.

MSC TRIAMINIC TABLETS
See *Antihistamines* (pheniramine and pyrilamine maleate), *Scopolamine*, and *Sympathomimetics* (phenylpropanolamine).

MUDRANE
See *Aminophylline*, *Phenobarbital* and *Ephedrine*.

MULTIFUGE
See *Anthelmintics* (Piperazine Citrate).

MULTIVITAMIN PREPARATIONS

Levodopa[686,715]
Pyridoxine in these preparations neutralizes the effects of levodopa.

MUMPSVAX LYOVAC
See *Neomycin* (each dose contains 25 mcg.) and *Vaccines, Live Virus, Attenuated*.

MUSCLE RELAXANTS, CENTRALLY ACTING

Include chlorzoxazone (Paraflex); the propanediol (meprobamate) type of agents like carisoprodol (Rela, Soma); chlorphenesin carbamate (Maolate); mephenesin; metaxolone (Skelaxin); methocarbamol (Robaxin); orphenedrine citrate (Norflex); orphenadrine HCl (Disipal).
Skeletal muscle relaxants act centrally or peripherally. Centrally acting skeletal muscle relaxants selectively act on the CNS to produce a prominent sedative action without loss of consciousness plus skeletal muscular relaxation. The peripherally acting drugs are either the depolarizing or nondepolarizing type. Some drug interactions are common to all types; others are specific and may have opposite effects with different types.

Amphotericin B[120] **(Fungizone)**
Amphotericin may cause a decrease in serum potassium, hypokalemia has been reported to cause muscular weakness and, potentially, may increase the toxicity of muscle relaxants.

MUSCLE RELAXANTS, CENTRALLY ACTING
(continued)

Barbiturates [65,555,558,576]
Barbiturates, through enzyme induction, inhibit certain centrally acting muscle relaxants, *e.g.*, carisoprodol. See also *CNS Depressants* below.

Benzodiazepines
See *Diazepam* under *Muscle Relaxants, Competitive Type.*

Chlorcyclizine [565] (Perazil)
Same as for *Barbiturates* above.

CNS depressants [166]
Centrally acting muscle relaxants may increase the sedation and respiratory depression produced by CNS depressants. This combination can be letahl with high dosages.

Diphenhydramine (Benadryl)
Same as for *Barbiturates* above.

MAO inhibitors [312]
MAO inhibitors, through enzyme inhibition, may potentiate these muscle relaxants.

Meprobamate [83,555-557,565]
Cross sensitization may occur between related structures. Thus, the allergic reactions of carisoprodol and meprobamate may be additive. Carisoprodol, by enzyme induction, decreases the tranquilizing action of meprobamate.

Phenothiazines [120,566]
Anticholinergic muscle relaxants (*e.g.*, benztropine mesylate, which has the anticholinergic properties of atropine and the antihistaminic properties of diphenhydramine) may relieve drug-induced parkinsonism symptoms produced by phenothiazines, but may intensify mental symptoms (possible toxic psychosis). Phenothiazines may potentiate muscle relaxants. Apnea may occur.

Propoxyphene [120,714] (Darvon)
See *Propoxyphene* under *Orphenadrine.*

Piminodine Ethanesulfonate [120]
(Alvodine Ethanesulfonate)
Muscle relaxants potentiate piminodine. See *CNS Depressants* and *Narcotic Analgesics.*

Pyridostigmine bromide [170]
A centrally acting muscle relaxant, methocarbamol (Robaxin), inhibited the action of pyridostigmine bromide administered to a patient for myasthemia gravis.

Reserpine [120]
Anticholinergic muscle relaxants (*e.g.*, benztropine mesylate) may relieve drug-induced parkinsonism symptoms produced by reserpine but may intensify mental symptoms (possible toxic psychosis).

MUSCLE RELAXANTS, PERIPHERALLY ACTING (Neuromuscular blocking agents)
See also *Neuromuscular Blocking Antibiotics* under *Antibiotics.* Neuromuscular blocking agents include the curariform (competitive, nondepolarizing, stabilizing) agents like gallamine (Flaxedil) triethiodide, dimethyl tubocurarine iodide (Metubine, Mesotrin), and *d*-tubocurarine; the depolarizing agents like decamethonium (Syncurine) and succinylcholine (Anectine) chloride; and agents with these combined actions like benzoquinonium (Mytolon).

All 3 types of peripherally acting muscle relaxants may interact with the following drugs as indicated but some drug interactions are specific for either the competitive or depolarizing type of relaxants and some drugs interact with each type in the opposite manner. Thus anticholinesterases such as isoflurophate and neostigmine antagonize curare and potentiate decamethonium. Competitive agents may be antagonistic to the depolarizing agents. Thus tubocurarine is antagonistic to decamethonium. Drug interactions that are more specific for the competitive and depolarizing agents are covered separately in sections following this one.

Aminoglycoside antibiotics [146,560,1448,1706,1890,1916]
(Gentamicin, Kanamycin, Neomycin, Paromomycin, Streptomycin, Tobramycin)
Neuromuscular blockade is dangerously potentiated (apnea, respiratory muscle paralysis) when one of these antibiotics is injected concomitantly with a neuromuscular blocking agent. See also *Neuromuscular Blocking Antibiotics* under *Antibiotics* and *Colistin* below.

Amphotericin B [28]
Amphotericin B, by producing hypokalemia, potentiates skeletal muscle relaxants.

Antiarrhythmics
See lidocaine under *Local Anesthetics* below.

Antibiotics [28]
The potentiating effect of neuromuscular blocking antibiotics is discussed below under *Colistin.* Also see *Neuromuscular Blocking Antibiotics* under *Antibiotics.*

Anticholinesterases [168,198]
(DFP, Parathion, etc.)
Anticholinesterases such as the decurarizing agents edrophonium and neostigmine inhibit the competitive type of peripheral acting muscle relaxants (dimethyl tubocurarine, gallamine, kanamycin, neomycin, streptomycin, tubocurarine, etc.) and may act as antidotes in curare type of overdosage, but they potentiate the depolarizing type (collistimethate, decamethonium, gramicidin, polymyxin, succinylcholine). Potentiation may lead to respiratory paralysis, and possibly death. The organophosphate insecticides and phospholine iodide (Echothiophate) are also anticholinesterases with similar actions.

Bacitracin
See *Colistin* below.

Benzodiazepines (Librium, Valium, etc.)
See *Muscle Relaxants* under *Benodiazepines.*

Cathartics [28]
Cathartics, by producing hypokalemia, potentiate skeletal muscle relaxants.

Cholinergics
See *Anticholinesterases* above.

Cinchona alkaloids
See *Quinidine* below.

Colistin and derivatives [120,146,178,432,442,500-507,560-563,890] (Coly-Mycin, etc.)
The peripheral acting muscle relaxants function by blocking nerve transmission at the neuromuscular junction. Since colistin also nas this activity, and since the muscle relaxants appear to sensitize the neuromuscular junction to this effect of the antibiotic, the combination should be used with great caution and it may be contraindicated. Additive interference with transmission may result in prolonged respiratory muscle paralysis and reversible or irreversible apnea. Other antibiotics that are depolarizing or competitive agents which may also potentiate neuromuscular blockade include bacitracin, dihydrostreptomycin, gentamicin, gramicidin, kanamycin, neomycin, polymyxin B, streptomycin, and viomycin. See under *Antibiotics* and *Neomycin.*

Cyclophosphamide
See *Succinylcholine* under *Cyclophosphamide*

Dihydrostreptomycin
See *Colistin* above.

Diuretics [28]
Diuretics, by producing hypokalemia, potentiate skeletal muscle relaxants.

Echothiophate
See *Succinylcholine* under *Echothiophate.*

Ethacrynic acid [28,433] **(Edecrin)**
Ethacrynic acid potentiates polarizing muscle relaxants.

Ether [168]
Ether anesthesia potentiates the polarizing peripheral acting muscle relaxants.

**Fluorophosphates
(insecticides, Echothiopate, Floropryl, etc.)**
See *Anticholinesterases* above.

Furosemide [433] **(Lasix)**
Prolonged paralysis of respiratory muscles may occur. Persistent curarization. Potassium depletion may be involved.

Gentamicin (Garomycin)
See *Aminoglycoside Antibiotics* above.

Gramicidin
See *Colistin* above.

Insecticides
See *Anticholinesterases* above.

Kanamycin (Kantrex)
See *Aminoglycoside Antibiotics* above.

Lidocaine
See *Muscle Relaxants* under *Lidocaine.*

Local anesthetics [435,579,790,878] **(Novocain, etc.)**
Local anesthetics (procaine, lidocaine, etc.) prolong apnea from succinylcholine chloride; intravenous procaine injections may potentiate the effect of succinylchloline by displacing it from protein binding.

Magnesium salts [1037,1444,1650]
Concomitant use of magnesium salts with neuromuscular blocking muscle relaxants (decamethonium, succinylcholine, tubocurarine, etc.) potentiates the blockade. Exercise caution with this combination and be prepared to relieve excessive neuromuscular blockade.

MAO inhibitors [855]
Muscle relaxants are potentiated by MAO inhibitors.

Methotrimeprazine
See *Muscle Relaxants* under *Methotrimeprazine*

Narcotic analgesics
See *Muscle Relaxants, Centrally Acting* under *Narcotic Analgesics.*

Neomycin
See *Aminoglycoside Antibiotics* above.

**Organophosphate cholinesterase inhibitors
(Antiglaucoma agents, insecticides, etc.)**
See *Anticholinesterases* above.

Paromomycin
See *Aminoglycoside Antibiotics* above.

Polymyxin B (Aerosporin)
See *Colistin* above.

Procaine
See *Succinylcholine* under *Procaine.*

Procainamide [120,564,619,790] **(Pronestyl)**
Procainamide potentiates succinylcholine and other peripherally acting muscle relaxants; enhanced neuromuscular blocking effect.

Propranolol [790,1186,1961]
Propranolol potentiates and prolongs the neuromuscular blocking action of succinycholine, tubocurarine, etc. See below under *Muscle Relaxants, Competitive Type.*

Quinidine [390]
Increased intensity and prolonged duration of the action of peripherally acting muscle relaxants, when used with quinidine, may lead to respiratory depression and apnea. The neuromuscular blocking effect of quinidine seems to be a curariform type of activity as well as a depression of muscle action potential.

Streptomycin
See *Aminoglycoside Antibiotics* above.

Thiamine [1829]
Thiamine may enhance the response of patients to muscle relaxants.

Thiazide diuretics [120,433,1448,1829]
Prolonged paralysis of respiratory muscles may occur with gallamine and tubocurarine. Persistent curarization. Potassium depletion may be involved.

Tobramycin
See *Aminoglycoside Antibiotics* above.

Trasylol (Aprotinin) [567]
Trasylol, a kallikrein inhibitor, produces apnea in patients who have just received neuromuscular blocking drugs such as succinylcholine and tubocurarine.

MUSCLE RELAXANTS, PERIPHERALLY ACTING, COMPETITIVE TYPE
(Curare, Gallamine, *d*-Tubocurarine, etc.)

Acetazolamide [330]
Acetazolamide potentiates muscle relaxants like gallamine.

Anesthetics, general [120]
(Fluoromar, Fluothane, Penthrane, etc.)
Many anesthetics (cyclopropane, ether, fluroxene, methoxyflurane) potentiate tubocurarine and its dosage must be reduced.

Anticholinesterases
See *Anticholinesterases* above.

Benzodiazepines (Librium, Valium, etc.)
See *Muscle Relaxants* under *Benzodiazepines.*

Carbon dioxide [1075]
Excess CO_2 potentiates *d*-tubocurarine.

Chlorthalidone [330] **(Hygroton)**
Chlorthalidone potentiates muscle relaxants like gallamine. Take necessary preoperative and postoperative precautions.

Colistin [120,146,563]
See the general statement under *Colistin* above. Potentiation and respiratory paralysis. See page 540.

Cyclopropane [878] **(Trimethylene)**
Same as for *Ether* below. Potentiation.

Diazepam [166,781,782,1331,1891] **(Valium)**
Neuromuscular block may be produced with this combination, *e.g.*, diazepam plus tubocurarine. Malignant hyperthermia. Some studies indicate that diazepam prolongs the duration of action of gallamine and decreases succinylcholine activity. Diazepam has centrally acting muscular relaxant activity, but this interaction has not been elucidated.

Dihydrostreptomycin
See *Colistin* above. Potentiation.

Diuretics [120] **(Lasix, thiazides, etc.)**
Sulfonamide diuretics potentiate tubocurarine.

Edrophonium (Tensilon)
Same as for *Neostigmine* below.

Epinephrine [168]
Epinephrine, possibly by increasing release of acetylcholine at nerve terminals, inhibits the effect of competitive agents like *d*-tubocurarine.

Ethacrynic acid [330] **(Edecrin)**
Ethacrynic acid potentiates muscle relaxants like gallamine.

MUSCLE RELAXANTS, PERIPHERALLY ACTING, COMPETITIVE TYPE
(continued)

Ether[878]
Ether acts synergistically with the competitive, neuromuscular blocking muscle relaxants, including benzoquinonium. The dosage of the muscle relaxants should be reduced accordingly.

Fluroxene (Fluoromar)
Same as for *Ether* above.

Furosemide[330] (Lasix)
Furosemide potentiates the gallamine type of muscle relaxant.

Halothane[878,1930] (Fluothane)
Same as for *Ether* above. Halothane and *d*-tubocurarine produce a hypotensive reaction.

Insecticides
See *Anticholinesterases* above.

Kanamycin (Kantrex)
See *Colistin* above (page 540).

MAO inhibitors[198]
MAO inhibitors potentiate the muscle relaxant action of tubocurarine.

Methotrimeprazine (Levoprome)
See *Muscle Relaxants* under *Methotrimeprazine*.

Methoxyflurane (Penthrane)
Same as for *Ether* above.

Neomycin[442]
See *Colistin* above (page 540).

Neostigmine[36,168]
Neostigmine, an anticholinesterase agent, can counteract the ganglionic blocking paralysis produced by competitive agents such as *d*-tubocurarine (decurarizing in overdosage) but not benzoquinonium which may even be potentiated.

Norepinephrine
Same as for *Epinephrine* above.

Polymyxin
See *Colistin* above (page 540).

Propranolol[790,1186,1961]
Propranolol may intensify and prolong the neuromuscular blockade produced by both depolarizing and nondepolarizing muscle relaxants by enhancing the depression of motor nerve terminal activity and by acting as a membrane stabilizer which renders the postjunctional membrane insensitive to acetylcholine.

Quinidine[324,390,447]
Quinidine prolongs the neuromuscular blockade produced by tubocurarine. See *Muscle relaxants* under *Quinidine*.

Quinethazone[330] (Hydromox)
Quinethazone potentiates the gallamine type of muscle relaxant.

Reserpine[1930]
Reserpine antagonizes *d*-tubocurarine, possibly by increasing excitability of the endplate.

Streptomycin[330,654]
See *Colistin* above (page 540).

Thiazide diuretics[120,330]
Thiazide diuretics potentiate the gallamine and tubocurarine type of muscle relaxants.

MUSCLE RELAXANTS, PERIPHERALLY ACTING, DEPOLARIZING
(Decamethonium [Syncurine] Succinylcholine [Anectine, Sucostrin], etc.)
See *Neuromuscular Blocking Antibiotics* under *Antibiotics*.

Acetylcholine[168]
See *Muscle Relaxants* under *Acetylcholine*.

Alkalinizing agents
See *Sodium Thiopental* below.

Anesthetics, fluorine[120] (Fluothane, Penthrane, etc.)
Fluorine anesthetics potentiate depolarizing muscle relaxants. Potentially very hazardous.

Antibiotics
See *Colistin and Derivatives* under *Muscle Relaxants, Peripherally Acting* above and *Neuromuscular Blocking Antibiotics* under *Antibiotics*.

Anticholinesterases[421]
Potentiation. See *Anticholinesterases* above under *Muscle Relaxants, Peripherally Acting*.

Antineoplastics[1925]
Cyclophosphamide, thiotepa, and nitrogen mustards, which reduce plasma cholinesterase, potentiate succinylcholine. Reduce the dosage of the muscle relaxant to avoid apnea, cardiac arrhythmias, and possible cardiac arrest. See *Succinylcholine* under *Cyclophosphamide* and *Thiotepa*.

Bacitracin[421]
Potentiation. See *Colistin* above (page 540).

Colistin[421]
Potentiation. See *Colistin* above in the general section on *Muscle Relaxants, Peripherally Acting* (page 540).

Cyclophosphamide (Cytoxan, Endoxan)
See *Succinylcholine* under *Cyclophosphamide*.

Dexpanthenol[421] (Cozyme, Ilopan, etc.)
Dexpanthenol potentiates the depolarizing muscle relaxants. It should not be given within one hour after the muscle relaxant. See *Succinylcholine* under *Pantothenic Acid*.

Digitalis glycosides
See *Succinylcholine* under *Digitalis*.

Dihydrostreptomycin[421]
See *Colistin* above (page 540). Potentiation.

Echothiophate[427,519] (Phospholine iodide)
Prolonged paralysis of respiratory muscles and a protracted apnea may occur with the combination of this anticholinesterase and a depolarizing muscle relaxant. Echothiophate can depress activity of serum cholinesterase to dangerously low levels on prolonged use and thus depress metabolism of succinylcholine. See also *Anticholinesterases* under *Muscle Relaxants, Peripherally Acting*.

Edrophonium[204] (Tensilon)
Same as for *Neostigmine* below.

EDTA[161] (Edetates, Versine, etc.)
EDTA increases intestinal absorption of decamethonium.

Fluorine anesthetics[421]
Potentiation.

Furosimide
See *Muscle Relaxants* under *Furosimide*.

Gramicidin[421]
Potentiation. See *Colistin* above (page 540).

Halothane[657,658] (Fluothane)
Malignant hyperpyrexia may occur.

Hexafluorenium[421] (Mylaxen)
Hexafluorenium, a pseudocholinesterase inhibitor and a competitive neuromuscular blocking agent, by prior administration greatly potentiates the muscle relaxation produced by the depolarizing type of peripheral acting muscle relaxants, *e.g.* succinylcholine chloride.

Kanamycin [421] **(Kantrex)**
See *Colistin* above. Potentiation and respiratory paralysis.

Lidocaine [421,435,640] **(Xylocaine)**
Same as for *Procaine* below. Potentiation. See *Muscle Relaxants* under *Lidocaine*.

MAO inhibitors
See *Succinylcholine* under *MAO Inhibitors*.

Methotrimeprazine (Levoprome)
See *Muscle Relaxants* under *Methotrimeprazine*.

Neomycin [322,421]
See *Colistin*   Potentiation, respiratory paralysis.

Neostigmine [421] **(Prostigmin)**
Neostigmine, an anticholinesterase, potentiates depolarizing muscle relaxants like succinylcholine. See *Anticholinesterases* above. See under *Muscle Relaxants, Peripherally Acting, Competitive Type*, for the opposite effect with curariform drugs.

Organophosphate insecticides [204]
Potentiation by the anticholinesterases. Use of organophosphate insecticides should be discontinued 6 weeks prior to surgery.

Phenothiazines [566]
Potentiation may occur. See *Promazine* below.

Polymyxin B [421]
See *Colistin* above   Potentiation.

Procaine [385,421,435,640] **(Novocaine)**
Procaine IV, especially in large doses, potentiates depolarizing peripherally acting muscle relaxants. Thus it increases the duration of apnea induced by succinylcholine. The increased effect may be due to competition for unspecific binding sites on plasma proteins and for specific sites on plasma cholinesterase with subsequent inhibition of plasma cholinesterase by the local anesthetic. This inhibits the metabolism of the muscle relaxant.

Quinidine [324,390,447,564]
See *Muscle relaxants* under *Quinidine*.

Promazine [566] **(Sparine)**
Prolonged apnea, respiratory depression, and paralysis may occur.

Propranolol
See *Propranolol* above under *Muscle Relaxants, Peripherally Acting, Competitive Type*.

Sodium thiopental (Pentothal Sodium) [120]
Sodium thiopental forms strongly alkaline solutions that hydrolyze succinylcholine. Inject the drugs separately.

Streptomycin [421]
See *Colistin* above (page 540). Potentiation.

Thiotepa
See *Succinylcholine* under *Thiotepa*.

d-Tubocurarine [168]
The effects of curariform muscle relaxants must be allowed to wear off before succinylcholine is administered.

Urea [1121]
A 30% infusion of urea decreased or prevented the increase in intraocular tension induced by succinylcholine (in the rabbit).

MUSHROOMS
See under *Alcohol*.

M.V.I.
See *Dietary Supplements*.

MYADEC
See *Dietary Supplements*.

MYAMBUTOL
See *Ethambutol*.

MYCHEL
See *Chloramphenicol*.

MYCOLOG
See *Triamcinolone*.

MYCOSTATIN
See *Nystatin*.

MYLANTA
See *Antacids* (magnesium hydroxide and aluminum hydroxide), also contains *Simethicone*.

MYLERAN
See *Busulfan*.

MYOCARDIAL DEPRESSANTS [1161]
See *Propranolol, Barbiturates, Chloroform, Ether, Morphine*

MYOCHOLINE
See *Parasympathomimetics* (Bethanechol Chloride).

MYODIGIN
See *Digitalis* (Digitoxin).

MYSOLINE
See *Anticonvulsants* (Primidone).

MYSTECLIN-F (Capsules and Syrup)
See *Amphotericin B* and *Tetracyclines*.

MYTELASE
See *Anticholinesterases* (Ambenonium).

NAFCILLIN (Unipen)
See *Penicillins*.

Acetylsalicylic acid [267-269]
Aspirin potentiates nafcillin by displacing it from protein binding sites.

Aminohippuric acid [433] **(PAHA)**
PAHA elevates serum levels of penicillin and increases toxicity.

Ampicillin [382] **(Alpen, Polycillin, etc.)**
Synergistic antibacterial effect *in vitro*.

Benzylpenicillin [382] **(Penicillin G)**
Synergistic antibacterial effect *in vitro*.

Sulfinpyrazone [267-269] **(Anturane)**
Sulfinpyrazone potentiates nafcillin by displacing it from protein binding sites.

Sulfonamides [267-269]
Sulfonamides such as sulfaethylthiadiazole, sulfamethoxypyridazine, sulfasymazine, and sulfisoxazole, potentiate nafcillin by displacing it from protein binding sites.

NALIDIXIC ACID (NegGram)

Acidifying agents [325,870]
Urinary acidifiers enhance the antibacterial effect of nalidixic acid by decreasing its excretion rate. They also increase its toxicity.

Alcohol [486]
This combination may decrease alertness, judgment and motor coordination.

NALIDIXIC ACID (NegGram) *(continued)*

Alkalinizing agents [198,421]
Urinary alkalinizers inhibit naladixic acid by increasing its excretion rate. May potentiate urinary antiseptic activity.

Antacids [28,202,633,1155]
Antacids may inhibit nalidixic acid because of decreased gastrointestinal absorption through increased ionization. Paradoxically, sodium bicarbonate appears to increase absorption of nalidixic acid.

Anticoagulants, oral [784]
Nalidixic acid potentiates oral anticoagulants like warfarin by displacing them from serum albumin binding sites.

EDTA [360,421]
EDTA potentiates nalidixic acid against *Ps. aeruginosa* by increasing the gastrointestinal absorption rate.

Nitrofurantoin [202,416,1704] **(Furadantin)**
Nitrofurantoin inhibits nalidixic acid as an antibacterial agent with 44 out of 53 strains of *Enterobacteriaceae*. Avoid concomitant use.

NALLINE
See *Nalorphine.*

NALORPHINE (Nalline)

Alcohol
See *CNS Depressants* below.

Barbiturates
See *CNS Depressants* below.

CNS depressants [166]
Nalorphine may add to the depressant effects of CNS depressants such as alcohol, anesthetics, barbiturates, hypnotics, sedatives, tranqulilizers, etc.

Codeine
See *Narcotic Analgesics* below.

Heroin
See *Narcotic Analgesics* below.

Fentanyl [120,166] **(Sublimaze)**
Nalorphine antagonizes the respiratory depression and the analgesic effect of fentanyl.

Meperidine [120] **(Demerol, etc.)**
Nalorphine is a specific antidote for the respiratory depression caused by meperidine overdosage or hypersensitivity to the drug.

Levorphanol tartrate (Levo-Dromoran Tartrate)
See *Narcotic Analgesics* below.

Methadone
See *Narcotic Analgesics* below.

Morphine
See *Narcotic Analgesics* below.

Naloxone [166]
Naloxone antagonizes psychotomimetic effects of nalorphine.

Narcotic analgesics [39,166]
Nalorphine as a narcotic antagonist reverses the respiratory depression produced by narcotic analgesics; however, it does not reverse respiratory depression caused by sedatives, hypnotics, anesthetics, etc. It is a potent antagonist of the depressant effects of all known synthetic narcotic analgesics. It may precipitate an acute abstinence syndrome in patients physically dependent on semisynthetic opiates, methadone, phenazocine, levorphanol, and related synthetics.

Narcotics, synthetics and semisynthetic
See *Narcotic Analgesics* above.

Phenazocine HBr (Prinadol HBr)
See *Narcotic Analgesics* above.

Propoxyphene [120,166] **(Darvon)**
Nalorphine is an antidote for lethal doses of propoxyphene.

Scorpion venom [421]
Nalorphine enhances the toxicity of scorpion venom.

NALORPHINE PLUS METHYLENE BLUE

Propoxyphene [951] **(Darvon)**
Nalorphine plus methylene blue antagonizes the toxicity of propoxyphene; it is an antidote for lethal dose of propoxyphene.

NALORPHINE PLUS TOLONIUM CHLORIDE

Propoxyphene [120] **(Darvon)**
Nalorphine plus tolonium chloride antagnizes the toxicity of propoxyphene; it is an antidote for lethal doses of propoxyphene.

NALOXONE

Cyclazocine [166,237]
Naloxone, a narcotic antagonist, antagonizes the miosis, respiratory depression, and psychotomimetic behavioral effects produced by cyclazocine and other narcotic antagonists as well as the effects of narcotic analgesics.

Nalorphine
See *Cyclazocine* above.

Narcotic analgesics [166]
Naloxone reverses the respiratory despression caused by narcotic analgesics. See also *Cyclazocine* above.

Pentazocine
See *Cyclazocine* and *Narcotic Anagesics* above.

NANDROLONE PHENPROPIONATE (Durabolin)
See *Anabolic Agents.*

NAPROXEN

Salicylates
See *Naproxen* under *Salicylates.*

NAQUA
See *Thiazide Diuretics* (Trichlormethiazide).

NAQUIVAL
See *Reserpine* and *Thiazide Diuretics* (Trichlormethiazide).

NARCOTIC ANALGESICS
(Alphaprodine [Nisentil] HCl, anileridine [Leritine], codeine, dextromoramide [Palfium], dihydrocodeine [Paracodin], dihydromorphinone [Dilaudid] HCl, dipipanone [Pipadone], fentanyl citrate [Sublimaze], hydrocodone [Hycodan], levorphanol [Levo-Dromoran] tartrate, meperidine [Demerol] HCl, metopon, methadone [Adanon, Amidone, Dolophine] HCl, morphine HCl or sulfate, opium alkaloids, oxycodone, oxymorphone [Numorphan] HCl, phenadoxone [Heptalgin], phenazocine [Prinadol], pholcodine [Ethnine, Pholdine], piminidone [Alvodine] ethanesulfonate, nalorphine [Nalline] HCl, etc.)

Acidifying agents [325,870]
Acidifying agents increase the urinary excretion of narcotic analgesics (weak bases) and thereby inhibit them.

β-Adrenergic blocking agents [698]
Propranolol, a beta-adrenergic blocking agent, has been shown to have synergistic CNS depressant action with morphine. This synergistic action may occur with other beta-adrenergic blocking agents.

Alcohol [121,311,421,634]
See *CNS Depressants* below.

Alkalinizing agents [325,870]
Alkalinizing agents decrease the urinary excretion of narcotic analgesics (weak bases) and thereby potentiate them.

Analeptics [120,968]
Analeptics should not be used to treat narcotic overdosage; fatal convulsions may be produced.

Anticoagulants, oral [120]
Prolonged use of narcotic analgesics may enhance the anticoagulant effect.

Anticonvulsants
See *CNS Depressants* below.

Antidepressants, tricyclic [120,421]
Tricyclic antidepressants increase the CNS depressant effects of narcotic analgesics; narcotic analgesics potentiate the sedation produced by tricyclic antidepressants.

Antihistamines
See *CNS Depressants* below.

Antipyretic analgesics
See *CNS Depressants* below.

Barbiturates
See *CNS Depressants* below.

Benzodiazepines [120,421]
See *CNS Depressants* below.

Calcium salts [166]
The intracisternal injection of calcium ions antagonizes the analgesic action of narcotic analgesics (opioids).

Chlordiazepoxide [283] (Librium)
See *CNS Depressants* below.

p-Chlorophenylalanine [421]
p-Chlorophenylalanine reverses the analgesic activity of narcotic analgesics.

Chlorpromazine [120] (Thorazine)
See *CNS Depressants* below.

CNS depressants [120,166,421,1235]
Narcotic analgesics potentiate all CNS depressants including the general depressants (alcohol, barbiturates, general anesthetics, hypnotics and sedatives) and the specific depressants (anticonvulsants, antipyretic and narcotic analgesics, antihistamines, centrally acting muscle relaxants, psychochemicals, etc.). If the potentiation (additive effect) is strong enough (large enough doses), then severe respiratory depression, profound coma, hypopyrexia, and death may ensue.

CNS Stimulants [2047]
Narcotic-induced supersensitivity of dopamine receptors may contribute to the residual effects of chronic intoxication with stimulants such as amphetamines.

Cyclazocine [166]
Cyclazocine is a narcotic antagonist.

Cyproheptadine [421] (Periactin)
Cyproheptadine reverses the analgesic activity of narcotic analgesics.

Diazepam (Valium)
See *CNS Depressants* above.

Diuretics [120,166]
Orthostatic hypotension may be potentiated.

Furazolidone [120]
Should be used in reduced dosages and with caution. See *MAO inhibitors* below.

General anesthetics
See *CNS Depressants* above.

Haloperidol [120,421]
Narcotic analgesics increase sedative effects of haloperidol. See *CNS Depressants* above.

Hydrochlorothiazide [120] (Hydrodiuril)
Orthostatic hypotension that can occur with hydrochlorothiazide may be potentiated by narcotics.

Hypnotics
See *CNS Depressants* above.

Isoniazid [330]
Isoniazid potentiates narcotics.

Levallorphan [120,166] (Lorfan)
Levallorphen reverses the respiratory depression produced by narcotic analgesics without abolishing analgesia.

MAO inhibitors [120,198,330,421]
MAO inhibitors potentiate narcotic analgesics. They interfere with detoxification of some narcotics (especially meperidine), causing a prolongation and intensification of CNS depression (hypotension and respiratory depression). Narcotics potentiate the hypotension produced by MAO inhibitors. May be contraindicated or used at much lower dosages. Potentially very hazardous.

Methotrimeprazine [120] (Levoprome)
Additive effects; the dose of one or both agents should be reduced when methotrimeprazine and a narcotic analgesic are given concurrently.

Methysergide [421] (Sansert)
Methysergide reverses the analgesic activity of narcotic analgesics.

Muscle relaxants, centrally acting
See *CNS Depressants* above. Potentiation of respiratory depression with this combination may be hazardous. Use caution.

Naloxone [166]
Naloxone, a narcotic analgesic without agonist activity, reverses the respiratory depression caused by narcotic analgesics. See *Nalorphine* below.

Nalorphine HCl [39,166] (Nalline HCl)
Nalorphine, a narcotic antagonist, reverses the respiratory depression produced by narcotic analgesics; however, it does not reverse the respiratory depression caused by sedatives, hypnotics, anesthetics, and other CNS depressants. Nalorphine is a potent antagonist of the depressant effects of all known synthetic narcotic analgesics. It may precipitate an acute abstinence syndrome in patients physically dependent on semisynthetic opiates, methadone, phenazocine, levorphanol, and related synthetics.

Pantothenyl alcohol [120,1814,1929] (Ilopan, panthenol)
Pantothenyl alcohol, when used with narcotics, may cause allergic reactions.

Pargyline (Eutonyl)
See *MAO inhibitors* above.

Pentazocine lactate [166] (Talwin)
Pentazocine is weakly antagonistic to narcotic analgesics. It can precipitate narcotic withdrawal symptoms in patients who have been receiving opiates.

Phenothiazines [120,198,421]
Narcotic analgesics potentiate phenothiazines. See *CNS Depressants* above. Some phenothiazines potentiate and prolong the depressant action of morphine.

NARCOTIC ANALGESICS *(continued)*

Procarbazine HCl[330] **(Matulane, Natulan)**
Narcotics should be used with caution with this enzyme inhibitor.

Psychotherapeutic agents
See *CNS Depressants* above.

Rauwolfia alkaloids
See *CNS Depressants* above.

Scorpion venom[421]
Narcotic analgesics enhance the toxicity of scorpion venom.

Sedatives and hypnotics
See *CNS Depressants* above.

Thiazide diuretics[120]
Narcotic analgesics may potentiate the orthostatic hypotension caused by thiazide diuretics.

Tranquilizers[120,166]
Enhanced activity. See *CNS Depressants* above.

Tricyclic antidepressants[120,421]
Narcotic analgesics potentiate the sedative effect of tricyclic antidepressants; tricyclic antidepressants increase the effect of narcotic analgesics.

Urinary acidifiers
See *Acidifying Agents* above.

Urinary alkalinizers
See *Alkalinizing Agents* above.

NARCOTIC ANTAGONISTS
See *Cyclazocine, Levallorphan, Nalorphine, Naloxone, Pentazocine,* etc.

NARCOTICS
See *Narcotic Analgesics* and specific drugs.

NARDIL
See *Phenelzine* and *MAO Inhibitors.*

NARINE TYROCAPS
See *Antihistamines* (chlorpheniramine), *Phenylephrine,* and *Scopolamine Methylbromide.*

NARONE
See *Dipyrone.*

NASAL DECONGESTANTS

Antihypertensives[950]
Nasal decongestants antagonize antihypertensives.

NATURETIN
See *Thiazide Diuretics* (bendroflumethiazide)

NAVANE
See *Thiothixene.*

NEGGRAM
See *Antibiotics* (nalidixic acid).

NEMBUTAL
See *Barbiturates* (pentobarbital).

NEOBIOTIC
See *Neomycin.*

NEOCYLATE
See *p-Aminobenzoic Acid* and *Salicylates.*

NEOCYTEN
See *p-Aminobenzoic Acid* and *Salicylates.*

NEO-HOMBREOL
See *Testosterone.*

NEOMYCIN
See *Aminoglycoside Antibiotics.*

Alkalinizing agents[578]
Alkalinizing agents that raise the urinary pH potentiate the antibacterial activity of neomycin.

Amobarbital[360]
Apnea, muscle weakness; enhanced neuromuscular blockage by the antibiotic. See *Antibiotics* below.

Anesthetics, general[37,120,146,322,499,503,504,507,750]
This antibiotic may cause neuromuscular paralysis with respiratory depression and apnea when given parenterally to patients who have been given anesthetics. See *Antibiotics* (ototoxic and neuromuscular blocking) below.

Antibiotics, ototoxic and neuromuscular blocking[120,653,813]
Dihydrostreptomycin, ethacrynic acid, kanamycin, neomycin, ristocetin, streptomycin, vancomycin, and other ototoxic drugs like furosemide may have progressive cumulative effects, possibly delayed, that can be additive and cause permanent deafness. Bacitracin, dihydrostreptomycin, gentamicin, gramicidin, kanamycin, polymyxin B, streptomycin, viomycin, and other neuromuscular blocking drugs, including neomycin may have additive effects and induce neuromuscular paralysis with respiratory depression, muscle weakness and apnea. This may be particularly pronounced with curariform agents, depolarizing muscle relaxants, anesthetics such as barbiturates (thiopental), ether, procainamide, promethazine, quinidine, and sodium citrate.

Anticholinesterases[178]
Anticholinesterases (cholinergics) antagonize the neuromuscular blocking effects of neomycin.

Anticoagulants, oral[193,234]
Neomycin potentiates the effects of oral coumarin anticoagulants. It may prolong the prothrombin time by interfering with vitamin K production by gut bacteria.

Bacitracin
Synergistic prophylaxis in surgery. Neomycin, used in combination with bacitracin as an irrigating solution during surgery, may cause respiratory depression. See *Antibiotics* above.

Blood cholesterol lowering agents[421]
Neomycin potentiates blood cholesterol lowering agents by blocking cholesterol absorption.

Calcium[178,494-498]
Calcium reduces the neuromuscular blocking effect of the antibiotic. See *Antibiotics* above.

Clofibrate (Atromid-S)
See *Blood Cholesterol Lowering Agents* above.

Colistimethate
See *Antibiotics* above.

Coumarin anticoagulants
See *Anticoagulants, Oral* above.

Curare and curariform compounds[358,656]
See *Muscle Relaxants* below. Respiratory arrest with intraperitoneal injection of these antimicrobials.

Decamethonium[168,421]
See *Muscle Relaxants* below.

Digitalis[1582]
See *Neomycin* under *Digitalis Glycosides.*

Dimenhydrinate[120] **(Dramamine)**
Dimenhydrinate may mask ototoxic symptoms caused by this antibiotic. Extra alertness is essential to detect the side effect.

Dimethyl sulfoxide[788] **(DMSO)**
Dimethyl sulfoxide potentiates the toxic effects of neomycin.

Edrophonium [178,494-498] **(Tensilon)**
Edrophonium antagonizes the curariformlike effects of neomycin.

EDTA [360,421]
EDTA potentiates neomycin.

Ethacrynic Acid (Edecrin)
See *Aminoglycoside Antibiotics* under *Edecrynic Acid.*

Ether [358,507,551,815-817]
Ether may cause respiratory paralysis due to potentiation of the neuromuscular blocking effects of neomycin.

Gallamine
See *Muscle Relaxants* below.

Gentamicin [120] **(Garamycin)**
See *Antibiotics* above. Gentamicin possesses cross-resistance with neomycin.

Kanamycin (Kantrex)
See *Antibiotics* above.

Methoxyflurane (Penthrane)
See under *Methoxyflurane.*

Muscle relaxants
(curare, succinylcholine, etc.) [37,120,146,322,330,358,499,503,504,507,656,856,858-860]
Neomycin potentiates the neuromuscular blockade induced by muscle relaxants. Prolonged paralysis of the respiratory muscles may cause prolonged respiratory depression and often irreversible apnea when the antibiotic is given while muscular relaxation is being maintained by a depolarizing agent. Previous prolonged administration of a depolarizing agent sensitizes the neuromuscular junction to the effect of antibiotics which also have neuromuscular blocking properties. See *Antibiotics* above.

Neomycin [120,179]
The ototoxic effect of neomycin is additive and its sequential use should be employed with full knowledge of this potential adverse effect. See also *Antibiotics* above.

Neostigmine [178,322,494-498]
Neostigmine, a parasympathetic stimulant, antagonizes the neuromuscular blockade produced by neomycin.

Organophosphate cholinesterase inhibitors [178]
These anticholinesterases antagonize the neuromuscular blocking effect of neomycin.

Ototoxic antibiotics
See *Antibiotics, Ototoxic* above.

Penicillins, oral [421,1287]
Neomycin inhibits the antibacterial action of penicillins by blocking their absorption. See *Antibiotics* under *Penicillins.*

Polymyxin B
See *Antibiotics* above.

Procainamide [619] **(Pronestyl)**
Procainamide may enhance the neuromuscular blockade produced by neomycin and thus may induce apnea and muscle weakness.

Promethazine [360] **(Phenergan)**
Promethazine may enhance the neuromuscular blockade produced by neomycin and thus may induce apnea and muscle weakness.

Quinidine [447,559]
Quinidine may enhance the neuromuscular blockade produced by neomycin and thus may induce apnea and muscle weakness.

Streptomycin
See *Antibiotics* above.

Succinylcholine [322]
This combination may induce respiratory paralysis. See *Antibiotics* and *Muscle Relaxants* above.

Triiodothyronine [421] **(Cytomel, liothyronine)**
Neomycin potentiates triiodothyronine.

***d*-Tubocurarine** [358,656,858-860]
This combination may induce respiratory paralysis. See *Antibiotics* and *Muscle Relaxants* above.

Vitamin B$_{12}$
See *Neomycin* under *Vitamin B$_{12}$.*

NEOSTIGMINE (Prostigmin) Bromide
See also *Anticholinesterases, Bromides,* and *Parasympathomimetics.*

Anticholinergics [120,168,754] **(Atropine, etc.)**
Anticholinergics may slow intestinal motility and decrease absorption of orally administered neostigmine. Atropine effectively blocks the cholinergic side effects of the anticholinesterase neostigmine used in myasthenia gravis by antagonizing its actions at muscarinic receptor sites. Atropine is an effective antidote in cholinergic crisis resulting from overdosage of anticholinesterases. Also atropine inhibits but does not abolish the intestinal and other muscarinic side effects of neostigmine; neostigmine counteracts the inhibition of gastric tone and motility induced by atropine. Atropine, administered to a patient pretreated with neostigmine may produce cardiac arrhythmias. Fatal cardiac arrest has occurred in *anesthetized patients* given both atropine and neostigmine for reversal of curarization.

Colistimethate [120,421] **(Coly-Mycin)**
Anticholinesterases like edrophonium and neostigmine are potentiated by colistimethate.

Decamethonium [168,421]
Neostigmine may potentiate the neuromuscular blocking effects of decamethonium.

Dihydrostreptomycin [120,421,656]
Neostigmine antagonizes the neuromuscular blockade induced by dihydrostreptomycin and other aminoglycoside antibiotics.

Kanamycin [120,421,656] **(Kantrex)**
Neostigmine reduces the neuromuscular blockade toxicity of aminogylcoside antibiotics. See *Antibiotics* under *Neomycin* above.

Meperidine [204]
Neostigmine increases the intensity and duration of analgesia produced by meperidine.

Methadone [204]
Neostigmine increases the intensity and duration of analgesia produced by methadone.

Morphine [204]
Neostigmine enhances the stimulatory effect of morphine and increases the intensity and duration of analgesia produced by the narcotic.

Muscle relaxants [36,168,421]
Neostigmine counteracts the paralysis produced by the curariform agents (decurarizing in overdosage), but potentiates depolarizing muscle relaxants like succinylcholine. See under *Muscle Relaxants.*

Neomycin [178,322,494-498]
The neuromuscular blocking effects of neomycin are antagonized by neostigmine.

Parasympathomimetic agents [168]
The effects with other parasympathomimetics may be additive.

NEOSTIGMINE (Prostigmin) Bromide
(continued)

Polymyxin B [312,619,656,882]
Neostigmine does not antagonize the noncompetitive neuromuscular blockade causing paralysis with polymyxin. It may potentiate the paralysis caused by the antibiotic.

Streptomycin [178]
The neuromuscular blocking effects of streptomycin (particularly intraperitoneally), used concomitantly with a nondepolarizing muscle relaxant like *d*-tubocurarine, are counteracted by neostigmine in the presence of adequate ventilation.

Succinylcholine [421]
The muscular relaxant effect of succinylcholine can be potentiated by neostigmine.

***d*-Tubocurarine** [168]
Neostigmine reverses the neuromuscular blockade produced by *d*-tubocurarine and can be used as an antidote for the curariform agent.

Vasopressin
See *Neostigmine* under *Vasopressin.*

NEO-SYNEPHRINE
See *Phenylephrine.*

NEO-SYNEPHRINE EYE DROPS

Guanethidine
Prolonged mydriasis.

NEOTRIZINE
See *Sulfonamides* (sulfadiazine, sulfamerazine, and sulfamethazine).

NEPHROTOXIC ANTIBIOTICS
See under *Antibiotics.*

NEPTAZANE
See *Carbonic Anhydrase Inhibitors* and *Sulfonamides* (methazolamide).

NESACAINE
See *Anesthetics, Local* (chloroprocaine).

NEUROMUSCULAR BLOCKING AGENTS
See *Muscle Relaxants* and *Neuromuscular Blocking Antibiotics* under *Antibiotics.*

NEVENTAL
See *Barbiturates* (nealbarbitone).

NIALAMIDE (Niamid)
See *MAO Inhibitors.*

NIAMID
See *MAO Inhibitors* (nialamide).

NICONYL
See *Isoniazid.*

NICOTINE (Smoking)

Acidifying agents [325,870]
Acidifying agents inhibit the effects of nicotine by increasing its urinary excretion.

Alkalinizing agents [325,870]
Opposite effects to *Acidifying Agents* above.

Corticosteroids [421]
Nicotine (smoking) increases the blood levels of endogenous corticosteroids and may thus have an additive effect with administered corticosteroids.

NICOTINIC ACID

Antidiabetics [191,888]
Large doses of nicotinic acid can increase blood glucose levels and thus antagonize antidiabetics.

NICOZIDE
See *Isoniazid.*

NIFUROXIME (Micofur)

Alcohol [121]
Nifuroxime, an enzyme inhibitor, prevents the oxidation of acetaldehyde, a metabolite of alcohol, and thus produces a disulfiram type of reaction.

NIKETHAMIDE (Coramine, Nikorin, etc.)
See *CNS Stimulants.*

NILEVAR
See *Norethandrolone.*

NILODIN
See *Lucanthone.*

NISENTIL
See *Analgesics.*

NITRATES AND NITRITES
(Organic nitrates and nitrites and the nitrite ion, including amyl nitrite, erythrityl tetranitrate, isosorbide dinitrate, mannitol hexanitrate, nitroglycerin, pentaerythritol tetranitrate, sodium nitrite, and trolnitrate phosphate)

Acetylcholine [170] **(Cholinergics)**
Organic nitrates and nitrites and inorganic nitrites are antagonistic physiologically to acetylcholine. See *Smooth Muscle Activators* below.

β-Adrenergic blockers (Inderal, etc.)
β-Adrenergic blockers like propranolol tend to potentiate the hypotensive effect of nitrates and nitrites.

Alcohol [48,120,421,634]
Nitrates and nitrites with alcohol mutually potentiate the vasodilator effects; may result in severe hypotension and cardiovascular collapse (disulfiramlike reaction with nitroglycerin).

Anticholinergics [421]
Nitrates and nitrites may potentiate some of the anticholinergic side effects. Hazardous in glaucoma.

Antidepressants, tricyclic [166,421]
Nitrates and nitrites potentiate the hypotensive and anticholinergic effects of tricyclic antidepressants.

Antihistamines [421]
Nitrates and nitrites may potentiate anticholinergic effects of the antihistamines.

Antihypertensives [5]
Severe hypotension may occur with this combination. Potentially very hazardous.

Cholinergics [170]
Cholinergics physiologically antagonize the effect of nitrates and nitrites. See *Smooth Muscle Activators* below.

Epinephrine [170]
Nitrates and nitrites are antagonistic physiologically to epinephrine, and can counteract the marked pressor effects of large doses of epinephrine.

Histamines [170]
Nitrates and nitrites are antagonistic physiologically to histamine.

Isosorbide dinitrite (Isordil, Sorbitrate)
Cross-tolerance may occur between this nitrate and other nitrates and nitrites.

MAO inhibitors[421]
This combination may produce a false sense of ability and cardiac strength.

Meperidine and close derivatives[421,633]
Nitrates and nitrites may potentiate the hypotensive effects of meperidine and related narcotics.

Nitrates and nitrites[170]
Additive effects and cross tolerance may occur with other nitrates and nitrites. See *Pentaerythritol Tetranitrate* under *Nitroglycerin.*

Norepinephrine[170]
A nitrate can act as a physiological antagonist to norepinephrine. The response may vary from maximal contraction to maximal relaxation with variations in the relative concentrations of the members of any such pair.

Pentaerythritol tetranitrate[120] (Peritrate, PETN, etc.)
Cross-tolerance may occur.

Smooth muscle activators[170]
Acetylcholine, histamine, norepinephrine and other agents that can activate pertinent smooth muscle, can act as physiological antagonists to organic nitrates and organic and inorganic nitrites which relax smooth muscle (biliary tract, bronchial, gastrointestinal tract, ureteral, uterine, and vascular).

Sympathomimetics[170]
Nitrates and nitrites that relax smooth muscle are physiologically antagonistic to the pressor (vasoconstrictor) effects of sympathomimetics like histamine and levarterenol.

Tricyclic antidepressants[166,421]
See *Antidepressants, Tricyclic* above.

NITRAZEPAM (Mogadon)
See *CNS Depressants* and *Sedatives and Hypnotics.*

NITROFURANS
See *Furazolidine* and *Nitrofurantoin.*

NITROFURANTOIN (Furadantin)

Acidifying agents[578]
Nitrofurantoin is potentiated by acidifiers (decreased excretion). It is most active against urinary tract infections when the pH of the urine is 5.5 or less.

Alcohol[28]
Nitrofurantoin, by inhibiting the oxidation of acetaldehyde, a metabolite of alcohol, produces a disulfiramlike reaction.

Alakinizing agents[28,202,421,633]
Agents that raise the pH of the urine inhibit nitrofurantoin by decreasing reabsorption and increasing its rate of excretion. The anti-infective is most active in an acid urine.

Antacids[198,421,633,870]
Antacids inhibit nitrofurantoin. See *Alkalinizing Agents* above.

Nalidixic acid[201]
Nalidixic acid inhibits nitrofurantoin because of decreased absorption.

Phenobarbital[120]
Phenobarbital inhibits nitrofurantoin.

Probenecid[120,1958] (Benemid)
Probenecid potentiates nitrofurantoin toxicity and decreases its effectiveness as a urinary anti-infective by decreasing its renal clearance.

Urinary acidifiers[325,870]
Agents that lower the pH of the urine potentiate nitrofurantoin; most effective in urinary pH less than 5.5. The mechanism is the reverse of that given for *Alkalinizing Agents* above.

NITROGEN MUSTARDS

Succimylcholine[1925]
See *Antineoplastics* under *Muscle Relaxants, Peripherally Acting, Depolarizing*

NITROGLYCERIN

Alcohol[48,198,634]
When taken together, these drugs may cause hypotension (increased vasodilation) and cardiovascular collapse; the reaction may be mistakenly attributed to coronary insufficiency or occlusion.

Pentaerythritol tetranitrate[120] (Peritrate)
Cross tolerance may occur following chronic administration. Thus nitroglycerin may lose some of its effectiveness in patients on long-acting nitrates such as Peritrate.

NITROUS OXIDE

Fluroxene (Fluoromar)[879]
Combined use of these two general anesthetics increases cardiac output and central venous pressure.

Halothane[166]
Anesthesia with 50:50 nitrous oxide and oxygen mixtures together with halothane or methoxyflurane in low concentration causes an increase in inspired tension of nitrous oxide and may produce appreciable depression of blood pressure, heart rate, and muscle tone.

Methadone[951]
Synergistic analgesic activity.

Methoxyflurane
See *Halothane* above.

Norepinephrine
Nitrous oxide, 80% in oxygen, slightly increases the response of vascular smooth muscle to the sympathetic mediator norepinephrine.

NOCTEC
See *Chloral Hydrate* and *Hypnotics*

NORADRENALINE
See *Levarterenol.*

NORBOLETHONE (Genabol)

Anticoagulants, oral[819] (Dicumarol, etc.)
The anabolic agent inhibits oral anticoagulants like bishydroxycoumarin.

NOREPINEPHRINE
See *Levarterenol.*

NORETHANDROLONE (Nilevar)

Coumarin anticoagulants[394,421,633,673] (Dicumarol, etc.)
The activity of the coumarin anticoagulants may be increased by some anabolic agents, particularly norethandrolone.

NORTRIPTYLINE (Aventyl)
See *Antidepressants, Tricyclic.*

NOVAHISTINE
See *Analgesics* (acetaminophen), *Antihistamines* (chlorphenpyridamine), and *Sympathomimetics* (phenylephrine).

NOVOBIOCIN (Albamycin)

Tetracyclines[201,619]
Tetracyclines diminish the effectiveness of novobiocin; physical inhibition.

NOVOCAIN
See *Anesthetics, Local* (procaine).

NYLIDRIN (Arlidin)

Phenothiazine tranquilizers[489]
Nylidrin, a β-receptor stimulator acting as a vasodilator, potentiates the antipsychotic effect of these tranquilizers clinically. It displaces the phenothiazines from secondary binding sites.

Propranolol[1181]
Propranolol inhibits nylidrin-induced gastric acid secretion. See *Nylidrin* under *Propranolol.*

OBEDRIN-LA
See *Methamphetamine.*

MAO inhibitors[120]
Contraindicated. Concomitant use with MAO inhibitors may potentiate the amphetamine in this preparation. Potentially lethal. See *Amphetamines* under *MAO Inhibitors* and *MAO Inhibitors* under *Sympathomimetics.*

OBESA-MEAD
See *Barbiturates* (amobarbital), *Homatropine,* and *Methamphetamine.*

MAO inhibitors[120]
Same as for *Obedrin* above.

OBETROL
See *Amphetamines.*

MAO inhibitors[120]
Same as for *Obedrin* above.

OBNATAL
See *Dietary Supplements.*

OBOTAN
See *Amphetamines.*

OBRON-6
See *Dietary Supplements.*

OGEN
See *Estrogens, Conjugated* (estrone).

OLEANDOMYCIN
See *Antibiotics.*

Penicillins[70,201,666,864]
Penicillin activity is inhibited by this bacteriostatic antibiotic. See *Antibiotics* under *Penicillins.*

OMNIPEN
See *Ampicillin.*

OMNI-TUSS
See *Antihistamines,* (chlorpheniramine), *Codeine, Ephedrine, Guaiacol Carbonate,* and *Phenyltoloxamine.*

ONCOVIN
See *Vincristine.*

ONIONS

Anticoagulants, oral[895]
Two ounces or more of boiled or fried onions added to a fat-enriched meal significantly increases fibrinolytic activity, and thus potentiates anticoagulants.

OPIATES, SEMI-SYNTHETIC
See *Narcotic Analgesics.*

OPIUM ALKALOIDS
See *Narcotic Analgesics.*

OPIDICE
See *Anorexigenics, Iron Salts,* and *Methamphetamine.*

OPTILETS
See *Dietary Supplements.*

ORACON
See *Oral Contraceptives* (ethinyl estradiol and dimethisterone).

ORAMINIC SPANCAP
See *Antihistamines* (chlorpheniramine maleate), *Atropine,* and *Phenylpropanolamine.*

ORASPAN
See *Dietary Supplements.*

ORAL ANTICOAGULANTS
See *Anticoagulants, Oral.*

ORAL CONTRACEPTIVES (OCs)
(Demulen, Enovid, Norinyl, Norlestrin, Ortho-Novum, Ovulen, etc.; combinations of a progestogen such as ethynodiol diacetate, norethindrone or norethynodrel with an estrogen such as ethinyl estradiol or mestranol). Agents like norethynodrel are enzyme inhibitors.
See also *Estrogens* and *Progestogens.*

Aminocaproic acid[901,1341,1390]
Aminocaproic acid, an antifibrinolytic, and oral contraceptives, which induce blood clotting problems (thromboembolism, etc.), when used concomitantly may enhance the probability of coagulation problems. Exercise caution. With large doses of aminocaproic acid, however, incoagulability may occur in some patients.

Androgens[181]
(Dianabol, Metandren, Nilevar, Oreton, etc.)
Estrogen-progestogens antagonize the anticancer effects of androgens.

Anticoagulants coumarin[673,814,905]
Oral contraceptives decrease the hypoprothrombinemic response to coumarin anticoagulants. Women taking oral contraceptives may require increased dosage of anticoagulant in order to produce the desired effect because the estrogen content may cause increased levels of clotting factors. In some patients some oral contraceptives have potentiated anticoagulants.

Antidepressants, tricyclic[1231,1536,1714,1821]
Accumulating evidence indicates that estrogens (in OCs), particularly in higher doses, may depress the metabolism of some tricyclic antidepressants and increase their toxic effects.

Antidiabetics[181,886]
Oral contraceptives may cause slightly decreased glucose tolerance and an increase in blood glucose levels; increased doses of hypogylcemic agent may be necessary.

Antihistamines[78]
Antihistamines may reduce the effectiveness of oral contraceptives by enzyme induction.

Antihypertensives[1137]
Oral contraceptives tend to elevate blood pressure and some cases of rapidly progressing hypertension have been seen in

some patients on OCs. These drugs are therefore at time antagonistic to antihypertensives.

Antipyrine [1279,1676-7,1822]

Oral contraceptives (estrogens) may inhibit the metabolism of antipyrine and increase its toxicity.

Barbiturates [28,78,83,222,287,812,1507]

Barbiturates, by means of enzyme induction, increase the metabolism of estrogens, and thus can decrease the effectiveness of oral contraceptives. Concern is being created by the decreased effectiveness of oral contraceptives especially those with low doses in women receiving barbiturates and other drugs that cause enzyme induction. Consider other forms of contraception when drugs that induce enzymes are being prescribed.

Blood cholesterol lowering agents [421]

Oral contraceptives may antagonize blood cholesterol lowering agents.

Chlorcyclizine [198] (Perazil)

Oral contraceptives are inhibited by chlorcyclizine. See *Enzyme Inducers* below.

Clofibrate [120,1746] (Atromid-S)

Oral contraceptives may antagonize the blood cholesterol lowering effect of clofibrate. Monitor patients with hyperlipidemia closely for elevation of serum cholesterol and triglycerides if OCs are being used.

Corticosteroids

See *Estrogens* under *Corticosteroids*.

o,p'-DDD [78]

See *Enzyme Inducers* below.

Enzyme inducers [78,222]
(Antihistamines, barbiturates, o,p'-DDD, phenytoin, sedatives, tranquilizers, etc.)

Concern is being created by the possible ineffectiveness of oral contraceptives in women receiving barbiturates, sedatives, tranquilizers, and other drugs that cause enzyme induction. See *Barbiturates* above.

Folic acid [28,924]

Malabsorption of folate has been associated with oral contraceptives. OCs could, therefore, potentiate folic acid antagonists such as the antineoplastic methotrexate.

Guanethidine [80] (Ismelin)

Satisfactory control of hypertension with guanethidine is difficult or impossible when oral contraceptives are being used. In 80% of cases, when oral contraceptives are withdrawn the dosage requirements of guanethidine are substantially decreased. See *Antihypertensives* above.

Halogenated insecticides [78,287,330,812,1059]
(Chlordane, DDT, etc.)

Halogenated insecticides induce not only the metabolism of cortisol, but also that of estrogens, androgens, and progesterone. These halogenated compounds decrease the uterotropic effects of both exogenous and endogenous estrogens.

Insulin [120,181]

Oral contraceptives may cause a significant increase in glucose levels. See *Antidiabetics* above.

Meperidine [92,1308,1830] (Demerol, pethidine, etc.)

Oral contraceptives increase urinary excretion of unchanged meperidine and decrease urinary ecretion of its metabolites. OCs thereby potentiate the analgesic (enzyme inhibition).

Meprobamate [78] (Equanil, Miltown)

Meprobamate may reduce the effectiveness of oral contraceptives by enzyme induction.

Methotrexate

See under *Folic Acid* above.

Mineral oil [28,1841]

Mineral oil may decrease intestinal absorption of OCs and thereby decrease their effectiveness. This also applies to estrogens. Prostatic carcinoma in patients being treated with estrogens was exacerbated when mineral oil was taken concomitantly.

Pesticides [287,330,812]

See *Halogenated Pesticides* above.

Phenobarbital [198,633]

Phenobarbital (enzyme inducer) inhibits oral contraceptives. See *Barbiturates* above.

Phenothiazines [1394]

Estrogens may increase plasma levels of phenothiazines by some inhibiting mechanism and thus potentiate their side effects.

Phenylbutazone [198,633]

Phenylbutazone inhibits oral contraceptives (enzyme induction).

Phenytoin [78]

See *Enzyme Inducers* above.

Promazine [92] (Sparine)

Oral contraceptives decrease the urinary excretion of promazine and its metabolites, and thereby potentiate the ataractic (enzyme inhibition).

Rifampin

See *Contraceptives, Oral* under *Rifampin*.

Smoking [862]

Smoking may increase the likelihood of thromboembolism with oral contraceptives.

Thyroid hormones [1598,1904]

In athyrotic patients, estrogens (and thus OCs with estrogen) inhibit thyroid hormones by increasing TBG (thyroxine-binding globulin), the plasma protein binder. In patients with sufficient thyroid function the increased binding of, and thus the tendency to decrease, free (active) thyroxine is offset by a compensating increase in thyroxine output by the thyroid gland. Triiodothyronine (Cytomel), which is bound much less by TBG, is not affected as much as thyroxine by this interaction. Monitor patients on OCs for possible need for increased thyroid hormone.

Triiodothyronine [421]

Estrogen-progestogens decrease triiodothyronine levels. See *Thyroid Hormones* above.

Tuberculin skin test [24]

The sensitivity of this test may be depressed by oral contraceptives.

Vitamins [848,1279]

Patients receiving oral contraceptives containing estrogens which cause a folic acid deficiency may require folic acid and supplements. Oral contraceptives inhibit the metabolism of D_3. Lower the dose.

ORAL MEDICATIONS

Inhibitors of absorption [1791]

Many drugs, including atropine and other anticholinergics, chloroquine, codeine, morphine, etc., delay gastric emptying and thus depress intestinal absorption of other drugs.

ORBIFERROUS

See *Dietary Supplements*.

ORENZYME

See *Chymotrysin-trypsin*.

ORETIC

See *Thiazide Diuretics* (hydrochlorothiazide).

ORETON
See *Testosterone.*

ORGANIC SOLVENTS

Anticoagulants, oral [433]
Hypoprothrombinemia may result with coumarin anticoagulants. See *Carbon Tetrachloride.*

ORGANIDIN (Iodinated Glycerol)
See *Iodine.*

ORGANOPHOSPHATE CHOLINESTERASE INHIBITORS (Organophosphorous insecticides, etc.)
See *Anticholinesterases.*
These insecticides have the same interactions with dexpanthenol, phenothiazines, polymyxin, procainamide, streptomycin, etc. as those given under *Anticholinesterases.*

Phenothiazines [120]
Some phenothiazines may antagonize and some may potentiate the toxic anticholinesterase effects of these insecticides.

Succinylcholine [120,204]
Use of any cholinesterase inhibtor should be discontinued 6 weeks before surgery since anticholinesterases potentiate succinylcholine.

ORINASE
See *Tolbutamide.*

ORNADE SPANSULE
See *Antihistamines* (chlorpheniramine maleate) and *Phenylpropanolamine.*

ORPHENADRINE (Disipal, Norflex, Norgesic)

Aminopyrine [555]
Orphenadrine, by enzyme induction, inhibits the action of this drug.

Anticholinergics [120]
Orphenadrine potentiates anticholinergics (additive effects).

Chlorpromazine [528,1858] **(Thorazine)**
Hypoglycemic coma, sweating, dryness and paresthesia have been reported in patients who were given orphenadrine with chlorpromazine.

Griseofulvin [529] **(Grifulvin)**
Orphenadrine, an enzyme inducer, causes a decreased griseofulvin effect.

Hexobarbital [555]
Same as for *Aminopyrine* above.

Orphenadrine [529]
Orphenadrine stimulates its own metabolism. Tolerance may develop.

Perphenazine [482] **(Trilafon)**
This combination may have a synergistic toxic effect on chromosomes.

Phenothiazines
See *Orphenadrine* under *Phenothiazines.*

Phenylbutazone [555]
Same as for *Aminopyrine* above.

Physostigmine [2000]
Orphenadrine overdosage (1.2-1.5 Gm.), causing severe agitation, hallucinations, delusions and paranoia, can be successfully treated with physostigmine, an antidote for anticholinergics.

Propoxyphene [120,421,528,714,1259,1903,1929] **(Darvon)**
When orphenadrine is used concurrently with propoxyphene, tremors, mental confusion and anxiety may result, according to the literature, possibly due to additive hypoglycemic effects, but this interaction has been questioned.

ORTHO-NOVUM
See *Oral Contraceptives* (mestranol and norethindrone).

OS-CAL (Calcium plus Minerals and Vit. D)
See *Calcium Salts* and *Iron Salts.*

OS-CAL-GESIC
See *Salicylamide.*

OS-CAL-MONE
See *Calcium Salts, Estradiol,* and *Testosterone.*

OTC MEDICATIONS
See *Cold, Hay Fever, Reducing, and Other OTC Remedies* and also *Cold and Cough Remedies.*

OTOTOXIC DRUGS
See *Antibiotics with Ototoxic Effects* under *Neomycin.*
Ototoxic drugs include ethacrynic acid, furosemide, kanamycin, neomycin, ristocetin, streptomycins, and vancomycin.

Ethacrynic acid [120,653,813]
Ethacrynic acid administered to patients also receiving ototoxic drugs has caused permanent deafness.

Furosemide [120]
Transient deafness is more likely to occur in patients with severe impairment of renal function and in patients who are also receiving drugs known to be ototoxic.

OTRIVIN
See *Sympathomimetics* (xylometazoline HCl).

OUABAIN
See *Cardiac Glycosides.*

OVOCYLIN
See *Estradiol.*

OVRAL TABLETS
See *Oral Contraceptives* (norgestrel with ethinyl estradiol).

OVULEN-28
See *Oral Contraceptives* (ethynodiol diacetate with mestranol).

OXACILLIN (Prostaphlin)
See *Penicillins.*

OXAINE M (Suspension)
See *Aluminum Hydroxide* and *Magnesium Hydroxide.* Also contains a local anesthetic (oxethazaine).

OXANDROLONE (Anavar)
See *Androgens* (anabolic agent).

OXAZEPAM (Serax)
See *Chlordiazepoxide* and *Diazepam.*
The drug interactions for these three benzodiazepines are similar. [120]

OX BILE

Vitamin A [165]
Absorption of vitamin A is enhanced if bile salts are also administered.

Vitamin K [165]
Absorption of vitamin K in patients with jaundice is enhanced if bile salts are also administered.

OXPRENOLOL
See *β-Adrenergic Blockers* and *Methyldopa* under *Phenylpropanolamine.*

OXTRIPHYLLINE
(Choledyl, choline theophyllinate)

Other xanthine preparations [120]
Concurrent use of this xanthine bronchodilator with other xanthine preparations (caffeine, theobromine, etc.) may lead to adverse reactions, particulary CNS stimulation in children.

OXYCODONE
See *Narcotic Analgesics* (dihydrohydroxycodeinone).

OXY-KESSO-TETRA
See *Tetracyclines* (oxytetracycline HCl)

OXYLIDINE (3-Quinuclidinol)

Aminopyrine [951]
Aminopyrine potentiates oxylidine.

OXYPHENBUTAZONE (Tandearil)
See also *Pyrazolone Compounds* and *Phenylbutazone*.
Oxyphenbutazone is an active metabolite (parahydroxy derivative) of phenylbutazone and the drug interactions for both of these highly potent drugs are therefore similar. Both drugs are highly toxic and must be very carefully administered only in severe inflammatory conditions, acute exacerbations of chronic arthritides, and specifically indicated conditions. [120]

Anabolic steroids
See *Oxyphenbutazone* under *Anabolic Agents*.

Androgens [257,421,448,633,1502] **(Anabolic agents)**
Potentiation (increased plasma level and possibly adverse effects) of oxyphenbutazone may occur with concomitant methandrostenolone therapy. Probably caused by enzyme inhibition (of glucuronyl transferase) or displacement of the anti-inflammatory drug from its binding sites on serum albumin. See also *Androgens* under *Phenylbutazone*.

Anticoagulants, oral [120,150,330,434,448,852]
See *Anti-inflammatory Agents* under *Anticoagulants, Oral*. Oxyphenbutazone also slows the clearance of Dicumarol from the plasma.

Antidiabetics, oral [120,191]
Oxyphenbutazone potentiates the hypoglycemic effect of the sulfonylurea antidiabetic agents (interference with excretion of active metabolite).

Cholestyramine
See *Cholestyramine* under *Phenylbutazone*.

Desipramine [85,863] **(Norpramin, Pertofrane)**
Desipramine reduces absorption of oxyphenbutazone (in the rat) and thus inhibits its activity.

Imipramine [85]
Same as for *Desipramine* above.

Insulin [120]
Pyrazole compounds, like oxyphenbutazone, potentiate insulin.

Methandrostenolone [198,330,448,852] **(Dianobol)**
See *Androgens* above.

Other chemotherapeutic agents [120]
Oxyphenbutazone is contraindicated in patients receiving other potent chemotherapy because of the possibility of increased toxic reactions.

Penicillins [198]
Oxyphenbutazone potentiates penicillin by decreasing its renal excretion.

Phenylbutazone [120] **(Butazolidin)**
Patients may experience cross-sensitivity to both oxyphenbutazone and phenylbutazone.

Salicylates [28,359,614]
In treating arthritic patients combined use of oxyphenbutazone and salicylates should be avoided because of the increased danger of gastrointestinal ulceration. See also *Salicylates* under *Phenylbutazone*.

Sulfamethoxypyridazine (Kynex)
See *Sulfonamides* below.

Sulfonamides [120,359]
Highly bound agents such as oxyphenbutazone are able to displace the longlasting albumin-bound sulfonamides from plasma protein. These sulfas are not rapidly metabolized or excreted. Thus, displaced molecules diffuse from plasma into skeletal muscle, cerebral spinal fluid, and other brain tissues. The potentiation causes increased toxicity as well as enhanced antibacterial activity.

Sulfonylurea antidiabetics
See *Antidiabetics, Oral* above.

Warfarin
See *Anticoagulants, Oral* below.

OXYTETRACYCLINE (Terramycin)
See *Tetracyclines*.

Antidiabetics, Oral
See *Oxytetracycline* under *Antidiabetics, Oral*.

OXYTOCICS
(Ergonovine [Ergotrate] maleate, methylergonovine maleate [Methergine], oxytocin [Pitocin, Syntocinon])

Anesthetics, local [120]
If hypotension occurs during an obstetrical procedure, the use of oxytocics concomitantly with a vasoconstrictor, such as may be present in a local anesthetic, may result in severe persistent hypertension. See *Vasoconstrictors* below.

Citrates [421]
When citrates are given concomitantly the effects are erratic and unpredictable.

Cyclophosphamide [421] **(Cytoxan)**
Oxytocin is potentiated by cyclophosphamide.

Ephedrine
See *Vasoconstrictors* below.

Estrogens [173]
In the presence of adequate estrogen, oxytocin augments the electrical and contractile activity of uterine smooth muscle; when estrogen levels are low, the effect of oxytocin is much reduced.

Methoxamine (Vasoxyl)
See *Vasoconstrictors* below.

Phenylephrine
See *Vasoconstrictors* below.

Sparteine [951]
Synergistic oxytocic activity.

Sympathomimetics [421,609]
See *Vasoconstrictors* below.

Tannates [421]
When tannates are given concomitantly the effects are erratic and unpredictable.

Triacetyloleandomycin (TAO, troleandomycin) [359]
This combination may cause ergotism with the ergot alkaloids (inhibition of metabolism).

Vasoconstrictors [173,609,611]
(Vasopressors)
Severe, persistent hypertension, with rupture of cerebral blood vessels may occur because of the synergistic and additive vasoconstrictive effects. Vasopressin blocks the increase in renal blood flow caused by oxytocin infusion. A potentially lethal interaction.

PABA
See *p-Aminobenzoic Acid.*

PABALATE
See *p-Aminobenzoic Acid* and *Salicylates* (sodium salicylate).

PABIRIN
See *p-Aminobenzoic Acid, Ascorbic Acid,* and *Salicylates* (aspirin).

PAGITANE
See *Muscle Relaxants, Centrally Acting* (cycrimine).

PAMAQUINE (Aminoquin, Plasmoquine, etc.)

Quinacrine [298, 421, 1028] (Mepacrine)
Quinacrine potentiates pamaquine by displacing it from binding sites in the liver and other storage tissues.

PAMISYL
See *p-Aminosalicylic Acid.*

PANCREATIN (Pancreatic extracts)

Cimetidine (Tagamet) [2064]
Cimetidine, a gastric secretion inhibitor by means of β_2-receptor blockade, improves the efficacy of pancreatin in pancreatic insufficiency or pancreatectomy. However, a combination of the inhibitor and an antacid seems to be necessary for satisfactory digestion in patients with pancreatic exocrine insufficiency.

Iron Salts
See *Pancreatic Extracts* under *Iron Salts.*

PANHEPRIN
See *Heparin* (Sodium heparin injection).

PANMYCIN
See *Tetracyclines.*

PANTOPON
See *Narcotic Analgesics* (opium alkaloid hydrochlorides).

PANTOTHENIC ACID, ITS SALTS, AND DEXPANTHENOL
(Ilopan, pantothenyl alcohol)

Barbiturates
See *Pantothenyl Alcohol* under *Barbiturates.*

Narcotic analgesics
See *Pantothenyl Alcohol* under *Narcotic Analgesics.*

Parasympathomimetics [120]
Dexpanthenol should not be given until 12 hours after use of a parasympathomimetic (neostigmine or other enterokinetic drug) used in paralytic ileus because of the possibility of hyperperistalsis.

Probenecid [120]
Probenecid inhibits renal tubular transport of pantothenic acid and prolongs its plasma levels.

Succinylcholine [120, 1814, 1965]
Dexpanthenol (pantothenyl alcohol), used in surgery for postpartum and postoperative intestinal and ureteral atony, is converted to pantothenic acid which enters into the formation of coenzyme A, which then induces formation of acetylcholine. The latter potentiates depolarizing muscle relaxants and thus dexpanthenol may potentiate succinylcholine (respiratory depression) and it should not be given within one hour after succinylcholine administration. However, only one such interaction, somewhat doubtful, appears in the literature up to 1978.

PANWARFIN
See *Anticoagulants, Oral* (warfarin).

Vitamin E
See *Warfarin* under *Vitamin E.*

PAPAIN

Anticoagulants, oral [198, 421]
Oral anticoagulants are enhanced by papain. Concurrent use is not recommended.

PAPASE
See *Papain.*

PAPAVERINE (Analog: ethaverine)

Histamine [120, 951]
Papaverine enhances the increase in capillary permeability and the hypotensive effect produced by histamine.

Levodopa [2001]
Papaverine reduces the efficacy of levodopa.

Morphine [619]
Morphine antagonizes the relaxing effect of papaverine.

PARA-AMINOBENZOIC ACID
See *p-Aminobenzoic Acid*

PARA-AMINOSALICYLIC ACID
See *p-Aminosalicylic Acid*

PARACETAMOL
See *Acetaminophen.*

PARACORT
See *Prednisone.*

PARACORTOL
See *Prednisolone.*

PARAFLEX
See *Muscle Relaxants, Centrally Acting* (chlorzoxazone).

PARALDEHYDE
See *CNS Depressants.*
Alcohol and other CNS depressants potentiate paraldehyde.

Disulfiram [120]
Disulfiram, an inhibitor of acetaldehyde dehydrogenase, should *not* be used concurrently with paraldehyde, a polymer of acetaldehyde. High blood levels of acetaldehyde produce the toxic disulfiram reaction.

Sulfonamides [433]
Antagonism of antibacterial activity due to increase in rate of metabolism of sulfonamide and possible crystalluria. Metabolism of sulfonamides involves acetylation. Acetylated compounds can crystallize in kidney tubules. Paraldehyde can supply an acetylation moiety and thus increase danger of crystalluria.

Tolbutamide [678] (Orinase)
Tolbutamide potentiates the hypnotic effect of paraldehyde.

PARASAL
See *p-Aminosalicylic Acid.*

PARASPAN
See *Anticholinergics* (methscopolamine nitrate).

PARASYMPATHOMIMETIC AGENTS
See also *Acetylcholine, Anticholinesterases, Neostigmine,* and *Pilocarpine,* etc.
Combined use of parasympathomimetic agents of various types may yield additive toxic or side effects.

Dexpanthenol and pantothenic acid[421]
Dexpanthenol should not be given for 12 hours after use of a parasympathomimetic because of the possibility of hyperperistalsis.

PARATHORMONE (Parathyroid injection)

Androgens[181]
Androgens antagonize parathormone. Parathyroid hormone promotes the mobilization of calcium from bone whereas androgens foster retention of calcium in the bones.

Calcitonin[181]
The hypocalcemic effect of calcitonin antagonizes the hypercalcemic effect of parathormone. Calcitonin also antagonizes the inhibitory effects of parathormone on pyrophosphatase activity.

Corticosteroids[181]
Corticosteroids antagonize parathormone induced hypercalcemia.

PAREDRINE
See *Amphetamines* and *Vasopressors* (hydroxyamphetamine).

PARGYLINE (Eutonyl)
See *MAO Inhibitors*.

Alcohol
Avoid this combination. See *MAO Inhibitors* under *Alcohol*.

Lidocaine[120] **(Xylocaine)**
Some patients receiving pargyline for a prolonged period of time become refractory to the nerve blocking effects of lidocaine.

PARNATE
See *MAO Inhibitors* (Tranylcypromine).

PAROMOMYCIN (Humatin)
See *Aminoglycoside Antibiotics*.

Dimenhydrinate (Dramamine)
See *Aminoglycoside Antibiotics* under *Dimenhydrinate*.

Ethacrynic Acid (Edecrin)
See *Aminoglycoside Antibiotics* under *Ethacrynic Acid*.

Gentamicin[120]
Gentamicin has been shown to possess cross-resistance between itself and paromomycin.

Methoxyflurane (Penthrane)
See under *Methoxyflurane*.

Muscle relaxants
See *Neuromuscular Blocking Antibiotics* under *Antibiotics*.

Penicillins
These bacteriostatic antibiotics inhibit penicillin activity. See under *Antibiotics*.

Sucrose[929]
Paromomycin causes malabsorption of sucrose.

Xylose[929]
Paromomycin causes malabsorption of xylose.

PARSIDOL
See *Antiparkinsonism Drugs* (ethopropazine).

PARSTELIN
See *MAO Inhibitors* (Parnate) and *Phenothiazines* (Stelazine).

PAS
See *p-Aminosalicylic Acid*.

PAS-C (Pascorbic)
See *Ascorbic Acid* and *p-Aminosalicylic Acid*.

PASNA PACK GRANULES
See *p-Aminosalicylic Acid* (sodium aminosalicylate).

PASNA TRI-PACK GRANULES
See *Isoniazid, p-Aminosalicyclic Acid*, and *Vitamin B Complex*.

PATHIBAMATE
See *Meprobamate* and *Anticholinergics* (tridihexethyl chloride)

PAVABID
See *Papaverine*.

P-B SAL-C
See *p-Aminobenzoic Acid, Ascorbic Acid*, and *Salicylates* (sodium salicylate).

PEDAMETH
See *Urinary Acidifiers* (*dl*-methionine).

PEDIAMYCIN
See *Erythromycin* (ethylsuccinate).

PEGANONE
See *Anticonvulsants* (ethotoin).

PEMPIDINE (Perolysen Tenormal hydrogen tartrate)
See *Ganglionic Blocking Agents*.

Acidifying agents[325,870]
Acidifying agents decrease absorption and increase the urinary excretion of pempidine and related compounds and decrease their activity.

Alkalinizing agents[325,870]
Alkalinizing agents increase absorption and decrease urinary excretion of pempidine and related ganglionic blocking agents and enhance their activity.

Levarterenol[117]
Pempidine potentiates the pressor effects of levarterenol.

Thiazide diuretics[120,633]
Synergistic antihypertensive activity.

PENBRITIN
See *Ampicillin*.

PENICILLAMINE (Cuprimine)

Benorylate[1984] **(Benoral)**
Benorylate, an ester of acetaminophen and aspirin, when given with D-penicillamine for rheumatoid arthritis, produced hepatotoxicity (hemorrhagic centrilobar necrosis). Perhaps D-penicillamine excretion as L-cysteine-D-penicillamine disulfide exhausted hepatic cysteine, a precursor of glutathione, and reduced the levels of the latter to the point where detoxification of acetaminophen metabolites was inadequate to prevent nephrotoxic effects.

Isoniazid[421]
Penicillamine, an effective chelator and therefore antidote for copper, lead, mercury and zinc, may potentiate the neurotoxicity (peripheral neuritis) and other adverse effects of isoniazid resembling pyridoxine deficiency. See *Pyridoxine* below and under *Isoniazed*.

Pyridoxine[175]
The adverse effects of the L and DL isomers, but probably not D-penicillamine, are prevented by pyridoxine which inhibits enzymes that are pyridoxal dependent. Thus, dietary supplementation of pyridoxine is desirable, even with the D isomer. See also under *Isoniazid* and *Isoniazid* above.

PENICILLINS

See also *Ampicillin, Carbenacillin,* etc.

Acidifying agents[178]

Penicillins may be decomposed by aqueous acid media. Gastric secretions rapidly destroy penicillin G, but ampicillin is acid stable. Stability varies with the structure of the penicillin.

Actinomycin D (Cosmegan)

Actinomycin D inhibits the bactericidal activity of penicillins. See *Antibiotics.*

Alkalinizing agents[78,201,633]

Antacids may increase ionization of oral penicillins and thus decrease absorption and therefore the effectiveness of some penicillins. On the other hand antacids also tend to protect penicillin from destruction by gastric acid. Further investigation is needed to determine the clinical significance of this interaction.

Allopurinol[1254,1260,1775]

Allopurinol may increase the frequency with which patients experience ampicillin rashes.

p-Aminobenzoic acid[268,269] (PABA)

PABA potentiates penicillins by displacing them from inactive binding sites.

Aminoglycoside Antibiotics

See *Neomycin* below.

Aminohippuric acid[433] (PAHA)

Aminohippuric acid increases penicillin concentration in the cerebrospinal fluid and blood; reduced concentration in the brain (inhibition of urinary excretion).

Amisometradine[121] (Rolicton)

Penicillins diminish the effectiveness of amisometradine by interfering with the carrier transport mechanism which facilitates its passage into cells.

Analgesics[198,267-269,359]

Some analgesics (salicylates like aspirin and pyrazolone derivatives like aminopyrine, antipyrine, oxyphenbutazone, phenylbutazone, etc.) potentiate penicillins by displacing them from secondary binding sites, and slowing renal excretion.

Antacids[78,201,633]

Antacids inhibit oral penicillins by reducing absorption. See *Alkalinizing Agents* above.

Antibiotics

See *Antibiotics* under *Antibiotics*

Anticoagulants, oral[120]

Penicillin potentiates coumarin anticoagulants.

Aspirin[267-269]

See *Analgesics* above.

Bacitracin

Bacitracin enhances the therapeutic effect of penicillin (in animals) against certain organisms.

Cephalosporins[120,233]
(Kafacin, Keflin, Loridine, etc.)

Cross-sensitivity occurs between the penicillins and cephalosporins. See also *Antibiotics* under *Antibiotics.*

Cheese[433]

Blue cheese inhibits the action of penicillin.

Chloramphenicol[240,301,444,492,633,864]
(Chloromycetin)

See *Antibiotics* under *Antibiotics.*

Chlorphenesin (Maolate)

Chlorphenesin reduces hypersensitivity to penicillin.

Chlortetracycline

See *Antibiotics* under *Antibiotics.*

Chymotrypsin, oral[27]

Chymotrypsin elevates blood levels of penicillin through enhanced absorption.

Cloxacillin

Same as for *Methicillin* below.

Dactinomycin

See *Antibiotics* under *Antibiotics.*

Erythromycin (Erythrocin, Ilotycin)[31,70,301,419,811]

Erythromycin inhibits the bactericidal activity of penicillins against most penicillin sensitive organisms but potentiates the activity against resistant strains of *Staph. aureus.*

Heparin[433]

Penicillin inhibits heparin. Withdrawal of penicillin IV may cause severe hemorrhage.

Kanamycin[210,233,239] (Kantrex)

See *Antibiotics* under *Antibiotics.* Kanamycin usually inhibits other antibiotics but against some organisms may potentiate the penicillins, *e.g.,* against *Brucella abortus.*

Methicillin[382]

Synergistic activity against *Str. pyogenes* and *Staph. aureus.*

Nafcillin

Same as for *Methicillin* above.

Neomycin[421,1287]

See *Antibiotics* under *Antibiotics.* Neomycin orally, by producing a malabsorption syndrome, inhibits considerably the absorption of penicillin V (Compocillin, Pen-Vee, V-Cillin) and probably other oral penicillins.

Oleandomycin

See *Antibiotics* under *Antibiotics.*

Oxyphenbutazone[198]

See *Analgesics* above.

Oxytetracycline[864]

See *Antibiotics* under *Antibiotics.*

Paromomycin (Humatin)

May antagonize the activity of penicillin. See *Antibiotics* under *Antibiotics.*

Phenylbutazone[198,633] (Butazolidin)

See *Analgesics* above.

Probenecid[43,160,269,619] (Benemid)

Probenecid potentiates penicillins by interfering with excretion and thus elevating and prolonging penicillin blood levels.

Pyrazolone derivatives[198,421]

See *Analgesics* above.

Salicylates[198,421]

See *Analgesics* above.

Streptomycin[178,210,233,239,492]

This combination is synergistically antimicrobial in subacute bacterial endocarditis, bacteremia, brain abscess, meningitis, and urinary tract infections caused by enterococci.

Sulfinpyrazone[267-269] (Anturane)

Sulfinpyrazone potentiates penicillins probably by displacing them from secondary binding sites.

Sulfonamides[267-269,1525]

Some sulfonamides may potentiate some penicillins by displacing them from secondary binding sites. Some combinations, however, may have an additive, indifferent, or inhibitory effect, depending on the sulfonamide and the penicillin. Sulfonamides, *e.g.,* sulfamethoxypyridazine, may lower the serum concentration of total penicillin but increase the concentration of unbound, antimicrobially active drug in serum and body fluids. Relatively large doses of sulfonamides can reduce the protein binding of penicillins and thus potentiate them.

Tetracyclines [233,238,285,301,633,666,1437,1520,1627]
See *Antibiotics* under *Antibiotics.*

PENTAERYTHRITOL TETRANITRATE (Peritrate, PETN, etc.)

Acetylcholine [120]
PETN acts as a physiological antagonist to acetylcholine, histamine, norepinephrine (levarterenol), and many other drugs.

Alcohol [120]
Alcohol may enhance the hypotensive effects of the nitrite and severe responses (nausea, vomiting, weakness, pallor, restlessness, perspiration, and collapse) may occur.

Histamine [120]
See *Acetylcholine* above.

Levarterenol
See *Acetylcholine* above.

Nitroglycerin [120]
The intake of nitroglycerin for angina pectoris can be reduced when PETN is used concomitantly. See also *Nitrates and Nitrites* below.

Nitrates and nitrites [120]
Cross-tolerance can develop between PETN and other nitrates and nitrites.

PENTAZOCINE (Talwin)

Methylphenidate [120,166] **(Ritaline)**
The respiratory depression caused by pentazocine is reversed by methylphenidate.

Naloxone [120,166] **(Narcan)**
Naloxone antagonizes the respiratory depression produced by pentazocine.

Narcotic analgesics [120,166]
Pentazocine weakly antagonizes the analgesic effects of meperidine, morphine and phenazocine, and it incompletely reverses the behavioral, cardiovascular and respiratory depressions produced by meperidine and morphine.

Smoking [1054]
Higher dosage of pentazocine is required in about 60% of city dwellers or smokers because of pollutants that are enzyme inducers.

PENTIDS
See *Penicillins.*

PENTOBARBITAL (Nembutal)
See *Barbiturates.*

PENTOLINIUM (Ansolysen)

Alcohol [120]
Alcohol potentiates this ganglionic blocker (enhanced hypotension).

Amphetamines [421]
Amphetamines inhibit the hypotensive action of the ganglionic blocking agent, pentolinium.

Anesthetics [421]
Pentolinium potentiates the CNS depressant action of anesthetics.

Anticholinergics [120]
Combined use may cause an exaggerated response to both drugs.

Ethacrynic acid [421]
Pentolinium potentiates ethacrynic acid.

Levarterenol [117]
Pentolinium (ganglionic blocker) potentiates the pressor effects of levarterenol.

MAO inhibitors [421]
MAO inhibitors potentiate the effects of pentolinium.

Reserpine [120]
Potentiated hypotensive action with this combination permits reduced dosage (fewer side effects).

Spironolactone [421] **(Aldactone)**
Pentolinium potentiates the hypotensive action of spironolactone.

Sympathomimetics [421]
Sympathomimetic pressor agents antagonize the hypotensive action of pentolinium and their response may be potentiated by the ganglionic blockader.

Thiazide diuretics [421]
Pentolinium potentiates the hypotensive action of the thiazide diuretics and vice versa.

Tricyclic antidepressants [421]
The tricyclic antidepressants antagonize the hypotensive action of pentolinium.

PENTOTHAL
See *Barbiturates* (thiopental).

PENTYLENETETRAZOL (Metrazol, etc.)

Alcohol [166]
Contraindicated. Alcohol suppresses convulsions induced by pentylenetetrazol but only in amounts that cause general depression of the CNS.

Barbiturates [120]
Pentylenetetrazol, a CNS stimulant, is used as an antidote to counteract the respiratory depression or failure caused by poisoning with barbiturates, meprobamate, etc.

Local anesthetics [167]
Local anesthetics, with their anticonvulsant properties, protect against convulsions produced by pentylenetetrazol.

Meprobamate
See *Barbiturates* above.

Phenothiazines [120,166]
Pentylenetetrazol should not be used as a CNS stimulating agent in treating overdosage of phenothiazines since it may cause convulsions with these drugs which lower the convulsive threshold. Drugs like chlorpromazine do not protect against the convulsant action of pentylenetetrazol.

Thioxanthenes [120,166] **(Taractan, etc.)**
Pentylenetetrazol should not be used as a stimulating agent in treating overdosage of thioxanthenes since it may cause convulsions with these drugs. Same actions as those given above for *Phenothiazines.*

PEN-VEE
See *Penicillins* (phenoxymethyl penicillin).

PEN-VEE K
See *Penicillins* (penicillin V potassium).

PERANDREN
See *Testosterone.*

PERAZIL
See *Antihistamines* (chlorcyclizine).

PERCOBARB
See *Barbiturates* (hexobarbital), *Caffeine, Homatropine, Narcotic Analgesics* (oxycodone), *Phenacetin,* and *Salicylates* (aspirin).

PERCODAN
See same as *Percobarb* without the barbiturate.

PERCORTEN
See *Desoxycorticosterone.*

PERIACTIN
See *Antihistamines* (cyproheptadine).

PERMITIL
See *Phenothiazines* (fluphenazine).

PERPHENAZINE (Trilafon)
See *Phenothiazines.*

l-Glutavite
l-Glutavite potentiates the psychotropic activity of perpenazine.

Heparin [764]
Perphenazine, in large doses, antagonizes the anticoagulant action of heparin.

Lysergide [482] **(LSD)**
Perphenazine with LSD induces major chromosome abnormalities (breaks, gaps, and hypodiploid cells).

Orphenadrine [482] **(Disipal)**
This combination (orphenadrine plus perphenazine) may have a synergistic toxic effect on chromosomes.

Pargyline and other MAO inhibitors [162,330]
Potentiation of hypotensive effects.

Rauwolfia alkaloids [421,633] **(Reserpine, etc.)**
Potentiation of hypotensive and sedative effects.

PERTROFRANE
See *Antidepressants, Tricyclic* (desipramine).

PESTICIDES
(Chlorinated hydrocarbons, Chlordane, DDT, etc.)

Androgens [78,83,485]
These pesticides stimulate the metabolism of androgens and thus decrease their effectiveness.

Estrogen-progestogens [78,83,485]
(Oral contraceptives)
Pesticides stimulate the metabolism of estrogen-progestogens and thus decrease their effectiveness.

Glucocorticoids [83,271,485]
Pesticides stimulate the metabolism of glucocorticoids and thus decrease their effectiveness.

PETHIDINE
See *Meperidine.*

PETN
See *Pentaerythritol Tetranitrate.*

PHELANTIN
See *Methamphetamine, Phenobarbital,* and *Phenytoin*

PHENACEMIDE (Phenurone)

Ethotoin [120] **(Peganone)**
Caution is advised since paranoid symptoms have been reported during therapy with this combination of the hydantoin (ethotoin) and the other anticonvulsant, phenacemide.

Other anticonvulsants [120]
Extreme caution is essential if phenacemide is administered with other anticonvulsants that cause similar toxic effects or administered to patients with a history of allergy associated with other anticonvulsants.

PHENACETIN (Acetophenetidin)

Phenobarbital [83,166]
Phenobarbital inhibits phenacetin.

Polysorbate [359]
The absorption of phenacetin is accelerated in the presence of polysorbate.

Sorbitol [359]
The absorption of phenacetin is accelerated in the presence of sorbitol.

PHENAGLYCODOL (Ultran)
See *CNS Depressants* and *Tranquilizers.*

Alcohol [121,166]
Phenaglycodol is potentiated by alcohol.

PHENAPHEN PLUS
See *Antihistamines* (pheniramine maleate), *Hyoscyamine, Phenacetin, Phenobarbital, Phenylephrine,* and *Salicylates* (aspirin).

PHENAZOCINE (Prinadol)
See *Narcotic Analgesics.*

Nalorphine [166]
Nalorphine can precipitate an acute abstinence syndrome in patients physically dependent on phenazocine.

PHENDIMETRAZINE (Bacarate, Bontril)
Phendimetrazine, an anorectic used in obesity, has effects similar to amphetamine (CNS stimulation, elevated blood pressure, etc.). See *Amphetamines* for drug interactions; alters insulin requirements in diabetes mellitus, [120] decreases hypotensive effect of guanethidine, [120] etc. Impairs ability of patient to engage in potentially hazardous activities (operating machinery, driving an automobile, etc.).

PHENELZINE (Nardil)
See *MAO inhibitors.*

PHENERGAN
See *Antihistamines* (promethazine) and *Phenothiazines.*

PHENERGAN VC EXPECTORANT
See *Antihistamines* (promethazine), *Chloroform, Ipecac, Phenothiazines, Phenylephrine,* and *Potassium Guaiacolsulfonate.*

PHENETHICILLIN
(Darcil, Maxipen, Syncillin, etc.)
See *Penicillins.*

Chymotrypsin [27]
Chymotrypsin potentiates phenethicillin.

PHENFORMIN (DBI)
This antidiabetic, the only biguanide made available, was removed from the market by FDA in 1977 after it had caused thousands of deaths from lactic acidosis, a condition with 50% mortality. The interaction with alcohol was particularly dangerous in this regard. Later, by 1978, FDA permitted the manufacturer to distribute the drug to a very few patients who could not tolerate any other antidiabetic agent including insulin.

PHENINDIONE (Danilone, Hedulin)

Clofibrate (Atromid-S)
Blood coagulation irregularities and hemorrhagic episodes may occur. See *Anticoagulants, Oral* under *Clofibrate.*

Haloperidol [340,703,814] (Haldol)

Haloperidol (enzyme inducer) decreases the anticoagulant effect of phenindione.

Phenyramidol [705] (Analexin)

Phenyramidol potentiates phenindione.

PHENIRAMINE (Trimeton)

See *Antihistamines.*

PHENMETRAZINE (Preludin)

Chlorpromazine [765]

Chlorpromazine and certain other phenothiazines inhibit the anorexic activity of phenmetrazine.

CNS stimulants [120]

Phenmetrazine should not be used with other CNS stimulants. Excessive additive effects.

MAO inhibitors [120]

Potentiation. The anorexiant should not be used with the MAO inhibitors (CNS stimulation).

Phenothiazines

See *Chlorpromazine* above.

PHENOBARBITAL

See *Barbiturates.* These inhibit the activity of many drugs.

Acetaminophen

See *Phenobarbital* under *Acetaminophen.*

Acetophenetidin

See *Phenacetin* below.

Acidifying agents [28,325,579,870]

The excretion of phenobarbital is decreased and its action potentiated by lowered urinary pH.

Actinomycin D [709]

Actinomycin D abolishes the induction of microsomal drug metabolizing enzymes by phenobarbital.

Alcohol [166,241,244,311,633,634,730,737,738]

A hazardous, potentially lethal CNS depressant combination. See *CNS Depressants.*

Alkalinizing agents [28,579,870]

The excretion of phenobarbital is markedly increased and its action strongly inhibited in alkaline urine.

dl-Amphetamine [359]

dl-Amphetamine delays intestinal absorption of phenobarbital, followed by synergistic anticonvulsant activity.

Androgens [83,198,330,421]

Phenobarbital increases androsterone and testosterone metabolism (hydroxylation) and thus inhibits androgenic activity.

Androsterone

See *Androgens* above.

Anticoagulants, oral [63-65,78,96,183,278,296,297,375,633,677,865,867]

(Coumadin, Dicumarol, Panwarfin, Sintrom, etc.)

Phenobarbital inhibits the effects of oral coumarin anticoagulants by stimulating the hepatic microsomal enzymes responsible for their metabolism: decreases plasma half-life. Serious and sometimes fatal hemorrhages have been reported after withdrawal of phenobarbital in patients on oral anticoagulants. Oral anticoagulants, *e.g.,* dicumarol, inhibit the metabolism (*p*-hydroxylation) of phenobarbital and potentiate the sedative effect. Phenindione does not interfere.

Antihistamines [633]

Phenobarbital and antihistamines inhibit each other. Enhanced sedation but enzyme induction by both tends to reduce effectiveness over a longer period of time.

Anti-inflammatory drugs [78,421]

Phenobarbital inhibits anti-inflammatory drugs.

Antipyrine [198]

Phenobarbital inhibits antipyrine.

Aspirin [83,275]

Phenobarbital inhibits the analgesic activity of aspirin.

Bishydroxycoumarin [96] (Dicumarol)

See *Anticoagulants, Oral* above.

Carisoprodol [120] (Rela, Soma)

Phenobarbital decreases relaxant effects of carisoprodol due to enhanced metabolism via enzyme induction.

Chloramphenicol [83] (Chloromycetin)

Phenobarbital inhibits chloramphenicol.

Chlordiazepoxide [120] (Librium)

Potentiation of CNS depressant effects. See *CNS Depressants.*

Chlorpromazine [83] (Thorazine)

The hypnotic effect is potentiated by chlorpromazine. Phenobarbital, by enzyme induction inhibits the action of chlorpromazine. See *Antihistamines* above.

Cholestyramine

See *Phenobarbital* under *Cholestyramine.*

Corticosteroids [28,84,257,330,633]

Phenobarbital inhibits corticosteroids like cortisone by increasing their rate of metabolism.

Cortisol [84,330] (Hydroxycortisone)

See *Corticosteroids* above. Phenobarbital, by enzyme induction, increases the urinary excretion of 6-beta-hydroxycortisol, a metabolite of cortisol.

Cortisone [257] (Cortone)

See *Corticosteroids* above.

Coumarin Anticoagulants

See *Anticoagulants, Oral* above.

DDT [1044]

Phenobarbital reduces the storage of DDT in the body by enzyme induction.

Desoxycorticosterone [198]

Phenobarbital inhibits desoxycorticosterone by enzyme induction.

Diphenhydramine (Benadryl)

Diphenhydramine may interact with phenobarbital by mutual enzyme induction to produce (1) decreased antihistamine activity and (2) decreased barbiturate activity. Enhanced sedation through additive effect may occur initially. Monitor the net effect.

Dipyrone (Dimethone)

Phenobarbital decreases the potency of dipyrone (enzyme induction).

Estradiol

See *Estrogens* below.

Estrogens [83,287,330,812] (Estradiol, estrone, etc.)

Phenobarbital induces the metabolism of many steroids including the estrogens, and thus decreases the uterotropic effects of both exogenous and endogenous estrogens.

Estrogen-progestogens [198,287,330,812] (Oral contraceptives)

Phenobarbital may decrease the effectiveness of oral contraceptives. See *Steroids* below.

Griseofulvin [63,66,67,83,490,633,821] (Fulvicin)

Phenobarbital inhibits griseofulvin by enzyme induction and possibly by inhibiting absorption, and may thus lead to inadequate antifungal therapy due to a decrease in griseofulvin blood levels.

PHENOBARBITAL *(continued)*

Hexobarbital (hexobarbitone)[83,330]
(Cyclonal, Evipan, Sombucaps, Sombulex, etc.)
Phenobarbital and hexobarbital may mutually inhibit each other through enzyme induction and reduce the hypnotic action. Tolerance develops. Phenobarbital induces the metabolizing enzymes for hexabarbital so strongly that the activity of the drug may be abolished.

Folic acid antagonists[421]
Phenobarbital potentiates folic acid antagonists.

Hydantoins[63,64,78,83,96,640,647,866,1250,1268-9,1324,1436,1467,1476, 1548,1557-8,1652,1745,1823,1866]
(Dilantin, DPH, Mesantoin, Peganone, etc,)
The interaction between phenytoin (and probably other hydantoins) and phenobarbital (and probably other barbiturates) is very complex. Barbiturates and DPN have an additive CNS depressant effect. DPN potentiates phenobarbital at first possibly by inhibiting microsomal metabolism (it does this with hexobarbital), by competitive inhibition of their metabolizing microsomal enzymes (hydroxylation), and by inhibiting urinary excretion. A marked increase in blood levels of barbiturate is then followed by a decrease as induction of the enzymes occurs. Barbiturates primarily cause inhibition of DPN through enzyme induction but they have a variable effect on hydantoin metabolism because of the degree of induction already present as a result of prior therapy, duration of therapy, individual genetic predisposition that determines both rate of metabolism and maximum degree of induction possible, status of liver function, and other factors. The combined convulsant therapy effectiveness depends on dosage levels, duration of therapy, frequency, timing, and route of administration of both drugs and so many opposing actions that it is highly variable and unpredictable in any given patient. Monitor patients carefully, especially when one of the drugs is added to the regimen or withdrawn.

Hypnotics[78,166]
Phenobarbital inhibits hypnotics after an initial potentiation of CNS depressant effects.

Isoniazid[333]
Isoniazid, enzyme inhibitor, potentiates phenobarbital.

MAO inhibitors[633]
MAO inhibitors potentiate phenobarbital by inhibiting metabolizing enzymes.

Meperidine[83] (Demerol, etc.)
Phenobarbital, by enzyme induction, inhibits meperidine.

Meprobamate[198,421] (Equanil, Miltown)
The net effect of this interaction in a given patient is unpredictable. Potentiation may occur because of additive CNS depression and yet both drugs are enzyme inducers and tend to inhibit each other.

Methylphenidate[156]
Methylphenidate potentiates the anticonvulsant action of barbiturates.

Nitrofurantoin[120] (Furadantin)
Phenobarbital, by enzyme induction, inhibits the action of nitrofurantoin.

Oral contraceptives
See *Estrogen-Progestogens* above.

Phenacetin[83,166] (Actophenetidin)
Phenobarbital, by enzyme induction, inhibits phenacetin and increases the formation of the metabolite 2-hydroxyphenetidin, a methemoglobin producer.

Phenobarbital[695]
Patients develop tolerance to phenobarbital by enzyme induction of its own metabolizing enzymes.

Phenothiazines[633]
(Compazine, Mellaril, Thorazine, etc.)
Phenobarbital and phenothiazines have an additive CNS depressant effect which is unpredictable.

Phenylbutazone[330]
Phenobarbital, through enzyme induction, increases the rate of metabolism of phenylbutazone; its dosage requirements are thus increased.

Phenytoin (Dilantin
See *Hydantoins* above.

Procaine (Novocain)[83,120]
Phenobarbital inhibits the action of procaine. See, however, *Procaine* under *Barbiturates*.

Progesterone[83,330]
Phenobarbital inhibits progesterone. See *Steroids* below.

Puromycin[709]
Puromycin inhibits the induction of microsomal drug metabolizing enzymes by phenobarbital.

Quinidine
See *Anticonvulsants* under *Quinidine*.

Salicylates[83,198,275,421]
Phenobarbital decreases the analgesic effect of salicylates due to enzyme induction.

Sodium bicarbonate[161,325,1092]
Administration of sodium bicarbonate to mice decreases the anesthetic effects of phenobarbital; gastrointestinal absorption may be decreased and urinary excretion increased with increased pH.

Steroids[78]
Phenobarbital, through microsomal enzyme induction, inhibits steroids including *Androgens, Corticosteroids, Estrogens, Progesterone*, etc.

Sulfonamides[83]
Phenobarbital, by enzyme induction, inhibits sulfadimethoxine and probably other sulfonamides.

Sulfonylureas[633]
(Diabinese, Dymelor, Orinase, Tolinase, etc.)
Sulfonylureas may potentiate phenobarbital.

Testosterone[83,198,330,421]
See *Androgens* and *Steroids* above.

Thyroxine[421]
Thyroxine decreases rate of metabolism of phenobarbital.

Tranquilizers, minor[633]
Phenobarbital and the tranquilizers like Librium, Serax, and Valium have an additive effect which is unpredictable.

Urinary acidifiers[579]
Acid urinary pH potentiates phenobarbital. See *Acidifying Agents* above.

Warfarin[83,296,297,375,867] (Coumadin)
See *Anticoagulants, Oral* above.

Zoxazolamine[83,184] (Flexin)
Phenobarbital markedly stimulates the rate of metabolism of zoxazolamine (no longer available in the US).

PHENOBARBITONE (Phenobarbital)
See *Barbiturates* and *Phenobarbital*.

Hexobarbitone[83,330] (Hexobarbital)
Phenobarbital so accelerates the metabolism of subsequent doses of hexobarbital that it abolishes almost completely its pharmacological activity. Mutual inhibition.

PHENOLSULFONPHTHALEIN (Phenol red, PSP)

Probenecid[120]
Probenecid inhibits the urinary excretion of PSP and elevates its plasma levels.

PHENOTHIAZINES
(Chlorcyclizine [Perazil], chlorpromazine [Thorazine], mesoridazine [Serentil], prochlorperazine [Compazine], thioridazine [Mellaril], etc.)

See also *Antihistamines, Antinauseants,* etc.

β-Adrenergic blockers [421]

β-Adrenergic blockers may increase the adrenergic blocking activity of phenothiazines.

Adrenergics [120,421,619]

Some phenothiazines decrease the pressor effect of adrenergics (sympathomimetics), others increase the effect.

Alcohol [121,148,311,633,634,731,937]

Alcohol increases the sedative effects of phenothiazines, phenothiazines potentiate CNS depression by alcohol (coma and death may occur). Alcohol blocks parkinsonism side effects of phenothiazines. Phenothiazines do not inhibit the enzyme (dehydrogenase) responsible for alcohol oxidation but presumably increase CNS sensitivity.

Amphetamines [166,922,1097,1644]

Antipsychotic phenothiazines such as chlorpromazine, used to treat amphetamine overdosage, when given in sufficient dosage antagonize the central action of amphetamine by inhibiting catecholamine uptake in adrenergic nerve endings. If amphetamines are prescribed for treatment of obesity, avoid phenothiazines concurrently. See *CNS Stimulants* below.

Analgesics [166]

Phenothiazines potentiate the CNS depression produced by analgesics.

Anesthetics [120,399,615]

Phenothiazines exert additive CNS depressant effects with anesthetics. See *CNS Depressants.*

Antacids [1407-8,1428]

Antacids taken orally, particularly aluminum hydroxide and magnesium trisilicate, may inhibit gastrointestinal absorption of phenothiazines.

Anticholinergics [120,198,400,488,1741]

Phenothiazines tend to potentiate the side effects (blurred vision, dry mouth, sedation, etc.) produced by anticholinergics. Urinary retention or glaucoma may be induced. Anticholinergics antagonize the parkinsonism effects of some phenothiazines. This latter desirable action may be due to lowered plasma levels of phenothiazine since anticholinergics such as trihexyphenidyl (Artane) slow gastric motility and emptying, depress intestinal motility, allow more metabolism to occur in the gut, and thus decrease blood levels of the phenothiazines. This has been used as an argument against the use of anticholinergics with phenothiazines.

Anticoagulants, oral [330,421,453]

Some phenothiazines (enzyme inducers) may inhibit oral anticoagulants.

Anticholinesterases [488]

Anticholinesterases extend the tranquilizing action of phenothiazines and this interaction is reversed by anticholinergics.

Anticonvulsants [120,330]

Some phenothiazines may lower the convulsive threshold in susceptible individuals; increased dosage of anticonvulsants may be necessary. Drugs like chlorpromazine do not potentiate the anticonvulsant action of barbiturates and certain other anticonvulsants. Do not reduce their dosages when starting therapy with the phenothiazine.

Antidepressants, tricyclic [78,400,1395,1456-7]

Tricyclic antidepressants potentiate the sedative and anticholinergic (atropinelike) effects of phenothiazines and phenothiazines potentiate tricyclic antidepressants. Additive CNS depression, sedation, orthostatic hypotension, urinaria reten-

tion, glaucoma, disorders of oral and nasal areas, etc. may occur unless dosages are adjusted. Apparently these drugs mutually inhibit the metabolism of each other. Combinations of amitriptyline and perphenazine (Triavil and Etrafon) are being marketed for anxiety and depression. Closely supervise patients to avoid the numerous drug interactions reported for both types of drugs. Such combinations may contribute to the development of chronic tardive dyskinesia syndrome.

Antidiabetics, oral [191,421,1928]

Phenothiazines may potentiate the hypoglycemic effects of oral antidiabetics (phenothiazine diabetes). See *Phenothiazines* under *Antidiabetics, Oral.*

Antihistamines [78,198,421]

Additive CNS depression; potentiated sedation. Urinary retention or glaucoma may be induced when both drugs have anticholinergic (atropinelike) effects.

Antihypertensives [78,231,1007]

Phenothiazines may potentiate antihypertensives. Do not use concurrently. Profound hypotension may occur. Since phenothiazines block α-receptors, and not β-receptors, reversal of pressor action may occur when such hypotension is treated with an agent like epinephrine which acts on both α and β receptors.

Antiparkinsonism agents [120,400]

Antiparkinsonism agents such as anticholinergics are frequently given with phenothiazines to control extrapyramidal symptoms. See also *Anticholinergics* above.

Aspirin [166]

This combination has additive CNS depressant effects.

Atropine [78]

Atropine potentiates phenothiazines in psychiatric treatment and counteracts the extrapyramidal symptoms produced by them. See *Anticholinergics* above. Urinary retention or glaucoma may be induced when the phenothiazine also has anticholinergic (atropinelike effects).

Attapulgite [1043]

Antidiarrheal mixtures containing activated attapulgite decrease the effectiveness of some phenothiazines, *e.g.,* promazine, by inhibiting gastrointestinal absorption.

Barbiturates [78,120,565,633,640,1313,1428]

Phenothiazines (antihistamines such as chlorcyclizine, psychochemicals such as chlorpromazine, etc.) potentiate the sedative (CNS depressant) effects but not the anticonvulsant effects of barbiturates; reduce dosage. Barbiturates antagonize the parkinsonism produced by phenothiazines; barbiturates with continued use, in higher dosages may increase the metabolism of phenothiazines through enzyme induction. Barbiturates also increase urinary excretion of the phenothiazines (chlorpromazine) and thus tend to inhibit them. Chlorpromazine is also an enzyme inducer. With low doses of phenobarbital and chlorpormazine, however, tolerance does not appear to develop. The combination in higher doses has been effective in refractory mental patients. But do not use barbiturates and phenothiazines together without close monitoring of the patient because of the potential for CNS depression and alterations in dosage required by mutual inhibition through enzyme induction.

Benzodiazepines [166,330,421]
(Librium, Serax, Valium)

Benzodiazepines increase the sedative effects of phenothiazines, and vice versa. Severe atropinelike reactions may occur.

Chloral Hydrate [166]

Some phenothiazines may potentiate the CNS depressant action of hypnotics.

PHENOTHIAZINES *(continued)*

Chlordiazepoxide (Librium)
See *CNS Depressants* below and *Benzodiazepines* above.

Chlorphentermine[765] (Pre-Sate)
Phenothiazines antagonize the action of the antiobesity agent.

CNS stimulants[166,1097]
Phenothiazines like chlorpromazine antagonize the central nervous system stimulant activity of amphetamines but do not protect against the convulsive action of pentylenetetrazol, picrotoxin and strychnine.

CNS depressants[78]
Phenothiazines exert additive effects and potentiate CNS depressants. See page 467. Enhanced sedation, severe hypotension, urinary retention, seizures, severe atropinelike reactions, etc. may occur depending on the combination.

Diazepam[78,120,166,330] (Valium)
See *CNS Depressants* above. Additive or super-additive effects may occur with diazepam. Also see *Benzodiazepines* above.

Diazepine derivatives (Librium, Serax, Valium)
See *CNS Depressants* and *Benzodiazepines* above.

Diphenhydramine[120] (Benadryl)
Diphenydramine antagonizes the parkinsonism symptoms produced by phenothiazines.

Dipyrone[421] (Dimethone, etc.)
Dipyrone potentiates the hypothermic effect of phenothiazines.

Epinephrine[120,231,619]
Some phenothiazines like chlorpromazine with α-adrenergic blocking activity antagonize peripheral vasoconstriction produced by epinephrine and certain other pressor agents with both α- and β-adrenergic activity, but they do not block the β-activity which then predominates, *e.g.*, causes vasodilation and increased hypotension. Some phenothiazines may thus reverse the pressor effects of epinephrine. Epinephrine may not decrease the hypotension produced by some phenothiazines. Epinephrine should not be used with drugs like chlorpromazine and methotrimeprazine when a vasopressor is required since a paradoxical decrease in blood pressure may result.

Flurothyl[935] (Indoklon)
See under *Flurothyl*.

Furazolidone[202,633] (Furoxone)
Furazolidone, a MAO inhibitor, potentiates phenothiazines through inhibition of metabolizing enzymes.

Glutethimide[120] (Doriden)
Potentiation. See *CNS Depressants* above.

Griseofulvin[822] (Grifulvin, Grisactin)
This combination may possibly precipitate acute porphyria.

Guanethidine[198,421,633] (Ismelin)
Phenothiazines may potentiate the hypotension produced by guanethidine. Others like *Chloropromazine* (see under *Guanethidine*) antagonize the hypotensive agent.

Hallucinogenic agents[120,619] (LSD, mescaline, psilocybin, etc.)
Some phenothiazines reduce the mydriasis and the unusual visual experiences of these agents. The CNS depressant action of the tranquilizer antagonizes the CNS stimulant action of the hallucinogenic agent.

Haloperidol[421] (Haldol)
Potentiation. See *CNS Depressants* above.

Heparin[764]
Large doses of phenothiazines antagonize the anticoagulant action of heparin.

Hydroxyzine[120,1756] (Atarax, Vistaril)
Hydroxyzine may have additive antiemetic, antihistaminic and antiemetic effects with some phenothiazines. It may also potentiate the drowsiness, dry mouth, and other symptoms produced by some phenothiazines. It may inhibit the therapeutic effects of some phenothiazines.

Hypnotics[120]
Potentiation. See *CNS Depressants* above.

Insulin[421]
Phenothiazines potentiate the hypoglycemic effect of insulin. Hypoglycemic episodes may occur.

Levarterenol[421] (Levophed)
Levarterenol antagonizes the hypotensive effect of phenothiazines.

Levodopa[724,922,923,1510,1648,1918-9,2001] (Dopar, Larodopa)
Phenothiazines may defeat the therapeutic effects of levodopa in Parkinson's syndrome by interfering with dopamine synthesis or blocking its receptors. Avoid this combination.

Lithium carbonate[120,1921] (Eskalith, Lithane, Lithonate)
Lithium carbonate and phenothiazines may have additive hyperglycemic effects. Monitor blood glucose.

MAO inhibitors[162,184,311,312,1007]
Additive effects. MAO inhibitors potentiate the hypotensive and other CNS depressant effects of some phenothiazines. In overdosage of MAO inhibitors, a phenothiazine tranquilizer may bring the agitation, anxiety, and manic symptoms under control. MAO inhibitors may also produce severe extrapyramidal reactions and hypertension with some phenothiazines.

Meperidine[78,633,844-846] (Demerol)
Some phenothiazines like chlorpromazine markedly potentiate the sedation and respiratory depression produced by meperidine. Fetal death may occur. Collapse may occur with parenteral administration. Reduce meperidine dosage.

Morphine[120,198,421,633]
Some phenothiazines like chlorpromazine potentiate the miotic and sedative effects of morphine. Mutual potentiation of CNS depressant effects. Reduce the morphine dosage to $\frac{1}{4}$ to $\frac{1}{2}$.

Mephenesin[166]
Phenothiazines potentiate the CNS depressant effects. See *CNS Depressants*.

Methyldopa
See *Phenothiazines* under *Methyldopa*.

Muscle relaxants[120,566,1829]
Phenothiazines such as promazine potentiate muscle relaxants such as succinylcholine, perhaps by inhibiting the metabolizing enzyme, pseudocholinesterase. Prolonged apnea may occur. Anticholinergic muscle relaxants (e.g., benztropine mesylate, which has the anticholinergic properties of atropine and the antihistaminic properties of diphenhydramine) may relieve drug-induced parkinsonism symptoms produced by phenothiazines, but may intensify mental symptoms (possible toxic psychosis). Exercise caution. Monitor patients closely.

Narcotics[120,198,421] (Narcotic analgesics)
Potentiation of sedative effects. See *CNS Depressants* above.

Norepinephrine[421]
The hypotensive effect of phenothiazines is antagonized by norepinephrine.

Nylidrin[489] (Arlidin)
See *Phenothiazine Tranquilizers* under *Nylidrin* and *Nylidrin* under *Tranquilizers*.

Oral contraceptives [92]

Oral contraceptives may potentiate promazine by decreasing the urinary excretion of the ataractic and its metabolites.

Organophosphate insecticides [120] (Parathion, TEPP, etc.)

Some phenothiazines may antagonize the toxic anticholinesterase effects of these insecticides, but others may potentiate the toxicity, *e.g.*, promazine may have caused the death of one patient exposed to parathion and phosdrin, perhaps because of cholinesterase inhibition by the phenothiazine (additive effect).

Orphenadrine [528,1427] (Norflex)

Hypoglycemia has been reported after use of orphenadrine with chlorpromazine.

Pargyline (Eutonyl)

See *MAO inhibitors* above.

Pentylenetetrazol [120,166]

Phenothiazines should not be used as agents in overdosage treatment since they fail to protect against the convulsant action of pentylenetetrazol.

Phenmetrazine [765] (Preludin)

Some phenothiazines like chlorpromazine inhibit the anorexic activity of phenmetrazine.

Phenobarbital [633]

Phenobarbital and phenothiazines like Compazine, Mellaril, and Thorazine have additive sedative and other CNS depressant effects. Because of enzyme inhibition the net effect is unpredictable.

Phenothiazines [951]

Some phenothiazines potentiate the antipsychotic effect of other phenothiazines in psychiatric treatment.

Phenylephrine [120] (Neo-Synephrine, etc.)

Phenylephrine antagonizes the hypotensive effect of phenothiazines.

Phenytoin [884] (Dilantin)

Phenothiazines have rarely been reported to potentiate phenytoin (enzyme inhibition?).

Phosphorous insecticides

See *Organophosphate Insecticides* above.

Picrotoxin

Same as for *Pentylenetetrazol* above.

Piminodine [120,619] (Alvodine)

Phenothiazines potentiate the CNS depressant actions of the synthetic narcotic analgesic, piminodine. See *CNS Depressants* and *Narcotic Analgesics*.

Piperazine [619,660,766] (Antepar, Pipizan Citrate, etc.)

Piperazine combined with a phenothiazine may precipitate violent, possibly fatal convulsions but this has been questioned. Propylalkylpiperazines (Compazine, Permitil, Proketazine, Stelazine, Tindal, Trilafon, etc.) which are derivatives of phenothiazine may increase the extrapyramidal effects of other drugs with the same actions (additive effects). See *Piperazine* under *Chlorpromazine*.

Procarbazine [120] (Matulane)

Phenothiazines should be used cautiously with this MAO inhibiting antineoplastic agent because of the possibility of synergistic CNS depression.

Progesterone [620]

Oral contraceptives and other drugs containing progesterone potentiate phenothiazines by inhibiting metabolizing enzymes, possibly by impeding their entry into the hepatic cells.

Propranolol [1182-3]

Additive hypotensive and EKG effects. See *Phenothiazines* under propranolol.

Quinidine

See *Phenothiazines* under *Quinidine*.

Rauwolfia alkaloids [198,421,633] (Reserpine, etc.)

Phenothiazines potentiate the CNS depressant effects of the Rauwolfia alkaloids.

Reserpine [198,421,633]

See *CNS Depressants* above.

Scopolamine [120] (Hyoscine)

This anticholinergic solanaceous alkaloid, like atropine, may have additive effects (blurred vision, constipation, dry mouth, etc.) with phenothiazines.

Sedatives [120,166,198,421]

In combination, the sedative effects of both the phenothiazines and the sedatives (barbiturates, etc.) are potentiated initially. See *CNS Depressants*. Possibly mutual inhibition with prolonged use because of enzyme induction.

Strychnine

Same as for *Pentylenetetrazol* above.

Succinylcholine [566,1829] (Anectine, Quelicin)

See *Muscle Relaxants* above.

Sympathomimetics [166,231,619]

The hypotensive effects of phenothiazines like chlorpromazine are counteracted by the pressor effects of sympathomimetics like levarterenol. Some phenothiazines potentiate the pressor effect of epinephrine, others reverse the effect. See *Epinephrine* above.

Thiazide diuretics [78,421,633] (Diuril, Hydrodiuril, etc.)

Thiazide diuretics given to the patient receiving a phenothiazine have been known to cause severe hypotension and shock. When attempts to reverse this with metaraminol were made, the phenothiazine blocked the metaraminol and caused increased hypotension.

Thiopental [116]

Potentiation of thiopental anesthesia has occurred from preoperative administration of phenothiazines.

Tranquilizers, minor [120,421,633]

Additive CNS depression and tranquilizing effects. See *CNS Depressants*.

Tricyclic antidepressants [421]

See *Antidepressants, Tricyclic* above.

Trihexyphenidyl [1741] (Artane)

See *Anticholinergics* above.

PHENOTHIAZINE-ORPHENADRINE COMBINATIONS

Antidiabetics, oral [120]

Phenothiazine-orphenadrine combinations potentiate oral antidiabetics.

PHENOXENE

See *Antiparkinsonism Drugs* (chlorphenoxamine).

PHENOXYBENZAMINE HCl (Dibenzyline)

Epinephrine [120]

Epinephrine is contraindicated as a treatment for shock induced by the phenoxybenzamine α-adrenergic blockade of the sympathetic nervous system and of the circulating epinephrine. Because epinephrine stimulates both α and β adrenergic receptors, the net effect is vasodilation and a further drop in blood pressure (epinephrine reversal).

PHENOXYBENZAMINE HCl (Dibenzyline)
(continued)

Levarterenol [117,619] **(Levophed, Norepinephrine)**
Phenoxybenzamine blocks hyperthermia production by levarterenol.

Propranolol [120] **(Inderal)**
α-Adrenergic blocking agents like phenoxybenzamine should be used with β-adrenergic blocking agents like propranolol during surgical treatment of pheochromocytoma to diminish the risk of excessive hypertension (they do not prevent excessive cardiac stimulation with catecholamines).

Reserpine [1]
Phenoxybenzamine blocks hypothermia production by reserpine.

PHENPROCOUMON (Liquamar)
See *Anticoagulants, Oral.*

PHENTERMINE (Adipex-P)
An anorexiant with pharmacologic properties like *Amphetamines.*

PHENTOLAMINE (Regitine)

Anesthetics [529]
Phentolamine antagonizes sensitization of the myocardium to anesthetics by adrenergics.

Antidiabetics [1992]
In acute juvenile diabetics, the highly overactive adrenergic system that inhibits insulin secretion in the pancreatic β-cells can be counteracted by an α-adrenergic blocker such as phentolamine which increases β-cell insulin secretion and inhibits adrenergic increase of lipolysis in fat cells and of glycogenolysis in muscle and liver tissues. A precipitous drop in blood sugar levels may be achieved even before insulin is administered.

Epinephrine and norepinephrine [117,619]
Phentolamine, an α-adrenergic blocking agent, antagonizes responses to circulating epinephrine and norepinephrine and antagonizes adrenergic sensitization of the myocardium to anesthetics. Epinephrine is contraindicated as a treatment for shock induced by phentolamine. See *Phenoxybenzamine* above for the reason.

Levarterenol [117,619] **(Levophed, Norepinephrine)**
Phentolamine reduces the hyperthermia produced by levarterenol. Levarterenol and not epinephrine should be used as the antidote for shock induced by overdosage of or hypersensitivity to phentolamine.

MAO inhibitors [120,166]
Hypertensive crises caused by MAO inhibitors may be counteracted by phentolamine.

Propranolol [120] **(Inderal)**
See *Propranolol* under *Phenoxybenzamine.* Phentolamine is also an α-adrenergic blocker.

Reserpine
Phentolamine blocks the hypothermia produced by reserpine.

PHENYLALANINE

Chloramphenicol [230,920]
Phenylalanine ameliorates the bone marrow depression caused by chloramphenicol.

PHENYLBUTAZONE (Butazolidin)
See also *Oxyphenbutazone.*

Acetohexamide [121,141,330,680,768,1315,1382,1479,1689,1807,1845]
See *Antidiabetics, Oral* below.

Acidifying agents [28,325,870]
Acidifying agents potentiate phenylbutazone because of decreased ionization, increased tubular reabsorption, and decreased urinary excretion.

Alkalinizing agents [28,325,870]
Alkalinizing agents antagonize phenylbutazone because of increased ionization, decreased tubular reabsorption, and increased urinary excretion.

Aminopyrine [16,63,96,133,555,694,701,704] **(Pyramidon)**
Phenylbutazone inhibits aminopyrine by enzyme induction, and possibly vice versa.

Androgens [257,330,421,448,470,633,852,1029,1502]
(See Androgens for names)
Phenylbutazone inhibits testosterone by enzyme induction. Phenylbutazone tends to be potentiated by methandrostenolone and certain other androgens. But the half lives of phenylbutazone and of its active metabolite oxyphenbutazone are individual pharmacogenetic characteristics. Methandrostenolone increases the plasma levels of the metabolite when it is given as a drug. When phenylbutazone is given as the drug, however, both it and its metabolite compete for protein binding sites and because the parent drug has a stronger affinity for albumin binding sites, it displaces the metabolite. Levels of the latter are also increased through enzyme inhibition and change in volume of distribution. Initially phenylbutazone levels are elevated. However, prolonged therapy with phenylbutazone may produce no change in its plasma levels perhaps because the drug displaces its active metabolite. But prolonged therapy with these inflammatory agents is hazardous and should be avoided. Also, in alcoholics an increase in plasma levels of both phenylbutazone and its metabolite tend to occur rather than the expected decrease (prolonged half-lives), probably because of decreased metabolism due to liver dysfunction.

Androstenedione
See *Androgens* above.

Antacids [198,633]
Antacids, if sodium free, may decrease the ulcerogenic and other gastrointestinal disturbances but they inhibit phenylbutazone by decreasing gastrointestinal absorption and perhaps increasing urinary excretion.

Anticoagulants, oral
See *Anti-inflammatory Agents* under *Anticoagulants, Oral.* See also *Oxyphenbutazone,* the metabolite of phenylbutazone.

Antidepressants, tricyclic [85,359,863]
Tricyclics like imipramine and desipramine may inhibit the intestinal absorption of phenylbutazone and thus inhibit its action.

Antidiabetics, oral [192,197,359,647,679,680,1689]
Enhanced hypoglycemic effect; displacement from protein binding sites may be involved in these interactions. In some Africans phenylbutazone has the opposite effect and tends to decrease hypoglycemia (racial, genetic differences as with G6PD). Phenylbutazone potentiates the hypoglycemic effect of acetohexamide, by inhibiting the renal excretion of its active metabolite (hydroxyhexamide). Increased plasma insulin and decreased blood glucose as a result of higher circulating levels of acetohexamide have resulted in deep hypoglycemic coma. Monitor patients receiving this combination closely. Since phenylbutazone should be given only for short periods, dosage adjustment of acetohexamide will probably be required not only when phenylbutazone is started but also a short time later when it is withdrawn.

Antihistamines [64,485]
Decreased effectiveness. Both are enzyme inducers. See *Antihistamines.*

Antipyrine [951]
Phenylbutazone inhibits antipyrine by enzyme induction.

Aspirin[28,359,614]
Aspirin inhibits the anti-inflammatory effect of phenylbutazone. See *Salicylates* below. Phenylbutazone inhibits the uricosuria induced by aspirin.

Barbiturates[330,555]
Barbiturates increase the rate at which phenylbutazone is metabolized; their rate of metabolism is also increased by phenylbutazone. Both drugs inhibit each other.

Bishydroxycoumarin (Dicumarol)
See *Anticoagulants, Oral* above.

Chlorcyclizine[64,485]
Chlorcyclizine decreases the effectiveness of phenylbutazone by enzyme induction.

Chlorinated insecticides (Chlordane, etc.)
See *Halogenated Insecticides* below.

Chloroquine[120]
Phenylbutazone and other agents known to cause drug sensitization and dermatitis should not be given concurrently with chloroquine or hydroxychloroquine.

Cholestyramine[769] **(Cuemid, Questran)**
Cholestyramine inhibits the absorption of phenlybutazone. Ingest latter drug at least 1 hour before or 4–6 hours after cholestyramine.

Colors[1977]
Phenylbutazone, in the dark is stable in solution alone or with various lakes (amaranth, erythosine sodium, FD & C yellow No. 6, and tartrazine) but in the light, erythrosine sodium solution rapidly decomposes the anti-inflammatory drug. It is stable in solution in the light with the other colors. This illustrates the fact that drugs can be affected by so-called inert ingredients of pharmaceutical dosage forms.

Corticosteroids[198,359,421]
The anti-inflammatory action of phenlybutazone may be due in part to its ability to displace corticosteroids from their plasma protein binding sites and allow their more ready dispersal into tissues. The metabolism of steroids like cortisol (urinary excretion of the metabolite 6-beta-hydroxycortisol) may be stimulated by inducing agents such as phenylbutazone and thus their activity diminished. The net effect of these two mechanisms determines dosage (immediate effect is potentiation).

Cortisol (Hydroxycortisone)
See *Corticosteroids* above.

Cortisone (Cortone)
See *Corticosteroids* above.

Coumarin anticoagulants
See *Anticoagulants, Coumarin* above.

Desipramine
See *Antidepressants, Tricyclic* above.

Desoxycorticosterone[198,421]
Phenylbutazone inhibits desoxycorticosterone by enzyme induction.

Digitalis glycosides (Digitoxin, digoxin)
Phenlybutazone markedly decreases the steady state level of digitoxin. See *Phenylbutazone* under *Digitalis*.

Diphenhydramine[64,485] **(Benadryl)**
Diphenhydramine and phenylbutazone mutually decrease their effectiveness by enzyme induction.

Dipyrone[694,695] **(Dimethone, etc.)**
Phenylbutazone inhibits dipyrone by increasing its rate of metabolism.

Estradiol[633]
Phenylbutazone inhibits estradiol by enzyme induction.

Estrogen-Progestogens[633] **(Oral contraceptives)**
Phenylbutazone may decrease the effectiveness of oral contraceptives by increasing their rate of metabolism.

Glucocorticoids[198,359,421]
Phenylbutazone potentiates glucocorticoids by displacing them from their protein binding sites. See *Corticosteroids* above.

Griseofulvin[64,65,490]
Phenylbutazone decreases the effectiveness of griseofulvin by enzyme induction.

Halogenated insecticides[83,485]
(Chlordane, DDT, etc.)
Insecticidal sprays containing chlordane stimulate the metabolism of phenylbutazone in test animals up to 5 months after withdrawal of the chlordane.

Hexobarbital[555]
See *Barbiturates* above.

Hydrocortisone
See *Corticosteroids* above.

Imipramine (Tofranil)
See *Antidepressants, Tricyclic* above.

Indomethacin[120] **(Indocin)**
Potentiation of the ulcerogenic effect.

Insulin[120]
Phenylbutazone potentiates insulin by displacement from protein binding sites.

Levodopa
See *Phenylbutazone* under *Levodopa*.

Methandrostenolone
See *Androgens* above.

Oral contraceptives[198,633]
Phenylbutazone inhibits oral contraceptives.

Other chemotherapeutic agents[120]
Phenylbutazone and oxyphenbutazone are contraindicated in patients receiving other potent chemotherapeutic agents because of the possibility of increased toxic reactions.

Oxyphenbutazone[120] **(Tandearil)**
Cross-sensitivity between phenylbutazone and oxyphenbutazone may be experienced by patients.

Penicillins[198,359]
Phenylbutazone potentiates penicillin by displacement from protein binding sites and slowing renal excretion.

Pentobarbital (Nembutal)
See *Barbiturates* above.

Phenobarbital[330]
See *Barbiturates* above.

Phenylbutazone[64,555] **(Butazolidin)**
Tolerance to phenylbutazone develops by induction of its own metabolizing enzymes.

Phenytoin[192,294,359,652,676] **(Dilantin)**
Phenylbutazone potentiates phenytoin by displacing it from protein binding sites, thus causing increased serum levels of the drug; this may lead to an increased incidence of side effects and toxicity.

Progesterone
Phenylbutazone inhibits progesterone. See *Corticosteroids* above.

Propranolol[586] **(Inderal)**
β-Adrenergic blocking agents like propranolol interfere with the anti-inflammatory effects of various drugs.

PHENYLBUTAZONE (Butazolidin) *(continued)*

Salicylates [28,359,433,614,1288]
The therapeutic effect of phenylbutazone is antagonized by salicylates. Aspirin, ingested prior to phenylbutazone, increases the affinity of the latter for human serum albumin. [1288] Also, both of these agents have an additive ulcerogenic effect on gastric mucosa and should not be used simultaneously. Phenylbutazone suppresses salicylate-induced uricosuria.

Steroids [198,359,421]
Phenylbutazone antagonizes steroids by enzyme induction. See *Corticosteroids* above.

Sulfamethoxypyridazine (Kynex)
See *Sulfonamides* below.

Sulfonamides [21,28,198,359,433,661]
Phenylbutazone potentiates sulfonamides. Enhances antibacterial activity and increases toxicity by displacing them from plasma protein binding sites.

Sulfonylureas [120,198,633]
(Diabinese, Dymelor, Orinase, etc.)
Phenylbutazone potentiates these hypoglycemics by displacement from protein binding sites.

Testosterone [198,421]
Phenylbutazone inhibits testosterone by enzyme induction. See *Androgens* above.

Tolbutamide (Orinase)
See *Antidiabetics, Oral* above.

Warfarin Sodium (Coumadin, Panwarfin)
See *Anticoagulants, Oral* above.

Zoxazolamine [555] (Flexin)
Phenylbutazone inhibits zoxazolamine (no longer marketed in the US) by enzyme induction.

PHENYLEPHRINE (Neo-Synephrine)

Antidepressants, Tricyclic
See *Phenylephrine* under *Antidepressants, Tricyclic.*

Debrisoquin
Hypertensive crisis possible. See *Phenylephrine* under *Debrisoquin.*

Epinephrine [120]
Phenylephrine should not be administered with epinephrine or other vasopressor sympathomimetic amines. Serious cardiac arrhythmias or death from hypertensive crisis can result.

Furazolidone [136] (Furoxone)
Contraindicated. See *MAO Inhibitors* below.

Guanethidine [553] (Ismelin)
Phenylephrine may decrease the hypotensive effect of guanethidine and may induce cardiac arrhythmias because guanethidine augments the response to vasopressors. Guanethidine may delay the reversal of mydriasis.

Haloperidol [120] (Haldol)
Phenylephrine antagonizes the hypotensive effects of haloperidol.

Halothane [820] (Fluothane)
The vasopressor with the anesthetic may induce cardiac arrhythmias.

Isocarboxazid (Marplan)
See *MAO Inhibitors* below.

Levodopa [717] (Dopar, Larodopa)
Levodopa (or its metabolites), by producing a competitive α-adrenergic receptor blockade, reduces the mydriatic action of phenylephrine.

MAO Inhibitors [25,37,45,99,120,136,162,217,305,312,356,532,533,546]
(Eutonyl, Furoxone, Marplan, Nardil, Niamid, Parnate, etc.)
MAO inhibitors and sympathomimetics may cause an acute hypertensive crisis with possible intracranial hemorrhage, hyperthermia, convulsions, coma and in some cases death. MAO is irreversibly inhibited and metabolism of monoamines is blocked; this causes their accumulation. This enzyme inhibition also prolongs and potentiates the action of ephedrine, tyramine, and many other sympathomimetic amines which release stored norepinephrine. This accumulation, release, and central additive stimulation cause the hypertensive crisis.

Nialamide (Niamid)
See *MAO Inhibitors* above.

Oxytocics [173,609,611]
Because of the danger of serious pressor potentiation, oxytocics are contraindicated in obstetric patients if vasopressor drugs are used to correct hypotension or if they are added to local anesthetic solutions for their hemostatic effect.

Pargyline (Eutonyl)
See *MAO Inhibitors* above.

Phenothiazines [120]
Phenylephrine antagonizes the hypotensive effect of phenothiazines.

Phenelzine (Nardil)
See *MAO Inhibitors* above.

Procaine [120] (Novocain)
Phenylephrine given IM or IV counteracts the vasodepressant effects of procaine.

Tranylcypromine (Parnate)
See *MAO Inhibitors* above.

PHENYLETHYLBIGUANIDE
See *Phenformin.*

α-PHENYLETHYLHYDRAZINE
See *MAO Inhibitors* (mebanazine).

β-PHENYLETHYLHYDRAZINE
See *MAO Inhibitors* (phenelzine).

PHENYLPROPANOLAMINE (Propadrine)
See *Sympathomimetics.*
This ingredient of cold remedies has entered into particularly severe interactions with MAO inhibitors, antihypertensives such as methyldopa, β-blockers, etc.

Anticoagulants, oral [466,951]
Phenylpropanolamine may oppose the hypoprothrombinemic action of oral anticoagulants.

Antidiabetics, oral [549]
Phenylpropanolamine may oppose the hypoglycemic action of oral antidiabetics.

Antihypertensives
See *Ornade* and *Phenylpropanolamine* under *Antihypertensives.*

Bethanidine (Estabal)
See *Phenylpropanolamine* under *Bethanidine.*

Cheese [2033]
Tyramine in ripe cheeses may synergistically interact with phenylpropanolamine to produce a hypertensive crisis.

Insulin [549]
Phenylpropanolamine may antagonize insulin.

MAO inhibitors [99,115,305,431]
MAO inhibitors potentiate phenylpropanolamine and cause a rapid and potentially dangerous rise of blood pressure. See the mechanism under *Phenylephrine* above.

Mebanazine [431]
See *MAO Inhibitors* above.

Methyldopa [1934]

Sympathomimetics like phenylpropanolamine antagonize the antihypertensive effect of adrenergic blocking agents such as bethanidine, guanethidine and methyldopa. The blocking agents potentiate the pressor effect of sympathomimetics by blocking their uptake to inactive receptor sites. When Triogesic (acetaminophen plus phenylpropanolamine), for example, was prescribed to alleviate cold symptoms in a patient on combined methyldopa and oxprenolol antihypertensive therapy, a particularly severe hypertensive reaction occurred. The β-adrenergic blocker, by allowing an unopposed α-constriction response to adrenergic stimulation, intensified the hypertension.

Nialamide [115] **(Niamid)**
See *MAO Inhibitors* above.

Phenelzine [431] **(Nardil)**
See *MAO Inhibitors* above.

PHENYTOIN
(Dilantin, diphenylhydantoin, DPH, Epanutin, etc.)

Alcohol [120,674,1360,1872]

Alcohol may inhibit the anticonvulsant action of the hydantoin in alcoholics probably because of enzyme induction. Excessive use of alcohol in patients on the anticonvulsant could cause epileptic seizures, but abrupt discontinuance of alcohol by an alcoholic may also result in seizures. Monitor alcoholics closely.

p-Aminosalicylic acid [272,294,884,919] **(PAS)**

The metabolism (*p*-hydroxylation) of phenytoin is inhibited by PAS (potentiation and increased toxicity by enzyme inhibition). PAS may also elevate blood levels of isoniazid which is usually given with PAS in tuberculosis. The isoniazid also inhibits metabolism of the anticonvulsant and thus there may be a double inhibitory and potentiating effect. Monitor patients closely for toxic reactions.

dl-**Amphetamine** [359]

dl-Amphetamine delays intestinal absorption of phenytoin, followed by synergistic anticonvulsant activity.

Analeptics [120,619]

Analeptics may increase the rate of fatality in phenytoin overdosage.

Anticoagulants, oral [78,113,189,294,379,421,633,673,884]
(Coumarin anticoagulants)

Phenytoin increases the anticoagulant effect by displacing coumarin derivatives from plasma binding sites. Coumarin anticoagulants potentiate Dilantin by inhibiting its enzymatic degradation and may cause drug intoxication due to the increased serum concentration of the hydantoin.

Antidepressants tricyclic [359,421,1056,1317,1792]

High doses of a tricyclic antidepressant with phenytoin may precipitate grand mal seizures, even in nonepileptics, due to enhanced toxicity of the tricyclics. Dosage of the anticonvulsant may have to be changed due to decreased convulsive threshold and increased toxicity because of displacement of the tricyclics from secondary binding sites. The highly lipophilic basic antidepressants are highly bound (91-99%). Some patients (those with alcoholism, barbiturate withdrawal, brain damage, family history of epilepsy, and previous ECT) are more susceptible. Monitor patients on concomitant therapy closely.

Antidiabetics, oral [1957]

See *Phenytoin* under *Antidiabetics, Oral*. Under some conditions of potentiated toxicity phenytoin has produced intense hyperglycemia, hypotension and death.

Antihistamines [64]

Antihistamines may decrease effectiveness of the anticonvulsant by enzyme induction.

Antihypertensives [120,619]

Phenytoin may potentiate the hypotensive action of diuretics and other antihypertensives.

Antituberculosis drugs [272,273,789,916,919]

See *p-Aminosalicylic Acid* above and *Isoniazid* and *Cycloserine* below. These may induce ataxia, nsystagmus, blood dyscrasias, and the other toxic effects possible with the anticonvulsant.

Aspirin [113,294]

Large doses of aspirin may enhance the anticonvulsant effect and toxicity of phenytoin. See *Salicylates* below.

Barbiturates
See *Hydantoins* under *Phenobarbital*.

Benzodiazepines [884,1529,1559,1861,1873]
(Dalmane, Librium, Serax, Tranxene, Valium)

Benzodiazepines potentiate phenytoin, similar to *Phenothiazines* below, by inhibiting the metabolizing enzymes. Monitor for phenytoin toxicity.

Bishydroxycoumarin [916] **(Dicumarol)**

Bishydroxycoumarin inhibits the microsomal enzymatic parahydroxylation of phenytoin and thus potentiates the activity and toxicity of the anticonvulsant.

Carbamazepine (Tegretol) [1289,1474]

Carbamazepine decreases the action of phenytoin by inducing the microsomal enzymes of the liver. Phenytoin is also an enzyme inducer and has the same type of antagonistic effect on carbamazepine. Adjust doses if necessary.

Chloramphenicol (Cloromycetin) [676,1225,1716]

Cloromycetin, by enzyme inhibition, potentiates the anticonvulsant action and toxic effects of phenytoin. Its half-life may be doubled. Use another antibiotic if possible or adjust dosage of phenytoin downward.

Chlorcyclizine [199] **(Perazil)**

See *Hydantoins* under *Phenobarbital*. Chlorcyclizine, an antihistamine (see above), may decrease the effectiveness of phenytoin by enzyme induction.

Chlordiazepoxide
See *Benzodiazepines* above.

Chloromycetin [676,1225,1716]
See *Chloramphenicol* above.

Chlorpromazine [884] **(Thorazine)**
See *Phenothiazines* below.

CNS depressants [120,619]

Phenytoin may have additive effects with other CNS depressants.

Contraceptives, oral [78,222,884,1400,1490,1559,1607]

Phenytoin, by means of enzyme induction, may increase the rate of metabolism of oral contraceptives and decrease their efficacy. The steroids in OCs may displace phenytoin from protein binding sites and increase its action and toxicity. The estrogens in OCs may also potentiate phenytoin through inhibition of metabolizing enzymes. Fluid accumulation from OC effects may possibly increase seizures. Although proof for all of these interactions is lacking, monitor patients on this combination carefully.

Corticosteroids [78,84,330,359,450-1,878,1232,1477,1518,1733,1897]
(Cortisol, cortisone, Cortone, dexamethasone, hydrocortisone, Hydrocortone, etc.)

Phenytoin stimulates the metabolism of corticosteroids by enzyme induction and thus reduces the activity of the steroids, *i.e.*, inhibits their capacity to suppress endogenous hydrocortisone. The induction occurs in adults but not in neonates who have been exposed to phenytoin throughout gestation.

PHENYTOIN *(continued)*

Cortisol [222,230] (Hydrocortisone, Hydrocortone)
See *Corticosteroids* above. Phenytoin increases urinary excretion of 6-beta-hydroxycortisol, a metabolite of cortisol.

Cycloserine [919]
The antituberculosis drug, cycloserine, potentiates the activity and toxicity of phenytoin.

Dalmane
See *Benzodiazepines* above.

DDT [1044]
Phenytoin tends to reduce the storage of DDT in the body (enzyme induction).

Dexamethasone (Decadron)
See *Corticosteroids* above.

Diazepam (Valium)
See *Benzodiazepines* above.

Dicumarol
See *Bishydroxycoumarin* above.

Digitalis glycosides [786,1818-9]
Phenytoin may enhance digitalis effects (bradycardia), and then on continued use, by enzyme induction, may markedly decrease the plasma concentration of the glycoside. In one report a patient had ataxia, nystagmus, and rigidity suggesting permanent brain damage, and was unable to walk, after receiving the combination. Monitor patients closely for underdigitalization and increased toxicity.

Digitoxin [786]
See *Digitalis Glycosides* above.

Diphenhydramine [199] (Benadryl)
Diphenhydramine may decrease the effectiveness of phenytoin by enzyme induction and vice versa.

Disulfiram [113,192,258,294,342,343,359,916] (Antabuse)
Disulfiram increases phenytoin toxicity by inhibition of the microsomal enzymes that metabolize the anticonvulsant. The serum concentration of phenytoin is elevated rapidly and urinary excretion of its metabolite is inhibited. Levels may not return to normal for about 3 weeks after withdrawal of disulfiram. Monitor patients closely for toxic effects.

Diuretics
See *Antihypertensives* above.

Estrogens [884]
Estrogens potentiate phenytoin (enzyme inhibition).

Excipient [113,294,1119]
When the excipient of Dilantin was changed from calcium sulfate to lactose in 1967, an "epidemic" of Dilantin overdosage occurred because of enhanced absorption (blood levels 2 to 5 times higher). This type of problem is encountered periodically and must be taken into consideration by prescribing physicians.

Fluroxene [1732,1835] (Fluoromar)
Phenytoin used concomitantly with the general anesthetic may produce necrosis of the liver. The anticonvulsant, by enzyme induction, stimulates metabolism of the anesthetic and forms a hepatotoxic metabolite.

Folic acid and its antagonists [198,444,633,880,1091,1229]
Phenytoin depresses folic acid levels in the body. This is at least partially responsible for its anticonvulsant action. It therefore potentiates folic acid antagonists (methotrexate, etc.) which may become very hazardous. Folic acid may reverse the antiepileptic effects of phenytoin and increase fit-frequency on a short-term basis due to increased parahydroxylation of the anticonvulsant with consequent loss of active agent and decreased efficacy. On a long-term basis, folic acid therapy may decrease phenytoin activity by slowly building up levels in the CNS. See *Folic Acid* under *Anticonvulsants.*

Furosemide (Lasix) [2063]
Epileptics on chronic phenytoin therapy have diminished response to furosemide because the anticonvulsant causes malabsorption of the diuretic.

Glutethimide [198] (Doriden)
Glutethimide antagonizes phenytoin by enzyme induction.

Griseofulvin [201,619]
Phenytoin may potentiate griseofulvin by displacing the antifungal from protein binding sites.

Halothane [1530] (Fluothane)
Concomitant use of phenytoin and halothane produces enhanced hepatotoxicity with impaired phenytoin metabolism. Elevated plasma levels of the anticonvulsant produce toxic effects. Monitor patients given hepatotoxic drugs with phenytoin closely.

Hydrocortisone [222,330,633]
Phenytoin inhibits hydrocortisone. See *Corticosteroids* above.

Insulin
See *Diphenylhydantoin* under *Insulin.*

Isoniazid [28,202,272,294,333,359,789,884,916,919,1398,1968,1981] (INH)
Isoniazid potentiates phenytoin by enzyme inhibition and decreases urinary excretion of its metabolite. Increased phenytoin toxicity and increased likelihood of thromboembolism result. The toxic effects are more severe in slow acetylators of isoniazid (ataxia, slurred speech, clouded consciousness, bizarre limb movements, and inability to stand, with hyperglycemia, hypertension, and hepatotoxicity). Death has occurred.

Librium
See *Benzodiazepines* above.

Lidocaine
See *Phenytoin* under *Lidocaine.*

Methotrexate
Phenytoin enhances methotrexate toxicity. See *Folic Acid* above.

Methylphenidate HCl [28,156,192,359,1555,1641] (Ritalin)
Methylphenidate, through enzyme inhibition, may produce potentially toxic blood levels of phenytoin and induce distressing reactions like ataxia, blood dyscrasias, diplopia, fatal toxic hepatitis, and nystagmus. This interaction probably is most significant with high dosage of the anticonvulsant.

Metyrapone (Metopirone) [1615,1898]
Phenytoin, by inducing microsomal enzymes that metabolize metyrapone and by inhibiting its gastrointestinal absorption, considerably reduces blood levels of the agent and interferes with its diagnostic value in determining pituitary response to reduced levels of plasma cortisol and its use in treating hypercortisolism from adrenal neoplasms.

Oxyphenbutazone (Tandearil)
Same as for *Phenylbutazone* below.

Phenobarbital [28,192]
See *Hydantoins* under *Phenobarbital.*

Phenothiazines [884,1559] (Compazine, Thorazine)
In rare instances, chlorpromazine and prochlorperazine have lowered the tolerance to phenytoin by impairing its metabolism (enzyme inhibition). Monitor patients closely for toxicity.

Phenylbutazone [192,294,359,569,652,676,1214] (Butazolidin)
Phenylbutazone and its metabolite oxyphenbutazone may enhance the effects of phenytoin by inhibition of *p*-hydroxylation and by displacement from protein binding sites (phenytoin intoxication). Carefully monitor patients receiving these drugs concomitantly.

Phenyramidol [198,413,421,633,916] **(Analexin)**
Phenyramidol inhibits the metabolism and increases the anticonvulsant and toxic effects of phenytoin; high plasma concentrations of phenytoin have been associated with nystagmus, ataxia, and brain damage. Phenyramidol has been withdrawn from the U.S. market.

Phetharbital
Phetharbital (enzyme inducer) decreases the effect of phenytoin. See *Hydantoins* under *Phenobarbital.*

Primidone (Mysoline) [1423,1529,1873,1906]
Primidone has drug interactions similar to those of *Barbiturates* since one of its major metabolites is phenobarbital. Phenytoin, through enzyme induction that hastens this conversion, and possibly through competitive inhibition of barbiturate metabolism, considerably elevates phenobarbital blood levels. The synergistic anticonvulsant effect may be of value but monitor patients closely for overdosage. See *Hydantoins* under *Phenobarbital.*

Prochlorperazine [486] **(Compazine)**
Prochlorperazine potentiates phenytoin. See *Phenothiazines* above.

Propoxyphene
See *Phenytoin* under *Propoxyphene.*

Propranolol [619,1152] **(Inderal)**
Phenytoin potentiates the action of propranolol. See *Phenytoin* under *Propranolol.*

Quinidine [619,1998]
Phenytoin may potentiate quinidine antiarrhythmic effects. But also see *Anticonvulsants* under *Quinidine.*

Ritalin
See *Methylphenidate* above.

Salicylates [652,1856]
Large doses of aspirin potentiate phenytoin by displacing it from protein binding sites and elevating plasma levels of unbound anticonvulsant. Monitor patients or this combination closely for toxicity.

Sedatives and hypnotics [198,421]
(Chloral hydrate, Doriden, phenobarbital, etc.)
Many sedatives and hypnotics inhibit phenytoin by enzyme induction.

Serax
See *Benzodiazepines* above.

SKF 525-A [391] **(Proadifen)**
SKF 525-A, by inhibiting microsomal enzymes, potentiates phenytoin.

Sulfafurazole [652] **(Gantrisin, sulfisoxazole)**
Potentiation of phenytoin. Same as for *Phenylbutazone and Salicylates* above. See *Sulfonamides* below.

Sulfaphenazole [202,294] **(Orisul)**
Sulfaphenazole enhances the effect of phenytoin by inhibiting its metabolism (phenytoin intoxication).

Sulthiame [190,192,294,1529,1651,1735] **(Ospolot, Trolone)**
Sulthiame may potentiate phenytoin considerably by increasing its blood levels through enzyme inhibition. Monitor patients closely for toxicity and reduce dosage as necessary.

Sulfonamides [202,294,652]
Some sulfonamides may produce potentially toxic blood levels of phenytoin and induce distressing reactions like ataxia, blood dycrasias, diplopia, fatal toxic hepatitis, and nystagmus. Sulfisoxazole (Gantrisin) displaces phenytoin from plasma protein binding sites and at least two sulfonamides—sulfamethizole (Thiosulfil) and sulfaphenazole (Sulfabid)—inhibit the enzymes that metabolize phenytoin. These interactions may double the half-life of the anticonvulsant. Monitor closely for excessive anticonvulsant effects and toxicity.

Tetracyclines [1660,1700]
Phenytoin, through enzyme induction, stimulates the metabolism of at least one tetracycline—doxycycline (Vibramycin)—and possibly others. Increase the tetracycline dosage as necessary.

Thyroid hormones [1434]
Phenytoin, by displacing thyroxine from plasma protein binding sites, elevates blood levels of unbound hormone and potentiates its therapeutic and toxic effects. Atrial flutter and supraventricular tachycardia, especially in athyrotic patients, may be encountered.

Tranxene
See *Benzodiazepines* above.

Triamcinolone [330,450,451] **(Aristocort)**
Phenytoin by microsomal enzyme induction and possibly a more complicated type of interaction, causes reduction in the activity of triamcinolone.

Tubocurarine [790]
Phenytoin potentiates tubocurarine.

Vaccines
See *Immunosuppressants* under *Vaccines.*

Valium
See *Benzodiazepines* above.

Vitamin D
See *Vitamin D* under *Anticonvulsants.*

pHOS-pHAID
See *Urinary Acidifiers.*

PHOSPHOLINE IODIDE (Echothiophate)
See *Anticholinesterases (Miotic Eyedrops).*

PHOSPHORUS INSECTICIDES
See *Insecticides, Organophosphorus.*

PHYSOSTIGMINE

Aminoglycosides
See *Antibiotics,* below.

Antibiotics [951]
Physostigmine antagonizes the curarelike effect of aminoglycoside antibiotics.

Antidepressants, tricyclic [166]
Physostigmine, which crosses the blood brain barrier, effectively reverses the anticholinergic CNS effects of tricyclic antidepressant poisoning.

Atropine [168]
Poisoning by atropine can be reversed by physostigmine (initial adult dose 0.5-2 mg.).

Orphenadrine
See *Physostigmine* under *Orphenadrine.*

Procaine [168]
Physostigmine and procaine have antagonistic actions at neuromuscular junctions.

PHYTIC ACID
See *Cereals* under *Iron Salts.*

PHYTONADIONE (Konakion)
See *Vitamin K* also.

Anticoagulants, oral [48,120,180]
Phytonadione restores prothrombin to the blood and thus tends to antagonize coumarin anticoagulants.

PICROTOXIN

Phenothiazines [120]
Picrotoxin should not be used as stimulating agent in treating overdosage of phenothiazines since it may cause convulsions. See also remarks under *Phenothiazines.*

Thioxanthenes
Same as for *Phenothiazines* above.

PICKLED HERRING
See *Tyramine-rich Foods*.

PIL-DIGIS
See *Digitalis*.

PILOCARPINE
See *Parasympathomimetics*.

Alcohol [951]
Pilocarpine prolongs the action of ethyl alcohol in the brain.

Anticholinergics [1221]
Same as for *Chlorpromazine* below.

Antidepressants, tricyclic [1221]
Same as for *Chlorpromazine* below.

Atropine [168]
Atropine displaces pilocarpine from receptors at parasympathetic nerve endings and thus acts as a competitive antagonist.

Chlorpromazine [1221]
The drug-induced oral and pharyngeal dryness produced by chlorpromazine and similar phenothiazines, as well as anticholinergics, tricyclic antidepressants, and certain other drugs with this side effect, is counteracted with pilocarpine nitrate syrup.

Echothiophate [120] (Phospholine Iodide)
Prior pilocarpine administration may have a protective effect with respect to the action of echothiophate anticholinesterase therapy on the lens.

PIPANOL
See *Antiparkinsonism Drugs* and *Trihexyphenidyl*.

PIPERAZINE (Antepar, etc.)

Phenothiazines [660,766] (Thorazine, etc.)
See *Piperazine* under *Chlorpromazine*.

PIPERIDOLATE HCl (Dactil)
See *Anticholinergics*.
This gastrointestinal spasmolytic resembles *Atropine*.

PIPERONYL BUTOXIDE

Various drugs [82]
(Antipyrine, barbiturates, griseofulvin, etc.)
This insecticide potentiator potentiates many drugs by enzyme inhibition.

PIPRADROL (Meratran)

Guanethidine [417] (Ismelin)
Pipradol, a CNS stimulant, may antagonize the hypotensive effect of guanethidine.

PITRESSIN
See *Vasopressors (Vasopressin)*.

PLACIDYL
See *Hypnotics* (ethchlorvynol).

PLAQUENIL
See *Antimalarials* (hydroxychloroquine).

PLASTICS

Medications [26,303]
Plastic containers may interact with drugs.

POLARAMINE
See *Antihistamines* (dexchlorpheniramine).

POLOXALKOL (Magcyl, Polykol)

Mineral oil
Poloxalkol, a surface-active agent may increase the absorption of mineral oil and should not be given with it for prolonged periods.

POLYCILLIN
See *Penicillins*.

POLYMECHANISTIC DRUGS
Some drug interactions appear to be paradoxical. See page 378.

POLYMIXIN B

Heparin
Incompatible in parenteral mixtures. See Chapter 7.

POLYMYXIN B SULFATE (Aerosporin)
See also *Neuromuscular Blocking Antibiotics* under *Antibiotics*

Aminoglycosides [633]
(Kanamycin, Neomycin, Streptomycin, etc.)
See *Neomycin* below.

Anticholinesterases [178]
Anticholinesterases potentiate the skeletal muscle relaxing and paralyzing effect of polymyxin B.

Colistin [120] (Coly-Mycin)
Same as for *Neomycin* below. Complete cross-resistance between colistin and polymyxin B exists.

Curariform agents [184,330,421]
(Curare, Gallamine, Tubocurarine)
Polymyxin potentiates these agents (additive muscle relaxant effect).

Dihydrostreptomycin [120]
Same as for *Neomycin* below.

Kanamycin [120] (Kantrex)
Same as for *Neomycin* below.

Muscle relaxants [120,184,330,421,547,881,1546,1706,1711]
See *Curariform Agents* above and *Succinylcholine* below. Polymyxin B which itself produces neuromuscular blockade may potentiate the blocking action of skeletal muscle relaxants and produce apnea, respiratory depression, muscle weakness, coma, and possibly death. See *Neuromuscular Blocking Antibiotics* under *Antibiotics; Aminoglycoside Antibiotics* under *Muscle Relaxants, Peripherally Acting;* and *Colistin* under the same heading. Low concentrations of calcium ions in the serum and loss of potassium from cells appear to be important factors in enhancing the neuromuscular blockade. Intravenous calcium may be useful if blockade occurs.

Neomycin [120,633]
Both neomycin and polymyxin B can interfere with nerve transmission at the neuromuscular junction; they should be used together only with great caution since increased interference of transmission may result in muscle weakness and apnea. The nephrotoxic effects may be aggravated. See also *Aminoglycoside Antibiotics*.

Neostigmine [506,656]
Neostigmine does not antagonize the muscle relaxant effect of polymyxin. It may potentiate the effect.

Organophosphates [178]
(cholinesterase inhibitors)
These inhibitors potentiate neuromuscular blocking effects of polymyxin.

Skeletal muscle relaxants
See *Muscle Relaxants* above.

Succinylcholine [120,421]
(Anectine, Quelicin, Sucostrin, etc.)
Polymyxin potentiates the muscle relaxant effect of succinylcholine. Contraindicated because prolonged respiratory paralysis is produced. See *Muscle Relaxants* above.

Streptomycin
Same as for *Neomycin* above.

***d*-Tubocurarine**
Same as for *Succinylcholine* above.

POLYSORBATE 80

Acetaminophen [359]
The gastrointestinal absorption of acetaminophen and some other drugs is accelerated in the presence of polysorbate 80, a surface active agent.

Phenacetin [359]
Same as for *Acetaminophen* above.

POLYVINYLPYROLIDONE

Tetracyclines [421]
Polyvinylpyrolidone prolongs the blood levels of tetracyclines.

PONSTEL
See *Mefenamic Acid.*

PONTOCAINE
See *Anesthetics, Local* (tetracaine).

PORFIROMYCIN
See *Antibiotics* (methylmitomycin C).

POTABA
See *p-Aminobenzoic Acid* (potassium salt).

POTASSIUM SALTS

Acetohexamide
See *Potassium Salts* under *Acetohexamide.*

Antidiabetics, oral
See *Potassium* under *Antidiabetics, Oral.*

Digitalis [120]
Hyperkalemia decreases the toxicity and effectiveness of digitalis. Hypokalemia produces the opposite effects.

Hydrochlorothiazide (Hydrodiuril)
See *Thiazide Diuretics* below.

Lithium carbonate
See *Potassium Iodide* under *Lithium Carbonate.*

Spironolactone [120] **(Aldactone)**
Spironolactone conserves potassium and increases the hyperkalemia produced by potassium salts.

Thiazide diuretics [120]
Thiazide diuretics tend to deplete potassium and cause hypokalemia. Enteric-coated dosage forms of potassium salts should be avoided, if possible, since ulceration of the small intestine may occur.

Triamterene
See *Potassium Salts* under *Triamterene.*

POTASSIUM TRIPLEX
See *Potassium Salts* (acetate, bicarbonate, and citrate).

PRALIDOXIME (Protopam)
See *Anticholinesterases.*

Anticholinesterases [168,619,1585]
(Organophosphate insecticides, echothiophate, etc.)
Pralidoxime antagonizes anticholinesterases by reactivating inhibited cholinesterase (if given early in poisoning cases) and elevating erythrocyte cholinesterase. Useful in poisoning with organophosphate insecticides, and other anticholinesterases, especially if given with atropine in carefully regulated dosage. Pralidoxime frees the enzyme from the anticholinesterase and tends to protect it from inhibition.

Contraindicated drugs [120]
(Aminophylline, morphine, succinylcholine, theophylline, or phenothiazine or reserpine types of tranquilizers)
These drugs are contraindicated when pralidoxime is used in poisoning with anticholinesterases. The reactivator of inhibited cholinesterase produces a depolarizing effect at the neuromuscular junction and it has an anticholinergic action.

Sevin [619]
Pralidoxime is contraindicated in poisoning with the carbamate insecticide, Sevin, since it increases the toxicity of the insecticide.

PREDNISOLONE
(Delta-Cortef, Hydeltra, Meticortelone, etc.)

Cyclophosphamide [359,1100] **(Cytoxan)**
Cyclophosphamide metabolism in the liver to an intermediate with potent alkylating activity is inhibited by prednisolone (in the rat). If a similar interaction happens in man, serious toxicity could develop if this or related steroids are discontinued while the dose of cyclophosphamide remains unchanged.

Salicylates [618]
Mutual enhancement of the anti-inflammatory effects of both substances. A combination of this kind is generally suited for long-term therapy. When prednisone and possibly other corticosteroids are withdrawn an excessive rise in blood salicylate levels may occur.

PREDNISONE
(Deltasone, Deltra, Meticorten, etc.)
See also *Prednisolone* and *Corticosteroids.*

Azathioprine [619,755] **(Imuran)**
The combination of the corticosteroid and azathioprine in prolonged therapy may cause negative nitrogen balance and muscle wasting; also possible development of reticulum cell sarcoma in homotransplantation.

Mercaptopurine [443] **(Purinethol)**
Hyperuricemia may occur with this combination.

PRELUDIN
See *Sympathomimetics* (phenmetrazine).

PRENYLAMINE (Segontin)

Epinephrine [170]
Prenylamine augments the response to epinephrine.

Isoproterenol [170] **(Isuprel, etc.)**
Prenylamine, a vasodilator, antagonizes isoproterenol and may reverse the pressor effect of the amine.

Levarterenol [170] **(Levophed)**
Prenylamine augments the response to levarterenol.

Reserpine [170]
Prenylamine possesses many of the effects of reserpine and may potentiate the hypotensive effects. See *Prenylamine* under *Reserpine.*

PRE-SATE
See *Sympathomimetics* (chlorphentermine).

PRESSONEX DISPOSABLE SYRINGES (Aramine, Pressorol)

See *Vasopressors* (metaraminol).

PRESSOR AGENTS

See *Sympathomimetics, Tyramine-rich Foods, Vasopressors,* etc.

PRILOCAINE (Citanest)

See *Anesthetics, Local.*

PRIMAQUINE

Quinacrine [120,177,202] (Atabrine, mepacrine)

Primaquine should not be given simultaneously with or to patients who have received quinacrine recently. Quinacrine increases the plasma concentration of primaquine from 5- to 10-fold, and may lead to toxic side reactions. This may occur even when primaquine is given as long as 3 months after the last dose of quinacrine.

PRIMIDONE (Mysoline)

Anticholinergics [120]

Primidone may potentiate the central depressant actions of anticholinergics (additive effect).

Anticoagulants, oral

See *Primidone* under *Anticoagulants, Oral.*

Anticonvulsants [120]

Primidone is often given with other anticonvulsants such as phenytoin, mephenytoin and mephobarbital for the synergistic effects. The transition from an anticonvulsant to primidone should not be completed in less than 2 weeks.

Barbiturates [120,165]

Since primidone is a barbiturate analog and its metabolites are phenobarbital and phenylethylmalonamide, patients receiving the drug should be monitored for possible barbiturate interactions.

Folic acid antagonists [421]

Folic acid may reverse the therapeutic anticonvulsant effect of primidone. Primidone may potentiate folic acid antagonists because it reduces plasma folate levels.

MAO Inhibitors

Since primidone is metabolized to barbiturate see *Barbiturates* above.

Methylphenidate [156,359] (Ritalin)

Methylphenidate potentiates the anticonvulsant action of primidone.

Phenytoin

See *Primidone* under *Phenytoin.*

PRINCIPEN

See *Penicillins.*

PROADIFEN

See *SKF 525-A.*

PRO-BANTHINE

See *Propantheline* under *Acetaninophen.*

PROBENECID (Benemid)

See *Uricosuric Agents.*

Acetohexamide [120] (Dymelor)

Probenecid may interfere with the excretion of the active metabolite hydroxyhexamide; as a result, increased sulfonylurea levels induce hypoglycemia.

Alkalinizers, urinary [325,870]

Urates tend to crystallize out of an acid urine; alkalinization decreases the possibility of formation of uric acid stones with probenecid, particularly with liberal fluid intake, and prevents acute attacks of gout in early stages of therapy.

Allopurinol [120,421]

Combined use of both uricosuric agents increases uricosuria (additive effect).

p-Aminobenzoic acid (PABA) [120]

Probenecid increases the plasma levels of PABA by decreasing its urinary excretion.

p-Aminohippuric acid (PAH) [43,120]

Probenecid increases the plasma levels of PAH by decreasing its urinary excretion.

p-Aminosalicylic acid (PAS) [120,925]

Probenecid decreases urinary excretion of PAS and increases the plasma levels of the antituberculosis agent up to 50% (potentiation).

Amisometradine (Rolicton) [950]

Amisometradine activity (diuresis) is diminished by probenecid through interference with the carrier transport mechanism which facilitates passage of amisometradine into cells.

Analgesics [198]

Analgesics (salicylates) antagonize probenecid and therefore tend to elevate serum uric acid through decreased uricosuric activity.

Antibiotics and other anti-infectives [120,1128]

Probenecid does not influence the plasma levels of chloramphenicol, chlortetracycline, neomycin, oxytetracycline, or streptomycin. It inhibits tubular reabsorption of erythromycin, and therefore decreases plasma levels and inhibits its action by increasing urinary excretion. On the other hand, probenecid strongly potentiates cephalosporins and penicillins (increases peak serum levels up to 300%) by inhibiting their urinary excretion (blocks renal tubular secretion) and promoting higher and more persistent plasma concentrations. See *Penicillins* below.

Anticoagulants, oral [147,930]

Probenecid may potentiate anticoagulants by promoting their accumulation.

Antidiabetics, oral [28,59,421]

Enhanced hypoglycemic response has been reported with probenecid; however, probenecid has little effect on the metabolism of tolbutamide. It may potentiate by inhibiting excretion. Also see *Acetohexamide* above.

Anti-infectives [120]

Probenecid prolongs the duration of action of some anti-infectives. See *Antibiotics and Other Anti-infectives* above.

Aspirin

See *Salicylates* below.

Cephalosporins (Loridine, Keflin, etc.)

See *Probenecid* under *Cephalosporins.*

Chlorothiazide

See *Thiazide Diuretics* below.

Cloxacillin

See *Penicillins* below.

Colchicine [120]

Colchicine is useful for preventing acute attacks of gout that may temporarily occur during early stages of uricosuric therapy with probenecid.

Dapsone [925] (Avlosulfon)

Probenecid potentiates dapsone by blocking its renal tubular excretion.

Erythromycin

See *Antibiotics and other Anti-infectives* above.

Ethacrynic acid [421] (Edecrin)

Ethacrynic acid antagonizes the uricosuric effect of probenecid. Probenecid tends to antagonize the diuretic action of ethacrynic acid.

Indomethacin [421,1048] **(Indocin)**
Probenecid potentiates indomethacin by interfering with its renal excretion. The uricosuric action of probenecid is not blocked.

Iodopyracet [120] **(Diodrast)**
Probenecid inhibits urinary excretion of iodopyracet and elevates its plasma level.

17-Ketosteroids [120]
Probenecid elevates the plasma levels of 17-ketosteroids by inhibiting their urinary excretion.

Methicillin
See *Antibiotics and other Anti-infectives* above.

Nitrofurantoin [120] **(Furadantin)**
Probenecid potentiates nitrofurantoin.

Oxacillin
See *Antibiotics and other Anti-infectives* above.

Pantothenic acid [120]
Probenecid inhibits the renal tubular transport of pantothenic acid and prolongs its plasma levels.

Penicillins [43,160,269,619]
Probenecid inhibits urinary excretion of penicillins, elevates penicillinemia 2- to 4-fold, and thus strongly potentiates the antibiotics (blocks their tubular excretion and decreases the volume of distribution of their derivatives).

Phenolsulfonphthalein [120] **(Phenol red, PSP)**
Probenecid inhibits urinary excretion of PSP and elevates its plasma levels. (Renal clearance is reduced to about ¼ the normal rate.)

Probenecid [64]
Probenecid stimulates its own metabolism on prolonged administration. Tolerance develops by this mechanism.

Pyrazinamide [1311]
Probenecid reduces the hyperuricemic action of pyrazinamide.

Rifampin
See *Probenecid* under *Rifampin.*

Salicylates [28,48,198,330,359,421,650]
Salicylates inhibit the uricosuric activity of probenecid by competition with tubular sites of secretion. Contraindicated during therapy with probenecid because of urate retention.

Sodium acetrizoate [120] **(Pyelokon-R, Salpix, etc.)**
Probenecid decreases renal excretion of sodium acetrizoate.

Sodium iodomethamate [120] **(Pyelecton, Uropac)**
Probenecid decreases the urinary excretion of the X-ray contrast medium.

Sulfinpyrazone [28,931] **(Anturane)**
Probenecid prolongs the uricosuric action of sulfinpyrazone and may increase its toxicity by inhibiting its renal excretion.

Sulfobromophthalein [120] **(Bromsulphalein, BSP)**
Probenecid inhibits both hepatic and urinary excretion of BSP and elevates its plasma level.

Sulfonamides [120,359,421,925]
Probenecid may potentiate the effects of sulfonamides, but does not appreciably increase unbound sulfonamide levels. Because it raises the plasma levels of conjugated sulfonamides, the levels should be determined periodically on long term combination therapy.

Sulfonylureas (Diabinese, Dymelor, Orinase, etc.)
See *Antidiabetics, Oral* above.

Tetracyclines
See *Antibiotics and other Anti-infectives* above.

Thiazide diuretics [120,421]
See *Thiazide Diuretics* for names.
Probenecid, a uricosuric, potentiates the diuretic effects of thiazides by decreasing their urinary excretion. Thiazide diuretics inhibit the action of probenecid; they tend to precipitate gout in patients with hyperuricemia.

Xanthines [421]
Xanthines (caffeine, theobromine, etc.) antagonize the uricosuric effect of probenecid.

PROCAINAMIDE (Pronestyl)

Acetazolamide [583,1153,1154,1332] **(Diamox)**
Acetazolamide, by alkalinizing the urine, tends to decrease procainamide excretion and thus may potentiate its action.

Acetylcholine [120,204]
Procainamide, with anticholinergic properties, antagonizes the depolarizing effects of acetylcholine and should be used with caution in patients with muscular weakness.

Alkalinizing agents [583,1153-4,1332]
Alkalinizing agents (molar sodium lactate or sodium bicarbonate, alone and in combination with sympathomimetic drugs) are useful in reversing the toxic effects of procainamide. However, alkalinizing the urine before procainamide injection tends to inhibit excretion and potentiates the action of the drug.

Antibiotics, neuromuscular blocking [120,619,790,1155]
Procainamide may potentiate the neuromuscular blocking activity of bacitracin, colistimethate, dihydrostreptomycin, gentamicin, gramicidin, kanamycin, neomycin, polymyxin B, streptomycin, and viomycin. The resulting respiratory depression can be hazardous. Caution must be exercised, to avoid apnea, muscle weakness, etc.

Anticholinergics [120,170,619]
Procainamide, which also has anticholinergic properties, enhances the anticholinergic effects (additive). Extreme caution must be exercised with such a combination.

Anticholinesterases [421]
Procainamide antagonizes the effect of anticholinesterases in myasthenia gravis. Paralysis returns.

Antihypertensives [120,619,1176,1177]
Procainamide may potentiate the hypotensive effects of thiazide diuretics and other antihypertensive agents. Adjustment of dosage may be necessary.

Bacitracin
See *Antibiotics* above.

Cholinergics [120,619]
See *Procainamide* under *Cholinergics.*

Digitalis [583,619]
Procainamide may have additive effects with the cardiotonic digitalis glycosides. May be useful in treating tachyarrhythmias of digitalis intoxication but must be used with caution in order to avoid ventricular fibrillation or excessive depression of cardiac function.

Dihydrostreptomycin
See *Antibiotics* above.

Gentamicin
See *Antibiotics* above.

Gramacidin
See *Antibiotics* above.

Kanamycin
See *Antibiotics* above.

Lidocaine [721] **(Lignocaine, Xylocaine, etc.)**
These two antiarrhythmic drugs have a synergistic effect on the CNS and may produce restless, noisy behavior with visual hallucinations.

PROCAINAMIDE (Pronestyl) *(continued)*

Magnesium salts[120,619]
Same caution as that given for *Antibiotics, Neuromuscular Blocking* above.

Muscle relaxants[120,564,619,790]
Same caution as that given for *Antibiotics, Neuromuscular Blocking* above. Procainamide potentiates the neuromuscular blocking action of skeletal muscle relaxants such as succinylcholine.

Neomycin
See *Antibiotics* above.

Organophosphate insecticides[120,421]
The anticholinesterases such as organophosphate insecticides antagonize the anticholinergic effects of procainamide and vice versa.

Polymyxin B
See *Antibiotics* above.

Pressor agents[120]
Levarterenol or phenylephrine may be used IV to counteract the hypotension produced by procainamide when given IP.

Procaine and aminobenzoic acid esters[120,170]
Procaine and aminobenzoic acid esters potentiate procainamide. Cross-sensitivity may occur.

Propranolol (Inderal)
See *Quinidine* below.

Quinidine[170,619]
Procainamide may have additive cardiac effects in depressing myocardial excitability, conduction in the atrium, ventricle, etc. Procainamide and quinidine both have some anticholinergic properties which may be additive. Lower the dosage of the individual drugs.

Sodium bicarbonate
See under *Alkalinizing Agents* above.

Sodium lactate
See under *Alkalinizing Agents* above.

Streptomycin
See *Antibiotics* above.

Sulfobromophthalein[120] **(Bromsulphalein, BSP)**
Procainamide increases BSP retention.

Thiazide diuretics[619]
Potentiated hypotensive effect. See *Antihypertensive* above.

Tubocurarine[790]
See *Muscle Relaxants* above.

Viomycin
See *Antibiotics* above.

PROCAINE (Novocain)
See *Anesthetics, Local.*

Acidifying agents[325,870]
Acidifying agents antagonize procaine because of increased urinary excretion.

Alkalinizing agents[78,870]
Alkalinizing agents potentiate procaine because of decreased urinary excretion.

Anticholineterases
See *Procaine* under *Anticholinesterases.*

Barbiturates[120]
Barbiturates (slow IV infusion, short-acting) protect against the toxicity of procaine. Use only if convulsions occur.

Conjugates[167]
Procaine forms highly insoluble conjugates with a number of drugs including heparin and penicillin, and thereby considerably prolongs their action.

Curare[168]
The neuromuscular blocking effects of procaine and curare are additive.

Echothiophate iodide (Phospholine iodide)
See *Procaine* under *Echothiophate Iodide.*

Ephedrine sulfate
Same as for *Phenylephrine* below.

Epinephrine[120] **(Adrenalin)**
Contraindicated in circulatory collapse. Ventricular fibrillation may occur in the presence of anoxia.

MAO inhibitors[120]
The effects of procaine may be enhanced with MAO inhibitors.

Muscle relaxants, depolarizing[421,435,640]
(Decamethonium, succinylcholine)
Intravenous injections of procaine may potentiate the muscle relaxant effect of succinylcholine. See below.

Pentylenetetrazol (Metrazol)[168]
Local anesthetics with their anticonvulsant properties alleviate convulsion caused by pentylenetetrazol.

Phenobarbital[83,120]
Phenobarbital, by enzyme induction, inhibits procaine. See also *Procaine* under *Barbiturates.*

Phenylephrine[120] **(Neo-Synephrine)**
Phenylephrine given IM or IV counteracts the vasodepressor effects of procaine.

Physostigmine[168]
Procaine and physostigmine actions at the neuromuscular junction are antagonistic.

Procainamide[120,170]
Procaine potentiates procainamide. Cross sensitivity may occur.

Succinylcholine[421,435,640]
When procaine is administered before or after succinylcholine, increased duration of apnea may be induced. This may be caused by competition for binding sites on plasma proteins and on plasma cholinesterase with subsequent increased inhibition of the cholinesterase.

Sulfonamides[167,178]
Procaine, a PABA derivative, antagonizes the antibacterial activity of sulfonamides. Contraindicated.

PROCARBAZINE (Matulane)
See also *MAO Inhibitors* and *Antineoplastics*

Alcohol[120,181,619]
Alcohol should not be used with procarbazine since there may be a disulfiramlike reaction as well as a potentially lethal CNS depression. See *CNS Depressants* below.

Antidepressants, Tricyclic[330,619]
Because procarbazine possesses MAO inhibiting properties, tricyclic antidepressants such as amitriplyline and imipramine should not be given concomitantly. Hyperpyretic crises and convulsive seizures can be fatal.

Antihistamines
See *CNS Depressants* below.

Antihypertensives[120]
Potentiated CNS depression may occur.

Barbiturates
See *CNS Depressants* below.

Bone marrow depressants[120]
(Antineoplastics, etc.)
One month should elapse after discontinuing medication with a chemotherapeutic agent known to have marrow-depres-

sant activity before beginning with procarbazine. The bone marrow depression may be additive.

CNS depressants [120,181,619]
Concomitant use of CNS depressants such as alcohol, antihistamines, barbiturates, hypnotics, hypotensives, meperidine, phenothiazines, sedatives, and tranquilizers with procarbazine, a MAO inhibitor, are often contraindicated because of the possibility of synergistic potentiation of CNS depression. Convulsions, hallucinations, blood pressure changes, apnea, etc. can be very severe. MAO inhibition with CNS depressants is potentially lethal.

Hypotensive agents
See *CNS Depressants* above.

Narcotics
See *CNS Depressants* above.

Phenothiazines
See *CNS Depressants* above.

Sympathomimetics [619]
(Pressor agents, tyramine-rich foods, etc.)
Because procarbazine possesses MAO inhibiting activity, sympathomimetics should not be given concomitantly. A hypertensive crisis may occur. See *MAO Inhibitors.*

Tyramine-containing foods, such as ripe cheese, bananas, etc.
See *Sympathomimetics* above and *Tyramine-rich Foods.*

PROCHLORPERAZINE (Compazine)
See *Phenothiazines.*

PROGESTERONE

Antihistamines [330]
Antihistamines inhibit progesterone.

Chlorcyclizine [330]
Chlorcyclizine may increase hydroxylation of the hormone and decrease its activity because of enzyme induction.

Phenobarbital [330]
Phenobarbital inhibits progesterone by means of enzyme induction.

Phenothiazines [620] (oral contraceptives, etc.)
Progesterone potentiates phenothiazines by enzyme inhibition.

Phenylbutazone [951]
Phenylbutazone inhibits progesterone (enzyme induction).

PROGESTOGENS

Sympathomimetics [538,620]
Progestational agents may inhibit catecholamines by increasing their metabolism.

PROGYNON
See *Estrogens* (Estradiol).

PROKLAR
See *Methenamine* (methenamine mandelate) and *Sulfonamides* (sulfacetamide).

PROLIXIN
See *Phenothiazines* (Fluphenazine).

PROLUTON
See *Progesterone.*

PROMAZINE HCL (Sparine)
See *Phenothiazines.*

PROMETHAZINE (Phenergan)
See *Antihistamines, CNS Depressants,* and *Phenothiazines.*

Streptomycin [360] and other neuromuscular blocking antibiotics.
Streptomycin, neomycin, or kanamycin in combination with promethazine may produce apnea and muscle weakness because of the enhanced neuromuscular blockade of antibiotics. See *Antibiotics* under *Neomycin* and *Neuromuscular Blocking Antibiotics* under *Antibiotics.*

Sulfonamides [421]
Promethazine potentiates the antibacterial action of sulfonamides.

PRONESTYL
See *Procainamide* and *Antiarrhythmics.*

PROPADRINE
See *Sympathomimetics* (phenylpropanolamine).

PROPANIDID

Atropine [527]
Marked peripheral vasodilation and severe hypotension may occur with a combination of intravenous atropine followed by propanidid.

PROPANTHELINE (Pro-Banthine)

Acetaminophen
See *Propantheline* under *Acetaminophen.*

Digitalis glycosides
See *Propantheline* under *Digitalis Glycosides.*

PROPIOMAZINE (Largon)
See *Phenothiazines.*

PROPITOCAINE (Citanest)
See *Anesthetics, Local* (prilocaine).

PROPOXYPHENE (Darvon)

Alcohol [28]
Alcohol potentiates propoxyphene. See *CNS Depressants.*

Amphetamines [120,421]
See *Analeptics* below.

Analeptics [120,421,968]
(Sodium benzoate and caffeine, amphetamine, etc.)
These analeptics should not be used to treat propoxyphene overdosage since fatal convulsions may be produced (CNS overstimulation).

Aspirin [120]
This combination may produce better analgesia than either drug alone.

Caffeine [120,421]
See *Analeptics* above.

Carbamazepine [2059] (Tegretol)
Propoxyphene strongly inhibits the metabolism of carbamazepine (increased plasma levels and decreased plasma clearance). Intoxication (ataxia, dizziness, headache, nausea, tiredness) may ensue.

Levallorphan [120] (Lorfan)
Same as for *Nalorphine* below.

Nalorphine [120,166] (Nalline)
Nalorphine antagonizes the toxicity of propoxyphene; an antidote of choice for lethal doses of propoxyphene.

Naloxone [1989] (Narcan)
Naloxone, a narcotic antagonist, reverses the toxic effects of propoxyphene overdosage. An effective antidote.

Orphenadrine [120,714] (Disipal, Norflex, Norgesic)
Contraindicated. See *Propoxyphene* under *Orphenadrine.*

Phenytoin [1559]
Propoxyphene is a strong inhibitor of phenytoin metabolism (tests in rats).

PROPRANOLOL (Inderal)

The interactions with propranolol may differ between oral and IV dosage. With oral propranolol an active metabolite (4-hydroxypropranolol) with a shorter half-life than the parent drug is formed whereas this metabolite is not formed with IV administration. The effect is greater orally than IV,[1292] with short term dosage, but on prolonged administration the disparity disappears as the effects are then those of the parent drug.

Acetohexamide (Dymelor)
See *Antidiabetics* below.

α-Adrenergic blockers[120] (Dibenzyline, Regitine)
These agents should be used with propranolol before and during surgical treatment of pheochromocytoma to diminish the risk of excessive hypertension.

Aminophylline[1156,1833]
Aminophylline, by inhibiting phosphodiesterase (inhibiting inactivation of cyclic AMP), simulates beta adrenergic activity and is therefore antagonistic to propranolol, a beta blocker. Propranolol attenuates the effects of aminophylline, *e.g.,* depression of growth hormone levels in the plasma and increase in levels of free fatty acids and insulin.

Aminopyrine
See *Anti-inflammatory Agents* below.

Anesthetics, general[120,698]
Synergistic CNS depression. Enhanced activity and toxicity of propranolol.

Antidepressants[120]
Propranolol is contraindicated for use with tricyclic antidepressant drugs with adrenergic properties and during 2 weeks following the withdrawal of these drugs.

Antidiabetics[1,42,263,681,1157,1158,1182,1283,1374,1645,2003]
Propranolol may produce prolonged hypoglycemia with undesirable effects in diabetics. It inhibits insulin release in response to glucose infusion. Use of propranolol and other β-adrenergic blockers is contraindicated in patients receiving insulin or oral antidiabetics. It dampens rebound of plasma glucose levels in hypogylcemia and may prevent the premonitory signs and symptoms of hypoglycemia from appearing. Propranolol may induce hypertensive crisis and decreased peripheral blood flow in hypertensive, insulin-dependent diabetics due to insulin-induced hypogylcemia plus endogenous catecholamine release. See also *Propranolol* under *Insulin.*

Antihistamines[421]
β-Adrenergic blocking agents like propranolol antagonize antihistamines.

Antihypertensives[120,1175]
Propranolol potentiates many antihypertensive agents, including isosorbide dinitrate, guanethidine, methyldopa, thiazides, and related diuretics (decreased heart rate and output and blood pressure). In one report propranolol increased the blood pressure in a hypertensive patient on methyldopa, following a cerebrovascular accident (stress situation). Under such a situation, when the beta-adrenergic stimulation of alpha-methyl-norepinephrine (accumulated in the storage sites of adrenergic neurons after administration of methyldopa) is blocked by propranolol, alpha-adrenergic stimulation is unopposed and pressor effects are increased. Also under stress situations other endogenous catecholamines are mobilized. The hypertensive reaction created by the propranolol/methyldopa interaction may be treated with phentolamine (Regitine) with care because this drug has caused cerebrovascular spasm and occlusion with shock following injection.

Anti-inflammatory agents[586]
β-Adrenergic blocking agents like propranolol inhibit or even abolish the anti-inflammatory effect of typical anti-inflammatory agents like aminopyrine, hydrocortisone, phenylbutazone, and salicylates.

Atropine[120,1160]
Atropine (and other anticholinergics) in acute myocardial infarction may prevent the unmasking of parasympathetic activity (bradycardia and decreased cardiac output by the beta adrenergic blocking action of propranolol.

Barbiturates[28,698]
Propranolol has potentiated the depressant effect of hexobarbital. See *Myocardial Depressants* below.

Catecholamines[42,165,263]
Propranolol inhibits the glycogenolytic action of catecholamines.

Chloroform[4c]
See *Myocardial Depressants* beolow.

Chlorpheniramine
Theoretically, this antihistamine could inhibit the β-adrenergic blockade produced by propranolol and enhance its quinidinelike effects.

Chlorpropamide (Diabinese)
See *Antidiabetics* above.

Cocaine
See *Propranolol* under *Cocaine.*

Digitalis[120,619,1162-4]
Bradycardia. Propranolol may act synergistically with cardiotonic glycosides (digoxin, digitoxin) to cause cardiac arrest in patients with pre-existing partial heart block due to digitalis. Also, digitalis which tends to augment contractility, is antagonistic to propranolol, a beta blocker, which reduces contractility. However, judicious use of digoxin with propranolol in angina pectoris reduces enlarged left heart dimensions and thus reduces myocardial oxygen demand even further and reduces frequency of the angina, whereas digoxin alone can aggravate the angina in patients with normal left-ventricular function and heart size.

Epinephrine[168,1157,1165,1169,1170]
Propranol potentiates the pressor effect of epinephrine. Administer epinephrine with caution to patients on propranolol. Blockage of the beta adrenergic epinephrine stimulation with propranolol may cause profound reflex bradycardia and atrioventricular block. See also *Isoproterenol* below. Epinephrine (adrenaline) release, caused by stresses such as anginal attacks, emotion, and hypoglycemia, produces vasodilation by activation of β_2-adrenergic receptors (net effect since epinephrine stimulates both α- and β-adrenergic receptors). Propranolol, a nonselective β-adrenergic blocker, blocks the vasodilation action and the epinephrine then produces vasoconstriction through its stimulation of α-receptors. The rise in blood pressure may be considerable, the blood flow decreased, and the vacular resistance increased. This situation does not occur significantly with a selective β-blocker like metoprolol.

Ergot alkaloids[1166-8,1204]
Propranolol, a beta blocker which blocks the vasodilating action of epinephrine, when given to some patients receiving potent vasoconstricting ergot alkaloids for migraine, may produce severe, painful peripheral vasoconstriction and may increase the frequency and severity of the migraine headaches. This somewhat rare interaction varies in severity with dosages involved. Use of propranolol in migraine is questionable and hazardous.

Ether
See *Myocardial Depressants* below and *Propranolol* under *Ether.*

Guanethidine (Ismelin)
See *Antihypertensives* above.

Hexobarbital[818]
Increased CNS depression. See *Propranolol* under *Hexobarbital*.

Hydralazine[1753]
An effective and logical combination. Propranolol obliterates the cardiac stimulation (palpitations, headache, etc.) associated with hydralazine regimens and potentiates the hypotensive response. Patients unresponsive to either drug alone may respond well to the combination.

Hydrocortisone
See *Anti-inflammatory Agents* above.

Hypoglcemics, oral[1,42]
(Diabinese, Dymelor, Orinase, etc.)
Propranolol potentiates oral hypoglycemics. See *Antidiabetics* above.

Indomethacin (Indocin)[2065]
By inhibiting endogenous prostaglandin synthesis (pgA and pgE are powerful hypotensives), indomethacin may abolish the antihypertensive action (diastolic pressure lowering effect) of propranolol and other β-adrenergic receptor blocking drugs.

Insulin[1,42,263,421,681]
Propranolol potentiates insulin and may prolong insulin hypoglycemia. See *Antidiabetics* above and *Propranolol* under *Insulin*.

Isoproterenol[330,1169,1170] (Isuprel, etc.)
Isoproterenol, a β-adrenergic agonist, antagonizes the β-adrenergic blocking effects of propranolol and vice versa. Beta-blocked patients on propranolol who develop an acute asthmatic attack or anaphylactic shock from some antigen may not respond adequately to epinephrine or isoproterenol (aminophylline or calcium gluconate or chloride are alternatives). See also *Epinephrine* above.

Isosorbide dinitrate[120] (Isordil)
Synergistic effects in treating angina pectoris have been reported; however, the potential benefit of using these agents in combination has been disputed. See also *Antihypertensives* above.

Levarterenol[120]
Propranolol blocks the hyperthermia produced by levarterenol and other β-adrenergic effects, particularly on the myocardium. See also *Catecholamines* above.

Levodopa[1171-4] (Dopar, Larodopa)
Propranolol may reinforce the antiparkinsonism action of levodopa. It also enhances the levodopa-induced stimulation of secretion of growth hormone to levels found in acromegaly. A favorable interaction in most instances is antagonism of the orthostatic hypotensive action of dopamine (formed from levodopa). By acting on the reticular formation of the tremorigenic neurohumoral system, propranolol may antagonize the beta-adrenergic actions of the dopamine formed from the levodopa. (Dopamine, a phenylalkylamine resembling tyramine may deplete norepinephrine by releasing it from adrenergic nerve endings. Such depletion explains the hypotesion produced.) Also, propranolol may block the positive inotropic effects of levodopa.

LSD[1130]
See *Propranolol* under *Lysergic Acid Diethylamide*.

MAO inhibitors[120,1179-80]
Propranolol should not to be used concurrently or during the 2 week withdrawal period following therapy with MAO inhibitors and other adrenergic-augmenting psychotropic drugs. Hazardous potentiation of the amine compound may occur. One report on one MAO inhibitor (mebenazine) discounts this interaction.

Metoprolol
See *Epinephrine* above.

Methyldopa (Aldomet)
See *Antihypertensives* above.

Morphine[698]
Propranolol has a synergistic CNS depressant action with morphine; this may occur with other β-adrenergic blocking agents. Death may occur.

Muscle relaxants
See *Propranolol* under *Muscle Relaxants, Peripherally Acting*.

Myocardial depressants[4c,198,698,818] (Chloroform, ether, etc.)
Use of propranolol to treat arrhythmias associated with anesthetics like ether, and its use with other myocardial depressants (barbiturates, morphine, etc.) are contraindicated. Hazardous potentiation of depression may occur; possibly death.

Narcotic analgesics[28,698]
See *Morphine* above.

Nitrates and nitrites[170]
β-Adrenergic blocking agents like propranolol tend to potentiate the hypotensive action of nitrates and nitrites. The tachycardia associated with nitrite hypotension is reduced.

Nylidrin[1181] (Arlidin)
Propranolol (beta-adrenergic receptor blocker), when administered prior to nylidrin (beta-adrenergic receptor stimulant) inhibits the increase in gastric acid secretion and volume produced by nylidrin.

Phenothiazines[1182-3]
Propranolol and phenothiazines have additive hypotensive effects. Propranolol reverses some of the EKG abnormalities produced by phenothiazines.

Phenoxybenzamine (Dibenzyline)
See *α-Adrenergic Blockers* above.

Phenylbutazone (Butazolidin)
See *Anti-inflammatory Agents* above.

Phenytoin[1152] (Dilantin)
Phenytoin potentiates the cardiac depressant action of propranolol (additive effects). Great caution must be exercised when the phenytoin is given IV, especially when the patient is susceptible to sinus arrest, when a beta blocker such as propranolol has already been given.

Psychotropic drugs[120]
Propranolol is contraindicated in patients on adrenergic-augmenting psychotropic drugs. See *MAO inhibitors* above.

Quinidine[585,932,1184-5,1885]
Synergistic activity in treatment of cardiac arrhythmia is useful, but an enhanced myocardial depressant effect (bradycardia) may occur.

Rauwolfia alkaloids[120] (Reserpine, etc.,)
The catecholamine blocking action added to the catecholamine depletion of the reserpine type of alkaloid may cause an excessive reduction of the resting sympathetic nervous activity (excessive sedation).

Salicylates
See *Anti-inflammatory Agents* above.

Skeletal muscle relaxants
See *d-Tubocurarine* below.

Smoking[587]
Combined use of nicotine and propranolol may considerably increase the blood pressure due to additive effects of β-adrenergic stimulation of heart rate, contractility and conduction velocity plus discharge of epinephrine from the adrenal medulla. Cardiac output is decreased.

PROPRANOLOL (Inderal) *(continued)*

Sulfonylureas (Diabinese, Dymelor, Orinase, etc.)
See *Antidiabetics* above.

Sympathomimetics[120]
β-Adrenergic blockers reverse the bronchial relaxing effect of sympathomimetics and exacerbate asthmatic conditions. The hypertensive effects are increased.

Thiazides and related diuretics
See *Antihypertensives*

***d*-Tubocurarine**[790,1186]
Propranolol potentiates tubocurarine.

Urethane[698]
Urethane increases the toxicity (CNS depressant action) of propranolol. Death may occur.

PROPYLTHIOURACIL

Anticoagulants, oral[147,330,912]
Propylthiouracil may enhance the anticoagulant effect by an antivitamin K action.

Warfarin[120] **(Coumadin)**
See *Anticoagulants, Oral* above.

PROSTAGLANDINS

Indomethacin (Indocin)
See *Indomethacin* under *Propranolol.*

Prostaglandin antagonists[2042]
Prostaglandins play roles in a wide variety of cell functions and conditions (asthma, fever, inflammation, lymphocyte formation, maintenance of patency of ductus arteriosus, platelet function, etc.) and are antagonized by a growing list of drugs—caffeine, chloroquine, clomipramine, procaine, quinidine, quinine, theophylline, etc.). Physicians should remain on the alert for adverse and beneficial interactions between newly marketed prostaglandins and prostaglandin antagonists.

PROSTIGMIN

See *Parasympathomimetics* (Neostigmine).

PROTAMINE SULFATE

Anticoagulants (Heparin)
See *Protamine Sulfate* under *Heparin.*

PROTEOLYTIC ENZYMES

See *Chymotrypsin, Papain,* and *Trypsin.*

PROTHIPENDYL

See *Phenothiazines.*

PROTHROMADIN

See *Anticoagulants, Oral* (sodium warfarin).

PROTRYPTILINE (Vivactil)

See *Antidepressants, Tricyclic.*

PROZINE

See *Meprobamate, Promazine,* and *Phenothiazines.*

PRYDON

See *Anticholinergics* (belladonna alkaloids).

PRYDONNAL

See *Anticholinergics* (belladonna alkaloids) and *Barbiturates* (phenobarbital).

PSEUDOEPHEDRINE (Sudafed)

Kaolin
See *Pseudoephedrine* under *Kaolin.*

PSILOCYBIN

See *Hallucinogenic Agents* (page 308).

Chlorpromazine[951]
Chlorpromazine antagonizes the mydriasis and visual distortion produced by psilocybin.

PSYCHOENERGIZERS (Psychic energizers)

See *Antidepressants, Tricyclic* and *MAO Inhibitors.*

PSYCHOPHARMACOLOGIC AGENTS (Antipsychotics, Psychotropic drugs, Psychochemicals, etc.)

See *Benzodiazepines; Butyrophenones; CNS Depressants; Dibenzazepines* (Antidepressants, Tricyclic); *Lithium Salts; MAO Inhibitors; Meprobamate; Phenothiazines; Reserpine;* and *Tranquilizers.*

Alcohol[71,116,120]
Psychotropic drugs may potentiate the CNS depressant effects of alcohol, and possibly cause severe hypothermia and possibly respiratory depression and death.

Amantadine[120] **(Symmetrel)**
Since amantadine may exhibit CNS and psychic side effects, it should be used cautiously in combination with psychotropic agents.

Propranolol
See *Psychotropic Drugs* under *Propranolol.*

PURGATIVES

See *Cathartics* and *Mineral Oil.*

PURINETHOL

See *Antineoplastics* (6-Mercaptopurine).

PURODIGIN

See *Digitalis.*

PUROMYCIN

See *Antibiotics.*
Puromycin prevents enzyme induction.[709,1095,1096]

Blood cholesterol lowering agents[421]
Puromycin potentiates blood cholesterol lowering agents.

Clofibrate[421] **(Atromid-S)**
Puromycin potentiates the blood cholesterol lowering effect of clofibrate.

Interferon
Interferon inhibits the antiviral activity of puromycin.

Phenobarbital[709]
Puromycin abolishes the induction of microsomal metabolizing enzymes by phenobarbital.

Triiodothyronine[421]
Puromycin potentiates triiodothyronine; blocks cholesterol absorption.

PYRAMIDON

See *Aminopyrine.*

PYRAZINAMIDE

ACTH[1311,1787]
ACTH reverses the hyperuricemic action of pyrazinamide, and produces a uricosuric action.

Aminosalicylic acid[1311]
Antagonistic to hyperuricemic action. See *Pyrazinamide* under *p-Aminosalicylic Acid.*

Antidiabetics, oral[619]
Diabetes mellitus may be more difficult to control during therapy with pyrazinamide. Doses of oral antidiabetics in patients on this tuberculostatic drug require careful monitoring.

Insulin
Same as for *Antidiabetics, Oral* above.

Probenicid [1311]
Antagonistic to hyperuricemic action. See *Pyrazinamide* under *Probenicid.*

PYRAZOLONE DERIVATIVES
See *Aminopyrine, Antipyrine, Azaproprazone, Oxyphenbutazone, Phenylbutazone,* and *Sulfinpyrazone.*

PYRIBENZAMINE
See *Antihistamines* (tripelennamine).

PYRICTAL
See *Barbiturates* (phenetharbital).

PYRIDOSTIGMINE (Mestinon)
See *Anticholinesterases.*

Atropine [120]
In the event of cholinergic crisis induced by excessive dosage of pyridostigmine, atropine should be given immediately as an antidote. But atropine used to control gastrointestinal muscarinic side effects of pyridostigmine can lead to inadvertent induction of cholinergic crisis by masking signs of overdosage.

Edrophonium [120] **(Tensilon)**
Edrophonium may have to be used to differentiate between myasthenic crisis, which requires more intensive therapy with an anticholinesterase like pyridostigmine, and cholinergic crisis which requires prompt withdrawal of the drug.

Muscle relaxants
See *Pyridostigmine Bromide* under *Muscle Relaxants, Centrally Acting.*

PYRIDOXINE

Anticholinergics
See *Pyridoxine* under *Anticholinergics*

Antidepressants, tricyclic
See *Pyridoxine* under *Antidepressants, Tricyclic.*

Chloramphenicol [120] **(Chloromycetin)**
Pyridoxine may prevent chloramphencol induced optic neuritis.

Isoniazid [120]
Pyridoxine reduces the neurotoxicity of isoniazid.

Levodopa (Dopar, Larodopa)
Pyridoxine reverses the antiparkinsonism effects of levodopa. Vitamin preparations containing pyridoxine may be contraindicated. See *Pyridoxine* under *Levodopa.*

PYRILGIN
See *Dipyrone.*

PYRIMETHAMINE (Daraprim)
See *Antimalarials.*

p-Aminobenzoic Acid [201,619,1209] **(PABA)**
PABA interferes with the antiplasmodial and antitoxoplasmic effects of pyrimethamine which depends on causing a folic acid deficiency for the microorganisms involved. The protozoa do not have the ability to utilize exogenous folate and must have PABA to synthesize their own. Thus PABA deficiency would be additive to the antifolate action (inhibition of dihydrofolate reductase) by pyrimethamine.

Barbiturates [120]
A barbiturate followed by folinic acid may be used as the antidote for overdosage of pyrimethamine (CNS stimulation, convulsions.)

Chloroguanide [619] **(Paludrine)**
Cross-resistance may occur.

Cyanocobalamin [619]
Cyancobalamin accentuates the hematologic deficiency produced by pyrimethamine.

Folic acid [120,177,1209,1629,1860] **(Folvite)**
Folic acid may be contraindicated in malaria for use with pyrimethamine, a folic acid antagonist because it interferes with the mechanism of pyrimethamine action. See *p-Aminobenzoic Acid* above. However, the very high dose of pyrimethamine used in toxoplasmosis (10 to 20 times the antimalarial dose) may induce a folic or folinic acid deficiency. Folinic acid may be administered IM for a few days to correct depressed platelet and leukocyte counts. It is also recommended to prevent the hematologic toxicity that may occur with continued daily use of the antiprotozoal drug, also for use with pyrimethamine for treatment of toxoplasmosis during pregnancy even though it may be teratogenic. This is a case where teratogervic effects from the drug must be weighed carefully against the risks of permanent damage to the fetus from the disease.

Folinic acid [120,177,619] **(Leucovorin)**
Folinic acid may be used as adjunctive therapy to reverse depressed platelet and leukocyte counts caused by folic acid deficiency without destroying the effectiveness of pyrimethamine. See *Folic Acid* above.

Quinine (Quinidine) [330]
When these drugs are given simultaneously in conventional doses, severe quinine toxicity (cinchonism, neutropenia) may be produced, since pyrimethamine increases quinine blood levels by displacing it from plasma protein binding sites.

Sulfonamides [120,177,619]
(Sulfadiazine, Trisulfapyrimidines)
Sulfonamides that are synergistic with pyrimethamine in toxoplasmosis and in malaria caused by *P. falciparum,* should be used conjointly in treating the parasitic infection. Less than 1/10 of the curative dose of pyrimethamine and less that 1/4 of the curative dose of sulfadiazine are then required when used concomitantly. Development of resistant strains is also inhibited.

PYRROBUTAMINE (Co-Pyronil)
See *Antihistamines.*

Q CAPS
See *Amphetamines* (dextroamphetamine) and *Barbiturates* (amobarbital).

QUAALUDE
See *Methaqualone* and *CNS Depressants.*

QUADAMINE
See *Amphetamines* (dextroamphetamine), *Ascorbic Acid, Barbiturates, Iodides, Iron Salts* (ferrous sulfate), and *Vitamins* (A, D, B_1, B_2, niacinamide). Also contains cobalt, copper, molybdenum and zinc.

QUADRINAL
See *Barbiturates* (phenobarbital), *Ephedrine, Lodides,* and *Theophylline.*

QUANTRIL
See *Benzquinamide.*

QUELICIN
See *Succinylcholine Chloride.*

QUESTRAN
See *Chloestyramine.*

QUIBRON
See *Glyceryl Guaiacolate* in Chapter 7 and *Theophylline.*

QUIDE
See *Phenothiazines* (piperacetazine).

QUIESS
See *Barbiturates* (butabarbital, pentobarbital and phenobarbital).

QUINACRINE (Atabrine, Mepacrine)

Acidifying agents [325,870]
Urinary acidifying agents increase the urinary excretion of quinacrine and thus decrease its effectiveness.

Alcohol [28,121]
Quinacrine, by inhibiting aldehyde dehydrogenase, may prevent oxidation of acetaldehyde, a metabolite of alcohol, and thus produces the disulfiram type of reaction.

Alkalinizing agents [325,870]
Urinary alkalinizing agents shift a large proportion of the drug to the noninoized and therefore lipid-soluble form which is more readily reabsorbed by the tubules and only small quantities appear in the urine. Thus sodium bicarbonate, used to offset nausea and vomiting, given concurrently in large enough doses tends to potentiate the drug and produce toxicity.

8-Aminoquinolines [177]
(Primaquine, Quinocide, etc.)
Contraindicated. Quinacrine greatly increases the toxicity of primaquine (and related antimalarials) because it increases the plasma concentration from 5- to 10-fold and prolongs the length of time it remains in the body. This phenomenon is observed even when primaquine is given as long as 3 months after the last dose of quinacrine.

Heprin [180,1208]
Quinacrine, a basic drug, may react with heparin, an acidic drug, and inhibit its anticoagulant activity. Monitor carefully.

MAO inhibitors [74,433]
Quinacrine, an anthelmintic and antimalarial of low toxicity, is stored in large quantities for prolonged periods in the liver. Since MAO inhibitors inhibit hepatic enzyme systems, they may potentiate the adverse effects of the drug, including explosive eczematoid skin reactions and other severe dermatitides, aplastic anemia and other severe blood dyscrasias, psychotic episodes, retinal damage, etc.

Pamaquine [298,1028]
Quinacrine potentiates pamaquine by displacing it from storage sites.

Primaquine
See *8-Aminoquinolines* above.

Quinocide
See *8-Aminoquinolines* above.

QUINAGLUTE
See *Quinidine*.

QUINETHAZONE (Hydromox)
See *Diuretics*.

ACTH
See *Digitalis* below.

Anesthetics [120]
Quinethazone decreases arterial responsiveness to norepinephrine and thus potentiates the hypotensive effects of anesthetics and preanesthetic agents. Their dosage should be reduced in emergency surgery when the diuretic cannot be withdrawn well before surgery.

Antihypertensives [120,619]
Quinethazone potentiates the hypotensive effect of the antihypertensives including ganglionic blocking agents, hydrala-

zine, and veratrum alkaloids, and their dosage should be reduced to avoid a sudden drop in blood pressure.

Corticosteroids
See *Digitalis* below.

Digitalis [120]
Quinethazone, particularly during concomitant use of ACTH and corticosteroids, may induce hypokalemia. If digitalis or one of its glycosides is then administered, its toxicity is considerably increased.

Gallamine
See *Tubocurarine* below.

Ganglionic blocking agents [120,619]
See *Antihypertensives* above.

Glucose [120]
Quinethazone decreases glucose tolerance and may aggravate or provoke diabetes mellitus with hyperglycemia and glycosuria.

Hydralazine [619]
See *Antihypertensives* above.

Hydrochlorothiazide [619]
Cross photosensitivity has occurred between quinethazone and hydrochlorothiazide.

Tubocurarine [120]
Quinethazone may increase the responsiveness to curariform agents like tobucurarine and gallamine.

Veratrum alkaloids [619]
See *Antihypertensives* above.

QUINIDEX
See *Quinidine*.

QUINIDINE (α-Isomer of quinine)

Acetazolamide [325,1187-8] (Diamox)
Acetazolamide (carbonic anhydrase inhibitor), by alkalinizing the urine, tends to increase quinidine tubular absorption and thus decrease its excretion, raise its blood levels, and potentiate its action.

Acetylcholine [168,1205]
Quinidine may antagonize the depolarizing effects of acetylcholine.

Acidifying agents [325,581,870]
Acidifying agents inhibit quinidine because of increased urinary excretion.

Alcohol
See *Quinine* under *Alcohol*.

Alkalinizing agents [325,581,870,1187-90] (Antacids)
Alkalinizing agents, such as sodium bicarbonate, magnesium hydroxide (Milk of Magnesia), Titrilac (calcium carbonate plus glycine), and Maalox and Mylanta (aluminum and magnesium hydroxide)—but not aluminum hydroxide (Amphojel) or dihydroxyaluminum glycinate (Robalate)—potentiate quinidine because of increased renal tubular absorption and because of increased blood levels. Large quantities of citrus fruits also tend to alkalinize the urine.

Aluminum hydroxide [1959]
Antacids containing aluminum hydroxide and related antacids tend to delay intestinal absorption of quinidine and a variety of other drugs and thus decrease their pharmacologic activity. See also *Alkalinizing Agents* above.

Antibiotics [447,559]
Quinidine may increase the neuromuscular blocking action of antibiotics like kanamycin, neomycin, streptomycin and other aminoglycosides and produce apnea and muscle weakness. Hazardous.

Anticholinergics [170,619]
Enhanced (additive) anticholinergic effects. Any combination of quinidine (vagal blocker) and an anticholinergic drug must be administered with caution.

Anticoagulants, oral [260,582,630,1192]
Quinidine, by depressing prothrombin formation or inhibiting synthesis of vitamin K sensitive clotting factors in the liver, tends to potentiate the anticoagulant effect of coumarin derivatives. The hemorrhagic tendency is increased.

Anticonvulsants [1998]
Phenobarbital and phenytoin (Dilantin) reduce the half-life of quinidine by about 50%, probably due to enzyme induction, and possibly also to decreased absorption. Monitor patients carefully for this significant decrease in quinidine effectiveness. Exercise particular caution when an anticonvulsant is discontinued, especially phenytoin for it is an antiarrhythmic like quinidine. Potentiated quinidine toxicity, arrhythmias, etc. may be produced.

Antihypertensives [170,619,1176]
Quinidine may potentiate the hypotensive effect of thiazides, related diuretics, and other antihypertensive agents. Dosages should be adjusted accordingly.

Barbiturates
See *Anticonvulsants* above.

Cholinergics [170]
Quinidine with its anticholinergic properties may antagonize cholinergics.

Cinchona alkaloids [1205]
The other alkaloids of cinchona may potentiate the effects of quinidine.

Curariform agents
See *Muscle Relaxants* below.

Decamethonium
See *Muscle Relaxants* below.

Digitalis [619] **and its glycosides**
Enhanced (additive) digitalis effect. Avoid overdosage. Use extreme caution. Bradycardia may occur.

Edrophonium [177,1205] **(Tensilon)**
Quinidine, with its curarelike action, antagonizes edrophonium.

Gallamine
See *Muscle Relaxants* below.

Heparin
See *Quinine* under *Heparin*.

Kanamycin
See *Antibiotics* above.

Magnesium salts
See *Muscle Relaxants* below.

Muscle relaxants [324,390,447,564,1205]
(Anectine, Flaxedil, Mecostrin, Metubine, Sucostrin, Suxcert, Syncurine, Tubarine, magnesium salts, etc.)
Quinidine potentiates the neuromsular blocking effect of skeletal muscle relaxants, both the curariform and depolarizing types, including the neuromuscular blocking antibiotics. Respiratory depression may cause apnea. "Recurarization" may occur when quinidine is administered again later. See also *Neuromuscular Blocking Antibiotics* under *Antibiotics*.

Neomycin
See *Antibiotics* above.

Neostigmine [177,1205] **(Prostigmin)**
Quinidine antagonizes neostigmine, physostigmine, and related drugs. In patients with myasthenia gravis who are well

controlled by neostigmine, quinine causes the symptoms to return.

Phenobarbital
See *Anticonvulsants* above.

Phenothiazines [166,330,1194-6]
Phenothiazines have a quinidinelike action on myocardial conducting and pacemaking tissue. These drugs and quinidine have additive cardiac depressant effects. Ventricular tachycardia induced by phenothiazines should not be treated with quinidine but should be treated like quinidine toxicity. A contraindicated combination.

Phenytoin [619] **(Dilantin)**
Phenytoin may potentiate the antiarrhythmic action of quinidine (additive effects). But see also under *Anticonvulsants* above.

Procainamide [170,619] **(Pronestyl)**
Additive effects permit lower dosage of the individual drugs. See *Quinidine* under *Procainamide*.

Propranolol [585,932,1184-5] **(Inderal)**
Quinidine effects may be additive with those of propranolol. Bradycardia may occur. Caution. See *Quinidine* under *Propranolol*.

Pyrimethamine [1109] **(Daraprim)**
When these drugs are given simultaneously in conventional doses, severe quinine (quinidine) toxicity (cinchonism, neutropenia) is produced (displacement by pyrimethamine).

Rauwolfia alkaloids [120,691,1960]
This combination should be used cautiously since cardiac arrhythmias caused by quinidine are increased by reserpine.

Reserpine
See *Rauwolfia alkaloids* above.

Sodium bicarbonate [325,1187-8]
See *Alkalinizing agents* above.

Streptomycin
See *Antibiotics* above.

Suxamethonium chloride
(Anectine, succinylcholine chloride, Sucostrin)
See *Muscle Relaxants* above.

Tubocurarine
See *Muscle Relaxants* above.

Urethane [697]
Urethane increases the toxicity of quinidine.

Veratrum alkaloids [120,619]
Caution should be observed when quinidine is used with veratrum alkaloids. Cardiac arrhythmias may develop.

Warfarin (Coumadin)
See *Anticagulants, Oral* above.

QUININE
See *Quinidine*.
Since quinidine is the dextroisomer of quinine, the actions and interactions of these drugs are similar and their effects differ usually only in intensity.

Alcohol
See *Quinine* under *Alcohol*.

Heparin
See *Quinine* under *Heparin*.

Pyrimethamine
See *Quinine* under *Pyrimethamine* and *Pyrimethamine* under *Quinidine*.

QUINORA
See *Quinidine*.

RADIATION
See *X-radiation*

RADIOACTIVE COMPOUNDS (Radiopharmaceuticals)

Anticoagulants, coumarin [9,180,861]
Radioactive compounds may prolong prothrombin time and may therefore increase the activity of these anticoagulants; hemorrhage may occur if they are added to a stabilized anticoagulant regimen.

RADIOIODINE TREATMENT

Iodine [54]
Small doses of iodine cause euthyroid patients, previously treated with radioiodine for the diffuse toxic goiter of Graves disease, to become hypothyroid. A defect in organic binding induced by radioiodine can result in a further enhancement of susceptibility to iodide myxedema.

RADIOPAQUE MEDIA (Radiographic or radiologic contrast media)

Antihistamines [632]
Antihistamines, *e.g.*, chlorpheniramine maleate are commonly injected to reduce side effects of radiopaque media.

RAUDIXIN
See *Rauwolfia Alkaloids* (whole root).

RAUJA
See *Rauwolfia Alkaloids* (whole root).

RAULEN
See *Rauwolfia Alkaloids* (whole root).

RAU-SED
See *Reserpine.*

RAUSERFIA
See *Rauwolfia Alkaloids* (whole root).

RAUSERPA
See *Rauwolfia Alkaloids* (whole root)

RAUTENSIN
See *Rauwolfia Alkaloids* (whole root).

RAUTINA
See *Rauwolfia Alkaloids* (whole root).

RAUVAL
See *Rauwolfia Alkaloids* (whole root).

RAUVERAT
See *Rauwolfia Alkaloids* and *Vertrum Viride Alkaloids.*

RAUVERID
See *Rauwolifa Alaloids* (whole root) and *Veratrum Viride Alkaloids* (extract).

RAUWILOID
See *Rauwolfia Alkaloids* (alseroxylon).

RAUWOLDIN
See *Rauwolfia Alkaloids* (whole root).

RAUWOLFIA ALKALOIDS (Ajmaline, Alseroxylon, rescinnamine, reserpine, whole powdered root)
See *Antihypertensives, Ajmaline,* and *Reserpine.*

RAUZIDE
See *Rauwolfia Alkaloids* (whole root) and *Thiazide Diuretics* (bendroflumethiazide).

RAVOCAINE
See *Anesthetics, Local* (propoxycaine).

REACTROL
See *Antihistamines* (clemizole).

RECTALAD AMINOPHYLLINE
See *Aminophylline.*

REGITINE
See *Phentolamine.*

REGROTON
See *Antihypertensives* (reserpine) and *Diuretics* (chlorthalidone).

RELA
See *Carisoprodol.*

RENACIDIN
See *Urinary Acidifiers* (citric, malic and gluconic acids).

RENALTABS-SC
See *Atropine, Hyoscyamine,* and *Methenamine.*

RENELATE
See *Methenamine.*

RENESE
See *Thiazide Diuretics* (polythiazide).

RENOGRAFIN
See *Radiopaque Media* (meglumine diatrizoate).

RENOVIST
See *Radiopaque Media* (diatrizoates).

REPOISE
See *Phenothiazines* (butaperazine).

RESCINNAMINE
See *Rauwolfia Alkaloids.*

RESERPINE (Prototype of Rauwolifa alkaloids; reserpine derivatives)
See *Antihypertensive* also.

β-Adrenergic blockers [120]
β-Adrenergic blockers increase the activity of reserpine (excessive sedation).

Adrenergics [633]
See *Sympathomimetics* below.

Alcohol [121,421]
Mutual potentiation (addition) of CNS depressant effects.

Amitriptyline
See *Antidepressants, Tricyclic* below.

Amphetamine [600,601]
In reserpine-treated animals, the response to pressor agents (tyramine) is blocked by amphetamine. See also *Sympathomimetics* below.

Anesthetics [120,198,421,633,634,751,752,1623]
Anesthetics potentiate the hypotensive effect of reserpine and its Rauwolfia derivatives and the combination causes bradycardia and possibly circulatory collapse. The anesthesiologist should be made aware of the patient's reserpine intake and consider this in the over-all management. Anticholinergics (see below) or adrenergics (metaraminol, norepinephrine) may be administered to counteract adverse circulatory effects.

Anticholinergics [421]
Reserpine and its derivatives antagonize the antisecretory ef-

Reserpine and its derivatives antagonize the antisecretory effects of anticholinergics. Anticholinergics given concomitantly counteract the abdominal cramps and diarrhea resulting from the increased gastrointestinal motility and tone produced by reserpine.

Anticoagulants, oral [180,193,453]
Reserpine potentiates coumarin anticoagulants with long-term therapy but antagonizes them with short-term therapy.

Anticonvulsants [120]
Reserpine may lower the convulsive threshold in susceptible individuals; an increase in the dosage of the anticonvulsant may be necessary.

Antidepressants, tricyclic [120,399,633,941,946,1516]
These antidepressants inhibit reserpine and may block or reverse the depressive effects of the drug and produce mania. They also increase blood glucose utilization, and elevate blood lactic acid and free fatty acids (desipramine in reserpinized rats) and reverse reserpine-induced hypothermia (produce hyperthermia). Although they are used in combination for endogenous depression refractory to imipramine alone, caution and very close monitoring are essential. The mechanism for this interaction is porbably the same as that of guanethidine. See *Antidepressants, Tricyclic* under *Guanethidine.*

Antihistamines
Increased CNS depression.

Antihypertensives, other [120]
Other antihypertensive agents such as hydralazine and thiazide diuretics enhance the hypotensive effect; reduced dosages of the hypotensive agents are frequently necessary.

Atropine [120]
Vagal blocking agents like atropine are used to prevent and treat vagal circulatory responses in patient receiving reserpine when emergency surgery must be performed. See also *Anticholinergics* above.

Barbiturates [120]
Reserpine potentiates the CNS depressant action of the barbiturates (bradycardia and hypotension).

Cardiac glycosides
See *Digitalis* below.

Catecholamines [168]
Reserpine and its derivatives reduce tissue levels of catecholamines. See page 378.

Chlorothiazide (Diuril)
See *Thiazide Diuretics* below.

Chlorpromazine (Thorazine)
See *Phenothiazines* below.

Desipramine (Pertofrane)
See *Antidepressants, Tricyclic* above.

Desoxycholic acid [603]
Desoxycholic acid may increase the blepharoptotic and other effects of reserpine by enhancing its rate of gastrointestinal absorption.

Dextrothyroxine [590] (Choloxin)
Reserpine abolishes the angina induced by dextrothyroxine in patients with coronary artery disease.

Digitalis [110,120,226,330,635,1754-5]
Reserpine enhances the toxicity of digitalis glycosides; digitalis glycosides enhance reserpine effects on the heart. Bradycardia and cardiac arrthythmias may occur. Use the combination with caution, particularly if reserpine is started in patients already stablized on a digitalis product, since both release catecholamines.

Digoxin
See *Digitalis* above.

Diuretics
See *Thiazide Diuretics* below.

Electroconvulsive therapy [794,795]
Apnea, respiratory depression, paralysis and death may be caused by combined reserpine electroshock therapy. Discontinue reserpine 2 weeks before ECT is employed.

Ephedrine [168,636,1624,1815]
Reserpine, a depletor of norepinephrine, antagonizes the pressor and mydriatic effects of ephedrine, which as an indirectly acting sympathomimetic depends for its effects on norepinephrine release. Since ephedrine also has a direct effect on receptors, however, the outcome of this interaction will obviously vary with dosages, patient's condition, etc. Monitor carefully since ephedrine may still exert substantial effects in reserpine-treated patients.

Flurothyl [935] (Indoklon)
See *Reserpine* under *Flurothyl.*

Furazolidone [633] (Furoxone)
See *MAO Inhibitors* below.

Ganglionic blocking agents [117]
Reserpine potentiates the hypotensive action of ganglionic blocking agents.

Guanethidine [120,421] (Ismelin)
Concomitant use of guanethidine and reserpine may exaggerate orthostatic hypotension, bradycardia, and psychic depression.

Hydralazine
See *Reserpine* under *Hydralazine.*

Imipramine (Tofranil)
See *Antidepressants, Tricyclic* above.

Levarterenol [117,198,330,421,633] (Norepinephrine)
Reserpine and its derivatives in the initial IV doses potentiates levarterenol by release of norepinephrine, and then continues to potentiate 2- to 3-fold by preventing its binding to inactive sites.

Levodopa [724,922,1240,1648,2001]
Reserpine, by uptake blockage and depletion of dopamine, can defeat the therapeutic purpose of levodopa in parkinsonism. Avoid this combination if possible.

LSD [166]
Reserpine aggravates the symptoms produced by LSD (lysergic acid diethylamide). Avoid this combination.

MAO inhibitors [104,120,162,166,633,637-640]
Parenteral reserpine may initially cause hypertensive reactions from sudden release of catecholamines (norepinephrine, dopamine). Through enzyme inhibition, MAO inhibitors may prolong the quantity and duration of the neurotransmitters and thereby potentiate the pressor effects (excitation, hypertension and tachycardia) of these amines. Thus reserpine tends initially to potentiate the antidepressant effect of MAO inhibitors. If MAO inhibitors are continued with reserpine the latter may be potentiated and severe psychic depression, possibly suicide, and gastrointestinal activity (cramps, diarrhea, acid secretion) may occur. See *Polymechamisms* (page 378). Use of reserpine is contraindicated for at least one week following treatment with a MAO inhibitor.

Mecamylamine [619] (Inversine)
An advantageous combination. Mecamylamine dosage may be reduced because of additive hypotensive effects.

Mephentermine [198,633,636] (Wyamine)
Reserpine (hypotensive which depletes norepinephrine) antagonizes mephentermine (pressor which acts by releasing norepinephrine) after an initial hypertension due to the release of norepinephrine by reserpine. See under *Reserpine* (page 378).

RESERPINE *(continued)*

Metaraminol [198,633,640] (Aramine)
See *Polymechanistic Drugs* (page 378).

Methamphetamine [117] (Desoxyn, Methedrine, etc.)
Reserpine, through its norepinephrine depleting action, abolishes the pressor response to methamphetamine which acts by releasing norepinephrine from its storage sites. See also *Mephentermine* above.

Methotrimeprazine [120] (Levoprome)
The orthostatic hypotension produced by methotrimeprazine is additive to the hypotensive action of reserpine. Avoid this combination. See *CNS Depressants* under *Methotrimeprazine*.

Morphine [643]
Reserpine inhibits the analgesic activity of morphine.

Muscle relaxants, centrally acting [120]
Anticholinergic muscle relaxants (*e.g.*, benztropine mesylate) may relieve drug-induced parkinsonism symptoms produced by reserpine but may intensify mental symptoms (possible toxic psychosis).

Nialamide (Niamid)
See *MAO Inhibitors* above.

Norepinephrine
See *Levarterenol* above.

Nortriptyline (Aventyl)
See *Antidepressants, Tricyclic* above.

Pargyline (Eutonyl)
See *MAO Inhibitors* above.

Perphenazine [421,633] (Trilafon)
Potentiation of CNS effects (hypotension, sedation) of reserpine.

Phenothiazines [198,421,633]
Phenothiazines potentiate the sedative and hypotensive effects of reserpine and its derivatives.

Phenoxybenzamine [1] (Dibenzyline)
Phenoxybenzamine blocks the production of hypothermia by reserpine.

Phentolamine (Regitine) [168]
Phentolamine blocks the production of hypothermia by reserpine.

Phenylpropanolamine
See *Methyldopa* under *Phenylpropanolamine* and *Sympathomimetics* below.

Prenylamine [170] (Segontin)
Additive hypotensive effect may occur. Prenylamine produces many of the same actions and effects as reserpine, *e.g.* depletes central and peripheral stores of norepinephrine, depresses amine uptake and norepinephrine synthesis by storage granules, depresses responses to tyramine, augments responses to epinephrine and norepinephrine, induces peripheral vasodilation, antagonizes response to isoproterenol, and may reverse the depressor effect of this latter agent to pressor.

Propranolol [120] (Inderal)
The addition of the β-adrenergic blocking action of propranolol to the norepinephrine depleting action of reserpine may cause excessive reduction of resting sympathetic nervous activity (excessive sedation and tranquilization).

Quinidine [120]
This combination should be used cautiously in combination since cardiac arrhythmias may occur.

Salicylates [951]
Reserpine inhibits the analgesic activity of salicylates.

Stress [120,619,794]
Sudden stress such as electroshock therapy or surgery may cause acute cardiovascular collapse in patients whose body stores of catecholamines have been depleted by Rauwolfia therapy, and death may occur.

Sympathomimetics [30,117,198,421,633]
Theoretically, sympathomimetics tend to inhibit the hypotensive and sedative effects of reserpine and its derivatives. However, timing and the specific nature of the given drug are important. Directly acting vasopressor agents like levarterenol are potentiated by reserpine (also by guanethidine, methyldopa) because it prevents uptake of the pressor agents by inactive storage sites. Indirectly acting agents like amphetamine, ephedrine, and mephentermine on the other hand are potentiated only by large initial IV doses of reserpine (also guanethidine, methyldopa). Both reserpine and the indirectly acting sympathomimetics release norepinephrine from its storage sites. Later, they are inhibited or their action may be abolished entirely if the norepinephrine, upon whose release they depend for their effects, has been depleted. See *Polymechanistic Drugs* (page 378) and *Methyldopa* under *Phenylpropanolamine*.

Thiazide diuretics [117,1352]
These agents synergistically potentiate the hypotensive effects of reserpine and minimize side effects. Reduction of the dosages of the hypotensive agent is frequently necessary (by as much as 50%). Reserpine plus hydrochlorothiazide is very effective combination for reducing high diastolic blood pressures.

Thiopental (Pentothal)
See *Barbiturates*.

Trifluoperazine (Stelazine)
See *Phenothiazines* above.

d-Tubocurarine
See *Reserpine* under *Muscle Relaxants, Peripherally Acting, Competitive Type*.

Tyramine [554,1624]
Reserpine diminishes and may completely prevent the pressor effect of tyramine. The alkaloid depletes the stores of norepinephrine through which tyramine indirectly exerts its pressor effect by release of transmitter. See *Reserpine* under *Tyramine-rich Foods*.

Tyramine-rich foods
See *Tyramine* above and *Reserpine* under *Tyramine Rich Foods*.

Vasodilators [950]
Vasodilators enhance the hypotensive effect of reserpine. Reduced dosage of the hypotensive agents is frequently necessary.

Vasopressors [120]
See *Sympathomimetics*.

RESERPOID
See *Reserpine*.

RHEOMACRODEX
See *Dextran*.

RHINEX
See *Aluminum Salts, Antihistamines* (chlorpheniramine), *Magnesium Salts* and *Sympathomimetics* (phenylephrine).

RIBOFLAVIN

Chloramphenicol [491]
Riboflavin ameliorates chloramphenicol-induced bone marrow depression; reduced incidence of chloramphenicol-induced optic neuritis.

RIFAMPIN
(Rifampicin, rifamycin derivative, Rifadin, Rifomycin, Rimactane)

Aminosalicylic acid
See *Rifampin* under *p-Aminosalicylic Acid.*

Anticoagulants, oral
See *Rifampin* under *Anticoagulants, Oral.*

Antidiabetics, oral
See *Rifampin* under *Antidiabetics, Oral.*

Contraceptives, oral [1201,1298,1375,1666]
Rifampin, by enzyme induction, increases the metabolism of oral contraceptives and decreases their effectiveness. An increased number of unplanned pregnancies and breakthrough bleeding, spotting, etc. have occurred in women on OCs who were given rifampin. Avoid this combination.

Corticosteroids and estrogens [178,2040]
Rifampin, through enzyme induction, enhances the metabolism of a number of steroids and decreases their effectiveness. Progressive deterioration of renal function occurred in renal transplant patients on glucocorticoids (methylprednisolone or prednisolone) during treatment with rifampin. Enhanced metabolism of the steroids (enzyme induction by rifampin) adversely affected protein catabolism and allograft function. When long-term rifampin therapy was stopped signs of steroid toxicity (sharp rise in BUN, severe peptic esophagitis and fluid retention) developed.

Disulfiram [1138]
See *Rifampin* under *Isoniazid*

Halothane [1654] **(Fluothane)**
Concomitant use of rifampin and halothane may produce hepatotoxicity. Do not give the tuberculostatic drug just before or just after the anesthetic.

Isoniazid [1306,1564]
See *Rifampin* under *Isoniazid.*

Methadone [1973]
See *Rifampin* under *Methadone.*

Probenecid [1206,1884] **(Benemid)**
Probenecid may strongly potentiate rifampin (may double the blood levels) by competition for hepatic uptake. Use of probenecid may be a cost effective way of reducing rifampin dosage.

Rifampin
Rifampin is a strong enzyme inducer that increases its own metabolism thus making the usual therapeutic doses less effective as the therapy is continued.

Tuberculin [178,1948]
Rifampin suppresses cutaneous sensitivity to tuberculin.

Warfarin
See *Rifampin* under *Anticoagulants, Oral*

RIOPAN
See *Antacids* (hydrated magnesium aluminate).

RITALIN
See *Methylphenidate.*

ROBALATE
See *Antacids* (dihydroxyaluminum aminoacetate).

ROBAXIN
See *Muscle Relaxants* (methocarbamol). Also contains *Glyceryl Guaiacol Carbonate.*

ROBAXISAL
See *Muscle Relaxants* (methocarbamol) and *Salicylates* (aspirin).

ROBINUL
See *Anticholinergics* (glycopyrrolate).

ROBINUL-PH
See *Anticholinergics* (glycopyrrolate) and *Barbiturates* (phenobarbital).

ROBITUSSIN-AC
See *Codeine* (phosphate), and *Glyceryl Guaiacolate.*

ROLAIDS
See *Aluminum Salts* (dihydroxy aluminum sodium carbonate)

ROMILAR CAPSULES
See *Acetaminophen, Antihistamines* (chlorpheniramine maleate), *Dextromethorphan,* and *Sympathomimetics* (phenylephrine)

Phenelzine [1792] **(Nardil)**
A 15-year old girl, receiving phenelzine, consumed several Romilar capsules for "kicks" and died. The MAO inhibitor plus the sympathomimetic produced a hypertensive crisis.

RONDOMYCIN
See *Antibiotics* and *Tetracyclines* (methacycline).

RUBBER
Medicaments [68]
Rubber stoppers may react with drugs.

RYNATAN
See *Antihistamines* (chlorpheniramine and pyrilamine tannates), *Sympathomimetics* (phenylephrine tannate) and *Vasoconstrictors.*

RYNATUSS
See *Antihistamines* (chlorpheniramine tannate), *Sympathomimetics* (ephedrine and phenylephrine tannates) and *Vasopressors.* Also contains *Carbetapentane.*

SALAMIDE
See *Salicylates.*

SALRIN
See *Salicylates* (salicylamide).

SALICYLAMIDE
See *Salicylates. An enzyme inhibitor.*

SALICYLATES
(Aspirin, sodium salicylate, etc.)

Acenocoumarol [120] **(Sintrom)**
See *Anticoagulants, Oral* below.

Acetazolamide
See *Salicylates* under *Acetazolamide.*

Acetohexamide (Dymelor)
See *Antidiabetics* below.

Acidifiers, urinary [275,325,870,1099,1577]
Urinary acidifiers decrease the urinary excretion rate of salicylates (salicylic acid) and potentiate them (increased tubular reabsorption). Salicylism may result from small decreases in pH. Thus ammonium chloride, a urinary acidifier, elevates salicylate blood levels significantly.

Alcohol [645,711]
Alcohol increases the incidence and intensity of gastric hemorrhage (occult blood loss) caused by salicylates such as aspirin. See *Salicylates* under *Alcohol.*

Alkalinizers, urinary [275,325,870,1099]
Urinary alkalinizers increase the urinary excretion rate of salicylates (salicylic) acid and thus inhibit them. Increasing the pH less than one unit (from 5.8 to 6.5) may decrease plasma levels of salicylate by 50%.

SALICYLATES *(continued)*

Allopurinol [120] (Zyloprim)

Salicylates interfere with the tubular urinary excretion of *oxypurines* (uric acid, etc.) and renal precipitation of oxypurines may occur with the combined therapy. Uricosuric agents (salicylates, sulfinpyrazone, etc.) may also lower the degree of inhibition of xanthine oxidase by allopurinol and thus enhance *oxypurinol* excretion.

p-Aminobenzoic acid [644,1812] (PABA)

PABA potentiates salicylates by interfering with their metabolism and excretion.

p-Aminosalicylic acid [78,166,178,198,202,421,633] (PAS)

Salicylates potentiate the activity and toxicity (gastric hemorrhage, peptic ulceration, etc.) of PAS, possibly by inhibiting its urinary excretion or displacing it from plasma protein binding sites. Also, aspirin blocks active transport of PAS from the cerebrospinal fluid to blood. Increased salicylate toxicity also may occur. Avoid if possible.

Ammonium chloride [1099,1577]

See *Acidifiers, Urinary* above.

Antacids [78,1416]

Antacids inhibit salicylate by decreasing their gastrointestinal absorption. See also *Alkalinizers, Urinary* above. Oral antacids such as aluminum and magnesium hydroxides (Maalox) may also expedite release of salicylates (and other drugs) from enteric-coated tablets as well as hasten gastric emptying. Therapeutic blood levels of salicylate are achieved more rapidly but gastric irritation may not be circumvented as intended with enteric coating.

Anticoagulants, oral

See *Salicylates* under *Anticoagulants, Oral.*

Antidepressants, tricyclic [48,219]

Death has occurred with this combination. The outcome was fatal for a patient who ingested an overdose of aspirin while receiving imipramine, in spite of every effort to revive her.

Antidiabetics, oral

See *Sulfonylureas* below.

Ascorbic acid [325,616,870,1099,1577] (Vitamin C)

Salicylates can increase the rate of urinary excretion of ascorbic acid (inhibition of the vitamin). Ascorbic acid, by lowering urinary pH, decreases the urinary excretion of salicylates (potentiation of salicylate analgesics).

Barbiturates [83,275]

Barbiturates, through microsomal enzyme induction, may inhibit the analgesic effect of aspirin and other salicylates.

CNS depressants [120,166]

Aspirin may have additive CNS depressant effects with CNS depressants. See *CNS Depressants*.

Chlorpropamide [120,633] (Diabinese)

In large doses salicylates may have an additive or synergistic effect with chlorpropamide in lowering the blood glucose level.

Clofibrate [28] (Atromid-S)

Clofibrate may interfere with the uricosuric action of salicylates.

Codeine [166]

Aspirin and codeine have a supra-additive analgesic effect and possibly additive CNS depressant effect.

Corticosteroids [421,618]

Both salicylates and corticosteroids have an ulcerogenic effect on the gastrointestinal mucosa (additive effect and increased danger of ulceration). Corticosteroids may increase the clearance rate of salicylates and withdrawal of the steroids with continued salicylate medication may lead to signs of salicylate intoxication. Salicylates potentiate the anti-inflammatory action of corticosteroids due to their ability to displace the steroids from their plasma protein binding sites and thus allow their more ready dispersal into tissues.

Dicumarol

See *Anticoagulants, Oral* above.

Fenoprofen [1761] (Nalfon)

Do not prescribe fenoprofen to patients in whom aspirin induces symptoms of asthma, rhinitis, or urticaria because of potential cross-hypersensitivity. Avoid drugs where these effects may be additive. Also, salicylates inhibit fenoprofen by decreasing its plasma half-life.

Flufenamic acid [120] (Arlef)

Aspirin inhibits the anti-inflammatory effect of flufenamic acid.

Furosemide [120] (Lasix)

Patients receiving high doses of salicylates in conjunction with furosemide may experience salicylate toxicity because of competition for renal excretory sites.

Folic acid antagonists

See *Methotrexate* below.

Heparin [1322,1661]

In patients receiving heparin, avoid use of aspirin which reduces platelet function and increases hemorrhagic potential, especially in thrombocytopenia. Substitution of another analgesic and antipyretic such as acetaminophen is recommended.

Imipramine [48] (Tofranil)

See *Antidepressants, Tricyclic* above. A very hazardous, potentially lethal combination.

Indomethacin [120,708,1284,1583,1761,1920] (Indocin)

Both salicylates and indomethacin have an ulcerogenic effect on the gastric mucosa and their combined use may therefore be especially dangerous, even fatal. Aspirin interferes with the gastrointestinal absorption of indomethacin, increases its fecal excretion, and decreases its anti-inflammatory action. No interaction occurs if aspirin is given orally and indomethacin is given rectally.

Insulin [421]

Salicylates enhance the hypoglycemic effect of insulin.

6-Mercaptopurine [470] (Purinethol)

Salicylates (aspirin) potentiate 6-mercaptopurine, probably by displacing it from secondary binding sites, and thus may induce pancytopenia. Very hazardous.

Methotrexate [197,198,330,421,512,633]

Salicylates potentiate the antineoplastic, antipsoriatic, and toxic effects of methotrexate through displacement from albumin binding sites and blocking of metabolism. Severe blood dyscrasias including pancytopenia have resulted and the interaction may be lethal.

Methotrimeprazine [120] (Levoprome)

Additive analgesic effects; dose of one or both agents may have to be reduced.

Naproxen [1778] (Naprosyn, Naxen)

Aspirin depresses naproxen plasma levels slightly, probably through competition for plasma protein binding sites and enhanced urinary excretion.

Oxyphenbutazone (Tandearil)

See *Phenylbutazone* below.

Penicillins [198,421]

Salicylates potentiate the anti-infective effect of penicillins by displacing them from protein binding sites.

Phenistix

Salicylates give a false PKU test with phenistix. For other clinical laboratory test interferences see Chapter 7.

Phenobarbital [83,198,275,421]
Phenobarbital inhibits the analgesic effects of salicylates due to enzyme induction.

Phenothiazines [120,166]
See *CNS Depressants* above and under main heading.

Phenylbutazone [28,120,359,614,1244] **(Butazolidin)**
Urate retention (hyperuricemia) may be produced by this combination. Phenylbutazone appears to compete successfully against urate and salicylate for tubular secretion and salicylate competes with phenylbutazone for plasma protein binding sites. This combination of drugs produces mutual suppression of uricosuric action and aspirin inhibits the anti-inflammatory effect of phenylbutazone. Combined use should be avoided or very carefully monitored because of the increased danger of gastrointestinal ulceration. Both drugs are ulcerogenic.

Phenytoin [652]
Large doses of aspirin have been reported to potentiate the effect of phenytoin, perhaps through displacement of the anticonvulsant from secondary binding sites.

Prednisolone and prednisone
See *Corticosteroids* above.

Probenecid [48,120,174,198,650,1244,1695,1750,1811] **(Benemid)**
Probenecid potentiates salicylates by inhibiting their renal tubular transport. But salicylates inhibit the uricosuric activity of probenecid through competition for plasma protein binding sites. Avoid this combination.

Propoxyphene [120,166] **(Darvon, etc.)**
The combination of aspirin plus Darvon appears to have synergistic analgesic effects.

Propranolol [586] **(Inderal)**
β-Adrenergic blocking agents like propranolol inhibit or abolish the anti-inflammatory effect of salicylates.

Pyrazolone derivatives [467,614]
(Anturane, Butazolidin, Tandearil)
Same effect for these drugs as for *Phenylbutazone* above.

Reserpine [951]
Reserpine inhibits analgesic activity of salicylates.

Spironolactone (Aldactone)
Spironolactone effects (diuresis and reduction of edema and of hypertension by blocking the sodium-retaining action of aldosterone on the distal convoluted tubule of the nephron) may be reversed by large doses of salicylates. See *Salicylates* under *Spironolactone*.

Sulfamethoxypyridazine [433] **(Kynex)**
See *Sulfonamides* below.

Sulfinpyrazone [120,421,467,651] **(Anturane)**
Salicylates inhibit the uricosuric activity of sulfinpyrazone. Same precautions as those given for *Phenylbutazone* above.

Sulfonamides [21,83,198,421]
Salicylates enhance the antibacterial activity and increase the toxicity of sulfonamides. Highly bound agents such as salicylic acid are able to displace the albumin bound sulfonamides from plasma protein. The long-lasting sulfas like sulfamethoxypyridazine that are not rapidly metabolized or excreted diffuse from plasma into tissues with increased antibacterial activity and possibly enhanced toxicity.

Sulfonylureas [3,141,166,197,418,421,646,649]
(Diabinese, Dymelor, Orinase, Tolinase etc.)
Salicylates potentiate these hypoglycemics by displacing them from secondary binding sites, possibly by inhibiting their metabolism, and by an additive hypoglycemic effect. Large doses of salicylates in certain individuals may have an antagonistic effect because they cause hyperglycemia and glycosuria by reducing aerobic metabolism of glucose and

by depleting liver and muscle glycogen through release of epinephrine induced by activation of hypothalamic sympathetic centers. However, in diabetic patients, salicylates, the first oral antidiabetic agents, have a hypoglycemic effect by increasing utilization of glucose by peripheral tissues in addition to the above potentiating effects. In such patients potentiation occurs (hypoglycemia) due to an additive effect.

Tobutamide (Orinase)
See *Sulfonylureas* above.

Uricosuric agents [28,120,467,651]
Salicylates inhibit the uricosuric action of some agents (sulfinpyrazone, other pyrazolons).

Vitamin C
See *Ascorbic Acid* above.

Warfarin (Coumadin)
See *Sulfonylureas* above.

SALICYLATES, BUFFERED

Alcohol [645]
Buffering reduces gastric hemorrhage from alcohol and salicylate.

SALICYLIC ACID
Same as for *Salicylates* above.

SALPHENYL
See *Acetaminophen, Antihistamines* (chlorpheniramine), *Salicylates* (salicylamide), and *Sympathomimetics* (phenylephrine).

SALRIN
See *Salicylates* (salicylamide).

SALURON
See *Thiazide Diuretics* (hydroflumethiazide).

SALUTENSIN
See *Reserpine, Thiazide Diuretics* (hydroflumethiazide), and *Veratrum Alkaloids* (protoveratrine A)

SANDOPTAL
See *Barbiturates* (butalbital)

SANDRIL
See *Reserpine*.

SANSERT
See *Methysergide*.

SANTONIN
See *Hexylresorcinol*.

SARCOLYSINE
See *Antineoplastics* (merphalan).

SAROXIN
See *Digitalis* (digoxin).

SCOLAMINE
See *Hyoscine*.

SCOPOLAMINE
See *Hyoscine* and *Solanaceous Alkaloids*.

SCORPION VENOM

Levallorphan tartrate [120] **(Lorfan)**
Levallorphan tartrate enhances toxicity of scorpion venom.

Nalorphine [120] **(Nalline)**
Nalorphine enhances toxicity of scorpion venom.

Narcotic analgesics [421]
Narcotic analgesics enhance toxicity of scorpion venom.

SECOBARBITAL (Seconal)
See *Barbiturates.*

SECONAL
See *Barbiturates* (secobarbital).

SECO-SYNATAN
See *Amphetamines* (dextroamphetamine) and *Barbiturates* (secobarbital)

SEDATIVES AND HYPNOTICS
See the general classes such as *Anesthetics, Anticonvulsants, Antihistamines, Barbiturates, Bromides, Diazepine Derivatives, Parasympatholytics, Phenothiazines, Tranquilizers, Ureides,* etc. and the specific drugs such as *Alcohol, Chloral Hydrate, Chlordiazepoxide, Diazepam, Ethchlorvynol, Ethinamate, Glutethimide, Meprobamate, Methyprylon, Paraldehyde, Phenaglycodol, Propiomazine, Tybamate,* etc. See also *CNS Depressants.*

Sedatives that inhibit motor activity in modest doses are usually hypnotic when potentiated by a drug interaction or when given in larger doses. The drug interactions for sedatives and hypnotics are covered under the general classes, under certain of the individual drugs, and under the general heading of *CNS Depressants.* The major drug interactions caused by these drugs are (1) inhibition of the actions of other drugs by enzyme induction, *e.g.,* by barbiturates, chloral hydrate, and glutethimide, (2) additive CNS depression, and (3) potentiation of the action of other drugs by displacement from inactive binding sites, *e.g.,* chloral hydrate in some instances. Timing and net effects are important.

Alcohol [120,619,633]
Contraindicated. Additive CNS effects can seriously impair coordination and may be lethal due to depressed cardiac activity and respiratory failure.

Analgesics [619]
Inhibition by the *Enzyme Inducers* (see below). Potentiated CNS depressant effects. See *CNS Depressants.*

Anticoagulants, oral [198,421]
Inhibited by the *Enzyme Inducers* (see below), except that chloral hydrate potentiates. Its metabolite, trichloracetic acid, displaces the oral anticoagulants from inactive binding sites. See *Chloral Hydrate, Barbiturates,* etc. under *Anticoagulants, Oral.*

Antidepressants [166,421]
(Dibenzazepines, Aventyl, Elavil, Nardil, Sinequan, Tofranil)
Both the MAO inhibitor antidepressants and the tricyclic antidepressants potentiate the CNS depressant action of sedatives and hypnotics. Contraindicated. Potentially very hazardous.

Antidiabetics [78] (Diabinese, Dymelor, Orinase)
The sulfonylurea antidiabetics potentiate the sedatives and hypnotics by means of enzyme inhibition.

Antihistamines [619]
Antihistamines may increase the depth and duration of narcosis with sedatives and hypnotics, but there may eventually be mutual inhibition through enzyme induction by both the antihistamines and the *Enzyme Inducers* (see below). See *CNS Depressants.*

Anti-inflammatory agents [78,421]
Inhibition by the *Enzyme Inducers* (see below).

Barbiturates [120,166,619]
Barbiturates initially potentiate the CNS depressant effects of other sedatives, but later, by enzyme induction, tend to inhibit and induce tolerance. Respiratory depression may be severe initially. See *CNS Depressants.*

Benzodiazepines [421] (Librium, Serax, Valium)
Inhibition by the *Enzyme Inducers* (see below). See *CNS Depressants.*

Chlorpromazine [120,166] (Thorazine)
Potentiation (additive CNS depression) with analgesics, sedatives, hypnotics, etc. See *CNS Depressants.*

Chlorpropamide [120] (Diabinese)
Chlorpropamide may prolong the sedative or hypnotic effect.

Chlorprothixene [120,166] (Taractan)
Same as for *Phenothiazines* below.

CNS depressants
Other CNS depressants may have an additive or superadditive effect. See *CNS Depressants.* Also see *Barbiturates* and *Antihistamines* above and *Enzyme Inducers* below.

Corticosteroids [198,421]
Inhibition by the *Enzyme Inducers* (see below). Some sedatives and hypnotics inhibit corticosteroids. Corticosteroids potentiate sedatives and hypnotics.

Enzyme Inducers [166]
(Barbiturates, chloral hydrate, glutethimide, etc.)
These agents affect the activity of a large number of other drugs by inducing the microsomal drug metabolizing enzymes and thus increasing the rate of metabolism of the other drugs. When the metabolites are less active, enzyme induction inhibits the drug action. When the metabolites are more active, enzyme induction potentiates the drug action. Induction of their own metabolizing enzymes leads to tolerance.

Furazolidone (Furoxone)
See *MAO inhibitors* below.

Glutethimide [78,120] (Doriden)
See *Enzyme Inducers* above. Also possible additive CNS depressant effects.

Griseofulvin [198,421] (Grifulvin)
Inhibition of griseofulvin by the *Enzyme Inducers* above.

Haloperidol [120] (Halodol)
Potentiation (additive effects). See *CNS Depressants.*

Hypnotics [198]
Inhibition of other hypnotics by the *Enzyme Inducers* above. Potentiation with other sedatives (additive effects). See *CNS Depressants.*

Hypotensives [198]
Mutual potentiation.

Insecticides, chlorinated [83,485,1053]
These insecticides inhibit barbiturates, etc. by enzyme induction.

Isoniazid [330]
Isoniazid potentiates sedatives (enzyme inhibition).

MAO inhibitors [120,330,421]
MAO inhibitors potentiate sedatives and hypnotics by enzyme inhibition. May be hazardous.

Mechlorethamine [120] (Mustargen)
Chlorpromazine, alone or with barbiturates, given prior to mechlorethamine helps control any nausea and vomiting it causes.

Mephenesin [120,166] (Tolserol, etc.)
Mephenesin and sedatives taken concomitantly may cause deep sedation and respiratory depression. See *CNS depressants.*

Meprobamate [166] (Equanil, Miltown)
Inhibition by the *Enzyme Inducers* above. Potentiation with other sedatives (additive effects). See *CNS Depressants.*

Narcotic analgesics [120,166]
Potentiation (additive effects). See *CNS Depressants.*

Phenothiazines [120,166,421]
Inhibition by the *Enzyme Inducers* above. Potentiation with other sedatives (additive effects). See also *Antihistamines* above.

Phenytoin (Dilantin)
Inhibition by the *Enzyme Inducers* (see above).

Pyrazolone derivatives [198,330]
(Butazolidin, Tandearil, etc.)
Inhibition by the *Enzyme Inducers* (see above).

Sedatives and hypnotics [120,166]
The group of *Enzyme Inducers* (see above) antagonize themselves and each other. This leads to tolerance. Additive CNS depression may be produced with combinations of sedatives and hypnotics. See *CNS Depressants.*

SEMETS NASAL SPRAY
See *Antihistamines* (pheniramine maleate) and *Sympathomimetics* (phenylephrine).

SEMIKON
See *Antihistamines* (methapyrilene HCl).

SEMOXYDRINE
See *Amphetamines* (methamphetamine HCl).

SENNA (Senakot)
See *Cathartics.*

SEPTRA
See *Sulfonamides* (sulfamethoxazole) and *Trimethoprim.*

SER-AP-ES
See *Hydralazine, Reserpine,* and *Thiazide Diuretics* (hydrochlorothiazide).

SERAX
See *Tranquilizers* (oxazepam).

SERC
See *Betahistine.*

SERENTIL
See *Tranquilizers* (mesoridazine).

SERFIN
See *Reserpine.*

SEROMYCIN
See *Cycloserine.*

SEROTONIN

Methylphenidate [853] **(Ritalin)**
Methylphenidate potentiates blood pressure response to serotonin.

SERPASIL
See *Reserpine.*

SERPASIL-APRESOLINE
See *Hydralazine* and *Reserpine.*

SERPASIL-ESIDRIX
See *Reserpine* and *Thiazide Diuretics* (hydrochlorothiazide).

SERPILOID
See *Reserpine.*

SILAIN-GEL
See *Alkalinizing Agents* (aluminum hydroxide and magnesium carbonate).

SINGOSERP
See *Antihypertensives* (syrosingopine).

SINOGRAFIN
See *Radiopaque Media* (meglumine diatrizoate and meglumine iodipamide).

SINTROM
See *Anticoagulants, Oral* (acenocoumarol).

SINUTAB
See *Acetaminophen* and *Sympathomimetics* (phenylpropanolamine).

Phenelzine [1976] **(Nardil)**
A single Sinutab in a patient taking the MAO inhibitor phenelzine produced an irregular pulse and palpitation (atrioventricular Wenckebach phenomenon). The pulse rate was 40 on admission to the hospital.

SITOSTEROLS

Anticoagulants, oral [330,619,910]
Sitosterols and other cholesterol-lowering agents may potentiate anticoagulants by interfering with vitamin K transport to the liver.

Blood cholesterol lowering agents [421]
Sitosterols potentiate blood cholesterol lowering agents.

Clofibrate [421] **(Atromid-S)**
Sitosterols potentiate clofibrate.

SKELAXIN TABLETS
See *Metaxalone.*

SKELETAL MUSCLE RELAXANTS
See *Muscle Relaxants, Centrally Acting.*

SKF 525-A
(Proadifen; β-dimethylaminoethyl diphenylpentanoate HCl)
Proadifen is the most extensively studied inhibitor of drug metabolism. It competitively or noncompetitively interferes with the binding of substrates to and the reduction of cytochrome P-450. It prolongs the action of other drugs by inhibiting their inactivation or decreasing the effects of active metabolites.

Barbiturates [65]
Proadifen prolongs the sedative effect of barbiturates by enzyme inhibition initially. See *Hexobarbital* below.

Hexobarbital [65] **(Sombucaps)**
SKF 525-A and some other enzyme inhibitors inhibit the metabolism of certain drugs initially but when administered chronically induce the metabolizing enzymes. Thus SKF 525-A at first potentiates the hypnotic action of hexobarbital and then with chronic administration drastically reduced this action.

Phenytoin [391]
SKF 525-A, by inhibiting microsomal enzymes, potentiates phenytoin.

SLEEPING PILLS
See page 308.
Sleeping pills such as Compoz and Sominex which are sold freely without a prescription may enter into many drug reactions with prescribed medications due to their content of antihistamines, anticholinergics and other drugs. [78]

SMALLPOX VACCINE

Corticosteroids [120,619]
Corticosteroids affect immune response to smallpox vaccination. See *Vaccines.*

SMALLPOX VACCINE   *(continued)*

Indomethacin [1594]
This anti-inflammatory drug may increase the severity of reactions to smallpox vaccination, including production of hemorrhage.

Methotrexate
See *Immunosuppressants* under *Vaccines.*

X-radiation
See *X-radiation* under *Vaccines.*

SMOKING
(charcoal broiled meats, tobacco smoke, etc.)

Anticoagulants, oral [633]
Same as for *Barbiturates* below.

Antipyrine [2037]
Antipyrine half-life is significantly shorter in smokers than in nonsmokers. The mean disappearance rate of the drug in one group increased by 23%. Cigarette smoking contributes to the large variation in rates of drug metabolism among individuals.

Barbiturates [78, 1093]
Tobacco smoke contains the environmental carcinogen benzpyrene which is also an enzyme inducer in the gastrointestinal tract as well as in the hepatic microsomes. Smoking therefore can inhibit the action of barbiturates and other medications, possibly at times so intensely that the drugs may exert little systemic effect. The same is true for charcoal broiled meats, coal tar, etc.

Oral contraceptives [862]
Smoking may increase the probability of thromboembolism in individuals taking oral contraceptives. Smoking markedly increases the risk of experiencing serious cardiovascular side effects from OC use, especially in women over 35 years of age. Women who use OCs should not smoke. [120]

Pentazocine [1054] (Talwin)
Higher dosage of pentazocine is required in about 60% of city dwellers or smokers because of enzyme inducing pollutants in the tobacco smoke and city atmosphere.

Phenacetin [2043]
Feeding charcoal-broiled beef (contains benzopyrene and other enzyme inducing hydrocarbons) to humans for as long as 4 days resulted in a 59 to 82% decrease in the mean concentrations of phenacetin in the plasma from 1-7 hours after the drug was given.

Propranolol [587]
Combined use of nicotine and propranolol may considerably increase the blood pressure. See under *Propranolol.*

SOAP

Acrisorcin [120] (Akrinol)
Soap should be completely removed after bathing from the area of application since it can considerably reduce the antifungal activity of acrisorcin against *Malassezia furfur* in tinea versicolor.

SODA LIME

Trichloroethylene [184] (Trilene)
Death has occurred due to phosgene formation during anesthesia.

SODIUM ACID PHOSPHATE
See *Urinary Acidifiers.*

SODIUM BICARBONATE
See *Alkalinizing Agents.*

Amphetamines
See *Alkalinizing Agents* under *Amphetamines.*

Barbiturates [161]
Sodium bicarbonate elevates pH, ionizes barbiturates, and thereby decreases their effectiveness by decreasing gastrointestinal absorption and increasing urinary excretion.

Calcium salts (chloride, glucoheptonate, etc.)
Incompatible in IV solutions. See Chapter 8.

Cephalothin (Keflin)
Incompatible in IV solutions. See Chapter 8.

Chlorpromazine (Thorazine)
Incompatible in IV solutions. See Chapter 8.

Codeine
Incompatible in IV solutions. See Chapter 8.

Dextrose solutions
Incompatible in IV solutions. See Chapter 8.

Hydromorphone
Incompatible in IV solutions. See Chapter 8.

Lactated Ringer's solution
Incompatible in IV solutions. See Chapter 8.

Lithium carbonate (Eskalith, Lithane, Lithonate)
See *Sodium Bicarbonate* under *Lithium Carbonate.*

Mecamylamine [325, 529, 726, 870]
Sodium bicarbonate as an alkalinizing agent potentiates mecamylamine by elevating pH and thereby increasing absorption and decreasing urinary excretion.

Methenamine
See *Alkalinizing Agents* under *Methenamine.*

Milk [61, 1085]
Prolonged intake of combination of milk and absorbable alkali (sodium bicarbonate) produces hypercalcemia, renal insufficiency with azotemia, alkalosis, and an ocular lesion resembling band keratitis. Antacids such as aluminum hydroxide and aluminum phosphate gels do not cause this problem, but calcium salts may induce a similar condition.

Oxytetracycline (Terramycin)
Incompatible in IV solutions. See Chapter 8. Also see *Bicarbonate of Soda* under *Tetracyclines.*

Phenobarbital [161]
Administration of sodium bicarbonate with phenobarbital decreases the sedative effects by decreasing gastrointestinal absorption and increasing urinary excretion.

Quinidine
See *Alkalinizing Agents* under *Quinidine.*

Tetracycline [472]
See *Bicarbonate of Soda* under *Tetracyclines.*

SODIUM BIPHOSPHATE
See *Urinary Acidifiers.*

SODIUM CHLORIDE

Lithium carbonate
See *Sodium Chloride* under *Lithium Carbonate.*

SODIUM CITRATE
See *Neuromuscular Blocking Antibiotics* under *Antibiotics.*

SODIUM DIATRIZOATE
See *Radiopaque Media.*

SODIUM NITROPRUSSIDE

Tolbutamide
See *Sodium Nitroprusside* under *Tolbutamide.*

SODIUM POLYSTYRENE SULFONATE (Kayexalate)

Antacids, oral
See *Sodium Polystyrene Sulfonate* under *Antacids*.

SODIUM SALTS
See *Sodium Salts* under *Diuretics*.

SODIUM THIOSULFATE

Mechlorethamine (Mustargen) [619]
A 2% solution of sodium thiosulfate neutralizes the vesicant effect of mechlorethamine on dermatomucosal surfaces.

SODIZOLE
See *Sulfonamides* (sulfisoxazole).

SOLANACEOUS ALKALOIDS
(Atropine [*dl*-hyoscyamine], hyoscine [scopolamine], and *l*-hyoscyamine)
These drugs are cholinergic blocking (antimuscarinic) agents which produce respiratory stimulation, selective sedation, and antagonism of anticholinesterases. They also depress smooth muscle (decreased gastrointestinal motility, mydriasis, loss of accommodation, bronchial and biliary dilatation, urinary retention, and tachycardia) and inhibit secretory glands (dryness of mucous membranes, decreased sweating.) [168,303]
The drug interactions of this group of alkaloids are in general those of the *Anticholinergics*. See also *Hyoscine* and *Atropine*. Drug interactions either potentiate or inhibit the actions and effects given above.

SOMA
See *Muscle Relaxants, Centrally Acting* (carisoprodol).

SOMBUCAPS
See *Barbiturates* (hexobarbital) and *CNS Depressants*.

SOMBULEX
See *Barbiturates* (hexobarbital) and *CNS Depressants*.

SOMINEX
See *Sleeping Pills* and page 308.

SOMNOS
See *Chloral Hydrate* and *CNS Depressants*.

SONILYN
See *Sulfonamides* (sulfachlorpyridazine).

SOPOR
See *CNS Depressants* (methaqualone).

SORBITOL

Acetaminophen [359] **(Paracetamol)**
The absorption of acetaminophen is accelerated in the presence of sorbitol. See *Polysorbate 80* and *Sorbitol* under *Acetaminophen*.

Phenacetin [359]
The absorption of phenacetin is accelerated in the presence of sorbitol.

SOY BEAN PREPARATIONS

Thyroid [48]
Use caution in patients taking thyroid medication as soy bean products are apparently goitrogenic.

SPARINE
See *Phenothiazines* (promazine) and *Tranquilizers*.

SPARTEINE
See *Oxytocics*.

Oxytocin [951]
Synergistic oxytocic activity.

SPARTOCIN
See *Oxytocics* (sparteine).

SPIRONOLACTONE (Aldactone)

Ammonium chloride [1602]
Acidifying doses of ammonium chloride, given concomitantly with spironolactone, may induce systemic acidosis. Inhibition of aldosterone by this diuretic may inhibit hydrogen ion secretion by the kidneys and in edematous patients with renal insufficiency induce significant hyperkalemia. Monitor patients on this combination carefully for acidosis.

Anesthetics [120]
Exercise caution in the management of patients subjected to general or regional anesthesia; spironolactone reduces vascular responsiveness to norepinephrine.

Anticoagulants, oral [819] **(Dicumarol, etc.)**
Spironolactone inhibits anticoagulants like bishydroxycoumarin.

Antihypertensives [120,421]
(Hydralazine, mecamylamine, pentolinium, veratrum alkaloids, etc.)
Potentiation of hypotensive effect of other antihypertensive agents may occur with spironolactone. Reduce the dose of these agents, particularly the ganglionic blocking agents, at least 50%.

Antipyrine [1493,1847]
Spironolactone may inhibit the activity of antipyrine through enzyme inducing activity.

Carbenoxolone [1329]
Spironolactone may inhibit the activity of carbenoxolone in healing gastric and duodenal ulcers. Avoid this combination if possible.

Clopamide [120] **(Aquex, Brinaldix)**
Clopamide, a diuretic, potentiates spironolactone (additive effect).

Digitalis glycosides [120,396] **((Digoxin, digitoxin)**
Spironolactone is a potassium-conserving diuretic; hyperkalemia may lead to decreased effectiveness of digitalis and interfere with digitalization. (Note that severe hyperkalemia in the presence of renal impairment has caused death.) Spironolactone counteracts digitalis glycoside toxicity by competitive inhibition of aldosterone. A potent antidote. Often given together to cardiac patients, but special monitoring of electrolyte balance is essential.

Diuretics, other [120,172]
Spironolactone is frequently combined with a thiazide or mercurial diuretic to reduce potassium loss caused by the other diuretics and to obtain an additive and more prompt effects. However, hyponatremia may be caused or aggravated by such combinations (drowsiness, dry mouth, lethargy, thirst). Sometimes glucocorticoids are also added as a third component of the regimen to increase the glomerular filtration rate.

Ganglionic blocking agents
See *Antihypertensives* above.

Hydralazine [421] **(Apresoline)**
Spironolactone potentiates the hypotensive effect of hydralazine. See *Antihypertensives* above.

Hydrochlorothiazide [433] **(Hydrodiuril)**
Combination of spironolactone and thiazides facilitates management of hypertension. The two drugs act independently and additively in their antihypertensive effect.

Hypotensive agents
See *Antihypertensives* above.

Levarterenol (Norepinephrine)
See under *Anesthetics* above.

SPIRONOLACTONE (Aldactone) *(continued)*

Mecamylamine (Inversine)
See *Antihypertensives* above.

Mercury salts[1120]
See *Toxic Drugs* below.

Pentolinium (Ansolysen)
See *Antihypertensives* above.

Potassium salts[330,1460,1522,1602,1788]
Spironolactone, a potassium conserver, increases the hyperkalemia produced by potassium salts, especially in patients with impaired renal function. Caution must be exercised as this interaction produces acidosis and has been lethal. Monitor closely.

Salicylates[951,1197,1393,1488,1868]
Salicylates in large doses, may reverse the therapeutic effect of spironolactone (inhibits sodium excretion by the aldosterone antagonist). Possibly salicylate displaces spironolactone from receptor sites where it has acted as a competitive antagonist of aldosterone.

Toxic drugs[1120]
Spironolactone, by enzyme induction and other mechanism, protects rats against intoxication with various drugs, including anesthetics, digitoxin, indomethacin, and mercuric chloride.

Triamterene[120,226] **(Dyrenium)**
Hazardous hyperkalemia may result with spironolactone and triamterene in combination.

Veratrum alkaloids
See *Antihypertensives* above.

SPIRONOLACTONE HYDROCHLORO-THIAZIDE (Aldactazide)
See also *Spironolactone* above.

Furosemide[443] **(Lasix)**
This combination may produce severe electrolyte imbalance.

STANOZOLOL (Winstrol)
See *Anabolic Agents*.

Anticoagulants, oral
See *Stanozolol* under *Anticoagulants, Oral.*

STANZAMINE
See *Antihistamines* (tripelennamine).

STAPHCILLIN
See *Penicillins* (methicillin).

STATUSS
See *Antihistamines* (chlorpheniramine).

STECLIN
See *Tetracyclines.*

STELAZINE
See *Phenothiazines* (trifluoperazine) and *Tranquilizers.*

STENTAL
See *Barbiturates* (phenobarbital).

STEPS
See *Nitrates* and *Nitrites* (pentaerythritol tetranitrate).

Other nitrates, nitrites[120]
Tolerance to this drug, and cross-tolerance to other nitrites and nitrates may occur.

STERANE
See *Prednisolone.*

STERAZOLIDIN
See *Phenylbutazone.*

STEROIDS (Desoxycortisterone, estradiol, steroid hormones, testosterone, etc.)
See *Anabolic Agents, Corticosteroids, Estrogens,* etc.

Enzyme inducers[65] **(chlorcyclizine, phenytoin, phenobarbital, phenybutazone, etc.)**
Enzyme inducers stimulate hydroxylation of the steroids in the liver and decrease their effectiveness.

STEROIDS, OVARIAN

Barbiturates[257,617]
Because of the resulting acceleration of the metabolism of ovarian steroids, administration of barbiturates to some patients may be contraindicated.

Chloral hydrate[198]
Steroids are inhibited by chloral hydrate (enzyme induction).

STEROLONE
See *Prednisolone.*

STIMAHIST
See *Antihistamines* (chlorpheniramine).

STOXIL
See *Antiviral Agents* (iodoxuridine).

STRASCOGESIC
See *Acetaminophen, Amphetamines* (raphetamine), *Atropine* (metropine), and *Salicylates* (salicylamide).

STREPTOKINASE-STREPTODORNASE (Varidase)

Anticoagulants, oral[120]
Streptokinase IM enhances fibrinolytic activity and thus may potentiate anticoagulants.

Antibiotics[120]
Streptokinase IM should be accompanied by administration of a broad-spectrum antibiotic.

STREPTOMYCIN
See *Aminoglycoside Antibiotics,* also *Neuromuscular Blocking Antibiotics* under *Antibiotics.*

Alcuronium chloride[432]
Streptomycins potentiate this muscle relaxant.

Alkalinizing agents[578]
Alkaline urinary pH potentiates streptomycin; alkalinization is probably only necessary when streptomycin is used to treat urinary tract infections caused by *E. coli* and *Proteus* organisms.

p-Aminosalicylic acid[181] **(PAS)**
PAS activity against the tubercle bacillus is potentiated.

Amobarbital[360]
Streptomycin in combination with amobarbital may produce apnea and muscle weakness because of enhanced neuromuscular blockade due to the antibiotic.

Ampicillin[210,492]
Streptomycin potentiates the bactercidal activity of ampicillin against *Enterococci.*

Anesthetics[37,226,500,505,561]
Neuromuscular paralysis with respiratory depression may occur when streptomycin is administered concurrently with anesthetics; streptomycin should not be administered until the patient has fully recovered from the effects of the anesthetic.

Antibiotics[120]
See *Antibiotics, Ototoxic* and *Neuromuscular Blocking* under *Neomycin.*

Anticholinesterases [421]
Anticholinesterases antagonize the neuromuscular blocking effects of streptomycin.

Calcium [178]
Calcium may reduce neuromuscular blockade produced by streptomycin.

Cephalothin [252,253] **(Keflin)**
Synergistic activity against *Str. viridans* and *Str. faecalis.*

Chloramphenicol [178] **(Chloromycetin)**
This combination is effective against *K. penumoniae* in biliary tract infection, osteomyelitis, pneumonia, and urinary tract infection.

Colistin [120,619] **(Colistimethate, Coly-Mycin)**
Both streptomycin and colistin can interfere with nerve transmission at the neuromuscular junction. Muscle weakness and apnea may occur. See *Neuromuscular Blocking Antibiotics* under *Antibiotics.*

Curare [421]
Streptomycin potentiates curare. See *Aminoglycoside Antibiotics* under *Muscle Relaxants, Peripherally Acting.*

Decamethonium [421]
Mutual potentiation of neuromuscular blockade. See *Muscle Relaxants* and *Neuromuscular Blocking Antibiotics* under *Antibiotics.*

Dimenhydrinate [120] **(Dramamine)**
Dimenhydrinate masks aural symptoms of streptomycin toxicity until they have reached a dangerous level. Caution.

Edrophonium [421]
Edrophonium antagonizes the neuromuscular blocking effect of streptomycin.

EDTA [360]
Streptomycin with EDTA may produce apnea and muscle weakness because of enhanced neuromuscular blockade.

Ethacrynic acid (Edecrin)
Ototoxicity potentiated. See *Aminoglycoside Antibiotics* under *Ethacrynic Acid.*

Erythromycin [178] **(Erythrocin, Ilotycin)**
This combination is effective against enterococcus in endocarditis.

Gallamine [330,654]
Streptomycin potentiates neuromuscular blockade by gallamine; prolonged paralysis of respiratory muscles may occur.

Isoniazid [120]
Synergistic activity against the tubercle bacillus.

Kanamycin [120]
Ototoxicity. Cumulative effect. See *Ototoxic Drugs* under *Kanamycin.*

Methoxyflurane (Penthrane)
See under *Methoxyflurane.*

Methylthymol blue [951]
Methylthymol blue potentiates the antibacterial activity of streptomycin against *Ps. aeruginosa.*

Muscle relaxants [146,421,432,502]
See *Muscle Relaxants* and *Neuromuscular Blocking Antibiotics* under *Antibiotics.*

Neomycin [178]
Ototoxicity. Cumulative effect. See *Aminoglycoside Antibiotics.*

Neostigmine [36,178]
Neostigmine in the presence of adequate ventilation reduces the neuromuscular blockade produced by the antibiotic (particularly intraperitoneally) with nondepolarizing muscle relaxants such as *d*-tubocurarine.

Organophosphate cholinesterase inhibitors [312,520]
These anticholinesterases antagonize the neuromuscular blocking effect of streptomycin.

Penicillin [178,210,233,239,492]
Streptomycin potentiates penicillin activity against enterococcus in urinary tract infections, endocarditis, bacteremia, brain abscess, and meningitis. See also *Antibiotics* under *Penicillins.*

Polymyxin B [178]
See *Neuromuscular Blocking Antiobiotics* under *Antibiotics.*

Promethazine [360] **(Phenergan)**
Streptomycin in combination with promethazine may produce apnea and muscle weakness because of enhanced neuromuscular blockade.

Streptomycin [178]
Ototoxicity. Cumulative effect.

Procainamide [619]
Same as for *Quinidine* below.

Quinidine [447,559]
Quinidine may enhance the neuromusclar blocking effect of streptomycin and thus may induce apnea and muscle weakness.

Succinylcholine [421]
Contraindicated. Streptomycin potentiates the neuromuscular blockade produced by succinylcholine. See *Muscle Relaxants* and *Antibiotics.*

Tetracyclines [178,1106]
Synergistic activity in bacteremic brucellosis.

Tubocurarine [137,330,421,505,654-656]
Respiratory insufficiency, paralysis.

STRESS

Reserpine [120,619]
Sudden stress, such as electroshock therapy or surgery, may cause acute cardiovascular collapse in patients whose stores of catecholamines have been depleted by Rauwolfia therapy, and death may occur.

STRONTIUM SALTS

Tetracyclines [421]
Strontium forms a complex with all tetracyclines and thus inhibits their gastrointestinal absorption. See *Complexing Agents.*

STROPHANTHIN
See *Cardiac Glycosides.*

SUCARYL
See *Cyclamates.*

SUCCINYLCHOLINE
See *Muscle Relaxants, Peripherally Acting, Depolarizing.*

MAO inhibitors
See *Succinylcholine* under *MAO Inhibitors.*

Pantothenic acid
See *Succinylcholine* under *Pantothenic Acid.*

SUCCINYLSULFATHIAZOLE
See *Sulfonamides.*

SUCOSTRIN
See *Muscle Relaxants* (succinylcholine chloride).

SUCROSE

Paromomycin [929]
Paromomycin causes malabsorption of sucrose.

SUDAFED
See *Ephedrine* and *Pseudoephedrine*.

SUGRACILLIN
See *Penicillins*.

SULFABID
See *Sulfonamides* (sulfaphenazole).

SULFACETAMIDE
See *Sulfonamides*.

SULFADIAZINE
See *Sulfonamides*.

SULFADIMETHOXINE (Madribon)
See *Sulfonamides*.

SULFADIMETINE (Elkosin)
See *Sulfonamides* (sulfisomidine).

SULFAETHIDOLE
(Sul-Spansion, Sul-Spantab)
See *Sulfonamides*.

SULFAETHYLTHIADIAZOLE
See *Sulfonamides* (sulfaethidole).

SULFAFURAZOLE (Gantrisin)
See *Sulfonamides* (sulfisoxazole).

    Colistin [951] **(Coly-Mycin)**
Synergistic bactercidal activity against *Proteus* species.

SULFAMERAZINE
See *Sulfonamides*.

SULFAMETER
See *Sulfonamides* (sulfametin).

SULFAMETHAZINE
See *Sulfonamides*.

SULFAMETHIZOLE
See *Sulfonamides*.

SULFAMETHOMIDINE
See *Sulfonamides*.

    Colistin [951]
Sulfamethomidine potentiates colistin activity against *P. vulgaris*.

SULFAMETHOXAZOLE (Gantanol)
See *Sulfonamides*.

SULFAMETHOXYDIAZINE (Sulla)
See *Sulfonamides* (sulfametin).

SULFAMETHOXYPYRIDAZINE (Kynex)
See *Sulfonamides*.

SULFAMETIN
See *Sulfonamides*.

SULFANILAMIDE
See *Sulfonamides*.

SULFAPHENAZOLE (Orisul, Sulfabid)
See *Sulfonamides*.

SULFAPYRIDINE
See *Sulfonamides*.

SULFASUXIDINE
See *Sulfonamides* (succinysulfathiazole).

SULFASYMAZINE
See *Sulfonamides*.

SULFATHALIDINE
See *Sulfonamides*.

SULFINPYRAZONE (Anturane)
Sulfinpyrazone, a pyrazolone derivative, is structurally related to aminopyrine, antipyrine, oxyphenbutazone, and phenylbutazone. Some of the drug reactions for these are similar or identical.

Alkalinizing agents [120,325,870]
Urinary alkalinizers are given with sulfinpyrazone to increase its solubility and thus to prevent urolithiasis and renal colic. But, elevation of pH decreases the activity of sulfinpyrazone.

Allopurinol [120] **(Zyloprim)**
See *Sulfinpyrazone* under *Allopurinol*.

Anticoagulants, oral
See *Sulfinpyrazone* under *Anticoagulants, oral*

Antidiabetics
See *Sulfinpyrazone* under *Antidiabetics, Oral*.

Aspirin and other salicylates [120,467,613,651]
See *Sulfinpyrazone* under *Salicylates*.

Citrates [120,421]
Citrates antagonize the uricosuric effect of sulfinpyrazone.

Insulin [120]
Sulfinpyrazone may potentiate the hypoglycemic effect of insulin.

Penicillins [267-269]
    (Cloxicillin, nafcillin, penicillin G, etc.)
Sulfinpyrazone may potentiate penicillin by displacement from protein binding sites.

Probenecid [28,931]
See *Sulfinpyrazone* under *Probenecid*

Salicylates [120,421,467,613,651] **(Aspirin, etc.)**
See *Sulfinpyrazone* and *Phenybutazone* under *Salicylates*.

Sulfamethoxypyridazine (Midicel)
See *Sulfonamides* below.

Sulfonamides [21,57,120,173,433,1217]
    (Gantrisin, Kynex, Sulfadiazine, etc.)
Sulfinpyrazone may potentiate the activity and toxicity of the sulfonamides by decreasing their renal excretion. Highly bound agents such as sulfinpyrazone are also able to displace the albumin-bound sulfonamides from plasma protein. The long-lasting sulfas, not rapidly metabolized or excreted, diffuse from plasma into the brain and other tissues with increased antibacterial activity and potential for toxic effects such as Stevens-Johnson syndrome.

Sulfonylureas [120,173,409]
    (Diabinese, Dymelor, Orinase, etc.)
Sulfinpyrazone potentiates the hypoglycemic action of the sulfonylureas.

Xanthines [421]
Xanthines inhibit the uricosuric activity of sulfinpyrazone.

SULFISOXAZOLE (Gantrisin, etc.)
See *Sulfonamides*.

SULFOBROMOPHTHALEIN
(Bromsulphalein, BSP)

Interfering drugs [120]
Procainamide increases BSP retention. Anabolic steroids, androgens, estrogens, and oral contraceptives interfere with BSP excretion. Amidone, MAO inhibitors, meperidine, and morphine give elevated readings. See Chapter 7.

SULFONAMIDES

Acenocoumarol [120,193] (Sintron)
Sulfonamides potentiate acenocoumarol. See *Anticoagulants, Oral* below.

Acetohexamide [120,173,330,409] (Dymelor)
See *Antidiabetics, Oral* below. Potentiation of the oral antidiabetic.

Acidifying agents [22,198,421,433,870]
(Ammonium chloride, ammonium nitrate)
Acidifying agents tend to enhance the gastrointestinal absorption and decrease the urinary excretion of weak acids like the sulfonamides. Thus the systemic activity and toxicity are potentiated, and prolonged. This may be hazardous if a severe reaction occurs. Also, lowering the pH of the urine with acidifying agents decreases the solubility of sulfonamides and tends to promote crystalluria.

Alcohol [121,202,399]
Sulfonamides potentiate the psychotoxic effects of alcohol by inhibiting oxidation of acetaldehyde (disulfiramlike reaction). Increases hazard of driving under the influence of alcohol.

Alkalinizing agents [22,28,198,325,633,870]
(Antacids, sodium bicarbonate, etc.)
Alkalinizing agents by increasing ionization of weakly acid sulfonamides tend to inhibit their gastrointestinal absorption and increase their urinary excretion. Thus the systemic activity and toxicity are decreased and shortened while the urinary levels are elevated and the urinary antibacterial activity enhanced. Elevating the pH of the urine with alkalinizing agents increases the solubility of the sulfonamides and tends to prevent crystalluria. See also *Alkalinizing Agents.*

p-Aminobenzoic acid [28,167,178,202,421,433,1211,1368] (PABA)
PABA and its analogs inhibit sulfonamides. Sulfonamides are effective antibacterials because they compete with PABA and prevent its normal utilization by microorganisms, thus an increased concentration of PABA decreases the activity of the sulfonamides. Local anesthethics that have a PABA nucleus exhibit the same effect. Procaine infiltration has resulted in local infection in spite of adequate sulfonamide dosage. Desirable to use local anesthetics without the PABA moiety (dibucaine, diperodon, lidocaine, etc.) when patients are on sulfonamides.

6-Aminonicotinamide [951]
These drugs act synergistically as teratogens in test animals.

p-Aminosalicylic acid [421] (PAS)
Aminosalicylic acid antagonizes the antibacterial action of sulfonamides.

Ammonium chloride
See *Acidifying Agents* above.

Ammonium nitrate
See *Acidifying Agents* above.

Ampicillin (Alpen, Omnipen, Polycillin, etc.)
See *Penicillins* below.

Analgesics [21,198]
Analgesics (oxyphenbutazone, phenybutazone, salicylates) potentiate sulfonamides through displacement of the sulfonamides from secondary binding sites. Both effectiveness and toxicity of the sulfonamides may be increased.

Anesthetics, local [28,167,178,202,433,1211,1368]
Local anesthetics which are derivatives of PABA inhibit sulfonamides. See *p-Aminobenzoic Acid* above.

Antacids [176,470]
See *Alkalinizing Agents* above. Note that some antacids are not alklalinizers systemically, notably the aluminum hydroxide compounds. Also repeated use of sodium bicarbonate and other alkalies stimulates gastric HCl output.

Antibiotics
See *Colistin* and *Penicillins* below.

Anticoagulants, oral [21,78,120,193,198,421,633,647,1974]
(Coumadin, Dicumarol, Tromexan, etc.)
Sulfonamides potentiate some anticoagulants and highly bound agents such as ethyl biscoumacetate displace sulfonamides from plasma protein (increased antibacterial activity and toxicity). See *Sulfonamides* under *Anticoagulants, Oral.*

Antidiabetics, oral [198,202,330,409,421,619,633]
(Diabinese, Dymelor, Orinase, etc.)
Sulfonamides potentiate oral antidiabetics. Hypoglycemic shock may occur. Sulfaphenazole increased the half-life of tolbutamide from 5 to 21½ hours and induced a large increase in free tolbutamide because of high affinity for the albumin binding sites in the plasma. Oral antidiabetics may improve the antibacterial action of sulfonamides.

Antipyretics [198]
Same as for *Analgesics* above.

Ascorbic acid [274,531,870]
Sulfonamides increase the excretion of ascorbic acid (inhibition of the vitamin). Ascorbic acid decreases excretion of sulfonamides (potentiation of the antimicrobials). The acidified urine increases the potential for crystalluria with the antimicrobials.

Barbiturates [1309,1310,1770]
Some barbiturates may be displaced from plasma protein binding sites by some sulfonamides. Thus less thiopental (Pentothal) was required for anesthesia when sulfisoxazole (Gantrisin) was given concomitantly. Phenobarbital may increase the biliary and decrease urinary excretion of salicylazosulfapyridine (Azulfidine) which is bacterially cleaved in the colon to *m*-aminosalicylic acid and sulfapyridine. Phenobarbital increases hydroxylation and decreases acetylation of the latter drug. Thus serum and urine levels of Azulfidine are affected by the barbiturate.

Bishydroxycoumarin (Dicumarol)
See *Anticoagulants, Oral* above.

Chlorpropamide (Diabinese)
See *Antidiabetics, Oral* above.

Cloxacillin (Tegopen)
See *Penicillins* below.

Colistin [883,1107] (Coly-Mycin)
Synergistic antibacterial activity against some organisms (*Proteus* and *Pseudomonas*).

Coumarin anticoagulants
See *Anticoagulants, Oral* above.

Dibucaine (Nupercaine)
See *p-Aminobenzoic Acid* above.

Dicloxacillin (Dynapen, Pathocil, Veracillin)
See *Penicillins* below.

Dicumarol
See *Anticoagulants, Oral* above.

Ethyl biscoumacetate [202] (Tromexan)
See *Anticoagulants, Oral* above.

Folic acid antagonists [421]
Sulfonamides potentiate folic acid antagonists. See *Methotrexate* below.

Furosemide [120] (Lasix)
Cross-sensitivity with other sulfonamides may occur.

Insulin [120]
Some sulfonamides may enhance the hypoglycemic effect of insulin.

SULFONAMIDES *(continued)*

Iophenoxic acid [21,202,359] (Teridax)
Highly bound agents such as iophenoxic acid are able to displace the long-lasting, albumin-bound sulfonamides from plasma protein. These sulfas are not rapidly metabolized or excreted. Thus displaced molecules diffuse from plasma into tissues with increased antibacterial activity and toxicity.

Isoniazid [443] (Niconyl, Nydrazide, etc.)
Combined use may give rise to an untoward drug interaction causing acute, hemolytic anemia.

Lidocaine (Xylocaine)
See *p-Aminobenzoic Acid* above.

6-Mercaptopurine [470] (Purinethol)
Sulfonamides potentiate 6-mercaptopurine and induce pancytopenia.

Methenamine [28,280,433,662] (Methenamine mandelate, etc.)
With this combination renal blockade may occur. Formaldehyde, liberated from methenamine in the urine, forms an insoluble precipitate with sulfonamides.

Methicillin (Staphcillin)
See *Penicillins* below.

Methotrexate [120,202,330,421,512,633,1581]
Methotrexate displacement from plasma protein by sulfonamides (including not only anti-infective ones but also sulfonylurea oral antihyperglycemics, thiazide diuretics, etc. with a sulfonamide moiety) may lead to serious toxic reactions: anorexia, weight loss, bloody diarrhea, leukopenia, pancytopenia and coma; symptomatic of fatal intoxication with this antineoplastic agent. Some sulfonamides may also inhibit renal tubular secretion of methotrexate. Use extreme caution with this potentially highly toxic combination.

Mineral oil [120,178,421]
Mineral oil inhibits the antibacterial action of sulfonamides in GI tract infections, probably by mechanically segregating the anti-infectives sulfas that are nonabsorbable.

Oxacillin [267-269] (Prostaphlin)
See *Penicillins* below.

Oxyphenbutazone [21,359,433] (Tandearil)
The antibacterial activity of sulfonamide may be enhanced by oxyphenbutazone. See *Analgesics* above.

Paraldehyde [433,1211,1465]
Paraldehyde may inhibit the antibacterial activity of sulfonamides due to enzyme induction. Also, paraldehyde can provide a moiety which can be used in acetylation of sulfonamides and thus increase danger of crystalluria. The more recently marketed sulfonamides are much more soluble than some of the earlier ones which have been removed from the U.S. market and crystalluria seldom occurs.

Penicillins [267-269,433] (Alpen, Dynapen, Omnipen, Pathocil, Penicillin G, O, or V, Polycillin, Prostaphlin, Tegopen, Viracillin, etc. and their salts)
Combination may have effect of being additive, indifferent, or inhibitory, depending on the sulfonamide and the penicillin. Sulfonamides, *e.g.*, sulfamethoxypyridazine, may lower the serum concentration of total penicillin but increase the concentration of unbound, antimicrobially active drug in serum and body fluids. Relatively large doses of sulfonamides can reduce the protein binding of penicillins and thus potentiate them.

Phenylbutazone [21,78,198,202,359] (Butazolidin)
Phenylbutazone potentiates sulfonamides by displacement from protein binding sites. See *Analgesics* above.

Phenytoin [28,222,359,433] (Dilantin)
Some sulfonamides (sulfaphenazole, etc.) may produce potentially toxic blood levels of phenytoin through inhibition of

p-hydroxylation by microsomal enzymes and induce distressing reactions like ataxia, blood dyscrasias, diplopia, fatal toxic hepatitis, and nystagmus.

Probenecid [120,421] (Benemid)
Probenecid increases total plasma levels of sulfonamides by decreasing renal excretion of conjugated sulfonamides. Not always a potentiation, however, as only unbound sulfonamide is active. Probenecid may possibly displace sulfonamides from plasma protein binding sites also. Check for excessive levels of sulfonamides.

Promethazine [421] (Phenergan)
Promethazine potentiates the antibacterial action of sulfonamides.

Procaine (Novocain)
See *p-Aminobenzoic Acid* above.

Pyrazolon derivatives [421] (Aminopyrine, Antipyrine, Anturane, Butazolidin, Tandearil, etc.)
Pyrazolon derivatives improve antibacterial action of sulfonamides by drug displacement. See specific drugs and *Analgesics* above.

Pyrimethamine [177] (Daraprim)
Sulfonamides potentiate pyrimethamine in the suppression and treatment of falciparum infections. See *Sulfonamides* under *Pyrimethamine*.

Salicylates [21,78,83,198,421] (Aspirin, etc.)
Salicylates improve antibacterial action of sulfonamides by drug displacement. See *Sulfonamides* under *Salicylates*.

Sulfinpyrazone [21,120,173,202,1046,1211] (Anturane)
Sulfinpyrazone potentiates action of certain sulfonamides by displacing them from plasma protein binding sites. It may also decrease renal excretion of sulfonamides. Use with caution and monitor sulfa blood levels. See *Sulfonamides* under *Sulfinpyrazone*.

Sulfonylureas [198,330,633] (Diabinese, Dymelor, Orinase)
Sulfonamides potentiate these hypoglycemics. See *Antidiabetics, Oral* above.

Tetracyclines [178,1041]
This combination is the drug of choice against *Nocardia* in brain abscess, lesions of various organs, and pulmonary lesions; against the organism causing lymphogranuloma venereum; and against the organism causing trachoma. A case of allergic myocarditis occurred with the combination of sulfaethidole and tetracycline (2 tablets).

Thenamine [48]
See *Methenamine*.

Thiotepa [120]
Sulfonamides potentiate thiotepa and increased depression of bone marrow may result.

Tolbutamide [137,202,409] (Orinase)
Sulfonamides potentiate tolbutamide and may cause a hypoglycemic reaction. See *Antidiabetics, Oral* above.

Trimethoprim [421,933] (Syraprim)
Trimethoprim improves the antibacterial action of sulfonamides against *S. pneumoniae, S. Pyogenes, N. gonorrhea, E. coli*.

Vitamin C [274,531]
Sulfonamides can cause increased excretion of vitamin C. See *Ascorbic Acid* above.

Warfarin
See *Sulfonamides* under *Anticoagulants, Oral*.

SULFONES
See *Dapsone*.

SULFONYLUREAS
See *Antidiabetics, Oral.*

SUL-SPANSION
See *Sulfonamides* (sulfaethidole).

SUL-SPANTABS
See *Sulfonamides* (sulfaethidole).

SULTACOF
See *Sulfonamides* (sulfamethazine).

SULTHIAME (Ospolot, Trolone)
Diphenylhydantoin [190,192,294] **(Dilantin)**
See *Sulthiame* under *Phenytoin*

SUMYCIN
See *Tetracyclines.*

SURBEX
See *Vitamin B Complex.*

SURFADIL
See *Antihistamines* (methapyrilene) and *Anesthetics, Local* (cyclomethycaine).

SUS-PHRINE
See *Epinephrine.*

SUXAMETHONIUM CHLORIDE
See *Muscle Relaxants* (succinycholine chloride).

SUX-CERT
See *Muscle Relaxants* (succinylcholine chloride).

SWEETA
See *Cylcamates.*

SWEET BIRCH OIL
See *Methyl Salicylate.*

SWEETENERS, ARTIFICIAL
See *Cyclamates.*

SYMMETREL
See *Amantadine.*

SYMPATHOMIMETICS
(Direct-acting catecholamines such as dopamine, epinephrine, isoproterenol, levarterenol or norepinephrine, isoetharine, nordefrin, and protokylol; other direct-acting drugs, with hydroxy groups that are not *ortho,* located either on the ring or on the ring and one on the side chain, such as fenoterol, isoxsuprine, metaproterenol, metaraminol, nylidrin, phenylephrine, ritodrine, salbutamol, soterenol, and terbutaline; indirect-acting norepinephrine releasers such as amphetamines, ephedrine, and mephentermine; CNS stimulants used as anorexians such as benzphetamine, phentermine, diethylpropion, phenmetrazine, and phendimetrazine; local vasoconstrictors such as cyclopentamine, naphazoline, oxymetazoline, phenylpropanolamine, propylhexedrine, tetrahydrozoline, tuaminoheptane, xyloylometazoline, etc.)
See also *Amphetamines, Epinephrine, Metaraminol, Mephentermine, Methamphetamine, Methylphenidate, Levarterenol,* etc.

Acidifying agents [325,330,421,870]
Acidifying agents tend to decrease gastrointestinal absorption and increase urinary excretion of sympathomimetics and thus inhibit them.

β-Adrenergic blockers [330,421] **(Propanolol, etc.)**
β-Adrenergic blocking agents reverse the bronchial relaxing effect of sympathomimetics and exacerbate asthmatic conditions. The hypertensive effects are increased.

Alcohol [537]
Alcohol potentiates the adrenergic effects of sympathomimetics (hypertension, etc.) by increasing adrenal secretion.

Alkalinizing agents [325,870]
Alkalinizing agents tend to increase gastrointestinal absorption and decrease urinary excretion of sympathomimetics and thus potentiate them.

Anesthetics, halogenated [664,684,799,806]
(Fluothane, Fluoromar, Penthrane, etc.)
Anesthetics increase the cardiac arrhythmia effects of sympathomimetics. Halogen anesthetics sensitize the ventricular conducting tissue to the actions of catecholamines. Potentially hazardous.

Anticholinergics [168,421]
(Atropine, Banthine, Disipal, Panparnit, Pathilon, etc.)
Contraindicated in glaucoma; the combination is hazardous because of enhanced mydriasis. Bronchial relaxation is potentiated.

Anticholinesterases [168,421]
(Floropryl, Mestinon, Mytelase, Phospholine Iodide, Tensilon, etc.)
Anticholinesterases antagonize the mydriatic effects of sympathomimetics. Sympathomimetics antagonize the miotic effect of anticholinesterases in glaucoma.

Antidepressants, tricyclic [120,194,242,424,433,541,941]
(Aventyl, Elavil, Pertofrane, Sinequan, Tofranil, Vivactil)
Because the tricyclic antidepressants have anticholinergic properties and because they potentiate the pressor effects of norepinephrine and the hypothermic response to epinephrine, isoproterenol, levodopa, and norepinephrine, their use concomitantly with sympathomimetics may be hazardous and such use must be carefully monitored. Enhanced activity of either tricyclic antidepressants or sympathomimetic agent may result. Careful adjustment of dosages is essential. Do not use in glaucoma.

Antidiabetics [4,5]
Sympathomimetics with a glycogenolytic effect may alter the dosage requirements of antidiabetics.

Antihistamines [169,232,235,242,400,483]
Antihistamines may potentiate the pressor effect of sympathomimetics. See under Levarterenol.

Antihypertensives [198,421]
(Methyldopa, reserpine, etc.)
The pressor activity of sympathomimetics is antagonized by the hypotensive activity of the antihypertensives and vice versa. See, however, *Polymechanistic Drugs* (page 378).

Cholinergics [421]
(Carcholin, Floropryl, Humorsol, Miochol, Phospholine Iodide, Physostigmine, Pilocarpine, etc.)
Cholinergics (miotics) antagonize the mydriatic effects of sympathomimetics and vice versa. Thus cholinergics should not be administered when a sympathomimetic like phenyl-

SYMPATHOMIMETICS *(continued)*

ephrine is being used in uveitis and sympathomimetics should not be administered when a cholinergic like echothiopate is being used in glaucoma. See also *Anticholinesterases.*

Cocaine [167]
Cocaine, which inhibits uptake of norepinephrine by nerve terminals, potentiates the mydriatic and vasoconstrictor effects of sympathomimetics as well as the pressor and pyrogenic effects. Cardiac arrhythmias and convulsions may occur. Acute glaucoma may be precipitated.

Colchicine [226]
Colchicine may enhance the response to sympathomimetics.

Corticosteroids [120,421,728,940]
Corticosteroids used chronically with sympathomimetics may increase ocular pressure; a dangerous combination in glaucoma or in a patient with incipient glaucoma. Aerosols of sympathomimetics with corticosteroids may be lethal in asthmatic children. Drugs like hydrocortisone sensitize the vascular smooth muscle to catecholamines.

Desipramine (Pertofrane)
See *Antidepressants, Tricyclic* above.

Digitalis and its glycosides [619]
Digitalis glycosides with adrenergics such as ephedrine and epinephrine (pressor agents) predispose the patient to cardiac arrhythmias. See *Sympathomimetics* under *Digitalis.*

Doxapram [120] (Dopram)
Sympathomimetics should be used cautiously with doxapram, a respiratory and CNS stimulant since an enhanced pressor effect may occur.

Doxepin (Sinequan)
See *Antidepressants, Tricyclic* above.

Epinephrine [6,120,185,313,370,547,693]
Excessive use of sympathomimetic amines, particularly in asthma, is hazardous because of the potential for production of dangerously high blood pressure, cardiac arrhythmias, and severe paradoxical airway resistance. Administration of epinephrine for status asthmaticus in a patient who has been using excessive amounts of other sympathomimetics may be lethal.

Ergot alkaloids [120]
(Cafergot, Ergotrate, Gynergen, etc.)
Extremely high elevations of blood pressure may occur when sympathomimetic vasoconstrictors are given concomitantly with ergot alkaloids.

Furazolidone [202,356,633] (Furoxone)
Furazolidone, a MAO inhibitor, potentiates sympathomimetics; hazardous hypertension may occur. See *MAO Inhibitors* below.

Guanethidine [120,633,871,872] (Ismelin)
Hypertension may be produced by this combination. Vasopressors tend to produce cardiac arrhythmias in patients receiving guanethidine; the drug potentiates response to pressor drugs like levarterenol that reverse the hypotensive effect of guanethidine which blocks uptake of norepinephrine by secondary receptors. See discussion on *Sympathomimetics* under *Reserpine.* Guanethidine in ophthalmic drops antagonizes the mydriatic action of amphetamine, dopamine, ephedrine, hydroxyamphetamine, phenmetrazine, and tyramine ophthalmic solutions. It potentiates the mydriatic action of epinephrine, methoxamine, and phenylephrine ophthalmic solutions. See also *Polymechanistic Drugs* (page 378).

Haloperidol [120,421] (Haldol)
Haloperidol blocks the vasopressor action of epinephrine which should not be used, therefore, in hypotension induced by haloperidol.

Halothane (Fluothane)
See *Anesthetics, Halogenated* above.

Hydralazine [120,421] (Apresoline)
Sympathomimetics antagonize the hypotensive effect of hydralazine. Hydralazine reduces the pressor response to epinephrine.

Imipramine (Tofranil)
See *Antidepressants, Tricyclic* above.

Insulin [549,805]
Epinephrine (hyperglycemic) antagonizes the antidiabetic drugs. Insulin modifies the cardiac and hypoglycemic effects of epinephrine.

Isocarboxazid (Marplan)
See *MAO Inhibitors* below.

Isoniazid [202,619]
Isoniazid, with certain adrenergic drugs, produces enhanced hazardous CNS stimulation, probably by enzyme inhibition.

Isoproterenol [6,48,120,185,547] (Isuprel)
Isoproterenol, a β-adrenergic agent, potentiates the bronchial dilating effects of other sympathomimetics. See *Sympathomimetics, Other* below.

MAO inhibitors [25,37,45,48,78,99,115,117,120,136,162,211,217,305,312,356,399,404,431,532,533,546,1245]
Contraindicated. May be lethal. MAO inhibitors potentiate the cardiac, central, metabolic and peripheral actions of sympathomimetics even after the MAOI have been withdrawn. Concurrent use has resulted in cardiac arrhythmias, increased mydriasis (hazardous in glaucoma), postanesthetic respiratory depression, and acute hypertensive crisis (elevated blood pressure with possible intracranial hemorrhage, severe headache, tachycardia hyperthermia, nausea, vomiting, neck stiffness, convulsions, coma, and in some cases death). Hypertensive crisis with MAO inhibitors plus tyramine-rich foods and other commonly encountered sympathomimetics is especially likely to occur in so-called "acting-out" adolescents who by the very nature of this psychopathology are unlikely to observe the precautions stated by their physician.[1792] The crisis can be immediately reversed by administration of an α-adrenergic blocking agent such as phentolamine. MAO inhibitors remain in the blood (in sufficient quantities to cause the interaction) for 7-10 days after their administration is discontinued. Some reports state that MAO inhibitors do not produce severe hypertension with the endogenous catecholamines, epinephrine and norepinephrine. However, iproniazid and levarterenol produced myocardial injury. Drug metabolizing enzymes may be irreversibly inhibited. Metabolism of monoamines is blocked, thus causing their accumulation. This prolongs and potentiates action of agents which release norepinephrine (see *MAO Inhibitors* under *Amphetamines*), as well as directly acting sympathomimetics. Note that many over-the-counter cold remedies, hay fever preparations, and nasal decongestants as well as anorexiants and other prescribed medications contain sympathomimetics. All are contraindicated for use with MAO inhibitors, except injected levarterenol, inhaled isoproterenol (isoprenaline), and epinephrine (*e.g.*, in local anesthetics). These may not be importantly affected by some MAO inhibitors since exogenous catecholamines are largely destroyed by COMT (catechol-O-methyl-transferase). MAOI do not increase the hazards of inhalation of isoproterenol in bronchial asthma.

Mecamylamine [168,198,421,633] (Inversine)
Mecamylamine, a ganglionic blocker, potentiates the pressor response to catecholamines and other vasopressors, Sympathomimetics, given to reduce the hypotensive effects of mecamylamine, must be given in reduced dosage.

Methyldopa [168,198,633] (Aldomet)
Sympathomimetics tend to inhibit the hypotensive effect of methyldopa. Methyldopa, in small doses, potentiates re-

sponses to the indirect-acting sympathomimetics such as amphetamine, ephedrine, and mephentermine. Hypertension may occur. In large doses, methyldopa antagonizes these sympathomimetics. See the discussion under *Polymechanistic Drugs* (page 378).

Methylphenidate[421] (Ritalin)
Methylphenidate potentiates the mydriatic and pressor effects of sympathomimetics. The combination is hazardous in glaucoma and it may induce severe hypotension.

Miotics
See *Anticholinesterases* and *Cholinergics* above.

Morphine
See *Narcotic Analgesics* below.

Narcotic analgesics[643]
Dopamine and tyramine antagonize the analgesic effects of morphine which depletes catecholamines.

Nialamide (Niamid)
See *MAO inhibitors* above.

Nitrates and nitrites[170,421]
Nitrates and nitrites are physiologic antagonists of norepinephrine and other sympathomimetics that activate smooth muscle. The net effect of such a combination may vary widely, from strong contraction to total relaxation depending on the relative concentration of the agents present.

Nortriptyline[120] (Aventyl)
Either the tricyclic antidepressant or sympathomimetic agent may be potentiated. See *Antidepressants, Tricyclic* above.

Oral contraceptives
See *Progestogens*.

Organophosphates[421]
(DFP, Parathion, Malathion, TEPP, Phospholine Iodide, etc.)
Sympathomimetics which are mydriatic antagonize the miotic effects of the cholinesterase inhibiting organophosphates.

Oxytocics[120,173]
(Ergotrate, Methergine, Pitocin, Spartocin, Syntocinon, Tocosamine, etc.)
Sympathomimetics given concomitantly with oxytocics of the ergot alkaloid type may cause severe prolonged hypertension. On the other hand a large dose of oxytocin as in therapeutic abortion or uterine surgery causes marked hypotension which is antagonistic to the pressor effects of sympathomimetics. Continous infusion of large doses, however, causes an initial hypotension followed by a small sustained hypertension which may be potentiated by sympathomimetic pressors.

Pargyline (Eutonyl)
See *MAO Inhibitors* above.

Pentolinium[168,421] (Ansolysen)
Sympathomimetic drugs can overcome the hypotensive effect due to ganglionic blockade by pentolinium. Response to sympathomimetics is frequently potentiated when administered to a patient subjected to ganglionic blockade. See *Mecamylamine* above.

Phenothiazines[120,330,421,619]
The hypotensive effects of phenothiazines like chlorpromazine are counteracted by the pressor effects of sympathomimetics like levarterenol. Some phenothiazines potentiate the pressor effect of epinephrine, others antagonize the effect by blocking α-receptors.

Phentolamine[120,619] (Regitine)
Phentolamine reduces the myocardial sensitization to sympathomimetics produced by certain anesthetics (chloroform, cyclopropane, etc.)

Phenelzine (Nardil)
See *MAO Inhibitors* above.

Procarbazine[120,659] (Matulane)
Sympathomimetics are contraindicated for use with the antineoplastics procarbazine because of its monoamine oxidase inhibiting action. See *MAO Inhibitors* above.

Progestogens[538,620]
Progestational agents may inhibit catecholamines by increasing their metabolism.

Rauwolfia alkaloids[198,421,633] (Reserpine, etc.)
Sympathomimetics tend to antagonize these hypotensives but timing and the agent are important. Directly acting agents like levarterenol are potentiated with reserpine because it prevents uptake of the pressor agents by inactive sites. Indirectly acting agents like amphetamine; ephedrine, metaraminol and mephentermine on the other hand are potentiated only by initial doses of reserpine when it is releasing norepinephrine from storage sites. Later, they are inhibited and their action may be abolished entirely if the norepinephrine, upon whose release they depend for their effects, has been depleted. See *Polymechanistic Drugs* (page 378).

Sympathomimetics, other[6,78,120,185,313,370,547,693]
Combinations of sympathomimetics may be desirable. Thus isoproterenol is synergistically beneficial with cyclopentamine, ephedrine, or phenylephrine in asthma (addtive bronchial dilating effects). Other combinations of sympathomimetics may be hazardous. Excessive use of various sympathomimetics as antiasthmatics, cardiac stimulants, decongestants, pressor agents, etc., may induce cardiac arrhythmias, dangerously high blood pressure, and severe paradoxical airway resistance. Administration of epinephrine for status asthmaticus in a patient who has been using excessive amounts of sympathomimetics may be lethal. Combined use of sympathomimetics with potent pressor effects, *e.g.*, epinephrine and isoproterenol, has caused death or led to conditions like ileus and unnecessary surgery.

Thiazide diuretics[120]
Thiazide diuretics enhance the hypotensive effect of adrenergic blocking drugs. The dosage of the latter must be reduced by at least 50%.

Tranylcypromine (Parnate)
See *MAO Inhibitors* above.

Veratrum alkaloids[421]
Sympathomimetics antagonize the hypotensive effects of veratrum alkaloids.

Xanthines[120]
(Caffeine, Coffee, Cola drinks, Tea, Theobromine, Theophylline, etc.)
Sympathomimetics with a bronchial relaxing effect are synergistically useful with xanthine drugs like the theophylline derivative, aminophylline, in asthma. Sympathomimetics such as amphetamines, ephedrine, isoproterenol and protokylol, with CNS stimulating properties may produce excessive CNS stimulation in conjunction with xanthines (arrhythmias, emotional disturbances, insomnia, nervousness, tachycardia, etc.).

SYNALAR
See *Corticosteroids* (fluocinolone).

SYNALGOS
See *Antihistamines* (promethazine), *Caffeine*, *Phenacetin*, and *Salicylates* (aspirin).

SYNALGOS-DC
In addition to items under *Synalgos*, see also *Codeine* (this combination contains dihydrocodeine).

SYNATE-M
See *Barbiturates* (secobarbital), *Iodides* (potassium iodide), *Nicotinic Acid* (nacinamide), *Sympathomimetics* (racephedrine), and *Theophylline* (theophylline sodium glycinate).

SYNCILLIN
See *Penicillins* (phenethicillin).

SYNCURINE
See *Muscle Relaxants* (decamethonium).

SYNKAYVITE
See *Vitamin K*.

SYNOPHYLATE
See *Theophylline* (theophylline sodium glycinate).

SYNTHROID
See *Thyroxine* (sodium levothyroxine).

SYNTOCINON
See *Oxytocics* (oxytocin).

SYROSINGOPINE (Singoserp)
See *Antihypertensives* and *Reserpine*.

SYTOBEX
See *Cyanocobalomin*.

TACARYL
See *Antihistamines* (methdilazine) and *Phenothiazines*.

TACE
See *Estrogens* (chlorotrianisene).

TAGAMET
See *Cimetidine*.

Pancreatin
See *Cimetidine* under *Pancreatin*.

TALBUTAL (Lotusate)
See *Barbiturates*.

TALWIN
See *Analgesics* and *Pentazocine*.

TANDEARIL
See *Oxyphenbutazone*.

TANNATES

Oxytocin [421]
This combination produces erratic and unpredictable results.

TAO
See *Antibiotics* (triacetyloleandomycin).

TARACTAN
See *CNS Depressants* and *Tranquilizers* (chlorprothixene).

TEA
See *Caffeine*.

TEDRAL
See *Ephedrine*, *Sympathomimetics*, and *Xanthines* (theophylline).

TEGOPEN
See *Penicillins* (sodium cloxacillin).

TEGRETOL
See *Carbamazepine*.

TELDRIN
See *Antihistamines* (chlorpheniramine maleate).

TELEPAQUE
See *Radiopaque Media* (iopanoic acid).

TEM
See *Antineoplastics* (triethylenemelamine).

TEMARIL
See *Antihistamines*, *CNS Depressants*, and *Phenothiazines* (trimeprazine).

TEMPRA
See *Acetaminophen*.

TENSILON
See *Parasympathomimetics* (edrophonium).

TENSODIN
See *Barbiturates* (phenobarbital), *Papaverine* (ethaverine), and *Xanthines* (theophylline calcium salicylate).

TENUATE
See *Sympathomimetics* (diethylpropion).

TEPANIL
See *Sympathomimetics* (diethylpropion).

TERFONYL
See *Sulfonamides*.

TERRA-CORTRIL
See *Corticosteroids* (hydrocortisone) and *Tetracyclines* (oxytetracycline).

TERRAMYCIN
See *Tetracyclines* (oxytetracycline).

TEST-ESTRIN
See *Testosterone* and *Estrogens* (ethinyl estradiol).

TESTOSTERONE
See also *Anabolic Agents* and *Androgens*.

Aminopyrine [555]
Aminopyrine inhibits testosterone by increasing its rate of metabolism (enzyme induction).

Antihistamines [65,479,485]
Antihistamines inhibit testosterone (enzyme induction).

Chlorcyclizine [198,421] **(Perazil)**
Chlorcyclizine inhibits testosterone by increasing its rate of metabolism (enzyme induction, increased hydroxylation).

Chlorzoxazone (Paraflex) [951]
Testosterone inhibits chlorzoxazone.

Hexobarbital [83,198,330,421] **(Sombucaps, Sombulex)**
Hexobarbital inhibits testosterone by enzyme induction and vice versa.

Phenobarbital [83,330,421]
Phenobarbital inhibits testosterone by increasing its rate of metabolism.

Phenylbutazone [198,421] **((Butazolidin)**
Phenylbutazone inhibits testosterone by increasing its rate of metabolism (enzyme induction).

Radiophosphorus [951] **(^{32}P)**
Potentiation of relief from pain and osseous metastasis in metastatic prostatic carcinoma.

TETANUS TOXOID

Chloramphenicol [633]
This antibiotic interferes with the immune response to the toxoid.

Cytarabine
See *Tetanus Toxoid* under *Cytarabine*.

TETD (Tetraethylthiuram Disulfide)
See *Disulfiram*.

TETRABENAZINE (Nitoman)

Antidepressants, tricyclic [399]
Tricyclic antidepressants inhibit the depression induced by tetrabenazine.

MAO inhibitors [874]
This combination of serotonin antagonist and MAO inhibitor may produce agitation and delirium.

TETRACAINE
See *Anesthetics, Local*.

TETRACHEL
See *Tetracyclines*.

TETRACHLOROETHYLENE (Perchloroethylene)

Alcohol [711,1387,1752]
Tetrachloroethylene, which is slightly absorbed from the gastrointestinal tract, can cause symptoms of inebriation: Alcohol may enhance these effects and should not be ingested 24 hours before or after use of the anthelmintic.

TETRACYCLINES
(Chlortetracycline [Aureomycin], demeclocycline [Declomycin], doxycyline [Vibramycin], methacycline [Rondomycin], oxyletracycline [Terramycin], and tetracycline [Achromycin])

Acidifying agents [578]
Tetracyclines are most active against urinary tract infections when the pH of the urine is 5.5 or less.

Acenocoumarol
See *Anticoagulants* below.

Alcohol [951]
Alcohol potentiates tetracyclines.

Aluminum Salts
(Aluminum carbonate, hydroxide, and phosphate; dihydroxy aluminum aminoacetate, etc.)
See *Complexing Agents* below. Aluminum ions inhibit tetracycline absorption from the intestine.

Ampicillin [157,208,301,433]
(Alpen, Omnipen, Polycillin, etc.
Antagonism. See *Penicillins* below.

Antacids [78,120,178,472,633,665,1376,1794]
Antacids containing divalent or trivalent ions inhibit tetracycline absorption from the intestine. See *Complexing Agents* and *Sodium Bicarbonate* below.

Anticoagulants [120,193,234,259,334,898,909,972]
Tetracyclines enhance the effect of anticoagulants due to interference with the synthesis of vitamin K by microorganisms in the gut.

Antidiabetics, oral
See *Oxytetracycline* and *Tetracycline* under *Antidiabetics, Oral*.

Barbiturates [1660]
Barbiturates, by inducing the microsomal enzymes responsible for tetracycline metabolism, antagonize the anti-infectives. This has been reported for phenobarbital and doxycycline (Vibramycin) and may be true for a wide variety of barbiturates and tetracyclines. Monitor blood levels and clinical response closely.

Calcium salts [107]
Calcium salts inhibit absorption of tetracyclines. See *Complexing Agents* below.

Carbamazepine (Tegretol)
Carbamazepine has the same action as *Barbiturates* above. It too induces the metabolizing enzymes for doxycyline.

Cephalothin (Keflin)
Incompatible in parenteral mixtures. See Chapter 8.

Cholestyramine
See *Tetracyclines* under *Cholestyramine*.

Chymotrypsin, oral [306,508]
This enzyme may elevate the antibiotic blood level by improving absorption.

Citric acid [107,270,696]
Citric acid elevates the blood levels of tetracyclines through enhanced absorption.

Cloxacillin (Tegopen)
See *Penicillins* below.

Complexing agents [48,120,178,472,509,619,665,1104,1376,1794]
A number of ionized divalent metals (calcium, iron, magnesium, strontium) and trivalent metals (aluminum, iron, bismuth) form tetracycline-metal complexes that are not readily absorbed from the gastrointestinal tract. Thus many antacids, dairy products (milk and milk products), dietary supplements, and a wide range of drug products inhibit tetracyclines. Do not administer oral tetracyclines within at least 1 hour before or 2 hours after these substances. Vibramycin (doxycycline) appears not to be markedly affected by milk; an exception.

Corticosteroids [1697]
Prolonged concomitant use of a corticosteroid with a tetracycline may lead to development of an infection resistant to tetracycline therapy. Thus a resistant *Proteus* infection developed with use of the combination in acne. Exercise caution when using corticosteroids, which decrease resistance to infection, with any antibiotic. A dangerous superinfection is always a possibility.

Dicloxacillin (Dynapen, Pathocil, Veracillin)
See *Penicillins* below.

Diuretics [1255,1844]
Both tetracyclines, with their antianabolic action, and diuretics have an additive BUN elevating effect which is an indication of a hazardous situation in renal impairment. Tetracycline levels may then increase and lead possibly to acidosis, azotemia, hyperphosphatemia, and even death, particularly in pregnancy.

Food [120,619]
Food interferes with absorption of tetracyclines. Give them 1 hour before or 2 hours after meals.

Heparin [120,1573]
Tetracyclines may partially decrease the anticoagulant effect of heparin.

Hepatotoxic drugs [120]
Tetracyclines have been known to cause hepatotoxicity; if they are given IV, other potentially hepatotoxic drugs should be avoided if possible.

Iron salts [359,1004,1228,1459,1603] **(Ferrous sulfate, etc.)**
Iron salts inhibit absorption of tetracyclines which reach only 10-50% of expected levels in the blood. See *Complexing Agents* above. Ferrous sulfate depresses the absorption of doxycycline (Vibramycin) and methacycline (Rondomycin) more than it does with oxytetracycline (Terramycin) and tetracycline (Achromycin, etc.). Enteric-coated ferrous sulfate does not depress absorption as strongly. Avoid concomitant

TETRACYCLINES *(continued)*

use of iron salts with tetracyclines or give as far apart timewise as possible (tetracycline 3 hours before or 2 hours after the iron).

Magnesium salts[48,421,665]
Magnesium salts inhibit absorption of tetracyclines by the cathartic action and by formation of a complex that inhibits absorption. See *Complexing Agents* above and *Cathartics*.

Methicillin (Staphcillin)
See *Penicillins* below.

Methoxyflurane[471,1191,1291,1307,1333,1429,1606,1794,1838]
(Penthrane)
Methoxyflurane anesthesia combined with tetracycline parenterally may produce severe nephrotoxicity, may seriously impair renal function, and lead to death. See also *Nephrotoxic Antibiotics* under *Antibiotics*.

Milk[201,665]
Decreased antibiotic blood level. See *Complexing Agents* above.

Novobiocin[201,619]
Tetracyclines diminish the effectiveness of novobiocin; physical inhibition.

Oxacillin[433] **(Prostaphlin)**
See *Penicillins* below.

Penicillins[70,157,178,208,285,301,402,421,433,633,666,1437]
(Alpen, Dynapen, Omnipen, Pathocil, Penicillin G, O, or V, Polycillin, Prostaphlin, Tegopen, Veracillin, etc. and their salts)
The penicillins which are bactericidal against multiplying bacteria only by virtue of formation of cell wall deficient (CWD) organisms are inhibited by the bacteriostatic tetracyclines. Antagonism is particularly intense with methicillin. See *Antibiotics* under *Antibiotics*.

Phenytoin
See *Tetracyclines* under *Phenytoin*.

Polyvinylpyrolidone[421]
Polyvinylpyrolidone prolongs blood levels of tetracyclines.

Probenecid[421]
See *Penicillins* under *Probenecid*.

Purgatives[28]
See *Magnesium Salts* above and *Cathartics*.

Riboflavin[509,641,642]
Riboflavin inhibits the antibiotic activity of tetracyclines.

Sodium bicarbonate[75,472,633,1392,1519]
Sodium bicarbonate reduces the gastrointestinal absorption of oral tetracyclines 50%. Do not give concomitantly. One theory put forth is that at elevated pH the capsule holding the drug becomes much less soluble in the intestinal fluid.

Streptomycin[178,1106]
Synergistic activity in bacteremic brucellosis.

Strontium salts[421]
Strontium salts inhibit absorption of tetracyclines. See *Complexing Agents* above.

Sulfaethidole[1041] **(Ethizole, Sul-Spantab, etc.)**
See *Tetracyclines* under *Sulfonamides*.

Sulfonamides[178]
See *Tetracyclines* under *Sulfonamides*.

Urinary acidifiers[509,578]
Acidifying agents potentiate tetracyclines.

Vitamin K[510]
Tetracyclines decrease vitamin K activity; altered intestinal bacterial flora.

TETRACYN
See *Tetracyclines*.

TETRAETHYLAMMONIUM
(Bromide or chloride)
See *Antihypertensives* and *Ganglionic Blocking Agents*.

Acetylcholine[168]
Tetraethylammonium displaces acetylcholine and acts as blocking agent at autonomic ganglia.

TETRAMETHYLAMMONIUM CHLORIDE
See *Antihypertensives* and *Ganglionic Blocking Agents*.

TETREX
See *Tetracyclines*.

THALFED
See *Barbiturates* (phenobarbital), *Sympathomimetics* (ephedrine), and *Xanthines* (aminophylline).

THAM-E
See *Alkalinizing Agents* and *Tromethamine*.

THEAMIN
See *Xanthines* (theophylline).

THEELIN
See *Estrogens* (estrone).

THENYLPYRAMINE
See *Antihistamines* (methapyrilene).

THEOCALCIN
See *Salicylates* and *Xanthines* (theobromine calcium salicylate).

THEO-GUAIA
See *Alcohol* and *Xanthines* (theophylline), also *Glyceryl Guaiacolate* under *HIAA* in Chapter 7.

THEOKIN
See *Iodides*, *Salicylates*, and *Xanthines* (theophylline calcium salicylate).

THEO-ORGANIDIN
See *Iodine* (iodopropylideneglycerol) and *Xanthines* (theophylline).

THEOPHYLLINE
See *Xanthines*.

THEOPHYLLINE ETHYLENEDIAMINE
See *Xanthines* (aminophylline).

THEO-SED L.A.
See *Barbiturates* (butabarbital), *Sympathomimetics* (pseudoephedrine) and *Xanthines* (theophylline).

THEO-SYL-R
See *Xanthines* (theophylline) and *Mercurial Diuretics* (sodium mersalyl).

THEPHORIN
See *Antihistamines* (phenindamine tartrate).

THIAMINE
Muscle relaxants
See *Thiamine* under *Muscle Relaxants, Peripherally Acting*.

THIAMYLAL
See *Barbiturates* and *CNS Depressants*.

THIAZIDE DIURETICS
(Bendroflumethiazide [Naturetin], benzthiazide [Aquatag, Exna], chlorothiazide [Diuril], cyclothiazide [Anhydron], hydrochlorothiazide [Esidrex, Hydrodiuril, Oretic], hydroflumethiazide [Saluron], methyclothiazide [Enduron], polythiazide [Renese], trichlormethiazide [Metahydron, Naqua], benzothiadiazides, etc.)

See *Antihypertensives* and *Diuretics*.

Interactions with thiazide (sulfonamide) diuretics result from the hypokalemia they produce, the hypotensive action, the inhibition of uric acid excretion, the hyperglycemic action, and the alkalinization of the urine.

Acetohexamide (Dymelor)
See *Antidiabetics* below.

Acidifying agents [325,870]
Acidifying agents potentiate thiazides (weak acids) by decreasing their urinary excretion.

ACTH
See *Corticosteroids* below.

Adrenergic-blocking drugs [120]
Thiazide diuretics enhance the hypotensive effect of adrenergic-blocking drugs. The dosage of the adrenergic blocker must be reduced by at least 50%.

Alcohol [120]
Alcohol may potentiate the orthostatic hypotension caused by the thiazide diuretics.

Allopurinol [421,2009] (Zyloprim)
Thiazide diuretics, by elevating serum uric acid, tend to antagonize the antihyperuricemic action of allopurinol. However, thiazides increase retention of allopurinol and its active metabolite alloxanthine (competition for same urinary excretion pathway) and therefore tend to potentiate the action of both the drug and its active metabolite as well as their toxic effects (interference with pyrimidine synthesis in patients that is mediated by oxypurinol ribonucleotide, another metabolite of allopurinol).

Ammonium chloride [120]
Ammonium chloride should not be used to correct hypochloremic alkalosis (caused by the diuretic) in patients with hepatic insufficiency. See also *Acidifying Agents* above.

Antidepressants, tricyclic [120,172,194,325,870,952]
Since the tricyclics may cause orthostatic hypotension, caution should be observed when thiazides that also lower the blood pressure are given concurrently. Since the thiazides alkalinize the urine, these weak bases, the tricyclic antidepressants, are potentiated by the decrease in urinary excretion.

Antidiabetics [120,191,421]
Thiazide-type diuretics may modify the diabetic state (cause hyperglycemia and glycosuria in latent diabetics) and alter the dosage of antidiabetic required. Depending on the patient, the requirements may be increased, unaltered, or decreased. Careful monitoring is essential.

Antihypertensives [78,421]
(Guanethidine, methyldopa, ganglionic blocking agents, etc.)
These diuretics potentiate antihypertensives. Adjust dosage. Withdraw these antihypertensives well before surgery. Agents like guanethidine and methyldopa persist for 7-10 days.

Barbiturates [120]
Barbiturates may potentiate the orthostatic hypotension caused by thiazide diuretics.

Cardiac Glycosides
See *Digitalis* below.

Chlorisondamine Chloride (Ecolid Chloride)
See *Ganglionic Blocking Drugs* below.

Cholestyramine [120,769] (Cuemid, Questran)
Cholestyramine inhibits the action of the acidic thiazide diuretics by binding them in the intestinal tract and decreasing absorption. Administer the diuretics at least an hour before or 4 to 6 hours after the anion exchange resin is given.

Colestipol [1531] (Colestid)
Colestipol, a bile acid sequestering resin with similar actions and interactions as *Cholestyramine* above produces a more than 50% decrease in the intestinal absorption of thiazides.

Corticosteroids [120,1853] (ACTH, etc.)
Excessive potassium depletion may occur since these agents and the diuretics can both cause hypokalemia. See *Corticosteroids* under *Diuretics*.

Corticotropin (ACTH)
See *Corticosteroids* above.

Curare [16,30,311]
Thiazide diuretics, by causing hypokalemia, enhance the muscle relaxant action of curare.

Diazoxide [117] (Hyperstat)
Thiazide diuretics enhance the diabetogenic effect of diazoxide. Thiazide diuretics potentiate diazoxide (enhanced hypotension, hyperglycemia, acidosis, hirsutism).

Digitalis [16,30,311,633] (Digitoxin, Digoxin, etc.)
Thiazide diuretics potentiate digitalis glycosides. Diuretics can cause hypokalemia; if the potassium loss is not corrected the heart can become more sensitive to the effects of digitalis, possibly resulting in digitalis toxicity.

Furazolidone [120,633] (Furoxone)
Furazolidone potentiates these diuretics. See *MAO Inhibitors* below. Mutual potentiation of the hypotensive effect.

Gallamine [16,30,311,330]
Thiazide diuretics potentiate gallamine.

Ganglionic blocking drugs [120,633]
(Ansolysen, Arfonad, Ecolid, Inversine, etc.)
Thiazide diuretics enhance the hypotensive effect of ganglionic blocking drugs.

Guanethidine (Ismelin)
See *Thiazide Diuretics* under *Guanethidine*.

Hexamethonium
See *Ganglionic Blocking Drugs* above.

Hydralazine [198,421,633] (Apresoline)
These diuretics potentiate the hypotensive action of hydralazine.

Insulin [120]
Insulin requirements may be increased with this combination. See *Antidiabetics* above.

Levarterenol [421]
Thiazide diuretics inhibit the hypertensive effect of levarterenol. Arterial responsiveness to norepinephrine may be decreased.

Licorice [151,186,326,667,1088,1089,1993]
Licorice, taken for long periods before or during administration of thiazides may produce severe hypokalemia and paralysis. See also *Antihypertensives* under *Glycyrrhiza*.

Lithium carbonate
See *Lithium Carbonate* under *Diuretics*.

MAO inhibitors [198,421,633]
Thiazide diuretics potentiate the hypotensive action of MAO inhibitor antihypertensives. MAO inhibitors increase diuresis by potentiation (enzyme inhibition) of the thiazides. Pargyline and methyclothiazide have been used in combination for the enhanced hypotensive effect.

THIAZIDE DIURETICS *(continued)*

Mecamylamine [198,421,633] (Inversine)
These diuretics potentiate the hypotensive effect of mecamylamine.

Methyldopa [117,120] (Aldomet)
Thiazide diuretics enhance the hypotensive effect of methyldopa. The diuretic also counteracts weight gain and edema which may occur with methyldopa therapy.

Muscle relaxants [120,330,1448,1829]
Prolonged paralysis of respiratory muscles may occur when thiazide diuretics enhance the effects of curariform, nondepolarizing muscle relaxants such as gallamine and tubocurarine, possibly in part due to diuretic-induced hypokalemia, as well as decreased arterial responsiveness to norepinephrine. Persistent curarization may develop. Discontinue thiazides 2-3 days prior to surgery.

Narcotics [120]
Narcotics may potentiate the orthostatic hypotension caused by thiazide diuretics.

Norepinephrine
See *Levarterenol* above.

Pargyline (Eutonyl)
See *MAO Inhibitors* above.

Pempidine [120,633] (Perolysen, Tenormal)
Synergistic antihypertensive activity.

Pentolinium [421] (Ansolysen)
Thiazide diuretics potentiate the hypotensive effect of this ganglionic blocking agent.

Phenothiazines [78,198,421,633]
Thiazide diuretics potentiate the orthostatic hypotension produced by phenothiazines and may cause shock. When attempts to reverse this with metaraminol have been made, the phenothiazine has partly blocked the metaraminol and caused increased hypotension.

Potassium salts [120]
Potassium salts are frequently given to correct diuretic-induced hypokalemia. Use of enteric-coated dosage forms of potassium salts should be avoided, if possible, since ulceration of the small intestine may occur.

Pressor amines [120]
Thiazide diuretics decrease arterial responsiveness to pressor amines. Withdraw the diuretics at least one week prior to surgery.

Probenecid [120,421] (Benemid)
Probenecid potentiates thiazide diuretics. The diuretics inhibit the action of probenecid; they tend to precipitate gout in patients with hyperuricemia.

Procainamide [619] (Pronestyl)
Procainamide potentiates the hypotensive effect of thiazides.

Reserpine [117,1352]
Synergistic hypotensive effect. See *Thiazide Diuretics* under *Reserpine*.

Spironolactone [120] (Aldactone)
Spironolactone is a potassium-conserving diuretic and may be combined with thiazide diuretics to reduce potassium loss and to enhance the diuretic effect.

Sulfonylureas [198,421,633]
(Diabinese, Dymelor, Orinase, etc.)
Thiazide diuretics may potentiate the hypoglycemic effect of sulfonylureas. See also *Antidiabetics* above and *Antidiabetics, Oral* under *Sulfonamides* (thiazides contain a sulfonamide moiety).

Tetraethylammonium chloride (TEA)
See *Ganglionic Blocking Drugs* above.

Triamterene [120,172] (Dyrenium)
Triamterene is a potassium-conserving diuretic and may be combined with thiazide diuretics to reduce potassium loss and to enhance the diuretic effect.

Trimethaphan Camsylate (Arfonad)
See *Ganglionic Blocking Drugs* above.

Trimethidinium Methosulfate (Ostensin)
See *Ganglionic Blocking Drugs* above.

Tubocurarine [120,198,330] (Metubine)
See *Muscle Relaxants* above.

Uricosuric agents [421] (Benemid, Zyloprim, etc.)
Thiazide diuretics antagonize uricosuric agents.

Veratrum alkaloids [421,619]
Thiazides potentiate the hypotensive effect of veratrum alkaloids.

6-THIOGUANINE

Kethoxal [951]
Synergistic activity against sarcoma 180 ascites tumor.

Mitomycin [951]
Synergistic activity against ascites cell neoplasms.

THIOMERIN
See *Diuretics* (mercaptomerin).

THIOPENTAL (Pentothal)
See *Barbiturates*.

Meprobamate
See *Barbiturates* under *Meprobamate*.

Phenothiazines [116]
Some phenothiazines (promazine, propriomazine, prothipendyl) more than doubled the hypnotic effect of thiopental, others (levomepromazine, methdilazine) and imipramine increased the effect by more than 50%.

Reserpine
See *Reserpine* under *Barbiturates*.

THIOPROPAZATE (Dartal)
See *CNS Depressants* and *Tranquilizers*.

THIORIDAZINE (Mellaril)
See *CNS Depressants*, *Phenothiazines*, and *Tranquilizers*.

Antiarrhythmics [1195]
Procainamide, propranolol, or quinidine have no effect on thioridazine-induced arrhythmias.

Mandrax [623]
(Methaqualone and diphenhydramine)
Thioridazine side effects (dryness of mouth, swelling of tongue, cracking of the angles of the mouth, dizziness, disorientation) are potentiated by Mandrax. Symptoms subside upon withdrawal of Mandrax even when the psychotropic drug is continued. Diphenhydramine has anticholinergic properties and may be the potentiating component of Mandrax.

THIOSULFIL
See *Sulfonamides* (sulfamethizole).

THIOTEPA
See *Alkylating Agents*.

Bone marrow depressors [120]
Thiotepa should not be administered after therapy with nitrogen mustards, X-ray, or other radiomimetic or bone marrow depressing medication until the full effects of such therapy have been carefully evaluated. Concomitant administration of these agents may cause anemia, bleeding, fever, leukopenia, and thrombocytopenia, and may lead to death.

Chloramphenicol [120] (Chloromycetin)
Increased depression of the bone marrow may result. See *Bone Marrow Depressors* above.

Succinylcholine [1646,1814,1888,1917,1925] (Anectine, Quelicin)
Thiotepa, like other antineoplastics, decreases plasma levels of the enzyme pseudocholinesterase which metabolizes succinylcholine. Inhibition of the enzyme thus potentiates the muscle relaxant. Use this combination with extreme caution.

Sulfonamides [120]
Increased depression of the bone marrow may result. See *Bone Marrow Depressors* above.

Uricosurics [120] (Probenecid, sulfinpyrazone, etc.)
Thiotepa, which tends to produce hyperuricemia with uric acid nephropathy, may be antagonistic to uricosurics such as allopurinol (Zyloprim), probenecid (Benemid), and sulfinpyrazone (Anturane). Such drugs may be given to prevent and control these adverse effects of thiotepa.

THIOTHIXENE (Navane, Navarone)
See *CNS Depressants, Tranquilizers* and *Thioxanthenes.*

Guanethidine
See *Thiothixene* under *Guanethidine Sulfate.*

THIOURACILS
See *Thiouracils* under *Anticoagulants, Oral.*

THIOXANTHENES
(Clopenthixol [Sordinol], chlorprothixene [Taractan], and thiothixene [Navane], etc.)
See *CNS Depressants.*
Because of the structural similarity to the phenothiazines, the thioxanthenes have many of the same potential drug interactions. All of the precautions associated with phenothiazine therapy should be considered.

Alcohol [120]
Since thioxanthenes may precipitate convulsions they should not be given during withdrawal of alcohol, because it may lower the convulsive threshold. See also *CNS Depressants.*

Anesthetics, general [120]
Thioxanthenes potentiate the CNS depressant effects of anesthetics. See *CNS Depressants.*

Anticholinergics [120,421,619]
Thioxanthenes, which have weak anticholinergic action, may potentiate the anticholinergics (additive effects).

Anticonvulsants [120]
Thioxanthenes may inhibit the anticonvulsants since they lower the convulsive threshold in susceptible patients. The dosage of the anticonvulsant may have to be increased.

Antidepressants, tricyclic [166]
Tricyclics and phenothiazines are frequently used in combination in treating agitated forms of depressions.

Antihypertensives [120]
Thioxanthenes may potentiate the hypotensive action. See *CNS Depressants.*

Antiparkinsonism agents [120]
Antiparkinsonism agents are frequently given concurrently to control the extrapyramidal symptoms that are sometimes caused by thioxanthenes.

Atropine [120]
See *Anticholinergics* above.

Barbiturates [120]
See *CNS Depressants* below.

CNS Depressants [120]
Thioxanthenes and other CNS depressant drugs have additive effects. Thus the dosage of barbiturates, narcotics, and other CNS depressant drugs should be reduced when given concomitantly. See *CNS Depressants.*

Epinephrine [120,619,1354]
Epinephrine and pressor agents other than levarterenol, metaraminol or phenylephrine should not be used to treat hypotension caused by thioxanthenes since they may reverse the pressor action, resulting in further lowering of blood pressure. See *Epinephrine* under *Phenothiazines.*

Guanethidine
See *Thiothixene* under *Guanethidine Sulfate.*

Hypotensives [120] (including diuretics)
The hypotensive effect may be enhanced (additive effect).

Insecticides, [120] (organophosphorous)
Thioxanthenes may potentiate the toxic effects of these insecticides.

Levarterenol [120]
See *Metaraminol* below.

Levodopa [2001]
See *Thioxanthenes* under *Levodopa.*

Metaraminol [120] (Aramine)
Hypotension caused by thioxanthenes responds to metaraminol or levarterenol. See *Epinephrine* above.

Narcotics [120]
See *CNS Depressants* above.

Pentylenetetrazol [120,166] (Metrazol)
Do not use pentylenetetrazol as a stimulating agent in treating overdosage since it may cause convulsions with thioxanthenes.

Phenothiazines [120]
Cross sensitivity between the phenothiazines and thioxanthenes may exist.

Picrotoxin [120]
Picrotoxin should not be used as a stimulating agent in treating overdosage since it may cause convulsions with thioxanthenes.

Piperazines [660,766]
Exaggeration of the extrapyramidal effects may occur when a piperazine is administered, since this occurs with phenothiazines. See *Piperazine* under *Phenothiazines.*

Toxic drugs [120]
Since thioxanthenes have antiemetic properties they may mask overdosage of toxic drugs.

THIPHENAMIL
See *Anticholinergics.*

THORAZINE
See *Phenothiazines* (chlorpromazine).

THYRAR
See *Thyroid Preparations.*

THYROBEX
See *Thyroid Preparations* and *Vitamins* (B complex, B_{12}).

THYROID PREPARATIONS
(Levothyroxine, liothyronine, liotrix, thyroid gland; Cytomel, Euthroid, Letter, Levoid, Proloid, Synthroid, Thyrolar, etc.)
See also *Dextrothyroxine.*

Acidifying agents [421]
Acidifying agents decrease the urinary excretion of, and thus potentiate, weak acids like thyroxine and its analogs.

THYROID PREPARATIONS *(continued)*

Adrenergic neuron blocking agents[590] (Ismelin, reserpine, etc.)
These blocking agents antagonize the augmentation of epinephrine and norepinephrine response and the resulting angina induced by thyroxine.

Adrenocortical hormones[120]
See *Corticosteroids* below.

Amitriptyline (Elavil)
See *Antidepressants, Tricyclic* below.

Anticoagulants, oral[120,393,394,401,408,411,673]
Thyroid replacement therapy may potentiate anticoagulants such as warfarin or bishydroxycoumarin, possibly by increasing their affinity for receptors. Reduction of anticoagulant dosage by one-third may be necessary. Faster turnover of clotting factors has also been proposed as a mechanism. See also *Dextrothyroxine* and *Thyroid Preparations* under *Anticoagulants, Oral.*

Antidepressants, tricyclic[456,670,934,1337,1486,1715,1901]
Mutual enhancement of activity of both medications may occur. Transient cardiac arrhythmias have been observed in some instances. T_3 (L-triiodothyronine) increases receptor sensitivity and enhances imipramine antidepressant activity. The tricyclics inhibit catecholamine uptake by adrenergic neurons and the excess catecholamine plus thyroid preparations may precipitate an episode of coronary insufficiency. When carefully used, though, in reduced dosage, potentiation of the antidepressants may produce better response by patients.

Antidiabetics, oral[120,421]
In patients with diabetes mellitus, addition of thyroid hormone therapy may cause an increase in blood sugar levels and thus may require an increase in the usual dosage of oral hypoglycemic agents. Decreasing the dose of thyroid hormone may possibly cause hypoglycemic reactions if the dose of the oral agents is not adjusted. Antidiabetics may enhance the effects of the thyroid preparations.

Barbiturates[330]
Increased barbiturate dosage is required when thyroid hormonal therapy is initiated (increased metabolism).

Catecholamines
See *Epinephrine* below.

Chlordane[421]
Chlordane decreases the rate of metabolism of thyroxine and thereby potentiates it.

Cholestyramine resin[28,672] (Cuemid, Questran)
This resin inhibits the action of thyroid hormone by reducing its gastrointestinal absorption. Cholestyramine binds thyroxine and triiodothyronine almost irreversibly. Administer the resin at least 4 or 5 hours after or before a thyroid product.

Clofibrate[421,589] (Atromid-S)
Some blood cholesterol lowering agents potentiate thyroxine by drug displacement or by enzyme inhibition.

Corticosteroids[120]
Thyroid preparations increase tissue demands for adrenocortical hormones and may cause an acute adrenal crisis in patients with adrenocortical insufficiency. Correct adrenal insufficiency with corticosteroids before administering thyroid hormones.

Desipramine[120] (Pertofrane)
See *Antidepressants, Tricyclic* above.

Dextrothyroxine[120] (Choloxin)
Dosage of other thyroid preparations may have to be altered.

Digitalis[330,619,787]
Thyroid preparations may potentiate the toxic effects of digitalis. Increased digitalis dosage is required when thyroid hormonal replacement therapy is initiated (increased metabolism).

Doxepin (Sinequan)
See *Antidepressants, Tricyclic* above.

Epinephrine[120,529]
See *Levarterenol* below.

Goitrogenic medications and foods[100,181,357]
Avoid the goitrogenic substances listed in Table 8-3 (page 259) as they may act as physiological antagonists to thyroid preparations.

Guanethidine[590] (Ismelin)
See *Adrenergic Neuron Blocking Agents* above.

Halofenate (Livipas)
See *Thyroid Hormones* under *Halofenate.*

Imipramine (Tofranil)
See *Antidepressants, Tricyclic* above.

Indomethacin[120] (Indocin)
This combination may cause cardiovascular toxicity; transient cardiac arrhythmia.

Insulin[120]
In patients with diabetes mellitus, addition of thyroid hormone therapy may cause an increase in the required dosage of hypoglycemic agents. Decreasing the dose of thyroid hormone may possibly cause hypoglycemic reactions if the dose of insulin is not adjusted.

Ketamine[1528] (Ketajet, Ketalar)
The parenteral anesthetic ketamine, when administered to patients on a thyroid preparation may cause hypertension and tachycardia. Use caution and be prepared to treat hypertension if necessary.

Levarterenol[120,539,590] (Levophed, norepinephrine)
Injection of catecholamines such as epinephrine and norepinephrine into patients receiving thyroid preparations increases the risk of precipitating an episode of coronary insufficiency, especially in patients with coronary artery disease. Thyroxine increases the adrenergic effect of these agents. Careful observation is required.

Meperidine[951] (Demerol, etc.)
Dextrothyroxine potentiates meperidine.

Nortriptyline (Aventyl)
See *Antidepressants, Tricyclic* above.

Oral Contraceptives
See *Thyroid Hormones* under *Oral Contraceptives.*

Phenobarbital[421]
Thyroxine metabolism is decreased by phenobarbital.

Phenytoin (Dilantin, etc.)
See *Thyroid Hormones* under *Phenytoin.*

Protriptyline (Vivactil)
See *Antidepressants, Tricyclic* above.

Reserpine[590] (Serpasil, etc.)
See *Adrenergic Neuron Blocking Agents* above.

Soy bean preparations[48,357] (Mull-Soy, etc.)
Use caution in the use of soy bean preparations in patients requiring thyroid medication as soy bean products may be goitrogenic.

Warfarin (Coumadin)
See *Anticoagulants, Oral* above.

THYROLAR
See *Thyroid Preparations* (liotrix).
Liotrix is a combination of sodium levothyroxine and L-triiodothyronine (liothyronine).

THYROXINE
See *Dextrothyroxine* and *Thyroid Preparations.*

TINDAL MALEATE

See *Phenothiazines* and *Tranquilizers* (acetophenazine maleate).

TITRALAC

See *Antacids* and *Calcium Salts.*

TITROID

See *Thyroid Preparations* (levothyroxine).

TOBACCO

See *Nicotine* and *Smoking.*

TOBRAMCYIN

Dimenhydrinate (Dramamine)

See *Aminoglycoside Antibiotics* under *Dimenhydrinate.*

Ethacrynic Acid (Edecrin)

See *Aminoglycoside Antibiotics* under *Ethacrynic Acid.*

Methoxyflurane (Penthrane)

See under *Methoxyflurane.*

TOCOSAMINE

See *Oxytocics* (sparteine).

TOFRANIL

See *Antidepressants, Tricyclic* (imipramine).

TOLAZAMIDE (Tolinase)

See *Antidiabetics, Oral.*

TOLAZOLINE (Priscoline)

See also *Antihypertensives.*

Alcohol [28]

Same interactions as with disulfiram. Tolazoline prevents the oxidation of acetaldehyde, a metabolite of alcohol, producing uncomfortable symptoms. Hazardous.

TOLBUTAMIDE (Orinase)

See also *Antidiabetics, Oral.*

Alcohol [48,120,254,674,675]

Tolbutamide prevents the oxidation of acetaldehyde, a metabolite of alcohol, and thus produces a disulfiramlike reaction; also increased vasodilation. The half-life of tolbutamide is reduced more than 2-fold in alcoholics. Prolonged heavy intake of alcohol increases microsomal enzyme activity responsible for metabolism of the drug. Effectiveness may be greatly reduced in diabetics if they consume alcohol. See also *Alcohol* under *Antidiabetics, Oral.*

Anticoagulants, oral

See *Antidiabetics, Oral* as well as *Tolbutamide* under *Anticoagulants, Oral.*

Antidiabetics, sulfonylurea [181]
(Diabinese, Dymelor, Orinase)

Some patients may develop a tolerance to a given sulfonylurea, through enzyme induction or increasing rate of excretion. Such "secondary" failure may sometimes be overcome by switching to another sulfonylurea.

Aspirin [359,412,647]

Potentiation of hypoglycemic effect. The metabolism of tolbutamide may be abnormally slow in a patient who develops hypoglycemia while taking aspirin. See *Salicylates* below.

Chloramphenicol [676]

Potentiation of tolbutamide through microsomal enzyme inhibition by chloramphenicol. The half-life of tolbutamide is prolonged when it is administered simultaneously.

Clofibrate [120]

Clofibrate may cause hypoglycemia in patients receiving tolbutamide (probably displacement from protein binding sites). Reduce the dosage.

Cortisone

Cortisone, which is diabetogenic, may antagonize tolbutamide. See *Corticosteroids* under *Antidiabetics, Oral.*

Diazoxide

See *Tolbutamide* under *Diazoxide.*

Hydralazine [1514]

Tolbutamide inhibits the hypotensive and oliguric effects of hydralazine.

Mao inhibitors [181]

Potentiation of hypoglycemic action. MAO inhibitors inhibit tolbutamide metabolism.

Methyldopa [421] (Aldomet)

Blood dyscrasias may be produced by this combination.

Paraldehyde [678]

Tolbutamide potentiates the hypnotic effect of paraldehyde, probably by inhibition of the metabolizing enzymes.

Pentolinium [1514]

Tolbutamide inhibits the hypotensive and oliguric effects of pentolinium.

Phenformin [181] (DBI)

The combination of a sulfonylurea and phenformin may be effective in maturity-onset diabetics who fail to respond to a single oral agent but see *Phenformin.*

Phenylbutazone [76,181,197,647,679]

Potentiation of hypoglycemic action. Phenylbutazone may induce hypoglycemia through displacement of tolbutamide from plasma portein binding sites.

Phenyramidol [359,412,647]

Tolbutamide is potentiated. Its metabolism is slowed by phenyramidol.

Propranolol [263,421,681] (Inderal)

Propranolol may cause hypoglycemia. The potential danger may be increased because propranolol may prevent the premonitory signs and symptoms of acute hypoglycemia.

Salicylates [181,197,649]

Large doses of salicylates may have an additive or synergistic effect with tolbutamide in lowering blood glucose levels.

Sodium nitroprusside [1514]
(Sodium nitroferricyanide)

Tolbutamide decreases the hypotensive and oliguric effects of sodium nitroprusside.

Sulfaphenzole [76,197,640,647,680] (Orisul, Sulfabid)

Sulfaphenazole, like other *Sulfonamides* (see below) prolongs the half-life of tolbutamide from 5 to 6-fold leading to a protracted hypoglycemic condition; more apt to occur in patients with largely regular endogenous insulin synthesis.

Sulfisoxazole [409] (Gantrisin)

Hypoglycemic reaction. See *Sulfonamides* below.

Sulfonamides [181,202,409,458]

Potentiation of hypoglycemic action with this combination may produce coma and a prolonged crisis. Strongly bound sulfonamides such as sulfadimethoxine (no longer available in US because of its toxicity) potentiate tolbutamide by displacing the antidiabetic drug from tissue and plasma binding sites and by inhibiting its oxidation. The sulfonylurea, tolbutamide, potentiates sulfonamides by decreasing their metabolism (competition for same metabolizing enzymes).

Tolbutamide [257,695]

Tolerance to tolbutamide may develop as the drug induces its own metabolizing enzymes. The dosage may have to be increased gradually.

TORECAN

See *Phenothiazines* (thiethylperazine maleate).

TOXIC DRUGS

Antiemetics [120]

Since some phenothiazines and thioxanthenes and other drugs with antiemetic properties may mask overdosage of toxic drugs, an irreversible state may go undetected.

TRANCOGESIC

See *CNS Depressants, Muscle Relaxants, Salicylates* (aspirin) and *Tranquilizers* (chlormezanone).

TRANCOPAL

See *CNS Depressants, Muscle Relaxants,* and *Tranquilizers* (chlormezanone).

TRANCOPRIN

Same as for *Trancogesic* above.

TRANQUILIZERS

(Acetophenazine maleate [Tindal], azacyclonol [Frenquel] HCl, buclizine [Softran], captodiame [Suvren] HCl, butaperazine [Repoise] maleate, carphenazine [Proketazine] maleate, chlordiazepoxide HCl [Librium], chlormezanone [Trancopal], chlorpromazine [Thorazine], chlorprothixene [Taractan], diazepam [Valium], droperidol [Inapsine], fluphenazine [Prolixin], haloperidol [Haldol], hydroxyphenamate [Listica], hydroxyzine [Atarax, Vistaril], meprobamate [Equanil, Miltown], mesoridazine besylate [Serentil], oxanamide [Quiactin], oxazepam [Serax], perphenazine [Trilafon], phenaglycodol [Ultran], prochlorperazine [Compazine], piperacetazine [Quide], promazine [Sparine] HCl, thiopropazate [Dartal] HCl, thioridazine HCl [Mellaril], thiothixene [Navane], trifluoperazine [Stelazine], triflupromazine [Vesprin] HCl, tybamate [Solacen], etc.)

See also *CNS Depressants, Butyrophenones, Benzodiazepines, Meprobamate* and its congeners, *Phenothiazines,* etc.

Alcohol [78,120,619]

Lowered tolerance to alcohol. Potentiation of CNS depression. Severe hypotension and deep sedation may occur. See *CNS Depressants* and also below.

Analgesics [619,878]

Potentiated CNS depressant effects. See *CNS Depressants* below.

Anesthetics, general [120,619]

See *CNS Depressants* below.

Anticholinergics [120,619,633]

Tranquilizers like certain benzodiazepines and phenothiazines potentiate the side effects (blurred vision, dry mouth, urinary retention, etc.) of anticholinergics (additive effects). Sedative effects are also potentiated.

Antidepressants, Tricyclic [194,198,619]

(Aventyl, Elavil, Pertofane, Sinequan, Tofranil, Vivactil)

Tricyclic antidepressants potentiate the anticholinergic and sedative effects of certain tranquilizers (benzodiazepines, phenothiazines). May lower convulsive threshold and potentiate seizures. Additive effects.

Antihistamines [120,619]

Potentiated CNS depressant effects. See *CNS Depressants* below.

Barbiturates

See *CNS Depressants* below.

CNS depressants [78,120,198,619,633]

(Alcohol, anesthetics, antihistamines, barbiturates, narcotic analgesics, hypnotics and sedatives, narcotics, etc.)

Considerable caution must be exercised when any combination of a tranquilizer and another CNS depressant is administered. Many such combinations are contraindicated because of excessive potentiation of CNS depression. The effect may vary from excessive sedation, hypnosis, and general anesthesia to coma and death with some combinations, to accentuated anticholinergic (atropinelike) effects with seizures, excitement, and rage with other combinations. See *CNS Depressants.*

Furazolidone (Furoxone)

See *MAO Inhibitors* below.

Heparin [764]

Phenothiazine tranquilizers antagonize the anticoagulant action of heparin.

Hypnotics and sedatives

See *CNS Depressants* above.

Imipramine (Tofranil)

See *Antidepressants, Tricyclic* above.

Isocarboxazid (Marplan)

See *MAO Inhibitors* below.

Levodopa [724] (Dopar, Larodopa)

The phenothiazine tranquilizers are capable of defeating the therapeutic purpose of levodopa in Parkinson's syndrome.

MAO inhibitors [74,433,633]

MAO inhibitors potentiate tranquilizers. The enhanced sedation may be potentially hazardous.

Meperidine [78,633,844-846] (Demerol, etc.)

Severe hypotension. With some phenothiazines (chlorpromazine, perphenazine and trifluoperazine) enhanced extrapyramidal symptoms and hypertension may occur. Death has occured. See *CNS Depressants,* above.

Methotrexate [198,512,619]

Tranquilizers may enhance methotrexate toxicity by displacing the antineoplastic from protein binding sites.

Narcotic analgesics

See *CNS Depressants* above.

Nialamide (Niamid)

See *MAO Inhibitors* above.

Nylidrin [489] (Arlidin)

Nylidrin, a vasodilator, potentiates the antipsychotic effect of the phenothiazine tranquilizers clinically. It displaces the phenothiazines from secondary binding sites.

Pargyline (Eutonyl)

See *MAO Inhibitors* above.

Phenelzine (Nardil)

See *MAO Inhibitors* above.

Phenobarbital

See *CNS Depressants* above.

Phenothiazines

See *CNS Depressants* above.

Phenytoin [884] (Dilantin)

Chlordiazepoxide may potentiate phenytoin by enzyme inhibition. Chlorpromazine may lower the convulsive threshold.

Thiopental [116]
Potentiation of thiopental anesthesia has occurred from preoperative administration of minor tranquilizers.

Tranylcypromine (Parnate)
See *MAO Inhibitors* above.

TRANYLCYPROMINE (Parnate)
See *MAO Inhibitors.*

TRASYLOL (Aprotinin)

Muscle relaxants [567]
Trasylol, a kallikrein inhibitor, potentiates muscle relaxants such as succinylcholine and tubocurarine and may produce apnea.

T-RAU
See *Rauwolfia alkaloids* (whole root).

TRECATOR
See *Ethionamide.*

TREMIN
See *Antiparkinsonism Drugs* (trihexyphenidyl).

TRIACETYLOLEANDOMYCIN (troleandomycin)
See *Antibiotics.*

Ergotamine [682]
Triacetyloleandomycin may inhibit the metabolism of ergotamine and precipitate acute ergotism.

TRIAMCINOLONE (Aristocort)
See also *Corticosteroids.*

Phenytoin [330,450,451]
Phenytoin, through microsomal enzyme induction and possibly a more complicated type of interaction, inhibits the activity of triamcinolone.

TRIAMINIC
See *Antihistamines* (pheniramine, pyrilamine), and *Sympathomimetics* (phenylpropanolamine).

TRIAMINICIN
See *Antihistamines* (chlorpheniramine), *Aspirin, Caffeine,* and *Sympathomimetics* (phenylpropanolamine).

TRIAMINICOL
See *Antihistamines* (pheniramine and pyrilamine) and *Sympathomimetics* (phenylpropanolamine), *Dextromethorphan,* and *Ammonium Chloride.*

TRIAMTERENE (Dyrenium)
See also *Diuretics.*

Acetazolamide (Diamox)
See *Amiloride* and *Acetazolamide.*

Antidiabetics [421]
Triamterene inhibits oral antidiabetics.

Antihypertensives [421]
Triamterene potentiates antihypertensives.

Digitalis [120]
Triamterene is a potassium-conserving diuretic; hyperkalemia may result, leading to decreased effectiveness of digitalis.

Diuretics, other [79,120]
Triamterene, a potassium conserver, is frequently combined with a thiazide diuretic to reduce potassium loss and to enhance the diuretic effect.

Hydralazine [421] **(Apresoline)**
Triamterene potentiates the hypotensive action of hydralazine.

Hydrochlorothiazide [120,172]
This combination has synergistic activity in diuresis and sodium excretion, with minimal potassium excretion. It reduces hypokalemic metabolic acidosis produced by hydrochlorothiazide, and hyperkalemic metabolic acidosis produced by triamterene.

Hypotensive agents [226]
Enhanced hypotensive effect.

Mecamylamine [421] **(Inversine)**
Triamterene potentiates the hypotensive action of mecamylamine.

Methotrexate [951]
Triamterene potentiates methotrexate.

Potassium salts [1686]
Concomitant use of triamterene, a conserver of potassium, and potassium supplements can be lethal if not closely monitored. The resulting hyperkalemia has caused pacemaker failure. See also *Potassium Salts* under *Spironolactone.*

Spironolactone [120,226] **(Aldactone)**
Severe, hazardous hyperkalemia may result with spironolactone and triamterene, both of which are potassium conservers, in combination.

Thiazide diuretics
See *Diuretics, Other* above.

Veratrum alkaloids [421]
Triamterene potentiates the hypotensive action of veratrum alkaloids.

TRIAVIL
See *Antidepressants, Tricyclic* (amitriptyline) and *Phenothiazines* (perphenazine).

TRICHLORMETHIAZIDE (Metahydrin, Naqua)
See *Thiazide Diuretics.*

TRICHLOROETHYLENE

Epinephrine [683,684]
Cardiac arrhythmias and death may occur with this combination.

Soda lime [184]
Death has occurred due to phosgene formation during anesthesia.

TRICLOFOS
See *Chloral Hydrate* under *Alcohol.*

TRICOFURON
See *MAO Inhibitors* (furazolidone).

TRICYCLAMOL
See *Anticholinergics.*

TRICYCLIC ANTIDEPRESSANTS
See *Antidepressants, Tricyclic.*

TRIDAL
See *Anticholinergics* (pipenzolate, piperidolate).

TRIDIHEXETHYL (Pathilon)
See *Anticholinergics.*

TRIDIONE
See *Anticonvulsants* (trimethadione).

TRIFLUOPERAZINE (Stelazine)
See *Phenothiazines* and *Tranquilizers.*

TRIFLUPERIDOL (Triperidol)
See also *Tranquilizers.*

Anticoagulants, oral [147]
This butyrophenone tranquilizer antagonizes oral anticoagulants by enzyme induction.

TRIFLUPROMAZINE (Vesprin)
See *Phenothiazines* and *Tranquilizers.*

TRIHEXYPHENIDYL (Artane)
See *Anticholinergics.*

Antihistamines [120]
Additive anticholinergic (atropinelike) effects. Causes very dry mouth with possible loss of teeth and suppurative parotitis.

Phenothiazines [1741]
See *Anticholinergics* under *Phenothiazines.*

TRIIODOETHIONIC ACID
See *Radiopaque Media* (iophenoxic acid).

TRIIODOTHYRONINE (Cytomel)
See also *Thyroid Preparations* (liothyronine).

Anticoagulants, oral [120,330,421,673]
Triiodothyronine increases anticoagulant effect of coumarin derivatives by increasing their affinity for receptors and displacing them from protein binding sites. Reduction of anticoagulant dosage by one-third may be necessary.

Imipramine [456] **(Tofranil)**
The speed and efficacy of imipramine in the treatment of clinical depression may be enhanced by the addition of triiodothyronine to the treatment program.

Neomycin [421]
Neomycin potentiates the hypocholesterolemic action of triiodothyronine.

Oral contraceptives [421]
See *Thyroid Hormones* under *Oral Contraceptives.*

Puromycin [421]
Puromycin potentiates the hypocholesterolemic action of triiodothyronine.

TRILAFON
See *Phenothiazines* (perphenazine).

TRILENE
See *Trichloroethylene.*

TRIMEPRAZINE (Temaril)
See *Phenothiazines.*

TRIMETHAPHAN (Arfonad) Camsylate
See *Antihypertensives* and *Ganglionic Blocking Agents.*

TRIMETHIDINIUM (Ostensin) Methosulfate
See *Antihypertensives* and *Ganglionic Blocking Agents.*

TRIMETHOPRIM (Syraprim)

Sulfonamides [421,933]
Trimethoprim improves antibacterial action of sulfonamides against *S. pneumoniae, S. pyogenes, N. gonorrhoeae, E. coli.*

TRIMETON
See *Antihistamines* (pheniramine).

TRIOGESIC
See *Sympathomimetics* and under *Phenylpropanolamine,* and *Acetominophen.*

TRIPELENNAMINE (Pyribenzamine).
See *Antihistamines.*

TRIPERIDOL
See *Trifluperidol.*

TRIPROLIDINE (Actidil)
See *Antihistamines.*

TRISOGEL
See *Antacids, Aluminum Salts,* and *Magnesium Salts.*

TROMETHAMINE (Tham-E)

Anticoagulants [120,147]
Tromethamine may produce an anticoagulant effect which is additive.

Dextran [951]
Dextran may prolong the action of tromethamine.

TROMEXAN
See *Anticoagulants, Oral* (ethyl biscoumacetate).

Barbiturates [685]
Barbiturates inhibit the anticoagulant action of tromexan.

Glutethimide [436]
Glutethimide inhibits the anticoagulant action of tromexan.

TRYPSIN

Anticoagulants, oral [198,421]
Proteolytic enzymes like trypsin potentiate the anticoagulant action of these agents.

TRYPTIZOL
See *Antidepressants, Tricyclic* (amitriptyline).

TRYPTOPHAN

Mao inhibitors
See *Tryptophan* under *MAO Inhibitors.*

Vinblastine [165]
Tryptophan interferes with the antitumor activity of vinblastine.

TUAMINE
See *Sympathomimetics* (tuaminoheptane).

TUBERCULIN (PPD) SKIN TEST

Corticosteroids [486]
Corticosteroids temporarily depress tuberculin response.

Measles, virus vaccine, live attenuated [120] **(Attenuvax, etc.)**
Live attenuated measles virus, when added to PPD sensitive lymphocytes, significantly reduces the response of these cells to PPD. The skin test should not be given concomitantly.

Mumps vaccine [716]
The tuberculin reaction is significantly depressed by live, attenuated mumps virus vaccine.

Rifampin
See *Tuberculin* under *Rifampin.*

TUBOCURARINE
See *Muscle Relaxants, Peripherally Acting, Competitive Type.*

TUINAL
See *Barbiturates* (amobarbital, secobarbital), and *CNS Depressants.*

TUSSAGESIC
See *Acetaminophen, Antihistamines* (pheniramine, pyrilamine), *Narcotics* (dextromethorphan), and *Sympathomimetics* (phenylpropanolamine).

TUSSAMINIC
Similar to *Tussagesic* without Acetaminophen.

TUSSANIL
See *Antihistamines* (chlorpheniramine, pyrilamine) and *Sympathomimetics* (phenylephrine, phenylpropanolamine).

TUSSAR-2
See *Antihistamines* (chlorpheniramine) and *Narcotic Analgesics* (codeine). Also contains carbetapentane, glyceryl guaiacolate, and alcohol.

TUSSAR SF
Similar to *Tussar-2,* but sugar free.

TUSSEND
See *Narcotics* (hydrocodone) and *Sympathomimetics* (phenylephrine).

TUSSI-ORGANIDIN
See *Alcohol, Antihistamines* (chlorpheniramine), *Iodine* (iodinated glycerol), and *Narcotic Analgesics* (codeine).

TUSSI-ORGANIDIN-DM
Same as above except dextromethorphan is substituted for codeine.

TUSS-ORNADE
See *Anticholinergics* (caramiphen, isopropamide), *Antihistamines* (chlorpheniramine), and *Sympathomimetics* (phenylpropanolamine).

TWEEN 80
See *Polysorbate 80.*

TYLENOL
See *Acetaminophen.*

TYRAMINE
See *Sympathomimetics* and *Tyramine-rich Foods.*

Reserpine [554]
Reserpine diminishes the pressor effect of tyramine because reserpine depletes the stores of norepinephrine through which tyramine indirectly exerts its pressor effect by release of the transmitter.

MAO inhibitors [161,218,687]
MAO inhibitors enhance and prolong the stimulatory effects of tyramine on blood pressure and the contractile force of the heart. Severe headache, hypertension, subarachnoid hemorrhage, perhaps death. See also *Tyramine-rich Foods.*

TYRAMINE-RICH AND PRESSOR-CONTAINING FOODS
(Avocados, beer, Brie, caviar, Cheddar, Camembert, Emmenthaler, Gruyere, Stilton, and other ripe cheeses, beef and chicken livers, chocolate, fermented products such as fermented bolognas and salamis, pepperoni and summer sausage, canned figs, kippered or pickled herring, Chianti and possibly other red wines, meat extracts such as Bovril, yeast extracts such as Marmite, etc.) and foods containing other pressor precursors or principles such as caffeine (coffee, tea, and cola drinks), dopa (broad bean pods and fava beans), histamine (some alcoholic beverages) and serotonin (bananas, pineapples, plums)

Amphetamines [529,533,534]
This combination may cause a hypertensive crisis.

Eutonyl
See *MAO Inhibitors* below.

Furazolidone [356] (Furoxone)
See *MAO inhibitors* below.

Guanethidine [117,633] (Ismelin)
Tyramine antagonises the hypotensive effect of guanethidine.

Isocarboxazid (Marplan)
See *MAO Inhibitors* below.

MAO Inhibitors [25,41,45-7,49,56,95,102,105,120,137,161,213,218,265,330,338,352,459,463,634,687,757,758,759,1357]

(Eutonyl, Furoxone, Marplan, Matulane, Nardil, Parnate, etc.)
Death may result from a combination of a MAO inhibitor (used in hypertension, infections, and psychiatric disorders) and a food containing tyramine in high enough concentration. Tyramine, a pressor principle which acts indirectly (epinephrine and norepinephrine releaser) and which is normally inactivated by MAO in the liver and gut, is potentiated by inhibition of catecholamine metabolism. A hypertensive crisis may occur (severe occipital headache radiating frontally, soreness or stiffness of the neck, palpitation with either bradycardia or tachycardia, nausea, vomiting, fever either with a cold, clammy skin or profuse sweating, constricting chest pain, dilated pupils, photophobia, coma, and subarachnoid hemorrhage). MAO inhibitors cause both tyramine and norepinephrine to accumulate. Use a short-acting α-adrenergic blocking agent such as phentolamine (Regitine) to treat a hypertensive crisis caused by these foods (and the others listed above) with an MAOI.

Morphine [643]
Tyramine antagonizes the analgesic effects of morphine which depletes catecholamines.

Nialamide (Niamid)
See *MAO Inhibitors* above. Discontinued in US.

Pargyline (Eutonyl)
See *MAO Inhibitors* above.

Phenelzine (Nardil)
See *MAO Inhibitors* above.

Procarbazine [120,619] (Matulane)
Contraindicated because the antineoplastic procarbazine is a MAO inhibitor. See above.

Reserpine [529,554]
Reserpine diminishes the pressor action of tyramine and may even completely nullify this action which depends on rapid, brief release of norepinephrine from adrenergic terminals. Reserpine initially produces a sympathomimetic effect as it begins to deplete the catecholamine from its adrenergic terminal storage sites but through this depleting effect removes catecholamine so that indirectly acting sympathomimetics like tyramine can no longer exert their action. Thus the major effect of reserpine is adrenergic blockade.

Tranylcypromine [137] (Parnate)
See *MAO Inhibitors* above.

ULACORT
See *Prednisolone.*

ULCIMINS
See *Antacids* and *Acetaminophen.*

ULO
See *Antitussives* (chlophedianol).

ULTANDREN
See *Androgens* (fluoxymesterone).

ULTRAN
See *CNS Depressants* and *Tranquilizers* (phenaglycodol).

ULVICAL AND ULVICAL PLUS
See *Dietary Supplements*.

UNIPEN
See *Antibiotics* (sodium nafcillin).

UNITENSEN
See *Antihypertensives* (cryptenamine).

URACIL MUSTARD
See *Alkylating Agents*.

URAMINE
See *Anticholinergics* (atropine, hyoscyamine), and *Methenamine*.

UREA

Anticoagulants [619]
Urea, with its fibrinolytic activity, may potentiate anticoagulants.

Lithium carbonate [120, 1851]
Urea antagonizes lithium carbonate by increasing its excretion.

Succinylcholine [1121]
A 30% infusion of urea prevents or decreases the rise in intraocular pressure induced by succinylcholine (in the rabbit).

URECHOLINE
See *Parasympathomimetics* (bethanechol).

URETHAN (Urethane)

Quinidine [697]
Urethan increases the toxicity of quinidine.

Hexobarbital [695]
Urethan (enzyme inducer) inhibits hexobarbital.

U.R.I. DELACAPS
See *Antihistamines* (chlorpheniramine) and *Sympathomimetics* (phenylephrine, phenylpropanolamine).

URICOSURIC AGENTS
(Probenecid [Benemid], oxyphenbutazone [Tandearil], phenylbutazone [Butazolidin], Sulfinpyrazone [Anturane], etc.)
See also under *Allopurinol* (antigout drug, not uricosuric), *Probenecid*, and *Sulfinpyrazone*. See *Antigout Drugs*.

URIFON
See *Sulfonamides* (sulfamethizole).

URINARY ACIDIFIERS
(Ammonium chloride, ammonium nitrate, calcium chloride, *dl*-methionine, etc.)
See also *Acidifying Agents*.
Acidification of the urine tends to convert weak acids into reabsorbable nonionized forms and thus potentiates them. The reverse is true for weak bases. [18, 36, 325, 870]

Adrenergics [529]
(Amphetamines, pressor amines, sympathomimetics, etc.)
Acidifiers inhibit these weak bases by accelerating their urinary excretion.

Amitriptyline [325, 870] (Elavil)
This weakly basic tricyclic is inhibited.

Amphetamines [486, 529]
Amphetamines (weakly basic amines) are inhibited by acidifiers.

Anticholinergics [165, 325, 870]
These weak bases are inhibited by urinary acidifiers.

Anticoagulants, oral [78, 325, 870]
These weak acids are potentiated by urinary acidifiers.

Antidepressants, tricyclic [28, 194, 579, 870]
(Aventyl, Elavil, Norpramin, Pertofrane, Tofranil, Triavil, Vivactil, etc.)
These weak bases are inhibited by urinary acidifiers.

Antihistamines [325, 870]
Antihistamines (weak bases) are inhibited.

Antimalarials [325, 870]
(Aralen, Atabrine, Avochlor, Daraprim, Malocide, Syraprim, etc.)
Antimalarials (weak bases) are inhibited.

Antipyrine [325, 870]
Antipyrine, a weak base, is inhibited.

Aspirin [78, 325, 870]
Salicylate analgesia is potentiated.

Barbiturates [28, 325, 870]
Barbiturates are potentiated.

Carbonic anhydrase inhibitors [173]
(Cardrase, Daranide, Diamox, Ethamide, Neptazane)
Acidifying agents tend to supply H^+ ions and thus antagonize the action of the carbonic anhydrase inhibitors which is alkalinization through depression of CO_2 hydration and inhibition of bicarbonate reabsorption.

Diuretics, mercurial [325, 870]
These diuretics are potentiated.

Ethacrynic acid [325, 870] (Edecrin)
Ethacrynic acid is potentiated.

Mecamylamine [325, 529, 726] (Inversine)
Mecamylamine is inhibited.

Methenamine [120, 578]
The antibacterial action of methenamine is potentiated. See *Acidifiers, Urinary* under *Methenamine*.

Methyldopa [325, 870]
Urinary acidifiers inhibit the hypotensive activity of the weak base, methyldopa, by increasing its rate of renal excretion.

Narcotic analgesics [325, 870]
Narcotic analgesics are inhibited.

Nitrofurantoin [578] (Furadantin)
Nitrofurantoin is potentiated.

Phenobarbital [28, 325, 870]
All barbiturates are potentiated.

Quinidine [325, 581, 870]
Quinidine is inhibited.

Salicylates [275, 325, 870]
Salicylates are potentiated.

Sulfonamides [198]
Sulfonamides are potentiated. Antibacterial activity is enhanced and excretion is retarded, but the likelihood of crystalluria is increased.

Tetracyclines [578]
Tetracyclines are excreted more readily in an acid pH but their antibacterial activity is enhanced.

URINARY ALKALINIZERS
(Sodium Bicarbonate, Sodium Citrate, Sodium Lactate, etc.)

See also *Alkalinizing Agents*.

The urinary alkalinizers have the opposite actions of the urinary acidifiers above. [18,36]

Amphetamines [325,870]

Urinary alkalinizers enhance the activity of amphetamine due to decreased rate of excretion.

Anticholinergics [205,325,870]

Enhanced anticholinergic effect.

Erythromycin [120] **(Ethrocin, Ilotycin)**

The antibacterial activity of erythromycin is enhanced when the urinary pH is more alkaline.

Kanamycin [120] **(Kantrex)**

Alkaline urinary pH potentiates the urinary antibacterial action of kanamycin.

Mecamylamine [325,726,870] **(Inversine)**

Mecamylamine is potentiated.

Methenamine [421]

An acidic urine is necessary for methenamine to liberate formaldehyde and be effective; alkalinization of the urine will decrease its effectiveness.

Nalidixic Acid [198]

Naladixic acid is inhibited by urinary alkalinizers; increased excretion in alkaline pH.

Neomycin-Kanamycin-Streptomycin [578]

An alkaline urinary pH enhances the urinary antibacterial activity of these three agents. Alkalinization is probably only necessary when streptomycin is used to treat urinary tract infections.

Phenobarbital [28,579] **(Phenobarbitone)**

All barbiturates are inhibited by the alkalinizers. The elimination of phenobarbital is accelerated by alkalinizing the urine.

Quinacrine [325] **(Atabrine)**

Antimalarials related to quinacrine are potentiated by alkalinizers. Toxic effects may be severe.

Salicylates [275,325,870]

Alkalinizers decrease the analgesic and antipyretic actions of salicylate due to increased rate of excretion.

Streptomycin [578]

An alkaline urinary pH enhances urinary antibacterial activity; alkalinization is probably necessary when streptomycin is used to treat urinary tract infections caused by *E. coli* and *Proteus* organisms.

Sulfonamides [22,870]

With some of the older sulfonamides (sulfadiazine, etc.) it was necessary to alkalinize the urine to prevent crystalluria. Since the sulfonamides are weak acids, alkalinization of the urine will increase the rate of excretion and possibly decrease the effectiveness of the drug. See also *Acidifying Agents* under *Sulfonamides*.

URISED

See *Anticholinergics* (atropine, hyoscyamine) and *Methenamine*.

UROBIOTIC

See *Sulfonamides* (sulfamethizole) and *Phenazopyridine* (see *Interferences in Clinical Laboratory Testing of Urine* in Chapter 7). See also *Antibiotics* (oxytetracycline).

UROKINASE

Anticoagulants, oral [901,904]

Urokinase, with its thrombolytic action, may potentiate anticoagulants and cause hemorrhage.

UROPEUTIC

See *Anticholinergics* (hyoscyamus), *Methenamine*, and *Sulfonamides* (sulfamethizole).

URO-PHOSPHATE

See *Urinary Acidifiers* (sodium acid phosphate) and *Methenamine*.

UROQID-ACID

See *Methenamine* and *Urinary Acidifiers* (sodium acid phosphate).

URSINUS

See *Antihistamines* (pheniramine, pyrilamine), *Calcium Salts*, *Salicylates* (calcium carbaspirin carbamide) and *Sympathomimetics* (phenylpropanolamine).

VACCINES,
(Live Virus, Attenuated (measles, mumps, rabies, smallpox, yellow fever, etc.)

Alkylating agents

See *Immunosuppressants* below.

Antimetabolites

See *Immunosuppressants* below.

Antineoplastics

See *Immunosuppressants* below.

Corticosteroids

See *Immunosuppressants* below.

Corticotropin (ACTH)

See *Immunosuppressants* below.

Immunosuppressants [120,198,203,312,377,486,619,1132,1199]
(Alkylating agents, antimetabolites such as methotrexate, other antineoplastics, corticosteroids, phenytoin, etc.)

Vaccines should not be administered to patients receiving immunosuppressant drugs which depress resistance to disease and reduce the effectiveness of the vaccination. Serious and possibly fatal illness may develop. Generalized vaccinia has developed following smallpox vaccination of a patient on immunosuppressant (methotrexate, prednisone, etc.) therapy. Phenytoin may produce low immunoglobulin A, inability to develop antibodies, absence of delayed hypersensitivity to antigens, etc. It suppresses both cellular and humoral immune responses, *e.g.*, patients failed to develop antibodies to tetanus toxoid.

Inactivated measles virus vaccine [1051,1083]

Dermal hypersensitivity reactions to skin tests with measles and polio vaccines are delayed in recipients of inactivated measles virus vaccine. Severe reactions (high fever, prodromal cough, and pulmonary consolidation) may occur in recipients of "killed" measles vaccine if they later receive live attenuated measles vaccine or if they are exposed to natural measles virus.

Indomethacin

See under *Smallpox Vaccine*.

Tuberculin test [716,1052]

The tuberculin reaction is significantly depressed by live, attenuated mumps vaccine and by live measles virus.

X-radiation [120,377,1990]

Virus vaccines are contraindicated in patients receiving irradiation. X-radiation tends to produce pancytopenia and atrophy of the bone marrow with decreased resistance to infection. A very dangerous combination (potentially lethal).

VALETHAMATE (Murel)

See *Anticholinergics*.

VALIUM
See *CNS Depressants* and *Tranquilizers* (diazepam).

VALLESTRIL
See *Estrogens* (methallenestril).

VALPIN
See *Anticholinergics* (anisotropine).

VANCOCIN
See *Antibiotics* (vancomycin).

VAPONEFRIN
See *Sympathomimetics* (epinephrine).

VAPO-N-ISO
See *Sympathomimetics* (isoproterenol).

VASOCONSTRICTORS
See also *Sympathomimetics.*

Anesthetics [120]
If hypotension from anesthetics occurs during obstetrical procedures use of an oxytocic with a vasoconstrictor may result in severe persistant hypertension.

Oxytocics [609-611]
Severe, persistent hypertension, with rupture of cerebral blood vessels may occur. Synergistic and additive vasoconstrictive effects of both drugs.

VASODILAN
See *Vasodilators* (isoxsuprine).

VASODILATORS
(Amyl nitrite, cyclandelate [Cyclospasmol], dioxyline [Paveril] phosphate, erithrityl tetranitrate [Cardilate], glyceryl trinitrate, isosorbid dinitrate [Isordil], isoxsuprine [Vasodilan], mannitol hexanitrate [Nitranitol], pentaerythritol tetranitrate [Peritrate], trolnitrate phosphate [Metamine, Nitretamin], etc.)

Antihypertensives [120]
(Aldomet, Apresoline, Arfonad, Capla, Inversine, Ismelin, Rauwolfia alkaloids, Regitine, Veratrum viride alkaloids)
Vasodilators also lower the blood pressure and there may be an enhanced hypotensive effect. Reduced dosage of the hypotensive agent is frequently necessary.

VASOPRESSIN (ADH, Pitressin)
See also *Vasopressors.*

Acetaminophen [421] (Tempra, Tylenol)
Acetaminophen potentiates vasopressin.

Acetohexamide (Dymelor)
See *Antidiabetics, Oral* below.

Anesthetics [173]
Anesthetics potentiate vasopressin.

Antidiabetics, oral [421,722,723]
(Diabinese, Dymelor, Orinase)
Oral antidiabetics (sulfonylureas) potentiate the antidiuretic action of vasopressin (small amounts).

Chlorpropamide [421]
See *Antidiabetics, Oral* above.

Cyclophosphamide [421] (Cytoxan)
Cyclophosphamide increases excretion of vasopressin and this inhibits its action.

Ganglionic blocking agents [173]
Ganglionic blocking agents markedly increase sensitivity to pressor effects of vasopressin.

Lithium carbonate [171,1913]
(Eskalith, Lithane, Lithonate)
Lithium carbonate may block the renal response to vasopressin by inhibiting its action on renal adenylate cyclase, and thus decreasing its stimulation of tubular reabsorption of water.

Neostigmine [172] (Prostigmin)
Neostigmine, a cholinergic, potentiates the action of vasopressin in relieving intestinal paresis and distention.

Phenformin [421] (DBI)
Phenformin (withdrawn from U.S. market) potentiates vasopressin. See *Phenformin.*

Tolbutamide
See *Antidiabetics, Oral* above.

VASOPRESSORS
(Angiotensin, ephedrine, epinephrine, levarterenol, Metaraminol, nicotine in tobacco, tyramine and dopa in certain foods, etc. See *Tyramine-rich Foods*).

Antihypertensives [78]
This combination on physiologically antagonistic agents increases the likelihood that cardiac arrhythmias may occur.

Ergonovine [120]
This combination of ergot alkaloid and pressor amine may result in excessively high blood pressure.

Furazolidone (Furoxone)
See *MAO Inhibitors* below.

Furosemide [120] (Frusemide, Lasix)
Sulfonamide diuretics like furosemide have been reported to decrease arterial responsiveness to pressor amines.

Guanethidine [30,117,120] (Ismelin)
Cardiac arrhythmias may occur with this combination. See the discussion on *Sympathomimetics* under *Reserpine.*

MAO inhibitors [633]
Contraindicated. MAO inhibitors may strongly potentiate the pressor amines and cause a hypertensive crisis, possibly death. Cold, hay fever, and weight reducing medications, nasal decongestants, and other products containing vasopressors, many obtainable over-the-counter, are contraindicated.

Methyldopa (Aldomet)
See the discussion on *Sympathomimetics* under *Reserpine.*

Methylergonovine [120]
Excessively high blood pressure may result.

Methylphenidate [120,619] (Ritalin)
Use cautiously with pressor agents. Its use is contraindicated with epinephrine and levarterenol since it strongly potentiates their actions.

Oxytocics [173,609,611]
(Ergotrate, Methergine, Pitocin, etc.)
Synergistic vasoconstriction. Excessively high blood pressure may result. The increase in renal blood flow caused by oxytocin infusion is blocked by vasopressin.

Pargyline [633]
See *MAO Inhibitors* above.

Procainamide [120]
Levarterenol or phenylephrine may be used IV to counteract the hypotension produced by procainamide given IV.

Reserpine
See the discussion on *Sympathomimetics* under *Reserpine.*

Veratrum alkaloids[120]
Vasopressors such as ephedrine and phenylephrine counteract any excessive hypotension produced by veratrum alkaloids.

VASOXYL
See *Sympathomimetics* (methoxamine) and *Vasopressors.*

V-CILLIN
See *Penicillins.*

VCR
See *Vincristine.*

VEGETABLES, GREEN LEAFY
See *Vitamin K* under *Anticoagulants, Oral.*

VELACYCLINE
See *Tetracyclines.*

VELBAN
See *Vinblastine.*

VENTILADE
See *Antihistamines* (methapyrilene, pheniramine, pyrilamine) and *Sympathomimetics* (phenylpropanolamine).

VERACILLIN
See *Penicillins* (sodium dicloxacillin).

VERATRUM ALKALOIDS
(Alkavervir [Veriloid], cryptenamine [Unitensin], protoveratrines A and B, etc.)
See also *Antihypertensives.*

Amphetamines[421]
Amphetamines inhibit the hypotensive action of veratrum alkaloids.

Anesthetics, general[421]
General anesthetics potentiate the hypotensive and central depressant actions of these alkaloids (additive effects). Withdraw the alkaloids two weeks before surgery.

Anesthetics, local[170]
Local anesthetics inhibit the action of veratrum on excitable cells.

Antidepressants, tricyclic[421]
Tricyclic antidepressants diminish the hypotensive action of these alkaloids.

Atropine sulfate[120,170]
Atropine sulfate abolishes the bradycrotic effect of cryptenamine and diminishes the hypotensive effect.

Digitalis[120,170]
Ectopic cardiac arrhythmias are likely to occur in patients receiving digitalis concurrently with veratrum alkaloids. Veratrum has a digitalislike action on the heart.

Ethacrynic acid[421] **(Edecrin)**
Ethacrynic acid potentiates the hypotensive action of veratrum alkaloids.

MAO inhibitors[421]
MAO inhibitors potentiate antihypertensives. Since both types of agents lower the blood pressure, there may be an enhanced hypotensive effect. Reduced dosage may be necessary.

Morphine and related drugs[120,619]
Morphine and related drugs act additively with veratrum alkaloids to produce bradycardia.

Pentobarbital[619]
Pentobarbital sodium IV controls the emesis produced by veratrum alkaloids.

Quinidine[120,619]
Caution should be observed when quinidine is used with veratrum alkaloids. Cardiac arrhythmias may develop.

Reserpine[120]
Reserpine and protoveratrines potentiate each other. This permits reduced dosages and fewer side effects.

Saluretic agent[120]
Concomitant treatment of hypertensive patients with cryptenamine or its formulations and a saluretic agent (*e.g.,* thiazide diuretics), results in a greater reduction of blood pressure than does treatment with either agent alone. Use lower doses of both agents.

Spironolactone[421]
Spironolactone potentiates the hypotensive action of veratrum alkaloids.

Sympathomimetics[421]
Sympathomimetics inhibit the hypotensive action of veratrum alkaloids.

Thiazide diuretics[421,619]
Thiazide diuretics potentiate the hypotensive action of veratrum alkaloids.

Triamterene[421]
Triamterene potentiates the hypotensive action of veratrum alkaloids.

Vasopressors[120]
Vasopressors such as ephedrine and phenylephrine counteract excessive hypotension produced by veratrum alkaloids.

VERCYTE
See *Antineoplastics* (pipobroman).

VERILOID
See *Veratrum Alkaloids* (alkavervir).

VERMIZINE
See *Piperazine.*

VERSENATE
See *EDTA.*

VESPRIN
See *Phenothiazines* (triflupromazine) and *Tranquilizers.*

VIBRAMYCIN
See *Tetracyclines.*

VINBARBITAL
See *Barbiturates.*

VINBLASTINE (Velban)
See also *Antineoplastics.*

Amino acids[179]
Several amino acids reverse the effects of vinblastine on leukemia.

Aspartic acid[120]
Aspartic acid protects test animals from lethal doses of vinblastine, but is not effective in reversing the antitumor action.

Glutamic acid[120,179]
Glutamic acid blocks both the toxic and antineplastic activity of vinblastine. It also protects test animals from lethal doses of the antineoplastic.

Tryptophan[120,179]
Tryptophan interferes with the antitumor activity of vinblastine.

VINCRISTINE (Oncovin)
See also *Antineoplastics*.

Glutamic acid [120,179]
See under *Vinblastine* above.

Methotrexate [433]
This combination may cause melena, hypotension.

VIOCIN
See *Antibiotics* (viomycin).

VISTARIL
See *Hydroxyzine*.

VI-SYNERAL
See *Dietary Supplements*.

VITAMIN A
See also *Vitamins, Fat-Soluble*.

Bile salts [165,176]
Absorption of vitamin A is enhanced if bile salts are also administered.

Corticosteroids [486]
Topically applied vitamin A overcomes the antihealing effect of corticosteroids and promotes wound healing by enhancing tissue lysosome production of healing enzymes.

Mineral oil [2026]
Timing of intake of mineral oil strongly influences its effect on body levels of vitamin A. If it is taken with food the oil absorbs the dietary source of A, carotene, which is converted to vitamin A in the liver and also stored there. If the oil is given at bedtime on an empty stomach it does not deplete the body of carotene. The pure vitamin A, either produced synthetically or ingested in foods containing A produced in animal livers (dairy products, eggs, fish liver oils, etc.) is an alcohol that is not absorbed by mineral oil.

VITAMIN B$_1$
See *Thiamine*.

VITAMIN B$_2$
See *Riboflavin*.

VITAMIN B$_6$
See *Pyridoxine*.

VITAMIN B$_{12}$ (Cyanocobalamin)

Alcohol [876]
Alcohol causes malabsorption of vitamin B$_{12}$.

***p*-Aminosalicylic acid** [202,880,1469,1481,1572,1692] **(PAS)**
PAS inhibits intestinal absorption and urinary excretion of vitamin B$_{12}$. See *Vitamin B$_{12}$* and *p-Aminosalicylic Acid*.

Chloramphenicol [491]
Vitamin B$_{12}$ prevents chloramphenicol induced optic neuritis.

Colchicine
See *Vitamin B$_{12}$* under *Colchicine*.

Neomycin [880,1405,1505]
Neomycin inhibits the gastrointestinal absorption of vitamin B$_{12}$. Administration of colchicine increases this malabsorption. Probably a significant interaction only when large doses are given for prolonged periods.

Potassium chloride [1062]
Potassium chloride impairs absorption of vitamin B$_{12}$ and may lead to a deficiency of the vitamin because of lowered intestinal pH. Below pH 5.5 vitamin B$_{12}$ is not absorbed.

Pyrimethamine [619] **(Daraprim)**
Cyanocobalamin accentuates the hematologic deficiency produced by pyrimethamine.

Vitamin C [1323,1495]
Vitamin B$_{12}$ is destroyed by vitamin C; 500 mg. of vitamin C may destroy 50–95% of B$_{12}$ in meals, in vitamin supplements,

the alimentary tract, and the enterohepatic circulation. Vitamin B$_{12}$ is protected to a large extent by iron and by taking the C at least 2 hours before or after meals. The manufacturers of vitamin C have contested this finding.

VITAMIN B COMPLEX
See also *Pyridoxine*.

Anticoagulants, oral [147]
Vitamin B complex increases prothrombin time and may cause hemorrhage with anticoagulants.

Cycloserine [880]
Cycloserine increases urinary excretion of vitamin B.

Isoniazid [178,202,619,880]
Isoniazid has an antipyridoxine effect. Pyridoxine decreases the toxic effects of isoniazid.

Mineral oil [28,35,198]
Mineral oil inhibits the absorption of many of the vitamins, particularly oil soluble A, D, E, K.

VITAMIN C (Ascorbic acid)
See *Acidifying Agents*.
Large doses of vitamin C (as in the common cold fad) enhance excretion of weak bases and inhibit excretion of weak acids. [962]

Aminosalicylic Acid
See *Ascorbic Acid* under *p-Aminosalicylic Acid*.

Anticoagulants, oral [963] **(Coumadin, etc.)**
See *Vitamin C* under *Anticoagulants, Oral*.

Antipyrine [325,616]
Vitamin C increases excretion of antipyrine (inhibition) and vice versa.

Atropine [325,616]
Vitamin C increases excretion of atropine (inhibition) and vice versa.

Barbiturates [270,325,616,692]
Vitamin C decreases excretion of barbiturates (potentiation of the sedative). Barbiturates increase the excretion of vitamin C.

Chenodeoxycholic acid
See *Vitamin C* under *Chenodeoxycholic Acid*.

Disulfiram
See *Ascorbic Acid* under *Disulfiram*.

Ferrous iron [180]
Vitamin C in dose of 1 gram or more enhances absorption of ferrous iron (potentiation).

Mineral oil [486]
Mineral oil may inhibit absorption of vitamin C.

Quinidine [962]
Vitamin C inhibits quinidine by increasing its urinary excretion.

Salicylates [274,325,616,870,1099,1577]
Salicylates increase excretion of vitamin C. Vitamin C decreases salicylate excretion (potentiation of analgesic and its toxicity).

Sulfonamides [616,962]
Vitamin C decreases excretion of sulfonamides (potentiation) and sulfonamides increase excretion of vitamin C (inhibition of the vitamin). The acidified urine increases the potential for crystalluria with the antibacterials, and also the precipitation of cystine, oxalate, and urate stones in the urinary tract.

Vitamin B$_{12}$ [1323,1495]
Vitamin B$_{12}$ is destroyed by vitamin C. See *Vitamin C* under *Vitamin B$_{12}$*.

Warfarin
See *Vitamin C* under *Anticoagulants, Oral.*

VITAMIN D
See *Vitamins, Fat-Soluble.*

Barbiturates[2030]
Barbiturates accelerate and alter the metabolism of vitamin D (conversion of cholecalciferol to metabolites other than the active 25-hydroxycalciferol). The drug-induced deficiency of vitamin D that is produced reduces serum calcium levels (osteomalacia). Intake of D should be increased during anticonvulsant therapy.

Hydantoins (Phenytoin, ethotoin, mephenytoin).
Inactivate the vitamin. See *Vitamin D* under *Anticonvulsants.*

Mineral Oil
See *under Vitamin K* below.

Primidone
Inactivates the vitamin. See *Vitamin D* under *Anticonvulsants.*

VITAMIN E
See *Vitamins, Fat-Soluble.*

Iron salts
See *Vitamin E* under *Iron Salts.*

Warfarin[1178] (Coumadin, Panwarfin)
Vitamin E reduces the levels of vitamin-K-dependent coagulation factors in patients on warfarin sodium and those with vitamin-K deficiency may risk hemorrhage if they take vitamin E.

VITAMIN G
See *Riboflavin.*

VITAMIN K
(Menadiol sodium diphosphate [Kappadione, Synkayvite], menadione [Vitamin K₃], menadione sodium bisulfite [Hykinone], phytonadione [AquaMephyton, Konakion, Mephyton, Mono-Kay, Phytomenadione, vitamin K₁], etc.)

Antibiotics [182,234,259,433,434,673,898,909,972]
Antibiotics, by their antibacterial action, inhibit production of vitamin K by the intestinal flora. This tends to potentiate anticoagulants and decreases the hepatic synthesis of prothrombin and blood clotting factors VII, IX and X. Severe deficiency of vitamin K, by causing hypoprothrombinemia, may lead to bleeding (gastrointestinal, nasal, intracranial, etc).

Anticoagulants, oral [120,330,673]
Vitamin K inhibits anticoagulants by encouraging formation of prothrombin and blood clotting factors.

Bile salts [165]
Absorption of vitamin K is enhanced by bile salts.

Cholestyramine [198]
Absorption of fat-soluble vitamins may be impaired by cholestyramine.

Mineral oil [28,35,176,616]
Mineral oil, by sequestering lipid-soluble vitamins, inhibits their absorption and thus reduces the various types of action. Reduction of vitamin K absorption may cause hypoprothrombinemia. Absorption of mineral oil may be increased; should not be given concurrently for long periods.

Tetracyclines [510]
See *Antibiotics* above.

VITAMINS, FAT-SOLUBLE
(Vitamins A, D, E, and K)
See also *Vitamin K.*

Cholestyramine resin [198]
Cholestyramine resin antagonizes fat-soluble vitamins. See under *Vitamin K* above.

Desoxycholic acid [603]
Desoxycholic acid, by virtue of its ability to form inclusion compounds (clathrates) and because of its surface activity, enhances the rate of absorption of the fat-soluble vitamins.

Mineral oil [35,274,616]
See under *Vitamin K* above.

Oral Contraceptives
See *Vitamins* under *Oral Contraceptives.*

VIVACTIL
See *MAO Inhibitors* (protriptyline).

VONTROL
See *Diphenidol.*

WARFARIN (Coumadin, Panwarfin, etc.)
See *Anticoagulants, Oral.*

Chlorinated Insecticides
See *Warfarin* under *Chlorinated Insecticides.*

Isoniazid
See *Isoniazid* under *Anticoagulants, Oral.*

Phenylbutazone
See under *Anticoagulants, Oral.*

Vitamin E [1178]
See *Warfarin* under *Vitamin E.*

WILPO, WILPOWR
See *CNS Stimulants* (phentermine).

WINES
See *Alcohol* and *Tyramine-rich Foods.*

WINGEL
See *Antacids, Aluminum Salts,* and *Magnesium Salts.*

WINSTROL
See *Anabolic Agents* and *Androgens* (stanozolol).

WINTERGREEN OIL
See *Salicylates* (methyl salicylate).

WOLFINA
See *Rauwolfia Alkaloids* (whole root).

WYAMINE
See *Sympathomimetics* (mephentermine).

WYCILLIN
See *Penicillins.*

WYDASE
See *Hyaluronidase.*

XANTHINES
(Caffeine including beverages made from coffee, cola, maté and tea; theobromine including cocoa; theophylline including aminophylline, Choledyl, Glucophylline, Lufyllin, and Neothylline).
See also *CNS Stimulants* (caffeine), and *Diuretics* (theophylline, theobromine).
The interactions of the methylxanthines (caffeine, theobromine, theophylline) depend on their CNS stimulant, cardiovascular, renal, respiratory, and smooth muscle actions. Xanthines stimulate insulin secretion, lipolysis, glycogenolysis and gluconeogenesis.[1769] Coffee and tea are enzyme inducers.[1094]

XANTHINES *(continued)*

Acidifying agents[870]
Acidifying agents, by increasing urinary excretion of weak bases like the xanthines, inhibit their action.

Alkalinizing agents[870]
Alkalinizing agents, by decreasing urinary excretion of weak bases like the xanthines, potentiate their action.

Allopurinol[421] (Zyloprim)
Xanthines antagonize the antihyperuricemic action of allopurinol.

Anticoagulants, oral[166]
The methylxanthines increase blood levels of prothrombin and fibrinogen, shorten the prothrombin time, and thus antagonize the effects of coumarin anticoagulants.

Ephedrine
See *Theophylline* under *Ephedrine*.

Other xanthine preparations[120]
Combined use of several xanthines may cause excessive CNS stimulation.

Oxtriphylline[120] (Choledyl)
Concurrent use of oxtriphylline, a theophylline derivative, with other xanthine preparations may lead to adverse reactions, particularly CNS stimulation in children.

Probenecid[421] (Benemid)
Xanthines antagonize the uricosuric action of probenecid.

Pyrazolon derivatives[421] (Sulfinpyrazone, etc.)
Xanthines antagonize the uricosuric activity of pyrazolon derivatives.

Sulfinpyrazone[120] (Anturane)
Xanthines antagonize the uricosuric action of sulfinpyrazone.

Sympathomimetics[120]
Combined use of xanthines such as caffeine with sympathomimetics like amphetamines may cause excessive CNS stimulation. Sympathomimetics with a bronchial relaxing effect are synergistically useful with xanthine drugs like aminophylline in asthma.

X-RADIATION

Actinomycin D[5,101,120]
See *Roentgen Radiation* under *Actinomycin D*.

Adriamycin
See *Radiation* under *Adriamycin*.

Anticoagulants, oral
Hemorrhage may occur if X-radiation is added to a stabilized anticoagulant regimen. See *Radioactive Compounds* under *Anticoagulants, Oral*.

Antineoplastics[120,198]
Mutual potentiation (additive cytotoxic effects).

Barbiturates[951]
X-ray accelerates onset and prolongs duration of hypnosis by barbiturates.

Chloroquine[1125]
Chloroquine protects against lethality of X-rays.

Metronidazole[2002] (Flagyl)
Metronidazole, an effective radiosensitizer and a directly toxic agent for hypoxic mammalian cells, may improve the results of radiation antitumor therapy.

X-RAY CONTRAST AGENTS FOR BRONCHOGRAPHY

Ether[951]
Decerebration-type syndromes may occur in children anesthetized with ether and subjected to these agents.

XYLOCAINE (lidocaine).
See *Anesthetics, Local* and *Antiarrhythmics*

XYLOSE

Paromomycin[929]
Paromomycin causes malabsorption of xylose.

YEAST EXTRACTS
See *Tyramine-rich Foods*.

MAO inhibitors[47]
MAO inhibitors potentiate the pressor action of tyramine.

YOGURT

MAO inhibitors[486]
Hypertension has been reported with this combination, although not likely in most people because of its very low tyramine content.

ZACTANE
See *Analgesics* (ethoheptazine).

ZACTIRIN
See *Analgesics* (ethoheptazine) and *Salicylates* (aspirin).

ZARONTIN
See *Anticonvulsants* (ethosuximide).

ZYLOPRIM
See *Allopurinol*.

Selected References

1. Abramson EA, Arky RA, Woeber KA: Effects of propranolol on the hormonal and metabolic responses to insulin-induced hypoglycaemia. *Lancet* 2:1386-1388 (Dec 24) 1966; Role of beta-adrenergic receptors in counterregulation to insulin-induced hypoglycemia. *Diabetes* 17:141-6 (Mar) 1968.

2. Adverse effects of topical antiglaucoma drugs. *Med Let Drugs Ther* 9:92 (Nov 17) 1967.

3. Aggeler PM, O'Reilly RA, et al: Potentiation of anticoagulant effect of warfarin by phenylbutazone. *N Engl J Med* 276:496-501 (Mar 2) 1967.

4. AMA Department of Drugs: *AMA Drug Evaluations,* ed 3, Littleton, MA, Publishing Sciences Group, Inc, 1977.

4a. *ibid:* pp 582-98.

4b. *ibid:* p 725-32.

4c. *ibid:* p 19.

4d. *ibid:* p 1080.

5. AMA Council on Drugs: *New Drugs,* ed 3, Chicago, Ill., American Medical Association, 1967, p 264.

6. Anon.: Adrenaline and isoprenaline in myocardial failure. *Lancet* 2:122 (July 17) 1965.

7. Anon.: Alcohol and anticoagulants. *Br. Med J* 2:1615, 1960.

8. Anon.: Anaesthesia during hypotensive therapy. *Lancet* 2:269-270 (July 30) 1966.

9. Anon.: Anticoagulants: Drug interactions. *Clin-Alert* No. 103, (May 8) 1968.

10. Anon.: Anticoagulants: multiple drug therapy. *Clin-Alert* No. 122 (May 7) 1964; 299 (Nov 24) 1965; 224 (Aug 31); 238 (Sep 17); 284 (Nov 4) 1966; 165 (Aug 5) 1967; 274 (Dec 11) 1968; 111 (May 6) 1970.

11. Anon.: Death after eating cheese. *Pharm J* 194:374, 1965.

12. Anon.: Doxepin (Sinequan) and other drugs for anxiety and depression. *Med Let Drugs Ther* 12:21-23 (Mar 6) 1970.

13. Anon.: Drug interactions. *Drug Intell Clin Pharm* 3:179 (June) 1969.

14. Anon.: Drug interactions that can affect your patient. *Patient Care* 1:32 (Nov) 1967.

15. Anon.: Measurement of drug effects. *Lancet* 1:1334-1335 (June 20) 1970.

16. Anon.: Interaction of drugs. *Br Med J* 1:811-812 (Apr 2) 1966.

17. Anon.: The interaction of drugs. *Lancet* 1:82-84 (Jan 8) 1966.

18. Anon.: Urine pH and drug excretion. *Lancet* 1:1256 (June 4) 1966.

19. Anon.: When drugs interact. *Hosp Pract* (Oct) 1966.

20. Antlitz, AM, et al: Effect of butabarbital on orally administered anticoagulants. *Current Therap Res* 10: 70-73 (Feb) 1968.

21. Anton, AH: A drug-induced change in the distribution and renal excretion of sulfonamides. *J Pharmacol Exp Ther* 134:291-303, 1961.

22. Arita T, Hori R, et al: Transformation and excretion of drugs in biological systems I. Renal excretion mechanisms of sulfonamides. *Clin Pharm Bull* 17:2526-2532 (Dec) 1969.

23. Arky RA, Veverbrants E, Abramson EA: Irreversible hypoglycemia: a complication of alcohol and insulin. *JAMA* 206:575-578 (Oct 14) 1968.

24. Arnason BG: Is tuberculin skin test sensitivity depressed by oral contraceptives? *JAMA* 212:1530 (June 1) 1970.

25. Asatoor AM, et al: Tranylcypromine and cheese. *Lancet* 2:733, 1963.

26. Autian J: Interaction between medicaments and plastics. *J Mondial Pharm* pp. 316-341 (Oct-Dec) 1966.

27. Avakian S, Kabacoff BL: Enhancement of blood antibiotic levels through the combined oral administration of phenethicillin and chymotrypsin. *Clin Pharmacol Ther* 5:716 (Nov-Dec) 1964.

28. Azarnoff DL, Hurwitz A: Drug interactions. *Pharmacol Physicians* 4:1-7 (Feb) 1970.

29. Babiak W: Case fatality due to overdosage of a combination of tranylcypromine (Parnate) and imipramine (Tofranil). *Can Med Assoc J* 85:377 (Aug 12) 1961.

30. Balmer V: Antihypertensive drugs and general anaesthesia. *Med J Austral* 1:143-148 (Jan 30) 1965.

31. Barber M: Drug combinations in antibacterial chemotherapy. *Proc Roy Soc Med* 58:990-995 (Nov) 1965.

32. Barnes BA: Drug interactions. NARD convention, Las Vegas, Nev, Oct 15, 1969.

33. Barr WH: Hazards of drug interactions. *Short Course on Adverse Drug Reactions and Drug Interactions,* Buffalo, NY, State University of New York, School of Pharmacy, 1969.

34. Beasley EW: Hypertensive reaction to pargyline and cheese. *Lancet* 2:586-587 (Sep 12) 1964.

35. Becker GL: The case against mineral oil. *Am J Dig Dis* 19:344-348 (Nov) 1952.

36. Beckett AH, Rowland M, Turner P: Influence of urinary pH on excretion of amphetamine. *Lancet* 1:303, 1965.

37. Belam OH: Anaesthesia and therapeutic drugs. *Postgrad Med J* 42:374-377 (June) 1966.

38. Bell DS: Dangers of treatment of status epilepticus with diazepam. *Br Med J* 1:159-161 (Jan 18) 1969.

39. Bellville JW, Fleischli G: The interaction of morphine and nalorphine on respiration. *Clin Pharmacol Ther* 9:152-161 (Mar-Apr) 1968.

40. Best CH, Taylor N: *The Physiological Basis of Medical Practice,* ed 8. Baltimore, Williams & Wilkins Co, 1966.

41. Bethune HC, et al: Vascular crisis associated with monoamine-oxidase inhibitors. Am J Psychiat 121:245-248 (Sep) 1964.

42. Bewsher PD: Propranolol, bloodsugar, and exercise. *Lancet* 1:104 (Jan 14) 1967.

43. Beyer KH, Russo HF, et al: Benemid, *p-* (di-*n*-propylsulfamyl)-benzoic acid: its renal affinity and its elimination. *Am J Physiol* 166:625-640 (Sep) 1951.

44. Binns TB: *Absorption and Distribution of Drugs.* Baltimore, Williams & Wilkins Co, 1964.

45. Blackwell B: Tranylcypromine. *Lancet* 2:414 (Aug 24) 1963.

46. ———: Hypertensive crisis due to monoamine-oxidase inhibitors. *Lancet* 2:849-857, 1963.

47. Blackwell B, Marley E, Taylor D: Effects of yeast extract after monoamine-oxidase inhibition. *Lancet* 1:1166 (May 29) 1965.

48. Block LH, Lamy PP: Therapeutic incompatibilities of legend drugs with o-t-c drugs. *J Am Pharm Assoc* NS8:66-68, 82-84 (Feb) 1968.

49. Blomley DJ: Monoamine-oxidase inhibitors. *Lancet* 2:1181-1182, 1964.

50. Borrie P, Clark PA: Megaloblastic anaemia during methotrexate treatment of psoriasis. *Br Med J* 1:1339 (May) 1966.

51. Bower BF, McComb R, Ruderman M: Effect of penicillin on urinary 17-ketogenic and 17-ketosteroid excretion. *N Engl J Med* 277:530-532 (Sep 7) 1967.

52. Boyd EM: Diet and drug toxicity. *Clin Toxicol* 2:423-433 (Dec) 1969.

53. Brachfeld J, Wirtshafter A, Wolfe S: Imipramine-tranylcypromine incompatibility. *JAMA* 186:1172-1173 (Dec 28) 1963.

54. Braverman LE, Woeber KA, Ingbar SH: Induction of myxedema by iodide in patients euthyroid after radioiodine or surgical treatment of diffuse toxic goiter. *N Engl J Med* 281:816-821 (Oct 9) 1969.

55. Brazil OV, Corrado AP: Curariform action of streptomycin. *J Pharmacol Exp Ther* 120:452-459 (Aug) 1957.

56. Breakstone IL: Hypertensive reaction to two monamine oxidase inhibitors. *Am J Psychiat* 122:104, 1965.

57. Brodie BB: Displacement of one drug by another from carrier or receptor sites. *Proc Roy Soc Med* 58:946-955 (Nov) 1965.

58. ———: Physico-chemical factors in drug absorption in Binns TB (ed): *Absorption and Distribution of Drugs.* Baltimore, Williams & Wilkins Co, 1964, p. 16-48.

59. Brook R, Schrogie JJ, Solomon HM: Failure of probenecid to inhibit the rate of metabolism of tolbutamide in man. *Clin Pharmacol Ther* 9:314-317 (May-June) 1968.

60. Brownlee G, Williams GW: Potentiation of amphetamine and pethidine by monoamine-oxidase inhibitors. *Lancet* 1:669 (Mar 23) 1963.

61. Burnett CH, Commons RR, et al: Hypercalcemia without hypercalcuria or hypophosphatemia, calcinosis and renal insufficiency. *N Engl J Med* 240:787-794, 1949.

62. Burns JJ, et al: Drugs effects on enzymes, in Siegler PE, Moyer JH, (eds.); *Pharmacologic Techniques in Drug Evaluation.* Chicago, Year Book, 1967.

63. Burns JJ: Implications of enzyme induction for drug therapy. *Am J Med* 37:327-331, 1964.

64. Burns JJ, Cucinell SA, et al: Application of drug metabolism to drug toxicity studies. *Ann N Y Acad Sci* 123:273-286 (Mar 12) 1965.

65. Burns JJ, Conney AH: Enzyme stimulation and inhibition in the metabolism of drugs. *Proc Roy Soc Med* 58:955-960 (Nov) 1965.

66. Busfield D, Child KJ, Atkinson RM, et al: An effect on phenobarbitone on blood-levels of griseofulvin in man. *Lancet* 2:1042-1043, 1963.

67. Busfield D, Child KJ, Tomich EG: An effect of phenobarbitone on griseofulvin metabolism in the rat. *Br. J Pharmacol* 22:137-142 (Feb) 1964.

68. Capper KR: Interaction of rubber with medicaments. *J Mondial Pharm* pp. 305-315 (Oct-Dec) 1966.

69. Catalano PM, Cullen SI: Warfarin antagonism by griseofulvin. *Clin Res* 14:266 (Apr) 1966.

70. Chang TW, Weinstein L: Inhibitory effects of other antibiotics on bacterial morphologic changes induced by penicillin G. *Nature* 211:763-765 (Aug 13) 1966.

71. Chappell AG: Severe hypothermia due to combination of psychotropic drugs and alcohol. *Br Med J* 1:356 (Feb) 1966.

72. Chatton MJ, et al: *Handbook of Medical Treatment,* ed. 10. Los Altos, California, Lange Medical Publications, 1966, p. 498.

73. Cherner R, Groppe CW, Rupp, JJ: Prolonged tolbutamide-induced hypoglycemia. *JAMA 185: 883-884* (Sep 14) 1963.

74. Chiles VK: Drug interactions and the pharmacist. *Can Pharm J* 101:241-247 (July) 1968.

75. Christensen EK, et al: Influence of gastric antacids on the release *in vitro* of tetracycline hydrochloride. *Pharm Weekblad* 102:463-473 (May 26) 1967.

76. Christensen LK, Hansen JM, Kristensen M: Sulfaphenazole-induced hypoglycaemic attacks in tolbutamide-treated diabetics. *Lancet* 2:1298-1301 (Dec 21) 1963.

77. Clark JB: Hospital pharmacy patient records and drug interactions. Drug Interaction Seminar, New Brunswick, N.J., Mar. 27, 1969.

78. Clark TH, Conney AH, Harpole BP, et al: Drug interactions that can affect your patients. *Patient Care* 1:33-71 (Nov) 1967.

79. Clegg H: *Today's Drugs.* New York, Grune and Stratton, Inc., p. 145, 1965.

80. Clezy TM: Oral contraceptives and hypertension: The effect of guanethidine. *Med J Austral* 1:638-640 (Mar 28) 1970.

81. Cluff LE: Problems with drugs. *Proceedings,* Conference on Continuing Education for Physicians in the Use of Drugs, Washington, D.C., Feb., 1969.

82. Conference on drug metabolism in man. *Proceedings,* The New York Academy of Sciences, June 29-July 1, 1970. *Ann NY Acad Sci* 179:9-773 (July 6) 1971.

88. Conney AH: Microsomal enzyme induction by drugs. *Pharmacol Physicians* 3:1-6 (Dec) 1969; Pharmacological implications of microsomal enzyme induction. *Pharmacol Rev* 19:317-366 (Sep) 1967.

84. Conney AH, Jacobson M, Schneidman K, et al: Induction of liver microsomal cortisol 6β-hydroxylase by diphenylhydantoin or phenobarbital: An explanation for the increased excretion of 6-hydroxycortisol in humans treated with these drugs. *Life Sci.* 4:1091-1098 (May) 1965.

85. Consolo S: An interaction between desipramine and phenylbutazone. *J Pharm Pharmacol* 20:574-575 (July) 1968.

86. Cooper AJ, Ashcroft G: Modification of insulin and sulfonylurea hypoglycemia by monoamine-oxidase inhibitor drugs. *Diabetes* 16:272-274 (Apr) 1967.

87. ———: Potentiation of insulin hypoglycaemia by MAOI antidepressant drugs. *Lancet* 1:407-409 (Feb 19) 1966.

88. Cooper AJ, Keddie KMG: Hypotensive collapse and hypoglycaemia after mebanazine—a monoamine-oxidase inhibitor. *Lancet* 1:1133-1135 (May 23) 1964.

89. Cooper J: Interaction between medicaments and containers. *J Mondial Pharm* pp 259-281 (Oct-Dec) 1966.

90. Cooper P: Dangerous drug combinations. *Pharm Dig* 28:166, 1964.

91. Crandell D: The anesthetic hazards in patients on antihypertensive therapy. *JAMA* 179:495-500, 1962.

92. Crawford JS, Rudofsky S: Some alterations in the pattern of drug metabolism associated with pregnancy, oral contraceptives, and the newly-born. *Br J Anaesth* 38:446-454, 1966.

93. Cremer RJ, Perryman PW, Richards DH: Influence of light on the hyperbilirubinaemia of infants. *Lancet* 1:1094-1097 (May 24) 1958.

94. Crocker J, Morton B: Tricyclic (antidepressant) drug toxicity. *Clin Tox* 2:397-402 (Dec) 1969.

95. Cronin D: Monoamine-oxidase inhibitors and cheese. *Br Med J* 2:1065, 1965.

96. Cucinell SA, Conney AH, Sansur MS: Drug interactions in man. Lowering effect of phenobarbital on plasma levels of bishydroxycoumarin (Di-cumarol) and diphenylhydantoin (Dilantin). *Clin Pharmacol Therap* 6:420-429, 1965.

97. Cucinell SA, Odessky L, Weiss M, et al: The effect of chloral hydrate on bishydroxycoumarin metabolism. *JAMA* 197:366-368 (Aug 1) 1966.

98. Cullen SI, Catalano PM: Griseofulvin-warfarin antagonism. *JAMA* 199:582-583 (Feb 20) 1967.

99. Cuthbert MF, et al: Cough and cold remedies: a potential danger to patients on monoamine oxidase inhibitors. *Br Med J* 1:404-406 (Feb 15) 1969.

100. Cutting WC: *Handbook of Pharmacology,* ed 4. New York, Appleton-Century-Crofts, 1969.

101. D'Angio GJ, et al: The enhanced response of the Ridgway osteogenic sarcoma to roentgen radiation combined with actinomycin D. *Cancer Res* 25:1002-1007 (Aug) 1965.

102. Davies EB: Tranylcypromine and cheese. *Lancet* 2:691-692, (Sep 28) 1963.

103. Davies G: Side-effects of phenelzine. *Br Med J* 2:1019 (Oct 1) 1960.

104. Davies TS: Monoamine oxidase inhibitors and rauwolfia compounds. *Br Med J* 2:739-740 (Sep 3) 1960.

105. Davis JG: Cheese and tranylcypromine. *Lancet* 2:1168 (Nov 30) 1963.

106. Dayton PG, Tarcan Y, et al: The influence of barbiturates on coumarin plasma levels and prothrombin response. *J Clin Invest* 40:1797-1802, 1961.

107. Dearborn EH, Litchfield JT, Jr., et al: The effects of various substances on the absorption of tetracycline in rats. *Antibiot Med Clin Ther* 4:627-641 (Oct) 1957.

108. Death from aspirin hypersensitivity. *Pharm J* 192:167 (Feb 22) 1964.

109. Deichmann WB, Gerarde HW: *Toxicology of Drugs and Chemicals,* ed 4. New York, Academic Press, 1969.

110. Dick HL, McCawley EL, Fisher WA: Reserpine-digitalis toxicity. *Arch Int Med* 109:503-506 (May 1962).

111. Dinel B, Latiolais CJ: Drug interaction-enzyme induction. *Hosp Form Manage* 2:35 (Oct) 1967.

112. Di Palma, JR: The why and how of drug interactions. *RN* 33:63-69 (Mar); 67-73 (Apr); 69-73 (May) 1970.

113. Diphenylhydantoin overdosage. *Clin-Alert* No. 287 (Dec 31) 1968.

114. Dixon RL: Effect of chlordan pretreatment on the metabolism and lethality of cyclophosphamide. *J Pharm Sci* 57:1351-1354 (Aug) 1968.

115. D'Mello A: Interaction between phenylpropanolamine and monoamine oxidase inhibitors. *J Pharm Pharmacol* 21:577-580 (Sep) 1969.

116. Dobkin A: Potentiation of thiopental anesthesia by derivatives and analogues of phenothiazine. *Anesthesiol.* 21:292-296 (May-June) 1960.

117. Dollery CT: Physiological and pharmacological interactions of antihypertensive drugs. *Proc Roy Soc Med* 58:983-987 (Nov) 1965.

118. Douglas JF, Ludwig BJ, Smith N: Studies on the metabolism of meprobamate. *Proc Soc Exp Biol Med* 112:436-438, 1963.

119. Dresdale FC, et al: Potential dangers in the combined use of methandrostenolone and sodium

warfarin. *J Med Soc NJ* 64:609–612 (Nov) 1967.

120. Drug package insert (FDA approved official brochure) and other labeling based on sponsored clinical investigations and New Drug Application data.

121. Dunphy TW: The pharmacist's role in the prevention of adverse drug interactions. *Am J Hosp Pharm* 26:366–377 (July) 1969.

122. Dunworth RD, Kenna FR: Incompatibility of combinations of medications in intravenous solutions. *Am J Hosp Pharm* 22:190–191 (Apr) 1965.

123. Eagle H, Fleischman R: Therapeutic activity of bacitracin in rabbit syphilis, and its synergistic action with penicillin. *Proc Soc Exp Biol Med* 68:415–417, 1948.

124. Ebel JA: Steps to a successful drug interaction program. *Hosp (JAHA)* 43:130–138 (Sep 1) 1969.

125. Edelson J, Douglas JF: Benactyzine inhibition of microsomal meprobamate metabolism. *Biochem Pharmacol* 16:2050–2052 (Oct) 1967.

126. Editorial: Anaesthesia during hypotensive therapy. *Lancet* 2:269–270, 1966.

127. ———: Drug-drug interaction. *JAMA* 208:1898 (June 9) 1969.

128. ———: Drug interactions. *Pharm J* 192:161–162 (Feb 22) 1964.

129. ———: Intravenous additives, polypharmacy and patient safety. *Drug Intell* 2:143 (June) 1968.

130. ———: Oral contraceptives and immune responses. *JAMA* 209:410, 1969.

131. ———: Pressor attacks during treatment with monoamine-oxidase inhibitors. *Lancet* 1:945–946 (May 1) 1965.

132. Effect of pH of the urine on antimicrobial therapy of urinary tract infections. *Med Let* 9:47–48 (June 16) 1967.

133. Eisen MJ: Combined effect of sodium warfarin and phenylbutazone. *JAMA* 189:64–65 (July 6) 1964.

134. Elias RA: Effect of various drugs on anticoagulant dosage, in Nichol E.S., et al, (eds.): *Anticoagulant Therapy in Ischemic Heart Disease.* New York, Grune and Stratton, 1965.

135. Elion GB, Callahan S, et al: Potentiation by inhibition of drug degradation: 6-substituted purines and xanthine oxidase. *Biochem Pharmacol* 12:85–93 (Jan) 1963.

136. Elis J, Laurence DR, et al: Modification by monoamine oxidase inhibitors of the effect of some sympathomimetics on blood pressure. *Br Med J* 2:75–78 (Apr 8) 1967.

137. Ellenhorn MJ, Sternad FA: Problems of drug interactions. *J Am Pharm Assoc* NS6:62–65 (Feb) 1966.

138. Fass RJ, Perkins RL, Saslow S: Positive direct Coombs' tests associated with cephaloridine therapy. *JAMA* 213:121–123 (July 6) 1964.

139. Fatal drug combinations. *Pharm J* 192:167 (Feb 22) 1970.

140. Fekete M, Macsek I: The effect of imipramine cocaine, and neostigmine on the hyperglycaemic response to noradrenaline and adrenaline. *J Pharm Pharmacol* 20:327–328, 1968.

141. Field JB, Ohta M, et al: Potentiation of acetohexamide hypoglycemia by phenylbutazone. *N Engl J Med* 277:889–894 (Oct 26) 1967.

142. Fildes P: A rational approach to research in chemotherapy. *Lancet* 238:955–957, 1940.

143. Fingl E, Woodbury DM: Factors modifying drug effects, in Goodman LS, Gilman A, (eds.): *The Pharmacological Basis of Therapeutics* ed., 4. New York, Macmillan, 1970, p. 25.

144. FitzGerald MG, Gaddie R, Malins JM, et al: Alcohol sensitivity in diabetics receiving chlorpropamide. *Diabetes* 2:40, 1962; 11:40–43 (Jan-Feb) 1962.

145. Foldes FF: The pharmacology of neuromuscular blocking agents in man. *Clin Pharmacol Ther* 1:345–395 (May-June) 1960.

146. Foldes FF, Lunn JN, Benz, HG: Prolonged respiratory depression caused by drug combinations. Muscle relaxants and intraperitoneal antibiotics as etiologic agents. *JAMA* 183:672–673 (Feb 23) 1963.

147. Formiller M, Cohon MS: Coumarin and indandione anticoagulants—potentiators and antagonists. *Am J Hosp Pharm* 26:574–582 (Oct) 1969.

148. Forney RB, Hughes FW: *Combined Effects of Alcohol and Other Drugs.* Springfield, Ill., Charles C Thomas 1968.

149. Fouts JR: Drug interactions: Effects of drugs and chemicals on drug metabolism. *Gastroenterol* 46:486–490 (Apr) 1964.

150. Fox SL: Potentiation of anticoagulants caused by pyrazole compounds. *JAMA* 188:320–321 (Apr 20) 1964.

151. Freycon F, Bertrand J, Levrat R, et al: Intoxication à la réglisse. *Lyon Med* 12:745, 1964, through *Presse Méd* 72:2231, 1964.

152. Lasix. *Med Let Drugs Ther* 9:6–8 (Jan 27) 1967.

153. Gabor M, Antal A, Dirner Z: Effect of anticoagulants on the capillary resistance of internal organs of rats. *J Pharm Pharmacol* 19:488 (July) 1967.

154. Gaddum JH: Theories of drug antagonism. *Pharmacol Rev* 9:211–218, 1957.

155. Garrettson LK: Hazards of drug interactions. *Short Course on Adverse Drug Reactions and Drug Interactions,* Buffalo, N.Y., State University of New York, School of Pharmacy, 1969.

156. Garrettson LK, Perel JM, Dayton PG: Methylphenidate interaction with both anticonvulsants and ethyl biscoumacetate. *JAMA* 207:2053–2056 (Mar 17) 1969.

157. Garrod LP, Waterworth PM: Methods of testing combined antibiotic bactericidal action and the significance of the results. *J Clin Pathol* 15:328–338 (July) 1962.

158. Gazzaniga AB, Stewart DR: Possible quinidine-induced hemorrhage in a patient on warfarin sodium. *N Engl J Med.* 280:711–712 (Mar 27) 1969.

159. Gibaldi M: Mechanisms of drug interactions. *Short Course on Adverse Drug Reactions and Drug Interactions,* Buffalo, N.Y., State University of New York, School of Pharmacy, 1969.

160. Gilbaldi M, Schwartz MA: Apparent effect of probenecid on the distribution of penicillins in man. *Clin Pharmacol Ther* 9:345–349 (May-June) 1968.

161. Gillette JR: Theoretical aspects of drug interaction, in Siegler PE, Moyer JH (eds): *Pharmacolog-*

ic *Techniques in Drug Evaluation,* vol 2. Chicago, Year Book, 1967.

162. Goldberg LI: Monoamine oxidase inhibitors. *JAMA* 190:456-462 (Nov 2) 1964.

163. Goldberg SR, Schuster CR: Nalorphine: increased sensitivity of monkeys formerly dependent on morphine. *Science* 166:1548-1549, 1969.

164. Goldner MG, Zarowtiz H, Akgun S: Hyperglycemia and glycosuria due to thiazide derivatives administered in diabetes mellitus. *N Engl J Med* 262:403-405 (Feb 25) 1960.

165. Goodman LS, Gilman A: *The Pharmacological Basis of Therapeutics.* New York, Macmillan 1975 pp 1-46.

166. *Ibid.,* Section II pp 46-378

167. *Ibid.,* Section III pp 379-403

168. *Ibid.,* Section IV pp 404-588

169. *Ibid.,* Section V pp 589-652

170. *Ibid.,* Section VI pp 653-752

171. *Ibid.,* Section VII pp 753-808

172. *Ibid.,* Section VIII pp 809-866

173. *Ibid.,* Section IX pp 867-880

174. *Ibid.,* Section X pp 881-911

175. *Ibid.,* Section XI pp 912-945

176. *Ibid.,* Section XII pp 946-1017

177. *Ibid.,* Section XIII pp 1018-1089

178. *Ibid.,* Section XIV pp 1090-1247

179. *Ibid.,* Section XV pp 1248-1308

180. *Ibid.,* Section XVI pp 1309-1368

181. *Ibid.,* Section XVII pp 1369-1543

182. *Ibid.,* Section VIII pp 1544-1704

183. Goss JE, Dickhaus DW: Increased bishydroxycoumarin requirements in patients receiving phenobarbital. *N Engl J Med* 273:1094-1095 (Nov 11) 1965.

184. Grosshandler SL, Henschel EO, Kampine J: Toxic reactions due to drug synergism and antagonism. *Anesth Analg Cur Res* 47:345-349 (July-Aug) 1968.

185. Greenberg MJ: Isoprenaline in myocardial failure. *Lancet* 2:442-443 (Aug 28) 1965.

186. Gross EG, Dexter JD, Roth RG: Hypokalemic myopathy with myoglobinuria associated with licorice ingestion. *N Engl J Med* 274:602-606 (Mar 17) 1966.

187. Gupta KK, Lillicrap CA: Guanethidine and diabetes. *Br Med J* 2:697-698 (June 15) 1968.

188. György L, Dóda M, Bite A: Guanethidine and carbachol on the isolated frog rectus: a noncompetitive interaction. *J Pharm Pharmacol* 20:575-577, 1968.

189. Hansen JM, Kristensen M, Skovsted L, et al: Dicoumarol-induced diphenylhydantoin intoxication. *Lancet* 2:265-266 (July 30) 1966.

190. Hansen JM, et al: Sulthiame (Ospolot) as inhibitor of diphenylhydantoin metabolism. *Epilepsia* 9:17-22 (Mar) 1968.

191. Hansten PD: Antidiabetic drug interactions. *Hosp Form Manag* 4:30-32 (Feb) 1969; Chlorpropamide and chloramphenicol. *Lancet* 1:1173 (May 30) 1970.

192. ———: Diphenylhydantoin drug interaction. *Hosp Form Manag* 4:28-29 (May) 1969.

193. ———: Oral anticoagulant drug interactions. *Hosp Form Manag* 4:20-22 (Jan) 1969.

194. ———: Tricyclic antidepressants: drug interactions. *Hosp Form Manag* 4:25-27 (Oct) 1969.

195. Harmel MH: Postanesthetic apnea—Causes and management. *NY State J Med* 57:4039-4041 (Dec) 1957.

196. Hartshorn EA: Drug interaction. *Drug Intell* 2:5-7 (Jan) 1968.

197. *Ibid.,* 2:58-65 (Mar) 1968.

198. *Ibid.,* 2:174-180 (July) 1968.

199. *Ibid.* 2:198-201 (Aug) 1968.

200. *Ibid.,* 3:14-20 (Jan) 1969.

201. *Ibid.,* 3:70-81 (Mar) 1969.

202. *Ibid.,* 3:130-137 (May) 1969.

203. *Ibid.,* 3:196-197 (July) 1969.

204. *Ibid.,* 4:60-63 (Mar) 1970.

205. *Ibid.,* 4:88-89 (Apr) 1970.

206. Hartshorn EA: Physiological states altering response to drugs. *Wisc Pharm* p. 453-460 (Dec) 1969.

207. Hedberg DL, Gordon MW, et al: Six cases of hypertensive crisis in patients on tranylcypromine after eating chicken livers. *Am J Psychiat* 122:933-937, 1966.

208. Herrell WE: Antibiotics and chemotherapy: yesterday, today and tomorrow. *Clin Med* 75:17-23 (July) 1968.

209. Herxheimer A: Drug interactions. *Prescriber's* 9:65 (Aug) 1969.

210. Hewitt WL, Seligman SJ, Deigh RA: Kinetics of the synergism of penicillin-streptomycin and penicillin-kanamycin for enterococci and its relationship to L-phase variants. *J Lab Clin Med* 67:792 (May) 1966.

211. Hirsch MS, Walter RM, Hasterlik RJ: Subarachnoid hemorrhage following ephedrine and MAO inhibitor. *JAMA* 194:1259 (Dec 13) 1965.

212. Hirschman JL, Maudlin RK: The DIAS rounds. *Drug Intell Clin Pharm* 4:129-131 (May) 1970.

213. Hodge JV, Nye ER, Emerson GW: Monoamine-oxidase inhibitors, broad beans, and hypertension. *Lancet* 1:1108, 1964.

214. Hoffbrand BI, Kininmonth DA: Potentiation of anticoagulants. *Br Med J* 2:838-839 (June 24) 1967.

215. Hogben CAM, Tocco DJ, et al: On the mechanism of intestinal absorption of drugs. *J Pharmacol Exp Ther* 125:275-282 (Apr) 1959.

216. Horita A, West TC, Dille JM: Cardiovascular responses during amphetamine tachyphylaxis. *J Pharmacol Exp Ther* 108:224-232 (June) 1953.

217. Horler AR, Wynne NA: Hypertensive crisis due to pargyline and metaraminol. *Br Med J* 2:460-461 (Aug 21) 1965.

218. Horwitz D, Lovenberg W, et al: Monoamine oxidase inhibitors, tyramine, and cheese. *JAMA* 188:1108-1110 (June 29) 1964.

219. Howarth E: Possible synergistic effects of the new thymoleptics in connection with poisoning. *J Mental Sci* 107:100-103, 1961.

220. Howieson WE: Cheese and migraine. *Lancet* 2:1063 (Nov 16) 1963.

221. Hrdina P, and Garattini S: Desipramine and potentiation of noradrenaline in the isolated perfused renal artery. *J Pharm Pharmacol* 18:259-260 (Feb 3) 1966.

222. Hunninghake DB: Drug interactions. *Postgrad Med* 47:71-75 (Jan.) 1970.

223. Hunninghake DB, Azarnoff DL: Drug interactions with warfarin. *Arch Int Med* 121:349-352 (April) 1968.

224. Hussar DA: Mechanisms of drug interactions *J Am Pharm Assoc* NS9:208-209, 213 (May) 1969.

225. ———: Oral anticoagulants—their interactions. *J Am Pharm Assoc* NS10:78-82 (Feb) 1970.

226. ———: Tabular compilation of drug interactions. *Am J Pharm* 141:109-156 (July-Aug) 1969.

227. ———: Therapeutic incompatabilities: drug interactions. *Am J Pharm* 139:215-233 (Nov-Dec) 1967.

228. ———: Therapeutic incompatibilities: drug interactions. *Hosp Pharm* 3:14 (Aug) 1968.

229. Hygroton: diabetogenic effect. *Clin-Alert* 204 (July 27) 1965.

230. Ingall D, Sherman JD, et al: Amelioration by ingestion of phenylalanine of toxic effects of chloramphenicol on bone marrow. *N Engl J Med* 272:180-185 (Jan 28) 1965.

231. Inglis JM, Barrow MEH: Premedication, a reassessment. *Proc Roy Soc Med* 58:29-32 (Jan) 1965.

232. Innes IR: Sensitization of the heart and nictitating membrane of the cat to sympathomimetic amines by antihistamine drugs. *Br J Pharmacol* 13:6-10, 1958.

233. Interactions between antimicrobial drugs. *Drug Therap Bull* 6:49-51 (June 21) 1968.

234. Interactions of oral anticoagulants with other drugs. *Med Let Drugs Ther* 9:97 (Dec 1) 1967.

235. Isaac L, Goth A: Interaction of antihistaminics with norepinephrine uptake: a cocaine-like effect. *Life Sci* 4:1899-1904, 1965.

236. Juchau MR, Gram TE, Fouts JR: Stimulation of hepatic microsomal drug-metabolizing enzyme systems in primates by DDT. *Gastroenterol* 51:213-218 (Aug) 1966.

237. Jasinski DR, Martin WR, et al: Antagonism of the subjective, behavioral, pupillary, and respiratory depressant effects of cyclazocine by naloxone. *Clin Pharmacol Therap* 9:215-222 (Mar-Apr) 1968.

238. Jawetz, E.: The use of combinations of antimicrobial drugs. *Ann Rev Pharmacol* 8:151-170, 1968.

239. Jawetz E, Gunnison JB: Antibiotic synergism and antagonism: an assessment of the problem. *Pharmacol Rev* 5:175-192, 1953.

240. Jawetz E, Gunnison JB, et al: Studies on antibiotic synergism and antagonism. The interference of chloramphenicol with the action of penicillin. *Arch Int Med* 87:349-359 (Mar) 1951.

241. Jetter WW, McLean R: Poisoning by the synergistic effect of phenobarbital and ethyl alcohol. *Arch Path* 36:112-122, 1943.

242. Jori A: Potentiation of noradenaline toxicity by drugs with antihistamine activity. *J Pharm Pharmacol* 18:824, 1966.

243. Jori A, Carrara MC: On the mechanism of the hyperglycaemic effect of chlorpromazine. *J. Pharm Pharmacol* 18:623-624 (Sep) 1966.

244. Joyce CRB, Edgecombe PCE, et al: Potentiation by phenobarbitone of effects of ethyl alcohol on

human behavior. *J Ment Sci* 105:51-60 (Jan) 1959.

245. Kabat HF: *Clinical Pharmacy Handbook.* Philadelphia, Lea & Febiger, 1970.

246. Kaijser L, Perman ES: Cardiac symptoms after alcohol in a patient treated with chlorpropamide. *Opuscula Med* 12:329-331 (Aug) 1967.

247. Kakemi K, Sezaki H, Kondo T: Absorption and excretion of drugs XLI. *Clin Pharm Bull* 17:1864-1870 (Sep.) 1969, and previous papers in the series.

248. Kakemi K, Sezaki H, Konishi R, et al: Effect of bile salts on the gastrointestinal absorption of drugs. *Clin Pharm Bull* 18:275-280 (Feb) 1970.

249. Kanamycin and neomycin. *Med. Let. Drugs Ther* 9:61-63 (Aug 11) 1967.

250. Kanamycin sulfate injection and kanamycin sulfate capsules. *Fed Reg* 35:397-399 (FR Doc 70:347) 1970.

251. Kane FJ, Jr: Toxic reactions to antidepressant drugs. *Southern Med J* 57:691-693, 1964.

252. Kaplan D, Koch W: Synergistic effect of combinations of cephalothin and kanamycin on strains of *E. coli. Nature* 218:1165-1166 (June 22) 1968.

253.———: Synergism of three antimicrobial drugs. *Nature* 209:718-719 (Feb 12) 1966.

254. Kater RMH, Tobon F, Iber FL: Increased rate of tolbutamide metabolism in alcoholic patients. *JAMA* 207:363-365 (Jan 13) 1969.

255. Katzung BG, Way WL: Potentiation of the neuromuscular blockade by quinidine. *Fed Proc* 25:718 (Mar-Apr) 1966.

256. Keller B, Bennett R: The responsibility of the pharmacist in detecting drug interactions. Paper presented at 1969 Convention of American Pharmaceutical Association, Montreal, Canada.

257. King TM, Burgard JK: Drug interaction. *Am J Obstet Gynecol* 98:128-134 (May) 1967.

258. Kiorboe E: Phenytoin intoxication during treatment with Antabuse (disulfiram). *Epilepsia* 7:246, 1966.

259. Klippel AP, Pitsinger B: Hypoprothrombinemia secondary to antibiotic therapy and manifested by massive gastrointestinal hemorrhage. *Arch Surg* 96:266-268 (Feb) 1968.

260. Koch-Weser J: Quinidine-induced hypoprothrombinemic hemorrhage in patients on chronic warfarin therapy. *Ann Int Med* 68:511-517 (Mar) 1968.

261. Kolodny AL: Side effects produced by alcohol in a patient receiving furazolidone. *Maryland Med J* 11:248, 1962.

262. Koshy KT, Troup AE, et al: Acetylation of acetaminophen in tablet formulations containing aspirin. *J Pharm Sci* 56:1117-1121, 1967.

263. Kotler MN, Berman L, Rubenstein AH: Hypoglycaemia preciptiated by propranolol. *Lancet* 2:1389-1390 (Dec 24) 1966.

264. Kreek MJ, Sleisenger MH: Reduction of serum-unconjugated-bilirubin with phenobarbitone in adult congenital non-haemolytic unconjugated hyperbilirubinaemia. *Lancet* 2: 73-78 (July 13) 1968.

265. Krikler DM, Lewis B: Dangers of natural foodstuffs. *Lancet* 1:1166 (May 29) 1965.

266. Kristensen M, Hansen JM: Potentiation of the

tolbutamide effect by dicoumarol. *Diabetes* 16:211-214 (Apr) 1967.

267. Kunin CM: Clinical pharmacology of the new penicillins I. The importance of serum protein binding in determining antimicrobial activity and concentration in serum. *Clin Pharmacol Ther* 7:166-179, 1966.

268. ———: Clinical pharmacology of the new penicillins II. Effect of drugs which interfere with binding to serum proteins. *Clin Pharmacol Ther* 7:180-188, 1966.

269. ———: Enhancement of antimicrobial activity of penicillins and other antibiotics in human serum by competitive serum binding inhibitors. *Proc Soc Exp Biol Med* 117-69 (Oct) 1964.

270. Kunin CM, Jones WF Jr., Finland M: Enhancement of tetracycline blood levels. *N Engl J Med* 259:147 (July 24) 1958.

271. Kupfer D, Peets L: The effect of o,p'-DDD on cortisol and hexobarbital metabolism. *Biochem Pharmacol* 15:573-581, 1966.

272. Kutt H, et al: Depression of parahydroxylation of diphenylhydantoin by antituberculosis chemotherapy. *Neurology* 16:594-602 (June) 1966.

273. ———: Inhibition of diphenylhydantoin metabolism in rats and rat liver microsomes by antitubercular drugs. *Neurology* 18:706-710 (July) 1968.

274. Lamy PP, Black DA: Therapeutic incompatibilities. *J Am Pharm Assoc* NS10:72-77 (Feb) 1970.

275. Lamy PP, Kitler ME: The actions and interactions of OTC drugs. *Hosp Form Manag* 4:17-23 (Nov) 1969; 4:25-29 (Dec) 1969; 5:19-26 (Jan) 1970.

276. Lasagna L: Drug interaction in the field of analgesic drugs. *Proc Roy Soc Med* 58:978-983 (Nov) 1965.

277. *Lasix. Med Let Drugs Ther* 9:6-8 (Jan 27) 1967.

278. Launchbury AP: Drug interactions. *Am J Hosp Pharm* 23:24-29 (Feb) 1966.

279. Laurence DR: Unwanted and dangerous interactions between drugs. *Prescriber's J* 3:46, 1963.

280. Lees B: Bizarre reactions. *Clin Med* 70:1977-1979, 1963.

281. Leishman AWD, Matthews HL, Smith AJ: Antagonism of guanethidine by imipramine. *Lancet* 1:112 (Jan 12) 1963.

282. Lemberg H: Compilation of pharmaceutical incompatibilities. *Hosp Pharm* 2:19, 22-25 (Aug) 1967.

283. *Librium and Valium. Med Let Drugs Ther* 11:81-84 (Oct 3) 1969.

284. Leonard JW, Gifford RW, Jr., Williams GH, Jr.: Pargyline and cheese. *Lancet* 1:883 (Apr 18) 1964.

285. Lepper MH, Dowling HF: Treatment of pneumococcic meningitis with penicillin compared with penicillin plus Aureomycin. *Arch Int Med* 88:489-494 (Oct) 1951.

286. Leszkovszky GP, Tardos L: Potentiation by cocaine and 3,3-di-(*p*-aminophenyl)-propylamine (TK 174) of the effect of isoprenaline and noradrenaline on isolated strips of cat spleen. *J Pharm Pharmacol* 20:377-380, 1968.

287. Levin W, Welch RM, Conney AH: Effect of phenobarbital and other drugs on the metabolism and uterotropic action of estradiol-17β and estrone. *J Pharmacol Exp Ther* 159:362-371, 1968.

288. Li MC, Whitmore W, Golbey R: Effect of combined drug therapy upon metastatic choriocarcinoma. *Proc Am Assoc Cancer Res* 3:37 (Mar) 1969.

289. Lloyd JTA, Walker, DRH: Death after combined dexamphetamine and phenelzine. *Br Med J* 2:168-169 (July 17) 1965.

290. Lockett MF, Milner G: Combining the antidepressant drugs. *Br Med J* 1:921 (Apr 3) 1965.

291. Lolli G, Balboni C, Ballatore C, et al: Wine in the diets of diabetic patients. *Q J Stud Alcohol* 24:412-416, 1963.

292. London WT, Vought RL, Brown FA: Bread—a dietary source of large quantities of iodine. *N Engl J Med* 273:381 (Aug 12) 1965.

293. Luby ED, Domino EF: Toxicity from large doses of imipramine and a MAO inhibitor in suicidal intent. *JAMA* 177:68-69 (July 8) 1961.

294. Lucas BG: Dilantin overdosage. *Med J Austral* 55:639-640 (Oct 12) 1968.

295. Luton CF: Carbon tetrachloride exposure during anticoagulant therapy. *JAMA* 194:1386-1387 (Dec 27) 1965.

296. MacDonald MG, Robinson DS: Clinical observations of possible barbiturate interference with anticoagulation. *JAMA* 204:97-100 (Apr 8) 1968.

297. MacDonald MG, Robinson DS, et al: The effects of phenobarbital, chloral betaine, and glutethimide administration on warfarin plasma levels and hypoprothrombinemic responses in man. *Clin Pharmacol Ther* 10:80-84 (Jan-Feb) 1969.

298. Macgregor AG: Clinical effects of interaction between drugs. Review of points at which drugs can interact. *Proc Roy Soc Med* 58:943-967 (Nov) 1965.

299. Magee PN: Toxicology and certainty. *New Scientist* pp 61-62 (April 9) 1970.

300. Majoor CLH: Aldosterone suppression by heparin. *N Engl J Med* 279:1172-1173 (Nov 21) 1968.

301. Manten A, Terra JI: The antagonism between penicillin and other antibiotics in relation to drug concentration. *Chemotherapia* 8:21-29, 1964.

302. Marcus FI, Pavlovich J, et al: The effect of reserpine on the metabolism of tritiated digoxin in the dog and in man. *J Pharmacol Exp Ther* 159:314-323 (Feb) 1968.

303. Martin EW: *Remington's Pharmaceutical Sciences.* Easton, Pa., Mack Publishing Co, 1966.

304. ———: *Techniques of Medication.* Philadelphia, Lippincott, 1969.

305. Mason A: Fatal reaction associated with tranylcypromine and methylamphetamine. *Lancet* 1:1073, 1962.

306. Mattila MJ, Tütinen H: Serum levels and urinary excretion of ethionamide and isoniazid after an oral intake of chymotrypsin. *Farm Aikakauslehti.* 76:294 (Nov-Dec) 1967.

307. Maurer HM, et al: Reduction in concentration of total serum-bilirubin in offspring of women treated with phenobarbitone during pregnancy. *Lancet* 2:122-124. 1968.

308. Mayer S, Maickel RP, Brodie, BB: Kinetics of penetration of drugs and other foreign compounds into cerebrospinal fluid and brain. *J Pharmacol Exp Ther* 127:205-211 (Nov) 1959.

309. McDougal MR: Interactions of drugs with aspi-

rin. *J Am Pharm Assoc* NS10:83-85 (Feb) 1970.

310. McGeer PL, Boulding JE, et al: Drug-induced extrapyramidal reactions. *JAMA* 177:665-670 (Sep 9) 1961.

311. McIver AK: Drug incompatibilities. *Pharm J* 195:609-612 (Dec 18) 1965.

312. ———: Drug interactions. *Pharm J* 199:205-210, 344, 360, 548 (Sep-Nov) 1967.

313. McManis AG: Adrenaline and isoprenaline: A warning. *Med J Austral* 51:76 (July 11) 1964.

314. Meyers DB: Drug interaction. *Tile & Till* 55:55 (Sep) 1969.

315. Meyers EL: Extemporaneous mixing of parenteral medication. *FDA Papers* 1:14-16 (June) 1967.

316. Meyler L: *Side Effects of Drugs* Vol I. Amsterdam, Excerpta Medica Foundation, 1957 (covers 1955-1956).

317. *Ibid.*, Vol 2, 1958 (covers 1956-1957).

318. *Ibid.*, Vol 3, 1960 (covers 1958-1960).

319. *Ibid.*, Vol 4, 1963 (covers 1960-1962).

320. *Ibid.*, Vol 5, 1966 (covers 1963-1965).

321. *Ibid.*, Vol 6, 1968 (covers 1965-1967). Baltimore, Williams & Wilkins and Amsterdam, Excerpta Medica Foundation.

322. Middleton WH, Morgan DD, Moyers J: Neostigmine therapy for apnea occurring after administration of neomycin. *JAMA* 165:2186-2187 (Dec 28) 1957.

323. Mielens ZE, Drobeck HP, et al: Interaction of aspirin with nonsteroidal anti-inflammatory drugs in rats. *J Pharm Pharmacol* 20:567-568 (July) 1968.

324. Miller RD, Way WL, Katzung BG: The potentiation of neuromuscular blocking agents by quinidine. *Anesthesiol* 28:1036-1041 (Nov-Dec) 1967.

325. Milne, MD: Influence of acid-base balance on efficacy and toxicity of drugs. *Proc Roy Soc Med* 58:961-963 (Nov) 1965.

326. Minvielle J, Cristol P, Badach L: L'abus de réglisse (glycyrrhizine). *Presse Méd* 71:2021-2024, 1963.

327. Mitchell JR, Arias L, Oates JA: Antagonism of the antihypertensive action of guanethidine sulfate by desipramine hydrochloride. *JAMA* 202:973-976 (Dec 4) 1967.

328. Molthan L, Reidenberg MM, Eichman MF: Positive direct Coombs tests due to cephalothin. *N Engl J Med* 277:123-125 (July 20) 1967.

329. Moore CB: Pitfalls in anticoagulant therapy for myocardial infarction. *Angiol* 15:27-34, 1964.

330. Morrelli HF, Melmon KL: The clinician's approach to drug interactions. *Calif Med* 109:380-389 (Nov) 1968.

331. Moser M, Brodoff B, et al: Experience with isocarboxazid. *JAMA* 176:276-280 (Apr 29) 1961.

332. Moser RH: *Diseases of Medical Progress: A Study of Iatrogenic Disease.* ed 3, Springfield, Ill, Charles C Thomas, 1969.

333. Murray FJ: Outbreak of unexpected reactions among epileptics taking isoniazid. *Am Rev Resp Dis* 86:729-732 (Nov) 1962.

334. Nelson E: Zero order oxidation of tolbutamide *in vivo. Nature* 193:76-77 (Jan 6) 1962.

335. Nelson MJ, Datta PR, Treadwell CR: Effects of residual DDT on *in vivo* and *in vitro* hepatic metabolism of selected non-barbiturate depressants in rats. *Clin Toxicol* 2:45-54 (Mar) 1969.

336. Nodine JH, Siegler PE: *Pharmacologic Techniques in Drug Evaluation.* Chap 6; Kinetics of absorption, distribution, excretion, and metabolism of drugs (Brodie BB). Chicago, Year Book, 1964.

337. Novick WJ, et al: The influence of steroids on drug metabolism in the mouse. *J Pharmacol Exp Ther* 151:139-142, 1966.

338. Nuessle WF, Norman FC, Miller HE: Pickled herring and tranylcypromine reaction. *JAMA* 192:726-727 (May 24) 1965.

339. Numeroff M, Perlmutter M, Slater S: Falsely elevated values for urinary 17-ketosteroids and 17-hydroxycorticoids associated with ingestion of triacetyloleandomycin. *J Clin Endocrinol Metab* 19:1350-1351 (Oct) 1959.

340. Oakley DP, Lautch H: Haloperidol and anticoagulant treatment. *Lancet* 2:1231 (Dec 7) 1963.

341. Oates JA: Drug-drug interaction: Interference with the delivery of drugs to their sites of action. *JAMA* 208:1898 (June 9) 1969.

342. Olesen OV: Disulfiramum (Antabuse) as inhibitor of phenytoin metabolism. *Acta Pharmacol* 24:317-322, 1966.

343. ———: The influence of disulfiram and calcium carbimide on the serum diphenylhydantoin. *Arch Neurol* 16:642-644 (June) 1967.

344. Oliver MF, et al: Effect of Atromid and ethyl chlorophenoxyisobutyrate on anticoagulant requirements. *Lancet* 1:143-144, 1963.

345. Olwin JH: *Anticoagulants and Fibrinolysins.* MacMillan RL, and Mustard, JF, (eds.), Philadelphia, Lea & Febiger, p. 250, 1961; Unusual experiences with anticoagulant therapy and the principles they represent. *Thrombosis and Embolism.* Proceedings of the First International Congress. (Eds: T Koller and WR Merz) pp 713-721. Basel, Benno Schwabe, 1955.

346. Owens JC, Neely WB, Owen WR: The effect of sodium dextrothyroxin in patients receiving anticoagulants. *N Engl J Med* 266:76-79, 1962.

347. Paterson JW, Dollery CT: Effect of propranolol in mild hypertension. *Lancet* 2:1148-1150 (Nov 26) 1966.

348. Paykel ES: Hallucinosis on combined methyldopa and pargyline. *Br Med J* 1:803 (Mar 26) 1966.

349. Payne JP, Rowe GG: The effects of mecamylamine in the cat as modified by the administration of carbon dioxide. *Br J Pharmacol* 12:457-460 (Dec) 1957.

350. Peaston MJT, Finnegan P: A case of combined poisoning with chlorpropamide, acetylsalicylic acid and paracetamol. *Br J Clin Pract* 22:30-31 (Jan) 1968.

351. Pelissier NA, Burger SL, Jr.: Guide to incompatibilities. *Hosp Pharm* 3:15-32 (Jan) 1968.

352. Penlington GN: Droperidol and monoamine oxidase inhibitors. *Br Med J* 1:483-484 (Feb 19) 1966.

353. Penna RP: A screening procedure for drug interactions *J Am Pharm Assoc* NS10:66-67 (Feb) 1970.

354. Perman ES: Intolerance to alcohol. *N Engl J Med* 273:114 (July 8) 1965.

355. Pettinger WA, Oates JA: Supersensitivity to tyra-

mine during monoamine oxidase inhibition in man: mechanism at the level of the adrenergic neuron. *Clin Pharmacol Ther* 9:341-344 (May-June) 1968.

356. Pettinger WA, Soyangco FG, Oates JA: Mono-amine-oxidase inhibition by furazolidone in man. *Clin Res* 14:258 (Apr) 1966; Inhibition of mono-amine oxidase in man by furazolidone. *Clin Pharmacol Ther* 9:442-447 (July-Aug) 1968.

357. Pinchera A, MacGillivray MH, Crawford JD, et al: Thyroid refractoriness in an athyreotic cretin fed soybean formula. *N Engl J Med* 273:83-87 (July 8) 1965.

358. Pittinger CB, Long JP, Miller JR: The neuromuscular blocking action of neomycin: a concern of the anesthesiologist. *Anesth Analg Cur Res* 37:276-282 (Sep-Oct) 1958.

359. Prescott LF: Pharmacokinetic drug interactions. *Lancet* 2:1239-1243 (Dec 6) 1969.

360. Preti M, Della Bella, D: Influence of certain drugs on the acute toxicity of specific antibiotics. *Boll Chimicofarm* 106:603 (Sep) 1967.

361. Propranolol: *Lancet* 1:939-940 (Apr 29) 1967.

362. ———: *Med Let Drugs Ther* 10:25-27 (Apr 5) 1968.

363. Protriptyline (Vivactil)—another antidepressant: *Med Let Drugs Ther* 10:17-18 (Mar 8) 1968.

364. Protein binding of drugs. *Lancet* 1: 73-74 (Jan 10) 1970.

365. Provost GP: Drug interactions in perspective. *Am J Hosp Pharm* 26:679 (Dec) 1969.

366. Pyorala K, Kekki M.: Decreased anticoagulant tolerance during methandrostenolone therapy. *Scand J Clin Lab Invest* 15:367-374, 1963.

367. Quinine potentiation of muscle relaxants: *Clin-Alert* 291, Dec 8, 1967.

368. Raftos J, Valentine PA: The prolonged use of alpha methyldopa in the treatment of hypertension. *Med J Austral* 51:837-842 (May 30) 1964.

369. Rechnitzer P: Digitalis and diuretics—a toxic drug combination. *Appl Ther* 6:217-218, 222, 1964.

370. Refshauge WD: Sympathomimetic drugs and bronchial asthma. *Med J Austral* 52:93-94 (Jan 16) 1965.

371. Reverchon F, Sapir M: Constatation clinique d'un antagonisme entre barbituriques et anticoagulants. *Presse Méd* 69:1570-1571, 1961.

372. Reynolds WA, Lowe FH: Mushrooms and a toxic reaction to alcohol. *N Engl J Med* 272:630-631 (May 25) 1965.

373. Roberts J, Ito R, et al: Influence of reserpine and beta TM10 on digitalis induced ventricular arrhythmia. *Circ Res* 13:149-158 (Aug) 1963.

374. Roberts RJ, Plaa GL: Effect of phenobarbital on the excretion of an exogenous bilirubin load. *Biochem Pharmacol* 16:827-835, 1967.

375. Robinson DS, MacDonald MG: The effect of phenobarbital administration on the control of coagulation achieved during warfarin therapy in man. *J Pharmacol Exp Ther* 153:250-253 (Aug) 1966.

376. Roos J, van Joost HE: The cause of bleeding during anticoagulant treatment. *Acta Med Scand* 178:129-131, 1965.

377. Rosenbaum EH, Cohen RA, Glatstein HR: Vaccination of a patient receiving immunosuppressive therapy for lymphosarcoma. *JAMA* 198:737-740 (Nov 14) 1966.

378. Rossi GV: The toxic constituents of pharmaceuticals. *Am J Pharm* 138:57-65 (Mar Apr) 1966.

379. Rothermich NO: Diphenylhydantoin intoxication. *Lancet* 2:640 (Sep 17) 1966.

380. Rouge J-C, Banner MP, Smith TC: Interactions of levallorphan and meperidine. *Clin Pharmacol Ther* 10:643-654 (Sep-Oct) 1969.

381. Royer R, Debry G, Lamarche M, et al: Sulfamides hypoglycémiants et effet antabuse. *Presse Med* 72:661-665, 1964.

382. Sabath LD, Elder HA, et al: Synergistic combinations of penicillins in the treatment of bacteriuria. *N Engl J Med* 277:232-238 (Aug 3) 1967.

383. Sachs BA, Wolfman L: Effect of oxandrolone on plasma lipids and lipoproteins of patients with disorders of lipid metabolism. *Metabolism* 17:400-410 (May) 1968.

384. Sadusk JF, Jr: Regulatory and medical aspects of public policy on home remedies. *Ann NY Acad Sci* 120: 868-871, 1965.

385. Salgado AS: Potentiation of succinylcholine by procaine. *Anesthesiol* 22:897-899 (Nov-Dec) 1961.

386. Samaan N, Dollery CT, Frazer R: Diabetogenic action of benzothiadiazines: serum-insulin-like activity in diabetes worsened or precipitated by thiazide diuretics. *Lancet* 2:1244-1247 (Dec 14) 1963.

387. Sartorelli AC, Booth BA: The synergistic antineoplastic activity of combinations of mitomycins with either 6-thioguanine or 5-flurouracil. *Cancer Res* 25:1393-1400 (Oct) 1965.

388. Saw-Lan Ip F: Pressor effect of 5-hydroxytryptamine. *Lancet* 1:91 (Jan 8) 1966.

389. Scherbel AL: Amine oxidase inhibitors. *Clin Pharmacol Ther* 2:559-566, 1961.

390. Schmidt JL, Vick NA, Sadove, MS: The effect of quinidine on the action of muscle relaxants. *JAMA* 183:669-671 (Feb 23) 1963.

391. Schrogie JJ: Drug interactions. *FDA Papers* 2:11-13 (Nov) 1968.

392. Schrogie JJ, Solomon HM, et al: Effect of oral contraceptives on vitamin K-dependant clotting activity. *Clin Pharmacol Ther* 8:670-675, 1967.

393. Schrogie JJ, Solomon HM: Hazards of multiple drug therapy in patients taking coumarin anticoagulants. *Circulation* 34 (Suppl. III):210-211 (Oct) 1966.

394. ———: The anticoagulant response to bishydroxycoumarin. II. The effect of D-thyroxin, clofibrate, and norethandrolone. *Clin Pharmacol Ther* 8:70-77 (Jan-Feb) 1967.

395. Schumacher GE: Toxic potential of some drug interactions. *Am J Hosp Pharm* 21:494-496 (Nov.) 1964.

396. Selye H, et al: Digitoxin poisoning: prevention by spironolactone. *Science* 164:842-843 (May 16) 1969.

397. Seneca H, Peer P: Enhancement of blood and urine tetracycline levels with a chymotrypsin-tetracycline preparation. *J Am Geriat Soc* 13: 708-717 (Aug) 1965.

398. Shafer N: Hypotension due to nitroglycerin combined with alcohol. *N Engl J Med* 273:1169, 1965.

399. Shepherd M: Psychotropic drugs (1). Interaction

between centrally acting drugs in man: Some general considerations. Clinically important examples of drug interaction. *Proc Roy Soc Med* 58:964-967 (Nov) 1965.

400. Sherrod TR, Loew ER, Schloemer, H.F.: Pharmacological properties of antihistamine drugs, Benadryl, Pyribenzamine, and Neoantergan. *J. Pharmacol Exp Ther* 89:247-255, 1947.

401. Sigell LT: Alleged adverse drug interactions reporyed in man. *Physician's Formulary,* Cincinnati General Hospital, p 11-19.

402. Simon C: Problem of antagonism with antibiotic combinations. *Chemotherapia* 11:43-62, 1966.

403. Singer W, Weston JK, et al.: Panel discussion. Drug interaction symposium for pharmacists and physicians, sponsored by Albany College of Pharmacy, its Southern Tier Alumni Group, and the Pharmaceutical Society of Broome County, Binghamton, N.Y., Sep 24, 1969.

404. Sjöqvist F: Psychotropic drugs (2). Interaction between monoamine-oxidase (MAO) inhibitors and other substances. *Proc Roy Soc Med* 58:967-978 (Nov) 1965.

405. Smith HE: Warning from ophthalmologist. *Utah Dig* p 12 (Nov) 1969.

406. Smith JW: A hospital adverse drug reaction reporting program. *Hosp (JAHA)* 40:90-6 (Feb 16) 1966.

407. Smith SLH: Drugs and investigations. *Br Med J* 2:1265 (Nov 14) 1964.

408. Sodium dextrothyroxine (Choloxin). *Med Let Drugs Ther* 9:103-104 (Dec 29) 1967.

409. Soeldner JS, Steinke J: Hypoglycemia in tolbutamide-treated diabetes. *JAMA* 193:398-399 (Aug 2) 1965.

410. Soffer A: The changing clinical picture of digitalis intoxication. *Arch Int Med* 107:681-688, 1961.

411. Solomon HM, Schrogie JJ: Changes in receptor site affinity: a proposed explanation for the potentiating effect of D-thyroxine on the anticoagulant response to warfarin. *Clin Pharmacol Ther* 8:797-799 (Nov-Dec) 1967.

412. ———: Effect of phenyramidol and bishydroxycoumarin on the metabolism of tolbutamide in human subjects. *Metabolism* 16:1029-1033 (Nov) 1967.

413. ———: The effect of phenyramidol on the metabolism of diphenylhydantoin. *Clin Pharmacol Ther* 8:554-556 (July-Aug) 1967.

414. Solomon J: The bitter sweeteners. *The Sciences* 9:20-25 (Sep) 1969.

415. Spiekerman RE, et al: Potassium-sparing effects of triamterene in the treatment of hypertension. *Circulation* 34:524-531 (Sep) 1966.

416. Stille W, Ostner KH: Antagonismus nitrofurantoin-nalidixinsäure. *Klin Wschr* 44:155-156, 1966.

417. Stone CA, Porter CC, et al: Antagonism of certain effects of catecholamine-depleting agents by antidepressant and related drugs. *J Pharmacol Exp Ther* 144:196-204, 1964.

418. Stowers JM, Constable LW, Hunter RB: A clinical and pharmacological comparison of chlorpropamide and other sulfonylureas. *Ann NY Acad Sci* 74:689-695 (Mar 30) 1959.

419. Strom J: Penicillin and erythromycin singly and in combination in scarlatina therapy and the interference between them. *Antibiot Chemother* 11:694-697, 1961.

420. Stuart DM: Drug metabolism Part 1. Basic fundamentals. *PharmIndex* 10:3-8 (Sep) 1968.

421. ———: Drug metabolism Part 2. Drug interactions. *PharmIndex* 10:4-16 (Oct) 1968.

422. Sugimoto I: Studies on Complexes XX. Effect of complex formation on drug absorption from alimentary tract. *Chem Pharm Bull* 18:515-526 (Mar) 1970.

423. Sulser F, Owens ML, Dingell JV: On the mechanism of amphetamine potentiation by desipramine (DMI). *Life Sci* 5:2005-2010 (Nov) 1966.

424. Svedmyr N: Potentiation risks in the administration of catecholamines to patients treated with tricyclic antidepressive agents. *Svenska Lakartidn* 65:72-76 (Suppl 1) 1968.

425. Taylor DC: Alarming reaction to pethidine in patients on phenelzine. *Lancet* 2:401-402 (Aug 25) 1962.

426. The choice of systemic antimicrobial drugs. *Med Let* 10:77 (Oct 4) 1968.

427. Thomas J: Some aspects of drug interactions. *Australasian J. Pharm* 48:S112-117 (Nov-Dec) 1967.

428. Thomas JCS: Monoamine-oxidase inhibitors and cheese. *Br Med J* 2:1406 (Nov 30) 1963.

429. Thorazine-hyperglycemia. *Clin.-Alert* 303 (Nov 3) 1964.

430. Tolis AD: Hypoglycemic convulsions in children after alcohol ingestion. *Pediat Clin N Am.* 12:423-425, 1965.

431. Tonks CM, Lloyd AT: Hazards with monoamine-oxidase inhibitors. *Br Med J* 1:589 (Feb 27) 1965.

432. Trubuhovich RV: Delayed reversal of diallyl-nor-toxiferine after streptomycin. *Brit J Anaesth* 38:843-844 (Oct) 1966.

433. Tuttle CB: Drug interactions. *Can J Hosp Pharm* 22:2-15 (May-June) 1969.

434. Udall JA: Recent advances in anticoagulant therapy. *GP* 40:117-121 (July) 1969; Don't use the wrong vitamin K. *Calif Med* 112:65-67 (Apr) 1970.

435. Usubiaga JE, Wikinski JA, et al: Interaction of intravenously administered procaine, lidocaine and succinylcholine in anesthetized subjects. *Anesth Analg* 46:39-45 (Jan-Feb) 1967.

436. van Dam FE, Overkamp M, Haanen C: The interaction of drugs. *Lancet* 2:1027 (Nov 5) 1966.

437. van Rossum JM: Potential danger of monoamine oxidase inhibitors and α-methyldopa. *Lancet* 1:950-951 (Apr 27) 1963.

438. Veldstra H: Synergism and potentiation with special reference to the combination of structural analogues. *Pharmacol Rev* 8:339-387 (Mar) 1956.

439. Vere DW: Errors of complex prescribing. *Lancet* 1:370-373 (Feb 13) 1965.

440. Vesell ES: Induction of drug-metabolizing enzymes in liver microsomes of mice and rats by softwood bedding. *Science* 157:1057-1058 (Sep 1) 1967.

441. Vigran IM: Dangerous potentiation of meperidine hydrochloride by pargyline hypochloride. *JAMA* 187:953-954 (Mar 21) 1964.

442. Viljoen JF: Parenteral neomycin and muscle re-

laxants. *S Afr Med J* 40:963-964 (Oct 29) 1966.

443. Visconti JA: Use of drug interaction information in patient medication records. *Am J Hosp Pharm* 26:378-387 (July) 1969.

444. Viukari NMA: Phenytoin, folates, and ATP ase. *Lancet* 1:1000-1001 (May 9) 1970.

445. Wallace JF, et al: Studies on the pathogenesis of meningitis VI. Antagonism between penicillin and chloramphenicol in experimental pneumococcal meningitis. *J Lab Clin Med* 70:408-18 (Sep) 1967.

446. Walton RP: Cardiac glycosides II: pharmacology and clinical use, in (Drill VA, ed): *Pharmacology in Medicine* ed 3 New York, McGraw-Hill 1965.

447. Way WL, Katzung BG, Larson CP, Jr: Recurarization with quinidine. *JAMA* 200:153-154 (Apr 10) 1967.

448. Weiner M, Siddiqui AA, et al: Drug interactions: The effect of combined administration on the half-life of coumarin and pyrazolone drugs in man. *Fed Proc* 24:153 (Mar-Apr) 1965.

449. Welch RM, et al: An experimental model in dogs for studying interactions of drugs with bishydroxycoumarin. *Clin Pharmacol Ther* 10:817-825 (Nov) 1969.

450. Werk EE, Jr, Choi Y, et al: Interference in the effect of dexamethasone by diphenylhydantoin. *N Engl J Med* 281:32-34, 1969.

451. Werk EE, Jr, et al: Effect of diphenylhydantoin on cortisol metabolism in man. *J Clin Invest* 43:1824-1835 (Sep) 1964.

452. White AG: Methyldopa and amitriptyline. *Lancet* 2:441 (Aug 28) 1965.

453. Weiner M: Effect of centrally active drugs on the action of coumarin anticoagulants. *Nature* 212:1599-1600 (Dec 31) 1966.

454. Wier JK, Tyler VE, Jr: An investigation of *Corprinus altramentarius* for the presence of disulfiram. *J Am Pharm Assoc* 49:426-429, 1960.

455. Williams JT, Moravec DF: Intravenous therapy. *Hosp Form Manag* 1: 28-30 (Sep) 1966.

456. Wilson IC, Prange AJ, Jr, et al: Thyroid hormone enhancement of imipramine in nonretarded depressions. *N Engl J Med* 282:1063-1067 (May 7) 1970.

457. Winer BM, Lubbe WF, Colton T: Antihypertensive actions of diuretics. *JAMA* 204:775-779 (May 27) 1968.

458. Wishinsky H, Glasser EJ, Perkal S: Protein interactions of sulfonylurea compounds. *Diabetes* 11:18-25 (Suppl) 1962.

459. Womack AM: Tranylcypromine. *Lancet* 2:463 (Aug 31) 1963.

460. Wood FC, Jr: Diabetes and alcoholism. *JAMA* 181:358 (July 28) 1962.

461. Woods DD: Relation of *p*-aminobenzoic acid to the mechanism of action of sulphanilamide. *Br J Exp Pathol* 21:74-90, 1940.

462. ———: The biochemical mode of action of the sulphonamide drugs. *J Gen Microbiol* 29:687-702, 1962.

463. Wortis J: Psychopharmacology and physiological treatment. *Am J Psychiat* 120:643-648 (Jan) 1964.

464. Wynn V, Doar JWH, Mills GL: Some effects of oral contraceptives on serum-lipid and lipoprotein levels. *Lancet* 2:720-723 (Oct 1) 1966.

465. Yanchik VA: Importance of drug interactions to pharmacists. *Tex Pharm* 12, 16, 21, 25, 29 (Oct) 1969.

466. ———: Drug interactions. *Wisc Pharm* pp 404-425 (Nov) 1969.

467. Yu TF, Dayton PG, Gutman AB: Mutual suppression of the uricosuric effects of sulfinpyrazone and salicylate. A study in interactions between drugs. *J Clin Invest* 42:1330-1339, 1963.

468. Zaharko DS, Bruckner H, Oliverio VT: Antibiotics alter methotrexate metabolism and excretion. *Science* 166:887-888 (Nov 14) 1969.

469. Zubrod CG: Combinations of drugs in the treatment of acute leukemias. *Proc Roy Soc Med* 58:988-990 (Nov) 1965.

470. Zupko AG: Drug interactions. *Pharm Times* pp 38-50 (Sep-Oct) 1969; *Hosp Form Manag* 5:17-21 (Apr); 16-19 (May); 18-22 (June) 1970.

471. Kuzucu EY: Methoxyflurane, tetracycline, and renal failure. *JAMA* 211:1162-1164 (Feb 16) 1970.

472. Barr WH, Adir J, Garretson L: Decrease of tetracycline absorption in man by sodium bicarbonate. *Clin Pharmacol Ther* 12:779-784, 1971.

473. Organic phosphate poisoning. *Morb Mort* 19:397, 404 (Oct 10) 1970.

474. Charcoal briquettes and other forms of charcoal: proposed declaration on hazardous substances that require special labeling. *Fed Reg* 35:13887-13888 (FR Doc 70-11551; Sep 2) 1970.

475. Nelson E: Pharmaceuticals of prolonged action. *Clin Pharmacol Ther* 4:283-292 (Feb) 1963.

476. Texter EC, Jr, et al: *Physiology of the Gastrointestinal Tract.* St. Louis, Mosby, 1968, p. 207.

477. Feuerstein RC, Finberg L, Fleishman E: The use of acetazoleamide in the therapy of salicylate poisoning. *Pediat* 25:215-227 (Feb) 1960.

478. Serrone DM, Fujimoto JM: The diphasic effect of N-methyl-3-piperidyl-(N', N')-diphenylcarbamate HCl (MPDC) in the metabolism of hexobarbital, *J Pharmacol Exp Ther* 133:12-17, 1961.

479. Conney AH, Schneidman K, Jacobsen M, et al: Drug-induced changes in steroid metabolism. *Ann NY Acad Sci* 123:98-109 (Mar) 1965.

480. Ellenhorn MJ, Sternad FA: Clinical look at problems of drug interactions. *J Am Pharm Assoc* NS6:62-64, 68 (Jan) 1966.

481. Cooney AH, et al: Stimulatory effect of chlorcyclizine on barbiturate metabolism. *J Pharmacol Exp Ther* 134:291, 1961.

482. Nielsen J, Friedrich U, Tsuboi T: Chromosome abnormalities in patients treated with chlorpromazine, perphenazine, and lysergide. *Br Med J* 3:634-636 (Sep 13) 1969.

483. Isaac L, Goth A: The mechanism of the potentiation of norepinephrine by antihistaminics. *J Pharmacol Exp Ther* 156:463-468 (June) 1965.

484. Peters G, Hodgson J, Donovan R: Effects of premedication with chlorpheniramine in reactions to methyl glucamine. *Allergy* 38:74 (Aug) 1966.

485. Conney AH, et al: Effects of pesticides on drug and steroid metabolism. *Clin Pharmacol Ther* 8:2-10 (Jan-Feb) 1967.

486. Cohen MS: *Therapeutic Drug Interactions.* Madison, Wis University of Wisconsin Medical Center, 1970.

487. Turner P: Antihistamine drugs and the central

nervous system. *Med News* 190:9 (May 27) 1968.

488. Gershon S, Neubauer H, Sundland DM: Interaction between some anticholinergic agents and phenothiazines; potentiation of phenothiazine sedation and its antagonism. *Clin Pharmacol Ther* 6:749–756 (Nov–Dec) 1965.

489. Chu J, Doering MF, Fogel EJ: The clinical determination of unique effect of potentiation of phenothiazine medication by nylidrin hydrochloride. *Intern J Neuropsychiat* 2:53–59 (Jan–Feb) 1966.

490. Lorenc E: A new factor in griseofulvin treatment failures: Case report. *Missouri Med* 64:32–33 (Jan) 1967.

491. Cocke JG, Jr: Chloramphenicol optic neuritis. *Am J Diseases Child* 114:424–426 (Oct) 1967

492. Jawetz E, Gunnison JB, Coleman VR: The combined action of penicillin with streptomycin or chloromycetin on enterococci *in vitro*. *Science* 111:254 (Mar 10) 1950.

493. Searle GD & Co: Dramamine package brochure (April 22) 1966

494. Freemon FR, Parker RL, Jr, Greer M: Unusual neurotoxicity of kanamycin. *JAMA* 200-410–411 (May 1) 1967.

495. Loder, RE, Walker GF: Neuromuscular-blocking action of streptomycin. *Lancet* 1:812, 1959.

496. Porth EJ: Critical analysis of intestinal antisepsis. *JAMA* 163:1317–1322 (Apr 13) 1957.

497. Sabawala PB, Dillon JB: The action of some antibiotics on the human intercostal nerve-muscle complex. *Anesthesiology* 20:659 (Sep–Oct) 1959.

498. Sikh SS, Sachdev KS: Duration of the neuromuscular blocking action of streptomycin. *Br J Anaesth* 37:158–160 (Mar) 1965.

499. Bell RW, Jenicek JA: Respiratory failure following intramural bowel injection of neomycin. Report of a case. *Med Ann DC* 35:603 (Nov) 1966.

500. Blake-Knox, PEA: Neuromuscular block with streptomycin. *Br Med J* 1:1319, 1961.

501. Bristol, Kanamycin Sulfate Injection: Bristol Laboratories Product Brochure, (Oct) 1967.

502. Bush GG: Prolonged neuromuscular block due to intraperitoneal streptomycin *Br Med J* 1:557 (Feb 25) 1961.

503. Doremus WP: Respiratory arrest following intraperitoneal use of neomycin. *Ann Surg* 149:546–548 (Apr) 1959.

504. Engel HL, Denson JS: Respiratory depression due to neomycin. *Surgery* 42:862–864 (Nov) 1957.

505. Fisk GC: Respiratory paralysis after a large dose of streptomycin. *Br Med J* 1:566-557, 1961.

506. Lindesmith LA, et al: Reversible respiratory paralysis associated with polymyxin therapy. *Ann Intern Med* 68:318 (Feb) 1968.

507. Pridgen JE: Respiratory arrest thought to be due to intraperitoneal neomycin. *Surgery* 40:571–574 (Sep) 1956.

508. MacDonald H, et al: Effect of chymotrypsin on absorption of tetracycline. *Antimicrob Agents Chemother* 173–178, 1964.

509. Kunnin CM, Finland M: Clinical pharmacology of the tetracycline antibiotics. *Clin Pharmacol Ther* 2:51–69 (Jan–Feb) 1961.

510. Krauer-Meyer B: Uber die Ursachen von Vitamin-K-Mangel-Zustanden. Theorie und Klinik (Vitamin K deficiency following antibiotic therapy). *Schweiz Med Wsch* 96/52:1746-1750 (Dec 31) 1966.

511. Lansdown FS, Beran M, Litwak T: Psychotoxic reaction during ethionamide therapy. *Am Rev Resp Dis* 95:1053-1055 (June) 1967.

512. Dixon RL, Henderson ES, Rall DP: Plasma protein binding of methotrexate and its displacement by various drugs. *Fed Proc* 24:454, 1965. (Abstract from paper at 49th Annual Meeting, 1965).

513. Kruger H-U: Hypoglycemic effect of cyclophosphamide in diabetic patients. *Klin MED* 61:1462-3 (Sep 16) 1966.

514. Cosmegan (Dactinomycin) Brochure, MSC, Dec, 1957.

515. Johnson RE, Brace KC: Radiation response of Hodgkin's disease recurrent after chemotherapy. *Cancer* 19:368-370 (Mar.) 1966.

516. Anon.: Drug Interactions. *Illinois Pharmacist* 34:336 (July) 1969.

517. Drachman DA, Skom JH: Procainamide—A hazard in myasthenia gravis. *Arch Neurol* 13:316-320 (Sep.) 1965.

518. Proctor CD, Denefield BA, Ashley LG: Extension of ethyl alcohol action by polocarpine. *Brain Res* 3:217-220 (Dec) 1966.

519. Ellis PP, Esterdahl M: Echothiophate iodide therapy in children. Effect upon blood cholinesterase levels. *Arch Ophthalmol* 77:598-601 (May) 1967.

520. Anon.: Topical treatment of chronic simple glaucoma. *Drug Therapy Bull.* 2:18, 1964.

521. Roman DT: Effect of variables on chemical and diagnostic specificity of laboratory tests, Memo to medical staff, Evanston Hospital.

522. McGavi DDM: Depressed levels of serum-pseudocholinesterase with ecothiophate-iodide eyedrops. *Lancet* 2:272-273 (Aug 7) 1965.

523. Seybold R, Brautigam KH: Prolonged succinyl-induced apnea as an indication of alkylphosphate poisoning. *Deut Med Wschr* 93:1405-1406 (July 19) 1968.

524. Arterberry JD, et al: Potentiation of phosphorus insecticides by phenothiazine derivatives. *JAMA* 182:848-850 (Nov 24) 1962.

525. Meyler L, Herxheimer A (eds): *Side Effects of Drugs* Vol. 6. Baltimore, Williams & Wilkins, 1968.

526. Eli Lilly and Co.: Package brochure, Darvon, May, 1969.

527. Kay B: Hypotensive reaction after propanidid and atropine. *Br Med J* 3:413 (Aug 16) 1969.

528. Buckle RM, Guillebaud J: Hypoglycaemic coma occurring during treatment with chlorpromazine and orphenadrine. *Br Med J* 4:599-600 (Dec 9) 1967.

529. Hartshorn EA: *Handbook of Drug Interactions.* Cincinnati, Ohio, Donald E. Francke, Editor and Publisher, 1970.

530. Anon.: Interaction of monoamine oxidase inhibitors and drugs used in dentistry. *Med J Austral* 53:1092 (June 18) 1966.

531. Block LH, Lamy PP: Drug interactions with emphasis on O-T-C drugs. *J Am Pharm Assoc* NS9:202-206 (May) 1969.

532. Bull C, et al: Hypertension with methionine in schizophrenic patients receiving tranylcypromine. *Am J Psychiat* 121:381-382 (Oct) 1964.

533. Eble JN, Rudzik AD: Tyramine and amphetamine. *Lancet* 1:766 (Apr 2) 1966.

534. ———: Amphetamine: Augmentation of pressor effects of tyramine in rats. *Proc Soc Exp Biol Med* 122:1059-1060 (Aug-Sep) 1966.

535. Mason AMS, Buckle RM: "Cold" cures and monoamine-oxidase inhibitors. *Br Med J* 1:845-846 (Mar 29) 1969.

536. Smith MC, Visconti JA: Adverse drug reactions . . . How community ℞ men can help prevent them. *Am Prof Pharmacist* 34:26 (Oct) 1968.

537. Bester JF: Potentiation of drugs by ethyl alcohol. *Am Assoc Indust Nurse J* 15:10 (Aug) 1967.

538. Grant ECC, Mears E: Mental effects of oral contraceptives. *Lancet* 2:945-946 (Oct) 1967.

539. Svedmyr N: The action of tri-iodothyronine on some effects of adrenaline and noradrenaline in man. *Acta Pharmacol* (Kobenhavn) 24:203-216, 1966.

540. Burns JJ, et al: Application of metabolic data on the evaluation of drugs. *Clin Pharmacol Ther* 10:607-634 (Sep-Oct) 1969.

541. Jori A, Garattini S: Interaction between imipramine-like agents and catecholamine-induced hyperthermia. *J Pharm Pharmacol* 17:480-488 (Aug) 1965.

542. Kimelberg H, Moran JF, Triggle JD: The mechanism of interaction of 2-halogenoethylamines at the noradrenaline receptor. *J Theoret Biol* 9:502-503 (Nov) 1965.

543. Anon.: Anaesthetics and the heart. *Lancet* 1:484-485 (Mar 4) 1967.

544. Dixon RL, Rogers LA, Fouts JA: Effects of norepinephrine treatment on drug metabolism by liver microsomes from rats. *Biochem Pharmacol* 13:623 (Apr) 1964.

545. Poyart C, et al: Depression of norepinephrine activity by acidosis: Its reversal by aminophylline. *Surg Forum* 17:41-42, 1966; metabolic effects of theophylline and norepinephrine in the dog at normal and acid pH. *Am J Physiol* 212:1247-1254 (June) 1967.

546. Mond E, Mack I: Cardiac toxicity of iproniazid (Marsilid): Report of myocardial injury in a patient receiving levarterenol. *J Am Heart Assoc* 59:134-139, 1960.

547. Parisi AF, Kaplan MH: Apnea during treatment with sodium colistimethate. *JAMA* 194:298-299 (Oct 18) 1965.

548. Low RF: Acute angle-closure glaucoma precipitated by miotics plus adrenaline eye-drops. *Med J Australia* 2:1037-1038 (Nov 26) 1966.

549. Anon.: Insulin and epinephrine. *S Afri Med J* 41:474 (May 13) 1967.

550. Day MD, Rand MJ: Antagonism of guanethidine by dexamphetamine and other related sympathomimetic amines. *J Pharm Pharmacol* 14:541-549 (Sep) 1962.

551. Kownacki VP, Serlin O: Intraperitoneal neomycin as a cause of apnea. *Arch Surg* 81:838-841, 1960.

552. Gaddum JH, Kwiatkowski H: The action of ephedrine. *J Physiol* 94:87-100 (Oct 14) 1938.

553. Cooper B: "Neo-Synephrine" (10%) eye drops. *Med J Australia* 55:420 (Aug 31) 1968.

554. Gelder MG, Vane JR: Interaction of the effects of tyramine, amphetamine and reserpine in man. *Psychopharmacologia* 3:231-241, 1962.

555. Conney AH, et al: Adaptive increases in drug-metabolizing enzymes induced by phenobarbital and other drugs. *J Pharmacol Exp Ther* 130:1-8 (Sep) 1960.

556. Kato R, Chiesara E: Increase of pentobarbitone metabolism induced in rats pretreated with some centrally acting compounds. *Br J Pharmacol* 18:29-38 (Feb) 1962.

557. Kato R, Vassanelli P: Induction of increased meprobamate metabolism in rats pretreated with some neutrotropic drugs. *Biochem Pharmacol* 11:779-794 (Aug) 1962.

558. Conney AH, Burns JJ: Biochemical pharmacological considerations of zoxazolamine and chlorzoxazone metabolism. *Ann NY Acad Sci* 86:167 (Mar) 1960.

559. Anon.: Quinidine potentiation of muscle relaxants. *Clin-Alert* 291 (Dec 8) 1967.

560. McQuillen MP, Cantor HE, O'Rourke JR: Myasthenic syndrome associated with antibiotics. *Arch Neurol* 18:402-415 (Apr) 1968.

561. Pinkerton HH, Muntro JR: Respiratory insufficiency associated with the use of streptomycin. *Scot Med J* 9:256 (June) 1964.

562. Vital Brazil O, Corrado AP: The curariform action of streptomycin. *J Pharmacol Exp Ther* 120:452-459 (Aug) 1957.

563. Weill MJ, Gauthier-Lafaye P, Dupuis J: Curarizing action of antibiotics and potentiation of curare by antibiotics. *Therapie* 23:879-884 (July-Aug) 1968.

564. Cuthbert MF: The effect of quinidine and procainamide on the neuromuscular blocking action of suxamethonium. *Br J Anaesthesia* 38:775-779 (Oct) 1966.

565. Kato R, Chiesara E, Vassanelli P: Further studies on the inhibition and stimulation of microsomal drug-metabolizing enzymes of rat liver by various compounds. *Biochem Pharmacol* 13:69-83 (Jan) 1964.

566. Regan AG, Aldrete JA: Prolonged apnea after administration of promazine hydrochloride following succinylcholine infusion: A case report. *Anesthesia Analgesia Current Res* 46:315-318 (May-June) 1967.

567. Chasapakis G, Dimas C: Possible interaction between muscle relaxants and the kallikrein-trypsin inactivator "Trasylol": Report of three cases. *Br J Anaesthesia* 38:838-839 (Oct) 1966.

568. Anon.: Interactions of oral anticoagulants with other drugs. *Med Let Drugs Ther* 9:97 (Dec 1) 1967.

569. Hansen JM, et al: Dicoumarol-induced diphenylhydantoin intoxication. *Lancet* 2:265-266 (July 30) 1966.

570. Rothstein E: Warfarin effect enhanced by disulfiram. *JAMA* 206:1574-1575 (Nov 11) 1968; 221:1052-3 (Aug 28) 1972.

571. Antlitz AM, et al: A double-blind study of acetaminophen used in conjunction with oral anticoagulant therapy. *Curr Ther Res* 11:360-361 (June) 1969.

572. ———: Potentiation of oral anticoagulant ther-

apy by acetaminophen. *Curr Ther Res* 10:501-507 (Oct) 1968.

573. Anon.: Warfarin sodium-quinidine. *Clin-Alert* 72, 1969.

574. Anon.: Oral contraceptives. *Clin-Alert* 233, 1967.

575. Sise HS: Potentiation of tolbutamide by dicumarol (editorial). *Ann Int Med* 67:460-461 (Aug) 1967.

576. Conney AH, Michaelson IA, Burns, JJ: Stimulatory effect of chlorcyclizine on barbiturate metabolism. *J Pharmacol Exp Ther* 132:202-206 (May) 1961.

577. Upjohn Company, brochure, neomycin sulfate (June) 1968.

578. Anon.: Effect of pH of the urine on antimicrobial therapy of urinary tract infections. *Med Let Drugs Ther* 9:47 (June 16) 1967.

579. Jenkins LC: The interaction of drugs. *Can Anaesth Soc J* 15:111-117 (Mar) 1968.

580. Nagata RE, Jr: Drug interactions-digitalis glycosides and kaliuresis. *Hosp Form Manag* 4:30-32 (Aug) 1969.

581. Gerhardt RE, Knouss RF, Thyrum PT, et al: Quinidine excretion in aciduria and alkaluria. *Ann Int Med* 71:927-933 (Nov) 1969.

582. Gassaniga AB, Stewart DR: Possible quinidine-induced hemorrhage in a patient on warfarin sodium. *N Engl J Med* 280:711 (Mar 27) 1969.

583. Castellanos A, Salhanick L: Electrocardiographic patterns of procaine amide cardiotoxicity. *Am J Med Sci* 253:52-60 (Jan) 1967.

584. Greene R, Oliver CC: Sensitivity to propranolol after digoxin intoxication. *Br Med J* 3:413-404 (Aug 17) 1968.

585. Stern S: Synergistic action of propranolol with quinidine. *Am Heart J* 72:569-570 (Oct) 1966.

586. Riesterer L, Jaques R: Interference with β-adrenergic blocking agents with the anti-inflammatory action of various drugs. *Helv Physiol Acta* 26:287-293, 1968.

587. Frankl WS, Soloff LA: The hemodynamic effects of propranolol hydrochloride after smoking. *Am J Med Sci* 254:623-628 (Nov) 1967.

588. Anon.: Evaluation of a hypocholesterolemic agent, dextrothyroxine sodium (Choloxin). *JAMA* 208:1014-1015 (May 12) 1969.

589. Best MM, Duncan CH: Effects of clofibrate and dextrothyroxine singly and in combination on serum lipids. *Arch Int Med* 118:97-102 (Aug) 1966.

590. Winters WL, Jr, Soloff LA: Observations on sodium d-thyroxine as a hypocholesteremic agent in persons with hypercholesteremia with and without ischemic heart disease. *Am J Med Sci* 243:458-459 (Apr) 1962.

591. Chang CC, Costa E, Brodie BB: Reserpine-induced release of drugs from sympathetic nerve endings. *Life Sci* 3:839-844, 1964.

592. ———: Interaction of guanethidine with adrenergic neurons. *J Pharmacol Exp Ther* 147:303 (Mar) 1965.

593. Day MD, Rand MJ: Antagonism of guanethidine and bretylium by various agents. *Lancet* 2:1282-1283 (Dec. 15) 1962.

594. Gulati OD, et al: Antagonism of adrenergic neuron blockage in hypertensive subjects. *Clin Pharmacol Ther* 7:510-514 (July-Aug) 1966.

595. Deshmanker BS, Lewis JA: Ventricular tachycardia associated with the administration of methylphenidate during guanethidine therapy. *Can Med Assoc J* 97:1166 (Nov 4) 1967.

596. Wilson R, Long C: Action of bretylium antagonized by amphetamine. *Lancet* 2:262 (July 30) 1960.

597. Kaumann A, Basso N, Aramendia P: The cardiovascular effects of N-(2-methylaminopropyl-iminodibenzyl)-HCl (Desmethylimipramine) and guanethidine. *J Pharmacol Exp Ther* 147:54-64 (Jan) 1965.

598. Skinner C, Coull DC, Johnston AW: Antagonism of the hypotensive action of bethanidine and debrisoquine by tricyclic antidepressants. *Lancet* 2:564-566 (Sep 13) 1969.

599. Kato R, Chiesara E, Vassanelli P: Mechanism of potentiation of barbiturates and meprobamate actions by imipramine. *Biochem Pharmacol* 12:357-364, 1963.

600. Yelnosky J, McGill JS, Mastrangelo AS: A comparison of the blood pressure effects of reserpine in dogs pretreated with amphetamine or tyramine. *Arch Int Pharmacodyn* 159:416-423 (Feb) 1966.

601. Eble JN, Rudzik AD: The blockade of the pressor response to tyramine by amphetamine in the reserpine-treated dog. *J Pharmacol Exp Ther* 153:62-69 (July 1966).

602. White RP, et al: Acute ergotropic response induced by reserpine and mephentermine. *Inter J Neuropharmacol* 5:143-154 (Mar) 1966.

603. Malone MH, Hockman HI, Nieforth KA: Desoxycholic acid enhancement of orally administered reserpine. *J Pharm Sci* 55:972-974 (Sep) 1966.

604. Anon.: A second report on levodopa. *Med Let Drugs Ther* 11:73-75 (Sep 5) 1969.

605. Roche Matulane (Procarbazine HCl), Roche literature (Aug) 1969.

606. Schelling J, Lasagna L: A study of cross tolerance to circulatory effects of organic nitrates. *Clin Pharmacol Ther* 8:256-260 (Mar-Apr) 1967.

607. Zupko G: "Drug Interactions" presentation to Lederle Pharmacy Consulting Board, Sep 15, 1969.

608. Lewis J: Introduction to Pharmacology, 3 ed, Baltimore, Williams & Wilkins, 1964, 348-349.

609. Casady GN, Moore DC, Bridenbaugh LD: Postpartum hypertension after the use of vasoconstrictor and oxytocic drugs. Etiology, incidence, complications and treatment. *JAMA* 172:1011-1015 (Mar 5) 1960.

610. Pedowitz P, Perell A: Aneurysms complicated by pregnancy II. Aneurysms of the cerebral vessels. *Am J Obstet Gynecol* 73:736-749 (Apr) 1957.

611. Sara C: Drugs that complicate the course of anaesthesia. *Med J Australia* 52:139-142 (Jan 30) 1965.

612. Martin HK: *Intern J Neurosurg* 24:317, 1966.

613. Yu TF, Dayton PG, Berger L, Gutman AB: Interactions of salicylate and sulfinpyrazone in man. *Federation Proc* 21:175, 1962.

614. Oyer JH, Wagner SL, Schmid FR: Supression of salicylate-induced uricosuria by phenylbutazone. *Am J Med Sci* 251:1-7 (Jan) 1966.

615. Zeppa R: Role of histamine in meperidine-induced hypotension. *J Surg Res* 2:26, 1962.

616. Ershoff BH: Conditioning factors in nutritional disease. *Physiol Rev* 28:107-137, 1948.

617. Werk EE: Drug-steroid interactions. From a symposium on drug interactions presented at Fall, 1966, meeting of the American Society for Pharmacology and Experimental Therapeutics, Mexico City, Mexico.

618. Klinenberg JR, Miller F: Effect of corticosteroids on blood salicylate concentration. *JAMA* 194:601-604 (Nov 8) 1965.

619. American Hospital Formulary Service. Washington, DC, American Society of Hospital Pharmacists.

620. Antonita SM: Necessary precautions when dispensing oral progestational drugs to inpatients. *Hosp Formulary Management* 3:34 (Feb) 1968.

621. Chelton LG, Whisnant CL: The combination of alcohol and drug intoxication. *South Med J* 59:393 (Apr) 1966.

622. Keats AS, Telford, J, Kurosu Y: "Potentiation" of meperidine by promethazine. *Anesthesiology* 22:34-41 (Jan-Feb) 1961.

623. Kessell A, et al: Side effects with a new hypnotic: Drug potentiation. *Med J Australia* 54:1194 (Dec 30) 1967.

624. Warnes H, Lehmann HE, Ban TA: Adynamic ileus during psychoactive medication: A report of three fatal and five severe cases. *Can Med Assoc J* 96:1112-1113 (Apr 15) 1967.

625. Schipior PG: An unusual case of antihistamine intoxication. *J Pediat* 71/4:589, 1967.

626. Gokhale SD, Gulati, OD, Udwadia BP: Antagonism of the adrenergic neurone blocking action of guanethidine by certain antidepressant and antihistamine drugs. *Arch Intern Pharmacodyn* 160:321-329 (Apr) 1966.

627. Sellers EM, Koch-Weser J: Potentiation of warfarin-induced hypoprothrombinemia by chloral hydrate. *N Engl J Med* 283:827-831 (Oct 15) 1970.

628. Lowenstein LM, Simone R, Boulter P, et al: Effect of fructose on alcohol concentrations in the blood in man. *JAMA* 213:1899-1901 (Sep 14) 1970.

629. Landauer AA, Milner G, Patman J: Alcohol and amitriptyline effects on skills related to driving behavior. *Science* 163:1467-1468 (Mar 28) 1969.

630. Udall JA: Quinidine and hypoprothrombinemia. *Ann Int Med* 69:403-404 (Aug) 1968.

631. Milner, G: Interaction between barbiturates, alcohol and some psychotropic drugs. *Med J Austral* 57:1204-1207 (June 13) 1970.

632. Marshall TR, Ling JT, Follis G, Rullell M: Pharmacological incompatibility of contrast media with various drugs and agents. *Radiology* 84:536-539, 1965.

633. Melmon K, Morelli HF, Oates JA, et al: Drug interactions that can affect your patients. *Patient Care* pp. 33-71 (Nov.) 1967. No documentation but a group of authorities have presented a useful panel discussion with very few errors. Updated in *Patient Care*, pp. 90 95-102 (Oct. 31) 1970.

634. Krantz JC, Jr: The problem of modern drug incompatibilities. *Am J Pharm* 139:115-121 (May-

June) 1967; *Curr Med Dig* pp. 1951-1956 (Dec) 1966.

635. Soffer A: Digitalis intoxication, reserpine, and double tachycardia. *JAMA* 191:777 (Mar 1) 1965.

636. Eger EL, II, Hamilton, WK: The effect of reserpine on the action of various vasopressors. *Anesthesiol* 20:641-645, 1959.

637. Chessin M, Kramer ER, Scott CC: Modifications of the pharmacology of reserpine and serotonin by iproniazid. *J Pharmacol Exp Ther* 119:453-460, 1957.

638. Chessin M, Dubnick B, Kramer ER, Scott CC: Modifications of pharmacology of reserpine and serotonin by iproniazid. *Fed Proc* 15:409 (Mar) 1956.

639. Pletscher A, Shore PA, Brodie BB: Serotonin as a mediator of reserpine action in brain. *J Pharmacol Exp Ther* 116:84-89 (Jan) 1956.

640. Jenkins LC: The interaction of drugs with particular reference to anesthetic practice. *Can Anaesthesiol Soc J* 15:111-117, 1968.

641. Dony-Crotheux J: Contributions à l'étude de l'inactivation des antibiotiques par les vitamines. *J. Pharm Belg* 12:179-184, 1957.

642. Im S, Latiolais CJ: Physico-chemical incompatibilities of parenteral admixtures—penicillin and tetracyclines. *Am J Hosp Pharm* 23:333-343, 1966.

643. Contreras E, Tamayo L: Effects of drugs acting in relation to sympathetic functions on the analgesic action of morphine. *Arch Intern Pharmacodyn* 160:312-320 (Apr) 1966.

644. Salassa RM, Bollman JL, Dry TJ: The effect of para-aminobenzoic acid on the metabolism and excretion of salicylate, *J Lab Clin Med* 33:1393-1401, 1948.

645. Goulston K, Cooke AR: Alcohol, aspirin, and gastrointestinal bleeding. *Br Med J* 4:664-665, 1968.

646. Douglas AS, McNicol GP: Toxicity of anticoagulant drugs. *Practitioner* 194:62-67, 1965.

647. Conney AH: Drug metabolism and therapeutics. *N Engl J Med* 280:653-660, 1969.

648. Shapiro S, Redish MH, Campbell HA: Studies on prothrombin IV. The prothrombinopenic effect of salicylate in man. *Proc Soc Exp Biol Med* 53;251-254, 1943.

649. Hecht A, Goldner MC: Reappraisal of the hypoglycemic action of acetylsalicylate. *Metabolism* 8:418-428, 1959.

650. Pascale LR, Dubin A, Bronsky D, Hoffman WS: Inhibition of the uricosuric action of Benemid by salicylate. *J Lab Clin Med* 45:771-777, 1955.

651. Ogryzlo MA, Digby JW, Montgomery DB, et al: The long term treatment of gout with sulfinpyrazone (Anturane). *10th Ann Cong Rheum,* Rome 1:3-8 1961.

652. Lunde PKM, Rane A, Yaffe SJ, et al: Plasma protein binding of diphenylhydantoin in man. Interaction with other drugs and the effect of temperature and plasma dilution. *Clin Pharmacol Ther* 11:846-855, 1970.

653. Mathog RH, Klein WJ, Jr: Ototoxicity of ethacrynic acid and aminoglycoside antibiotics in uremia. *N Engl J Med* 280:1223-1224, 1969.

654. Iwatsuki, K, Ueda T, Yamada A, et al: Effects of

streptomycin on muscle relaxants. *Med J Shinshu U* 3:299-310, 1958.

655. Bezzi G, Gessa GL: Neuromuscular blocking action of some antibiotics. *Nature* 184:905-906, 1959.

656. Timmerman JC, Long JP, Pittinger CB: Neuromuscular blocking properties of various antibiotic agents. *Toxicol Appl Pharmacol* 1:299-304, 1959.

657. Wilson RD, Dent TE, Traber DL, et al.: Malignant hyperpyrexia with anesthesia. *JAMA* 202:183-186, 1967.

658. Satnick JH: Hyperthermia under anesthesia with regional muscle flaccidity. *Anesthesiol* 30:472-474, 1969.

659. Mann AM, Hutchison JL: Manic reaction associated with procarbazine hydrochloride therapy of Hodgkin's disease. *Can Med Assoc J* 97:1350-1353, 1967.

660. Armbrecht BH: Reaction between piperazine and chlorpromazine. *N Engl J Med* 282:1490-1 (Jun 25) 1970; 283:11-14, 1970.

661. Anton AH: The relation between the binding of sulfonamides to albumin and their antibacterial efficacy. *J Pharmacol Exp Ther* 129:282-290, 1960.

662. Lipton JH: Incompatibility between sulfamethizole and methenamine mandelate. *New Engl J Med.* 268:92-93 (Jan. 10) 1963.

663. van Rossum JM, Hurkmans JA TM: Reversal of the effect of α-methyldopa by monoamine oxidase inhibitors. *J Pharm Pharmacol* 15:493-499, 1963.

664. Katz RL, Epstein RA: The interaction of anesthetic agents and adrenergic drugs to produce cardiac arrhythmias. *Anesthesiol* 29:763-784 (July-Aug) 1968.

665. Scheiner J, Altemeier WA: Experimental study of factors inhibiting absorption and effective therapeutic levels of Declomycin. *Surg Gynecol Obstet* 114:9-14, 1962.

666. Strom J: The question of antagonism between penicillin and chlortetracycline, illustrated by therapeutical experiments in scarlatina. *Antibiot Med* 1:6-12, 1955.

667. Pelner L: Licorice and hypertension. *JAMA* 208:1909, 1969.

668. Dundee JW, Scott WEB: The effect of phenothiazine derivates on thiobarbiturate narcosis. *Anesthesiol Analg* 37:12-19, 1958.

669. Sadove MS, Balagot RC, Reyes RM: The potentiating action of chlorpromazine. *Curr Res Anesth Analg* 35:165-181, 1956.

670. Prange AJ, Jr: Paroxysmal auricular tachycardia apparently resulting from combined thyroid-imipramine treatment. *Am J Psychiat* 119:994-995, 1963.

671. Oates JA, Arias L, Mitchell JR: Interaction of drugs with adrenergic neuron blockers. *Pharmacol* 9:79-80, 1967.

672. Northcutt RC, Stiel JN, Hollifield JW, Stant EG, Jr: The influence of cholestyramine on thyroxine absorption. *JAMA* 208:1857-1861, 1969.

673. Lubran M: The effects of drugs on laboratory values. *Med Clin N Am* 53:211-222, 1969.

674. Kater RMH, Roggin G, Tobon F, et al: Increased rate of clearance of drugs from the circulation of alcoholics. *Am J Med Sci* 258:35-39, 1969.

675. Podgainy H, Bressler R: Biochemical basis of the sulfonylurea-induced antabuse syndrome. *Diabetes* 17:679-683, 1968.

676. Christensen LK, Skovsted L: Inhibition of drug metabolism by chloramphenicol. *Lancet* 2:1397-1399, 1969.

677. Welch RM, Harrison YE, Conney AH, Burns, JJ: An experimental model in dogs for studying interactions of drugs with bishydroxycoumarin. *Clin Pharmacol Ther* 10:817-825, 1969.

678. Menon MM, Iyer KS: Potentiation of paraldehyde hypnosis by tolbutamide. *Ind J Physiol Pharmacol* 8:65-67 (Jan) 1964.

679. Gulbrandsen R: Potentiation of tolbutamide by phenylbutazone? *Tids Norski Laegeforen.* 79:1127-1128, 1959.

680. Christensen LK, Hansen JM, Kristensen M: Sulphaphenazole induced hypoglycaemic attacks in tolbutamide-treated diabetics. *Lancet* 2:1298-1301, 1963.

681. Byers SO, Friedman M: Insulin hypoglycemia enhanced by beta adrenergic blockade. *Proc Soc Exp Biol Med* 122:114-115, 1966.

682. Hayton AC: Precipitation of acute ergotism by triacetyloleandomycin. *New Zeal Med J* 69:42, 1969.

683. Katz RL: Epinephrine and PLV-2: cardiac rhythm and local vasoconstrictor effects. *Anesthesiol* 26:619-623, 1965.

684. Morris LE, Noltensmeyer MH, White JM, Jr: Epinephrine induced cardiac irregularities in the dog during anesthesia with trichloroethylene, cyclopropane, ethyl chloride and chloroform. *Anesthesiol* 14:153-158, 1953.

685. Avallareda M: Interferencia de los barbituricos en la acción del tromexan. *Medicina* 15:109-115, 1955.

686. Duvoisin RC: Confirms therapeutic effectiveness of L-dopa in Parkinson's disease. *Drug Topics* pp 17, 23 (Oct 13) 1969.

687. Blackwell B, Marley E, Price J, Taylor D: Hypertensive interactions between monoamine oxidase inhibitors and foodstuffs. *Br J Psychiat* 113:349-365, 1967.

688. Juchau MR, Gram TE, Fouts JR: Stimulation of hepatic microsomal drug-metabolizing enzyme systems in primates by DDT. *Gastroenterol* 51:213-218, 1966.

689. Modell W: *Drugs of Choice.* St. Louis, Mosby, 1970-1971.

690. Editorial: Teratology and carbonic anhydrase inhibition. *Arch Ophthal* 85:1-2 (Jan) 1971.

691. Interactions of drugs. *Med Let Drugs Ther* 12:93-96 (Nov 13) 1970.

692. McGavi DDM: Depressed levels of serum-pseudocholinesterase with echothiophate iodide eye drops. *Lancet* 2:272-273 (Aug 7) 1965.

693. Lockett MF: Dangerous effects of isoprenaline in myocardial failure. *Lancet* 2:104-106 (July 17) 1965.

694. Chen W, Vrindten PA, Dayton PG, Burns JJ: Accelerated aminopyrine metabolism in human subjects pretreated with phenylbutazone. *Life Sci* 2:35-42, 1962.

695. Remmer H: Drug tolerance, *in Ciba Foundation*

Symposium on Enzymes and Drug Action. De Reuck AVS, Mongar JL, (eds): Boston, 1962.

696. Sweeney WM, Hardy SM, Dornbush AC, Rueg-segger JM: Absorption of tetracycline in human beings as affected by certain excipients. *Antibiot Med Clin Ther* 4:642-656 (Oct) 1957.

697. Vikhlyaev YI, Avakumov VM: Mechanisms potentiating hypnotic action of certain barbiturates through the medium of chloracizin, spasmolytin (Trasentine) and chlorpromazine. *Farmakol Toksikol* 30:283-286, 1967.

698. Murmann W, Almirante L, Saccani-Guelfi M: Effects of hexobarbitone, ether, morphine, and urethane upon the acute toxicity of propranolol and D(−)INPEA. *J Pharm Pharmacol* 18:692-694, 1966.

699. Williams EE: Effects of alcohol on workers with carbon disulfide. *JAMA* 109:1472-1473 (Oct 30) 1937.

700. Cucinell SA, Koster R, Conney AH, Burns JJ: Stimulatory effect of phenobarbital on the metabolism of diphenylhydantoin. *J Pharmacol Exp Ther* 141:157-160, 1963.

701. Wilson GM: Ill health due to drugs. *Br Med J* 1:1065-1069 (Apr 30) 1966.

702. Churchill-Davidson HC: Anaesthesia and monoamine-oxidase inhibitors. *Br Med J* 1:520 (Feb 20) 1965.

703. When drugs interact. *Hosp Pract* pp 72-77 (Oct) 1966.

704. Burns JJ, Conney, AH, Koster R: Stimulatory effect of chronic drug administration on drug-metabolizing enzymes in liver microsomes. *Ann NY Acad Sci* 104:881-893 (Feb 4) 1963.

705. Carter S: Potentiation of the effect of orally administered anticoagulants by phenyramidol hydrochloride. *N Engl J Med* 273:423-426 (Aug 19) 1965.

706. Solomon HM, Schrogie JJ: The effect of phenyramidol on the metabolism of bishydroxycoumarin. *J Pharmacol Exp Ther* 154:660-666 (Oct Dec) 1966.

707. Warfarin sodium: quinidine. *Clin-Alert* 72 (Apr 25) 1969.

708. Jeremy R, Towson J: Interaction between aspirin and indomethacin in the treatment of rheumatoid arthritis. *Med J Austral* 57:127-129 (July 18) 1970.

709. Orrenius S, Ericsson JLE, Ernster L: Phenobarbital-induced synthesis of the microsomal drug-metabolizing enzyme system and its relationship to the proliferation of endoplasmic membranes. *J Cell Biol* 25:627-639 (June) 1965.

710. Koch-Weser J: Potentiation by glucagon of the hypoprothrombinemic action of warfarin. *Ann Int Med* 72:331-335 (Mar) 1970.

711. Parker WJ: Alcohol-drug interactions. *J Am Pharm Assoc* NS10:664-673 (Dec.) 1970.

712. Weiner M, Moses D: The effect of glucagon and insulin on the prothrombin response to coumarin anticoagulants. *Proc Soc Exp Biol Med* 127:761-763, 1968.

713. Pirk LA, Engelberg R: Hypoprothrombinemic action of quinine sulfate. *JAMA* 128:1093(1095 (Aug 11) 1945.

714. Pearson RE, Salter FJ: Drug interaction?—orphenadrine with propoxyphene. *N Engl J Med* 282:1215 (May 21) 1969.

715. Duvoisin R, et al.: Parkinsonism bows to levodopa—usually. *JAMA* 210:434-436 (Oct 20) 1969; Pyridoxine reversal of l-dopa effects in parkinsonism. *Trans Am Neurol Assoc* 94:81-84, 1969.

716. Kupers TA, Petrich JM, et al.: Depression of tuberculin delayed hypersensitivity by live attenuated mumps virus. *J. Pediat* 76:716-721 (May) 1970.

717. Godwin-Austen RB, Lind NA, Turner P: Mydriatic responses to sympathomimetic amines in patients treated with L-dopa. *Lancet* 2:1043-1044 (Nov 15) 1969.

718. Whittington HG, Grey L: Possible interaction between disulfiram and isoniazid. *Am J Psychiat* 125:1725-1729 (June) 1969.

719. Schnell RC, Miya TA: Altered drug absorption from the rat ileum induced by carbonic anhydrase inhibition. *Pharmacology* 11:292, 1969.

720. Henriksen FW, Way LW: The concept of potentiation. *Gastroenterol* 57:617-622 (Nov) 1969.

721. Ilyas M, Owens D, Kvasnicka G: Delirium induced by a combination of antiarrhythmic drugs. *Lancet* 2:1368-1369 (Dec 20) 1969.

722. Berndt WO, Miller M, Kettyle WM, Valtin H: Potentiation of the antidiuretic effect of vasopressin by chlorpropamide. *Endocrinol* 86:1028-1032 (May) 1970.

723. Miller M, Moses AM: Potentiation of vasopressin action by chlorpropamide *in vivo. Endocrinol* 86:1024-1027 (May) 1970.

724. Cotzias GC, Papavasiliou PS, Gellene R: L-Dopa in Parkinson's syndrome. *N Engl J Med* 281:272 (July 31) 1969.

725. Michot F, Burgi M, Buttner J: Rimactan (Rifampizin) und Antikoagulantientherapie. *Schweiz Med Wschr* 100:583-584, 1970.

726. Milne MD, Rowe GG, Somers K, et al.: Observations on the pharmacology of mecamylamkne. *Clin Sci* 16:599-614, 1957.

727. Chatterjea JB, Salomon L: Antagonistic effect of ACTH and cortisone on the anticoagulant activity of ethyl biscoumacetate. *Br Med J* 2:790-792, 1954.

728. Norman AP, Sanders S: Mortality in asthma in childhood. *Practitioner* 201:909-914, 1968.

729. Patman J, Landauer AA, Milner G: The combined effect of alcohol and amitriptyline on skills similar to motorcar driving. *Med J Austral* 56:946-949 (Nov 8) 1969.

730. Ramsey H, Haag HB: The synergism between the barbiturates and ethyl alcohol. *J Pharmacol Exp Ther* 88:313-322, 1946.

731. Zirkle GA, King PD, et al: Effects of chlorpromazine and alcohol on coordination and judgment. *JAMA* 171:1496-1499 (Nov 14) 1959.

732. Goldberg L: Behavioral and physiological effects of alcohol on man. *Psychosom Med* 28:570-595, 1966.

733. Zirkle GA, McAtee OB, King PD, Van Dyke R: Meprobamate and small amounts of alcohol. Effects on human ability, coordination, and judgment. *JAMA* 173:1823-1825, 1960.

734. Glasser J: Methotrexate and psoriasis. *JAMA* 210:1925 (Dec 8) 1969.

735. Winter D, Sauvard S, et al.: The influence of metronidazole and disulfiram on the pharmacologic action of ethanol. *Pharmacol* 2:27–31, 1969.

736. Lampo B: Treatment of alcoholism with metronidazole. *Minerva Med* 58:2531–2533, 1967.

737. Dille JM, Ahlquist RP: The synergism of ethyl alcohol and sodium pentobarbital. *J Pharmacol Exp Ther* 61:385–392, 1937.

738. Graham JDP: Ethanol and the absorption of barbiturate. *Toxicol Appl Pharmacol* 2:14–22, 1960.

739. Isaacs P: Alcohol and phenformin in diabetes *Br Med J* 3:773–774, 1970.

740. Alcoholic beverages and orally given hypoglycemic drugs. *JAMA* 173:128 (May 7) 1960.

741. Barboriak JJ: Drug reactions after ingestion of alcohol. *Wisc Med J* 63:213–214, 1964.

742. Meyer JF, McAllister K, Goldberg LI: Insidious and prolonged antagonism of guanethidine by amitriptyline. *JAMA* 213:1487–1488, 1970.

743. Domino EF, Sullivan TS, Luby ED: Barbiturate intoxication in a patient treated with a MAO inhibitor. *Am J Psychiat* 118:941–943, 1962.

744. Robinson DS, Sylwester D: Interaction of commonly prescribed drugs and warfarin. *Ann Intern Med* 72:853–856, 1970.

745. O'Dea K, Rand MJ: Interaction between amphetamine and monoamine oxidase inhibitors. *Europ J Pharmacol* 6:115–120, 1969.

746. Krisko I, Lewis E, Johnson JE: Severe hyperpyrexia due to tranylcypromine-amphetamine toxicity. *Ann Int Med* 70:559–564, 1969.

747. Zeck P: The dangers of some antidepressant drugs. *Med J Austral* 48:607–608, 1961.

748. Wehrle PF, Mathies AW, et al.: Bacterial meningitis. *Ann NY Acad Sci* 145:488–498, 1967.

749. Mullett RD, Keats AS: Apnea and respiratory insufficiency after intraperitoneal administration of kanamycin. *Surgery* 49:530–533, 1961.

750. Davidson EW, Modell JH, Moya F, Farmati O: Respiratory depression following use of antibiotics in pleural and pseudocyst cavities. *JAMA* 196:456–457, 1966.

751. Ziegler CH, Lovette JB: Operative complications after therapy with reserpine and reserpine compounds. *JAMA* 176:916–919, 1961.

752. Ominsky AJ, Wollman H: Hazards of general anesthesia in the reserpinized patient. *Anesthesiol* 30:443–446, 1969.

753. Drug interactions may need change in warfarin dose. *JAMA* 213:1251–1252, 1970.

754. Fielder DL, Nelson DC, Andersen TW, Gravenstein JS: Cardiovascular effects of atropine and neostigmine in man. *Anesthesiol* 30:637–641, 1969.

755. Doak PB, Montgomerie JZ, et al.: Reticulum cell sarcoma after renal homotransplantation and azathioprine and prednisone therapy. *Br Med J* 4:746–748, 1968.

756. Ayd FJ, Jr: Toxic somatic and psychopathologic reactions to antidepressant drugs. *J Neuropsychiat Suppl* 1:5119–5122 (Feb) 1961.

757. Boulton AA, Cookson B, Paulton R: Hypertensive crisis in a patient on MAOI antidepressants following a meal of beef liver. *Can Med Assoc J* 102:1394–1395, 1970.

758. Harper M: Toxic effects of monoamine-oxidase inhibitors. *Lancet* 2:312, 1964.

759. Sjoerdsma A: E. Catecholamine-drug interactions in man. *Pharmacol Rev* 18:673–683, 1966.

760. Sellers EM, Koch-Weser J: Potentiation of warfarin-induced hypoprothrombinemia by chloral hydrate. *N Engl J Med* 283:827–831 (Oct 15) 1970.

761. Levy AG: Further remarks on ventricular extrasystoles and fibrillation under chloroform. *Heart* 7:105–110, 1918.

762. Levy AG, Lewis T: Heart irregularities, resulting from the inhalation of low percentages of chloroform vapour, and their relationship to ventricular fibrillation. *Heart* 3:99–112, 1911.

763. Meek WJ, Hathaway HR, Orth OS: The effects of ether, chloroform and cyclopropane on cardiac automaticity. *J Pharmacol Exp Ther* 61:240–252, 1937.

764. Nelson RM, Frank CG, Mason JO: The antiheparin properties of the antihistamines, tranquilizers and certain antibiotics. *Surg Forum* 9:146–150, 1959.

765. Sletten IW, Ognjanov V, et al.: Weight reduction with chlorphentermine and phenmetrazine in obese psychiatric patients during chlorpromazine therapy. *Curr Ther Res* 9:570–575, 1967.

766. Boulos BM, Davis LE: Hazard of simultaneous administration of phenothiazine and piperazine. *N Engl J Med* 280:1245–1246, 1969.

767. Petitpierre B, Fabre J: Chlorpropamide and chloramphenicol. *Lancet* 1:789 (Apr 11) 1970.

768. Kristensen M, Hansen JM: Accumulation of chlorpropamide caused by dicoumarol. *Acta Med Scand* 183:83–86, 1968.

769. Gallo DG, Bailey KR, Sheffner AL: The interaction between cholestyramine and drugs. *Proc Soc Exp Biol Med* 120:60–65, 1965.

770. Benjamin D, Robinson DS, McCormack J: Cholestyramine binding of warfarin in man and *in vitro*. *Clin Res* 18:336, 1970.

771. Pickett RD: Acute toxicity of heroin, alone and in combination with cocaine or quinine. *Br J Pharmacol* 40:145P–146P, 1970.

772. Matteo RS, Katz RL, Papper EM: The injection of epinephrine during general anesthesia with halogenated hydrocarbons and cyclopropane in man. 3. Cyclopropane. *Anesthesiol* 24:327–330, 1963.

773. Johnstone M: Adrenaline and noradrenaline during anesthesia. *Anesthesia* 8:32–42, 1953.

774. Dresel PE, Sutter MC: Factors modifying cyclopropane-epinephrine cardiac arrhythmias. *Circ Res* 9:1284–1490, 1961.

775. Dresel PE, MacCannell KL, Nickerson M: Cardiac arrhythmias induced by minimal doses of epinephrine in cyclopropane-anesthetized dogs. *Circ Res* 8:948–955, 1960.

776. Price HL, Lurie AA, Jones RE, et al.: Cyclopropane anesthesia. II. Epinephrine and norepinephrine in initiation of ventricular arrhythmias by carbon dioxide inhalation. *Anesthesiol* 19:619–630, 1958.

777. Adelman MH: Sudden death during cyclopropane-ether anesthesia following the administra-

tion of epinephrine: case report. *Anesthesiol* 2:657:660, 1941.

778. Moore EN, Morse HT, Price HL: Cardiac arrhythmias produced by catecholamines in anesthetized dogs. *Circ Res* 15:77-82, 1964.

779. Rivers N, Horner B: Possible lethal reaction between Nardil and dextromethorphan. *Can Med Assoc J* 103:85, 1970.

780. Jones RJ, Cohen L: Sodium dextrothyroxine in coronary disease and hypercholesterolemia. *Circulation* 24:164-170, 1961.

781. Feldman SA, Crawley BE: Diazepam and muscle relaxants. *Br Med J* 1:691, 1970; Interaction of diazepam with the muscle-relaxant drugs. *Br Med J* 2:336-338, 1970.

782. Kalow W: Malignant hyperthermia. *Proc Roy Soc Med* 63:178-180, 1970.

783. Doughty A: Unexpected danger of diazepam. *Br Med J* 2:239, 1970.

784. Sellers EM, Koch-Weser J: Displacement of warfarin from human albumin by diazoxide and ethacrynic, mefenamic and nalidixic acids. *Clin Pharmacol Ther* 11:524-529, 1970.

785. Kleinman PD, Griner PF: Studies of the epidemiology of anticoagulant-drug interactions. *Arch Int Med* 126:522-523, 1970.

786. Viukari NMA, Oho K: Digoxinphenytoin interaction. *Br Med J* 2:51, 1970.

787. Phansalkar AG, Joglekar GV, et al.: A study of digoxin, thyroxine and reserpine interrelationship. *Arch Int Pharmacodyn* 182:44-48, 1969.

788. Herd JK, Cramer A, et al.: Ototoxicity of topical neomycin augmented by dimethyl sulfoxide. *Pediat* 40:905-907, 1967.

789. Brennan RW, et al.: Diphenylhydantoin intoxication attendant to slow inactivation of isoniazid. *Neurol* 20:687-693, 1970.

790. Harrah MD, Way WL, Katzang BG: The interaction of *d*-tubocurarine with antiarrhythmic drugs. *Anesthesiol* 33:406-410, 1970.

791. Rothstein E, Clancy DD: Toxicity of disulfiram combined with metronidazole. *N Engl J Med* 280:1006-1007, 1969.

792. Hunter KR, Boakes AJ, Laurence DR, Stern GM: Monoamine oxidase inhibitors and l-dopa. *Br Med J* 3:388, 1970.

793. Horwitz D, Goldberg LI, Sjoerdsma A: Increased blood pressure responses to dopamine and norepinephrine produced by monoamine oxidase inhibitors in man. *J Lab Clin Med* 56:747-753, 1960.

794. Bracha S, Hes JP: Death occurring during combined reserpine-electroshock treatment. *Am J Psychiat* 113:257, 1956.

795. Foster MW, Jr, Gayle RF, Jr: Dangers in combining reserpine (Serpasil) with electroconvulsive therapy. *JAMA* 159:1520-1522, 1955.

796. Stephen CR, Margolis G, et al.: Laboratory observations with fluothane. *Anesthesiol* 19:770-781, 1958.

797. Gulati OD, Dave BT, et al.: Antagonism of adrenergic neuron blockade in hypertensive subjects. *Clin Pharmacol Ther* 7:510-514, 1966.

798. Low-Beer GA, Tidmarsh D: Collapse after "parstelin." *Br Med J* 2:683-684, 1963.

799. Hall KD, Norris FH: Fluothane sensitization of dog heart to action of epinephrine. *Anesthesiol* 19:631-641, 1958.

800. Virtue RW, Payne KW, et al.: Observations during experimental and clinical use of Fluothane. *Anesthesiol* 19:478-487, 1958.

801. Andersen N, Johansen SH: Incidence of catecholamine-induced arrhythmias during halothane anesthesia. *Anesthesiol* 24:51-56, 1963.

802. Forbes AM: Halothane, adrenaline and cardiac arrest. *Anaesthesia* 21:22-27, 1966.

803. Hirshom WI, Taylor RC, Sheehan JC: Arrhythmias produced by combinations of halothane and small amounts of vasopressor. *Br J Oral Surg* 2:131-136, 1964-1965.

804. Varejes L: The use of solutions containing adrenaline during halothane anesthesia. *Anaesthesia* 18:507-510, 1963.

805. Hiatt N, Katz J: Modification of cardiac and hyperglycemic effects of epinephrine by insulin. *Life Sci* 8:551-558, 1969.

806. Israel JS, Criswick VG, Dobkin AB: Effect of epinephrine on cardiac rhythm during anesthesia with methoxyflurane (Penthrane) and trifluoroethyl vinyl ether (Fluoromar). *Acta Anaesth Scand* 6:7-11, 1962.

807. Bamforth BJ, Siebecker KL, et al: Effect of epinephrine on the dog heart during methoxyflurane anesthesia. *Anesthesiol* 22:169-173, 1961.

808. Chang FN, Weisblum B: The specificity of lincomycin binding to ribosomes. *Biochem* 6:836-843, 1967.

809. Griffith LJ, Ostrander WE, et al: Drug antagonism between lincomycin and erythromycin. *Science* 147:746-747, 1965.

810. Manten A, Wisse MJ: Antagonism between antibacterial drugs. *Nature* 192:671-672, 1961.

811. Manten A: Synergism and antagonism between antibiotic mixtures containing erythromycin. *Antibiot Chemother* 4:1228-1233, 1954.

812. Fahim MS, King TM, Hall DG: Induced alterations in the biologic activity of estrogen. *Am J Obstet Gynecol* 100:171-175, 1968.

813. Johnson AH, Hamilton CH: Kanamycin ototoxicity—possible potentiation by other drugs. *South Med J* 63:511-513, 1970.

814. Meyers FH, Javetz E, Goldfien A: *Review of Medical Pharmacology.* Los Altos, Cal, Lange, 1968, pp 647-663.

815. Pittinger CB, Long JP: Danger of intraperitoneal neomycin during ether anesthesia. *Surgery* 43:445-446, 1958.

816. ———: Neuromuscular blocking action of neomycin sulfate. *Antibiot Chemother* 8:198-203, 1958.

817. Stechishin O, Voloshin PC, Allard CA: Neuromuscular paralysis and respiratory arrest caused by intrapleural neomycin. *Can Med Assoc J* 81:32-33, 1959.

818. Murmann W, Almirante L, Saccani-Guelfi, M: Effects of hexobarbitone, ether, morphine, and urethane upon the acute toxicity of propranolol and D-(-)-INPEA. *J Pharm Pharmacol* 18:692-694, 1966.

819. Solymoss B, Varga S, et al: Influence of spironolactone and other steroids on the enzymatic decay

and anticoagulant activity of bishydroxycoumarin. *Thromb Diath Haemorrh* 23:562–568, 1970.

820. Leohning RW, Czorny VP: Halothane-induced hypotension and the effect of vasopressors. *Can Anaesth Soc J* 7:304–309, 1960.

821. Riegelman S, Rowland M, Epstein WL: Griseofulvin-phenobarbital interaction in man. *JAMA* 213:426–431, 1970.

822. Clinicopathologic conference. Unclassified pulmonary-renal syndrome. *Am J Med* 45:933–942, 1968.

823. Mitchell JR, Cavanaugh JH, Arias L, Oates JA: Guanethidine and related agents. III Antagonism by drugs which inhibit the norepinephrine pump in man. *J Clin Invest* 49:1596–1604 (Aug) 1970.

824. Guimaraes S, Sottomayor M, Castro-Tavares J: Modification of some actions of guanethidine by the acute administration of reserpine. *Naunyn Schmied Arch Pharm Exp Path* 286:119–130, 1970.

825. Weiner M, Dayton PG: Effect of barbiturates on coumarin activity. *Circulation* 20:783, 1959.

826. Aggeler PM, O'Reilly RA: Effect of heptabarbital on the response to bishydroxycoumarin in man. *J Lab Clin Med* 74:229–238, 1969.

827. Fouts JR, Brodie BB: On the mechanism of drug potentiation by iproniazid (2-isopropyl-1 isonicotinyl hydrazine). *J Pharmacol Exp Ther* 116:480–485, 1956.

828. Kane FJ, Jr, Freeman D: Nonfatal reaction to imipramine-MAO inhibitor combination. *Am J Psychiat* 120:79–80, 1963.

829. McCurdy RL, Kane FJ, Jr: Transient brain syndrome as a non-fatal reaction to combined pargyline imipramine treatment. *Am J Psychiat* 121:397–398, 1964.

830. Hills NF: Combining the antidepressant drugs. *Br Med J* 1:859, 1965.

831. Besendorf H, Pletscher A: Beeinflussung zentraler Wirkungen von Reserpin und 5-Hydroxytryptamin durch Isonicotinsaurehydrazide. *Helv Physiol Pharmacol Acta* 14:383–390, 1956.

832. Iwatsuki K, Ueda T, et al: Effects of kanamycin on the action of muscle relaxants. *Med J Shinshu U* 3:311–319, 1958.

833. Food and Drug Administration: Current drug information. *Ann Int Med* 73:445–448, 1970.

384. Denton PH, Borrelli VM, Edwards NV: Dangers of monoamine oxidase inhibitors. *Br Med J* 2:1752–1753, 1962.

835. Palmer H: Potentiation of pethidine. *Br Med J* 2:944, 1960.

836. Analgesics and monoamine oxidase inhibitors. *Br Med J* 4:284, 1967.

837. Blackwell B, Marley E, Ryle A: Hypertensive crisis associated with monoamine-oxidase inhibitors. *Lancet* 1:722–723, 1964.

838. Duby SE, Cotzias GC: Report on use of apomorphine with levodopa. Report to American Societies for Experimental Biology, Chicago, 1971.

839. Clement AJ, Benazon D: Reactions to other drugs in patients taking monoamine-oxidase inhibitors. *Lancet* 2:197–198, 1962.

840. Mitchell RS: Fatal toxic encephalitis occurring during iproniazid therapy in pulmonary tuberculosis. *Ann Int Med* 42:417–424, 1955.

841. Papp C, Benaim S: Toxic effects of iproniazid in a patient with angina. *Br Med J* 2:1070–1072, 1958.

842. Shee JC: Dangerous potentiation of pethidine by iproniazid, and its treatment. *Br Med J* 2:507–509, 1960.

843. Reid NC, Jones D: Pethidine and phenelzine. *Br Med J* 1:408, 1962.

844. Waghmarae D: Collapse after pethidine and promethazine. *Br Med J* 2:936, 1963.

845. Donaldson IA: Collapse after pethidine and promazine. *Br Med J* 2:1592, 1963

846. Amias AG, Fairbairn D: Foetal death after pethidine and promazine. *Br Med J* 2:432–433, 1963.

847. Stark DCC: Effects of giving vasopressors to patients on monoamine-oxidase inhibitors. *Lancet* 1:1405–1406, 1962.

848. Luhby AL, Shimizu N, et al: Women taking oral contraceptives containing estrogen analogues may need folic acid supplements. Report to Federation of American Societies for Experimental Biology, Chicago, April, 1971.

849. McLaren G: Sudden death in asthma. *Br Med J* 4:456, 1968.

850. Cooper AJ, Magnus RV, Rose MJ: A hypertensive syndrome with tranyicypromine medication. *Lancet* 1:527–529 1964.

851. Dally PJ: Fatal reaction associated with tranylcypromine and methylamphetamine. *Lancet* 1:1235–1236, 1962.

852. Weiner M, Siddiqui AA: Drug interactions: The effect of combined administration on the half-life of coumarin and pyrazolone drugs in man. *Fed Proc* 24:153, 1965.

853. Rutledge RA, Barrett WE, Plummer AJ: Alterations in the blood pressure response to serotonin caused by methylphenidate and reserpine. *Fed Proc* 18:441, 1959.

854. Craig DDH: Reaction to pethidine in patients on phenelzine. *Lancet* 2:559, 1962.

855. Bodley PO, Halwax K, Potts L: Low serum pseudocholinesterase levels complicating treatment with phenelzine. *Br Med J* 3:510–512, 1969.

856. Iwatsuki K, Ueda T, Yamada A, et al: Effects of neomycin on the action of muscle relaxants. *Med J Shinshu U* 3:321–330, 1958.

857. Cooper EA, Hanson R de G: Oral neomycin and anaethesia. *Br Med J* 2:1527–1528, 1963.

858. Grem FM: Case report No 203. *Am Soc Anesth Newsletter* 22:33–35, 1958.

859. Stanley VF, Giesecke AH, Jenkins MT: Neomycin-curare neuromuscular block and reversal in cats. *Anesthesiol* 31:228–232, 1969.

860. Emery ERJ: Neuromuscular blocking properties of antibiotics as a cause of post-operative apnoea. *Anesthesia* 18:57–65, 1963.

861. Vigran IM: *Clinical Anticoagulant Therapy.* Philadelphia, Lea & Febiger, 1965, pp. 143–145.

862. Frederiksen H, Ravenholt RT: Oral contraceptives and thromboembolic disease *Br Med J* 4:770, 1968.

863. Consolo S, Garattini S: Effect of desipramine on intestinal absorption of phenylbutazone and other drugs. *Europ J Pharmacol* 6:322–326, 1969.

864. Speck RS, Jawetz E: Antibiotic synergism and antagonism in a subacute experimental streptococ-

cus infection in mice. *Am J Med Sci* 223:280-285, 1952.

865. Corn M, Rockett JF: Inhibition of bishydroxycoumarin activity by phenobarbital. *Med Ann DC* 34:578-579, 588, 1965.

866. Garrettson LK, Dayton PG: Disappearance of phenobarbital and diphenylhydantoin from serum of children. *Clin Pharmacol Ther* 11:674-679, 1970.

867. Corn M: Effect of phenobarbital and glutethimide on biological half-life of warfarin. *Thromb Diath Haemorrh* 16:606-612, 1966.

868. Barth P, Kommerell B: Effect of clofibrate on blood coagulation. *Klin Med* 61:1466-1468, 1966.

869. Solomon HM, Schrogie JJ: The effect of various drugs on the binding of warfarin-14C to human albumin. *Biochem Pharmacol* 16:1219-1226, 1967.

870. Schanker LS: Mechanisms of drug absorption and distribution. *Ann Rev Pharmacol* 1:29-44, 1961; Passage of drugs across body membranes. *Pharmacol Rev* 14:501-530, 1962; *Adv Drug Res,* vol. 1 (ed: Harper, N.J., Simmonds, A.B.). London, 1964.

871. Sneddon TM, Turner P: The interactions of local guanethidine and sympathomimetic amines in the human eye. *Arch Ophthalmol* 81:622-627 (May) 1969.

872. Spiers ASD, Calne DB: Action of dopamine on the human iris. *Br Med J* 4:333-335 (Nov 8) 1969; Spiers ASD, Calne DB, Fayers PM: Miosis during L-dopa therapy. *Br Med J* 2:639-640 (June 13) 1970.

873. Patel AR, Paton AM, Rowan T, et al: Clinical studies on the effect of laevulose on the rate of metabolism of ethyl alcohol. *Scot Med J* 14:268-271 (Aug) 1969.

874. Monoamine oxidase inhibitors. *Br Med J* 2:35-37 (Apr 6) 1968.

875. Blomley DJ: Monoamine-oxidase inhibitors. *Lancet* 2:1181-1182 (Nov 28) 1964.

876. Lindenbaum J, Lieber CS: Alcohol-induced malabsorption of vitamin B_{12} in man. *Nature* 224:806 (Nov 22) 1969.

877. Analgesics and monoamine oxidase inhibitors. *Br Med J* 4:284 (Nov 4) 1967.

878. Ngai SH, Mark LC, Papper EM: Pharmacologic and physiologic aspects of anesthesiology. *N Engl J Med* 282:479-491 (Feb 26) 1970.

879. Heart output boosted by fluroxene, nitrous oxide. *JAMA* 210:1685 (Dec 1) 1969.

880. Visconti JA: Drug information—the influence of drugs on nutritional status. *Hosp Form Manag* 5:30-32 (Feb) 1970.

881. Levine RA: Polymycin B-induced respiratory paralysis reversed by intravenous calcium chloride. *J Mount Sinai Hosp, NY* 36:380-387 (Sep-Oct) 1969.

882. Davidson E, et al: Respiratory depression following use of antibiotics in pleural and pseudocyst cavities. *JAMA* 196:456-457 (May 2), 1966.

883. Simmons NA, McGillicuddy DJ: Potentiation of inhibitory activity of colistin on *Pseudomonas aeruginosa* by sulfamethoxazole and sulfamethizole. *Br Med J* 3:693-696 (Sep 20) 1969.

884. Kutt H, McDowell F: Management of epilepsy with diphenylhydantoin sodium. *JAMA* 203:969-972 (Mar 11) 1968.

885. Coon WW, Willis PW: Some aspects of the pharmacology of oral anticoagulants. *Clin Pharmacol Ther* 11:312-336 (May-June) 1970

886. Welch RM, Harrison YE, Conney AH, Burns, JJ: An experimental model in dogs for studying interactions of drugs with bishydroxycoumarin. *Clin Pharmacol Ther* 10:817-825 (Nov-Dec) 1969.

887. Kalkhoff RK, Kim H, Stoddard FJ: Acquired subclinical diabetes mellitus in women receiving oral contraceptive agents. *Diabetes* 17:307 (May) 1968

888. Molnar GD, Berge KG, et al: The effect of nicotinic acid in diabetes mellitus. *Metabolism* 13:181-190, 1964.

889. Ku LLJH, Ward CO, Sister Jane Marie Durgin: A clinical study of drug interaction and anticoagulant therapy. *Drug Intell Clin Pharm* 4:300-306 (Nov) 1970.

890. Beckman H: *Dilemmas in Drug Therapy.* Philadelphia, Saunders, 1967, p 102.

891. Moser KM, Hajjar GC: Effect of heparin on the one-stage prothrombin time—source of artifactual "resistance" to prothrombinopenic therapy. *Ann Int Med* 66:1207-1213 (June) 1967.

892. Cartwright GE: *Diagnostic Laboratory Hematology,* ed 3. New York, Grune & Stratton, 1963, p. 159.

893. Propylthiouracil: hypoprothrombinemia. *Clin-Alert* 270 (Oct) 1964.

894. Taylor PJ: Hemorrhage while on anticoagulant therapy precipitated by drug interaction. *Arizona Med* 24:697-699 (Aug) 1967.

895. Menon IS, et al: Effect of onions on blood fibrinolytic activity. *Br Med J* 3:351-352 (Aug 10) 1968.

896. Frost J, Hess H: Concomitant administration of indomethacin and anticoagulants. International Symposium on Inflammation. Freiburg Im Breisgau, Germany, May 4-6, 1966.

897. Spivack M: How anticoagulants interact with other drugs. *Med Times* 99: 129-133 (Jan) 1971.

898. Solomon HM: Pitfalls of drug interference with coumarin anticoagulants. *Hosp Pract* 3:51-55 (July) 1968.

899. Johnson HD: Pharmacology of blood coagulation. *Am J Hosp Pharm* 25:60-69 (Feb) 1968.

900. Bressler R: Combined drug therapy. *Am J Med Sci* 255:89-93 (Feb) 1968.

901. Ambrus JL, Ambrus CM, et al: Treatment of fibrinolytic hemorrhage with proteinase inhibition: a preliminary report. *Ann NY Acad Sci* 146:625-641 (June 28) 1968.

902. Miller DC: The unmourned demise of an insidious killer. *FDA Papers* 4: 4-8 (Dec-Jan) 1971.

903. Cauwenberge H van, Jaques LB: Haemorrhagic effect of ACTH with anticoagulants. *Can Med Assoc J* 79:536-540, 1968.

904. Susahara AA, Canilla JE, Belko JS, et al: Urokinase therapy in clinical pulmonary embolism. *N Engl J Med* 277:1168-1173 (Nov 20) 1967.

905. Weiner M: The rational use of anticoagulants. *Pharmacol Phys* 1:1-7 (Nov) 1967.

906. Poller L, et al: Progesterone oral contraception and blood coagulation. *Br Med J* 1:554-556 (Mar 1) 1969.

907. Juergens J: What drugs have an influence on the prothrombin level? *Germ Med Monthly* 9:37 (Jan) 1964.

908. Aggeler PM, O'Reilly RA: The pharmacological basis of oral anticoagulant therapy. *Thromb Diath Haemorrh Suppl* 21:227-256, 1966.

909. Searcy RL, Foreman JA, Myers HD, Bergquist LM, et al: Anticoagulant properties of tetracyclines. Third Interscience Conference on Antimicrobial Agents and Chemotherapy, Washington, D.C., Oct. 28-30, 1963, pp. 471-484.

910. Alcohol, general anesthetics influence level of anticoagulant dosage. *JAMA* 187:34-35 (Mar 7) 1964.

911. Solomon HM, Schrogie JJ: The effect of various drugs on the binding of warfarin-14C to human albumin. *Biochem Pharmacol* 16:1219-1226 (July) 1967.

912. Smith JW: *Manual of Medical Therapeutics*, ed 19, Boston, Little, Brown, 1966, pp 85-91.

913. Goldberg ME, Johnson HE: Potentiation of chlorpromazine-induced behavioral changes by anticholinesterase agents. *J Pharm Pharmacol* 16:60-61, 1964.

914. ———: Behavioral effects of a cholinergic stimulant in combination with various psychotherapeutic agents. *J Pharmacol Exp Ther* 145:367-372, 1964.

915. Laurence DR, Nagle RE: The effects of bretylium and guanethidine on the pressor responses to noradrenaline and angiotensin. *Br J Pharmacol* 21:403-413 (Dec) 1963.

916. Kutt H, Brennan R, Dehejia H, et al: Diphenylhydantoin intoxication. A complication of isoniazid therapy. *Ann Rev Resp Dis* 101:307-384 (Mar) 1970.

917. Doniach D: Cell-mediated immunity in halothane hypersensitivity. *N Engl J Med* 283:315-316 (Aug 6) 1970.

918. Braham J, Adjuvants to L-dopa for parkinsonism. *Br Med J* 2:540 (May 30) 1970.

919. Kutt H, Verebely K, McDowell F: Inhibition of diphenylhydantoin metabolism in rats and in rat liver microsomes by antitubercular drugs. *Neurology* 18:706-710 (July) 1968.

920. Burke HL, McCurdy PR: The effect of riboflavin on acute bone marrow toxicity due to chloramphenicol. *Clin Res* 16:41 (Jan) 1968.

921. Crounse RG: Effective use of griseofulvin. *Arch Dermatol* 87:176-178 (Feb) 1963.

922. Klawans HL, Jr: The pharmacology of parkinsonism. *Dis Nerv Syst* 29:805-816 (Dec) 1968.

923. Stern G: Parkinsonism. *Br Med J* 4:541-542 (Nov 29) 1969.

924. Necheles TF, Snyder LM: Malabsorption of folate polyglutamates associated with oral contraceptive therapy. *N Engl J Med* 282:858-859 (Apr 9) 1970.

925. Goodwin CS, Sparell G: Inhibition of dapsone excretion by probenecid. *Lancet* 2:884-885 (Oct 25) 1969.

926. Gleason MN, Gosselin RE, Hodge HC, Smith RP: *Clinical Toxicology of Commercial Products.* Baltimore, Williams & Wilkins, 1969.

927. Fenfluramine up to date. *Drug Ther Bull* 8:21-23 (Mar 13) 1970.

928. Hall GJL, Davis AE: Inhibition of iron absorption by magnesium trisilicate. *Med J Austral* 56:95-96 (July 12) 1969.

929. Keusch GT, Troncale FJ, Buchanan RD: Malabsorption due to paromomycin. *Arch Int Med* 125:273-276 (Feb) 1970.

930. *Martindale, The Extra Pharmacopoeia,* ed. 26 London, Pharmaceutical Press, 1972, pp. 860-6.

931. Perel JM, Dayton PG, et al: Studies of interactions among drugs in man at the renal level: probenecid and sulfinpyrazone. *Clin Pharmacol Ther* 10:834-840 (Nov-Dec) 1969.

932. Stern S, Eisenberg S: The effect of propranolol (Inderal) on the electrocardiogram of normal subjects. *Am Heart J* 77:192-195 (Feb) 1969.

933. Synergy of trimethoprim and sulfonamides. *Br Med J* 2:507 (May 24) 1969.

934. Prange AJ, Wilson IC, Rabon AM, Lipton MA: Enhancement of imipramine antidepressant activity by thyroid hormone. *Am J Psychiat* 126:457-469 (Oct) 1969; 127:191

935. Dolenz BJ: Flurothyl (Indoklon) side effects. *Am J Psychiat* 123:1453-1455 (May) 1967.

936. Brest AN, Onesti G, Swartz, C, et al: Mechanisms of antihypertensive drug therapy. *JAMA* 211:480-484 (Jan 19) 1970.

937. Brodie BB, Shore PA, Silver SL: Potentiating action of chlorpromazine and reserpine. *Nature* 175:1113-1134 (June 25) 1955.

938. Dixon LD, Fouts JR: Inhibition of microsomal drug metabolic pathways by chloramphenicol. *Biochem Pharmacol* 11:715-720, 1962.

939. Peters MA, Fouts JR: The inhibitory effect of Aureomycin (chlortetracycline) pretreatment on some rat liver microsomal enzyme activities. *Biochem Pharmacol* 18:1511-1517, 1969.

940. Besse JC, Bass AD: Potentiation by hydrocortisone of responses to catecholamines in vascular smooth muscle. *J Pharmacol Exp Ther* 154:224-238 (Nov) 1966.

941. Jori A, Carrara, MC, Garattini S: Importance of noradrenaline synthesis for the interaction between desipramine and reserpine. *J Pharm Pharmacol* 18:619-620 (Sep) 1966.

942. Murray KMF, Smith SE: Desipramine and hypertensive episodes. *Lancet* 2:591 (Sep 10) 1966.

943. MacCannell KL, Dresel PE: Potentiation by thiopental of cyclopropane-adrenaline cardiac arrhythmias. *Can J Physiol Pharmacol* 42:627-639 (Sep) 1964.

944. Rauzzino FJ, Seifter J: Potentiation and antagonism of biogenic amines. *J Pharmacol Exp Ther* 157:143-148 (July) 1967.

945. Winter CA: The potentiating effect of antihistaminic drugs upon the sedative action of barbiturates. *J Pharmacol Exp Ther* 94:7-11 (Sep) 1948.

946. Jori A, Paglialunga S, Garattini S: Adrenergic mediation in the antagonism between desipramine and reserpine. *J Pharm Pharmacol* 18:326-327, 1966.

947. Mantegazza P, Tyler C, Zaimis E: The peripheral action of hexamethonium and of pentolinium. *Br J Pharmacol* 13:480-484 (Dec) 1958.

948. Seneca H, Peer P: Effect of chymotrypsin on the absorption of tetracycline from the intestinal

tract. *Antimicrob Agents Chemother,* 3:657-661, 1963.

949. Kim JH, Eidinoff ML: Action of 1-β-D-arabinofuranosylcytosine on the nucleic acid metabolism and viability of HeLa cells. *Cancer Res* 25:698-702 (June) 1965.

950. This interaction may be predicted because of the pharmacology of the drugs involved or because the same interaction has occurred with structurally and pharmacodynamically similar drugs and is so widely accepted that documentation is unnecessary.

951. This interaction has appeared in the literature without adequate documentation and is presented merely to draw attention to a problem that requires further investigation in man.

952. Weiner IM, Mudge GH: Renal tubular mechanisms for excretion of organic acids and bases. *Am J Med* 36:743-762 (May) 1964.

953. Abdou FA: Elavil-Librium combination. *Am J Psychiat* 120:1204 (June) 1966.

954. Kane FJ, Taylor TW: A toxic reaction to combined Elavil-Librium therapy. *Am J Psychiat* 119:1179-1180 (June) 1963.

955. FDA: *Reports of Suspected Adverse Reactions to Drugs.* No. 680301-044-00401, 1968.

956. Jarecki HG: Combined amitriptyline and phenelzine poisoning. *Am J Psychiat* 120:189 (Aug) 1963.

957. Stimulant augments antidepressant. *JAMA* 208:1616 (June 2) 1969.

958. Gillette JR: Drug toxicity as a result of interference with physiological control mechanisms. *Ann NY Acad Sci* 123:42-54 (Mar 12) 1965.

959. Porter AMW: Body height and imipramine side-effects. *Br Med J* 2:406-407 (May 18) 1968.

960. Brodie BB: Physicochemical and biochemical aspects of pharmacology. *JAMA* 202:600-609 (Nov 13) 1967.

961. Borden EC, Rostand SG: Recovery from massive amitriptyline overdosage. *Lancet* 1:1256 (June 8) 1968.

962. Vitamin C—Were the trials well controlled and are large doses safe? *Med. Let. Drugs Ther* 13:46-48 (May 28) 1971.

963. Rosenthal G: Interaction of ascorbic acid with warfarin. *JAMA* 215:1671 (Mar 8) 1971.

964. Hornykiewicz O: Report to the Academy of Medicine, University of Toronto, Feb. 7, 1969.

965. Southren AL, Tochimoto S, Strom L, et al: Remission in Cushing's syndrome with o,p'-DDD. *J Clin Endocrinol* 26:268-278 (Mar) 1966.

966. Pesticide poisoning may appear anywhere. *Calif Med* 111:68-69 (July) 1969.

967. Current guidelines to anticoagulant therapy. *JAMA* 201:877-878 (Sep 11) 1967.

968. Eckenhoff JE, Richards RK: Pharmacologic limitations of analeptic therapy. *Physiol Pharmacol Physic* 1: 1-3 (Apr) 1966.

969. DeGraff AC: Guanethidine and local anesthetics. *Am Fam Phys* p. 103 (Aug) 1965.

970. Jenkins LC, Graves HB: Potential hazards of psycho-active drugs in association with anesthesia. *Can Anaesth Soc J* 12:121-128 (Mar) 1965.

971. Twrdy von E, Weissel W, Zimmermann E: Interactions of coumarin and barbiturates. *Munch Med Wschr* 109:1272-1275 (June 9) 1967.

972. McLaughlin GE, McCarty DJ, Jr, Segal BL: Hemarthrosis complicating anticoagulant therapy. *JAMA* 196:1020-1021 (June 13) 1966.

973. Van Itallie TB: Treatment of familial hypercholesterolemia. *JAMA* 202:996 (Dec 4) 1967.

974. Orgain ES, Bogdonoff MD, Cain C.: Clofibrate with androsterone effect on serum lipids. *Arch Int Med* 119:80-85 (Jan) 1967.

975. Katz RL: Clinical experience with neurogenic cardiac arrhythmias. *Bull NY Acad Med* 43:1106-1118 (Dec) 1967.

976. Spurny OM, Wolf JW, Devins GS: Protracted tolbutamide-induced hypoglycemia. *Arch Intern Med* 115: 53-56, 1965.

977. Weller JM, Borondy PE: Effects of benzothiadiazine drugs on carbohydrate metabolism. *Metabolism* 14:708-714 (June) 1965.

978. Nuessle WF, Norman FC, Miller HF: Pickled herring and tranylcypromine reaction. *JAMA* 192:726-727 (May 24) 1965.

979. Cavallaro RJ, Krumperman LW, Kugler F: Effect of echothiophate therapy on the metabolism of succinylcholine in man. *Anesth Analg* 47:570-574 (Sep-Oct) 1968.

980. Winer JA, Bahn S: Loss of teeth with antidepressant drug therapy. *Arch Gen Phychiat* 16:239-240 (Feb) 1967.

981. Santos GW: The pharmacology of immunosuppressive drugs. *Pharmacol Phys* 2:1-6 (Aug) 1968.

982. Menzel, J, Dreyfuss F: Effect of prednisone on blood coagulation time in patients on dicoumarol therapy. *J Lab Clin Med* 56:14-20, 1960.

983. Allopurinol may affect iron metabolism. Medical News, *JAMA* 200:39 (May 15) 1967.

984. Oates JA: Antihypertensive drugs that impair adrenergic neuron function. *Pharmacol Phys* 1:1-7 (June) 1967.

985. Katz RL, Gissen AJ: Neuromuscular and electromyographic effects of halothane and its interaction with d-tubocurarine in man. *Anesthesiol* 28:564-567 (May-June) 1967.

986. Kessler RH: The use of furosemide and ethacrynic acid in the treatment of edema. *Pharmacol Phys* 1:1-5 (Sep) 1967.

987. Fekety FR Jr: Clinical pharmacology of the new penicillins and cephalosporins. *Pharmacol Phys* 1:1-7 (Oct) 1967.

988. Doherty JE, Murphy ML: Recognition and management of the intermediate coronary syndrome. *Med Times* 95:391-401 (Apr) 1967.

989. Abramson EA, Arky RA: Role of beta-adrenergic receptors in counter-regulation to insulin-induced hypoglycemia. *Diabetes* 17:141-146 (Mar) 1968.

990. Drug interactions. *Med Sci* pp. 27-28 (May) 1967.

991. Kater RMH: Heavy drinking accelerates drugs' breakdown in liver. *JAMA* 206:1709 (Nov 18) 1968.

992. Rubin E, Lieber CS: Hepatic microsomal enzymes in man and rat: induction and inhibition by ethanol. *Science* 162:690-691 (Nov 8) 1968.

993. Gitelson S: Methaqualone-meprobamate poisoning. *JAMA* 201:977-979 (Sep 18) 1967.

994. Perkins HA: Concomitant intravenous fluids and blood. *JAMA* 206:2122 (Nov 25) 1968.

995. deVilliers, JC: Intracranial haemorrhage in patients with monoamineoxidase inhibitors. *Br J Psychiat* 112:109:118 (Feb) 1966.

996. Dubach VC, et al: Influence of sulfonamides on the blood-glucose decreasing effect of oral antidiabetics. *Schweiz Med Wschr* 96:1483-1486 (Nov 5) 1966.

997. Alcohol, general anesthetics influence level of anticoagulant dosage. *JAMA* 187:34-35 (Mar 7) 1964.

998. Tranquada RE: Diuretic for diabetic patient taking an oral hypoglycemic agent. *JAMA* 206:1580-1581 (Nov 11) 1968.

999. Hellemans J: Factors influencing the action of coumarin. *Belg Tijdschr Geneesk* 18:361 (Apr 15) 1962.

1000. Eiderton TE, Farmati O, Zsigmond EK: Reduction in plasma cholinesterase level after prolonged administration of echothiophate iodide eyedrops. *Canad Anaesth Soc J* 15:291-296 (May) 1968.

1001. Goldstein G: Gamma-globulin and active immunization. *JAMA* 193:254 (July 19) 1965.

1002. Frei E, III, Loo TL: Pharmacologic basis for the chemotherapy of leukemia. *Pharmacol Phys* 1:1-5 (May) 1967.

1003. Wessler S, Avioli, LV: Propranolol therapy in patients with cardiac disease. *JAMA* 206:357-361 (Oct 7) 1968.

1004. Asthma medication "often misused." *JAMA* 206:2639 (Dec 16) 1968.

1005. Pines KL: The pharmacologic basis for the use of oral hypoglycemic agents in diabetes. *Physiol Pharmacol Phys* (Feb) 1966.

1006. Bryant JM: Monoamine oxidase (MAO) inhibition—a therapeutic adjunct. *Med Times* 95:420-434 (Apr) 1967.

1007. Barsa J, Saunders JC: A comparative study of tranylcypromine and pargyline. *Psychopharmacol* 6:295-298 (Oct 14) 1964.

1008. Starke JC: Photoallergy to sandalwood (sandela) oil. *Arch Derm* 96:62-63 (July) 1967.

1009. Warfarin plus griseofulvin may lower prothrombin time. *JAMA* 197:37 (Aug 1) 1966.

1010. Council on Drugs: Evaluation of a new antipsychotic agent, haloperidol (Haldol). *JAMA* 205:577-578 (Aug 19) 1968.

1011. ———: A convulsant agent for psychiatric use, flurothyl (Indoklon). *JAMA* 196:29-30 (Apr 4) 1966.

1012. ———: Evaluation of a new antibiotic, sodium cephalothin (Keflin). *JAMA* 194:182-183 (Oct 11) 1965.

1013. ———: Evaluation of a new oral diuretic agent, furosemide (Lasix). *JAMA* 200:979-980 (June 12) 1967.

1014. ———: A nonnarcotic analgesic agent, methotrimeprazine (Levoprome). *JAMA* 204:161-162 (Apr 8) 1968.

1015. ———: Evaluation of a new antibacterial agent, cephaloridine (Loridine). *JAMA* 206:1289-1290 (Nov 4) 1968.

1016. ———: Current status of measles immunization. *JAMA* 194:1237-1238 (Dec 13) 1965.

1017. ———: Evaluation of a new antipsychotic agent, thiothixene (Navane). *JAMA* 205:924-925 (Sep 23) 1968.

1018. ———: Evaluation of a new antipsychotic agent, butaperazine maleate (Repoise Maleate). *JAMA* 206:2307-2308 (Dec 2) 1968.

1019. ———: An agent for the amelioration of vertigo in Meniere's syndrome, betahistine hydrochloride (Serc). *JAMA* 203:1122 (Mar 25) 1968.

1020. ———: Evaluation of two antineoplastic agents, pipobroman (Vercyte) and thioguanine. *JAMA* 200:619-620 (May 15) 1967.

1021. ———: Evaluation of a new antidepressant agent, protriptyline hydrochloride (Vivactil). *JAMA* 206:364-365 (Oct 7) 1968.

1022. ———: Evaluation of a new antiemetic agent, diphenidol (Vontrol). *JAMA* 204:253-254 (Apr 15) 1968.

1023. Nies AS, Melmon KL: Recent concepts in the clinical pharmacology of antihypertensive drugs. *Calif Med* 106:338-399 (May) 1967.

1024. Adnitt PI: Hypoglycemic action of monoamineoxidase inhibitors (MAOI's). *Diabetes* 17:628-633 (Oct) 1968.

1025. Muelheims GH, Entrup RW, Paiewonsky D, Mierzwaik DS: Increased sensitivity of the heart to catecholamine-induced arrhythmias following guanethidine. *Clin Pharmacol Ther* 6:757-762 (Nov-Dec) 1965.

1026. Dundee JW: Clinical pharmacology of general anesthetics. *Clin Pharmacol Ther* 8:91-123 (Jan-Feb) 1967.

1027. Consolo S, Dolfini E, Garattini S, et al: Desipramine and amphetamine metabolism. *J Pharm Pharmacol* 19:253-256 (Apr) 1967.

1028. Zubrod CG, Kennedy TJ, Shannon JA: Studies on the chemotherapy of the human malarias VIII: the physiological disposition of pamaquine. *J Clin Invest* 27:114-120 (May) 1948.

1029. Weiner M, et al: Effects of steroids on disposition of oxyphenbutazone in man. *Soc Exp Biol Med* 124:1170-1173 (Apr) 1967.

1030. Walts L, McFarland W: Effect of vagolytic agents on ventricular rhythm during cyclopropane anesthesia. *Anesth Analg* 44:429-432 (July-Aug) 1965.

1031. Kinyon GE: Anticholinesterase eye drops—need for caution. *N Engl J Med* 280:53 (Jan 2) 1969.

1032. Torda TAG, et al: The interactions of neuromuscular blocking agents in man: the role of hexafluorenium. *Anesthesiol* 28:1010-1019 (Nov-Dec) 1967.

1033. Katz RL: Neuromuscular effects of diethyl ether and its interaction with succinylcholine and *d*-tubocurarine. *Anesthesiol* 27:52-63 (Jan-Feb) 1966.

1034. DeConti RC, Calabrici P: Use of allopurinol for prevention and control of hyperuricemia in patients with neoplastic diseases. *N Engl J Med* 274:481-486 (Mar 3) 1966.

1035. Goldfinger S, Klinenberg JR, Seegmiller JE: The renal excretion of oxypurines *J Clin Invest* 44:623-628, 1965.

1036. Adriani J: Anesthesia problems in small hospitals. *Postgrad Med* 45: 116-123 (Feb) 1969.

1037. Ghoneim MM, Long JP: The interaction between magnesium and other neuromuscular blocking agents. *Anesthesiol* 32:23-27 (Jan) 1970.

1038. FDA: L-dopa. *Current Drug Information* (June) 1970.

1039. ———: Lithium carbonate. *Current Drug Information* (Apr.) 1970.

1040. Weiner M: Drug interaction. *N Engl J Med* 283:871-872 (Oct 15) 1970.

1041. Zakharov VN, Vasilevich MT: On medicinal disease with infarction-like allergic myocarditis. *Terapevt Arkh* 43:97-99, 1971 (through Ringdoc from USSR Ministry of Public Health).

1042. Wagner JG: Pharmacokinetics I. Definitions, modeling and reasons for measuring blood levels and urinary excretion *Drug Intell* 2:38-42, 1968.

1043. Sorby DL, Liu G: Effects of adsorbents on drug absorption II. Effect of an antidiarrhea mixture on promazine absorption. *J Pharm Sci* 55:504-510, 1966.

1044. Davies JE, et al: Effect of anticonvulsant drugs on dicophane (DDT) residues in man. *Lancet* 2:7-9, 1969.

1045. Dixon RL: Effect of chloramphenicol on the metabolism and lethality of cyclophosphamide in rats. *Proc Soc Exp Biol Med* 127:1151-1155, 1968.

1046. Anton AH: The effect of disease, drugs, and dilution on the binding of sulfonamides in human plasma. *Clin Pharmacol Ther* 9:561-567, 1968.

1047. Maickel RP, Miller FP, Brodie BB: Interaction of non-steroidal anti-inflammatory agents with corticosterone binding to plasma proteins in the rat. *Arzneimit Forsch* 19:1803-1805, 1969.

1048. Skeith MD, Simkin PA, Healey LA: The renal excretion of indomethacin and its inhibition by probenecid. *Clin Pharm Ther* 9:89-93, 1968.

1049. Kraines SH: Therapy of the chronic depressions. *Dis Nerv Syst* 28:577-584, 1967.

1050. Cheese "high" eases hypotension. *Med World News* 10:24 (May 30) 1969.

1051. Lennon RG, Isacson P, Rosales T, et al: Skin tests with measles and poliomyelitis vaccines in recipients of inactivated measles virus vaccine. Delayed dermal hypersensitivity. *JAMA* 200:275-280 (Apr 24) 1967.

1052. Smithwick EM, Berkovich S: *In vitro* suppression of the lymphocyte response to tuberculin by live measles virus. *Proc Soc Exp Biol Med* 123:276-278 (Oct) 1966.

1053. Hart LG, Shultice RW, Fouts JR: Stimulatory effects of chlordane on hepatic microsomal drug metabolism in the rat. *Toxicol Appl Pharmacol* 5:371-386, 1963.

1054. Keeri-Szanto M, Muir JM, Remington B: Smoking reduces the effectiveness of narcotics. *Clin Pharmacol Ther* 14:139 (Jan-Feb) 1973.

1055. O'Reilly RA, Aggeler PM: Effect of barbiturates on oral anticoagulants in man. *Clin Res* 17:153, 1969; *Pharmacol Rev* 22:35-96 (Mar) 1970.

1056. Borga O, Azarnoff DL, Forshell G P, Sjöqvist F: Plasma protein binding of tricyclic antidepressants in man. *Biochem Pharmacol* 18:2135-2143, 1969.

1057. Fouts JR, Rogers LA: Morphological changes in the liver accompanying stimulation of microsomal drug metabolising enzyme activity by phenobarbital, chlordane, benzpyrene, or methylchloranthrene in rats. *J Pharmacol Exp Ther* 147:112-119, 1965.

1058. Marshall WJ, McLean AEM: The effect of oral phenobarbitone on hepatic microsomal cytochrome P-450 and demethylation activity in rats fed normal and low protein diets. *Biochem Pharmacol* 18:153-157, 1969.

1059. Kolmodin B, Azarnoff DL, Sjöqvist F: Effect of environmental factors on drug metabolism: Decreased plasma half-life of antipyrine in workers exposed to chlorinated hydrocarbon insecticides. *Clin Pharmacol Ther* 10:638-642, 1969.

1060. Kato R, Chiesara E, Vassanelli P: Further studies on the inhibition and stimulation of microsomal drug-metabolizing enzymes of rat liver by various compounds. *Biochem Pharmacol* 13:69-83, 1964.

1061. Kato R, Vassanelli P, Chiesara E: Inhibition of some microsomal drug-metabolizing enzymes by inhibitors of cholesterol biosynthesis. *Biochem Pharmacol* 12:349-351, 1963.

1062. Palva IP, Salokannel SJ: Report to the International Congress of Hematology Munich 1971.

1063. Booth J, Gillette JR: The effect of anabolic steroids of drug metabolism by microsomal enzymes in rat liver. *J Pharmacol Exp Ther* 137:374-379, 1962.

1064. Brown RR, Miller JA, Miller EC: The metabolism of methylated aminoazo dyes IV. Dietary factors enhancing demethylation *in vitro*. *J Biol Chem* 209:211-222, 1954.

1065. Fouts JR: Factors influencing the metabolism of drugs in liver microsomes. *Ann NY Acad Sci* 104:875-880, 1963.

1066. Hoogland DR, Miya TS, Bousquet WF: Metabolism and tolerance studies with chlordiazepoxide-2-¹⁴C in the rat. *Toxicol Appl Pharmacol* 9:116-123, 1966.

1067. Juchau MR, Fouts JR: Effects of norethynodrel and progesterone on hepatic microsomal drug-metabolizing enzyme systems. *Biochem Pharmacol* 15:891-898, 1966.

1068. Kato R, Chiesara E, Frontino G: Influence of sex difference on the pharmacological action and metabolism of some drugs. *Biochem Pharmacol* 11:221-227, 1962.

1069. Remmer H: Die Verstäkung der Abbaugeschivindigkeit von Evipan durch Glykocorticoide. *Arch Exp Pathol Pharmakol* 233:184-191, 1958.

1070. Remmer H: Drugs as activators of drug enzymes. *Proc. 1st Int. Pharmacol. Mtg.,* Stockholm, vol 6, pp. 235-249, New York, Macmillan, 1962.

1071. Van Dyke RA: Metabolism of volatile anesthetics III. Induction of microsomal dechlorinating and ethercleaving enzymes. *J Pharmacol Exp Ther* 154:364-369, 1966.

1072. Wattenberg LW, Leong JL: Effects of phenothiazines on protective systems against polycyclic hydrocarbons. *Cancer Res* 25:365-370, 1965.

1073. Yamamoto I, Nagai K, Kimura H, Iwatsubo K: Nicotine and some carcinogens in special reference to the hepatic drug-metabolizing enzymes. *Jap J Pharmacol* 16:183-190, 1966.

1074. Courvoisier S, Fournel J, Ducrot R, et al: Propriétés pharmacodynamiques du chlorhydrate de chloro-3 (diméthylamino-z′ propyl)-10 phénothiazine (4.560 R.P.). *Arch Int Pharmacodyn* 92:305-361, 1953.

1075. Payne JP: Further studies of the influence of carbon dioxide on neuromuscular blocking agents in the rat. *Br J Anaesth* 32:202-205 (May) 1960.

1076. Trolle D: Decrease of total serumbilirubin concentration in newborn infants after phenobarbitone treatment. *Lancet* 2:705–708 (Sep 28) 1968.

1077. Straker M, Robertson DS: Combinations of pharmaceuticals. *Can Med Assoc J* 85:711–712 (Sep 16) 1961.

1078. The interaction of drugs. *Lancet* 1:82–84 (Jan 8) 1966.

1079. Dolger H: Alcoholic beverages and orally given hypoglycemic drugs. *JAMA* 173:1278 (July 16) 1960.

1080. Holland WC, Sekul A: Influence of K^+ and Ca^{++} on the effect of ouabain on Ca^{45} entry and contracture in rabbit atria. *J Pharmacol Exp Ther* 133:288–294 (Sep) 1961.

1081. Klepzig H: Caution in the use of gelatine-polymers (Haemaccel®) in the presence of full digitalization. *Germ Med Monthly* 10:165 (Apr) 1965.

1082. Misage JR, McDonald RH: Antagonism of hypotensive action of bethanidine by "common cold" remedy. *Br Med J* 4:347 (Nov 7) 1970.

1083. Measles virus vaccine, inactivated (killed); altered reactivity to measles virus. *Clin-Alert* 289 (Nov 26) 1970.

1084. Garb S: *Clinical Guide to Undesirable Drug Interactions and Interferences.* New York, Springer 1971.

1085. Antacids in peptic ulcer. *Med Let. Drugs Ther* 7:91–92 (Oct 22) 1965.

1086. Sargant W, Dally P: Treatment of anxiety states by antidepressant drugs. *Br Med J* 1:6–9 (Jan 6) 1962.

1087. Clark WC, Hulpieu HR: The disulfiram-like activity of animal charcoal. *J Pharmacol Exp Ther* 123:74–80, 1958.

1088. Chamberlain TJ: Licorice poisoning, pseudo-aldosteronism, and heart failure. *JAMA* 213:1343 (Aug 24) 1970.

1089. Conn JW, Rovner DR, Cohen EL: Licorice induced pseudoaldo-steronism. *JAMA* 205:492–496 (Aug 12) 1968.

1090. Koster M, David GK: Reversible severe hypertension due to licorice ingestion. *N Engl J Med* 278:1381–1383 (June 20) 1968.

1091. Viukari NMA: Folic acid and anticonvulsants. *Lancet* 1:980 (May 4) 1968.

1092. Mark LC, Papper EM: Changing therapeutic goals in barbiturate poisoning. *Pharmacol Physicians* 1:1–5 (Mar) 1967.

1093. Welch RM, Harrison YE, Conney AH, et al: Cigarette smoking: stimulatory effect on metabolism of 3, 4-benzpyrene by enzymes in human placenta. *Science* 160:541–542 (May 3) 1968.

1094. Mitoma C, Sorick TJ II, Neubauer SE: The effect of caffeine on drug metabolism. *Life Sci* 7:145–151 (Feb) 1968.

1095. Conney AH, Gilman AG: Puromycin inhibition of enzyme induction by 3-methylcholanthrene and phenobarbital. *J Biol Chem* 238:3682–3685 (Nov) 1963.

1096. Gelboin HV, Blackburn NR: The stimulatory effect of 3-methylcholanthrene on benzpyrene hydroxylase activity in several rat tissues: inhibition by actinomycin D and puromycin. *Cancer Res* 24:356–360 (Feb) 1964.

1097. Espelin DE, Done AK: Amphetamine poisoning: effectiveness of chlorpromazine. *N Engl J Med* 278:1361–1365 (June 20) 1968.

1098. Aderhold RM, Muniz CE: Acute psychosis with amitriptyline and furazolidone. *JAMA* 213:2080 (Sep 21) 1970.

1099. Levy G, Leonards JR: Urine pH and salicylate therapy. *JAMA* 217:81 (July 5) 1971.

1100. Hayakawa T, Kanai N, Yamada R, et al: Effect of steroid hormone on activation of Endoxan (cyclophosphamide). *Biochem Pharmacol* 18:129–135, 1969.

1101. Cavallito CJ, O'Dell TB: Modification of rates of gastrointestinal absorption of drugs II. Quaternary ammonium salts. *J Am Pharm Assoc Sci Ed* 47:169–173 (Mar) 1958.

1102. Poller L, Thomas JM: Clotting factors during oral contraception: further report. *Br Med J* 2:23–25 (July 2) 1966.

1103. Comstock EG: Glutethimide intoxication. *JAMA* 215:1668 (Mar 8) 1971.

1104. Editorial: Another drug interaction. *Br Med J* 4:509; Neuvonen PJ, Gothoni G, et al: Interference of iron with the absorption of tetracyclines in man. *Br Med J* 4:532–534 (Nov 28) 1970.

1105. Cairncross KD: On the peripheral pharmacology of amitriptyline. *Arch Int Pharmacodyn Thér* 154:438–448, 1965.

1106. Richardson M, Holt JN: Synergistic action of streptomycin with other antibiotics on intracellular *Brucella abortus* in vitro. *J Bact* 84:638–646, 1962.

1107. Gale GR, Odell CA: Antagonism of colistin-sulphonamide synergism by para-aminobenzoic acid. *Nature* 209:1357 (Mar 26) 1966.

1108. Wagner JG: Biopharmaceutics: absorption aspects. *J Pharm Sci* 50:359–387 (May) 1961.

1109. Blount RE: Management of chloroquine-resistant falciparum malaria. *Arch Int Med* 119:557–560 (June) 1967.

1110. Nagashima R, Levy G, O'Reilly RA: Comparative pharmacokinetics of coumarin anticoagulants IV. Application of a three-compartmental model to the analysis of the dosedependent kinetics of bishydroxycoumarin elimination. *J Pharm Sci* 57:1888–1895 (Nov) 1968.

1111. Almquist HJ: Vitamin K. *Physiol Rev* 21:194–216, 1941.

1112. Breckenride RT, Kellermeyer RW: A hemorrhagic syndrome due to Dicumarol poisoning masquerading as propythiouracil sensitivity. *Ann Int Med* 60:1066–1068 (June) 1964.

1113. Jarnum S: Cincophen and acetylsalicylic acid in anticoagulant treatment. *Scand J Clin Lab Invest* 6:91–93, 1954.

1114. Verstraete M, Vermylen J, Claeys H: Dissmilar effect of two antianginal drugs belonging to the benzofuran group on the action of coumarin derviatives. *Arch Int Pharmacodyn Thér* 176;33–41, 1968.

1115. Hrdina P, Kovalcík V: Influence of morphine and pethidine on the hypoprothrombinemic effect of indirect anticoagulants. *Int J Neuropharmacol* 2:135–141, 1963.

1116. Weiner M, Dayton PG: Induced "hyperprothrombinemia" in guinea pigs. *Fed Proc* 19:57, 1960.

1117. Baumann CA, Field JB, et al: Studies on hemorrhagic sweet clover disease X. Induced vitamin C excretion in the rat and its effect on the hypoprothrombinemia caused by 3,3'-methylenebis-(4-hydroxycoumarin). *J Biol Chem* 146:7-14 (Nov) 1942.

1118. Godfrey H: Dangers of dioctyl sodium sulfosuccinate in mixtures. *JAMA* 215:643 (Jan 25) 1971.

1119. Tyrer JH, Eadie MJ, Sutherland JM, Hooper WD: Outbreak of anticonvulsant intoxication in an Australian city. *Br Med J* 4:271-273 (Oct 31) 1970.

1120. Selye H: Mercury poisoning: prevention by spironolactone. *Science* 169:775-776 (Aug 21) 1970.

1121. Pecoldawa K: Urea effect on intraocular tension caused by succinylcholine. *Polish Med J* 7:958-988, 1968.

1122. Brumfitt W, Percival A: Antibiotic combinations. *Lancet* 1:387-390 (Feb 20) 1971.

1123. Conney AH, Klutch A: Increased activity of androgen hydroxylases in liver microsomes of rats pretreated with phenobarbital and other drugs. *J Biol Chem* 238:1611-1617 (May) 1963.

1124. Ditman KS, Gottlieb L: Transient diuresis from chlordiazepoxide and diazepam. *Am J Psychiat* 120:910-911 (Mar) 1964.

1125. Bielicky T, Zak M: Protective effect of chloroquine on the survival of mice following total body irradiation. *Casopis Lekaru Ceskych* 106:1001-1003, 1967. [*Int Pharm Abstr* 5:152 (Feb 15) 1968.]

1126. Gessner PK, Cabana BE: A study of the interaction of the hypnotic effects and of the toxic effects of chloral hydrate and ethanol. *J Pharmacol Exp Ther* 174:247-259, 1970; The kinetics of chloral hydrate metabolism in mice and the effect thereon of ethanol. *Ibid:* 260-275, 1970.

1127. Jacobsen E: Death of alcoholic patients treated with disulfiram (tetraethylthiuram disulfide) in Denmark. *Quart J Stud Alcohol* 13:16-26, 1952.

1128. Use of probenecid in antimicrobial therapy. *Med Let Drugs Ther* 13:88 (Oct 15) 1971.

1129. Acar JF, Sabath LD, Ruch PA: Antagonism of the antibacterial action of some penicillins by other penicillins and cephalosporins. *J Clin Invest* 55:446-53 (Mar) 1975.

1130. Linken A: Propranolol for LSD-induced anxiety states. *Lancet* 2:1039-1040 (Nov 6) 1971.

1131. Phillips GB: Effects of alcohol on glucose tolerance. *Lancet* 2:1317-1318 (Dec 11) 1971; alcoholic diabetes. *JAMA* 217:1513-1519 (Sep 13) 1971.

1132. Sorrell TC, Forbes IJ, Burness FR, Rischbieth RHC: Depression of immunological function in patients treated with phenytoin sodium (sodium diphenylhydantoin). *Lancet* 2:1233-1235 (Dec 4) 1971.

1133. Amador D, Gazdar A: Sudden death during disulfiram-alcohol reaction. *Quart J Stud Alcohol* 28:649-654, 1967.

1134. Aleyassine H, Lee SH: Inhibition by hydrazine, phenelzine and pargyline of insulin release from rat pancreas. *Endocrinol* 89:125-129 (July) 1971.

1135. Koch-Weser J, Sellers EM: Drug interactions with coumarin anticoagulants. *N Engl J Med* 285:487-498 (Aug 26), 547-558 (Sept 2) 1971.

1136. Hoffbrand AV: The role of malabsorption in the development of folate deficiency. *Clin Med* 79:19-22 (Jan) 1972.

1137. Kilpatrick R: Advances in medicine. *Practitioner* 207:411-421 (Oct) 1971.

1138. Rothstein E: Rifampin with disulfiram. *JAMA* 219:1216 (Feb 28) 1972.

1139. Tipton DL, Sutherland VC, et al: Effect of chlorpromazine on blood level of alcohol in rabbits. *Am J Physiol* 200:1007-1010 (May) 1961.

1140. Sutherland VC, Burbridge TN, et al: Cerebral metabolism in problem drinkers under the influence of alcohol and chlorpromazine hydrochloride. *J Appl Physiol* 15:189-196 (Feb) 1960.

1141. Frahm M, Lobkens, K, Soehring K: Der Einfluss subchroinischer Alkoholgaben auf die Barbiturat-Narkose von Meerschweinken. *Arzneimittelforschung* 12:1055-1056 (Nov) 1962.

1142. Hughes FW, Routree LB, Forney RB: Suppression of learned avoidance and discriminative responses in the rat by chlordiazepoxide (Librium) and ethanol chlordiazepoxide combinations. *Quart J Stud Alcohol* 26:136, 1965; *J Genet Psychol* 103:139-145, 1963.

1143. Wiberg GS, Coldwell BB, Trenholm HL: Toxicity of ethanolbarbiturate mixtures. *J Pharm Pharmacol* 21:232-236, 1969.

1144. Hume R, Johnstone JMS, Weyers E: Interaction of ascorbic acid and warfarin. *JAMA* 219:1479 (Mar 13) 1972.

1145. Cohen WJ, Cohen NH: Lithium carbonate, haloperidol, and irreversible brain damage. *JAMA* 230: 1283-7 (Dec 2) 1974.

1146. Osol A, et al: *The United States Dispensatory and Physicians' Pharmacology,* (ed 26). Philadelphia J.B. Lippincott Co, 1967.

1147. Dent CE, Richens A, Rowe DJF, et al: Osteomalacia with long-term anticonvulsant therapy in epilepsy. *Br Med J* 4:69-72 (Oct 10) 1970.

1148. Hunter J, Maxwell JD, Stewart DA, et al: Altered calcium metabolism in epileptic children on anticonvulsants. *Br Med J* 4:202-4 (Oct 23) 1971.

1149. Bleifeld W: Side effects of antiarrhythmic drugs. *Naunyn-Schmiedebergs Arch Pharmacol* 269:282-97 (Symposium II) 1971.

1150. Heinonen J, et al: Plasma lidocaine levels in patients treated with potential inducers of microsomal enzymes. *Acta Anaesth Scand* 14:89-95, 1970.

1151. Dunbar RW, Boettner RB, Haley JV, et al: The effect of diazepam on the antiarrhythmic response to lidocaine. *Anesth Analg* 50:685-92 (July-Aug) 1971.

1152. Wood RA: Sinoatrial arrest: an interaction between phenytoin and lignocaine. *Br Med J* 1:645 (Mar 20) 1971.

1153. Weily HS, Genton E: Clinical pharmacology of procainamide. *Ann Intern Med* 74:823, (May) 1971. 52nd Annual Session, American College of Physicians, Mar 29-Apr. 2, 1971, Denver, Co.

1154. Koch-Weser J: Pharmacokinetics of procainamide in man. *Ann NY Acad Sci* 179:370-82, 1971.

1155. Adam WR, Dawborn JK: Plasma levels and urinary excretion of nalidixic acid in patients with renal failure. *Aust NZ J Med* 2:126, 1971.

1156. Ensinck JW, Stoll RW, Gale CC, et al: Effect of aminophylline on the secretion of insulin, glucagon, luteinizing hormone and growth hormone in humans. *J Clin Endocrinol Metab* 31:153-61 (Aug) 1970.

1157. Berchtold P, Bessman AN: Propranolol. *Ann Intern Med* 80:119, 1974.

1158. McMurtry RJ: Propranolol, hypoglycemia and hypertensive crisis. *Ann Intern Med* 80:669-70, 1974.

1159. Goodman LS, Gilman A: *The Pharmacological Basis of Therapeutics.* New York, Macmillan, 1975, pp 686-96.

1160. Stannard M, Sloman G: Haemodynamic effects of propranolol. *Br Med J* 1:700 (Mar 18) 1967.

1161. Jones RV: Warfarin and Distalgesic interaction, *Br Med J* 1:460 (Feb. 21) 1976.

1162. O'Reilly M, Golberg E, Chaithiraphar S: Propranolol and digitalis. *Lancet* 1:138 (Jan 26) 1974.

11163. Crawford MH, Le Winter M, Kerliner JS, O'Rourke RA: Propranolol and digitalis. *Lancet* 1;457-8 (Mar 16) 1974; Propranolol, digoxin, and combined therapy in patients with angina pectoris. *Clin Pharmacol Ther* 15:203 (Feb) 1974.

1164. Watt DAL: Sensitivity to propranolol after digoxin intoxication. *Br Med J* 3:413-4 (Aug 17) 1968.

1165. Kram J, Bourne HR, Melmon KL, Maibach H: Propranolol. *Ann Intern Med* 80:282 (Feb) 1974.

1166. Baumrucker JF: Drug interaction—propranolol and Cafergot. *N Engl J Med* 288:916-7 (Apr 26) 1973.

1167. Diamond S: Propranolol and ergotamine tartrate. *N Engl J Med* 289:159 (July 19) 1973.

1168. Blank NK, Reider MJ: Paradoxical response to propranolol in migraine. *Lancet* 2:1336 (Dec 8) 1973.

1169. Corbascio AN: Propranolol. *Clin Pharmacol Ther* 12:559-61 (May-June) 1971.

1170. Stubbs D, Pugh D, Bell H: Combined use of isoproterenol and propranolol in cardiogenic shock. *Clin Pharmacol Ther* 11:244-50 (Mar-Apr) 1970.

1171. Kissel P, Jridon P, André JM: Levodopa-propranolol therapy in parkinsonian tremor. *Lancet* 1:403-4 (Mar 9) 1974.

1172. Camanni F, Massara F: Enhancement of levodopa-induced growth hormone stiumlation by propranolol. *Lancet* 1:942 (May 11) 1974.

1173. Whitsett TL, Cucinell EA, Goldberg LI: Propranolol blockade of positive inotropic effects of L-dopa in dog and man. *Pharmacologist* 12:213 (Aug. 24) 1970.

1174. Duvoisin RC: Hypotension caused by L-dopa. *Br Med J* 3:47 (July 4) 1970.

1175. Nies AS, Shand DG: Hypertensive response to propranolol in a patient treated with methyldopa—a proposed mechanism. *Clin Pharmacol Ther* 14:823-6 (Sep-Oct) 1973.

1176. Schwartz ML: Comparative antiarrhythmic effects of intravenously administered lidocaine and procainamide and orally administered quinidine. *Am J Cardiol* 26: 520-523 (Nov) 1970.

1177. Giardina EV: Intermittent intravenous procaine amide to treat ventricular arrhythmias. Correlation of plasma concentration with effect on arrhythmia, electrocardiogram, and blood pressure. *Ann Intern Med* 78:183-193, (Feb) 1973.

1178. Corrigan JJ, Marcus FI: Coagulopathy associated with vitamin E ingestion. *JAMA* 230:1300-1301 (Dec 2) 1974.

1179. Frieden J: Propranolol as an antiarrhythmic agent. *Am Heart J* 74:283, 1967.

1180. Barrett AM, Cullum VA: Lack of inter-action between propranolol and mebenazine. *J Pharm Pharmacol* 20:911-915 (Dec) 1968.

1181. Geumei A, Issa I, El-Gindi M, Abd-el-Samie Y: Beta-adrenergic receptors and gastric acid secretion. *Surgery* 66: 663-668 (Oct) 1967.

1182. Baker L, Barcai A, Kaye R, Haque N: Beta adrenergic blockade and juvenile diabetes: acute studies and long-term therapeutic trial. *J Pediatr* 75:19-29 (July) 1969.

1183. Arita M, Mashiba H: Effects of phenothiazine and propranolol on ECG. The effects of propranolol on the electrocardiographic abnormalities induced by phenothiazine derivatives. *Jap Circ J* 34:391-400 (May) 1970.

1184. Stern S: Haemodynamic changes following separate and combined administration of beta-blocking drugs and quinidine. *Eur J Clin Invest* 1:432, 1971.

1185. Dreifus LS, Lim HF, Watanabe Y, et al: Propranolol and quinidine in the management of ventricular tachycardia. *JAMA* 204:736-739 (May 20) 1968.

1186. Rozen MS, Whan FM: Prolonged curarization associated with propranolol. *Med J Aust* 1:467-468 (Mar 4) 1972.

1187. Knouss RF, Gebhardt RE, Thyrum PT, et al: Variation in quinidine excretion with changing urine pH. *Ann Intern Med* 68:1157 (May) 1968.

1188. Adams RD: Manic-depressive psychosis, involutional melancholia, and hypochondriasis in Wintrobe MM *et al* ed: *Harrison's Principles of Internal Medicine,* ed 6 New York, McGraw-Hill, 1970, p 1876.

1189. Zinn MB; Quinidine intoxication from alkali ingestion. *Texas Med* 66:64-66 (Dec) 1970.

1190. Gibaldi M, Grundhofer B, Levy G: Effect of antacids on pH of urine. *Cline Pharmacol Ther* 16:520-525 (Sep) 1974.

1191. Albers DD: Renal failure following prostatovesiculectomy related to methoxyflurane anesthesia and tetracycline-complicated by candida infection. *J Urol* 106:348-350 (Sep) 1971.

1192. Udall JA: Drug interference with warfarin therapy. *Am J Cardiol* 23:143 (Jan) 1969; *Clin Med* 77:20-25, (Aug) 1970.

1193. Sopher IM, Ming SC: Fatal corpus luteum hemorrhage during anticoagulant therapy. *Obstet Gynecol* 37:695-697 (May) 1971.

1194. Fletcher GF, Kazamias TM, Wenger NK: Cardiotoxic effects of Mellaril; conduction disturbances and supraventricular arrhythmias. *Am Heart J* 78:135-138 (July) 1969.

1195. Schoonmaker FW, Osteen RT, Greenfield JC: Thioridazine (Mellaril)-induced ventricular tachycardia controlled with an artificial pacemaker. *Ann Intern Med* 65:1076-1078 (Nov) 1966.

1196. Giles TD, Modlin RK: Death associated with ventricular arrhythmia and thioridazine hydrochloride. *JAMA* 205:108-110 (July 8) 1968.

1197. Connell PH: Central nervous system stimulant and antidepressant drugs in *Side Effects of Drugs.*

Amsterdam, Excerpta Medica Foundation, 6:28-29, 1968. Alberti RL (Searle Laboratories): Personal communication, July 21, 1975.

1198. Alexanderson B, et al: Steady state plasma levels of nortriptyline in twins: Influence of genetic-factors and drug therapy. *Br. Med J* 4:764-8 (Dec 27) 1969.

1199. Allison J: Methotrexate and smallpox vaccination (Letter). *Lancet* 2:1250 (Dec 7) 1968.

1200. Allison RD, Kraner JC, Roth GM: Effects of alcohol and nitroglycerin on vascular responses in man. *Angiology* 22:211-22 (Apr) 1971.

1201. Altschuler SL, Valenteen JW: Amenorrhea following rifampin administration during oral contraceptive use. *Obstet Gynecol* 44:771-2 (Nov) 1974.

1202. Ambre JJ, Fischer LJ: Effect of coadministration of aluminum and magnesium hydroxides on absorption of anticoagulants in man. *Clin Pharmacol Ther* 14:231-237 (Mar-Apr) 1973.

1203. *American Hospital Formulary Service:* Procainamide. 24:04, (Oct) 1968, Washington, DC American Society of Hospital Pharmacists.

1204. *ibid:* Propranolol. 24:04 (Jul) 1977.

1205. *ibid:* Quinidine. 24:04 (Sep) 1977.

1205. *ibid:* Isoniazid. 8:16 (Jul) 1972.

1207. *ibid:* Ethionamide. 8:16 (May) 1963.

1208. *ibid:* Heparin Sodium USP 20:12.04 (May) 1969.

1209. *ibid:* Pyrimethamine. 8:40 (April) 1960.

1210. *ibid:* Disulfiram. 92:00 (May) 1977.

1211. *ibid:* Sulfonamides. 8:24 (Nov) 1976.

1212. Aminu J, D'Mello A, Vere DW: Interaction between debrisoquine and phenylephrine *Lancet* 2:935-6 (Oct 31) 1970.

1213. Andreasen PB, et al: Abnormalities in liver function tests during long-term diphenylhydantoin therapy in epileptic outpatients. *Acta Med Scand* 194:261-264, 1973.

1214. Andreasen PB, et al: Diphenylhydantoin half life in man and its inhibition by phenylbutazone: the role of genetic factors. *Acta Med Scand* 193:561-564, 1973.

1215. Anggard E, Jonsson L-E, Hogmark A-L, et al: Amphetamine metabolism in amphetamine psychosis. *Clin Pharmacol Ther* 14:870-80 (Sep-Oct) 1973.

1216. *Anticoagulant Therapy*—A Selected Bibliography. Endo Laboratories, 1968, p. 49.

1217. Anton AH: Increasing activity of sulfonamides with displacing agents: a review. *Ann NY Acad Sci* 226:273-292, 1973.

1218. Arneson GA: Phenothiazine derivatives and glucose metabolism. *J Neuropsychiat* 5:181-5 (Feb) 1964.

1219. Arnold K, Gerber N: The rate of decline of diphenylhydantoin in human plasma. *Clin Pharmacol Ther* 11:121-34 (Jan-Feb) 1970.

1220. Aronow WS, Chesluk HM: Evaluation of nitroglycerin in angina in patients on isosorbide dinitrate. *Circulation* 42:61-3 (July) 1970.

1221. Ayd FJ Jr (ed): Rx tip: Relieving drug-induced oral and pharyngeal dryness. *Int Drug Ther Newsletter* 2:24 (June) 1967.

1222. Babb RR, Wilbur RS: Aspirin and gastrointestinal bleeding. An opinion. *Calif Med* 110:440-1 (May) 1969.

1223. Bailey RR: Renal failure in combined gentamicin and cephalothin therapy *Br Med J* 2:776-7 (June 30) 1973. See also ref 1432.

1224. Baker H: Intermittent high dose oral methotrexate therapy in psoriasis. *Br J Dermatol* 82:65-69 (Jan) 1970.

1225. Ballek RE, Reidenberg MM, et al: Inhibition of diphenylhydantoin metabolism by chloramphenicol. *Lancet* 1:150 (Jan 20) 1973.

1226. Barrett AM: Modification of the hypoglycaemic response to tolbutamide and insulin by mebanazine, an inhibitor of monoamine oxidase. *J Pharm Pharmacol* 17:19-27 (Jan) 1965.

1227. Barrow MV, et al: Salicylate hypoprothrombinemia in rheumatoid arthritis with liver disease. *Arch Int Med* 120:620-4 (Nov) 1967.

1228. Bateman FJA: Effects of tetracyclines *Br Med J* 4:802, (Dec 26) 1970.

1229. Baylis EM, Crowly JM, et al: Influence of folic acid on blood-phenytoin levels. *Lancet* 1:62-4 (Jan 9) 1971.

1230. Bazzano G, Bazzano GS: Digitalis intoxication: treatment with a new steroidbinding resin. *JAMA* 220:828-30 (May 8) 1972.

1231. Beaumont G: Drug interaction with clomipramine (Anafranil). *J Int Med Res* 1:480, 1973.

1232. Becker B, et al: Diphenylhydantoin and dexamethasone-induce changes of plasma cortisol: comparison of patients with and without glaucoma. *J Clin Endocrinol Metab* 32:669-70 (May) 1971.

1233. Beliles RP, Foster GV, Jr: Interaction of bishydroxycoumarin with chloral hydrate and trichloroethyl phosphate. *Toxicol Appl Pharmacol* 27:225-29 (Feb) 1974.

1234. Beller GA, Hood WB, et al: Correlation of serum magnesium levels and cardiac digitalis intoxication. *Am J Cardiol* 33:225-9 (Feb) 1974.

1235. Bellville JW, Cohen EN, et al: The interaction of morphine and d-tubocurarine on respiration and grip strength in man. *Clin Pharmacol Ther* 5:35-43 (Jan-Feb) 1964.

1236. Benn A, et al: Effect of intraluminal pH on the absorption of pteroylmonoglutamic acid. *Br Med J* 1:148-50 (Jan 16) 1971.

1237. Bergman H: Hypoglycemic coma during sulfonylurea therapy. *Acta Med Scand* 177:287-298 (Mar) 1965.

1238. Berns A, Rubinfeld S, et al: Hazard of combining allopurinol and thiopurine. *N Engl J Med* 286:730 (Mar 30) 1972.

1239. Bieger R, de Jonge H, et al: Influence of nitrazepam on oral anticoagulation with phenprocoumon. *Clin Pharmacol Ther* 13:361-5 (May-June) 1972.

1240. Bianchine JR, Sunyapridakul L: Interactions between levodopa and other drugs: significance in the treatment of parkinson's disease. *Drugs* 6:364-88 (May-June) 1973.

1241. Bianchine JR, et al: Levodopa and pyridoxine coadministration: Differential metabolic effect in parkinson and normal subjects. *Ann Intern Med* 78:830 (May) 1973.

1242. Birch AA Jr, Mitchell GD, Playbord GA, et al: Changes in serum potassium response to succinylcholine following trauma. *JAMA* 210:490-3 (Oct 20) 1969.

1243. Bleiweiss H: Salt supplements with lithium. *Lancet* 1:416 (Feb 21) 1970.

1244. Bluestone R, et al: Effect of drugs on urate binding to plasma proteins. *Br Med J* 4:590-3 (Dec 6) 1969.

1245. Boakes AJ, Lawrence DR, et al: Interactions between sympathomimetic amines and antidepressant agents in man. *Br Med J* 1:311-5 (Feb 10) 1973.

1246. Boakes AJ: Sympathomimetic amines and antidepressant agents *Br Med J* 2:114 (Apr 14) 1973.

1247. Boekhout-Mussert MJ, Loeliger EA: Influence of ibuprofen on oral anticoagulation with phenprocoumon. *J Int Med Res* 2:279-83 1974.

1248. Boger WP, Pitts FW: Influence of p-(Di-N-propylsulfamyl)-benzoic acid, "Benemid," on para-aminosalicylic acid (PAS) plasma concentrations. *Am Rev Tuberc* 61:862, 1950.

1249. Boman G, Borga O: Drug interaction: decreased serum concentrations of rifampicin when given with P.A.S. *Lancet* 1:800 (Apr. 17) 1971.

1250. Booker HE, et al: Concurrent administration of phenobarbital and diphenylhydantoin: lack of an interference effect. *Neurology* 21:383-5 (Apr) 1971.

1251. Bobrow SN, Jaffe E, Yong RC: Anuria and acute tubular necrosis associated with gentamicin and cephalothin. *JAMA* 222:1546-7 (Dec 18) 1972.

1252. Boston Collaborative Drug Surveillance Program: Interaction between chloral hydrate and warfarin. *N Engl J Med* 286:53-5 (Jan 13) 1972.

1253. *ibid:* Adverse reactions to the tricyclic antidepressant drugs. *Lancet* 1:529-31 (Mar 4) 1972.

1254. *ibid:* Excess of ampicillin rashes associated with allopurinol or hyperuricemia. *N Engl J Med* 286:505-7 (Mar 9) 1972.

1255. *ibid:* Tetracycline and drug-attributed rises in blood urea nitrogen. *JAMA* 220:377-79 (Apr 17) 1972.

1256. *ibid:* Allopurinol and cytotoxic drugs. Interaction in relation to bone marrow depression. *JAMA* 227:1036-40 (Mar 4) 1974.

1257. Bouchier IA, Williams HS: Determination of faecal blood-loss after combined alcohol and sodium-acetylsalicylate intake. *Lancet* 1:178-80 (Jan 25) 1969.

1258. Bowe JC, et al: Evaluation of folic acid supplements in children taking phenytoin. *Dev Med Child Neurol* 13:343, 1971 (References and Reviews, *JAMA* 217:1272, 1971).

1259. Brainerd H, et al: *Current Diagnosis and Treatment.* Los Altos, California, Lange Medical Publications, 1970, p. 621.

1260. Brauner GJ: Ampicillin rashes. *N Engl J Med* 286:1217 (June 1) 1972.

1261. Breckenridge A, Ormi ML, et al: Dose-dependent enzyme induction. *Clin Pharmacol Ther* 14:514-20 (July-Aug) 1973.

1262. Bressler R, Vargas-Cord M, Lehovitz HE: Tranylcypromine: a potent insulin secretagogue and hypoglycemic agent. *Diabetes* 17:617-24 (Oct) 1968.

1263. Bridgmen JF, et al: Complications during clofibrate treatment of nephrotic-syndrome hyperhypoproteinaemia. *Lancet* 2:506-509 (Sep 9) 1972.

1264. Brogan E, et al: Glucagon therapy in heart failure. *Lancet* 1:482-4 (Mar 8) 1969; 1157-8 (Jun 7) 1969.

1265. Brooks SM, et al: Adverse effects of phenobarbital on corticosteroid metabolism in patients with bronchial asthma. *N Engl J Med* 286:1125-28 (May 25) 1972.

1266. Brotherton PM, et al: A study of the metabolic fate of chlorpropamide in man. *Clin Pharmacol Ther* 10:505-514 (July-Aug) 1969.

1267. Brozovic M, Curd LJ: Prothrombin during warfarin treatment. *Br J Haematol* 24:579-88 (May) 1973.

1268. Buchanan RA, Allen RJ: Diphenylhydantoin and phenobarbital blood levels in epileptic children. *Neurology* 21:866-871 (Aug) 1971.

1269. Buchanan RA, Heffelfinger JC, Weiss CF: The effect of phenobarbital on diphenylhydantoin metabolism in children. *Pediatrics* 43:114-6 (Jan) 1969.

1270. Bullip NF: *American Drug Index.* Philadelphia, J.B. Lippincott Co. 1977.

1271. Burland WL, et al: Combining cephaloridine and streptomycin for the treatment and prophylaxis of neonatal infections. *Postgrad Med J* 46 (Suppl):85-89 (Oct-Dec) 1970.

1272. Burnett GB, Reading HW: Drug interactions in alcoholism treatment. *Lancet* 1:415 (Feb 22) 1969.

1273. Burrows GD, Davies B: Antidepressants and barbiturates *Br Med J* 4:113 (Oct 9) 1971.

1274. Busuttil AA, et al: Possible cephaloridine nephrotoxicity in a neonate. *Lancet* 1:264-5 (Feb 3) 1973.

1275. Calabro JJ, Castleman B: Case records of the Massachusetts General Hospital (Case 4-1972). *N Engl J Med* 286:205-212 (Jan 27) 1972.

1276. Caldwell JH, et al: Interruption of the enterohepatic circulation of digitoxin by cholestyramine. *J Clin Invest* 50:2638-44 (Dec) 1971.

1277. Carr DT, et al: Concentration of PAS and tuberculostatic potency of serum after administration of PAS with and without Benemid. *Proc Staff Meet Mayo Clin* 27:209-15 (May 21) 1952.

1278. Carter AB: Pyridoxine and parkinsonism *Br Med J* 4:236 (Oct 27) 1973.

1279. Carter D, et al: Effect of oral contraceptives on drug and vitamin D_3 metabolism *Clin Pharmacol Ther* 15:202 (Feb) 1974.

1280. Carulli N, et al: Alcohol drugs interaction in man: alcohol and tolbutamide. *Eur J Clin Invest* 1:421-4 (Sep) 1971.

1281. Casdorph HR: Safe uses of cholestyramine *Ann Intern Med* 72:759 (May) 1970.

1282. Casdorph HR: The efficacy and safety of cholestyramine therapy in hyperlipidemic patients *Ann Intern Med* 74:818 (May) 1971.

1283. Cerasi E, et al: Role of adrenergic receptors in glucose-induced insulin secretion in man. *Lancet* 2:301-2 (Aug 9) 1969.

1284. Champion GD, Paulus HE, et al: The effect of aspirin on serum indomethacin. *Clin Pharmacol Ther* 13:239-44 (Mar-Apr) 1972.

1285. Chaplin H, Jr., Cassell M: Studies on the possible relationship of tolbutamide to dicumarol in anticoagulant therapy. *Am J Med Sci* 235:706-716 (Jun) 1958.

1286. Chapman AH: Reaction to alcohol and chloral hydrate *JAMA* 167:273 (May 10) 1958.

1287. Cheng SH, White A: Effect of orally administered neomycin on the absorption of penicillin V. *N Engl J Med* 267:1269-7 (Dec 20) 1962.

1288. Chignell CF, Starkweather DK: Optical studies of drug-protein complexes. V. The interaction of phenylbutazone, flufenamic acid, and dicumarol with acetylsalicylic acid-treated human serum albumin. *Mol Pharmacol* 7:229-237 (May) 1971.

1289. Christiansen J, Dam M: Influence of phenobarbital and diphenylhydantoin on plasma carbamazepine levels in patients with epilepsy. *Acta Neurol Scand* 49:543, 1973.

1290. Chung D-K, Koenig MG: Reversible cardiac enlargement during treatment with amphotericin B and hydrocortisone. *Am Rev Resp Dis* 103:831-41 (Jun) 1971.

1291. Churchill D: Persisting renal insufficiency after methoxyflurane anesthesia. *Am J Med* 56:575-82 (Apr) 1974.

1292. Cleaveland CR, Shand DG: Effect of route of administration on the relationship between β-adrenergic blockade and plasma propranolol level. *Clin Pharmacol Ther* 13:181-5 (Mar-Apr) 1972.

1293. *Clin-Alert,* Anticoagulants-Drug Interactions. No. 103, May 8, 1968. See also ref no 223.

1294. Coe RO, Bull FE: Cirrhosis associated with methotrexate treatment of psoriasis. *JAMA* 206:1515-20 (Nov 11) 1968.

1295. Coffey JJ, et al: Effect of allopurinol on the pharmacokinetics of 6-mercaptopurine (NSC 755) in cancer patients. *Cancer Res* 32:1283-1289 (Jun) 1972.

1296. Cohen H: Mineral oil, vitamin A, and carotene. Genesis and correction of a common misconception. *J Med Soc NJ* 67:111-115 (Mar) 1970.

1297. Cohen PF, et al: A simple test for abnormal pseudocholinesterase. *Anesthesiology* 32:281-2 (Mar) 1970.

1298. Cohn HD: Rifampicin and the pill *JAMA* 228:828 (May 13) 1974.

1299. Coldwell BB, Thomas BH: Effect of aspirin on the fate of bishydroxycoumarin in the rat. *J Pharm Pharmacol* 23:226-7 (Mar) 1971.

1300. Conn JW: Hypertension, the potassium ion and impaired carbohydrate tolerance. *N Engl J Med* 273:1135-43 (Nov 18) 1965.

1301. Consolo S, et al: Delayed absorption of phenylbutazone caused by desmethylimipramine in Humans. *Eur J Pharmacol* 10:239-42 (May) 1970.

1302. Cotzias GC: Metabolic modification of some neurologic disorders. *JAMA* 210:1255-62 (Nov 17) 1969.

1303. Cotzias GC, Papavasiliou PS: Blocking the negative effects of pyridoxine on patients receiving levodopa. *JAMA* 215:1504-5 (Mar 1) 1971.

1304. Council on Drugs—Evaluation of mesoridazine (Serentil). *JAMA* 216:313-314 (Apr 12) 1971.

1305. *ibid:* Evaluation of a hypocholesterolemic agent. Dextrothyroxine sodium (Choloxin). *JAMA* 208:1014-1015 (May 12) 1969.

1306. *ibid:* Evaluation of a new antituberculous agent, Rifampin (Rifadin, Rimactane). *JAMA* 220:414-415 (Apr 17) 1972.

1307. Cousins MJ, Mazze RI: Tetracycline, methoxyflurane anaesthesia, and renal dysfunction. *Lancet* 1:751-752 (Apr 1) 1972.

1308. Crawford JS, Hooi HW: Binding of bromsulphthalein by serum albumin from pregnant women, neonates and subjects on oral contraceptives. *Br J Anaesth* 40:723-9 (Oct) 1968.

1309. Csogor SI, Papp J: Competition between sulphonamides and thiopental for the binding sites of plasma proteins. *Arzneim Forsch* 20:1925-27 (Dec) 1970.

1310. Csogor SI, Kerek SF: Enhancement of thiopentone anesthesia by sulpha furazole. *Br J Anaesth* 42:988-90 (Nov) 1970.

1311. Cullen JH, Levine M, Fiore JM: Studies of hyperuricemia produced by pyrazinamide. *Am J Med* 23:587-595 (Oct) 1957.

1312. Curran FJ, et al: Report of a severe case of tetanus managed with large doses of intramuscular succinylcholine. *Anesth Analg* 47:218-221 (May-June) 1968.

1313. Curry SH, et al: Factors affecting chlorpromazine plasma levels in psychiatric patients. *Arch Gen Psychiat* 22:209-15 (Mar) 1970.

1314. Cushard WG, et al: Blastomycosis of bone. Treatment with intramedullary amphotericin B. *J Bone Joint Surg* 51A:704, 1969.

1315. Dalgas M, et al: Hypoglycemic episodes induced by phenylbutazone in diabetic patients treated with chlorpropamide. *Ugeskr Laeg* 127:834, 1965.

1316. Dall JLC, et al: Hypogylcaemia due to chlorpropamide. *Scot Med J* 12:403-4 (Nov) 1967.

1317. Dallos V, Heathfield K: Iatrogenic epilepsy due to antedepressant drugs. *Br Med J* 4:80-82 (Oct 11) 1969.

1318. Davidson MB, et al: Phenformin, hypoglycemia and lactic acidosis. *N Engl J Med* 275:886-8 (Oct 20) 1966.

1319. Deckert FW: Ascorbic acid and warfarin. *JAMA* 223:440 (Jan 22) 1973.

1320. De Oya JC, et al: Decreased anticoagulant tolerance with oxymetholone in paroxysmal nocturnal haemoglobinuria *Lancet* 2:259 (July 31) 1971.

1321. De Titis F, et al: Chloramphenicol combined with ampicillin in treatment of typhoid. *Br Med J* 4:17-18 (Oct 7) 1972.

1322. Deykin D: The use of heparin. *N Engl J Med* 280:937-8 (Apr 24) 1969.

1323. Newmark HL, Scheiner J: Destruction of vitamin B_{12} by vitamin C. *Am J Clin Nutr* 30:299 (Mar) 1976.

1324. Diamond WD, Buchanan RA: A clinical study of the effect of phenobarbital on diphenylhydantoin plasma levels. *J Clin Pharmacol* 10:306-11 (Sep-Oct) 1970.

1325. Dietze F, Brushke G: Inhibition of iron absorption by pancreatic extracts. *Lancet* 1:424 (Feb 21) 1970.

1326. Difazio CA, Brown RE: Lidocaine metabolism in normal and phenobarbital-pretreated dogs. *Anesthesiology* 36:238-243 (May) 1972.

1327. Dobbing J: Faecal blood-loss after sodium acetylsalicylate taken with alcohol. *Lancet* 1:527-8 (Mar 8) 1969.

1328. Dodds MG, Foord RD: Enhancement by potent diuretics of renal tubular necrosis induced by cephaloridine. *Br J Pharmacol* 40:227-36 (Oct) 1970.

1329. Doll R, et al: Treatment of gastric ulcer with car-benoxolone: antagonistic effect of spironolactone. *Gut* 9:42-5 (Feb) 1968.

1330. McLean AEM: Treatment of paracetamol over-dose. *Lancet* 2:362, 1976.

1331. Dretchen K, et al: The interaction of diazepam with myoneural blocking agents. *Anesthesiology* 34:463-8 (May) 1971.

1332. Dreyfuss J, et al: Metabolism of procainamide in rhesus monkey and man. *Clin Pharmacol Ther* 13:366-71 (May-June) 1972.

1333. Dryden GE: Incidence of tubular degeneration with microlithiasis following methoxyflurane compared with other anesthetic agents. *Anesth Analg* 53:383-5 (May-Jun) 1974.

1334. Dubin HV, Harrell ER: Liver disease associated with methotrexate treatment of psoriatic patients. *Arch Dermatol* 102:498-503 (Nov) 1970.

1335. Dujovne CA, et al: The stomach as an important factor in the metabolism and effectiveness of L-DOPA in parkinsonian patients *Gastroenterology* 58:1039 (June) 1970.

1336. Eade NR, et al: Potentiation of bishydroxycou-marin in dogs by isoniazid and p-aminosalicylic acid. *Am Rev Resp Dis* 103:792-9 (June) 1971.

1337. Earle BV: Thyroid hormone and tricyclic antide-pressants in resistant depressions. *Am J Psychiat* 126:1667-9 (May) 1970.

1338. Eastham RD: Warfarin dosage influenced by clo-fibrate plus age. *Lancet* 1:1450 (June 23) 1973.

1339. Eastham RD, Griffiths EP: Reduction of platelet adhesiveness and prolongation of coagulation time of activated plasma by glyceryl guaiacolate. *Lancet* 1:795-6 (Apr 9) 1966.

1340. Editorial: Alcohol and hypoglycemic coma. *JAMA* 206:639 (Oct 14) 1968.

1341. Editorial: Aminocaproic acid in haemophilia and in menorrhagia. *Drug Ther Bull* 5:63-4 (Aug 4) 1967.

1342. Editorial: Analgesics and monoamine-oxidase in-hibitors. *Br Med J* 4:284 (Nov 4) 1967.

1343. Editorial: A second look at lincomycin (Lincocin). *Med Lett Drugs Ther* 11:107-8 (Dec 26) 1969.

1344. Editorial: Aspirin and bleeding *JAMA* 218:89 (Oct 4) 1971.

1345. Editorial: Aspirin and gastrointestinal bleeding. *JAMA* 207:2430-1 (Mar 31) 1969.

1346. Editorial: Chloral hydrate and oral anticoagu-lants. *Lancet* 1:524 (Mar 4) 1972.

1347. Editorial: Chlorpromazine—another guanethi-dine antagonist *JAMA* 220:1288-9 (June 5) 1972.

1348. Editorial: Clinicopathologic conference: Hyper-tension and the lupus syndrome. *Am J Med* 49:519-28 (Oct) 1970.

1349. Editorial: Doxapram (Dopram)—An Analeptic. *Med Lett Drugs Ther* 11:7-8 (Jan 24) 1969.

1350. Editorial: Drug interactions *Lancet* 1:904-5 (Apr 19) 1975.

1351. Editorial: Drug interactions may need change in warfarin dose *JAMA* 213:1251-2 (Aug 24) 1970.

1352. Editorial: Veterans Administration Cooperative Study on Antihypertensive agents. *Arch Intern Med* 106:81-96 (Jul) 1960: Effects of treatment on morbidity in hypertension. II. Results in patients

with diastolic blood pressure averaging 90 through 114 mm Hg. *JAMA* 213:1143-52 (Aug 17) 1970.

1353. Editorial: Evaluation of a new antibacterial agent. Cephaloridine (Loridine). *JAMA* 206:1289-90 (Nov 4) 1968.

1354. Editorial: Evaluation of a new antipsychotic agent. Thiothixene (Navane). *JAMA* 205:924-5 (Sep 23) 1968.

1355. Editorial: Evaluation of a new antituberculosis agent: rifampin (Rifadin, Rimactane). *JAMA* 220:414-5 (Apr 17) 1972.

1356. Editorial: FDA approves lithium for manic de-pression *JAMA* 212:558 (Apr 27) 1970.

1357. Editorial: Foods potentially harmful to patients taking MAO inhibitors. *Med Lett Drugs Ther* 18:32 (Mar 26) 1976.

1358. Editorial: General practitioner clinical trials. Chlordiazepoxide with amitriptyline in neurotic depression. *Practitioner* 202:437-40 (Mar) 1969.

1359. Editorial: Haloperiodol *Med Lett Drugs Ther* 9:70-72 (Sep 8) 1967.

1360. Editorial: Heavy drinking accelerates drugs' breakdown in liver. *JAMA* 206:1709 (Nov 18) 1968.

1361. Cholestyramine. *Med Lett Drugs Ther* 16:33-36 (Apr 12) 1974.

1362. Laiho K, et al: Death in the sauna bath following intake of quinine and alcohol. *Arch Toxik* 21:352-4, 1966.

1363. Editorial: Interactions of oral anticoagulants with other drugs. *Med Lett Drug Ther* 9:97, 1967.

1364. Svendsen T, Kristensen M, et al: The influence of disulfiram on the half-life and metabolic clearance rate of diphenylhydantoin and tolbutamide in man. *Eur J Clin Pharmacol* 9:439-41, 1976.

1365. Editorial: Metabolism of drugs. *Br Med J* 1:767-8 (Mar 28) 1970.

1366. Editorial: Methylphenidate (Ritalin). *Med Lett Drug Ther* 11:47-8 (May 30) 1969.

1367. Editorial: *New Drugs,* ed 3. Chicago, Council on Drugs of the American Medical Association, 1967, pp 32-37.

1368. Editorial: *New Drugs,* ed 3. Chicago, Council on Drugs of the American Medical Association, 1967, pp 183-187.

1369. Editorial: Official literature on new drugs: pro-triptyline HCl (Vivactil HCl). *Clin Pharmacol Ther* 9:409-12 (May-June) 1968.

1370. Editorial: Official literature on new drugs: So-dium dextrothyroxine. *Clin Pharmacol Ther* 8:629-36 (July-Aug) 1967.

1371. Editorial: Oral contraceptives and carbohydrate metabolism. *Br Med J* 3:726 (Sep 16) 1967.

1372. Editorial: Possible interaction occurs with aspirin and two drugs *JAMA* 214:39 (Oct 5) 1970.

1373. Editorial: Oral hypoglycemic agents. *Med Lett Drug Ther* 11:5-7 (Jan 24) 1969.

1374. Editorial: Propranolol. *Lancet* 1:939-40 (Apr 29) 1967.

1375. Editorial: Rifampicin, "pill" do not go well to-gether *JAMA* 227:608 (Feb 11) 1974.

1376. Editorial: Risk of drug interaction may exist in 1 of 13 prescriptions *JAMA* 220:1287-8 (June 5) 1972.

1377. Stowers J, et al: Pharmacology and mode of action of sulfonylureas in man. *Lancet* 1:278-83, 1958.

1378. Daubresse J, et al: Potentiation of hypoglycemic effect of sulfonylureas by clofibrate. *N Engl J Med* 294:613, 1976.

1379. Editorial: Scheduling avoids interaction problem *JAMA* 215:876 (Feb 8) 1971.

1380. Bonaccorsi A, et al: Studies on the hypoglycaemia induced by chlorpromazine in rats. *Br J Pharmacol* 23:93-100 (Aug) 1964.

1381. Schwartz L, Munoz R: Blood sugar levels in patients treated with chlorpromazine. *Am J Psychiat* 125:253-5 (Aug) 1968.

1382. Editorial: Therapeutic conferences. Drug Interaction. *Brit Med J* 1:389-91 (Feb 13) 1971.

1383. Ferrari C, et al: Potentiation of hypoglycemic response to intravenous tolbutamide by clofibrate. *N Engl J Med* 294:1184 (May 20) 1976.

1384. Jankelson OM, et al: Effect of coffee on glucose tolerance and circulating insulin in men with maturity-onset diabetes. *Lancet* 1:527-9 (Mar 11) 1967.

1385. Editorial: The safety of cyclamate—an artificial sweetener. *Med Lett Drug Ther* 11:85-87 (Oct 17) 1969.

1386. Sandberg H, et al: Coffee's effect on diabetes tested. *JAMA* 209:350 (Jul 21) 1969.

1387. Editorial: Thiabendazole (mintezol)—A new anthelmintic. *Med Lett Drug Ther* 9:99-102 (Dec 15) 1967.

1388. Editorial: Today's Drugs. Mefenamic acid. *Br Med J* 2:1506-7 (Dec 17) 1966.

1389. Edwards MS, Curtis JR: Decreased anticoagulant tolerance with oxymetholone *Lancet* 2:221 (July 24) 1971.

1390. Elgee NJ: Medical aspects of oral contraceptives. *Ann Intern Med* 72:409-18 (Mar) 1970.

1391. Elion GB, et al: Renal clearance of oxipurinol, the chief metabolite of allopurinol. *Am J Med* 45:69-77 (July) 1968.

1392. Elliott GR, Armstrong MF: Sodium bicarbonate and oral tetracycline *Clin Pharmacol Ther* 13:459 (May-June) 1972.

1393. Elliott HC: Reduced adrenocortical steroid excretion rates in man following aspirin administration. *Metabolism* 11:1015-18 (Sep) 1962.

1394. El-Yousef MK, Manier DH: Estrogen effects on phenothiazine derivative blood levels *JAMA* 228:827-8 (May 13) 1974.

1395. El-Yousef MK, Manier DH: Tricyclic antidepressants and phenothiazines. *JAMA* 229:1419 (Sep 9) 1974.

1396. Emmanuel JH, Montgomery RD: Gastric ulcer and the antiarthritic drugs. *Postgrad Med J* 47:227-32 (Apr) 1971.

1397. Emori W, et al: The pharmacokinetics of indomethacin in serum *Clin Pharmacol Ther* 14:134 (Jan-Feb) 1973.

1398. Engel J, et al: Phenytoin encephalopathy? *Lancet* 2:824-5 (Oct 9) 1971.

1399. Esbenshade JH, Jr, et al: A long-term evaluation of pargyline hydrochloride in hypertension. *Am J Med Sci* 251:81-5 (Jan) 1966.

1400. Espir M, et al: Epilepsy and oral contraception. *Br Med J* 1:294-5 (Feb 1) 1969.

1401. Evans-Prosser CDG: The use of pethidine and

morphine in the presence of monoamine oxidase inhibitors. *Br J Anaestheia* 40:279-82 (Apr) 1968.

1402. Eykyn S, et al: Gentamicin plus carbenicillin *Lancet* 1:545-6 (Mar 13) 1971.

1403. Fahn S: "On-off" phenomenon with levodopa therapy in parkinsonism. *Neurology* 24:431-41 (May) 1974.

1404. Falliers CJ: Corticosteroids and phenobarbital in asthma *N Engl J Med* 287:201 (July 27) 1972.

1405. Faloon WW, Chodos RB: Vitamin B_{12} absorption studies using colchicine, neomycin and continuous 57Co B_{12} administration *Gastroenterology* 56:1251 (June) 1969.

1406. Fann WE, et al: Chlorpromazine reversal of the antihypertensive action of guanethidine *Lancet* 2:436-7 (Aug 21) 1971.

1407. Fann WE: Chlorpromazine: effects of antacids on its gastrointestinal absorption. *J Clin Pharmacol* 13:388-90 (Oct) 1973.

1408. Fann WE, et al: The effects of antacids on the blood levels of chlorpromazine. *Clin Pharmacol Ther* 14:135 (Jan-Feb) 1973.

1409. Fausa O: Salicylate-induced hypoprothrombinemia. *Acta Med Scand* 188:403-8 (Nov) 1970.

1410. FDA: *Reports of Suspected Adverse Reactions to Drugs.* 1969, No. 690501-153-01301.

1411. FDA: *Reports of Suspected Adverse Reactions to Drugs.* 1970, No. 700201-056-00101.

1412. FDA: *Reports of Suspected Adverse Reactions to Drugs,* 1970, No. 700301-064-01001.

1413. FDA: Revised Labeling for Oral Contraceptives. *Fed Reg* 41:53630-42 (Dec 7) 1976.

1414. Feagin OT, et al: Uptake and release by guanethidine and bethanidine by the adrenergic neuron. *J Clin Invest* 48:23a (Abstracts) 1969.

1415. Feinstein DI, et al: Factor V inhibitor: Report of a case, with comments on a possible effect of streptomycin. *Ann Intern Med* 78:385-8 (Mar) 1973.

1416. Feldman S, Carlstedt BC: Effect of antacid on absorption of enteric-coated aspirin *JAMA* 227:660 (Feb 11) 1974.

1417. Fermaglich J, Chase TN: Methyldopa or methyldopahydrazine as levodopa synergists. *Lancet* 1:1261-2 (June 2) 1973.

1418. Fermaglich J, O'Doherty DS: Second generation of l-dopa therapy. *Neurology* 21:408-9 (Apr) 1971.

1419. Fermaglich J, O'Doherty DS: Effect of gastric motility on levodopa. *Dis Nerv Syst* 33:624-5 (Sep) 1972.

1420. Fernandez D: Another esophageal rupture after alcohol and disulfiram. *N Engl J Med* 286:610 (Mar 16) 1972.

1421. Fernandez PC, Kovnat PJ: Metabolic acidosis reversed by the combination of magnesium hydroxide and a cation exchange resin. *N Engl J Med* 286:23-4 (Jan 6) 1972.

1422. Fichman MP, et al: Diuretic-induced hyponatremia. *Ann Intern Med* 75:853-63 (Dec) 1971.

1423. Fincham RW, et al: The influence of diphenylhydantoin on primidone metabolism. *Arch Neurol* 30:259-62 (Mar) 1974.

1424. Finegold SM: Interaction of antimicrobial therapy and intestinal flora. *Am J Clin Nutr* 23:1466-71 (Nov) 1970.

1425. Fleischer N, et al: Chronic laxative-induced hyperaldosteronism and hypokalemia stimulating Bartter's syndrome. *Ann Intern Med* 70:791-8 (Apr) 1969.

1426. Flemenbaum A: Does lithium block the effects of amphetamine? *Am J Psychiat* 131:820-1 (July) 1974.

1427. Fleming P, et al: Levodopa in drug-induced extrapyramidal disorders. *Lancet* 2:1186 (Dec 5) 1970.

1428. Forrest FM, et al: Modification of chlorpromazine metabolism by some other drugs frequently administered to psychiatric patients. *Biol Psychiat* 2:53, 1970.

1429. Frascino JA: Tetracycline, methoxyflurane anaesthesia, and renal dysfunction *Lancet* 1:1127 (May 20) 1972.

1430. Freeman J, Schulman MP: Reactions of chloral hydrate and ethanol with alcohol dehydrogenase from human liver *Fed Proc* 29:275Abs, 1970 (Abstracts, 54th annual Meeting, FASEB, Atlantic City, NJ, Apr 12-17, 1970.)

1431. Frey HH, Kampmann E: Interaction of amphetamine with anticonvulsant drugs. II. Effect of amphetamine on the absorption of anticonvulsant drugs. *Acta Pharmacol Toxicol* 24:310, 1966.

1432. Fillastre JP, Laumonier R, et al: Acute renal failure associated with combined gentamicin and cephalothin therapy. *Brit Med J* 2:396-397 (May 19) 1973.

1433. Friend DG, Bell WR, Kline NS: The action of L-dihydroxyphenylalanie in patients receiving nialamide. *Clin Pharmacol Ther* 6:362-6 (May-June) 1965.

1434. Fulop M, et al: Possible diphenylhydantoin-induced arrhythmia in hypothyroidism. *JAMA* 196:454-6 (May 2) 1966.

1435. Gabriel R, et al: Reversible encephalopathy and acute renal failure after cephaloridine. *Br Med J* 4:283-4 (Oct 31) 1970.

1436. Gallagher BB, et al: Primidone, diphenylhydantoin and phenobarbital. Aspects of acute and chronic toxicity. *Neurology* 23:145-49 (Feb) 1973.

1437. Garrod LP: Causes of failure in antibiotic treatment. *Br Med J* 4:473-6 (Nov 25) 1972.

1438. Genton E: Guidelines for heparin therapy. *Ann Intern Med* 80:77-82 (Jan) 1974.

1439. Gershberg H, Hecht A: Antidiabetic effect of acetohexamide. Effect of potassium supplements. *NJ State J Med* 69:1287-91 (May 15) 1969.

1440. Gessner PK, Soble AG: Studies on the role of brain 5-hydroxytryptamine in the interaction between tranylcypromine and meperidine (abst). *Fed Proc* 29:685 Abs.

1441. Forrest WH, Jr, Brown BW, et al: Dextroamphetamine with morphine for the treatment of postoperative pain. *N Engl J. Med* 296:712-715 (Mar 31) 1977.

1442. Spanney J, et al: Hyperglycemic, hyperosmolar, nonketoacidotic diabetes; a complication of steroid and immunosuppressive therapy. *Diabetes* 18:107-10, 1969.

1443. Gibberd FB, Small E: Interaction between levodopa and methyldopa. *Br Med J* 2:90-91 (Apr 14) 1973.

1444. Giesecke AH, Jr, et al: Of magnesium, muscle re-

1445. laxants, toxemic parturients, and cats. *Anesth Analg* 47:689-95 (Nov-Dec) 1968.

1445. Glassner J: Methotrexate and psoriasis *JAMA* 210:1925 (Dec 8) 1969.

1446. Glatt MM: Drug interactions in alcoholism treatment *Lancet* 1:627-8 (Mar 22) 1969.

1447. Glazko AJ, et al: Metabolic disposition of diphenylhydantoin in normal human subjects following intravenous administration. *Clin Pharmacol Ther* 10:498-504 (July-Aug) 1969.

1448. Goddard JE, Jr, Phillips OC: The influence of nonanesthetic drugs on the course of anesthesia. *Penn Med J* 68:43-6 (June) 1965.

1449. Goldberg LI, Whitsett TL: Cardiovascular effects of levodopa. *Clin Pharmacol Ther* 12:376-82 (Mar-Apr) 1971.

1450. Goldfinger P: Hypokalemia, metabolic acidosis, and hypocalcemic tetany in a patient taking laxatives. *J Mt Sinai Hosp* 36:113-116 (Mar-Apr) 1969.

1451. Gooch AS, et al: Influence of exercise on arrhythmias induced by digitalis-diuretic therapy in patients with atrial fibrillation. *Am J Cardiol* 33:230-7 (Feb) 1974.

1452. Goodhue WW Jr: Disulfiram-metronidazole (well identified) toxicity. *N Engl J Med* 280:1482-3 (June 26) 1969.

1453. Goodpasture HC, et al: Clinical correlations during amphotericin B therapy (abst). *Ann Intern Med* 76:872 (May) 1972.

1454. Gould L, et al: Prothrombin levels maintained with meprobamate and warfarin. A controlled study. *JAMA* 220:1460-2 (June 12) 1972.

1455. Grace ND, et al: Effect of allopurinol on iron mobilization. *Gastroenterology* 59:103-8 (Jan) 1970.

1456. Gram LF, Overo KF: Drug interaction: Inhibitory effect of neuroleptics on metabolism of tricyclic antidepressants in man. *Br Med J* 1:463-5 (Feb 19) 1972.

1457. Gram LF, et al: Influence of neuroleptics and benzoliazepines on metabolism of tricyclic antidepressants in man. *Am J Psychiatr* 131:863-6 (Aug) 1974.

1458. Gram LF, Kefod B, et al: Imipramine metabolism: pH dependent distribution and urinary excretion. *Clin Pharmacol Ther* 12:239-44 (Mar-Apr) 1971.

1459. Greenberger NJ: Absorption of tetracyclines: interference by iron. *Ann Intern Med* 74:792-3 (May) 1971.

1460. Greenblatt DJ, Koch-Weser J: adverse reactions to spironolactone: A report from The Boston Colaborative Drug Surveillance Program. *Clin Pharmacol Ther* 14:136-7 (Jan-Feb) 1973.

1461. Griner PF, et al: Chloral hydrate and warfarin interaction: clinical significance? *Ann Intern Med* 74:540-3 (Apr) 1971.

1462. Gross L, Brotman M: Hypoprothrombinemia and hemorrhage associated with cholestyramine therapy. *Ann Intern Med* 72:95-6 (Jan) 1970.

1463. Gupta KK: Guanethidine and glucose tolerance in diabetics. *Br Med J* 3:679 (Sep 14) 1968.

1464. Gupta KK: The anti-diabetic action of guanethidine. *Postgrad Med J* 45:455-6 (July) 1969.

1465. Hadden JW, Metzner RJ: Pseudoketosis and hyperacetaldehydemia in paraldehyde acidosis. *Am J Med* 47:642-7 (Oct) 1969.

1466. Hague DE, Smith ME, Ryan JR, et al: The effect of methylphenidate and prolintane on the metabolism of ethyl biscoumacetate. *Clin Pharmacol Ther* 12:259-62 (Mar-Apr) 1971.

1467. Hahn TJ, et al: Effect of chronic anticonvulsant therapy on serum 25-hydroxycalciferol levels in adults. *N Engl J Med* 287:900-4 (Nov 2) 1972.

1468. Haider I: A comparative trial of Ro 4-6270 and amitriptyline in depressive illness. *Br J Psychiat* 113:993-8, 1967.

1469. Halsted CH, McIntyre PA: Intestinal malabsorption caused by aminosalicylic acid therapy. *Arch Intern Med* 130:935-9 (Dec) 1972.

1470. Ham JM: Hypoprothrombinaemia in patients undergoing prolonged intensive care. *Med J Aust* 2:716-8 (Oct 2) 1971.

1471. Hamblin TJ: Interaction between warfarin and phenformin. *Lancet* 2:1323 (Dec 11) 1971.

1472. Hammer W, Martins S, et al: A comparative study of the metabolism of desmethylimipramine, nortriptyline, and oxyphenbutazone in man. *Clin Pharmacol Ther* 10:44-9 (Jan-Feb) 1969.

1473. Hansen JM, Siersbaek-Nielson K, et al: Effect of diphenylhydantoin on the metabolism of dicumarol in man. *Acta Med Scand* 189:15-19 (Jan-Feb) 1971.

1474. Hansen JM, Siersbaek-Nielson K, et al: Carbamazepine-induced acceleration of diphenylhydantoin and warfarin metabolism in man. *Clin Pharmacol Ther* 12:539-43 (May-June) 1971.

1475. Hansten PD: Oral anticoagulant therapy in the patient with altered thyroid function. *Northwest Med J* 1:39-45 (April) 1974.

1476. Hansten PD: Interactions between anticonvulsant drugs: primidone, diphenylhydantoin and phenobarbital. *Northwest Med J* 1:17-23 (Oct) 1974.

1477. Haque N, et al: Studies on dexamethasone metabolism in man: effect of diphenylhydantoin. *J Clin Endocrinol Metab* 34:44-50 (Jan) 1972.

1478. Harley BJS, Davies RO: Propranolol in the office treatment of angina pectoris. *Can Med Assoc J* 99:527-30 (Sep 21) 1968.

1479. Harris EL: Adverse reactions to oral antidiabetic agents. *Br Med J* 3:29-30 (July 3) 1971.

1480. Hedberg DL, et al: Tranylcypromine-trifluoperazine combination in the treatment of schizophrema. *Am J Psychiat* 127:1141, 1971.

1481. Heinivaara O, Palva IP: Malabsorption of vitamin B_{12} during treatment with para-aminosalicylic acid: A preliminary report. *Acta Med Scand* 175:469-71 (Apr) 1964.

1482. Hill DF: Gold therapy for rheumatoid arthritis. *Med Clin Nam* 52:733-738, 1968.

1483. Heizer WD, et al: Protein-losing gastroenteropathy and malabsorption associated with factitious diarrhea. *Ann Intern Med* 68:839-52 (Apr) 1968.

1484. Hiatt N, Bonorris G: Insulin response in pancreatectomized dogs treated with oxytetracycline. *Diabetes* 19:307-10 (May) 1970.

1485. Hickman JW, Kirtley WR: Five year's experience with Dymelor. *J Indiana State Med Assoc* 61:1114-7 (Aug) 1968.

1486. Hoch FL: The pharmacologic basis for the clinical use of thyroid hormones. *Pharmacol Physicians* 4:1-5 (April) 1970.

1487. Hoffbrand BI: Interaction of nalidixic acid and warfarin. *Br Med J* 2:666 (June 22) 1974.

1488. Hofmann LM, et al: Interactions of spironolactone and hydrochlorothiazide with aspirin in the rat and dog. *J Pharmacol Exp Ther* 180:1-5 (Jan) 1972.

1489. Holmes EL: Pharmacology of the fenamates. IV. Toleration by normal human subjects. *Ann Phys Med* (Suppl) 9:36, 1967.

1490. Hooper WD, Bochner F, et al: Plasma protein binding of diphenylhydantoin. Effects of sex hormones, renal and hepatic disease. *Clin Pharmacol Ther* 15:276-282 (Mar) 1974.

1491. Houben PFM, et al: Anticonvulsant drugs and folic acid in young mentally retarded epileptic patients. *Epilepsia* 12:235, 1971.

1492. Huffman DH, Suk Han Wan, et al: Pharmacokinetics of methotrexate. *Clin Pharmacol Ther* 14:572-9 (July-Aug) 1973.

1493. Huffman DH, et al: The effect of spironolactone on antipyrine metabolism in man. *Pharmacology* 10:338-44, 1973.

1494. Humberstone PM: Hypertension from cold remedies *Br Med J* 1:846 (Mar 29) 1969.

1495. Herbert V, Jacob E: Destruction of vitamin B_{12} by ascorbic acid. *JAMA* 230:241-2 (Oct 14) 1974; Destruction of vitamine B_{12} by vitamin C; *Am J Clin Nutr* 30:297-9 (Mar) 1976; Vitamins C and B_{12}. *JAMA* 232:246 (Apr 21) 1975.

1496. Hunt TK, et al: Effect of vitamin A on reversing the inhibitory effect of cortisone on healing of open wounds in animals and man. *Ann Surg* 170:633-41 (Oct) 1969.

1497. Hunter KR, et al: Use of levodopa with other drugs. *Lancet* 2:1283-85 (Dec 19) 1970.

1498. American Pharmaceutical Association: *Evaluation of Drug Interactions,* 1973, pp 78-9.

1499. Hurtig HI, Dyson WL: Lithium toxicity enhanced by diuresis. *N Engl J Med* 290:748-9 (Mar 28) 1974.

1500. Hurwitz A, Schlozman DL: Effects of antacids on gastrointestinal absorption of isoniazid in rat and man. *Am Rev Resp Dis* 109:41-7 (Jan) 1974.

1501. Hurwitz A: The effects of antacids on gastrointestinal drug absorption. II. Effect on sulfadiazine and quinine. *J Pharmacol Exp Ther* 179:485-9 (Dec) 1971.

1502. Hvidberg EF, et al: Studies of the interaction of phenylbutazone, oxyphenbutazone and methandrostenolone in man. *Proc Soc Exp Biol Med* 129:438-43 (Nov) 1968.

1503. Itil TI, et al: Central effect of metronidazole. *Psychiatric Research Report 24,* American Psychiatric Assoc, March, 1968.

1504. Jablonski J: Guanethidine (Ismelin) as an adjuvant in pharmacological mydriasis. *Ophthalmologica* 168:27-38, 1974.

1505. Jacobson ED, et al: An experimental malabsorption syndrome induced by neomycin. *Am J Med* 28:524-33 (Apr) 1960.

1506. Jacoby GA: Carbenicillin and gentamicin. *N Engl J Med* 284:1096-7 (May 13) 1971.

1507. Janz D, Schmidt D: Anti-epileptic drugs and failure of oral contraceptives. *Lancet* 1:1113 (Jun 1)

1974; antiepileptika und die Sicherheit oraler Kontrazeptiva. *Bibl Psychiatr* 151:82-5, 1975.

1508. Jelliffe RW: Effect of serum potassium level upon risk of digitalis toxicity. *Ann Intern Med* 78:821 (May) 1973.

1509. Jelliffe RW, Blankenhorn DH: Effect of phenobarbital on digitoxin metabolism. *Clin Res* 14:160 (Jan) 1966.

1510. Jenkins RB, Groh RH: psychic effects in patients treated with levodopa. *JAMA* 212:2265 (June 29) 1970.

1511. Jensen ON, Olesen OV: Subnormal serum folate due to anticonvulsive therapy. *Arch Neurol* 22:181-2 (Feb) 1970.

1512. Jiji RM, et al: Chloramphenicol and its sulfamoyl analogue. Report of reversible erythropoietic toxicity in healthy volunteers. *Arch Int Med* 111:70-82 (Jan) 1963.

1513. Johansson S: Apparent resistance to oral anticoagulant therapy and influence of hypnotics on some coagulation factors. *Acta Med Scand* 184:297-300 (Oct) 1968.

1514. Johnson B, et al: Effect of tolbutamide on hypotensive and oliguric drugs *Clin Res* 17:248 (Apr) 1969.

1515. Johnson HK, Waterhouse C: Relationship of alcohol and hyperlactatemia in diabetic subjects treated with phenformin. *Am J Med* 45:98-104 (July) 1968.

1516. Jori A, et al: Metabolic effects induced by the interaction of reserpine with desipramine. *J Pharm Pharmacol* 20:862-6 (Nov) 1968.

1517. Jounela AJ, Kivimaki T: Possible sensitivity to meperidine in phenylketonuria. *N Engl J Med* 288:1411 (June 28) 1973.

1518. Jubiz W, et al: Effect of diphenylhydantoin on the metabolism of dexamethasone. Mechanism of the abnormal dexamethasone suppression in humans. *N Engl J Med* 283:11-14 (July 2) 1970.

1519. Juhl RP, Blaug SM: Factors affecting release of medicaments from hard gelatin capsules. *J Pharm Sci* 62:170 (Jan) 1973.

1520. Kabins SA: Interactions among antibiotics and other drugs. *JAMA* 219:206-12 (Jan 10) 1972.

1521. Kaegi A, Pineo GF, Shimizu A, et al: Arteriovenous-shunt thrombosis. Prevention by sulfinpyrazone. *N Engl J Med* 290:304-306 (Feb 7) 1974.

1522. Kalbian VV: Iatrogenic hyperkalemic paralysis with electrocardiographic changes. *South Med J* 67:342-5 (Mar) 1974.

1523. Kaldor A, et al: Enhancement of methyldopa metabolism with barbiturate. *Br Med J* 3:518-9 (Aug 28) 1971.

1524. Kale AK, Satoskar RS: Modification of the central hypotensive effect of α-methyldopa by reserpine, imipramine and tranylcypromine. *Eur J Pharmacol* 9:120-3 (Jan) 1970.

1525. Kampmann J, et al: Effect of some drugs on penicillin half-life in blood. *Clin Pharmacol Ther* 13:516-9 (July-Aug) 1972.

1526. Kaplan SR, Calabresi P: Immunosupressive agents *N Engl J Med* 289:852-5 (Nov 1) 1973.

1527. Kaplan HL, et al: Chloral hydrate and alcohol metabolism in human subjects. *J Forensic Sci* 12:295-304 (Jul) 1967.

1528. Kaplan JA, Cooperman LH: Alarming reactions to ketamine in patients taking thyroid medication—treatment with propranolo. *Anesthesiology* 35:229-30 (Aug) 1971.

1529. Kariks J, et al: Serum folic acid and phenytoin levels in permanently hospitalized epileptic patients receiving anticonvulsant drug therapy. *Med J Aust* 2:368-71 (Aug 14) 1971.

1530. Karlin JM, Kutt H: Acute diphenylhydantoin intoxication following halothane anesthesia. *J Pediat* 76:941-4 (June) 1970.

1531. Kauffman RE, Azarnoff DL: Effect of colestipol on gastrointestinal absorption of chlorothiazide in man. *Clin Pharmacol Ther* 14:886-90 (Sep-Oct) 1973.

1532. Kazmier FJ, Spittell JA: Coumarin drug interactions. *Mayo Clin Proc* 45:249-55 (Apr) 1970.

1533. Kelley DB: Diabetic emergencies: drug-induced hypoglycemia. *Med Clin N Amer* 53:465-467 (Mar) 1969.

1534. Kenyon IE: Unplanned pregnancy in an epileptic. *Br Med J* 1:686-7 (Mar 11) 1972.

1535. Kenwright S, Levi AJ: Impairment of hepatic uptake of rifamycin antibiotics by probenecid, and its therapeutic implications. *Lancet* 2:1401-5 (Dec 22) 1973.

1536. Khurana RC: Estrogen-imipramine interaction. *JAMA* 222:702-3 (Nov 6) 1972.

1537. Killian JM, Fromm GH: Carbamazepine in the treatment of neuralgia. Use and side effects. *Arch Neurol* 19:129-36 (Aug) 1968.

1538. Kinyon GE: Anticholinesterase eye drops—need for caution. *N Engl J Med* 280:53 (Jan 2) 1969.

1539. Klippel AP, Pitsinger B: Hypoprothrombinemia secondary to antibiotic therapy and manifested by massive gastrointestinal hemorrhage. *Arch Surg* 96:266-8 (Feb) 1968.

1540. Klastersky J, et al: Gram-negative infections in cancer. Study of empiric therapy comparing carbenicillin-cephalothin with and without gentamicin. *JAMA* 227:45-8 (Jan 7) 1974.

1541. Kleinknecht D, et al: Nephrotoxicity of cephaloridine. *Ann Intern Med* 80:421 2 (Mar) 1974.

1542. Kleinknecht D, et al: Acute renal failure after high doses of gentamicin and cephalothin. *Lancet* 1:1129 (May 19) 1973.

1543. Kline NS: Experimental use of monamine oxidase inhibitors with tricyclic antidepressants *JAMA* 227:807 (Feb 18) 1974.

1544. Kline NS: Psychochemotherapeutic drug combinations *JAMA* 210:1928 (Dec 8) 1969.

1545. Koch-Weser J: Hemorrhagic reactions and drug interactions in 500 warfarin-treated patients. *Clin Pharmacol Ther* 14:139 (Jan- Feb) 1973.

1546. Koch-Weser J, et al: Adverse effects of sodium colistimethate. Manifestations and specific reaction rates during 317 course of therapy. *Ann Intern Med* 72:857-68 (Jun) 1970.

1547. Kofman O: Treatment of Parkinson's disease with l-dopa: A current appraisal. *Can Med Assoc J* 104:483-7 (Mar 20) 1971.

1548. Kokenge R, et al: Neurological sequelae following Dilantin overdose in a patient and in experimental animals. *Neurology* 15:823-9 (Sep) 1965.

1549. Konickova L, Prat V: Effect of carbenicillin, gentamicin, and their combination on experimental

Pseudomonas aeruginosa urinary tract infection. *J Clin Path* 24:113-6 (Mar) 1971.

1550. Kontturi M, Sotaniemi E: Estrogen induced metabolic changes during treatment of prostatic cancer. *Scand J Lab Clin Invest* 25:45 (Suppl 113), 1970.

1551. Kott E, et al: Excretion of dopa metabolites. *N Engl J Med* 284:395 (Feb 18) 1971.

1552. Kreisberg RA, et al: Hyperlacticacidemia in man: ethanol-phenformin synergism. *J Clin Endocr* 34:29-35 (Jan) 1972.

1553. Kristensen M, et al: Barbiturates and methyldopa metabolism. *Br Med J* 1:49 (Jan 6) 1973.

1554. Kristensen M, et al: Plasma concentration of alfamethyldopa and its main metabolite, methyldopa-O-sulfate during long-term treatment with alfamethyldopa, with special reference to possible interaction with other drugs given simulataneously. *Clin Pharmacol Ther* 14:139-140 (Jan-Feb) 1973.

1555. Kupferberg HJ, Jeffery W, Hunninghake DB: Effect of methylphenidate on plasma anticonvulsant levels. *Clin Pharmacol Ther* 13:201-4 (Mar-Apr) 1972.

1556. Kurz M: Diamox and Manifestierung von Diabetes Mellitus, *Wien Med Wschr* 118:239-241 (Mar) 1968.

1557. Kutt H, et al: The effect of phenobarbital on plasma diphenylhydantoin level and metabolism in man and in rat liver microsomes. *Neurology* 19:611-6 (June) 1969.

1558. Kutt H, et al: The effect of phenobarbital upon diphenylhydantoin metabolism in man *Neurology* 15:274-5 (Mar) 1965.

1559. Kutt H, Verebely K: Metabolism of diphenylhydantoin by rat liver microsomes. I. Characteristics of the reaction. *Biochem Pharmacol* 19:675-86, 1970.

1560. Lacher J, Lasagna I: Phenformin and lactic acidosis. *Clin Pharmacol Ther* 7:477-81 (July-Aug) 1966.

1561. Lackner H, Hunt VE: The effect of Librium on hemostasis. *Am J Med Sci* 256:368-72 (Dec) 1968.

1562. Lader MH, et al: Interactions between sympathomimetic amines and a new monamine oxidase inhibitor. *Psychopharmacologia* 18:118-23, 1970.

1563. Lahti RA, Maichel RP: The tricyclic antidepressants—Inhibition of norepinephrine uptake as related to potentiation of norepinephrine and clinical efficacy. *Biochem Pharmacol* 20:482-6, 1971.

1564. Lal S, et al: Effect of rifampicin and isoniazid on liver function. *Br Med J* 1:148-50 (Jan 15) 1972.

1565. Landon J, et al: The effect of anabolic steroids on blood sugar and plasma insulin levels in man. *Metabolism* 12:924-35 (Oct) 1963.

1566. Laurie W: Alcohol as a cause of sudden unexpected death. *Med J Aust* 1:1224-7 (Jun 5) 1971.

1567. Lavigne J-G, Marchand C: Inhibition of the gastrointestinal absorption of p-aminosalicylate (PAS) in rats and humans by diphenhydramine. *Clin Pharmacol Ther* 14:404-412 (May-June) 1973.

1568. Leon AS, et al: Pyridoxine antagonism of levodopa in Parkinsonism. *JAMA* 218:1924-27 (Dec 27) 1971.

1569. Leonards JR: Absence of gastrointestinal bleeding following administration of salicylsalicylic acid. *J Lab Clin Med* 74:911-4 (Dec) 1969.

1570. Leonards JR, Levy G: Reduction or prevention of aspirin-induced occult gastrointestinal blood loss in man. *Clin Pharmacol Ther* 10:571-5 (July-Aug) 1969.

1571. Levine R: Mechanisms of insulin secretion. *N Engl J Med* 283:522-26 (Sep 3) 1970.

1572. Levine RA: Steatorrhea induced by para-aminosalicylic acid. *Ann Intern Med* 68:1265-70 (Jun) 1968.

1573. Levine WG: Anticoagulant, antithrombotic, and thrombolytic drugs. Goodman LS, Gilman A (eds): *The Pharmacological Basis of Therapeutics.* New York, Macmillan, 1975, pp 1350-1368.

1574. Malherbe C, et al: Effect of diphenylhydantoin on insulin secretion in man. *N Engl J Med* 286:339-42, 1972.

1575. Levison ME, Kaye D: Carbenicillin plus gentamicin. *Lancet* 2:45-6 (Jul 3) 1971.

1576. Levy G, et al: Pharmacokinetic analysis of the effect of barbiturate on the anticoagulant action of warfarin in man. *Clin Pharmacol Ther* 11:372-7, 1970.

1577. Levy G, Tsuchya T: Salicylate accumulation kinetics in man. *N Engl J Med* 287:430-2 (Aug 31) 1972.

1578. Levy J, Michel-Ber E: Difficulties and complications caused in man by monoamine oxidase (MAO) inhibitors, with special reference to their specific and secondary pharmacological effects. in *Toxicity and Side-effects of Psychotropic Drugs,* Amsterdam, Exerpta Medica Foundation, pp 223-245.

1579. Lewis RJ: Effect of barbiturates on anticoagulant therapy. *N Engl J Med* 274:110 (Jan 13) 1966.

1580. Lieber CS: Hepatic and metabolic effects of alcohol (1966 to 1973). *Gastroenterology* 65:821-46, 1973.

1581. Liegler DG, Henderson ES, et al: The effect of organic acids on renal clearance of methotrexate in man. *Clin Pharmacol Ther* 10:849-57 (Nov-Dec) 1969.

1582. Lindenbaum J, et al: Impairment of digoxin absorption by neomycin. *Clin Res* 20:410, 1972.

1583. Lindquist B, Jensen KM, et al: Effect of concurrent administration of aspirin and indomethacin on serum concentrations. *Clin Pharmacol Ther* 15:247-252 (Mar) 1974.

1584. Linnoila M, Hakkinen S: Effects of diazepam and codeine, alone and in combination with alcohol, on simulated driving. *Clin Pharmacol Ther* 15:368-73 (Apr) 1974.

1585. Lipson ML, et al: Oral administration of pralidoxime chloride in echothiophate iodide therapy. *Arch Ophthal* 82:830-5 (Dec) 1969.

1586. Desser KB: Effects of "speed" and "pot" on the juvenile diabetic *JAMA* 214:2065 (Dec 14) 1970.

1587. Loeliger EA, et al: The biological disappearance rate of prothrombin, factors VII, IX and X from plasma in hypothyroidism, hyperthyroidism, and during fever. *Thromb Diath Haemorrh* 10:267-77, 1964.

1588. Longridge RGM, et al: Decreased anticoagulant tolerance with oxymetholone *Lancet* 2:90 (Jul 10) 1971.

1589. Lucarotti RL, et al: Enhanced pseudoephedrine absorption by concurrent administration of aluminum hydroxide gel in humans. *J Pharm Sci* 61:903-5 (Jun) 1972.

1590. Lutz EE, Margolis AJ: Obstetric hepatosis: treatment with cholestyramine and interim response to steroids. *Obstet Gynecol* 33:64-71 (Jan) 1969.

1591. Lyon GM: Allopurinol and cytotoxic agents. JAMA 228:1371-2 (Jun 10) 1974.

1592. MacCallum WAG: Drug interactions in alcoholism treatment *Lancet* 1:313 (Feb 8) 1969.

1593. MacLeod I: Fatal reaction to phenelzine. *Br Med J* 1:1554 (Jun 12) 1965.

1594. Maddocks AC: Indomethacin and vaccination. *Lancet* 2:210-11 (July 28) 1973.

1595. Malims JM: Diuretics in diabetes mellitus *Practitioner* 201:529, 1968.

1596. Manninen V, et al: Effect of propantheline and metoclopramide on absorption of digoxin. *Lancet* 1:1118-19 (May 19) 1973.

1597. Manninen V, et al: Altered absorption of digoxin in patients given propantheline and metoclopramide. *Lancet* 1:398-400 (Feb 24) 1973.

1598. Margulis RR, Leach RG: Effect of oral contraceptives on thyroid function. *JAMA* 206:2326-7 (Dec 2) 1968.

1599. Mark LC, et al: Hypotension following use of monoamine oxidase inhibitor. *NY State J Med* 67:570-2 (Feb 15) 1967.

1600. Mars H. Levodopa, carbidopa, and pyridoxine in parkinson disease. Metabolic interactions. *Arch Neurol* 30:444, 1974.

1601. Martin WJ: Hemorrhagic diathesis induced by antimicrobials *JAMA* 205:192 (Jul 15) 1968.

1602. Mashford ML, Robertson MB: Spironolactone and ammonium and potassium chloride. *Br Med J* 4:298-9 (Nov 4) 1972.

1603. Mattila MJ, et al: Interference of iron preparations and milk with the absorption of tetracyclines. *Exerpta Medica International Congress Series No. 254,* Amsterdam, Exerpta Medica, 1972, pp 128-133.

1604. Matz GJ, Naunton RF: Ototoxic drugs and poor renal function. *JAMA* 206:2119 (Nov 25) 1968.

1605. Mawdsley C, Williams IR, Pullar IA, et al: Treatment of parkinsonism by amantadine and levodopa. *Clin Pharmacol Ther* 13:575-583, 1972.

1606. Mazze RI, et al: Renal dysfunction associated with methoxyflurane anesthesia. A randomized, prospective clinical evaluation. *JAMA* 216:278-88 (Apr 12) 1971.

1607. McArthur J: Oral contraceptives and epilepsy. *Br Med J* 3:162 (Jul 15) 1967.

1608. McCall CE, et al: Lincomycin: activity *in vitro* and absorption and excretion in normal young men. *Am J Med Sci* 254:144-55 (Aug) 1967.

1609. McGehee RF Jr, et al: Comparative studies of antibacterial activity in vitro and absorption and excretion of lincomycin and clinimicin. *Am J Med Sci* 256:279-92 (Nov) 1968.

1610. McIntosh TJ, et al: Increased sensitivity to warfarin in thyrotoxicosis. *J Clin Invest* 49:63a-63b, 1970.

1611. McLaughlin JE, Reeves DS: Gentamicin plus carbenicillin. *Lancet* 1:864-5 (Apr 24)

1612. McLaughlin JE, Reeves DS: Clinical and laboratory evidence for inactivation of gentamicin by carbenicillin. *Lancet* 1:261-4 (Feb 6) 1971.

1613. Medin S, Nyberg L: Effect of propantheline and metoclopramide on absorption of digoxin. *Lancet* 1:1393 (Jun 16) 1973.

1614. Mehar GS, et al: Interaction between alcohol, minor tranquilizers and morphine. *Int J Clin Pharmacol* 9:70-4 (Jan) 1974.

1615. Meikle AW, et al: Effect of diphenylhydantoin on the metabolism of metyrapone and release of ACTH in man. *J Clin Endocrinol Metab* 29:1553-8 (Dec) 1969.

1616. Melhorn DK, Gross S: Relationships between iron-dextran and vitamin E in an iron deficiency anemia in children. *J Lab Clin Med* 74:789-802 (Nov) 1969.

1617. Mellk HM, et al: Diphenylhydantoin metabolism in chronic uremia. *Ann Intern Med* 72:801 (May) 1970.

1618. Meriwether WD, et al: Deafness following standard intravenous dose of ethacrynic acid. *JAMA* 216:795-8 (May 3) 1971.

1619. Merriam TW: Aspirin and gastrointestinal bleeding. *J Maine Med Assoc* 59:237-9 (Dec) 1968.

1620. Meyers BR, Kaplan K, et al: Cephalexin-microbiological effects and pharmacologic parameters in man. *Clin Pharmacol Ther* 10:810-16 (Nov-Dec) 1969.

1621. Meyer JF, et al: Insidious and prolonged antagonism of guanethidine by amitriptyline. *JAMA* 213:1487-8 (Aug 31) 1970.

1622. Meyers FH, et al: *Review of Medical Pharmacology.* ed 3 Los Altos, California, Lange Medical Publications, 1972, pp 103-104.

1623. Meyers FH, et al: Op cit, pp 102.

1624. Meyers FH, et al: Op cit, pp 88-89.

1625. Meyers FH, et al: Op cit, pp 518-519.

1626. Meyers FH, et al: Op cit, pp 504-505.

1627. Meyers FH, et al: Op cit, pp 572-576.

1628. Meyers FH, et al: Op cit, pp 536-537.

1629. Meyers FH, et al: Op cit, pp 578-580.

1630. Meyers FH, et al: Op cit, pp 109-113.

1631. Meyler L (ed): *Side Effects of Drugs.* vol 4, Amsterdam. Exerpta Medica Foundation, 1964, pp. 137-141.

1632. Meyler L, Herxheimer A (eds): *Side Effects of Drugs.* vol 6, Amsterdam, Exerpta Medica Foundation. 1968, pp. 22-40.

1633. Mezey E, Robles EA: Effects of phenobarbital administration on rates of ethanol clearance and on ethanol-oxidizing enzymes in man. *Gastroenterology* 66:248-53 (Feb) 1974.

1634. Michalopoulos CD, Koutoulidis CV: Altered digoxin bioavailability. *Lancet* 1:167-8 (Feb 2) 1974.

1635. Middleton E, Finke SR: Metabolic response to epinephrine in bronchial asthma. *J Allerg* 42:288-99 (Nov) 1968.

1636. Miller JB: Hypoglycaemic effect of oxytetracycline. *Br Med J* 2:1007 (Oct 22) 1966.

1637. Miller RP, Bates JH: Amphotericin B toxicity. *Ann Intern Med* 71:1089-95 (Dec) 1969.

1638. Milner G, Landauer AA: The effects of doxepin, alone and together with alcohol, in relation to driving safety. *Med J Aust* 1:837-41 (Apr 28) 1973.

1639. Milner G: Gastro-intestinal side effects and psychotropic drugs. *Med J Aust* 2:153-5 (Jul 19) 1969.

1640. Milner G, Landauer AA: Alcohol, thioridazine and chlorpromazine effects on skills related to driving behaviour. *Br J Psychiatry* 118:351-2 (Mar) 1971.

1641. Mirkin BL, Wright F: Drug interactions: Effect of methylphenidate on the disposition of diphenylhydantoin in man. *Neurology* 21:1123-8 (Nov) 1971.

1642. Misra PS, et al: Increase of ethanol, meprobamate and pentobarbital metabolism after chronic ethanol administration in man and in rats. *Am J Med* 51:346-51 (Sep) 1971.

1643. Mitchell JR, Oates JA: Guanethidine and related agents. I. Mechanism of the selective blockade of adrenergic neurons and its antagonism by drugs. *J Pharmacol Exp Ther* 172:100-7 (Jan) 1970.

1644. Modell W, Hussar AE: Failure of dextroamphetamine sulfate to influence eating and sleeping patterns in obese schizophrenic patients. Clinical and pharmacological significance. *JAMA* 193:275-8 (Jul 26) 1965.

1645. Molnar GW, Read RC: Propranolol enhancement of hypoglycemic sweating. *Clin Pharmacol Ther* 15:490-6 (May) 1974.

1646. Mone JG, Mathie WE: Qualitative and quantitative defects of pseudocholinesterase activity. *Anaesthesia* 22:55-68 (Jan) 1967.

1647. Mones RJ: Evaluation of alpha methyl dopa and alpha methyl dopa hydrazine with L-dopa therapy. *NY State J Med* 74:47-51 (Jan) 1974.

1648. Morgan JP, Bianchine JR: The clinical pharmacology of levodopa. *Rational Drug Ther* 5:1-8 (Jan) 1971.

1649. Morowitz DA: Complications of long-term mineral oil intake. *JAMA* 204:937 (Jun 3) 1968.

1650. Morris R, Giesecke AH Jr: Potentiation of muscle relaxants by magnesium sulfate therapy in toxemia of pregnancy. *South Med J* 61:25-8 (Jan) 1968.

1651. Morselli PL, et al: Effect of sulthiame on blood and brain levels of diphenylhydantoin in the rat. *Biochem Pharmacol* 19:1846-7, 1970.

1652. Morselli PL, et al: Interaction between phenobarbital and diphenylhydantoin in animals and in epileptic patients. *Ann NY Acad Sci* 179:88-104 (Jul 6) 1971.

1653. Moss JM: Cocktails and diabetes *GP* 40:129 (Aug) 1969.

1654. Most JA, Markle GB. IV: A nearly fatal hepatotoxic reaction to rifampin after halothane anesthesia. *Am J Surg* 127:593-5 (May) 1974.

1655. Mould GP, et al: Interaction of glutethimide and phenobarbitone with ethanol in man. *J Pharm Pharmacol* 24:894-9 (Nov) 1972.

1656. Mould G: Faecal blood-loss after sodium acetylsalicylate taken with alcohol. *Lancet* 1:1268 (June 21) 1969.

1657. Muelheims GH, Entrup RW, et al: Increased sensitivity of the heart to catecholamine-induced arrhythmias following guanethidine. *Clin Pharmacol Ther* 6:757-62 (Nov-Dec) 1965.

1658. Murakami M, et al: Effects of anabolic steroids on anticoagulant requirements. *Jap Circ J* 29:243-50 (Mar) 1965.

1659. Nelson DH, et al: Potentiation of the biologic effect of administered cortisol by estrogen treatment. *J Clin Endocrinol Metab* 23:261-5 (Mar) 1963.

1660. Neuvonen PJ, Penttila O: Interaction between doxycycline and barbiturates. *Br Med J* 1:535-6 (Mar 23) 1974.

1661. Niclasson PM, et al: Thrombocytopenia and bleeding—complications in severe cases of meningococcal infection treated with heparin, dextran 70 and chlorpromazine. *Scand J Infect Dis* 4:183-91 1972.

1662. Nies AS, Oates JA: Clinicopathologic conference: Hypertension and the lupus syndrome—revisited. *Am J Med* 51:812-4 (Dec) 1971.

1663. Nimmo J, et al: Pharmacological modification of gastric emptying: effects of propantheline and metoclopramide on paracetamol absorption. *Br Med J* 1:587-9 (Mar 10) 1973.

1664. Nimmo J: The influence of metoclopramide on drug absorption. *Postgrad Med J* 49 Suppl 4: 25-9 (Jul) 1973.

1665. Noble J, Matthew H: Acute poisoning by tricyclic antidepressants: clinical features and management of 100 patients. *Clin Toxicol* 2:403-21 (Dec) 1969.

1666. Nocke-Finck L, et al: Effects of rifampicin on menstrual cycle and on estrogen excretion in patients taking oral contraceptives. *JAMA* 226:378, 1973.

1667. Nola GT, et al: Assessment of the synergistic relationship between serum calcium and digitalis. *Am Heart J* 79:499-507 (Apr) 1970.

1668. Noone P, et al: Renal failure in combined gentamicin and cephalothin therapy. *Br Med J* 2:776-7 (Jun 30) 1973.

1669. Noone P, et al: Acute renal failure after high doses of gentamicin and cephalothin *Lancet* 1:1387-8 (June 16) 1973.

1670. Nord HJ, et al: Treatment of congestive heart failure with glucagon. *Ann Intern Med* 72:649-3 (May) 1970.

1671. Norris JW, Pratt RF: A controlled study of folic acid in epilepsy. *Neurology* 21:659-64 (Jun) 1971.

1672. Oates JA: Effect of doxepin on the norepinephrine pump. A preliminary report. *Psychosomatics* 10:12-3 (May-Jun) 1969.

1673. Ober KF, Wang RIH: Drug interactions with guanethidine. *Clin Pharmacol Ther* 14:190-5 (Mar-Apr) 1973.

1674. O'Brien JR, et al: A comparison of an effect of different anti-inflammatory drugs on human platelets. *J Clin Pathol* 23:522-25 (Sep) 1970.

1675. O'Grady BA: The influence of drugs and diseases on the prothrombin time. *Canad J Med Techn* 28:140-60 (Aug) 1966.

1676. O'Malley K, et al: Increased antipyrine half-life in women taking oral contraceptives. *Scot Med J* 15:454-6 (Dec) 1970.

1677. O'Malley K, Stevenson IH, et al: Impairment of human drug metabolism by oral contraceptive steroids. *Clin Pharmacol Ther* 13:552-7 (July-Aug) 1972.

1678. Opitz A, et al: Akute Niereninsuffizienz nach

Gentamicin-Cephalosporin-Kombinationstherapie. *Med Welt* 22:434–8 (Mar) 1971.

1679. O'Reilly RA: Interaction of sodium warfarin and disulfiram (Antabuse ®) in man. *Ann Intern Med* 78:73–6 (Jan) 1973.

1680. O'Reilly RA: The binding of sodium warfarin to plasma albumin and its displacement by phenylbutazone. *Ann NY Acad Sci* 226:293–308 (Nov 26) 1973.

1681. O'Reilly RA, Aggeler PM: Determinants of the response to oral anticoagulant drugs in man. *Pharmacol Rev* 22:35–96 (Mar) 1970.

1682. O'Reilly RA, Levy G: Kinetics of the anticoagulant effect of bishydroxycoumarin in man. *Clin Pharmacol Ther* 11:378–84 (May-June) 1970.

1683. O'Reilly RA, et al: Impact of aspirin and chlorthalidone on the pharmacodynamics of oral anticoagulant drugs in man. *Ann NY Acad Sci* 179:173–86 (July 6) 1971.

1684. O'Reilly RA: Potentiation of anticoagulant effect by disulfiram. *Clin Res* 19:180 (abstr) 1971.

1685. O'Reilly RA: Interaction of sodium warfarin and rifampin. Studies in man. *Ann Intern Med* 81:337–40 (Sep) 1974.

1686. O'Reilly MV, et al: Transvenous pacemaker failure induced by hyperkalemia. *JAMA* 228:336–7 (Apr 15) 1974.

1687. Osol A, et al: *The United States Dispensatory and Physicians' Pharmacology.* ed 26, Philadelphia, Lippincott, 1967, p 526.

1688. Osol A, et al: Op cit, pp 549–556.

1689. Owusu SK, Ocran K: Paradoxical behaviour of phenylbutazone in African diabetics. *Lancet* 1:440–1 (Feb 19) 1972.

1690. Packham MA, et al: Alteration of the response of platelets to surface stimuli by pyrazole compounds. *J Exp Med* 126:171–188 (July 1) 1967.

1691. Pai SH, Werthamer S, Zale, FG: Severe liver damage caused by treatment of psoriasis with methotrexate. *NY State J Med* 73:2585–7 (Nov 1) 1973.

1692. Palva IP, et al: Drug-induced malabsorption of vitamin B_{12}. V. Intestinal pH and absorption of vitamin B_{12} during treatment with para-aminosalicylic acid. *Scand J Haematol* 9:5–7, 1972.

1693. Papavasiliou PS, et al: Levodopa in Parkinsonism: potentiation of central effects with a peripheral inhibitor. *N Engl J Med* 286:8–14 (Jun 6) 1972.

1694. Parkes JD, et al: Controlled trial of amantadine hydrochloride in Parkinson's disease. *Lancet* 1:259–62 (Feb 7) 1970; Treatment of Parkinson's disease with amantadine and levodopa. A one-year study. *Lancet* 1:1083–6 (May 29) 1971.

1695. Pascale LR, et al: Therapeutic value of probenecid (Benemid) in gout. *JAMA* 149:1188, 1952.

1696. Patel H, Crichton JU: The neurologic hazards of diphenylhydantoin in childhood. *J Pediat* 73:676–84 (Nov) 1968.

1697. Paver K: Complications from combined oral tetracycline and oral corticoid therapy in acne vulgaris. *Med J Aust* 1:1059–60 (May 23) 1970.

1698. Penick SB, et al: Metronidazole in the treatment of alcoholism. *Am J Psychiat* 125:1063–6 (Feb) 1969.

1699. Penttila O, et al: Interaction between doxycycline and some antiepileptic drugs. *Br Med J* 2:470–2 (Jun 1) 1974.

1700. Vivkari NMA, Oho K: Digoxin-phenytoin interaction. *Brit. Med J* 2:51, 1970.

1701. Petersen V, et al: Effect of prolonged thiazide treatment on renal lithium clearance. *Br Med J* 3:143–5 (Jul 20) 1974.

1702. Petitpierre B, et al: Behaviour of chlorpropamide in renal insufficiency and under the effect of associated drug therapy. *Int J Clin Pharmacol Ther Toxicol* 6:120–4, 1972.

1703. Pettinger WA, Korse A, et al: Debrisoquin, a selective inhibitor of intraneuronal monoamine oxidase in man. *Clin Pharmacol Ther* 10:667–74 (Sep-Oct) 1969.

1704. Piguet JD: L'action inhibitrice de la nitrofurantoïne sur le pouvoir bacteriostatique *in vitro* de l'acide nalidixique. [In vitro inhibitive action of nitrofurantoin on the bacteriostatic activity of nalidixic acid] *Ann Inst Pasteur* 116:43–8 (Jan) 1969

1705. Pillay VK, et al: Transient and permanent deafness following treatment with ethacrynic acid in renal failure. *Lancet* 1:77–9 (Jan 11) 1969.

1706. Pittinger CB, et al: Antibiotic-induced paralysis. *Anesth Analg* 49:487–501 (May-Jun) 1970.

1707. Pitts NE: The clinical evaluation of doxepin. A new psychotherapeutic agent. *Psychosomatics* 10:164–71 (May-Jun) 1969.

1708. Platman SR, Fieve RR: Lithium retention and excretion. The effect of sodium and fluid intake. *Arch Gen Psychiat* 20:285–9 (Mar) 1969.

1709. Podolsky S, et al: Effect of marijuana on the glucose-tolerance test. *Ann NY Acad Sci* 191:54–60 (Dec 31) 1971.

1710. Podrizki A: Methocarbamol and myasthenia gravis. *JAMA* 205:938 (Sep 23) 1968.

1711. Pohlmann G: Respiratory arrest associated with intravenous administration of polymyxin B sulfate. *JAMA* 196:181–3 (Apr 11) 1966.

1712. Postlethwaite AE, Kelly WN: Studies on the mechanism of ethambutol-induced hyperuricemia. *Arthritis Rheum* 15:403–9 (Jul-Aug) 1972.

1713. Poucher RL, Vecchio TJ: Absence of tolbutamide effect on anticoagulant therapy. *JAMA* 197:1069–70 (Sep 26) 1966.

1714. Prange AJ Jr, et al: Estrogen may well affect response to antidepressant. *JAMA* 219:143–4 (Jan 10) 1972.

1715. Prange AJ Jr, et al: Enhancement of imipramine by thyroid stimulating hormone: clinical and theoretical implications. *Am J Psychiat* 127:191–9 (Aug) 1970.

1716. Prater MS: Diphenylhydantoin metabolism. *Hosp Pharm* 9:158 (Apr) 1974.

1717. Prazma J, et al: Ethacrynic acid ototoxicity potentiation by kanamycin. *Ann Otol Rhinol Laryngol* 83:111–8 (Jan-Feb) 1974.

1718. Prescott LF: Pharmacokinetic drug interactions. *Lancet* 2:1239–43 (Dec 6) 1969.

1719. Prichard BNC, et al: Haemodynamic studies in hypertensive patients treated by oral propranolol. *Br Heart J* 32:236–40, 1970.

1720. Pullar-Strecker H: Drug interactions in alcoholism treatment. *Lancet* 1:735 (Apr 5) 1969.

1721. Hypoglycaemic effect of chlorpropamide. *Med J Aust* 2:539–40 (Oct 1) 1960.

1722. Pyorala K, et al: Absorption of warfarin from the stomach and small intestine. *Scand J Gastroenterol* (Suppl 9): 95-103, 1970.

1723. Quick AJ: Aspirin and gastric bleeding. *Br Med J* 4:173-4 (Oct 21) 1967.

1724. Raisfeld IH: Cardiovascular complications of antidepressant therapy. *Am Heart J* 83:129-33 (Jan) 1972.

1725. Ralston AJ, et al: Effects of folic acid on fit—frequency and behaviour in epileptics on anticonvulsants. *Lancet* 1:867-8 (Apr 25) 1970.

1726. Ravina A: Antidiuretic action of chlorpropamide. *Lancet* 2:203 (Jul 28) 1973.

1727. Reder JA, Tulgan H: Impairment of diabetic control by norethynodrel with mestranol. *NY State J Med* 67:1073-4 (Apr 15) 1967.

1728. Reimann HA, D'Ambola J: The use and cost of antimicrobials in hospitals. *Arch Environ Health* 13:631-6 (Nov) 1966.

1729. Reimann HA, D'Ambola J: Cost of antimicrobial drugs in a hospital. *JAMA* 205:537 (Aug 12) 1968.

1730. Remenchik AP, et al: Insulin secretion by hypertensive patients receiving hydrochlorothiazide. *JAMA* 212:869 (May 4) 1970.

1731. Reynolds EH: Anticonvulsants, folic acid, and epilepsy. *Lancet* 1:1376-8 (Jun 16) 1973; Schizophrenia-like psychoses of epilepsy and disturbances of folate and vitamin B_{12} metabolism induced by anticonvulsant drugs. *Brit J Psychiat* 113:911-9, 1967.

1732. Reynolds ES, et al: Massive hepatic necrosis after fluroxene anesthesia—a case of drug interaction? *N Engl J Med* 286:530-1 (Mar 9) 1972.

1733. Reynolds JW, Mirkin BL: Urinary corticosteroid and diphenylhydantoin metabolite patterns in neonates exposed to anticonvulsant drugs in utero. *Clin Pharmacol Ther* 14:891-97 (Sep-Oct) 1973.

1734. Rice AJ, et al: Decreased sensitivity to warfarin in patients with myxedema. *Am J Med Sci* 262:211-5 (Oct) 1971.

1735. Richens A, Houghton GW: Phenytoin intoxication caused by sulthiame. *Lancet* 2:1442-3 (Dec 22) 1973.

1736. Ritchie JM: The aliphatic alcohols, in Goodman LS, Gilman A (eds): *The Pharmacological Basis of Therapeutics*, ed 5, New York, Macmillan, 1975, pp 137-151

1737. Rickles FR, Griner PF: Chloral hydrate and warfarin. *N Engl J Med* 286:611-2 (Mar 16) 1972.

1738. Riff LJ, Jackson GG: Laboratory and clinical conditions for gentamicin inactivation by carbenicillin. *Arch Intern Med* 130:887-91 (Dec) 1972.

1739. Riff L, Jackson GG: Gentamicin plus carbenicillin. *Lancet* 1:592 (Mar 20) 1971.

1740. Ritchie JM: Central nervous system stimulants. The Xanthines in Goodman LS, Gilman A (ed): *The Pharmacological Basis of Therapeutics*. ed 5, New York, Macmillan, 1975, pp 359-366.

1741. Rivera-Calimlim L, et al: Effects of mode of management on plasma chlorpromazine in psychiatric patients. *Clin Pharmacol Ther* 14:978-86 (Nov-Dec) 1973.

1742. Rivera-Calimlim L, et al: L-Dopa absorption and metabolism by the human stomach (abst 379). *Pharmacologist* 12:269 (Aug 26) 1970.

1743. Rivera-Calimlim L, et al: L-Dopa absorption and metabolism by the human stomach (abst). *J Clin Invest* 49:79a (Jun) 1970.

1744. Rivera-Calimlim L, et al: L-Dopa treatment failure: Explanation and correction. *Br Med J* 4:93-4 (Oct 10) 1970.

1745. Rizzo M, et al: Further observations on the interactions between phenobarbital and diphenylhydantoin during chronic treatment in the rat. *Biochem Pharmacol* 21:449-54 (Feb) 1972.

1746. Robertson-Rintoul J: Raised serum-lipids and oral contraceptives. *Lancet* 2:1320-1 (Dec 16) 1972.

1747. Robinson BHB, et al: Decreased anticoagulant tolerance with oxymetholone. *Lancet* 1:1356 (Jun 26) 1971.

1748. Robinson DS, Amidon EL: Interaction of benzodiazepines with warfarin in man. Presented at the Annual Symposium on Benzodiazepines, Milan, Italy, November 2-4, 1971.

1749. Robinson DS, Benjamin DM, et al: Interaction of warfarin and nonsystemic gastrointestinal drugs. *Clin Pharmacol Ther* 12:491-5 (May-June) 1971.

1750. Robinson WD: Current status of the treatment of gout. *JAMA* 164:1670-4 (Aug 10) 1957.

1751. Roggin GM, Iber FL: The duration of accelerated drug removal after heavy alcohol ingestion (abst). *Clin Res* 17:309 (Apr) 1969.

1752. Rollo IM: Drugs used in the chemotherapy of helminthiasis in Goodman LS, Gilman A (ed): *The Pharmacological Basis of Therapeutics*, ed 5, New York, Macmillan, 1970, pp 1018-1044

1753. Rosenfeld MG (ed): *Manual of Medical Therapeutics*, ed 21, Boston, Little, Brown and Co., 1976, p 154.

1754. *Ibid*, pp 151.

1755. *Ibid*, pp 121-145.

1756. Ross EK, Priest RG: The effect of hydroxyzine on phenothiazine therapy. *Dis Nerv Syst* 31:412-4 (Jun) 1970.

1757. Millichap JG: Hyperglycemic effect of diphenylhydantoin. *N Engl J Med* 281:447 (Aug 21) 1969.

1758. Rowland M: Amphetamine blood and urine levels in man. *J Pharm Sci* 58:508-9 (Apr) 1969.

1759. Royds RB, Knight AH: Tricyclic antidepressant poisoning. *Practitioner* 204:282-6 (Feb) 1970.

1760. Ramos FH, Barròs B, Larrosa RA, et al: Present status of gold in the treatment of rheumatoid arthritis. *AIR* 6:105-112, 1963.

1761. Rubin A, et al: Interactions of aspirin with nonsteroidal antiinflammatory drugs in man. *Arthritis Rheum* 16:635-45 (Sep-Oct) 1973.

1762. Rubin, E, et al: Inhibition of drug metabolism by acute ethanol intoxication: A hepatic microsomal mechanism. *Am J Med* 49:801-6 (Dec) 1970.

1763. Sabath LD, et al: Excretion of erythromycin and its enhanced activity in urine against gram-negative bacilli with alkalinization. *J Lab Clin Med* 72:916-23 (Dec) 1968.

1764. Saidi P, et al: Effect of chloramphenicol on erythropoiesis. *J Lab Clin Med* 57:247-56 (Feb) 1961.

1765. Sargant W: Combining the antidepressant drugs. *Br Med J* 1:251 (Jan 23) 1965.

1766. Schick D, Scheuer J: Current concepts of therapy with digitalis glycosides. Part II. *Am Heart J* 87:391-6 (Mar) 1974.

1767. Schimpff S, et al: Empiric therapy with carbenicillin and gentamicin for febrile patients with cancer and granulocytopenia. *N Engl J Med* 284:1061-5 (May 13) 1971.

1768. Schneeweiss J, Poole GW: Hyperuricemia due to pyrazinamide. *Br Med J* 2:830-2 (Sep 17)

1769. Turtle JR, Littleton GK, Kipnis DM: Stimulation of insulin secretion by theophylline. *Nature* 213:727-8 (Feb 18) 1967.

1770. Schroder H, Lewkonia RM, et al: Metabolism of salicylazosulfapyridine in healthy subjects and in patients with ulcerative colitis. Effects of colectomy and of phenobarbital. *Clin Pharmacol Ther* 14:802-9 (Sep-Oct) 1973.

1771. Schroeder ET: Alkalosis resulting from combined administration of a "non-systemic" antacid and a cation-exchange resin. *Gastroenterology* 56:868-74 (May) 1969.

1772. Schuckit U, et al: Tricyclic antidepressants and monoamine oxidase inhibitors. Combination therapy in the treatment of depression. *Arch Gen Psychiat* 24:509-14 (Jun) 1971.

1773. Schwab RS, et al: Amantadine in the treatment of Parkinson's disease. *JAMA* 208:1168-70 (May 19) 1969.

1774. Schwartz GH, et al: Ototoxicity induced by furosemide. *N Engl J Med* 282:1413-21 (Jun 18) 1970.

1775. Schwartz HA: Ampicillin rashes. *N Engl J Med* 286:1217-8 (Jun 1) 1972.

1776. Scott RB, et al: Reduced absorption of vitamin B_{12} in two patients with folic acid deficiency. *Ann Intern Med* 69:111-4 (July) 1968.

1777. Searcy RL, et al: Evaluation of the blood-clotting mechanism in tetracycline-treated patients. *Antimicrob Agents Chemother*—1964. pp 179-183, 1965.

1778. Segre EJ, Chaplin M, et al: Naproxen-aspirin interactions in man. *Clin Pharmacol Ther* 15:374-9 (Apr) 1974.

1779. Self TH: Interaction of warfarin and aminosalicylic acid. *JAMA* 223:1285 (Mar 12) 1973.

1780. Seller RH, et al: Digitalis toxicity and hypomagnesemia. *Am Heart J* 79:57-68 (Jan) 1970.

1781. Sellers EM, Lang M, et al: Enhancement of warfarin-induced hypoprothrombinemia by triclofos. *Clin Pharmacol Ther* 13:911-15 (Nov-Dec) 1972.

1782. Sellers EM, Koch-Weser J: Protein binding and vascular activity of diazoxide. *N Engl J Med* 281:1141-5 (Nov 20) 1969.

1783. Sellers EM, Koch-Weser J: Kinetics and clinical importance of displacement of warfarin from albumin by acidic drugs. *Ann NY Acad Sci* 179:213-25 (Jul 6) 1971.

1784. Sellers EM, et al: Interaction of chloral hydrate and ethanol in man. I. Metabolism. *Clin Pharmacol Ther* 13:37-49 (Jan-Feb) 1972; II. Hemodynamics and performance. *Clin Pharmacol Ther* 13:50-8 (Jan-Feb) 1972.

1785. Seltzer HS, Allen EW: Hyperglycemia and inhibition of insulin secretion during administration of diazoxide and trichlormethiazide in man. *Diabetes* 18:19-28 (Jan) 1969.

1786. Shan MN, et al: Comparison of blood clearance of ethanol and tolbutamide and the activity of hepatic ethanol-oxidizing and drug metabolizing enzymes in chronic alcoholic subjects. *Am J Clin Nutr* 25:135-9 (Feb) 1972.

1787. Shapiro M, Hyde L: Hyperuricemia due to pyrazinamide. *Am J Med* 23:596-599 (Oct) 1957.

1788. Shapiro S, et al: Fatal drug reactions among medical inpatients. *JAMA* 216:467-72 (Apr 19) 1971.

1789. Sharpe J, et al: Idiopathic orthostatic hypotension treated with levodopa and MAO inhibitor: a preliminary report. *Can Med Assoc J* 107:296-300 (Aug 9) 1972.

1790. Shelburne RF, et al: Guanethidine in combination with hydralazine and with hydrochlorothiazide in hypertension. *Am J Med Sci* 247:307-12 (Mar) 1964.

1791. Shepherd M, Lader M, Rodnight R: *Clinical Psychopharmacology.* Philadelphia, Lea & Febiger, 1968, pp 141-152.

1792. Shamsic SJ, Barriga C: The hazards of use of monoamine oxidase inhibitors in disturbed adolescents. *Can Med Assoc J* 104:715 (Apr 17) 1971.

1793. Sherrod TR: The cardiac glycosides. *Hosp Practice* 2:56, 1967.

1794. Shils ME: Some metabolic aspects of tetracycline. *Clin Pharmacol Ther* 3:321-39 (May-June) 1962.

1795. Shirriffs GG, Bewsher PD: Hypothermia, abdominal pain, and lactic acidosis in phenformin-treated diabetic. *Br Med J* 3:506 (Aug 29) 1970.

1796. Shopsin B, et al: Iodine and lithium-induced hypothyroidism. Documentation of synergism. *Am J Med* 55:695-9 (Nov) 1973.

1797. Siersbaek-Nielsen K, Hansen JM, et al: Sulfamethizone-induced inhibition of diphenylhydantoin and tolbutamide metabolism in man (abst). *Clin Pharmacol Ther* 14:148 (Jan-Feb) 1973.

1798. O'Regan JB: Adverse interaction of lithium carbonate and methyldopa. *Can Med Assoc J* 115:385-6 (Sep 4) 1976

1799. Silverman G, Braithwaite R: Interaction of benzodiazepines with tricyclic antidepressants. *Br Med J* 4:111 (Oct 14) 1972.

1800. Silverman JL, Wurzel HA: The comparative effects of glyceryl guaiacolate and adenosine on the inhibition of ADP-induced platelet aggregation. *Am J Med Sci* 254:491-8 (Oct) 1967.

1801. Simmons AV, et al: Case of self-poisoning with multiple antidepressant drugs. *Lancet* 1:214-6 (Jan 31) 1970.

1802. Simpson IJ: Nephrotoxicity and acute renal failure associated with cephalothin and cephaloridine. *NZ Med J* 74:312-5 (Nov) 1971.

1803. Singer DL, Hurwitz D: Long-term experience with sulfonylureas and placebo. *N Engl J Med* 277:450-6 (Aug 31) 1967.

1804. Singh MM, Smith JM: Reversal of some therapeutic effects of an antipsychotic agent by an antiparkinsonism drug. *J Nerv Ment Dis* 157:50-8 (Jul) 1973.

1805. Sjoqvist F, et al: Plasma level of monomethylated tricyclic antidepressants and side-effects in man. *Toxicity and Side-effects of Psychotropic Drugs.* Amsterdam, Exerpta Medica Foundation 1968, pp 246-257.

1806. Sjoqvist F, Berglund F, et al: The pH-dependant excretion monomethylated tricylic antidepressants in dogs and man. *Clin Pharmacol Ther* 10:826-33 (Nov-Dec) 1969.

1807. Slade IH, Iosefa RN: Fatal hypoglycemic coma from the use of tolbutamide in elderly patients: report of two cases. *J Am Geriat Soc* 15:948-50 (Oct) 1967.

1808. Slone D, et al: Intravenously given ethacrynic acid and gastrointestinal bleeding. *JAMA* 209:1668-71 (Sep 15) 1969.

1809. Smith DB, Racusen LC: Folate metabolism and the anticonvulsant efficacy of phenobarbital. *Arch Neurol* 28:18-22 (Jan) 1973.

1810. Smith EC, et al: Interaction of ascorbic acid and warfarin. *JAMA* 221:1166 (Sep 4) 1972.

1811. Smith MJH, Smith PK: *The Salicylates.* A Critical Bibliographic Review, New York, Interscience Publishers, 1966, pp. 86-90.

1812. *Ibid,* pp 34-43.

1813. Smith RB: Cocaine and catecholamine interaction. A review. *Arch Otolaryngol* 98:139-41 (Aug) 1973.

1814. Smith RM, Jr, et al: Succinylcholine-pantothenyl alcohol: A reappraisal. *Anesth Analg Curr Res* 48:205-8 (Mar-Apr) 1969.

1815. Sneddon JM, Turner P: Ephedrine mydriasis in hypertension and the response to treatment. *Clin Pharmacol Ther* 10:64-71 (Jan-Feb) 1969.

1816. Solomon GE, et al: Coagulation defects caused by diphenylhydantoin. *Neurology* 22:1165-71 (Nov) 1972.

1817. Solomon HM, et al: Mechanisms of drug interaction. *JAMA* 216:1997-9 (Jun 21) 1971.

1818. Solomon HM, Abrams WB: Interactions between digitoxin and other drugs in man. *Am Heart J* 83:277-80 (Feb) 1972.

1819. Solomon HM, et al: Interactions between digitoxin and other drugs *in vitro* and *in vivo. Ann NY Acad Sci* 179:362-9 (Jul 6) 1971.

1820. Solomon RB, Rosner F: Massive hemorrhage and death during treatment with clofibrate and warfarin. *NY State J Med* 73:2002-3 (Aug 1) 1973.

1821. Somani SM, Khurana RC: Mechanism of estrogen-imipramine interaction. *JAMA* 223:560 (Jan 29) 1973.

1822. Sotaniemi EA, Kontturi MJ, et al: Drug metabolism and androgen control therapy in prostatic cancer. *Clin Pharmacol Ther* 14:413-17 (May-June) 1973.

1823. Sotaniemi E, et al: The clinical significance of microsomal enzyme induction in the therapy of epileptic patients. *Ann Clin Res* 2:223-7 (Sep) 1970.

1824. Sotaniemi E, et al: Increased clearance of tolbutamide from the blood of asthmatic patients. *Ann Allergy* 29:139-41 (Mar) 1971.

1825. Spaans F: No effect of folic acid supplement on CSF folate and serum vitamin B_{12} in patients on anticonvulsants. *Epilepsia* 11:403-11 (Dec) 1970.

1826. Spangler AS, et al: Enhancement of the anti-inflammatory action of hydrocortisone by estrogen. *J Clin Endocr* 29:650-5 (May) 1969.

1827. Spellacy WN, et al: Growth hormone alterations by a sequential-type oral contraceptive. *Obstet Gynec* 33:506-10 (Apr) 1969.

1828. Spergel G, et al: The effect of potassium on the impaired glucose tolerance in chronic uremia. *Metabolism* 16:581-5 (Jul) 1967.

1829. Sphire RD: Gallamine: A second look. *Anesth Analg* 43:690-5 (Nov-Dec) 1964.

1830. Stambaugh JE Jr, Wainer IW: Drug interactions I: meperidine and combination oral contraceptives. *J Clin Pharmacol* 15:46-51 (Jan) 1975.

1831. Starke K: Interactions of guanethidine and indirect-acting sympathomimetic amines. *Arch Int Pharmacodyn Ther* 195:309-14 1972.

1832. Starr KJ, Petrie JC: Drug interactions in patients on long-term oral anticoagulant and antihypertensive adrenergic neuron-blocking drugs. *Br Med J* 4:133-38 (Oct 21) 1972.

1833. Stauch M, et al: Effets hémodynamiques de la stimulation des bêta-récepteurs après blocage bêta-adrénergique et théophylline. *Ann Cardiol Angeiol* 20:71-2 (Jan-Feb) 1971.

1834. Stein HL, Hilgartner MW: Alteration of coagulation mechanism of blood by contrast media. *Am J Roentgen* 104:458-63 (Oct) 1968.

1835. Stenger RJ: Enhanced hepatotoxicity of fluroxene. *N Engl J Med* 286:1005-6 (May 4) 1972.

1836. Stephens FO, et al: Effect of cortisone and vitamin A on wound infection. *Am J Surg* 121:569-71 (May) 1971.

1837. Stevenson H, et al: Changes in human drug metabolism after long-term exposure to hypnotics. *Br Med J* 4:322-4 (Nov 11) 1972.

1838. Stoelting RK, Gibbs PS: Effect of tetracycline therapy on renal function after methoxyflurane anesthesia. *Anesth Analg* 52:431-6 (May-Jun) 1973.

1839. Sullivan JM, et al: Pharmacologic control of thromboembolic complications of cardiac-valve replacement. *N Engl J Med* 284:1391-4 (Jun 24) 1971.

1840. Sweet RD, Lee JE, et al: Methyldopa as an adjunct to levodopa treatment of Parkinson's disease. *Clin Pharmacol Ther* 13:23-27 (Jan-Feb) 1972.

1841. Swyer GIM: Liquid paraflin and oral contraception. *The Practitioner* 202:592 (Apr) 1969.

1842. Symchowicz S, et al: A comparative study of griseofulvin-^{14} C metabolism in the rat and rabbit. *Biochem Pharmacol* 16:2405-11 1967.

1843. Talbot JM, Meade BW: Effect of silicones on the absorption of anticoagulant drugs. *Lancet* 1:1292 (Jun 19) 1971.

1844. Tannenberg AM: Tetracycline and rises in urea nitrogen. *JAMA* 221:713 (Aug 14) 1972.

1845. Tannenbaum H, et al: Phenylbutazone-tolbutamide drug interaction. *N Engl J Med* 290:344 (Feb 7) 1974.

1846. Kaplan R, et al: Phenytoin, metronidazole and multivitamins in the treatment of alcoholism. *QJ Stud Alcohol* 33:94-104 (Mar) 1972; Swinson RP: Long term trial of metronidazole in male alcoholism. *Brit J Psychiat* 119:85-9 (Jul) 1971.

1847. Taylor SA, et al: Spironolactone—A weak enzyme inducer in man. *J Pharm Pharmacol* 24:578-9 (Jul) 1972.

1848. Thomas FB, et al: Inhibition of the intestinal absorption of inorganic and hemoglobin iron by cholestyramine. *J Lab Clin Med* 78:70-80 (Jul) 1971.

1849. Thompson WG: Altered absorption of digoxin in

patients given propantheline and metoclopramide. *Lancet* 1:783-4 (Apr 7) 1973.

1850. Thompson WG: Effect of cholestryamine on absorption of ³H digoxin in rats. *Am J Dig Dis* 18:851-6 (Oct) 1973.

1851. Thomsen K, Schou M: Renal lithium excretion in man. *Am J Physiol* 215:823-7 (Oct) 1968.

1852. Thonnard-Neumann E: Phenothiazines and diabetes in hospitalized women. *Am J Psychiat* 124:978-82 (Jan) 1968.

1853. Thorn GW: Clinical considerations in the use of corticosteroids. *N Engl J Med* 274:775-81 (Apr 7) 1966.

1854. Thune S: [Gastrointestinal bleeding and salicylates. A comparative study of acetylsalicylic acid and salicylsalicylic acid]. *Nord Med* 79:312-4 (Mar 14) 1968.

1855. Tjandramaga TB, Cucinell SA: Interaction of probenecid and allopurinol in gouty subjects. *Fed Proc* 30:392 (Abstract 1112) 1971.

1856. Toakley JG, et al: "Dilantin" overdosage. *Med J Aust* 2:639-640 (Oct 12) 1968.

1857. Tobias H, Auerbach R: Hepatotoxicity of long-term methotrexate therapy for psoriasis. *Arch Intern Med* 132:391-6 (Sep) 1973.

1858. Todd RG (ed): *Extra Pharmacopoeia—Martindale* ed. 26. London, The Pharmaceutical Press 1975, p 1814.

1859. *Ibid,* pp 102-4.

1860. Tong MJ, et al: Supplemental folates in the therapy of *Plasmodium falciparum* malaria. *JAMA* 214:2330-3 (Dec 28) 1970.

1861. Treasure T, Toseland PA: Hyperglycaemia due to phenytoin toxicity. *Arch Dis Child* 46:563-4 (Aug) 1971.

1862. Tuano SB, et al: Cephaloridine versus cephalothin: Relation of the kidney to blood level differences after parenteral administration. *Antimicrob Agents Chemother—1966*, pp 101-106, 1967.

1863. Tuck D, et al: Drug interactions: effect of chlorpromazine on the uptake of monoamines into adrenergic neurons in man. *Lancet* 2:492 (Sep 2) 1972.

1864. Tucker HA: *Oral Antidiabetic Therapy, 1956-1965* Springfield Ill. Charles C Thomas 1965, pp. 239-240.

1865. Tucker HSG, Hirsch JI: Sulfonamide-sulfonylurea interaction. *N Engl J Med* 286:110-11 (Jan 13) 1972.

1866. Tudhope GR: Advances in medicine. *Practitioner* 203:405-17 (Oct) 1969.

1867. Turtle JR, Burgess JA: Hypoglycemic action of fenfluramine in diabetes mellitus. *Diabetes* 22:858-67 (Nov) 1973.

1868. Tweeddale MG, Ogilvie RI: Antagonism of spironolactone-induced natriuresis by aspirin in man. *N Engl J Med* 289:198-200 (Jul 26) 1973.

1969. Udall JA: Chloral hydrate and warfarin therapy. *Ann Intern Med* 75-141-2 (Jul) 1971.

1870. Udall JA: Warfarin therapy not influenced by meprobamate. A controlled study in nine men. *Curr Ther Res* 12:724-8 (Nov) 1970.

1871. Vagenakis AG, et al: Enhancement of warfarin-induced hypoprothrombinemia by thyrotoxicosis. *John Hopkins Med J* 131:69-73 (Jul) 1972.

1872. Vaisrub S: Rum fits and dt's. *JAMA* 212:2112-2113 (June 22) 1970.

1873. Vajda FJE, et al: Interaction between phenytoin and the benzodiazepines. *Br Med J* 1:346 (Feb 6) 1971.

1874. Vall-Spinosa A, Lester TW: Rifampin: Characteristics and role in the chemotherapy of tuberculosis. *Ann Intern Med* 74:758-60 (May) 1971.

1875. Valsrub S: Alcohol-induced sensitivity and tolerance. *JAMA* 219:508-9 (Jan 24)

1876. van Cauwenberge H, Jaques LB: Haemorrhagic effect of ACTH with anticoagulants. *Can Med Assoc J* 79:536-40 (Oct.) 1958.

1877. Van Dam FE, et al: The interaction of drugs. *Lancet* 2:1027 (Nov 5) 1966.

1878. Van Rossum JM: Potential dangers of monoamineoxidase inhibitors and d-methyldopa. *Lancet* 1:950-1 (Apr 27) 1963.

1879. Vesell ES, et al: Impairment of drug metabolism in man by allopurinol and nortriptyline. *N Engl J Med* 283:1484 (Dec 31) 1970.

1880. Vesell ES, et al: Impairment of drug metabolism by disulfiram in man. *Clin Pharmacol Ther* 12:785-92 (Sep-Oct) 1971.

1881. Vesell ES, et al: Failure of indomethacin and warfarin to interact in normal human volunteers. *J Clin Pharmacol* 15:486-95 (Jul) 1975.

1882. Vieweg WVR, et al: Complications of intravenous administration of heparin in elderly women. *JAMA* 213:1303-6 (Aug 24) 1970.

1883. Vigran IM: Dangerous potentiation of meperidine hydrochloride by pargyline hydrochloride. *JAMA* 187:953-4 (Mar 21) 1964.

1884. Vitek V, Rysanek K: Interaction of D-cycloserine with the action of some monoamine oxidase inhibitors. *Biochem Pharmacol* 14:417-8, 1965.

1885. Waal HJ: Hypotensive action of propranolol. *Clin Pharmacol Ther* 7:588-98 (Sep-Oct) 1966.

1886. Wadman B, Werner I: Thromboembolic complications during corticosteroid treatment of temporal arteritis. *Lancet* 1:907 (Apr 22) 1972.

1887. Wagner JG: Aspects of pharmacokinetics and biopharmaceutics in relation to drug activity. *Am J Pharm* 141:5-20 (Jan-Feb) 1969.

1888. Walker IR, et al: Cyclophosphamide, cholinesterase and anaesthesia. *Aust NZ J Med* 22:247-51 (Aug) 1972.

1889. Walters MB: The relationship between thyroid function and anticoagulant therapy. *Am J Cardiol* 11:112-4 (Jan) 1963.

1890. Warner WA, Sanders E: Neuromuscular blockade associated with gentamicin therapy. *JAMA* 215:1153-4 (Feb 15) 1971.

1891. Webb SN, Bradshaw EG: Diazepam and neuromuscular blocking drugs. *Br Med J* 3:640 (Sep 11) 1971.

1892. Weinberger M, Bronsky E: Interaction of ephedrine and theophylline. *Clin Pharmacol Ther* 15:223 (Feb) 1974.

1893. Weiner M, Moses D: The effect of glucagon and insulin on the prothrombin response to coumarin anticoagulants. *Proc Soc Exp Biol Med* 127:761-3 (Mar) 1968.

1894. Weiner M: Species differences in the effect of chloral hydrate on coumarin anticoagulants. *Ann NY Acad Sci* 179:226-34 (Jul 6) 1971.

1895. Weinstein L: Drugs used in the chemotherapy of leprosy and tuberculosis in Goodman LS, Gilman A (ed): *The Pharmacological Basis of Therapeutics,* ed 5 New York, Macmillan 1975, pp 1201-23.

1896. Weintraub M, Griner PF: Warfarin and ascorbic acid: Lack of evidence for a drug interaction. *Toxicol Appl Pharmacol* 28:53-6 (Apr) 1974.

1897. Werk EE, Jr, et al: Cortisol production in epileptic patients treated with diphenylhydantoin. *Clin Pharmacol Ther* 12:698-703 (Jul-Aug) 1971.

1898. Werk EE, Jr, et al: Failure of metyrapone to inhibit 11-hydroxylation of 11-deoxycortisol during drug therapy. *J Clin Endocrinol Metab* 27:1358, 1967.

1899. Westervelt FB Jr, Atuk NO: Methyldopa-induced hypertension. *JAMA* 227:557 (Feb 4) 1974.

1900. Wharton RN, et al: A potential clinical use for methylphenidate with tricyclic antidepressants. *Am J Psychiat* 127:1619-25 (Jun) 1971.

1901. Wheatley D: Potentiation of amitriptyline by thyroid hormone. *Arch Gen Psychiat* 26:229-33 (Mar) 1972.

1902. Whitfield JB, et al: Changes in plasma γ-glutamyl transpeptidase activity associated with alterations in drug metabolism in man. *Br Med J* 1:316-8 (Feb 10) 1973.

1903. Wiedlerholt IC, et al: Recurrent episodes of hypoglycemia induced by propoxyphene. *Neurology* 17:703-6 (Jul) 1967.

1904. Wiener JD: Thyroid hormones and protein-bound iodine. *JAMA* 207:1717 (Mar 3) 1969.

1905. Williams RB, Jr, Sherter C: Cardiac complications of tricyclic antidepressant therapy. *Ann Int Med* 74:395-8 (Mar) 1971.

1906. Wilson JT, Wilkinson GR: Chronic and severe phenobarbital intoxication in a child treated with primidone and diphenylhydantoin. *J Pediat* 83:484-9 (Sep) 1973.

1907. Winston F: Combined antidepressant therapy. *Br J Psychiat* 118:301-4 (Mar) 1971.

1908. Winters RE, et al: Combined use of gentamicin and carbenicillin. *Ann Intern Med* 75:925-7 (Dec) 1971.

1909. Wodak J, et al: Review of 12 months' treatment with l-dopa in Parkinson's disease, with remarks on unusual side effects. *Med J Aust* 2:1277-82 (Dec 2) 1972.

1910. Wolff F: Diazoxide misunderstood. *N Engl J Med* 286:612 (Mar 16) 1972.

1911. Wolff H: Die hemmung der serumcholinesterase durch cyclophosphamid (Endoxan). *Klin Wschr* 43:819-21 (Aug 1) 1965.

1912. Wood PHN: Faecal blood-loss after sodium acetylsalicylate taken with alcohol. *Lancet* 1:677-8 (Mar 29) 1969.

1913. White MG, Fetner CD: Treatment of the syndrome of inappropriate secretion of antidiuretic hormone with lithium carbonate. *N Engl J Med* 292:390-392, 1975.

1914. Woodbury DM, Fingl E: Analgesic-antipyretics, anti-inflammatory agents, and drugs employed in the therapy of gout, in Goodman LS, Gilman A (ed): *The Pharmacological Basis of Therapeutics,* ed 5, New York Macmillan 1975, pp 325-358.

1915. Wosilait WD, Eisenbrandt LL: The side of oxyphenbutazone on the excretion of ¹⁴C-warfarin in the bile of rat. *Res Commun Chem Pathol Pharmacol* 4:413-20 (Sep) 1972.

1916. Wright EA, McQuillen MP: Antibiotic-induced neuromuscular blockade. *Ann NY Acad Sci* 183-358-68 (Sep 15) 1971.

1917. Yahr MD, et al: Treatment of parkinsonism with levodopa. *Arch Neurol* 21:343-54 (Oct) 1969.

1918. Yahr MD, Duvoisin RC: Drug therapy of Parkinsonism. *N Engl J Med* 287:20-4 (Jul 6) 1972.

1919. Yaryura-Tobias JA, et al: Action of l-dopa in drug-induced extrapyramidalism. *Dis Nerv Syst* 31:60-3 (Jan) 1970.

1920. Yesair DW, et al: Comparative effects of salicylic acid, phenylbutazone, probenecid and other anions on the metabolism, distribution and excretion of indomethacin by rats. *Biochem Pharmacol* 19:1591-1600, 1970.

1921. Zall H, et al: Lithium carbonate: A clinical study. *Am J Psychiat* 125:549-555 (Oct) 1968.

1922. Zaroslinski J, et al: Effect of sabacute administration of methaqualone, phenobarbital and glutethimide on plasma levels of bishydroxycoumarin. *Arch Int Pharmacodyn Ther* 195:185-91, 1972.

1923. Zeidenberg P, et al: Clinical and metabolic studies with imipramine in man. *Am J Psychiat* 127:1321-6 (Apr) 1971.

1924. Zinner SH, et al: Erythromycin plus alkalinization in treatment of urinary infections. *Antimicrob Agents Chemother 9th Conf.* 1969.

1925. Zsigmond EK, Robins G: The effect of a series of anticancer drugs on plasma cholinesterase activity. *Can Anaesth Soc J* 19:75-82 (Jan) 1972.

1926. Zsigmond EK, Eilderton TE: Abnormal reaction to procaine and succinylcholine in a patient with inherited atypical plasma cholinesterase. Case report. *Can Anaes Soc J* 15:498-500 (Sep) 1968.

1927. Zucker MB, Peterson J: Effect of acetylsalicylic acid, other nonsteroidal anti-inflammatory agents, and dipyridamole on human blood platelets. *J Lab Clin Med* 76:66-75 (Jul) 1970.

1928. Marinow A: Diabetes in chronic schizophrenia. *Dis Nerv Syst* 32:777-8 (Nov) 1971.

1929. Hansten PD: Personal observations of patients. *Drug Interactions* (ed 3). Philadelphia, Lea & Febiger, 1975, pp 25, 213.

1930. Dijl Wvan: Neuromuscular blocking agents, in Meyler L, Herxheimer A (eds): *Side Effects of Drugs,* vol. 7. Excerpta Medica, Amsterdam, pp 210-211, 1972.

1931. American Pharmaceutical Association: *Evaluations of Drug Interactions,* 1973, p 3.

1932. Stern IJ, Hollifield RD, Buzard JA: The antimonamine oxidase effects of furazolidone, a drug which does not itself inhibit monoamine oxidase. *J. Pharmacol Exp Ther* 156:492-9, 1967.

1933. Hussar DA: Drug interactions. *Clin Toxicol* 9:107-118 (Feb) 1976.

1934. McLaren EH: Severe hypertension produced by interaction of phenylpropanolamine with methyldopa and oxyarenolol. *Brit Med J* 1:283-4 (July 31) 1976.

1935. Crome P, Vale JA, et al: Methionine in acetaminophen poisoning. *N Engl J Med* 296:824 (Apr 7) 1977.

1936. Arky RA: Diphenylhydantoin and the beta cell. *N Engl J Med* 286:371-2 (Feb 17) 1972.

1937. Yamamoto T: Diabetes insipidus and drinking alcohol. *N Engl J Med* 294:55-6 (Jan 1) 1976.

1938. Webster B, Bain J: Antidiuretic effect and complications of chlorpropamide therapy in diabetes insipidus. *J Clin Endocrinol Metab* 30:215-27, 1970.

1939. AMA Dept of Drugs: *AMA Drug Evaluations*, ed 3 Acton, MA, Publishing Sciences Group, 1977.

1940. Aynsley-Green A, Illig R: Enhancement by ohlorpromazine of hyperglycemic action of diazoxide. *Lancet* 2:658-9 (Oct 4) 1971.

1941. Danforth E, Jr: Hyperglycemia after diazoxide. *N Engl J Med* 285:1487 (Dec 23) 1971.

1942. Appel GB, Neu HC: The nephrotoxicity of antimicrobial agents. *N Engl J Med* 296:663-70 (Mar 24); 722-8 (Mar 31); 784-7 (Apr 7) 1977.

1943. Jain AK, Ryan JR, McMahon FG: Potentiation of hypoglycemic effect of sulfonylureas by halofenate. *N Engl J Med* 293:1283-6 (Dec 18) 1975.

1944. Hughes JE, Steahly LP, Bier MM: Marihuana and the diabetic coma. *JAMA* 214:1113-4 (Nov 9) 1970.

1945. Syvalahti E, et al: Half-life of tolbutamide in patients receiving tuberculostatic agents. *Scand J Resp Dis* (Suppl) 88:17, 1974; Effect of tuberculostatic agents on the response of serum growth hormone and immunoreactive insulin to intravenous tolbutamide, and on the half-life of tolbutamide. *Int J Clin Pharmacol Biopharm* 13:83-9, 1976.

1946. Zilly W, Breimer D, Richter E: Induction of drug metabolism in man after rifampicin treatment measured by increased hexobarbital and tolbutamide clearance. *Eur J Clin Pharmacol* 9:219-27, 1975.

1947. Zilly W, et al: Effect of rifampicin on the pharmacokinetics of tolbutamide in healthy subjects. *Verk Dtsch Ges Inn Med* 80:1538-40, 1974.

1948. Mukerjee P, Schuldt S, Kasik JE: Effect of rifampin on cutaneous hypersensitivity to purified protein derivatives in humans. *Antimicrob Agents Chemother* 4:607-11, 1973.

1949. Miller JB: Hypoglycemic effect of oxytetracycline. *Brit Med J* 2:1007 (Oct 22) 1966.

1950. Sen S, Mukerjee A: Hypoglycemic action of oxytetracycline. *J Ind Med Assoc* 52:366-9, 1969.

1951. Van Meter JC, Oleson JJ: Effect of aureomycin on the respiration of normal rat liver homogenates. *Science* 113:273 (Mar 9) 1951.

1952. Prochazka P, Rokos J, et al: Localization and binding of chlortetracycline in pancreas. *Cas Lek Cesk* 104:743-4, 1965.

1953. Mahfouz M, et al: Potentiation of the hypoglycemic action of tolbutamide by different drugs. *Arzneim Forsch* 20:120-2, 1970.

1954. Solomon HM: Clinical disorders of drug interaction. *Adv Intern Med* 16:285-301, 1970.

1955. Wesseling H, et al: Interaction of diphenylhydantoin (DPH) and tolbutamide. *Eur J Clin Pharmacol* 8:75-8, 1975; Effect of sulfonylureas (tolazamide, tolbutamide and chlorpropamide) on the metabolism of dephenylhydantoin in the rat. *Biochem Pharmacol* 22:3033-40, 1973.

1956. Maronde RF, et al: Comparison of guanethidine and guanethidine plus a thiazide diuretic. *Am J Med Sci* 242:228-33 (Aug) 1961.

1957. Goldberg EM, Sanbar SS: Hyperglycemic nonketotic coma following administration of Dilantin (diphenylhydantoin). *Diabetes* 18:101-6 (Feb) 1969.

1958. Hubmann R, Bremer G: Die Ausscheidung von Furadantin bei manifester Niereninsuffizieng. *Med Welt* 19:1039-49 (May 8) 1965.

1959. Grote IW, Woods M: Studies on antacids IV. Adsorption effects of various aluminum antacids upon simultaneously administered drugs, *JAPhA, Sci Ed* 42:319-20 (May) 1953.

1960. Nye E, Roberts J: Effect of reserpine on the reactivity of atrial and ventricular pacemakers to guinidine. *Nature* 210:1376-7 (Jun 25) 1966.

1961. Usubiaga JE: Neuromuscular effects of beta adrenergic blockers and their interaction with skeletal muscle relaxants. *Anesthesiology* 29:484-92 (May-Jun) 1968

1962. Karliner JS: Intravenous diphenylkydantoin sodium (Dilantin) in cardiac arrhythmias. *Dis Chest* 51:256-69 (Mar) 1967.

1963. Lee PC, et al: Large and small doses of ascorbic acid in the absorption of ferrous iron. *Can Med Assoc J* 97:181-4 (Jul 22) 1967.

1964. Bloom WL, Brewer SS, JR: The independent yet synergistic effects of heparin and dextran. *Acta Chir Scand Suppl* 387:53, 1968.

1965. Stewart P: Case reports. *J Am Assoc Nurse Anesth* 28:56, 1960.

1966. Rubin E: Hepatic microsomal enzymes in man and rat: induction and inhibition by alcohol. *Science* 162:690-1 (Nov 8) 1968.

1967. Merrill J, et al: Adriamycin and radiation: synergistic radiotoxicity. *Ann Intern Med* 82:122-3 (Jan) 1975.

1968. Johnson J: Epanutin and isoniazid interaction. *Brit Med J* 1:152 (Jan 18) 1975.

1969. Romankiewicz JA, Ehrman M: Rifampin and warfarin: a drug interaction. *Ann Intern Med* 82:224-5 (Feb) 1975.

1970. Lutz EG: Lithium toxicity precipitated by diuretics. *J Med Soc NJ* 72:439-40 (May) 1975.

1971. Cabanillas F, et al: Nephrotoxicity of combined cephalothin-gentamicin regimen. *Arch Intern Med* 135:850-2 (June) 1975.

1972. Malach M, Berman N: Furosemide and chloralhydrate: adverse drug interaction. *JAMA* 232:638-9 (May 12) 1975.

1973. Garfield JW: Surprising side effect of rifampin: in patients on methadone, it causes withdrawal symptoms. *Med World News* 16:60 (July 28) 1975.

1974. Self TH, et al: Interaction of sulfisoxazole and warfarin. *Circulation* 52:528 (Sep) 1975.

1975. Byrd GJ: Methyldopa and lithium carbonate: suspected interaction. *JAMA* 233:320 (July 28) 1975.

1976. Jerry R, et al: Sinutab. *Med J Austral* 1:763 (Jan 14) 1975.

1977. Baugh R, Calvert RT, Fell JT: Stability of phenylbutazone in presence of pharmaceutical colors. *J Pharm Sci* 66:733-5 (May) 1977.

1978. Mathog RH, Matz GJ: Ototoxic effects of ethacrynic acid. *Ann Otol Rhinol Laryngol* 81:871-5 (Dec) 1972.

1979. Bruce DL: Anesthetic-induced increase in murine mortality from cyclophosphamide *Cancer* 31:361-3 (Feb) 1973.

1980. Prout MN, et al: Adriamycin cardiotoxicity in children. *Cancer* 39:62-65 (Jan) 1977.

1981. Johnson J, Freeman HL: Death due to isoniazid (INH) and phenytoin. *Brit J Psychiat* 129:511 (Nov) 1976.

1982. Loudon JB, Waring H: Toxic reactions to lithium and haloperidol. *Lancet* 2:1088 (Nov 13) 1976.

1983. Geisler A, Klysner R: Combined effect of lithium and fluxpenthiol on strital adenylate cyclase. *Lancet* 1:430-1 (Feb 19) 1977.

1984. Sacher M, Thaler H: Toxic hepatitis after therapeutic doses of benorylate and D-penicillamine. *Lancet* 1:481-2 (Feb 26) 1977.

1985. May L, Swoboda W: Bandrylat-Therapic bei rheumatischen Erkankungen im Kindesalter. *Z Rheumatol* 33:352-60, 1974.

1986. Brown TGK: Sodium bicarbonate and trycyclic-antidepressant poisoning. *Lancet* 1:375 (Feb 12) 1977.

1987. Gerber JG, et al: Effect of N-acetylcysteine on hepatic covalent binding of paracetamol (acetaminophen). *Lancet* 1:657 (Mar 19) 1977.

1988. Goonewardene A, Toghill PJ: Gross oedema ocurring during treatment for depression. *Brit Med J* 1:879-80 (Apr 2) 1977; Pathak SK: Gross oedema during treatment for depression. *Brit Med J* 1:1220 (May 7) 1977.

1989. Wiseman M, et al: Dextropropoxyphene overdosage and naloxone. *Brit Med J* 1:1159 (Apr 30) 1977.

1990. Kempe CH: Vaccinia, in Beeson PB, McDermott W, ed: *Cecil-Loeb Textbook of Medicine* Philadelphia, WB Saunders Co, 1967, p 47-51.

1991. Powell-Jackson PR: Interaction between azapropazone and warfarin. *Brit Med J* 1:1193-4 (May 7) 1977.

1992. Cegrell L: Phentolamine and juvenile diabetes. *Lancet* 2:1421 (Dec 30) 1972.

1993. Epstein MT, et al: Effect of eating liquorice on the renin-angiotensin-aldosterone axis in normal subjects. *Brit Med J* 1:488-90 (Feb 19) 1977.

1994. Smith CR, et al: Controlled comparison of amikacin and gentamicin. *N Engl J Med* 296:349-53 (Feb 17) (1977); Carey JT et al: Testing for ototoxicity: amikacin and gentamicin. *N Engl J Med* 296:1124 (May 12) 1977.

1995. Rappolt RT, Gay GR: Propranolol in the treatment of cardiopressor effects of cocaine. *N Engl J Med* 295:448 (Aug 19) 1976.

1996. Thornton WE: Dementia induced by methyldopa with haloperidol. *N Engl J Med* 294:1222 (May 27) 1976.

1997. Allen T, et al: Tetrahydrocannabinol and chemotherapy. *N Engl J Med* 294:168-9 (Jan 15) 1976; 293:795-7, 1975.

1998. Data JL, Wilkinson GR, Nies AS: Interaction of quinidine with anticonvulsant drugs. *N Engl J Med* 294:699-702 (Mar 25) 1976.

1999. Ginter E: Chenodeoxycholic acid, gallstones and vitamin C. *N Engl J Med* 295:1260-1 (Nov 25) 1976.

2000. Snyder BD, et al: Orphenadrine overdosage treated with physostigmine. *N Engl J Med* 295:1435 (Dec 16) 1976.

2001. Hausner R: Drugs that reduce efficacy of levodopa. *N Engl J Med* 295:1538 (Dec 30) 1976.

2002. Tannock I: Metronidazole as a radiosensitizer. *N Engl J Med* 295:901 (Oct 14) 1976.

2003. Feely J: Beta blockers for diabetics. *Lancet* 1:950 (Apr 30) 1977.

2004. Polacsek E, Barnes T, Turner N, et al: *Interaction of Alcohol and Other Drugs.* Toronto, Ontario, Addiction Research Foundation, 1972.

2005. Smithard DJ, Langman MJS: Vitamin C and drug metabolism. *Brit Med J* 1:1029-30 (Apr 16) 1977.

2006. Hongie C: Anticoagulant action of protamine sulphate. *Proc Soc Exp Biol Med* 98:130-3, 1958.

2007. King JC: *Guide to Parenteral Admixtures.* St. Louis, MO, Cutter Laboratories, Inc, 1978. Updated frequently by supplements.

2008. Dunlevy DLF: Phenelzine and oedema. *Brit Med J* 1:1353 (May 21) 1977.

2009. Wood MH, Sebel E, O'Sullivan WJ: Allopurinol and thiazides. *Lancet* 1:751 (Apr 1) 1972.

2010. Di Maggio G, Ciaceri G: The influence of meprobamate on binding of pentothal by plasma proteins. *Abstract of Communications,* 4th International Congress or Pharmacology, Basel, 1969, p 449.

2011. Kuck NA: Adjuvant effect of phoscolic acid on tetracycline in bacterial infections in mice. *Antimicrob Agents Chemother* 168-172, 1964.

2012. Kunin CM, Jones WF Jr, Finland M: Enhancement of tetracycline blood levels *N Engl J Med* 259:147-56 (July 24) 1957.

2013. Ludtike E: Uber die Beeinflussung der Rastinon belasting bei Diabetikern durch Chlorpromazin. *Klin Wschr* 41:163-4 (Dec 1) 1963.

2014. Wiezarek WD, Graupner K: Der Einfuss von Bestandteilen lytischer Mischungen auf die Wirkung blutzuckersenkender Substanzen. *Arch Int Pharmacodyn* 146:386-91 (Dec 1) 1963.

2015. Lancaster NP, Jones DH: Chlorpromazine and insulin in psychiatry. *Br Med J* 2:565-7, (Sept 4) 1954.

2016. LeBlanc JA: Potentiaion of chlorpromazine by insulin. *Proc Soc Exp Biol Med* 103:621-3, 1960.

2017. Bagdon WJ, Mann DE Jr: Promazine hyperthermia in young albino mice. *J Pharm Sci* 54:240-6 (Feb) 1965.

2018. Norman D, Hiestand WA: Glycemic effects of chlorpromazine in the mouse, hamster, and rat. *Proc Soc Exp Biol Med* 90:89-91. 1955.

2019. Ryall RW: Some actions of chlorpromazine. *Br J Pharm* 2:339-45, 1956.

2020. Manninen K, Pekkarinen A: Effect of drugs on urinary adrenaline secretion, blood glucose and body temperature during insulin shock in rats. *Acta Endocrinol* (Suppl 119:20 (Abstr)) 1967.

2021. Manninen, Pekkarinen *Acta Physiol Scand* 68 (Suppl 277): 131, 1966.

2022. Bhide MB, Tiwari NM, Balwani JH: Effect of chlorpromazine on peripheral utilisation of glucose. *Arc Int Pharmacodyn* 156:166-71 (Jul) 1965

2023. Tiwari NM, Bhide MB, Sen SC: Effect of chlorpromazine and related phenothiazines on epinephrine and insulin induced response on blood sugar. *J Exp Med Sci* 7:104-9, (Mar) 1964.

2024. Nybäck H, Borzecki Z, Sedvall G: Accumulation and disappearance of catecholamines formed from tyrosine-14C in mouse effect of some psychotyopic drugs. *Eur J Pharmacol* 4:395–403 (Nov) 1968.

2024. Alstott RL: Studies on the combined effects of caffeine and ethanol. PhD Thesis, Indiana University, 1970.

2025. Owen CA, Tyce GM, Flock EV, McCall JT: Heparin-ascorbic acid antagonism. *Mayo Clin Proc* 45:140–5 (Feb) 1970.

2026. Cohen H: Mineral oil vitamin A, and carotene. *J Med Soc NJ* 67:111–5 (Mar) 1970.

2027. Spiers ASD, Calne DB, Fayers PM: Miosis during L-dopa therapy. *Br Med J* 1:639 (Jun 13) 1970.

2028. Bellville JW, Forrest WH Jr, Shroff P, et al: The hypnotic effect of codeine and secobarbital and their interaction in man. *Clin Pharmacol Ther* 12:607–12, 1971.

2029. Carulli N, Manenti F, Gallo M, Salvioli GF: Alcohol-drug interaction in man: alcohol and tolbutamide. *Europ J Clin Invest* 1:421–4, 1971.

2030. Richens A, Rowe DJF: Anticonvulsant osteomalacia. *Br Med J* 2: (Dec 11) 1971.

2031. Arvela P, Karki NT, Nieminen L, et al: Effect of long-term levodopa treatment on drug metabolism in rat liver. *Lancet* 1:439–40 (Feb 19) 1972.

2032. Forney RB: The interactions of alcohol and other drugs including psychotomimetics. *Drug Info Bull* 6:59–63 (Jan–Jun) 1972.

2033. Gibson GJ, Warrell DA: Hypertensive crises and phenylpropanolamine. *Lancet* 2:492–3 (Sep 2) 1972.

2034. Binnion PF, McDermott M: Bioavailability of digoxin. *Lancet* 2:592 (Sep 16) 1972.

2035. Roland M: Warfarin. Stereochemical aspects of its metabolism and the interaction with phenylbutazone. *J Clin Invest* 53:1607–17 (Jun) 1974.

2036. Kipperman A, Fine EW: The combined abuse of alcohol and amphetamines. *Am J Psychiat* 131:1277–80, 1974.

2037. Hart P, Farrell GC, Cooksley WGE, Powell LW: Enhanced drug metabolism in cigarette smokers. *Br Med J* 2:147–9 (Jul 17) 1976.

2038. Deacon SP, Barnett D: Comparison of atenolol and propranolol during insulin-induced hypoglycaemia. *Br Med J* 2:272–3 (Jul 31) 1976.

2039. Roberts CJC, Mitchell JV, Donley AJ: Hyponatremia: adverse effect of diuretic treatment. *Br Med J* 1:210 (Jan 22) 1977.

2040. Buffington GA, Dominguez JH, Piering WF, et al: Interaction of rifampin and glucocorticoids. *JAMA* 236:1958–60 (Oct 25) 1976.

2041. Brown DD, Juhl RP: Decreased bioavailability of digoxin due to antacids and kaolin-pectin. *N Engl J Med* 295:1034–7 (Nov 4) 1976.

2042. Manku MS, Horrobin DF: Chloroquine, quinine, procaine, quinidine, tricyclic antidepressants and methylxanthines as prostaglandin agonists and antagonists. *Lancet* 2:1115–7 (Nov 20) 1976.

2043. Pantuck EJ, Conney AH, Garland WA, et al: Effect of charcoal-broiled beef on metabolism in man. *Science* 194: 1055–7 (Dec 3) 1976.

2044. Jeffery WH, Ahlin TA, Goren C, Hardy WR: Loss of warfarin effect after occupational insecticide exposure. *JAMA* 236:2881–2 (Dec 20) 1976.

2045. Reidenberg MM: Some extraneural interactions of drugs of abuse: an overview. *Ann NY Acad Sci* 281:1–10 (Dec 10) 1976.

2046. Vessell ES, Braude MC: Interactions of drug abuse. *Ann NY Acad Sci* 281:1–489 (Dec 10) 1976.

2047. Ellinwood, et al: Stimulants: interaction with chemically relevant drugs. *Ibid* 393–408.

2048. Forney, et al: Marihuana and dextroamphetamine. *Ibid* 162–70.

2049. Kreek, et al: Drug interactions with methadone. *Ibid* 350–71.

2050. Mizroch S, Yurasek M: Hypotension and bradycardia following diazoxide and hydralazine therapy. *JAMA* 237:2471–2 (Jun 6) 1977.

2051. Green AE, Hort JF, Korn HET, Leach H: Potentiation of warfarin by azapropazone. *Br Med J* 1:1532 (Jun 11) 1977.

2052. Janson PA, Watt JB, Hermos JA: Doxepin overdosage. Success with physostigmine and failure with neostigmine in reversing toxicity. *JAMA* 237:2632–2 (Jun 13) 1977.

2053. Rose JQ, Choi HK, Schentag JJ, et al: Intoxication caused by interaction of chloramphenicol and phenytoin. *JAMA* 237:2630–1 (Jun 13) 1977.

2054. Howard CW, Hanson SG, Wahed MA: Anabolic steroids and anticoagulants. *Br Med J* 1-1659–60 (Jun 23) 1977.

2055. Naylor GJ, McHarg A: Profound hypothermia on combined lithium carbonate and diazepam treatment. *Br Med J* 2:22 (Jul 2) 1977.

2056. Meinertz T, Gilfrich H-J, Bork R: Treatment of phenprocoumon intoxication with cholestyramine. *Br Med J* 2:439 (Aug 13) 1977.

2057. DeMots H, Rahimtoola SH: Digitalis and propranolol:together. *Mod Med* 45:68–69, 75, 79 (Aug 15) 1977.

2058. Dukes GE, Kuhn JG, Evens RP: Alcohol in pharmaceutical products. *Am Fam Phys* 15:97–103 (Sep) 1977.

2059. Dam M, Christiansen J: Interaction of propoxyphene with carbamazepine. *Lancet* 2:509 (Sep 3) 1977.

2060. Horder JM: Fatal chlormethiazole poisoning in chronic alcoholics. *Br Med J* 2:614 (Sep 3) 1977.

2061. Chambers G, Kerry RJ, Owen G: Lithium used with a diuretic. *Br Med J* 2:805–6 (Sep 24) 1977.

2062. Mitchell B, Grahame-Smith DG: Monoamine-oxidase inhibitors and caviar. *Lancet* 2:816 (Oct 15) 1977.

2063. Fine A, Henderson S, Morgan DR: Malabsorption of frusemide caused by phenytoin. *Br Med J* 2:1061–2 (Oct 22) 1977.

2064. Porro GB, Dolcini R, Grossi E, et al: Cimetidine in treatment of pancreatic insufficiency. *Lancet* 2:878–9 (Oct 22) 1977.

2065. Durão V, Prata MM, Gonçalves LMP: Modification of antihypertensive effect of β-adrenergic blocking agents by inhibition of endogenous prostaglandin synthesis. *Lancet* 2:1005–7 (Nov 12) 1977.

2066. Rosenthal AR, Self TH, Baker ED, Linden RA: Interaction of isoniazid and warfarin. *JAMA* 238:2177 (Nov 14) 1977.

2067. Sweet DL, Ultmann JE: Effects of anti-neoplastic agents on prothrombin time in patients taking coumarin. *JAMA* 238:2307 (Nov 21) 1977.

2068. Catravas JD, Waters IW, et al: Antidotes for cocaine poisoning. *N Engl J Med* 297:1238 (Dec 1) 1977.

Index

Numbers in italics indicate a figure; "t" in italics
following a page number indicates a table.